Cardiopulmonary
Critical Care

DANTZKER | SCHARF

Cardiopulmonary Critical Care

THIRD EDITION

David R. Dantzker, M.D.
Professor, Albert Einstein College of Medicine of
  Yeshiva University
Bronx

President, Long Island Jewish Medical Center
New Hyde Park, New York

Steven M. Scharf, M.D., Ph.D.
Professor, Albert Einstein College of Medicine of
  Yeshiva University
Bronx

Pulmonary and Critical Care Division
Long Island Jewish Medical Center
New Hyde Park, New York

W.B. SAUNDERS COMPANY
A Division of Harcourt Brace & Company
Philadelphia London Toronto Montreal Sydney Tokyo

W.B. SAUNDERS COMPANY
A Division of Harcourt Brace & Company

The Curtis Center
Independence Square West
Philadelphia, Pennsylvania 19106

Library of Congress Cataloging-in-Publication Data

Cardiopulmonary critical care / [edited by] David R. Dantzker,
Steven M. Scharf.—3rd ed.

p.   cm.

Includes bibliographical references and index.

ISBN 0–7216–6543–8

1. Respiratory intensive care.   2. Cardiopulmonary system—Diseases.
   I. Dantzker, David R.   II. Scharf, Steven M. [DNLM: 1. Lung
   Diseases—therapy.   2. Heart Diseases—therapy.   3. Critical Care.
   WF 600 C267 1998]

RC735.R48C37   1998   616.2′4—dc21

DNLM/DLC   96–36901

CARDIOPULMONARY CRITICAL CARE   ISBN 0–7216–6543–8

Printed in the United States of America.

Last digit is the print number: 9   8   7   6   5   4   3   2   1

To Sherrye Roberta for everything—*DRD*
To Barbara Jean for her unceasing love and support—*SMS*

Contributors

Tahir Ahmed, M.D.
Professor of Medicine, University of Miami
School of Medicine, Miami; Chief, Pulmonary
Division, Mount Sinai Hospital, Miami Beach,
Florida, United States

STATUS ASTHMATICUS

Qamar U. Arfeen, M.D.
Clinical Fellow, Division of Pulmonary and
Critical Care Medicine, University of Texas
Medical School at Houston, Houston, Texas,
United States

OXYGEN TRANSPORT AND UTILIZATION

Takao Ayuse, D.D.S., Ph.D.
Associate Professor, Department of Dental
Anesthesiology, Nagasaki University School of
Dentistry, Nagasaki, Japan

PERIPHERAL CONTROL OF VENOUS RETURN IN CRITICAL
ILLNESS: ROLE OF THE SPLANCHNIC VASCULAR
COMPARTMENT

Kenneth I. Berger, M.D.
Instructor of Medicine, New York University
School of Medicine; Director, Pulmonary
Function Laboratory, Tisch Hospital, New York,
New York, United States

CHRONIC OBSTRUCTIVE PULMONARY DISEASE

Monty M. Bodenheimer, M.D.
Professor of Medicine, Albert Einstein College of
Medicine of Yeshiva University, Bronx; Chief of
Cardiology, Long Island Jewish Medical Center,
New Hyde Park, New York, United States

ACUTE MYOCARDIAL INFARCTION

Bernard R. Borbely, M.D.
Postdoctoral Fellow in Pulmonary and Critical
Care Medicine, Division of Pulmonary and
Critical Care Medicine, Temple University
School of Medicine, Philadelphia, Pennsylvania,
United States

THE MUSCLES OF RESPIRATION

Noel G. Boyle, M.D., Ph.D.
Assistant Professor of Medicine, University of
California, Los Angeles, School of Medicine;
Co-Director, Cardiac Electrophysiology, UCLA
Medical Center, Los Angeles, California, United
States

CARDIAC RHYTHM DISORDERS IN THE CRITICAL CARE
SETTING: PATHOPHYSIOLOGY, DIAGNOSIS, AND
MANAGEMENT

Nicola Brienza, M.D.
Assistant Professor, Instituto di Anestesia e
Rianimazione, Universita' degli Studi di Bari,
Bari, Italy

PERIPHERAL CONTROL OF VENOUS RETURN IN CRITICAL
ILLNESS: ROLE OF THE SPLANCHNIC VASCULAR
COMPARTMENT

Roy G. Brower, M.D.
Associate Professor of Medicine, Pulmonary and
Critical Care Medicine, Johns Hopkins
University School of Medicine, Baltimore,
Maryland, United States

PATHOPHYSIOLOGY OF THE PULMONARY VASCULAR BED

Alejandro D. Chediak, M.D.
Associate Professor of Medicine, University of
Miami School of Medicine, Miami; Chief, Sleep
Disorder Center, and Associate, Pulmonary
Division, Mount Sinai Hospital, Miami Beach,
Florida, United States

STATUS ASTHMATICUS

Heidi V. Connolly, M.D.
Senior Instructor, Pediatric Critical Care Fellow,
Pediatric Pulmonology, University of Rochester
School of Medicine and Dentistry; Attending
Physician, Pediatric Intensive Care Unit, Strong
Memorial Hospital, Rochester, New York,
United States

THE MICROCIRCULATION AND TISSUE OXYGENATION

Gilbert E. D'Alonzo, D.O.
Professor of Medicine, Division of Pulmonary and Critical Care Medicine, Temple University School of Medicine; Attending Physician and Fellowship Program Director, Temple University Hospital, Philadelphia, Pennsylvania, United States

DEEP VENOUS THROMBOSIS AND PULMONARY EMBOLISM

David R. Dantzker, M.D.
Professor, Department of Medicine, Albert Einstein College of Medicine of Yeshiva University, Bronx; President, Long Island Jewish Medical Center, New Hyde Park, New York, United States

PULMONARY GAS EXCHANGE

Peter M. C. DeBlieux, M.D.
Clinical Assistant Professor of Medicine, Louisiana State University School of Medicine in New Orleans; Emergency Medicine Residency Program Director, Louisiana State University School of Medicine in New Orleans, New Orleans, Louisiana, United States

CARDIOPULMONARY RESUSCITATION

Steven J. Evans, M.D.
Assistant Professor of Medicine, Albert Einstein College of Medicine of Yeshiva University, Bronx; Director of Cardiac Electrophysiology, Long Island Jewish Medical Center, New Hyde Park, New York, United States

CARDIAC RHYTHM DISORDERS IN THE CRITICAL CARE SETTING: PATHOPHYSIOLOGY, DIAGNOSIS, AND MANAGEMENT

Jean K. Fleischman, M.D.
Assistant Professor of Medicine, Mount Sinai School of Medicine of the City University of New York, New York; Chief, Division of Pulmonary and Critical Care Medicine, Attending Physician, Division of Pulmonary and Critical Care Medicine, Queens Hospital Center, Jamaica, New York, United States

SMOKE INHALATION INJURY

Seán P. Gaine, M.B., B.Ch.
Senior Clinical Fellow, Pulmonary and Critical Care Medicine, Johns Hopkins University School of Medicine, Baltimore, Maryland, United States

PATHOPHYSIOLOGY OF THE PULMONARY VASCULAR BED

Thomas E. J. Gayeski, M.D., Ph.D.
Department of Anesthesiology, Pharmacology and Physiology, University of Rochester School of Medicine and Dentistry, Rochester, New York, United States

THE MICROCIRCULATION AND TISSUE OXYGENATION

Harly E. Greenberg, M.D.
Assistant Professor of Medicine, Albert Einstein College of Medicine of Yeshiva University, Bronx; Attending Physician, Division of Pulmonary and Critical Care Medicine, Long Island Jewish Medical Center, New York, United States

SMOKE INHALATION INJURY

Guillermo Gutierrez, M.D., Ph.D.
Professor of Medicine, University of Texas Medical School at Houston, Houston, Texas, United States

OXYGEN TRANSPORT AND UTILIZATION

Stephen R. Hayden, M.D.
Assistant Clinical Professor of Medicine, University of California, San Diego, School of Medicine, La Jolla; Attending Physician, Hyperbaric Medical Center, Assistant Director, Department of Emergency Medicine, UCSD Medical Center, San Diego, California, United States

HYPERBARIC MEDICINE

Peter G. Herman, M.D.
Professor of Radiology, Albert Einstein College of Medicine of Yeshiva University, Bronx; Chairman of Radiology, Long Island Jewish Medical Center, New Hyde Park, New York, United States

CRITICAL CARE RADIOLOGY

Irving Jacoby, M.D.
Clinical Professor of Medicine and Surgery, University of California, San Diego, School of Medicine, La Jolla; Associate Director, Hyperbaric Medicine Center, Assistant Director, Department of Emergency Medicine, UCSD Medical Center, San Diego, California, United States

HYPERBARIC MEDICINE

Philip C. Johnson, M.D.
Associate Professor and Associate Director,
Clinical Research Center, University of Texas
Medical School at Houston; Division Chief of
Service and Infectious Disease Consultant,
Hermann Hospital, Houston, Texas, United
States

HOSPITAL-ACQUIRED PNEUMONIA AND PNEUMONIA IN
THE IMMUNOSUPPRESSED HOST; COMMUNITY-
ACQUIRED PNEUMONIA

Steven G. Kelsen, M.D.
Professor of Medicine and Physiology, Division
of Pulmonary and Critical Care Medicine,
Temple University School of Medicine;
Attending Physician, Temple University
Hospital, Philadelphia, Pennsylvania, United
States

THE MUSCLES OF RESPIRATION

Arfa Khan, M.D.
Professor of Radiology, Albert Einstein College
of Medicine of Yeshiva University, Bronx;
Associate Chairperson, Department of Radiology,
Long Island Jewish Medical Center, New Hyde
Park, New York, United States

CRITICAL CARE RADIOLOGY

Marin H. Kollef, M.D.
Assistant Professor of Medicine, Department of
Internal Medicine, Washington University
School of Medicine; Director, Medical Intensive
Care Unit; Director, Respiratory Care Services,
Barnes Hospital and Jewish Hospital of St. Louis,
St. Louis, Missouri, United States

ACUTE RESPIRATORY DISTRESS SYNDROME

Stephen E. Lapinsky, M.B., B.Ch.
Assistant Professor of Medicine, University of
Toronto Faculty of Medicine; Associate Director,
Intensive Care Unit, Mount Sinai Hospital,
Toronto, Ontario, Canada

PRINCIPLES OF MECHANICAL VENTILATION AND
WEANING

Sheldon Magder, M.D.
Associate Professor of Medicine, McGill
University Faculty of Medicine; Director,
Critical Care Division, Royal Victoria Hospital,
Montreal, Quebec, Canada

HEART-LUNG INTERACTIONS IN SEPSIS

John J. Marini, M.D.
Professor of Medicine, University of Minnesota
Medical School—Minneapolis/St. Paul; Director
of Pulmonary and Critical Care Medicine, Saint
Paul-Ramsey Medical Center, St. Paul,
Minnesota, United States

PULMONARY MECHANICS IN CRITICAL CARE

Alan Multz, M.D.
Assistant Professor of Medicine, Albert Einstein
College of Medicine of Yeshiva University,
Bronx; Director, Critical Care, Pulmonary and
Critical Care Division, Long Island Jewish
Medical Center, New Hyde Park, New York,
United States

PHARMACOLOGIC AND VENTILATORY SUPPORT OF THE
CIRCULATION IN CRITICALLY ILL PATIENTS

Obi N. Nwasokwa, M.D., Ph.D.
Assistant Professor of Medicine, Albert Einstein
College of Medicine of Yeshiva University,
Bronx; Long Island Jewish Medical Center, New
Hyde Park, New York, United States

CARDIAC FUNCTION

David M. Rapoport, M.D.
Associate Professor of Clinical Medicine, New
York University School of Medicine; Medical
Director, Sleep Disorders Center, New York
University Medical Center; Associate Director,
Pulmonary Laboratory, Bellevue Hospital Center,
New York, New York, United States

CHRONIC OBSTRUCTIVE PULMONARY DISEASE

Jean-Pierre Revelly, M.D.
Service d'Anesthesiologie Centre, Hospitalier
Universitaire Vaudois, Lausanne, Switzerland

PERIPHERAL CONTROL OF VENOUS RETURN IN CRITICAL
ILLNESS: ROLE OF THE SPLANCHNIC VASCULAR
COMPARTMENT

James L. Robotham, M.D.
Professor, Department of Anesthesiology/Critical
Care Medicine, Johns Hopkins University
School of Medicine, Baltimore, Maryland,
United States

PERIPHERAL CONTROL OF VENOUS RETURN IN CRITICAL
ILLNESS: ROLE OF THE SPLANCHNIC VASCULAR
COMPARTMENT

George A. Sarosi, M.D.
Professor of Medicine, Indiana University School
of Medicine; Chief, Medical Service, Richard L.
Roudebush VA Medical Center, Indianapolis,
Indiana, United States

HOSPITAL-ACQUIRED PNEUMONIA AND PNEUMONIA IN
THE IMMUNOSUPPRESSED HOST; COMMUNITY-
ACQUIRED PNEUMONIA

Steven M. Scharf, M.D., Ph.D.
Professor of Medicine, Albert Einstein College of Medicine of Yeshiva University, Bronx; Pulmonary and Critical Care Division, Long Island Jewish Medical Center, New Hyde Park, New York, United States

MECHANICAL CARDIOPULMONARY INTERACTIONS IN CRITICAL CARE; PHARMACOLOGIC AND VENTILATORY SUPPORT OF THE CIRCULATION IN CRITICALLY ILL PATIENTS

Robert B. Schoene, M.D.
Professor of Medicine, Division of Pulmonary and Critical Care Medicine, University of Washington School of Medicine; Director of Pulmonary Function and Exercise Laboratory, Harborview Medical Center, Seattle, Washington, United States

PULMONARY FAILURE CAUSED BY HIGH ALTITUDE

Daniel P. Schuster, M.D.
Director, Critical Care Program, Department of Internal Medicine; Professor of Medicine and Radiology, Washington University School of Medicine; Barnes Hospital and Jewish Hospital of St. Louis, St. Louis, Missouri, United States

ACUTE RESPIRATORY DISTRESS SYNDROME

Peggy McGinnis Simon, M.D.
Consultant, Division of Pulmonary and Critical Care Medicine, Mayo Clinic, Rochester, Minnesota, United States

VENTILATORY CONTROL IN THE CRITICAL CARE SETTING

Richard H. Simon, M.D.
Professor of Internal Medicine, Pulmonary and Critical Care Medicine Division, University of Michigan Medical School; Associate Chair of Internal Medicine, University of Michigan Medical School, Ann Arbor, Michigan, United States

PATHOGENESIS OF ACUTE LUNG INJURY

Arthur S. Slutsky, M.D.
Professor of Medicine, University of Toronto Faculty of Medicine; Staff Physician, Mount Sinai Hospital, Toronto, Ontario, Canada

PRINCIPLES OF MECHANICAL VENTILATION AND WEANING

Warren R. Summer, M.D.
Howard A. Buechner Professor of Medicine, Louisiana State University School of Medicine in New Orleans; Section Chief, Louisiana State University School of Medicine in New Orleans; Director, Pulmonary Services, Medical Center of Louisiana at Charity Hospital; Section Chief, Pulmonary/Critical Care, Ochsner Clinic, New Orleans, Louisiana, United States

CARDIOPULMONARY RESUSCITATION

Ira L. Weg, M.D.
Assistant Professor of Medicine, Albert Einstein College of Medicine of Yeshiva University, Bronx; Director, Inpatient Cardiology, Harris Chasanoff Heart Institute, Long Island Jewish Medical Center, New Hyde Park, New York, United States

ACUTE MYOCARDIAL INFARCTION

Charles M. Wiener, M.D.
Assistant Professor of Medicine, Pulmonary and Critical Care Medicine, Johns Hopkins University School of Medicine, Baltimore, Maryland, United States

PATHOPHYSIOLOGY OF THE PULMONARY VASCULAR BED

Preface

The goal of the first edition of *Cardiopulmonary Critical Care* was to provide insight into the pathophysiology of disease processes that affect the heart and lungs. The second edition expanded the scope somewhat beyond this original goal. In this, the third edition, we reemphasize the goal of the first edition and concentrate on an up-to-date scholarly review of topics relevant to the care of patients with cardiopulmonary failure. In particular, this edition provides a detailed discussion of disease processes that are important and often difficult to manage, rather than a brief survey, such as that often found in larger comprehensive critical care textbooks. *Cardiopulmonary Critical Care* will therefore be useful to students, researchers, and practitioners.

An understanding of the pathophysiologic processes that underlie the failure of the circulatory and respiratory systems is the basis for the care of the most seriously ill patients. Advances in biomedical knowledge, technology, and pharmacology form the foundation for changes in critical care practice. To cope with our expanded scope of knowledge, chapters are extensively revised or rewritten. New contributors are added in order to achieve new perspectives on the subject matter. New chapters have been added on ventilator management, control of the peripheral circulation (in critically ill patients and in sepsis), inhalational lung injury, hyperbaric therapy, and high altitude pulmonary edema.

As in the previous editions, the stress is on understanding the basic pathophysiologic mechanisms that underlie the disease. This knowledge provides a solid foundation for diagnosis and therapy of the most seriously ill patients in our care. Further, a well-grounded knowledge base in pathophysiology of disease is the means by which the latest advances in medicine are incorporated into daily practice.

DAVID R. DANTZKER, M.D.
STEVEN M. SCHARF, M.D., PH.D.

Contents

SECTION **II**
PRINCIPLES OF TREATMENT

SECTION III
SPECIFIC DISORDERS

CHAPTER **26**

Hyperbaric Medicine   627

CHAPTER **27**

**Pulmonary Failure Caused by High
Altitude**   639

Index

I

PATHOPHYSIOLOGY

Pathogenesis of Acute Lung Injury

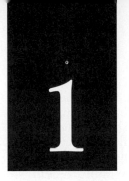

Richard H. Simon, M.D.

To function as a gas exchange organ, the lung must bring inspired air into close contact with pulmonary blood. The anatomy of the lung is well-suited for this purpose with its extensive capillary network coursing through thin alveolar walls. However, this close approximation between capillary blood and alveolar air is not without risk. Any pathologic process that disrupts the structural or functional properties of the capillary-alveolar wall leads to extravasation of fluid and impairment of gas exchange. When the process is severe and the areas of lung involvement are widespread, respiratory failure ensues.

Over the last several decades, an extensive amount of research has been directed toward understanding the etiology and pathophysiology of diseases that lead to alveolar injury and respiratory failure. Although there are substantial gaps in our knowledge, a number of pieces to the puzzle are beginning to fall into place. These discoveries are providing new approaches to prevent and treat severe pulmonary injury. In this chapter, the current state of knowledge regarding acute lung injury will be reviewed with emphasis being placed on those areas that hold promise for improving clinical outcomes.

BACKGROUND AND DEFINITION OF THE ADULT RESPIRATORY DISTRESS SYNDROME (ARDS)

In 1967, Ashbaugh, Bigelow, Petty, and Levine described 12 patients who acutely developed respiratory failure having had no prior history of lung disease (Ashbaugh et al, 1967). All 12 patients had serious acute illnesses that were not commonly thought to lead to diffuse lung damage. The patients' diagnoses included major trauma, pancreatitis, and drug overdose. Because many of the characteristics of the respiratory failure that occurred in these patients were similar to those seen in infant respiratory distress syndrome, the investigators named the newly recognized condition *adult respiratory distress syndrome*, or *ARDS*.

As originally described, ARDS is a syndrome with a set of defining clinical criteria. Attempts to find a simple laboratory test that can differentiate

ARDS from other causes of acute respiratory failure have been unsuccessful. Hence, the diagnosis of ARDS continues to be based upon the fulfillment of clinical criteria. These defining criteria were originally written so that only patients with very severe respiratory impairment were included. The published definitions of ARDS usually encompassed the following elements (Ashbaugh et al, 1967; Pepe et al, 1982; Fowler et al, 1983):

1. Acute onset of severe respiratory dysfunction.

   The respiratory impairment had to be severe enough to require endotracheal intubation and assisted mechanical ventilation. The progression to respiratory failure had to be rapid (hours to at most a few days).

2. Rapid appearance of bilateral alveolar infiltrates on chest roentgenogram.

   This criterion ensures that the respiratory failure be a result of widespread alveolar flooding and not localized lung disease. Patients with lung injury that is initially confined to one or several anatomic regions can later meet this criterion, but only after panlobar infiltrates appear on chest radiographs. The justification for excluding patients with severe but localized disease is based upon the premise that ARDS is the consequence of a generalized, systemic process that affects the lung diffusely. This assumption is still considered true, but computer-assisted tomography of the chest shows that the distribution of alveolar edema in ARDS is more heterogeneous than was initially appreciated from conventional radiographs (Maunder et al, 1986b).

3. Exclusion of cardiogenic factors as being solely responsible for the respiratory abnormalities.

   Many investigations of ARDS have included in their defining criteria the requirement that pulmonary artery occlusion pressure be 16 to 18 mm Hg or less. Although this criterion ensured that patients with pulmonary edema from cardiogenic sources be excluded, it also eliminated those patients who had both primary alveolar injury and impaired left ventricular function.

4. Decreased static lung compliance.

   The original article by Ashbaugh and colleagues reported that the lungs of their patients were stiff (Ashbaugh et al, 1967). Since then, many investigators have included this requirement in their definition.

However, the criterion adds relatively little to the definition of ARDS because it is unusual for patients to fulfill all the other criteria and still have normal lung compliance. Chapter 18 contains a detailed discussion of the mechanical abnormalities in ARDS.

5. Hypoxemia that responds poorly to administration of supplemental oxygen.

   This criterion eliminates patients with chronic obstructive pulmonary diseases because the hypoxemia in these patients is the consequence of hypoventilation and/or ventilation/perfusion mismatch, which respond well to supplemental oxygen. The hypoxemia of ARDS is caused by intrapulmonary shunting, which corrects poorly with increasing the concentration of inspired oxygen.

As mentioned, the patients described in earlier studies of ARDS had very severe pulmonary impairment. The same pathophysiologic processes that are associated with ARDS can cause milder lung injury. To accommodate these milder cases, a scoring system has been proposed that both defines and grades the severity of lung injury (Murray et al, 1988). Points are assigned to the following clinical variables: (1) extent of alveolar consolidation as seen on chest radiographs; (2) severity of hypoxemia; (3) level of positive end-expiratory pressure (PEEP) used to improve arterial oxygenation; and (4) respiratory system compliance. The values assigned to each of these variables are used to calculate a lung injury score. In 1994, the definition of ARDS was addressed by an American-European consensus conference (Bernard et al, 1994a). The attendees adopted a scoring system to define "acute lung injury" (Table 1–1). The term ARDS was reserved for the most severe form of acute lung injury.

PATHOLOGIC ABNORMALITIES IN ACUTE LUNG INJURY

For intravascular fluid to reach the alveolar airspaces, several physical barriers must be breached. The fluid must cross the capillary endothelium, the endothelial basement membrane, an interstitial space of varying width, the epithelial cell basement membrane, and finally the epithelial cell layer (Fig. 1–1). Any disease process that causes a severe and diffuse increase in permeability of the capillary-alveolar wall leads to ARDS.

In typical cases of ARDS, the consequences of alveolar injury can easily be observed by mi-

Table 1-1
American-European Consensus Conference Definitions

Acute Lung Injury

1. Acute onset of pulmonary impairment
2. PaO_2/FiO_2 <300 mm Hg (regardless of positive end-expiratory pressure)
3. Bilateral infiltrates seen on frontal chest radiograph
4. Pulmonary artery occlusion pressure <18 mm Hg when measured, or no clinical evidence of left atrial hypertension

Adult Respiratory Distress Syndrome

Same as acute lung injury, except PaO_2/FiO_2 <200 mm Hg

croscopy (Fig. 1–2). The alveolar spaces are flooded with a protein-rich edema fluid (Hill et al, 1982; Pratt, 1982). Hyaline membranes that consist largely of fibrin, plasma proteins, and cellular debris line the damaged alveoli. The interstitial space is often swollen with edema fluid.

Early investigations into the pathophysiology of ARDS concentrated on the role of the endothelium. Transmission electron micrographs revealed that capillary endothelial cells were frequently swollen and separated from their basement membrane (Schnells et al, 1980; Tomaschefski et al, 1983). In severely affected areas, endothelial cell necrosis was seen. These pathologic features have also been observed in various animal models of ARDS. Although not widely appreciated initially, the alveolar epithelium also shows signs of injury in ARDS (Nash et al, 1974; Bachofen and Weibel, 1977). Both the type I and type II alveolar epithelial cells can be damaged, with the thin, flattened type I alveolar epithelial cells appearing more susceptible to injury. In many areas of lung, type I cells are lifted off their basement membrane and appear necrotic. The cuboidal, surfactant-producing type II cells are more resistant to injury, although they occasionally have cytoplasmic swelling and evidence of cell death. In scattered areas, the basement membranes that belong to either or both the endothelium and epithelium appear interrupted. In short,

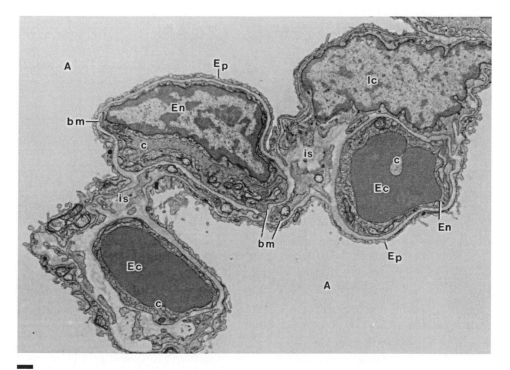

Figure 1-1
Transmission electron micrograph of normal human lung parenchyma. Blood erythrocytes (Ec) can be seen within the capillaries (c). Fluid within the capillary vessels is separated from the alveolar air spaces (A) by endothelial cells (En), basement membranes (bm), the interstitial space (is), and epithelial cells (Ep). The nucleus of an interstitial cell (Is) is also seen in this micrograph. (× 10,800.) (Courtesy of Theodore F. Beals, MD, Department of Pathology, University of Michigan.)

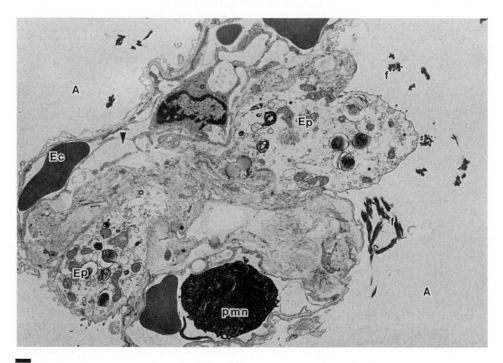

Figure 1–2
Transmission electron micrograph of rat lung following intratracheal instillation of an oxygen metabolite generating system (Johnson et al, 1981). Degenerating type II alveolar epithelial cells are present (Ep). Blebs can be seen in the endothelial cells (*arrowhead*). A polymorphonuclear leukocyte (pmn) is present within an injured capillary loop. Fibrin (f) is present within the alveolar spaces (A). Erythrocytes (Ec) are contained within the alveolar capillaries. (× 5800.) (Courtesy of Kent J. Johnson, MD, and Robin G. Kunkel, Department of Pathology, University of Michigan.)

there is widespread anatomic injury of lung parenchyma in ARDS.

PHYSIOLOGIC ABNORMALITIES

Both the endothelium and epithelium serve as semipermeability membranes. The flux of fluid across these barriers can be described by the Starling equation:

$$\text{Fluid flux} = K((P_i - P_o) - \sigma(\Pi_i - \Pi))$$

where K is the permeability coefficient of either the endothelium or epithelium; P_i and P_o are the hydrostatic pressures inside and outside the membrane of interest; σ is the membrane reflection coefficient, which is a measure of the permeability of the barrier for macromolecules; and Π_i and Π_o are the protein osmotic pressures of the fluid inside and outside the membrane of interest. In the normal lung, the hydrostatic pressures tend to drive fluid out of the capillary bed and into the alveolar space ($P_{capillary} > P_{interstitial} > P_{alveolar}$). The osmotic gradients tend to drive fluid the opposite direction ($P_{capillary} > P_{interstitial} > P_{alveolar}$). The over-

all balance of forces varies between lung regions, principally because of the changes in microvascular and interstitial hydrostatic forces. In addition, the lung is richly endowed with a lymphatic system designed to drain excess interstitial edema.

The endothelial barrier is more permeable to proteins compared with the epithelium. For example, the reflection coefficient, σ, of the endothelium for proteins the size of albumin is approximately 0.6, whereas that of the epithelium is 1.0 (Gorin and Stewart, 1979). This implies that in the normal lung, plasma continually leaks from the vascular space into the interstitial compartment. A buildup of fluid within the interstitial space is prevented by its removal via the lymphatic system. In contrast, the epithelium is a much tighter barrier and permits relatively fewer macromolecules to leak across it into the alveolar airspaces.

Loss of Endothelial Barrier Function

Various mechanisms contribute to accumulation of alveolar fluid in ARDS (Table 1–2). Several

Table 1–2
Causes of Alveolar Fluid Accumulation in ARDS

Increased permeability of the endothelial cell layer
Increased permeability of the epithelial cell layer
Decreased active ion transport by epithelial cells
Decreased surfactant activity

animal models have been used to assess the degree of the endothelial injury that occurs in various types of ARDS. One of the more intensively studied models uses sheep in which a lymphatic vessel that drains a region of lung is cannulated, allowing measurement of the fluid flux between the vascular space and interstitial compartment (Staub, 1979). Under basal conditions, the protein concentration of sheep lung lymph is approximately two-thirds that of plasma. However, if the permeability of the capillary endothelium is increased, both the flow rate and protein concentration of lymph increases. This is exactly the pattern of changes that are seen in sheep given acute lung injury (e.g., by intravascularly infusing *Pseudomonas* bacteria [Brigham et al, 1974] or *Escherichia coli* endotoxin [Brigham et al, 1979]). Thus, increased endothelial permeability appears likely to be an important component of the pathophysiology of ARDS.

Loss of Epithelial Barrier Function

The permeability of the alveolar epithelium has also been measured in ARDS. The clearance of the low-molecular-weight tracer technetium 199m (^{199m}Tc)-diethylenetriamine pentaacetate from the lung following aerosolized delivery to the alveoli has been used to measure epithelial permeability. Its rate of clearance from the lung serves as an indirect measurement of transport across the epithelial layer. In clinical studies of patients with ARDS, the clearance of ^{199m}Tc was found to be significantly more rapid compared with that of normal volunteers and with that of patients who had other lung diseases thought not to be associated with increased alveolar epithelial permeability (Mason et al, 1985).

Impaired Epithelial Cell Active Transport

In addition to acting as a passive barrier to macromolecules, the alveolar epithelial layer uses active ion transport to help maintain a dry alveolar space. Evidence supporting this conclusion was first obtained during studies of cultured monolayers of rat alveolar epithelial cells. The studies showed that epithelial cell monolayers actively

transported sodium from their apical (airspace) to their basolateral (interstitial) surfaces (Goodman and Crandall, 1982; Mason et al, 1982). This phenomenon very likely occurs within the intact lung and serves as a critical means to clear fluid that has leaked into the alveolar space (Matthay and Wiener-Kronish, 1990; Sakuma et al, 1994). Any pulmonary insult that diminishes this active transport function could either initiate or exacerbate alveolar edema. Furthermore, active transport is most likely needed to clear the alveolar space of fluid following successful repair of the epithelial cell layer.

Altered Alveolar Surface Tension

Pulmonary edema can also be caused or exacerbated by alterations in the surface tension of the fluid lining the alveolar spaces (Guyton and Moffatt, 1981). Under normal circumstances, surface tension within air-filled alveoli is kept low by surfactant, a secretory product of type II epithelial cells (Rooney, 1985). Any pulmonary injury that decreases the production of surfactant or lowers its surface active properties increases surface tension. When surface tension is high, the hydrostatic pressure of the fluid that is below the surface is reduced. This reduction in alveolar fluid pressure drives more fluid from the capillary bed, which is at higher pressure, into the lower pressure alveolar spaces (Albert et al, 1979).

The surface tension of fluid recovered from the lungs of patients with ARDS is abnormal (Lewis and Jobe, 1993). One likely reason is that the type II alveolar epithelial cells, which are the source of surfactant, are frequently injured in ARDS. Another reason is that existing surfactant becomes inactivated by proteins that leak into the alveolar space. Many plasma proteins, including hemoglobin, fibrinogen, fibrin degradation peptides, and albumin, inhibit the surface active properties of surfactant (Enhorning, 1989). Together, these abnormalities in surfactant activity are most likely causes of the atelectasis that is commonly seen in ARDS.

The surfactant abnormalities in ARDS are similar to those that are found in premature neonates who have the so-called infant respiratory distress syndrome. In this condition, surfactant deficiency appears to be the primary event leading to respiratory failure. Appreciation of this fact led to successful development of surfactant therapy for neonates with infant respiratory distress syndrome. Because of the many similarities between infant respiratory distress syndrome and ARDS, surfactant therapy has also been tested in ARDS. Unfortunately, the trials to date, using a totally artificial surfactant, have been disappointing (Anzueto et al, 1994). However, preliminary tests using a more natural surfactant have yielded some promising results (Gregory et al, 1994).

ETIOLOGY OF ARDS

It is apparent from the earlier discussion that maintaining an air-filled alveolar space depends upon the structural and functional integrity of many alveolar components. Disruption of endothelium or epithelium, inhibition of active transport processes, and/or alterations in alveolar surfactant can all lead to noncardiogenic pulmonary edema. Given the diversity of these possibilities, it should be no surprise that searches for the cause of ARDS have not converged on a single mechanism. In fact, multiple overlapping and interacting pathways most likely exist, with no single mechanism responsible for every case. The diversity of pathways is highlighted by inspecting the list of underlying diseases that are associated with ARDS (Table 1–3). Review of the list fails to suggest a single universal theme.

DIRECT LUNG INJURY

In a subgroup of patients, ARDS appears to be the result of toxic agents that directly damage

Table 1–3
Some Diseases Associated with ARDS

Shock of any etiology	Inhaled toxins
Infection	Oxygen toxicity
Sepsis syndrome	Smoke
Pneumonia (viral,	Corrosive chemicals
bacterial, or fungal)	(NO_2, Cl_2, NH_3,
Pneumocystis carinii	phosgene, cadmium)
Trauma	Hematologic disorders
Fat embolism	Diffuse intravascular
Lung contusion	coagulation
Major nonthoracic	Massive blood transfusion
trauma	Postcardiopulmonary
Head injury	bypass
Burns	Transfusion reaction
Liquid aspiration	Miscellaneous
Gastric juices	Pancreatitis
Near-drowning	Carcinomatosis
Hydrocarbon fluids	Eclampsia
	Radiation pneumonitis
Drug overdose or	Amniotic fluid or air
sensitivity	emboli
Narcotics	High altitude exposure
Aspirin	Collagen vascular diseases
Others	Uremia

lung tissue. Among the list of responsible agents are various inhaled gases (e.g., phosgene), ingested chemicals (e.g., paraquat [Deneke and Fanburg, 1980]), pharmaceuticals (e.g., the sedative-hypnotic ethchlorvynol [Fairman et al, 1981]), high tensions of inhaled oxygen (Deneke and Fanburg, 1980), and aspirated gastric fluids. Chapter 25 treats the topic of inhalation lung injury in great detail. Infectious organisms can also elaborate cytotoxins that are directly damaging to pulmonary parenchymal cells. Although each of these agents may be sufficient to cause lung damage, the full extent of injury may be contributed to by the indirect mechanisms discussed later.

INDIRECT LUNG INJURY

Although in some cases of ARDS, a toxin can be identified that is directly injurious to lung tissue, in the majority of situations this is not the case. Instead, developments outside the lung seem to set into motion a series of events that culminate in lung injury. There seems to be little in common among the various diagnoses associated with progression to ARDS. However, over the years there has accumulated an abundance of evidence that links inflammation to many cases of ARDS.

INFLAMMATORY CASCADES IN ARDS

Early investigations into the pathophysiology of ARDS revealed evidence that multiple inflammatory cascades were being activated during the disease process. These revelations led to the hypothesis that inflammation was a cause, and not merely a consequence, of ARDS. The formulation of this hypothesis was heavily influenced by the similarities between ARDS and two other conditions, namely systemic sepsis and multiorgan failure. In parallel with studies of ARDS, investigations of these other two conditions yielded evidence that inflammatory cascades were being activated. ARDS, sepsis, and multiorgan failure are further linked by their frequent occurrence in the same patient. Each of the three is often initiated by the same stimuli. For example, endotoxin, a product of bacteria, has been implicated in the pathogenesis of all three (see later). Moreover, there is evidence that similar to sepsis and multiorgan failure, ARDS is a systemic disease. Even in patients who appear to have isolated lung disease, sensitive techniques that detect vascular injury have revealed signs of extrapulmonary vascular damage (Kreuzfelder et al, 1988; Nuytinck et al, 1988). Because of the overlap between ARDS, sepsis, and multiorgan failure, any discussion of ARDS by necessity has to include data from studies of the other two conditions. However, this chapter focuses predominantly on ARDS. Sepsis and multiorgan failure are dealt with elsewhere and are mentioned only when the information contributes to the understanding of ARDS.

Of the various triggers that seem to be involved in the initiation of ARDS, endotoxin is the most extensively studied. One important pathway by which endotoxin activates inflammatory cascades involves its binding to a carrier protein called the lipopolysaccharide binding protein, or LBP (Beutler, 1995; Kuhns et al, 1995). Complexes of endotoxin/LBP interact with CD14, a receptor on the surface of macrophages. Binding to CD14 activates a number of macrophage-mediated processes that lead to the release of inflammatory mediators (discussed later, Fig. 1–3). Evidence supporting the involvement of this pathway can be found in bronchoalveolar lavage fluid from patients with ARDS in which both endotoxin/LBP complexes (Martin et al, 1994) and macrophage-derived inflammatory products are found (see later).

Although endotoxin may play an important role in ARDS, it must be acknowledged that endotoxin alone is insufficient to cause the syndrome. Only a minority of patients with bacterial infection and endotoxemia develop ARDS (Pepe et al, 1982; Fowler et al, 1983). Furthermore, the concentration of endotoxin in the blood of patients with sepsis does not correlate well with the subsequent development of lung injury (Parsons et al, 1989).

Before discussing individual inflammatory mediators, it is appropriate to emphasize the extensive interactions that occur between different inflammatory cascades. Shortly after the role of inflammation in ARDS became apparent, numerous groups attempted to identify a single pathway leading to lung injury. However, it rapidly became apparent that a single pathway was unlikely to exist. Almost without exception, every time a different inflammatory cascade was investigated, signs were found that it was activated in ARDS. The list of inflammatory cascades implicated in the pathogenesis of ARDS has now grown to

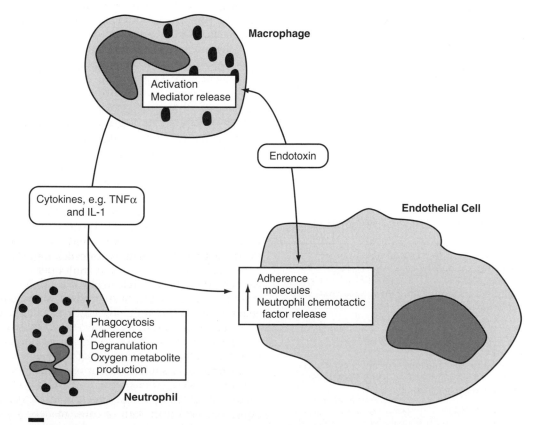

Figure 1–3
Effects of endotoxin on macrophages and endothelial cells that affect neutrophil behavior. The central roles of tumor necrosis factor and interleukin-1 are emphasized, although other cytokines (*not shown*) also participate in the modulation of neutrophil function.

include many systems. Similar to the situation with soluble mediators, there is a diversity of inflammatory cells that participate in ARDS including neutrophils, monocytes, macrophages, eosinophils, and platelets.

It is now apparent that very early in the pathogenesis of ARDS, there is a branching of pathways to encompass many different but interrelated inflammatory cascades. The complexity of this pattern makes it difficult to determine the relative contribution of a single system. In the final analysis, each cascade probably contributes to some extent to the lung injury. No single pathway is likely to be sufficient to account for all the manifestations of the disease.

NEUTROPHILS IN ARDS

An early hint that neutrophils were involved in ARDS came from histologic examinations of lung tissue taken from patients dying with ARDS (Table 1–4) (Bachofen and Weibel, 1977). Numerous neutrophils were found free within the alveolar space, in the interstitium, and as aggregates in the pulmonary capillaries. Subsequent studies reported that markedly increased numbers of neutrophils were found in bronchoalveolar lavage fluid from patients with ARDS (Lee et al, 1981; Fowler et al, 1982; McGuire et al, 1982). Normally, few neutrophils are present extravascularly in lungs. Only 1 to 3% of cells recovered in bronchoalveolar lavage are neutrophils, with the majority being macrophages with a few lymphocytes. However, in ARDS, 76 to 85% of the cells

Table 1–4
Evidence Supporting a Role for Neutrophils in ARDS

Human studies
   Neutrophils accumulate within lungs early in the disease process
   Circulating neutrophils show signs of *in vivo* activation
Animal studies
   Stimulated neutrophils injure lungs both *in vivo* and *ex vivo*
   Neutrophil products directly injure intact lungs
   Neutrophil depletion protects lungs from a variety of different types of injury
Cell culture studies
   Stimulated neutrophils damage lung epithelial and endothelial cells
   Neutrophil products directly damage cultured lung cells

recovered are neutrophils. As expected, tagged neutrophil studies have shown that the lung neutrophils come from circulating blood (Warshawski et al, 198).

Peripheral blood neutrophils of patients with ARDS show signs of activation. In vitro, these neutrophils produce elevated levels of oxygen metabolites (see later) and demonstrate increased responses to chemotactic agents (Zimmerman et al, 1983). Increased levels of lactoferrin, a secretory product of stimulated neutrophils, are found in sera of patients with ARDS (Hallgren et al, 1987). Evidence that neutrophils are more than innocent bystanders comes from studies of neutropenic patients receiving chemotherapy for cancer treatment (Rinaldo and Borovetz, 1985). In a subgroup of these patients who develop pulmonary dysfunction from infection or drug reactions, lung impairment often worsens if and when the bone marrow recovers and peripheral neutrophil counts increase. The implication is that bone marrow recovery provides greater numbers of neutrophils that migrate to the lung and cause injury.

Although the vast majority of published studies support a role for neutrophils in ARDS, there are exceptions. In particular, ARDS occasionally occurs in patients who lack circulating neutrophils (Laufe et al, 1986; Maunder et al, 1986a; Ognibene et al, 1986). Rather than disproving the importance of neutrophils in ARDS, these reports serve as reminders that the pathophysiology of ARDS is likely to involve multiple and diverse mechanisms. Neutrophils may play a role in many but clearly not all cases.

Much of the data supporting the role of neutrophils in lung injury is derived from animal studies. One of the earliest such investigations studied the pulmonary effects of hemorrhagic shock in dogs (Ratliff et al, 1971). The hypotensive animals were noted to become neutropenic due to sequestration of neutrophils within pulmonary capillaries. A commonly used approach to studying the contribution of neutrophils is to determine the effects of neutrophil depletion on the extent of lung injury. In one of the earlier studies, lung injury in rats was induced by infusing cobra venom factor, which activates the complement system (Till et al, 1982). Prior neutrophil depletion using an antineutrophil antibody reduced the lung damage. A similar pattern of results was seen in rats following cutaneous burns (Till et al, 1983) and in sheep infused with endotoxin (Heflin and Brigham, 1981). In both of these models, as well as many others, prior neutrophil depletion protected the animals from lung injury.

On the other hand, neutrophil depletion failed to protect the lungs of sheep that develop increased lung permeability following infusion of the sedative-hypnotic ethchlorvynol (Fairman et al, 1981). In another model, intratracheal instillation of phorbol myristate acetate into rats, which activates both neutrophils and macrophages, caused diffuse lung injury that was not reduced by prior neutrophil depletion (Johnson and Ward, 1982).

Ex vivo perfused animal lungs have also been used to study neutrophil-induced damage. When stimulated neutrophils are added to the perfusate in isolated rabbit lungs, the permeability of the capillary alveolar walls is increased (Shasby et al, 1982). Similar results have been found using lungs from other species (e.g., rats [Morganroth et al, 1986]). The susceptibility of various types of cultured cells to neutrophil-induced damage has also been studied. Relevant to the lung, stimulated neutrophils can kill cultured monolayers of endothelial cells (Sacks et al, 1978; Weiss et al, 1981) and pulmonary alveolar epithelial cells (Suttorp and Simon, 1982; Simon et al, 1986).

MECHANISMS BY WHICH NEUTROPHILS INJURE LUNG TISSUE

Neutrophils possess a wide variety of armaments that kill invading microorganisms (Table 1–5) (Haslett et al, 1989; Weiss, 1989; Smith, 1994). However, the same weapons that are so effective at killing foreign invaders can also injure surrounding normal tissues. Neutrophil-derived products that have been implicated in causing lung damage include oxygen metabolites, reactive lipid molecules, lysosomal enzymes, and lysosomal cationic peptides.

Oxygen Metabolites

The discovery that neutrophils release the superoxide radical generated intense interest in the role of oxygen metabolites in inflammatory tissue injury (Babior et al, 1973). *Oxygen metabolite* is a loosely defined term that applies to a group of molecules that are generated following the reduction of molecular oxygen (Fig. 1–4) (McCord, 1993; Halliwell and Cross, 1994; Kinnula et al, 1995). Neutrophils possess an enzyme, NADPH oxidase, that when activated transfers an electron from NADPH to oxygen. With its additional electron, oxygen becomes a free radical, superoxide anion, that has altered reactivity compared with oxygen.

Superoxide can interact directly with a variety of biomolecules, leading to their alteration. Alternatively, it can react with itself or with other molecules to generate additional toxic agents. For example, when two molecules of superoxide combine, they undergo a dismutation reaction to form hydrogen peroxide and oxygen. If a metal ion such as iron or copper is available and in the proper oxidation state, hydroxyl radical is formed. This radical is exceedingly reactive and interacts with most biologic molecules at diffusion-limited rates. Myeloperoxidase, a neutrophil granule enzyme, catalyzes the reaction between hydrogen peroxide and chloride to form hypochlorous acid. Under the proper conditions, various oxygen metabolites can peroxidize polyunsaturated fatty acids, oxidize sulfhydryl and amino groups, cleave nucleic acids, and alter carbohydrates. Oxygen metabolites are thus ideally suited to kill invading microorganisms, but unfortunately they can also damage normal tissues.

Another free radical was added to the list of potentially toxic agents in ARDS (Freeman et al, 1995). Nitric oxide, produced from arginine by the enzymatic activity of nitric oxide synthase, is generated by a number of cell types including neutrophils, macrophages, and endothelial cells. Although nitric oxide is best known as *endothelium-derived relaxing factor* for its control of vascular tone, it can also be cytotoxic. For example, when nitric oxide is produced in conjunction with superoxide, the two radicals interact to form peroxynitrite anion (Pryor and Squadrito, 1995). The acid form of peroxynitrite anion, peroxynitrous acid, directly oxidizes a variety of biologically relevant substrates including sulfides (e.g., cysteine, glutathione), amines (e.g., amino acids, proteins), lipids, nucleic acids, and ascorbate. Theoretically, peroxynitrous acid can also undergo homolysis to form hydroxyl radical. Although this pathway was thought to be involved in nitric oxide–induced tissue injury, there is a question as to whether this reaction occurs *in vivo* (Pryor and Squadrito, 1995).

Direct evidence that oxygen metabolites par-

Table 1–5
Neutrophil-derived Agents Associated With Lung Injury

Products derived from reduction
    of molecular oxygen
  Superoxide
  Hydrogen peroxide
  Hydroxyl radical
  Myeloperoxidase-derived agents
  Peroxynitrite radical
Proteases
Defensins
Leukotoxin
Others

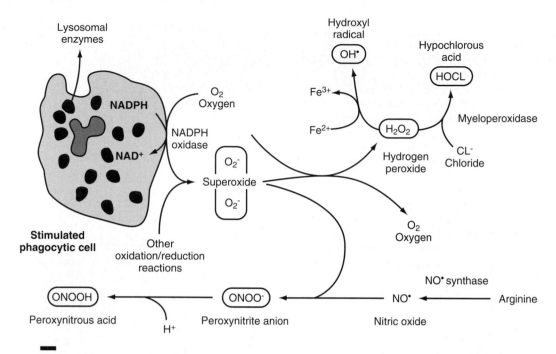

Figure 1–4
Phagocytic cell production of superoxide anion with subsequent generation of other potentially toxic molecules.

ticipate in human ARDS is limited. The hypothesis is supported most heavily by experiments using animal models or cells in tissue culture. However, there are several published human studies that provide evidence for oxidant stress during ARDS. In particular, α_1-antitrypsin, a protein normally present in bronchoalveolar lavage fluid, shows oxidative changes when recovered from patients with ARDS (Cochrane et al, 1983). Normal bronchoalveolar lavage fluid also contains glutathione, a molecule that serves as a substrate to scavenge hydrogen peroxide and repair oxidative damage to lipids and proteins (Cantin et al, 1987). In bronchoalveolar lavage fluid from patients with ARDS, glutathione levels are diminished and residual glutathione is found in its oxidized form (Bunnell and Pacht, 1993). More directly, oxygen metabolites have been detected in the lungs of patients with ARDS (Baldwin et al, 1986). In particular, when exhaled gases from ventilated patients were condensed and analyzed, hydrogen peroxide levels were found to be significantly higher in patients with ARDS than patients having other forms of respiratory failure.

The possibility that oxidant stress may play a role in ARDS has led to therapeutic trials of two agents that increase glutathione, namely N-acetylcysteine and 2-oxothiazolidine-4-carboxylate (OTC) (Jepsen et al, 1992; Bernard et al, 1994b; Suter et al, 1994). When administered to patients with ARDS, N-acetylcysteine and OTC reduced the progression to multiorgan failure, although overall survival was not affected.

The role of nitric oxide as a cytotoxic agent in ARDS is uncertain. Inhibitors of nitric oxide synthase are being studied as treatment for patients with septic shock (Petros et al, 1991; Cohen et al, 1996). Although the studies are designed to determine if inhibition of nitric oxide formation will reverse the hypotension of septic shock, data assessing its effect on tissue damage will likely become available. From the opposite perspective, nitric oxide has been tested as a therapeutic agent in ARDS. The rationale for its use is to function as endothelium-derived relaxing factor and reduce the pulmonary hypertension that occurs during ARDS. To date, these therapeutic studies have uncovered no evidence of lung injury when nitric oxide is delivered by inhalation.

In addition to the clinical studies mentioned earlier, the contribution of oxygen metabolites to inflammatory lung injury has been evaluated in a variety of experimental animal models. When generators of oxygen metabolites are instilled intratracheally into rats, lung injury occurs (Johnson et al, 1981).

Various evidence supports the conclusion

that lung damage can be caused by oxygen metabolites released by neutrophils. For example, experiments were performed in which a neutrophil-activating chemotactic peptide was instilled intratracheally into rabbits (Schraufstatter et al, 1984). The generation of oxygen metabolites was inferred by detecting hydrogen peroxide within the lungs of the rabbits using an indirect assay and by detecting decreases in glutathione concentrations. Neutrophil depletion reduced both the amount of hydrogen peroxide detected and the extent of lung injury. Superoxide dismutase, a scavenger of superoxide, also limited the depletion of glutathione. In two other experimental models, infusion of the oxygen metabolite scavengers superoxide dismutase and catalase reduced lung injury in rats that was induced by intravascular complement activation (Till et al, 1982) or by cutaneous burns (Till et al, 1983). Both of these models had been shown to be neutrophil-dependent.

Evidence linking neutrophils and oxygen metabolites in lung injury has been further strengthened by experiments using isolated perfused lungs (Shasby et al, 1982). Perfusion of rabbit lungs with solutions containing stimulated neutrophils was shown to cause lung edema. The resultant increase in alveolar wall permeability can be blocked by adding catalase to the perfusate. In similar model systems, isolated tissue cells maintained in culture have been used to study the mechanisms by which neutrophils injure normal cells (Weiss, 1989).

Many but not all of the studies conclude that oxygen metabolites are involved in the cytotoxic process. For example, neutrophil-induced injury of endothelial cells can be inhibited by adding catalase, a scavenger of hydrogen peroxide (Sacks et al, 1978; Weiss et al, 1981). Neutrophils from patients with chronic granulomatous disease, whose neutrophils cannot generate oxygen metabolites, fail to kill endothelial cells. Of the various species of oxygen metabolites, hydrogen peroxide frequently appears to have primary importance in causing cellular damage (Simon et al, 1981). Whether the tissue injury is caused by hydrogen peroxide or another species generated by hydrogen peroxide is unknown. Another candidate for causing injury is hydroxyl radical, which can be generated from hydrogen peroxide in the presence of metal ions. In various animal models and culture experiments, chelation of iron reduces oxygen metabolite–induced injury (Ward et al, 1983; Halliwell and Gutteridge, 1992).

Cytoplasmic Granule Contents
Proteases

Although neutrophil-generated oxygen metabolites have received much of the attention regarding mechanisms of lung injury in ARDS, there is abundant evidence to suggest that the contents of neutrophil granules also contribute. As mentioned earlier, myeloperoxidase can generate hypochlorous acid from hydrogen peroxide. Neutrophil cytoplasmic granules contain an assortment of degradative enzymes including proteases, lipases, nucleases, and saccharidases. Obviously, proteases can injure tissues by degrading cellular and extracellular proteins. However, they can also participate in a number of indirect and sometimes contradictory ways. For example, neutrophil-derived proteases can (1) activate or inactivate inflammatory mediators; (2) degrade cell surface receptors that are involved in upregulating or downregulating inflammatory pathways; (3) inactivate other proteases; and (4) destroy the ability of protease inhibitors to interfere with the activities of other proteases (Jochum et al, 1994).

Various proteases have been detected in bronchoalveolar lavage fluid from patients with ARDS. The proteases identified include elastase (Lee et al, 1981; Fowler et al, 1982; Idell et al, 1985; Wewers et al, 1988); collagenase (Christner et al, 1985); and cathepsins (Assfalg-Machleidt et al, 1990). Intratracheal instillation of neutrophil-derived proteases into animals induces acute alveolitis and tissue destruction (Marco et al, 1971). When adherent monolayers of cultured endothelial cells (Harlan et al, 1981) or alveolar epithelial cells (Ayars et al, 1984) are exposed to stimulated neutrophils, the monolayers detach from the culture dish. The loss of adherence has been attributed to the action of neutrophil elastase. In other experiments, neutrophils that are primed by low concentrations of endotoxin can be stimulated by chemotactic peptides to cause lysis of endothelial cells (Smedly et al, 1986). Again, a portion of the injury seems to be mediated by neutrophil elastase.

Defensins

Neutrophils contain within their cytoplasmic granules a group of cationic peptides called *defensins*. When released from the cells, defensins kill bacteria by creating pores within their cellular membranes. In addition to killing bacteria, defensins can also injure tissue cells. They have been shown to increase the permeability of cultured monolayers of epithelial cells (Nygaard et al, 1993), and under certain circumstances they kill a variety of cellular targets (Kagan et al, 1994). Although these data demonstrate a potential for defensins to be involved in tissue damage, their role in ARDS remains relatively unexplored.

Leukotoxin

Another toxic agent released by stimulated neutrophils is an oxidation product of linoleic acid called *leukotoxin* (9,10-epoxy-12-octadecenoate). Leukotoxin has been detected in bronchoalveolar lavage fluid obtained from patients with ARDS and from rats with lung injury caused by exposure to 100% oxygen (Ozawa et al, 1988). When infused intravascularly into isolated perfused lungs (Ishizaki et al, 1995) or intravenously into rats (Ozawa et al, 1988), leukotoxin causes acute edematous lung injury. Its contribution to the tissue damage in clinical ARDS has not been adequately assessed.

INTERACTIONS BETWEEN NEUTROPHIL-DERIVED TOXINS

Although neutrophil-derived enzymes and oxygen metabolites can directly and independently injure lung tissue, they can also cooperate to cause injury in a synergistic fashion. For example, oxygen metabolites alter structural proteins, increasing their susceptibility to proteolytic cleavage (Fligiel et al, 1984). Furthermore, oxygen metabolites can convert metalloproteinases to their active form (Weiss et al, 1985) and can potentiate the effects of proteases by inactivating protease inhibitors (Campbell et al, 1982; Cochrane et al, 1983; Ossanna et al, 1986).

INVOLVEMENT OF OTHER PHAGOCYTIC CELLS IN ARDS

Although the majority of investigations implicate neutrophils as being the major direct cause of tissue injury in ARDS, monocytes/macrophages and eosinophils may also participate.

MONOCYTES AND MACROPHAGES

Monocytes and macrophages possess many of the same toxic weapons that are found in neutrophils. Their cytoplasmic granules contain various degradative enzymes, and when stimulated, they generate and release oxygen metabolites.

Under certain circumstances, the proteases and oxygen metabolites produced by macrophages may be the primary cause of lung injury. An example of this is the occasional patient with extensive miliary tuberculosis whose lung damage is severe and diffuse enough to fulfill the criteria for ARDS (Huseby and Hudson, 1976).

In several animal models, oxygen metabolites generated by macrophages appear to be responsible for lung injury. For example, when phorbol myristate acetate is instilled intratracheally into rats, lung injury occurs (Johnson and Ward, 1982). Phorbol esters are potent inducers of oxygen metabolites from both neutrophils and macrophages. Scavenging hydrogen peroxide by catalase inhibits the lung injury in this model, but neutrophil depletion does not. One interpretation of these results is that macrophage-derived oxygen metabolites are responsible for the lung damage.

Another model of lung injury in which macrophages are implicated occurs when IgA immune complexes are formed within the lung (Johnson et al, 1984). Again, neutrophil depletion does not protect, whereas catalase does. Unfortunately, the role of macrophages cannot be more directly examined by depleting animals of macrophages before challenge. At present, there is no simple method to selectively eliminate macrophages without causing many other confounding effects.

EOSINOPHILS

Another cell type that has been implicated in ARDS is the eosinophil. Similar to neutrophils, eosinophils can injure pulmonary parenchymal cells *in vitro* via various mechanisms, including those involving oxygen metabolites and eosinophil granule contents (Davis et al, 1984). Bronchoalveolar lavage fluid from patients with ARDS contains elevated levels of eosinophil cationic protein, which is a major secretory product of stimulated eosinophils (Hallgren et al, 1987). In a small number of patients with ARDS, eosinophils appear in high numbers in bronchoalveolar lavage fluid (Allen et al, 1989). In this subgroup, administration of glucocorticoids appears to be therapeutic, whereas in the more typical case of ARDS they are not. When added to media perfusing isolated lungs, stimulated eosinophils cause a permeability-type injury similar to that seen with neutrophils (Rowen et al, 1990).

SOLUBLE MEDIATORS OF ARDS

Many agents have been suspected of contributing to the development of ARDS (Table 1–6). However, as mentioned earlier, it is difficult to determine which of them initiate the injury and which are a consequence of the presence of injured tissue. Furthermore, because inflammatory reactions are complex interacting cascades, activation of one leads to perturbation of others. One example of this interrelationship is the consequences of Hageman factor activation. Following its activation, Hageman factor rapidly activates the com-

---
Table 1–6
Classes of Soluble Mediators Implicated in ARDS

Complement
Arachidonic acid metabolites
Cytokines
Fibrinogen/fibrin-derived peptides
Histamine
Platelet activating factor
Serotonin
Kinins

---

plement, coagulation, kinin, and fibrinolytic systems. When viewed after the fact, it is difficult if not impossible to determine the order of activation.

COMPLEMENT COMPONENTS

The complement system was one of the first inflammatory cascades to be investigated in ARDS. Involvement of complement was first suspected because it was known that it can be activated by endotoxin, a common participant in ARDS. Furthermore, complement activation was recognized as causing neutrophil sequestration within the lung. A direct association between complement and ARDS was demonstrated when it was reported that a large percentage of patients with ARDS had activated complement fragments in their plasma (Hammerschmidt et al, 1980).

Subsequent studies confirmed the high prevalence of complement activation in patients with ARDS and spawned a considerable amount of investigative work using animal models. For example, intravascular infusion of cobra venom factor, a potent activator of complement, caused pulmonary neutrophil sequestration and injury in rats (Till et al, 1982). Plasma in which complement was activated by zymosan also caused neutrophils to accumulate in the lungs, with resulting hypoxemia (Hohn et al, 1980). Signs of complement activation are also present in several more clinically relevant models of lung injury such as cutaneous burns (Till et al, 1983) and streptococcal bacteremia (Hosea et al, 1980). Importantly, lung injury in each of these animal models was inhibitable by preventing complement activation.

Taken together, the information strongly suggests that complement activation is tightly linked to the development of ARDS. However, subsequent clinical studies of patients at risk for developing ARDS revealed that the active complement components C5a and C3a were frequently present in the plasma of patients who did not develop the full syndrome (Mayes et al, 1984). A reason for the lack of a tight correlation between ARDS and

complement activation was offered by data suggesting that only the terminal components of the complement cascade that make up the "attack complex" were important (Langlois and Gawryl, 1988). However, this suggestion was not supported by subsequent data (Parsons and Giclas, 1990).

Although complement activation is not sufficient to cause ARDS, it is likely to be an important participant, nonetheless. Of the various complement proteins, C5a has many properties that could contribute to the development of ARDS. In particular, C5a is chemotactic for neutrophils, causes neutrophil aggregation, and stimulates neutrophils to release toxic products. In some experiments, infusion of C5a causes lung injury that is preventable by prior neutrophil depletion (Shaw et al, 1980). However, the ability of C5a or complement activation to initiate lung injury by itself in animal models is uncertain. In one series of experiments, neither C5a, zymosan-activated plasma, nor cobra venom factor caused lung injury in awake, uninstrumented rabbits (Webster et al, 1982). C5a or complement activation was able to induce lung edema, but only if the animals were first experimentally manipulated by administering anesthesia, placing a tracheotomy, and inserting intravascular catheters. Apparently events initiated by these manipulations act in concert with C5a to cause lung injury.

ARACHIDONIC ACID METABOLITES

In a search for agents that mediate lung damage in ARDS, interest has been directed toward the products of arachidonic acid metabolism. Many cell types including macrophages, platelets, endothelial cells, epithelial cells, and neutrophils can release arachidonic acid and metabolize it to various bioactive products. The spectrum of effects caused by these arachidonic acid metabolites makes them attractive candidates for initiating or modulating some of the abnormalities that characterize ARDS. Thromboxane B_2 (the stable breakdown product of the biologically active vasoconstrictor thromboxane A_2) and 6-keto-prostaglandin $F_{1\alpha}$ (the degradation product of prostacyclin) have been detected in bronchoalveolar lavage fluid from patients with ARDS (Deby-Dupont et al, 1987). Ibuprofen, a cyclooxygenase inhibitor, reduced lung injury in an animal model of ARDS (see later). However, cyclooxygenase inhibitors have been tested in humans with the related condition, sepsis, and have not been shown to be beneficial (Haupt et al, 1991).

Much of the data implicating arachidonic acid metabolites come from results of animal and *in vitro* experiments. Endotoxin infusion into sheep initiates a two-phased response (Brigham et al, 1979). In the initial phase, pulmonary artery pressure and lymph flow increase. Because the concentration of protein in the lymph draining the lung is low, the increased lymph flow during the initial phase is not the result of increased lung permeability but rather is related to increased microvascular hydrostatic pressures. A role for cyclooxygenase products in the initial phase has been suggested by the observation that the increased lymph flow is prevented by cyclooxygenase inhibitors such as meclofenamate and indomethacin (Demling et al, 1981; Ogletree et al, 1982). Direct measurements of cyclooxygenase products in the lymph or plasma of the sheep during this phase reveal the presence of prostaglandin $F_{2\alpha}$ and thromboxane (Demling et al, 1981). Several hours after endotoxin infusion, a second elevation of pulmonary artery pressure occurs that is associated with a high permeability injury to the alveolar wall. Most cyclooxygenase inhibitors do not reduce the lung injury of this second phase, although ibuprofen does (Kopolovic et al, 1984). The mechanism by which ibuprofen blocks the injury is unknown but may involve modulating neutrophil function.

Leukotrienes are potent mediators of inflammation. For example, leukotriene B_4 has strong chemotactic activity. Leukotrienes C_4, D_4, and E_4 are a group of molecules that constitute what was formerly known as slow reacting substance of anaphylaxis. Leukotriene C_4 (Stephenson et al, 1988) and D_4 (Matthay et al, 1984; Stephenson et al, 1988) have been found to be elevated in the respiratory secretions of patients with ARDS. Ketaconazole, an antifungal antibiotic that inhibits thromboxane synthetase and 5-lipoxygenase, has been reported to prevent ARDS and improve survival in patients at risk due to severe trauma or sepsis (Slotman et al, 1988; Yu and Tomasa, 1993). The two studies reporting these results are small and confirmatory investigations are needed.

In animal experiments, administration of leukotrienes have been shown to have considerable hemodynamic and airway effects. Their elevation has been detected in various models of lung injury (Ogletree et al, 1982; Olson et al, 1987). With the development of stable analogues, more specific inhibitors, and transgenic animals lacking or overexpressing arachidonic acid metabolic enzymes, a more precise assessment of the activities of these agents in ARDS should be forthcoming.

CYTOKINES

Tumor Necrosis Factor (TNFα)

TNFα, a product of macrophages, may play a prominent role in many cases of ARDS (see Fig. 1–3) (Table 1–7). Bronchoalveolar lavage fluid and plasma from patients with ARDS often contain elevated levels (Millar et al, 1989; Marks et al, 1990; Hyers et al, 1991; Roten et al, 1991; Parsons et al, 1992; Suter et al, 1992; Antonelli et al, 1994). However, plasma TNFα has not been shown to be specific for ARDS because many patients with risk factors for ARDS and elevated TNFα do not go on to develop the syndrome. Although the presence of TNFα is not sufficient to cause ARDS, it most likely plays an important intermediary function in many cases.

Intravenous infusion of low doses of endotoxin into human volunteers causes a brief increase in circulating TNFα simultaneous with the appearance of systemic effects such as fever, tachycardia, and leukocytosis (Michie et al, 1988). In animals, TNFα infusion induces many of the systemic abnormalities that occur in septic shock (Beutler et al, 1985; Tracey et al, 1986). Included in this repertoire of effects is acute lung injury of a type similar to that which occurs in ARDS (Stephens et al, 1988). Electron microscopy of lung tissue obtained from sheep infused with TNFα reveal neutrophil accumulation, endothelial and epithelial damage, and edema (Johnson et al, 1991). If antibodies to TNFα are infused into animals before administration of endotoxin, the degree of organ injury, including that of the lungs, was less severe (Mathison et al, 1988; Tracey et al, 1988). Furthermore, transgenic mice producing excess murine TNFα in the lung develop chronic pulmonary injury with fibrosis (Miyazaki et al, 1995).

The linkage between TNFα and the systemic effects of endotoxin are just beginning to be dissected. TNFα can act directly to increase the adherence of neutrophils to endothelial cells (Gamble et al, 1985) and augment the production of potentially toxic agents by stimulated neutrophils (Klebanoff et al, 1986). TNFα can also

Table 1–7
Participation of Cytokines and Growth Factors in ARDS

Early responses
  Tumor necrosis factor α (TNFα)
  Interleukin-1 (IL-1)

Amplifiers
  Interleukin-8 (IL-8)
  Macrophage inhibitory peptide-1α (MIP-1α)

Repair/Scarring
  Transforming growth factor-β (TGF$_\beta$)
  Platelet-derived growth factor (PDGF)

serve as a pivotal point for generation of other inflammatory mediators. For example, it stimulates macrophages to release interleukin-1, interleukin-6, platelet-activating factor, arachidonic acid metabolites, and growth factors (Traccy ct al, 1989). Along with endotoxin and interleukin-1, TNFα can induce endothelial cells to release a chemotactic factor for neutrophils (Strieter et al, 1989). TNFα also stimulates the release of interleukin-1 from endothelial cells (Nawroth et al, 1986).

Synthesis and release of multiple cytokines may be coordinated in part at the level of gene transcription. Analysis of the nontranscribed sequences of the TNFα gene has uncovered a consensus sequence shared by other genes involved in various aspects of inflammation, including genes for lymphotoxin, interleukin-1, and fibronectin (Caput et al, 1986).

The linkage of TNFα with both sepsis and ARDS has fostered an intense effort to develop treatment strategies designed to interrupt TNFα effects. However, clinical studies using anti-TNFα antibodies (Fisher et al, 1993) or soluble TNFα receptors have not yet shown substantial clinical benefits in patients with sepsis.

Interleukin-1

Interleukin-1 (IL-1) is another early-response cytokine that has been linked to the pathogenesis of ARDS (see Fig. 1–3). Many of the stimuli that induce macrophages to release TNFα also cause IL-1 secretion. Furthermore, TNFα itself causes IL-1 synthesis and secretion. IL-1 shares many properties with TNFα. In particular, it induces neutrophil recruitment and activation. Like TNFα, IL-1 has been detected in increased amounts in bronchoalveolar lavage fluid obtained from patients with ARDS (Siler et al, 1989; Suter et al, 1992; Meduri et al, 1995). However, similar to TNFα, elevated levels of IL-1 have also been found in patients who have conditions placing them at risk for the developing of ARDS but who do not develop the full syndrome. Clinical trials of a naturally occurring protein inhibitor of IL-1, IL-1 receptor antagonist, have been performed in patients with sepsis. Despite initial encouraging results (Fisher et al, 1994), further data have not confirmed significant efficacy.

Interleukin-8

Early studies of bronchoalveolar lavage fluid from patients with ARDS revealed the presence of an otherwise unidentified peptide that accounted for a substantial portion of the measured chemotactic

activity of the fluid (Parsons et al, 1985). Subsequent work identified the peptide as the 8.4 kD, interleukin-8 (IL-8) (Jorens et al, 1992; Miller et al, 1992; Chollet-Martin et al, 1993; Donnelly et al, 1994b). IL-8, a member of the chemokine family, is a product of monocyte/macrophages, endothelial cells, fibroblasts, and epithelial cells. Its secretion is upregulated by TNFα and IL-1. Unlike TNFα and IL-1, which appear to be rapidly downregulated following activation, IL-8 levels remain elevated for longer periods. IL-8 has also been detected in the plasma of patients with ARDS (Meade et al, 1994). In a neutrophil-dependent model of ARDS in rats, an antibody to human IL-8 protected against lung injury (Mulligan et al, 1993a).

COAGULATION AND FIBRINOLYTIC SYSTEMS

Disordered fibrin metabolism is a prominent features of ARDS. Immunohistologic evaluation of lung tissue obtained from patients with ARDS shows that the hyaline membranes that are typically seen lining the damaged alveolar walls are made up of fibrin. Both histologic and angiographic studies show that the pulmonary vasculature of patients with ARDS is frequently plugged with thrombi (Tomaschefski et al, 1983; Greene et al, 1987) Fibrinogen dynamics are altered in ARDS, as demonstrated by abnormally rapid pulmonary uptake of iodine 125–labeled fibrinogen from the blood (Busch et al, 1975b). Circulating platelet counts in patients with sepsis and ARDS are often low early in the course of the disease (Fein et al, 1983; Rivkind et al, 1989). The low platelet number is caused by a shortened life span resulting from platelet sequestration within the lungs, liver, and spleen (Schneider et al, 1980).

Lung injury in animals can be induced by activation of the coagulation system. The simultaneous infusion of thrombin and an inhibitor of fibrinolysis into dogs causes acute alveolar damage (Saldeen, 1983). The mechanism of this injury is independent of neutrophils and platelets, because edema is not diminished by making the dogs both neutropenic and thrombocytopenic (Busch et al, 1975a). However, if the dogs are depleted of fibrinogen, alveolar injury is reduced.

In ARDS, fibrin dynamics are influenced by alterations in both coagulation and fibrinolysis. In many patients, the diagnosis of diffuse intravascular coagulation can be made (Bone et al, 1976). D-antigen, a product of fibrin/fibrinogen degradation, is found in the blood of patients with ARDS, although it is not specific for the disease (Haynes et al, 1980). Elevated levels have been reported in patients with major burns or traumatic injury whose disease does not progress to ARDS (Curreri et al, 1975). Likewise, many patients with diffuse intravascular coagulation do not go on to fulfill criteria for ARDS (Modig et al, 1983).

The coagulation and fibrinolytic profiles of the pulmonary extravascular compartment are also altered in ARDS. When plasma is introduced into a normal alveolar spaces, fibrin is rapidly formed (Simon et al, 1995). The coagulation cascade in the alveolus is triggered by tissue factor (McGee and Rothberger, 1985) that is produced by alveolar macrophages and epithelial cells. In ARDS, the levels of tissue factor recovered in bronchoalveolar lavage fluid are increased (Idell et al, 1989b). When lung injury is induced in mice by intratracheal bleomycin, tissue factor mRNA is increased (Olman et al, 1995). Under normal circumstances, fibrin is cleared from the alveolar space by plasmin that is activated from plasminogen. The enzyme responsible for activating plasminogen is urokinase that is secreted by both alveolar epithelial cells and macrophages (Chapman et al, 1986; Hasday et al, 1988). During ARDS, fibrinolysis is suppressed by increases in inhibitors such as plasminogen activator inhibitor-1 (PAI-1) (Chapman et al, 1986; Bertozzi et al, 1990).

In animal models of ARDS, similar changes are seen (Idell et al, 1988; Idell et al, 1989a; Idell et al, 1989c; Idell et al, 1992; Olman et al, 1995). The fibrin that forms in the alveolar space may be beneficial by reducing the leakage of plasma through damaged alveolar walls. However, its persistence may have adverse effects by serving as a scaffold on which fibroblasts invade to form collagenous scars.

A link has been demonstrated between the fibrinolytic system and fibrosis that follows lung inflammation (Eitzman et al, 1996). Transgenic mice with altered PAI-1 genes were given intratracheal saline or bleomycin, and the amount of lung collagen that formed was measured. In animals given bleomycin, those with reduced fibrinolytic activity due to overexpression of a PAI-1 transgene developed more lung scarring. Conversely, bleomycin-treated animals having accelerated fibrinolysis due to inactivation of PAI-1 genes accumulated less collagen.

OTHER SOLUBLE FACTORS

In addition to the mediators already discussed, there are many other agents that have been associated with ARDS. Administration of an antihistamine reduced lung edema in a sheep endotoxin model (Brigham and Owen, 1975a) and a rat

cutaneous burn model (Friedl et al, 1989), suggesting that histamine may have a role in acute lung injury. Platelet activating factor (acetyl glyceryl ether phosphoryl choline) is another agent that has the potential to contribute to the lung injury of ARDS. It augments a number of neutrophil activities including adherence, aggregation, chemotaxis, degranulation, and production of oxygen metabolites and arachidonic acid metabolites (McManus and Deavers, 1989).

Elevated levels of platelet activating factor have been detected in bronchoalveolar lavage fluid obtained from patients with ARDS (Matsumoto et al, 1992). Platelet activating factor can also cause pulmonary neutrophil accumulation and lung edema in rabbits (Worthen et al, 1983) and can be involved in the hemodynamic alterations and lung injury that follow endotoxin infusion into rats (Chang et al, 1987). In isolated perfused animal lungs, platelet activating factor causes lung edema in the presence (Heffner et al, 1983) or absence (Hamasaki et al, 1984) of platelets in the perfusate.

Other inflammatory pathways investigated in ARDS include serotonin (Brigham and Owen, 1975b) and the kallikrein-kinin system (Carvalho et al, 1988). Unfortunately, insufficient information is available at present to determine the contribution of these mediators to the various manifestations of ARDS.

ADHERENCE MOLECULES IN ARDS

An important step in the pathophysiology of ARDS is the accumulation of neutrophils within lung parenchyma. Under normal circumstances, a portion of circulating neutrophils exist as marginated, quiescent cells in the pulmonary capillary bed. Early in the pathogenesis of ARDS, mediators are released that alter neutrophil and/or endothelial cell behavior, causing a rapid increase in neutrophil sequestration. One proposed mechanism explaining neutrophil accumulation within the lung is that following activation, neutrophil stiffness increases. The cells are no longer able to deform and squeeze through the narrow pulmonary capillaries, leading to impaction and sequestration in the pulmonary vascular bed (Worthen et al, 1989).

In addition to changes in cell deformability, there are other adherence mechanisms that are likely to be operative. A complex system of cell surface molecules controls neutrophil adherence to endothelial cells. One group of molecules, the selectins, causes neutrophils to be slowed as they pass through the vascular bed (Bevilacqua and

Nelson, 1993; Tedder et al, 1995). By forming loose associations between endothelial cells and neutrophils, the neutrophils are slowed, causing them to appear to roll along the endothelial surface.

At present, three different but related selectin molecules have been characterized. L-selectin (also known as CD62L, LAM-1, MEL-14) is constitutively produced and expressed on the surface of hematopoietic cells, including neutrophils. Following exposure to inflammatory stimuli, the binding affinity of L-selectin is rapidly increased. However, the change in L-selectin conformation also renders the molecule susceptible to proteolytic cleavage, releasing a soluble form of L-selectin into the circulation. P-selectin (CD62P, PADGEM, GMP-140) is synthesized and stored in cytoplasmic bodies within endothelial cells. Exposure to inflammatory stimuli including thrombin, histamine, and complement components rapidly brings the P-selectin molecule to the endothelial cell surface where it can participate in tethering neutrophils. E-selectin (CD62E, ELAM-1) is found on the surface of endothelial cells and is upregulated by endotoxin, TNFα, and IL-1. The ligands that bind to the selectins consist of a spectrum of glycoproteins, some of which have terminal tetrasaccharides that are recognized as sialyl Lewis[x] or sialyl Lewis[a] antigens. Other phosphorylated mono- and polysaccharides and sulfated polysaccharides can also serve as ligands.

The different selectins appear to have overlapping roles in neutrophil accumulation at sites of inflammation. Depending on the inflammatory stimulus and the time following exposure, different selectin interactions contribute to slowing the transit of neutrophils through the endothelial bed. In ARDS, the expression of each of the selectins has been found to be altered. Plasma concentration of soluble P-selectin is elevated in patients with ARDS (Sakamaki et al, 1995). In patients at high risk for developing ARDS, circulating levels of soluble L-selectin are lower in the subgroup who go on to develop the full syndrome (Donnelly et al, 1994a).

Blocking selectins with antibodies has been found to reduce lung injury in some animal models. For example, an antibody directed against both E-selectin and L-selectin reduced pulmonary neutrophil accumulation and lung injury in pigs receiving *Pseudomonas* bacteria (Ridings et al, 1995). In neutrophil-dependent lung injury models in rats, antibodies to E-selectin, P-selectin, and L-selectin were also found to be protective (Mulligan et al, 1991; Mulligan et al, 1993b; Mulligan et al, 1994).

Tighter binding of neutrophils to the endo-

thelial surface is accomplished by pairs of other adhesion molecules, including the integrins. β$_2$-integrins are heterodimeric proteins found on the surface of activated neutrophils. They bind to endothelial cell intercellular adhesion molecules, ICAM-1 and ICAM-2. Stimulation of neutrophils with endotoxin, TNFα, or IL-1 causes the β$_2$-integrin molecules to migrate rapidly to the neutrophil surface. These same stimuli increase endothelial cell ICAM expression. Antibodies directed at various adhesion molecules have been used to evaluate their contribution to lung injury using animal models (Mulligan et al, 1995). The results of these studies demonstrate that the function of the different adhesion molecules in ARDS is complex and is likely to depend upon the stimulus, time after initiation of ARDS, and site of neutrophil interaction being studied (vascular vs. interstitium vs. airspace).

REPAIR PROCESSES IN ARDS

The outcome of ARDS is heavily dependent on the speed and completeness of lung repair processes. To regenerate normal anatomy and function following injury, a number of steps must take place. Cellular debris and excess plasma-derived proteins must be removed. The lungs possess several mechanisms to accomplish this. In particular, phagocytic cells including neutrophils and monocytes/macrophages engulf the material and degrade it, using their lysosomal enzymes. As mentioned previously, the fibrinolytic system is also responsible for breaking down fibrin that forms in the alveolar space. Failure of these processes leads to replacement of the lung with collagen tissue.

The fibrotic process represents a complex series of events that is orchestrated by a variety of inflammatory cells, pulmonary parenchymal cells, and soluble factors. Molecular biologic techniques have demonstrated the presence of increased amounts of a variety of cytokines and growth factors in lungs taken from patients with fibrotic lung diseases. These include transforming growth factor-β (Broekelmann et al, 1991) and platelet-derived growth factor (Antoniades et al, 1990). Evidence that collagen deposition occurs early in ARDS comes from studies measuring type III procollagen peptide in bronchoalveolar lavage fluid (Clark et al, 1995). Type III procollagen peptide is cleaved from nascent collagen molecules and its presence reflects recent collagen synthesis. The level of this procollagen peptide in bronchoalveolar lavage fluid has been found to correlate with a poor outcome in patients with ARDS. Although past studies of anti-inflammatory glucocorticoids given early in ARDS showed no benefit or that they caused harm, the question has been raised whether they may be beneficial in preventing fibrosis if given later in the course of the disease (Meduri et al, 1994).

To complete the repair process, plugged capillaries must be reopened and their surfaces relined with endothelial cells. This process is similar to that of angiogenesis. A number of cellular factors and receptors have been identified as playing a role in this process (Henke et al, 1991; Kovacs and DiPietro, 1994). In addition to repairing blood vessels, damaged alveolar epithelial cells must be replaced. Histologic studies using metabolic labeling of newly synthesized DNA show that damaged type I cells are replaced by proliferation of surviving type II cells that later differentiate into type I cells (Evans et al, 1973). If repair is not successful, the residual airspaces remain lined with hyperplastic type II cells that fail to differentiate into a type I cell phenotype.

A final stage in lung repair requires removal of excess inflammatory and interstitial cells. This process is under active investigation and most likely involves programmed cell death or apoptosis (Haslett et al, 1994). Part of this process induces changes in the plasma membrane of apoptotic neutrophils that signal macrophages to phagocytize and degrade them. It is likely, but unproved, that the excess hyperplastic type II epithelium and possibly the fibroblasts also undergo apoptosis.

SUMMARY

ARDS is a diverse group of conditions that have common clinical and physiologic manifestations. The pathologic processes that lead to ARDS include damage to both alveolar endothelium and epithelium. Based on experimental evidence, it is highly likely that neutrophils are responsible for much, but not all, of the damage in ARDS. Oxygen metabolites in conjunction with neutrophil granule contents most likely participate in the process of injury. The agents that initiate or perpetuate ARDS are multiple and include the complement system, arachidonic acid metabolites, and cytokines. A better understanding of these complex cascades will lead to improved prevention and treatment for ARDS.

REFERENCES

Albert RK, Lakshminarayan S, Hildebrandt J, et al: Increased surface tension favors pulmonary edema formation in anesthetized dogs' lungs. J Clin Invest 63:1015–1018, 1979.

Allen JN, Pacht ER, Gadek JE, et al: Acute eosinophilic pneumonia as a reversible cause of noninfectious respiratory failure [see comments]. N Engl J Med 321:569–574, 1989.

Antonelli M, Raponi G, Lenti L, et al: Leukotrienes and alpha tumor necrosis factor levels in the bronchoalveolar lavage fluid of patient at risk for the adult respiratory distress syndrome. Minerva Anestesiol 60:419–426, 1994.

Antoniades HN, Bravo MA, Avila RE, et al: Platelet-derived growth factor in idiopathic pulmonary fibrosis. J Clin Invest 86:1055–1064, 1990.

Anzueto A, Baughman R, Guntupalli K, et al: An international randomized, placebo-controlled trial evaluating the safety and efficacy of aerosolized surfactant in patients with sepsis-induced ARDS. Am J Resp Crit Care Med 149:A567, 1994.

Ashbaugh DG, Bigelow DB, Petty TL, et al: Acute respiratory distress in adults. Lancet 2:319–323, 1967.

Assfalg-Machleidt I, Jochum M, Nast-Kolb D, et al: Cathepsin B–indicator for the release of lysosomal cysteine proteinases in severe trauma and inflammation. Biol Chem Hoppe Seyler: 211–222, 1990.

Ayars GH, Altman LC, Rosen H, et al: The injurious effect of neutrophils on pneumocytes in vitro. Am Rev Respir Dis 130:964–973, 1984.

Babior BM, Kipnes RS, Curnutte JT: Biological defense mechanisms. The production by leukocytes of superoxide, a potential bactericidal agent. J Clin Invest 52:741–744, 1973.

Bachofen A and Weibel ER: Alterations of the gas exchange apparatus in adult respiratory insufficiency associated with septicemia. Am Rev Respir Dis 116:589–615, 1977.

Baldwin SR, Simon RH, Grum CM, et al: Oxidant activity in expired breath of patients with adult respiratory stress syndrome. Lancet 1:11–13, 1986.

Bernard GR, Artigas A, Brigham KL, et al: The American-European Consensus Conference on ARDS. Definitions, mechanisms, relevant outcomes, and clinical trial coordination. Am J Respir Crit Care Med 149:818–824, 1994a.

Bernard GR, Dupont W, Eden T, et al: Antioxidants in the acute respiratory distress syndrome. Am J Resp Crit Care Med 149:A241, 1994b.

Bertozzi P, Astedt B, Zenzius L, et al: Depressed bronchoalveolar urokinase activity in patients with adult respiratory distress syndrome. N Engl J Med 322:890–897, 1990.

Beutler B: TNF, immunity and inflammatory disease: Lessons of the past decade. J Invest Med 43:227–235, 1995.

Beutler B, Milsark IW, Cerami AC: Passive immunization against cachectin/tumor necrosis factor protects mice from lethal effect of endotoxin. Science 229:869–871, 1985.

Bevilacqua MP and Nelson RM: Selectins. J Clin Invest 91:379–387, 1993.

Bone RC, Francis PB, and Pierce AK: Intravascular coagulation associated with adult respiratory distress syndrome. Am J Med 61:585–589, 1976.

Brigham KL, Bowers RE, and Haynes J: Increased sheep lung vascular permeability caused by Escherichia coli endotoxin. Circ Res 45:292–297, 1979.

Brigham KL and Owen PJ: Increased sheep lung vascular permeability caused by histamine. Circ Res 37:647–657, 1975a.

Brigham KL and Owen PJ: Mechanism of the serotonin effect on lung transvascular fluid and protein movement in awake sheep. Circ Res 36:761–770, 1975b.

Brigham KL, Woolverton WC, Blake LH, et al: Increased sheep lung vascular permeability caused by pseudomonas bacteremia. J Clin Invest 54:792–804, 1974.

Broekelmann TJ, Limper AH, Colby TV, et al: Transforming growth factor beta 1 is present at sites of extracellular matrix gene expression in human pulmonary fibrosis. Proc Natl Acad Sci USA 88:6642–6646, 1991.

Bunnell E and Pacht ER: Oxidized glutathione is increased in the alveolar fluid of patients with the adult respiratory distress syndrome. Am Rev Respir Dis 148:1174–1178, 1993.

Busch C, Dahlgren S, Jakobson S, et al: The use of ^{125}I-labelled fibrinogen for determination of fibrin trapping in the lungs in patients developing the microembolism syndrome. Acta Anaesthesiol Scand [Suppl] 57:46–54, 1975a.

Busch C, Dahlgren S, Jakobson S, et al: The use of ^{125}I-labelled fibrinogen for determination of fibrin trapping in the lungs of patients developing the microembolism syndrome. Acta Anesthesiol Scand [Suppl] 57:45–54, 1975b.

Campbell EJ, Senior RM, McDonald JA, et al: Proteolysis by neutrophils. Relative importance of cell-substrate contact and oxidative inactivation of proteinase inhibitors in vitro. J Clin Invest 70:845–852, 1982.

Cantin AM, North SL, Hubbard RC, et al: Normal alveolar epithelial lining fluid contains high levels of glutathione. J Appl Physiol 63:152–157, 1987.

Caput D, Beutler B, Hartog K, et al: Identification of a common nucleotide sequence in the 3'-untranslated region of mRNA molecules specifying inflammatory mediators. Proc Natl Acad Sci USA 83:1670–1674, 1986.

Carvalho AC, DeMarinis S, Scott CF, et al: Activation of the contact system of plasma proteolysis in the adult respiratory distress syndrome. J Lab Clin Med 112:270–277, 1988.

Chang SW, Feddersen CO, Henson PM, et al: Platelet-activating factor mediates hemodynamic changes and lung injury in endotoxin-treated rats. J Clin Invest 79:1498–509, 1987.

Chapman HA, Allen CL, and Stone OL: Abnormalities in pathways of alveolar fibrin turnover among patients with interstitial lung disease. Am Rev Respir Dis 133:437–443, 1986.

Chollet-Martin S, Montravers P, Gibert C, et al: High levels of interleukin-8 in the blood and alveolar spaces of patients with pneumonia and adult respiratory distress syndrome. Infect Immunol 61:4553–4559, 1993.

Christner P, Fein A, Goldberg S, et al: Collagenase in the lower respiratory tract of patients with adult respiratory distress syndrome. Am Rev Respir Dis 131:690–695, 1985.

Clark JG, Milberg JA, Steinberg KP, et al: Type III procollagen peptide in the adult respiratory distress syndrome. Ann Intern Med 122:17–23, 1995.

Cochrane CG, Spragg R, and Revak SD: Pathogenesis of the adult respiratory distress. J Clin Invest 71:754–761, 1983.

Cohen R, Huberfeld S, Genovese J, et al: A comparison between the effects of nitric oxide syntase inhibition and fluid resuscitation on myocardial function and metabolism in endotoxemic dogs. J Crit Care 11:17–36, 1996.

Curreri PW, Wilterdink ME, and Baxter CR: Characterization of elevated fibrin split products following thermal injury. Ann Surg 181:157–160, 1975.

Davis WB, Fells GA, Sun XT, et al: Eosinophil-mediated injury to lung parenchymal cells and interstitial matrix. J Clin Invest 74:269–278, 1984.

Deby-Dupont G, Braun M, Lamy M, et al: Thromboxane and prostacyclin release in adult respiratory distress syndrome. Intensive Care Med 13:167–174, 1987.

Demling RJ, Smith M, Gunther R, et al: Pulmonary injury and prostaglandin production during endotoxemia in conscious sheep. Am J Physiol 240:H348–H53, 1981.

Deneke SM and Fanburg BL: Normobaric oxygen toxicity of the lung. N Engl J Med 303:76–86, 1980.

Donnelly SC, Haslett C, Dransfield I, et al: Role of selectins in development of adult respiratory distress syndrome. Lancet 344:215–219, 1994a.

Donnelly TJ, Meade P, Jagels M, et al: Cytokine, complement, and endotoxin profiles associated with the development of the adult respiratory distress syndrome after severe injury. Crit Care Med 22:768–776, 1994b.

Eitzman DT, McCoy RD, Fay WP, et al: Bleomycin-induced pulmonary fibrosis in transgenic mice that either lack or overexpress the murine plasminogen activator inhibitor-1 gene. J Clin Invest 97:232–237, 1996.

Enhorning G: Surfactant replacement in adult respiratory distress syndrome. Am Rev Respir Dis 140:281–283, 1989.

Evans MJ, Cabral LJ, Stephens RJ, et al: Renewal of alveolar epithelium in the rat following exposure to NO_2. Am J Pathol 70:175–198, 1973.

Fairman RP, Glauser FL, Falls R: Increases in lung lymph and albumin clearance with ethchlorvynol. J Appl Physiol 50:1151–1155, 1981.

Fein AM, Lippmann M, Holtzman H, et al: The risk factors, incidence, and prognosis of ARDS following septicemia. Chest 83:40–42, 1983.

Fisher CJ Jr, Opal SM, Dhainaut JF, et al: Influence of an anti-tumor necrosis factor monoclonal antibody on cytokine levels in patients with sepsis. The CB0006 Sepsis Syndrome Study Group. Crit Care Med 21:318–327, 1993.

Fisher CJ Jr, Slotman GJ, Opal SM, et al: Initial evaluation of human recombinant interleukin-1 receptor antagonist in the treatment of sepsis syndrome: A randomized, open-label, placebo-controlled multicenter trial. The IL-1RA Sepsis Syndrome Study Group. Crit Care Med 22:12–21, 1994.

Fligiel SE, Lee EC, McCoy JP, et al: Protein degradation following treatment with hydrogen peroxide. Am J Pathol 115:418–425, 1984.

Fowler AA, Hamman RF, Good JT, et al: Adult respiratory distress syndrome: Risk with common predispositions. Ann Intern Med 98:593–597, 1983.

Fowler AA, Walchak S, Giclas PC, et al: Characterization of antiproteinase activity in the adult respiratory distress syndrome. Chest 81:50S–51S, 1982.

Freeman BA, Gutierrez H, and Rubbo H: Nitric oxide: a central regulatory species in pulmonary oxidant reactions [editorial; comment]. Am J Physiol 268:L697–698, 1995.

Friedl HP, Till GO, Trentz O, et al: Roles of histamine, complement and xanthine oxidase in thermal injury of skin. Am J Pathol 135:203–217, 1989.

Gamble JR, Harlan JM, Klebanoff SJ, et al: Stimulation of the adherence of neutrophils to umbilical vein endothelium by human recombinant tumor necrosis factor. Proc Natl Acad Sci USA 82:8667–8671, 1985.

Goodman BE and Crandall ED: Dome formation in primary cultured monolayers of alveolar epithelial cells. Am J Physiol 243:C95–C100, 1982.

Gorin AB and Stewart PA: Differential permeability of endothelial and epithelial barriers to albumin flux. J Appl Physiol 47:1315–1324, 1979.

Greene R, Lind S, Jantsch H, et al: Pulmonary vascular obstruction in severe ARDS: Angiographic alterations after i.v. fibrinolytic therapy. AJR Am J Roentgenol 148:501–508, 1987.

Gregory TJ, Godek JE, Weiland JE, et al: Surfanta supplementation in patients with acute respiratory distress syndrome (ARDS). Am J Respir Crit Care Med 149:A567, 1994.

Guyton AC and Moffatt DS: Role of surface tension and surfactant in the transepithelial movement of fluid and in the development of pulmonary edema. Prog Respir Res 15:62–75, 1981.

Hallgren R, Samuelsson T, Venge P, et al: Eosinophil activation in the lung is related to lung damage in adult respiratory distress syndrome. Am Rev Respir Dis 135:639–642, 1987.

Halliwell B and Cross CE: Oxygen-derived species: Their relation to human disease and environmental stress. Environ Health Perspect 102 [Suppl] 10:5–12, 1994.

Halliwell B and Gutteridge JM: Biologically relevant metal ion-dependent hydroxyl radical generation. An update. FEBS Lett 307:108–112, 1992.

Hamasaki Y, Mojarad M, Saga T, et al: Platelet-activating factor raises airway and vascular pressures and induces edema in lungs perfused with platelet-free solution. Am Rev Respir Dis 129:742–746, 1984.

Hammerschmidt DE, Weaver LJ, Hudson LD, et al: Association of complement activation and elevated plasma-C5a with adult respiratory distress syndrome. Pathophysiological relevance and possible prognostic value. Lancet 1:947–949, 1980.

Harlan JM, Killen PD, Harker LA, et al: Neutrophil-mediated endothelial injury in vivo. J Clin Invest 68:1394–1403, 1981.

Hasday JL, Bachwich PR, Lynch JP, et al: Procoagulant and plasminogen activator activities of bronchoalveolar fluid in patients with pulmonary sarcoidosis. Exp Lung Res 14:261–278, 1988.

Haslett C, Savill JS, Meagher L: The neutrophil. Curr Opin Immunol 2:10–18, 1989.

Haslett C, Savill JS, Whyte MK, et al: Granulocyte apoptosis and the control of inflammation. Philos Trans R Soc Lond B Biol Sci 345:327–333, 1994.

Haupt JT, Jastremski MS, Clemmer TP, et al: Effect of ibuprofen in patients with severe sepsis: A randomized, double-blind, multicenter study. Crit Care Med 19:1339–1347, 1991.

Haynes JB, Hyers TM, Giclas PC, et al: Elevated fibrinogen) degradation products in the adult respiratory distress syndrome. Am Rev Respir Dis 122:841–847, 1980.

Heffner JE, Shoemaker SA, Canham EM, et al: Acetyl glyceryl ether phosphorylcholine-stimulated human platelets cause pulmonary hypertension and edema in isolated rabbit lungs. Role of thromboxane A_2. J Clin Invest 71:351–357, 1983.

Heflin C and Brigham KL: Prevention by granulocyte depletion of increased vascular permeability of sheep lung following endotoxemia. J Clin Invest 68:1253–1260, 1981.

Henke C, Knighton D, Wick M, et al: Mechanisms of alveolar fibrosis following acute lung injury. Presence of angiogenesis bioactivity in the lower respiratory tract. Chest 99:40S, 1991.

Hill JD, Ratliff JL, Parrott JCW, et al: Pulmonary pathology in acute respiratory insufficiency: Lung biopsy as a diagnostic tool. J Thorac Cardiovasc Surg 71:64–71, 1982.

Hohn DC, Meyers AJ, Gherini ST, et al: Production of acute pulmonary injury by leukocytes and activated complement. Surgery 88:48–58, 1980.

Hosea S, Brown E, Hammer C, et al: Role of complement activation in a model of adult respiratory distress syndrome. J Clin Invest 66:375–382, 1980.

Huseby JS and Hudson LD: Miliary tuberculosis and adult respiratory distress syndrome. Ann Intern Med 85:609–611, 1976.

Hyers TM, Tricomi SM, Dettenmeier PA, et al: Tumor necrosis factor levels in serum and bronchoalveolar lavage fluid of patients with the adult respiratory distress syndrome. Am Rev Respir Dis 144:268–271, 1991.

Idell S, James KK, and Coalson JJ: Fibrinolytic activity in bronchoalveolar lavage of baboons with diffuse alveolar damage: Trends in two forms of lung injury. Crit Care Med 20:1431–1440, 1992.

Idell S, James KK, Gillies C, et al: Abnormalities of pathways of fibrin turnover in lung lavage of rats with oleic acid and bleomycin-induced lung injury support alveolar fibrin deposition. Am J Pathol 137:387–389, 1989a.

Idell S, James KK, Levin EG, et al: Local abnormalities in coagulation and fibrinolytic pathways predispose to alveolar fibrin deposition in the adult respiratory distress syndrome. J Clin Invest 84:695–705, 1989b.

Idell S, Kucich U, Fein A, et al: Neutrophil elastase-releasing factors in bronchoalveolar lavage from patients with adult respiratory distress syndrome. Am Rev Respir Dis 132:1098–1105, 1985.

Idell S, Peters J, James K, et al: Local abnormalities in coagulation and fibrinolytic pathways that promote alveolar fibrin deposition in the lungs of baboons with diffuse alveolar damage. J Clin Invest 84:181–193, 1989c.

Idell S, Petersen BT, Gonzalez KK, et al: Local abnormalities of coagulation and fibrinolysis and alveolar fibrin deposition in sheep with oleic acid-induced lung injury. Am Rev Respir Dis 138:1282–1294, 1988.

Ishizaki T, Shigemori K, Nakai T, et al: Leukotoxin, 9,10-epoxy-12-octadecenoate causes edematous lung injury via activation of vascular nitric oxide synthase. Am J Physiol 269:L65–70, 1995.

Jepsen S, Herlevsen P, Knudsen P, et al: Antioxidant treatment with N-acetylcysteine during adult respiratory distress syndrome: A prospective, randomized, placebo-controlled study. Crit Care Med 20:918–923, 1992.

Jochum M, Gippner-Steppert C, Machleidt W, et al: The role of phagocyte proteinases and proteinase inhibitors in multiple organ failure. Am J Respir Care Med 150:S123–S130, 1994.

Johnson J, Brigham KL, Jesmok G, et al: Morphologic changes in lungs of anesthetized sheep following intravenous infusion of recombinant tumor necrosis factor alpha. Am Rev Respir Dis 144:179–186, 1991.

Johnson KJ, Fantone JC III, Kaplan J, et al: In vivo damage of rat lungs by oxygen metabolites. J Clin Invest 67:983–993, 1981.

Johnson KJ and Ward PA: Acute and progressive lung injury after contact with phorbol myristate acetate. Am J Pathol 107:29–35, 1982.

Johnson KJ, Wilson BS, Till GO, et al: Acute lung injury in rat caused by immunoglobulin A

immune complexes. J Clin Invest 74:358–369, 1984.

Jorens PG, Van Damme J, De Backer W, et al: Interleukin 8 (IL-8) in the bronchoalveolar lavage fluid from patients with the adult respiratory distress syndrome (ARDS) and patients at risk for ARDS. Cytokine 4:592–597, 1992.

Kagan BL, Ganz T, and Lehrer RI: Defensins: A family of antimicrobial and cytotoxic peptides. Toxicology 87:131–149, 1994.

Kinnula VL, Crapo JD, and Raivio KO: Generation and disposal of reactive oxygen metabolites in the lung. Lab Invest 73:3–19, 1995/

Klebanoff SJ, Vadas MA, Harlan JM, et al: Stimulation of neutrophils by tumor necrosis factor. J Immunol 136:4220–4225, 1986.

Kopolovic R, Thrailkill KM, Martin DT, et al: Effects of ibuprofen on a porcine model of acute respiratory failure. J Surg Res 36:300–305, 1984.

Kovacs EJ and DiPietro LA: Fibrogenic cytokines and connective tissue production. Faseb J 8:854–861, 1994.

Kreuzfelder E, Joka T, Keinecke HO, et al: Adult respiratory distress syndrome as a specific manifestation of a general permeability defect in trauma patients. Am Rev Respir Dis 137:95–99, 1988.

Kuhns DB, Alvord WG, and Gallin JI: Increased circulating cytokines, cytokine antagonists, and E-selectin after intravenous administration of endotoxin in humans. J Infect Dis 171:145–152, 1995.

Langlois PF and Gawryl MS: Accentuated formation of the terminal C5b–9 complement complex in patient plasma precedes development of the adult respiratory distress syndrome. Am Rev Respir Dis 138:368–375, 1988.

Laufe MD, Simon RH, Flint A, et al: Adult respiratory distress syndrome in neutropenic patients. Am J Med 80:1022–1026, 1986.

Lee CT, Fein AM, Lippmann M, et al: Elastolytic activity in pulmonary lavage fluid from patients with adult respiratory distress syndrome. N Engl J Med 304:192–196, 1981.

Lewis JF and Jobe AH: Surfactant and the adult respiratory distress syndrome. Am Rev Respir Dis 147:218–233, 1993.

McCord JM: Human disease, free radicals, and the oxidant/antioxidant balance. Clin Biochem 26:351–357, 1993.

McGee MP and Rothberger H: Tissue factor in bronchoalveolar lavage fluids. Evidence for an alveolar macrophage source. Am Rev Respir Dis 131:331–336, 1985.

McGuire WW, Spragg RG, Cohen AB, et al: Studies on the pathogenesis of the adult respiratory distress syndrome. J Clin Invest 69:543–553, 1982.

McManus LM and Deavers SI: Platelet activating factor in pulmonary pathobiology. Clin Chest Med 10:107–118, 1989.

Marco V, Mass B, Meranze DR, et al: Induction of

experimental emphysema in dogs using leukocyte homogenates. Am Rev Respir Dis 104:595–598, 1971.

Marks JD, Marks CB, Luce JM, et al: Plasma tumor necrosis factor in patients with septic shock. Mortality rate, incidence of adult respiratory distress syndrome, and effects of methylprednisolone administration. Am Rev Respir Dis 141:94–97, 1990.

Martin TR, Rubenfeld G, Steinberg KP, et al: Endotoxin, endotoxin-binding protein, and soluble CD14 are present in bronchoalveolar lavage fluid of patients with adult respiratory distress syndrome. Chest 105:55S–56S, 1994.

Mason GR, Effros RM, Uszler JM, et al: Small solute clearance from the lungs of patients with cardiogenic and noncardiogenic pulmonary edema. Chest 88:327–334, 1985.

Mason RJ, Williams MC, Widdicombe JH, et al: Transepithelial transport by pulmonary alveolar type II cells in primary culture. Proc Natl Acad Sci USA 79:6033–6037, 1982.

Mathison JC, Wolfson E, and Ulevitch RJ: Participation of tumor necrosis factor in the mediation of gram negative bacterial lipopolysaccharide-induced injury in rabbits. J Clin Invest 81:1925–1937, 1988.

Matsumoto K, Taki F, Kondoh Y, et al: Platelet-activating factor in bronchoalveolar lavage fluid of patients with adult respiratory distress syndrome. Clin Exp Pharmacol Physiol 19:509–515, 1992.

Matthay MA, Eschenbacher WL, and Goetzel EJ: Elevated concentrations of leukotriene D4 in pulmonary edema fluid of patients with adult respiratory distress syndrome. J Clin Immunol 4:479–483, 1984.

Matthay MA and Wiener-Kronish JP: Intact epithelial barrier function is critical for the resolution of alveolar edema in humans. Am Rev Respir Dis 142:1250–1257, 1990.

Maunder RJ, Hackman RC, Riff E, et al: Occurrence of the adult respiratory distress syndrome in neutropenic patients. Am Rev Respir Dis 133:313–315, 1986a.

Maunder RJ, Shuman WP, McHugh JW, et al: Preservation of normal lung regions in the adult respiratory distress syndrome. Analysis by computed tomography. JAMA 255:2463–2465, 1986b.

Mayes JT, Schreiber RD, and Cooper NR: Development and application of an enzyme-linked immunosorbent assay for the quantitation of alternative complement pathway activation in human serum. J Clin Invest 73:160–170, 1984.

Meade P, Shoemaker WC, Donnelly TJ, et al: Temporal patterns of hemodynamics, oxygen transport, cytokine activity, and complement activity in the development of adult respiratory distress syndrome after severe injury. J Trauma 36:651–657, 1994.

Meduri GU, Chinn AJ, Leeper KV, et al: Corticosteroid rescue treatment of progressive fibroproliferation in late ARDS. Patterns of response and predictors of outcome. Chest 105:1516–1527, 1994.

Meduri GU, Headley S, Kohler G, et al: Persistent elevation of inflammatory cytokines predicts a poor outcome in ARDS. Plasma IL-1 beta and IL-6 levels are consistent and efficient predictors of outcome over time. Chest 107:1062–1073, 1995.

Michie HR, Manogue KR, Spriggs DR, et al: Detection of circulating tumor necrosis factor after endotoxin administration. N Engl J Med 318:1481–1486, 1988.

Millar AB, Foley NM, Singer M, et al: Tumor necrosis factor in bronchopulmonary secretions of patients with adult respiratory distress syndrome. Lancet 2:712–714, 1989.

Miller EJ, Cohen AB, Nagao S, et al: Elevated levels of NAP-1/interleukin-8 are present in the airspaces of patients with the adult respiratory distress syndrome and are associated with increased mortality. Am Rev Respir Dis 146:427–432, 1992.

Miyazaki Y, Araki K, Vesin C, et al: Expression of a tumor necrosis factor-transgene in murine lung causes lymphocytic and fibrosing alveolitis. J Clin Invest 96:250–259, 1995.

Modig J, Borg T, Wegenius G, et al: The value of variables of disseminated intravascular coagulation in the diagnosis of adult respiratory distress syndrome. Acta Anaesthesiol Scand 27:369–375, 1983.

Morganroth ML, Till GO, Kunkel RG, et al: Complement and neutrophil-mediated injury of perfused rat lungs. Lab Invest 54:507–514, 1986.

Mulligan MS, Jones ML, Bolanowski MA, et al: Inhibition of lung inflammatory reactions in rats by an anti-human IL-8 antibody. J Immunol 150:5585–5595, 1993a.

Mulligan MS, Miyasaka M, Tamatani T, et al: Requirements for L-selectin in neutrophil-mediated lung injury in rats. J Immunol 152:832–840, 1994.

Mulligan MS, Paulson JC, De Frees S, et al: Protective effects of oligosaccharides in P-selectin-dependent lung injury. Nature 364:149–151, 1993b.

Mulligan MS, Vaporciyan AA, Warner RL, et al: Compartmentalized roles for leukocytic adhesion molecules in lung inflammatory injury. J Immunol 154:1350–1363, 1995.

Mulligan MS, Varani J, Dame MK, et al: Role of endothelial-leukocyte adhesion molecule 1 (ELAM-1) in neutrophil-mediated lung injury in rats. J Clin Invest 88:1396–1406, 1991.

Murray JF, Matthay MA, Luce JM, et al: An expanded definition of the adult respiratory distress syndrome. Am Rev Respir Dis 138:720–723, 1988.

Nash G, Foley FD, Langlinias PC: Pulmonary interstitial edema and hyaline membranes in adult burn patients. Hum Pathol 5:149–161, 1974.

Nawroth PP, Bank I, Handley D, et al: Tumor necrosis factor/cachectin interacts with endothelial cell receptors to induce release of interleukin 1. J Exp Med 163:1363–1375, 1986.

Nuytinck HK, Offermans XJ, Kubat K, et al: Whole-body inflammation in trauma patients. An autopsy study. Arch Surg 123:1519–1524, 1988.

Nygaard SD, Ganz T, Peterson MW: Defensins reduce the barrier integrity of a cultured epithelial monolayer without cytotoxicity. Am J Respir Cell Mol Biol 8:193–200, 1993.

Ogletree ML, Oates JA, Brigham KL, et al: Evidence for pulmonary release of 5-hydroxyeicosatetraenoic acid (5-HETE) during endotoxemia in unanesthetized sheep. Fed Proc 23:459–468, 1982.

Ognibene FP, Martin SE, Parker MM, et al: Adult respiratory distress syndrome in patients with severe neutropenia. N Engl J Med 315:547–551, 1986.

Olman MA, Mackman N, Gladson CL, et al: Changes in procoagulant and fibrinolytic gene expression during bleomycin-induced lung injury in the mouse. J Clin Invest 96:1621–1630, 1995.

Olson NC, Dobrowsky RT, and Fleisher LN: Hydroxyeicosatetraenoic acids are increased in bronchoalveolar lavage fluid of endotoxemic pigs. Prostaglandins 34:493–503, 1987.

Ossanna PJ, Test ST, Matheson NR, et al: Oxidative regulation of neutrophil elastase-alpha-1-proteinase inhibitor interactions. J Clin Invest 77:1939–1951, 1986.

Ozawa T, Sugiyama S, Hayakawa M, et al: Existence of leukotoxin 9,10-epoxy-12-octadecenoate in lung lavages from rats breathing pure oxygen and from patients with the adult respiratory distress syndrome. Am Rev Respir Dis 137:535–540, 1988.

Parsons PE, Fowler AA, Hyers TM, et al: Chemotactic activity in bronchoalveolar lavage fluid from patients with adult respiratory distress syndrome. Am Rev Respir Dis 132:490–493, 1985.

Parsons PE and Giclas PC: The terminal complement complex (sC5b-9) is not specifically associated with the development of the adult respiratory distress syndrome. Am Rev Respir Dis 141:98–103, 1990.

Parsons PE, Moore FA, Moore EE, et al: Studies on the role of tumor necrosis factor in adult respiratory distress syndrome. Am Rev Respir Dis 146:694–700, 1992.

Parsons PE, Worthen GS, Moore EE, et al: The association of circulating endotoxin with the development of the adult respiratory distress syndrome. Am Rev Respir Dis 140:294–301, 1989.

Pepe PE, Potkin RT, Reus DH, et al: Clinical predictors of the adult respiratory distress syndrome. Am J Surg 144:124–130, 1982.

Petros A, Bennett D, and Vallance P: Effect of nitric oxide synthase inhibitors on hypotension in patients with septic shock [see comments]. Lancet 338:1557–1558, 1991.

Pratt PC: Pathology of adult respiratory distress syndrome: Implications regarding therapy. Semin Respir Med 4:79–85, 1982.

Pryor WA and Squadrito GL: The chemistry of peroxynitrite: A product from the reaction of nitric oxide with superoxide. Am J Physiol 268:L699–L722, 1995.

Ratliff NB, Wilson JW, Mikat E, et al: The lung in hemorrhagic shock. IV. The role of neutrophilic polymorphonuclear leukocytes. Am J Pathol 65:325–334, 1971.

Ridings PC, Windsor AC, Jutila MA, et al: A dual-binding antibody to E- and L-selectin attenuates sepsis-induced lung injury. Am J Respir Crit Care Med 152:247–253, 1995.

Rinaldo JE and Borovetz H: Deterioration of oxygenation and abnormal lung microvascular permeability during resolution of leukopenia in patients with diffuse lung injury. Am Rev Respir Dis 131:579–583, 1985.

Rivkind AI, Siegel JH, Guadalupi P, et al: Sequential patterns of eicosanoid, platelet, and neutrophil interactions in the evolution of the fulminant post-traumatic adult respiratory distress syndrome. Ann Surg 210:355–372, 1989.

Rooney SA: The surfactant system and lung phospholipid biochemistry. Am Rev Respir Dis 131:439–460, 1985.

Roten R, Markert M, Feihl F, et al: Plasma levels of tumor necrosis factor in the adult respiratory distress syndrome. Am Rev Respir Dis 143:590–592, 1991.

Rowen JL, Hyde DM, and McDonald RJ: Eosinophils cause acute edematous injury in isolated perfused rat lungs. Am Rev Respir Dis 142:215–220, 1990.

Sacks T, Moldow CF, Craddock PR, et al: Oxygen radicals mediate endothelial cell damage by complement-stimulated granulocytes. An in vitro model of immune vascular damage. J Clin Invest 61:1161–1167, 1978.

Sakamaki F, Ishizaka A, Handa M, et al: Soluble form of P-selectin in plasma is elevated in acute lung injury. Am J Respir Crit Care Med 151:1821–1826, 1995.

Sakuma T, Okaniwa G, Nakada T, et al: Alveolar fluid clearance in the resected human lung. Am J Respir Crit Care Med 150:305–310, 1994.

Saldeen T: Clotting, microembolism, and inhibition of fibrinolysis in adult respiratory distress. Surg Clin North Am 63:285–304, 1983.

Schneider RC, Zapol WM, and Carvalho AC: Platelet consumption and sequestration in severe acute respiratory failure. Am Rev Respir Dis 122:445–451, 1980.

Schnells G, Voigt WH, Redl H, et al: Electron-microscopic investigation of lung biopsies in patients with post-traumatic respiratory insufficiency. Acta Chir Scand [Suppl] 499:9–20, 1980.

Schraufstatter IU, Revak SD, and Cochrane CG: Proteases and oxidants in experimental pulmonary inflammatory injury. J Clin Invest 73:1175–1184, 1984.

Shasby DM, Vanbenthuysen KM, Tate RM, et al: Granulocytes mediate acute edematous lung injury in rabbits and in isolated rabbit lungs perfused with phorbol myristate acetate: Role of oxygen radicals. Am Rev Respir Dis 125:443–447, 1982.

Shaw JO, Henson PM, Henson J, et al: Lung inflammation induced by complement-derived chemotactic fragments in the alveolus. Lab Invest 42:547–558, 1980.

Siler TM, Swierkosz JE, Hyers TM, et al: Immunoreactive interleukin-1 in bronchoalveolar lavage fluid of high-risk patients and patients with the adult respiratory distress syndrome. Exp Lung Res 15:881–894, 1989.

Simon RH, DeHart PD, and Todd RF III: Neutrophil-induced injury of rat pulmonary alveolar epithelial cells. J Clin Invest 78:1375–1386, 1986.

Simon RH, Edwards JA, and Sitrin RG: Fibrin is rapidly formed and lysed when plasma is introduced into the alveolar space of intact lungs. Am J Respir Crit Care Med 151:A344, 1995.

Simon RH, Scoggin CH, and Patterson D: Hydrogen peroxide causes the fatal injury to human fibroblasts exposed to oxygen radicals. J Biol Chem 256:7181–7186, 1981.

Slotman GJ, Burchard KW, D'Arezzo A, et al: Ketoconazole prevents acute respiratory failure in critically ill surgical patients. J Trauma 28:648–654, 1988.

Smedly LA, Tonnesen MG, Sandhaus RA, et al: Neutrophil-mediated injury to endothelial cells. Enhancement by endotoxin and essential role of neutrophil elastase. J Clin Invest 77:1233–1243, 1986.

Smith JA: Neutrophils, host defense, and inflammation: A double-edged sword. J Leukoc Biol 56:672–686, 1994.

Staub NC: Pathways for fluid and solute fluxes in pulmonary edema. In Fishman AP, Renkin EM (eds): Pulmonary Edema. Bethesda, American Physiological Society, 1979, pp 113-124.

Stephens KE, Ishizaka A, Wu ZH, et al: Granulocyte depletion prevents tumor necrosis factor-mediated acute lung injury in guinea pigs. Am Rev Respir Dis 138:1300–1307, 1988.

Stephenson AH, Lonigro AJ, Hyers TM, et al: Increased concentrations of leukotrienes in bronchoalveolar lavage fluid of patients with ARDS or at risk for ARDS. Am Rev Respir Dis 138:714–719, 1988.

Strieter RM, Kunkel SL, Showell HJ, et al: Endothelial cell gene expression of a neutrophil chemotactic factor by TNF-alpha, LPS, and IL-1 beta. Science 243:1467–1469, 1989.

Suter PM, Domenighetti G, Schaller MD, et al: N-acetylcysteine enhances recovery from acute lung injury in man. A randomized, double-blind, placebo-controlled clinical study. Chest 105:190–194, 1994.

Suter PM, Suter S, Girardin E, et al: High bronchoalveolar levels of tumor necrosis factor and its inhibitors, interleukin-1, interferon, and elastase, in patients with adult respiratory distress syndrome after trauma, shock, or sepsis. Am Rev Respir Dis 145:1016–1022, 1992.

Suttorp N and Simon LM: Lung cell oxidant injury. J Clin Invest 70:342–350, 1982.

Tedder TF, Steeber DA, Chen A, et al: The selectins: Vascular adhesion molecules. Faseb J 9:866–873, 1995.

Till GO, Beauchamp C, Menapace D, et al: Oxygen radical–dependent lung damage following thermal injury of rat skin. J Trauma 23:269–277, 1983.

Till GO, Johnson KJ, Kunkel R, et al: Intravascular activation of complement and acute lung injury. Dependency on neutrophils and toxic oxygen metabolites. J Clin Invest 69:1126–1135, 1982.

Tomaschefski JF, Davies P, Boggis C, et al: The pulmonary vascular lesions of the adult respiratory distress syndrome. Am J Pathol 112:112–126, 1983.

Tracey KJ, Buetler B, Lowry SF, et al: Shock and tissue injury induced by recombinant human cachectin. Science 234:470–474, 1986.

Tracey KJ, Lowry SF, and Cerami A: Cachetin/TNF-alpha in septic shock and septic adult respiratory distress syndrome. Am Rev Respir Dis 138:1377–1379, 1988.

Tracey KJ, Vlassara H, and Cerami A: Cachectin/tumour necrosis factor. Lancet 1:1122–1126, 1989.

Ward PA, Till GO, Kunkel R, et al: Evidence for role of hydroxyl radical in complement and neutrophil-dependent tissue injury. J Clin Invest 72:789–801, 1983.

Warshawski FJ, Sibbald WJ, Driedger AA, et al: Abnormal neutrophil-pulmonary interaction in the adult respiratory distress syndrome. Qualitative and quantitative assessment of pulmonary neutrophil kinetics in humans with in vivo 111 indium neutrophil scintigraphy. Am Rev Respir Dis 133:797–804, 1986.

Webster RO, Larsen GL, Mitchell BC, et al: Absence of inflammatory lung injury in rabbits challenged intravascularly with complement-derived chemotactic factors. Am Rev Respir Dis 125:335–340, 1982.

Weiss SJ: Tissue destruction by neutrophils [see comments]. N Engl J Med 320:365–376, 1989.

Weiss SJ, Peppin G, Ortiz X, et al: Oxidative autoactivation of latent collagenase by human neutrophils. Science 227:747–749, 1985.

Weiss SJ, Young J, LoBuglio AF, et al: Role of hydrogen peroxide in neutrophil-mediated destruction of cultured endothelial cells. J Clin Invest 68:714–721, 1981.

Wewers MD, Herzyk DJ, and Gadek JE: Alveolar fluid neutrophil elastase activity in the adult respiratory distress syndrome in complexed to alpha-2-macroglobulin. J Clin Invest 82:1260–1267, 1988.

Worthen GS, Goins AJ, Mitchel BC, et al: Platelet-activating factor causes neutrophil accumulation and edema in rabbit lungs. Chest 83:13S–15S, 1983.

Worthen GS, Schwab BI, Elson EL, et al: Mechanics of stimulated neutrophils: Cell stiffening induces retention in capillaries. Science 245:183–186, 1989.

Yu M and Tomasa G: A double-blind, randomized trial of ketoconazole, a thromboxane synthetase inhibitor, in the prophylaxis of the adult respiratory distress syndrome. Crit Care Med 21:1635–1644, 1993.

Zimmerman GA, Renzetti AD, and Hill HR: Functional and metabolic activity of granulocytes from patients with adult respiratory distress syndrome. Am Rev Respir Dis 127:290–300, 1983.

CHAPTER

Pulmonary Gas Exchange

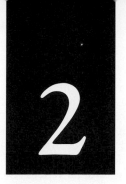

David R. Dantzker, M.D.

The major role of the lung, and by far its most unique contribution to the body's homeostasis, is the exchange of oxygen and carbon dioxide between the environment and the blood. Abnormal pulmonary gas exchange contributes to the morbidity and mortality of most critically ill patients, regardless of the underlying illness. Each different mechanism of abnormal gas exchange requires a separate therapeutic approach for optimal resolution. An overview of the normal physiology of pulmonary gas exchange is presented in this chapter. The abnormal mechanisms seen in clinical disease are discussed in detail, and a critical analysis is made of available techniques for differentiating and quantitating the degree of dysfunction as well as assessing longitudinal alterations in lung function.

Oxygen is required at a very low partial pressure by the mitochondria to accept electrons from cytochrome oxidase at the end of the cytochrome pathway. The elemental oxygen that is formed then combines with hydrogen ions to form water. Although the availability of sufficient oxygen is rarely a rate-limiting step to the production of energy, it may become so in situations of diminished oxygen delivery (see Chapter 8). The amount of oxygen used, the oxygen uptake or consumption ($\dot{V}O_2$), is normally determined by the body's energy requirements and can be quantified from the Fick equation:

$$\dot{V}O_2 = \dot{V}I \times FIO_2 - \dot{V}E \times FEO_2$$
$$= \dot{Q} (CaO_2 - C\bar{v}O_2)$$

where $\dot{V}I$ and $\dot{V}E$ are inspired and expired minute ventilations, FIO_2 and FEO_2 are the inspired and expired fractional concentrations of oxygen, $\dot{Q}$ is the cardiac output, and CaO_2 and $C\bar{v}O_2$ are the arterial and mixed venous O_2 contents.

In practice, the $\dot{V}O_2$ can be measured in three ways. It can be measured directly by rebreathing from a spirometer filled with O_2. The CO_2 is absorbed from the expired gas, and the change in the volume of the spirometer per unit time is the $\dot{V}O_2$. This technique is rarely used today, because even small leaks in the spirometer circuit lead to significant error. The other two techniques require that the patient be in steady state such that metabolic demands, $\dot{V}E$, and $\dot{Q}$, are all constant. Then the amount of oxygen taken up by the tissues is equal to the amount taken up in the lung, and the $\dot{V}O_2$ can be calculated from either the gas side of the system, measuring the difference between the amount of O_2 in the inspired and mixed expired gas, or the blood side as the product of the cardiac output and the arterial-venous O_2 difference. The method chosen in any particular clinical situation is conditioned by the limitations of each technique.

Measurement from the gas side is noninvasive but depends on the ability to accurately measure the FIO_2 and FEO_2. In a patient breathing room air, this measurement is easy and accurate. However, in patients breathing an increased FIO_2 the accuracy is limited by the consistency of the O_2 delivery system. This is particularly relevant in patients on mechanical ventilation in whom back pressure on the inspiratory side can vary the FIO_2 throughout the breath by as much as 1 to 2%. Although this is an inconsequential clinical problem, it markedly increases the error of the calculation. In patients with severe obstructive airway disease, extremely slow spaces within the lung may mean that extremely long (>30 min) equilibration times are necessary to accurately measure $\dot{V}O_2$ if there has been a change in FIO_2. Techniques for open-circuit measurement of $\dot{V}O_2$ in patients on mechanical ventilation are available to obviate some of the technical problems (Kappogoda et al, 1974) and are now being incorporated into clinically useful machines. Quantitation of $\dot{V}O_2$ from the blood side, although invasive, requiring measurement of cardiac output as well as the sampling of mixed venous and arterial blood, bypasses the problem of consistency of inspired O_2 and thus is a method commonly used in critically ill patients. Its major disadvantage is the large number of variables (partial pressure and saturation of arterial and mixed venous blood, hemoglobin concentration, and cardiac output) that must be measured, each of which is subject to error. When properly measured, all three of these methods should obviously result in the same value for $\dot{V}O_2$. The only systematic difference seen is a higher $\dot{V}O_2$ measured from the expired gas as compared with blood measurements in patients with marked lung inflammation. This finding has been ascribed to the excessive O_2 consumed by the high metabolic rate of the diseased lung (Smithies et al, 1991).

CO_2 is produced as a byproduct of metabolism. The amount of CO_2 produced ($\dot{V}CO_2$) depends, in addition to the energy requirements of the body, on the fuel being burned. When carbohydrate is the main source of energy, the $\dot{V}CO_2$ is equal to the $\dot{V}O_2$ and the respiratory exchange ratio, R ($\dot{V}CO_2/\dot{V}O_2$), is 1.0. By contrast, with protein the R is 0.8, and with fat the R is 0.7. Under anaerobic conditions, when glycolysis is used for energy production, CO_2 is produced by the buffering of the ensuing acidosis, and, because no O_2 is consumed, the R may actually exceed 1.0. One other clinical situation during which the R may exceed 1.0 is when fat is synthesized and stored in the body, which may occur when caloric intake exceeds metabolic requirements. This finding has been documented by Askanazi and associates (1980) in patients receiving excessive amounts of hyperalimentation.

The measurement of $\dot{V}CO_2$ is easier than that of $\dot{V}O_2$ because the inspired gas contains no CO_2. It is measured from a timed collection of the expired gas:

$$\dot{V}CO_2 = \dot{V}E \times FECO_2$$

Normally, $\dot{V}CO_2$ adds about 17,000 mEq/day of acid to the blood, which must be removed to maintain normal homeostasis.

The body has minimal O_2 and CO_2 stores and thus depends on continuous exchange with the environment to provide for its metabolic demands and to prevent the development of life-threatening acidosis. The efficiency with which this exchange takes place is mirrored in the arterial blood gases and reflects the culmination of several processes.

In its most simple form, the gas-exchanging unit of the lung can be considered as a tonometer into which the inspired air and venous blood are added at a rate equal to the alveolar ventilation ($\dot{V}A$) and cardiac output ($\dot{Q}_t$), respectively (Fig. 2–1). The gas and blood phases are separated by a thin membrane across which the gases move by diffusion. The resultant partial pressure of O_2 and CO_2 in the arterial blood (PaO_2 and $PaCO_2$) is dependent, in addition to the $\dot{V}A$ and $\dot{Q}_t$, on the gas composition in the inspired air (FIO_2) and mixed venous blood ($PvO_2 + PvCO_2$), the ability of the blood and gas phases to come into equilibration, and the adequacy with which the lung matches $\dot{V}A$ and $\dot{Q}_t$ in each lung unit, the ventilation-perfusion ratio ($\dot{V}A/\dot{Q}$) (West, 1977). An abnormality in any of these factors results in disordered gas exchange.

REDUCTION OF INSPIRED PO_2

In the absence of supplemental oxygen, the FIO_2 depends on atmospheric pressure, which decreases exponentially as we ascend above sea level. The PIO_2 (which is 150 mm Hg at sea level) falls to 120 mm Hg in Denver, to 70 mm Hg in villages high in the Andes, and to as low as 38 mm Hg

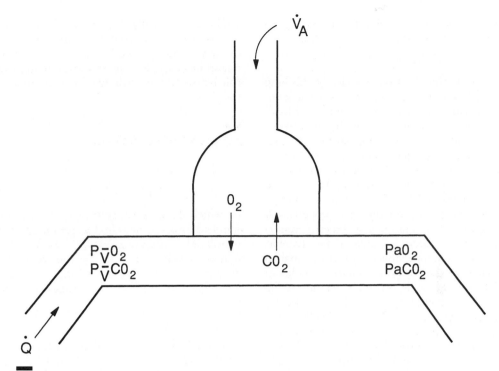

Figure 2–1
A simplified model of the basic gas-exchanging unit of the lung. The alveolar and thus end-capillary P_{O_2} and P_{CO_2} depend on cardiac output ($\dot{Q}$), alveolar ventilation ($\dot{V}_A$), the ratio of $\dot{V}_A$ and $\dot{Q}$ (the ventilation-perfusion ratio), and the mixed venous blood gases ($P\bar{v}_{CO_2}$).

on the summit of Mt. Everest. The effect of this reduction of the P_{IO_2} on oxygenation can be calculated from the alveolar gas equation in which P_{AO_2} is the alveolar P_{O_2},

$$P_{AO_2} = P_{IO_2} - P_{ACO_2} \times [F_{IO_2} + (1 - F_{IO_2})/R]$$

A simplified form of the alveolar gas equation is often used clinically:

$$P_{AO_2} = P_{IO_2} - P_{ACO_2}/R$$

Acute compensation for a decrease in F_{IO_2} is accomplished by a hypoxic-stimulated increase in minute ventilation, which reduces the P_{ACO_2} and correspondingly increases the P_{AO_2} (Luft, 1965). The result is an acute respiratory alkalosis, which is thought to contribute to the development of acute mountain sickness characterized by nausea, headache, dizziness, and insomnia. The failure of a vigorous respiratory response to hypoxia, as may be seen in subjects with a "low gain" respiratory center, limits an individual's ability to function at higher altitudes. Chronic compensation for the hypoxia of altitude occurs through a further increase in the red blood cell mass and thus the amount of O_2 carried at any P_{AO_2} (Hurtado et al, 1945). A shift in the oxyhemoglobin dissociation curve to the right, subsequent to an increase in

the concentration of 2,3-diphosphoglycerate (2,3-DPG), with resultant improved release of O_2 to the tissues, has been considered as an additional compensatory mechanism. However, the importance of this is now being questioned because the shift to the right is often balanced by the chronic respiratory alkalosis that shifts the curve in the opposite direction (Winslow et al, 1984). In addition, the efficacy of a shift to the right to improved tissue oxygenation is also unclear (see Chapter 8).

Although few physicians practice medicine at high altitudes, exposure of patients to a reduced F_{IO_2} is common. The cabins in commercial airplanes are usually pressurized to simulate altitudes as high as 10,000 feet and provide a P_{IO_2} as low as 100 mm Hg. In patients with underlying lung disease, the result may be a value of P_{AO_2} as low as 40 mm Hg. The hypoxemia in patients with lung disease may be further exaggerated in this setting because of the inability to augment minute ventilation to the same degree as normal subjects.

ABNORMAL DIFFUSION

O_2 and CO_2 move between the alveolar gas and the pulmonary capillary blood by diffusion across the alveolar-capillary membrane, according to Fick's first law of diffusion:

$$\text{Gas flow} = D_L (P_1 - P_2)$$

in which D_L is the diffusing capacity of the lung and P_1 and P_2 are the partial pressures of the gases in the alveolus and pulmonary capillary blood. Two resistances must be overcome by the physiologic gases, and both are encompassed in D_L. The first resistance is the movement of gas through alveolar gas, across the alveolar-capillary membrane, through the plasma layer, and across the membrane of the red blood cell. This membrane component depends on the diffusion properties of the gas in the membranes and is directly proportional to the cross-sectional area of the alveolar-capillary membrane and inversely proportional to the thickness of the pathway from the alveolus to the red blood cell. The second resistance to be overcome is the combination or release of the gas from the hemoglobin in the red blood cell, which depends on the volume of blood in the pulmonary capillaries and on the reaction rate for the chemical combination of O_2 and CO_2 with the available hemoglobin. In most clinical situations in which D_L is low, this latter factor, and more specifically a decreased pulmonary capillary blood volume, is responsible (Roughton and Forster, 1957).

Actual measurements of the D_L for the physiologic gases are impossible to obtain, especially in sick patients, and much of our knowledge about the role of abnormal diffusion in disease is based on theoretical calculations or on indirect assessment. The blood normally spends about 0.75 second within the pulmonary capillaries, and during this time it must equilibrate with the alveolar gas. Ordinarily this process takes only about one third of the available time, leaving a wide margin of safety. Because of this, even significant reductions in D_L do not lead to a failure of alveolar-end-capillary equilibration (i.e., a diffusion defect). Three factors may, however, stress the system sufficiently to cause abnormal gas exchange on the basis of abnormal diffusion: (1) an increase in the diffusion pathway, which may be seen with interstitial fibrosis; (2) a decrease in the time that the blood spends in the capillaries as a result of an increased cardiac output or reduction in the cross-sectional area of the bed; and (3) a reduction in the driving pressure ($P_1 - P_2$), which is seen at high altitude. At least two of these factors must apparently be present concurrently before a reduced D_L is likely to cause hypoxemia. Abnormal diffusion has been shown to contribute to hypoxemia in patients with severe interstitial fibrosis during exercise and in normal subjects exercising at altitude (Wagner,

1977). For critically ill patients, debates over the importance of abnormal diffusion as a mechanism of abnormal gas exchange are of secondary importance, because most diffusion impairments can be overcome easily with modest increases in the F_{IO_2}.

HYPOVENTILATION

The Pa_{CO_2} depends on the level of $\dot{V}_A$:

$$Pa_{CO_2} = Pa_{CO_2} = \dot{V}_{CO_2}/\dot{V}_A \times K$$

in which K is a constant usually 0.863 using standard units (mm Hg for pressure, l/min for ventilation, ml/min for $\dot{V}_{CO_2}$. $\dot{V}_A$ is less than the minute ventilation ($\dot{V}_E$) by the ventilation of dead space ($\dot{V}_D$), regions of lung that are ventilated but not perfused by pulmonary capillary blood:

$$\dot{V}_A = \dot{V}_E - \dot{V}_D$$

In normal subjects, the volume of the dead space ($\dot{V}_D$) consists mainly of the conducting airways, approximately 1 ml/lb of body weight and is thus a fixed proportion of $\dot{V}_E$ (Krogh and Lindhard, 1917). We can therefore consider $\dot{V}_E$ and Pa_{CO_2} to be inversely proportional (Fig. 2–2).

Hypoventilation can be defined most simply as a $\dot{V}_E$ (and thus $\dot{V}_A$) that is inadequate to maintain a normal Pa_{CO_2} for a given $\dot{V}_{CO_2}$. Hyperventilation is a minute ventilation in excess of metabolic needs. $\dot{V}_A$ may decrease with no change in $\dot{V}_E$ if the ventilatory pattern is altered so that respiratory frequency increases while tidal volume decreases. Because the $\dot{V}_D$ per breath stays essentially the same regardless of the tidal volume, the contribution of the tidal volume to $\dot{V}_A$ must fall. The $\dot{V}_A$ may also fall in the face of an unchanged or even increased $\dot{V}_E$ when ventilation-perfusion inequality develops. This change is referred to sometimes as an increase in alveolar dead space and is discussed subsequently.

The rise in Pa_{CO_2} seen with hypoventilation leads to a secondary fall in Pa_{O_2}, which is described by the alveolar gas equation. Thus, the hypoxemia associated with hypoventilation is not the result of an inefficiency of pulmonary gas exchange but of an inadequate ventilatory pump or, less commonly, an abnormality of the respiratory pattern. Under normal circumstances, the Pa_{CO_2} is constrained tightly by the central and peripheral chemoreceptors that set $\dot{V}_E$ at a level appropriate for the $\dot{V}_{CO_2}$. Hypercapnia resulting from hypoventilation is therefore seen characteristically in patients with a depressed central nervous system or in patients with neuromuscular or

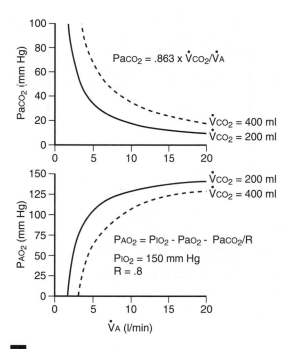

Figure 2–2
The effect of altering alveolar ventilation ($\dot{V}A$) on
arterial PCO_2 and alveolar PO_2. The different levels of
CO_2 production are demonstrated. As alveolar
ventilation falls, $PaCO_2$ increases at a rate determined
by the relationship $PaCO_2 = 0.863 \times \dot{V}CO_2/\dot{V}A$. The
effect of changes of $\dot{V}A$ on alveolar oxygen tension
can be calculated from the alveolar gas equation.
(From Dantzker DR: Pulmonary gas exchange. In
Scharf SM: Cardiopulmonary Physiology in Critical
Care. New York, Marcel Dekker, 1992, p 295. With
permission.)

skeletal abnormalities that result in a weakness
or dysfunction of the respiratory muscles. for
proper treatment, hypoventilation must be clearly
differentiated from disordered gas exchange due
to intrinsic lung disease. Although small increases
in the FIO_2 correct the hypoxemia of hypoventilation, the progression of the underlying disorder
leads eventually to respiratory failure and acidosis.
The differentiation of hypoventilation from other
causes of abnormal arterial blood gases can be
made by the finding of a normal alveolar-arterial
gradient for O_2 (see later).

VENTILATION-PERFUSION INEQUALITY

We have been considering the lung, up to now,
as a single homogeneous gas-exchanging unit,
whereas in reality it is made up of 300 million
gas-exchanging units perfused in parallel and ventilated both in parallel and in series. This complex
arrangement, along with gravitational and conformational influences on the regional distribution
of ventilation and blood flow, guarantees variation
in the matching of ventilation and blood flow.
The ventilation-perfusion ratio ($\dot{V}A/\dot{Q}$) may vary
from zero (perfused but not ventilated or shunt)
to infinity (ventilated but not perfused or dead
space) and is a major determinant of the alveolar
and thus end-capillary composition of both O_2
and CO_2 in any given lung unit (West, 1969).

Figure 2–3 shows the influence of the $\dot{V}A/\dot{Q}$
on both the partial pressures and contents of O_2
and CO_2 in the end-capillary blood of single lung
units. When the $\dot{V}A/\dot{Q}$ is low, there is little transfer of either O_2 or CO_2 and thus little modification of the alveolar gas or end-capillary blood
from the $P\bar{v}O_2$ and $P\bar{v}CO_2$. As the $\dot{V}A/\dot{Q}$ increases,
the alveolar and thus end-capillary PO_2 and PCO_2
rise toward the inspired levels. Because of the
different shapes of the oxyhemoglobin and CO_2
dissociation curves, changes in the $\dot{V}A/\dot{Q}$ affect
O_2 and CO_2 exchange differently (Fig. 2–4). The
O_2 content does not continue to increase despite
a progressive increase in PO_2 because of the plateauing of the oxyhemoglobin curve. By contrast,
the CO_2 content decreases continuously along
with the PCO_2 as the $\dot{V}A/\dot{Q}$ increases. The significance of this different behavior of O_2 and CO_2
is discussed subsequently. The arterial blood-gas
composition, of course, depends on the relative
number of lung units with differing $\dot{V}A/\dot{Q}$ present
in the lung (i.e., distribution of the $\dot{V}A/\dot{Q}$).

In young, normal subjects, the distribution of
$\dot{V}A/\dot{Q}$ ratios in the lung varies from about 0.6 to
3.0, and the distribution is usually centered on a
$\dot{V}A/\dot{Q}$ of 1.0 (Fig. 2–5) (Wagner et al, 1974).
With age, there is a gradual increase in the range
of $\dot{V}A/\dot{Q}$ units that are found (i.e., an increase in
the degree of $\dot{V}A/\dot{Q}$ inequality). When lung disease develops, the distribution of $\dot{V}A/\dot{Q}$ may become markedly abnormal, and lung units with
high and low $\dot{V}A/\dot{Q}$ may predominate (Fig. 2–6)
(Wagner et al, 1977). Lung units with low $\dot{V}A/\dot{Q}$
develop most often because of inadequate ventilation due to structural changes in the airway or
bronchospasm, as seen in chronic obstructive lung
disease, asthma, or interstitial fibrosis. A low $\dot{V}A/\dot{Q}$ unit can also result from overperfusion of a
normally ventilated lung. This cause of hypox-
emia is seen following a pulmonary embolism in
which blood flow from obstructed regions is diverted to the normal areas of the lung (Dantzker
et al, 1978). Conversely, lung regions served by
the obstructed pulmonary vessels may develop
into high $\dot{V}A/\dot{Q}$ units or dead space, depending
on the completeness of the vascular obstruction.

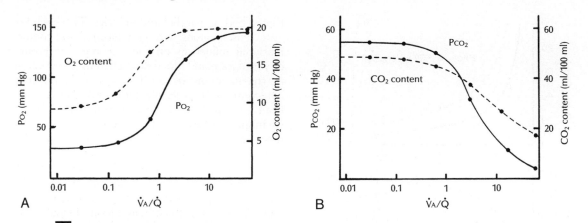

Figure 2–3
(A) The relationship between the end-capillary P_{O_2} and O_2 content and the ventilation-perfusion ratio. The major increase in oxygenation of the arterial blood takes place over a relatively narrow range of ventilation-perfusion ratios. (B) The relationship between the arterial P_{CO_2} and CO_2 content and the ventilation-perfusion ratio. There is a fall in the CO_2 content and partial pressure as the ventilation-perfusion ratio is increased. (From Dantzker DR: Critical Care: A Comprehensive Approach. Park Ridge, IL, American College of Chest Physicians, 1984, p 3. With permission.)

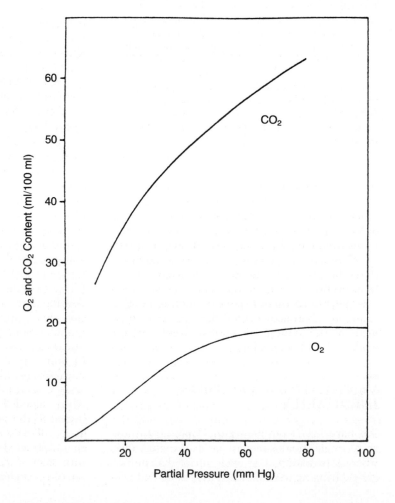

Figure 2–4
The oxyhemoglobin and carbon dioxide dissociation curves. The oxyhemoglobin curve is sigmoid-shaped, whereas the carbon dioxide curve is linear throughout the physiologic range.

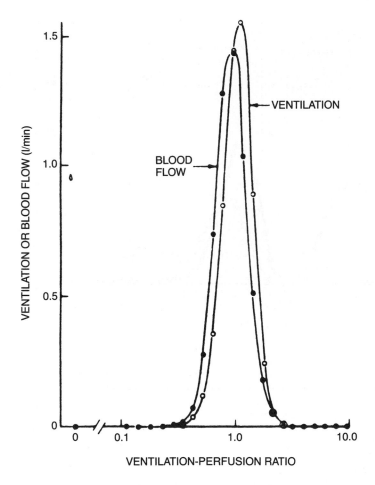

Figure 2–5
An example of a distribution of
ventilation-perfusion ratios in a young
normal subject, which were obtained by
the multiple inert gas technique. Most of
the ventilation and blood flow go to lung
units with ventilation-perfusion ratios
near 1. (From Wagner PD, Laravuso RB,
Uhl RR, et al: Continuous distributions
of ventilation-perfusion ratios in normal
subjects breathing air and 100% O_2. J
Clin Invest 54:54, 1974. Reproduced
from the Journal of Clinical Investigation
by copyright permission of the American
Society for Clinical Investigation.)

The most common cause of high $\dot{V}_A/\dot{Q}$ units is
emphysema, in which the reduction in perfusion
due to destruction of the alveolar walls is even
greater than the resultant decrease in ventilation
(Wagner et al, 1977). High $\dot{V}_A/\dot{Q}$ units may also
be seen subsequent to the diversion of blood flow
by high positive alveolar pressures generated during mechanical ventilation (Dantzker et al, 1979).

Conservative reflexes are present in the lung,
whose function is to minimize the degree of $\dot{V}_A/\dot{Q}$ inequality. A fall in the $\dot{V}_A/\dot{Q}$ leads to the
development of alveolar hypoxia, which, in turn,
results in vasoconstriction of the perfusing arteriole (Fishman, 1980). The mechanism by which
alveolar hypoxia is sensed and translated into
hypoxic vasoconstriction is unknown, but may
involve the release of one or more humoral messengers (see Chapter 3). The beneficial effect of
hypoxic vasoconstriction on pulmonary gas exchange comes from its ability to decrease the
denominator of the $\dot{V}_A/\dot{Q}$ ratio. Hypoxic vasoconstriction operates over a range of alveolar values
of P_{O_2} between 150 and 30 mm Hg (Barer et al,
1970). More severe hypoxia may actually have

a dilating effect on the pulmonary vasculature
(Sylvester et al, 1980).

Hypoxic vasoconstriction should have a
major beneficial role in the correction of regional
$\dot{V}_A/\dot{Q}$ inequality (Grant, 1982), but many factors
interfere with its efficient application. Certain
drugs abolish or interfere significantly with hypoxic vasoconstriction, including nitroglycerin,
nitroprusside, beta-agonists, calcium channel
blockers, and inhalational anesthetics (Bergofsky,
1979). In addition, elevation of left atrial pressure
and the presence of pulmonary infection or inflammation also interfere with hypoxic vasoconstriction (Staub, 1974).

When the entire lung is hypoxic, the advantages of hypoxic vasoconstriction may be over-
shadowed by the development of pulmonary hypertension. In the fetus, a generalized increase
in pulmonary vascular resistance is important to
ensure that most of the blood returning from the
placenta is shunted around the collapsed lungs.
However, in adults, a similar overall increase in
pulmonary vascular resistance may cause right
ventricular failure (Burrows et al, 1972). This

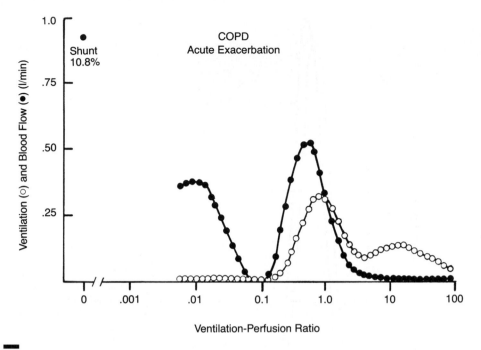

Figure 2–6
The ventilation-perfusion distribution of a patient with chronic obstructive pulmonary disease during an episode of acute bronchitis. The ventilation-perfusion ratio ($\dot{V}A/\dot{Q}$) of the lung units spans the range from shunt to high $\dot{V}A/\dot{Q}$ units. (From Dantzker DR: Chronic Obstructive Pulmonary Disease. New York, Churchill Livingstone, 1983. With permission.)

increase is the major cause of cor pulmonale in chronic respiratory failure and may be responsible for pulmonary edema at a high altitude (Grover et al, 1979). Selective dilation of vessels perfusing open alveoli has been demonstrated using inhaled nitric oxide in patients with adult respiratory distress syndrome. This can improve gas exchange by diverting blood flow from regions of shunt to well-ventilated regions of lung (Rossaint et al, 1993).

A second conservative reflex is hypocapnic bronchoconstriction. An increase in the $\dot{V}A/\dot{Q}$, which may occur subsequent to vascular obstruction, leads to alveolar hypocapnia and by some unknown mechanism to bronchoconstriction and subsequent decrease in ventilation to that lung region (Swenson et al, 1961). The role of hypocapnic bronchoconstriction in disease has been less well characterized than that of hypoxic vasoconstriction, but its aim is clearly to maintain the $\dot{V}A/\dot{Q}$ close to unity. Hypocapnic bronchoconstriction is a weak reflex and is overcome easily by increased tidal volume, which probably explains why decreased ventilation of embolized lung regions is rarely seen on ventilation-perfusion lung scans, because a vital capacity breath of xenon gas is the initial maneuver.

The development of $\dot{V}A/\dot{Q}$ inequality has a dramatic effect on pulmonary gas exchange and interferes with the transfer of both O_2 and CO_2 (Wagner et al, 1974). Thus, one might expect patients with $\dot{V}A/\dot{Q}$ inequality to always have both hypoxemia and hypercapnia (Fig. 2–7). However, even small increases in the $PaCO_2$ activate the chemoreceptors and stimulate minute ventilation. Because of the underlying lung pathology that caused the $\dot{V}A/\dot{Q}$ inequality in the first place, the bulk of the increased ventilation is directed most often to lung units that are already well ventilated. The increase in the $\dot{V}A/\dot{Q}$ in these units leads to an increase in the end-capillary PO_2; however, because of the shape of the oxyhemoglobin dissociation curve (see Fig. 2–4), this increased PO_2 results in only a minimal rise in the O_2 content. Thus, when combined with the desaturated blood coming from the still poorly ventilated lung units, there is little improvement in the PaO_2.

The carbon dioxide–hemoglobin dissociation curve, by comparison, is approximately linear throughout the physiologic range (see Fig. 2–4). Therefore, the decrease in end-capillary PCO_2 seen as the $\dot{V}A/\dot{Q}$ increases in the well-ventilated units is translated into a decrease in the content of CO_2 in the end-capillary blood. The greater excretion of CO_2 in the overventilated units can,

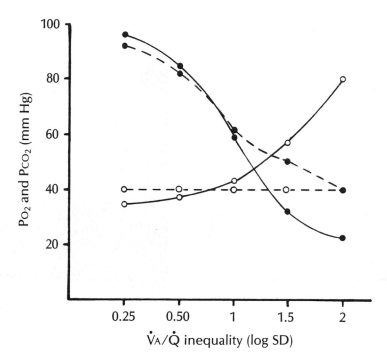

Figure 2–7
The effect of increasing ventilation-perfusion ($\dot{V}A/\dot{Q}$) inequality on arterial PO_2 and PCO_2. Ventilation-perfusion inequality has been increased by increasing the log standard deviation (SD) of a log normal distribution centered on a $\dot{V}A/\dot{Q}$ value of 1.0. The solid lines represent the situation when cardiac output and minute ventilation are held constant. Under these circumstances an increase in ventilation-perfusion inequality results in both hypoxemia and hypercapnia. The result of increasing $\dot{V}A/\dot{Q}$ inequality when ventilation is allowed to increase sufficiently to keep the arterial PCO_2 unchanged is shown by the dotted lines. Increased ventilation can normalize the PCO_2 without a significant impact on the PO_2. (From Dantzker DR: Chronic Obstructive Pulmonary Disease. New York, Churchill Livingstone, 1983. With permission.)

thus, compensate for the failure of CO_2 removal in the poorly ventilated ones. This accounts for the common finding in patients with lung diseases characterized by $\dot{V}A/\dot{Q}$ inequality of hypoxemia without hypercapnia.

As the $\dot{V}A/\dot{Q}$ inequality increases, so does the $\dot{V}E$ necessary to maintain a normal $PaCO_2$. The relationship between $\dot{V}E$ and $PaCO_2$ can be used as an index of the degree of $\dot{V}A/\dot{Q}$ inequality and is often quantitated by the measurement of the dead space–to-tidal volume ratio (VD/VT). Eventually, if the degree of $\dot{V}A/\dot{Q}$ inequality increases greatly (i.e., the proportion of the lung units with low $\dot{V}A/\dot{Q}$ becomes high enough), the increased ventilatory requirement may exceed the individual's maximal sustainable ventilation. This point is often reached when the work of breathing increases beyond the point that the patient is capable of maintaining. When this occurs, other than by improving lung function, the only way to eliminate the CO_2 produced by metabolism, and

thus prevent the development of progressive acidosis, is to allow the $PaCO_2$ to rise to a new steady-state value. This approach permits the elimination of CO_2 at a higher concentration per liter of minute ventilation and thus makes more efficient use of the existing ventilatory capacity.

The point at which hypercapnia develops in any individual patient depends on a complex interaction among the degree of $\dot{V}A/\dot{Q}$ inequality, the associated increased work of breathing, and the respiratory drive. For example, in obstructive lung disease, for the population as a whole, the $PaCO_2$ correlates inversely with the forced expiratory volume in 1 second (FEV_1) (Fig. 2–8) (Anthonisen and Cherniack, 1981). However, the variation from one individual to another is very large, and two patients with the same degree of abnormal lung mechanics may have a very different $PaCO_2$. This finding is thought to reflect, in part, differences in the gain control of the chemoreceptors, which influence an individual's toler-

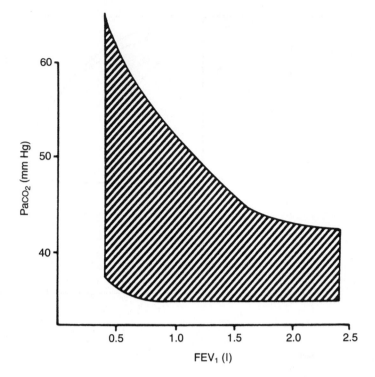

Figure 2–8
FEV$_1$ versus PaCO$_2$ relationship in chronic obstructive lung disease. The shaded area pertains to the range of PaCO$_2$ observed at any given level of obstruction. Although a relationship exists between the level of obstruction and the likelihood of hypercapnia, there is great variability from individual to individual. (From Anthonisen NR and Cherniack RM: Regulation of Breathing, Vol 2. New York, Marcel Dekker, 1981. With permission.)

ance to a rise in PaCO$_2$. A person with a very sensitive respiratory gain may continue to have an increase in $\dot{V}$E despite the increased work. In contrast, someone with a more sluggish response may minimize the work by allowing hypercapnia to develop. Differences in chemoreceptor gain may be partly genetically determined or may represent changes in chemoreceptor drive resulting from chronic airway obstruction (Greenberg et al, 1995). It is also influenced by factors that control the strength and endurance of the respiratory muscles, setting limits on the increase in ventilation that can be maintained without the development of fatigue (see Chapter 6).

The treatment of the abnormal gas exchange caused by $\dot{V}$A/$\dot{Q}$ inequality is directed ideally at correcting the underlying pulmonary pathology. However, the hypoxemia and hypercapnia must often be treated first to prevent organ disfunction, which may result from hypoxia or acidosis. The hypoxemia can always be eliminated by increasing the FIO$_2$ (Fig. 2–9). When the degree of $\dot{V}$A/$\dot{Q}$ inequality is mild, there is an almost linear increase in the PaO$_2$ with increases in FIO$_2$. As the $\dot{V}$A/$\dot{Q}$ inequality increases, the rate of rise becomes more resistant to a change in the FIO$_2$. When marked $\dot{V}$A/$\dot{Q}$ inequality is present, no significant improvement may be seen until the FIO$_2$ increases above 0.40.

Chronic hypercapnia with metabolic compensation for the respiratory acidosis is well tolerated, but acute and progressive hypercapnia must

be treated promptly by reducing the amount of $\dot{V}$A/$\dot{Q}$ inequality (e.g., by reversing bronchospasm) or by increasing minute ventilation, which usually requires mechanical ventilation. Drugs such as doxapram, which are direct stimulants to the central nervous system, can increase minute ventilation (Moser et al, 1973). However, they also have many side effects (in particular, seizures) and are rarely given. Other drugs such as theophylline and progesterone also stimulate central respiratory drive, although to a considerably lesser degree (Lyons and Huang, 1968; Stroud et al, 1955). Almitrine has its stimulatory effect on the peripheral chemoreceptors and improves the distribution of $\dot{V}$A/$\dot{Q}$ by increasing the sensitivity to hypoxic vasoconstriction (Naeij et al, 1981). Unfortunately, none of these drugs has proved to be clinically useful on a large scale.

Oxygen therapy in the patient with marked $\dot{V}$A/$\dot{Q}$ inequality and hypercapnia often leads to further elevations of PaCO$_2$. This finding has previously been attributed entirely to the suppression of hypoxic drive in a patient whose CO$_2$ drive has been blunted by chronic hypercapnia. Aubier and associates (1980), however, showed that only a portion of the increased PaCO$_2$ can be explained by a reduction in $\dot{V}$E. These investigators postulated adverse effects on $\dot{V}$A/$\dot{Q}$ relations within the lung to explain elevated PaCO$_2$ in patients receiving O$_2$ therapy. The increase in PaO$_2$ also shifts the carboxyhemoglobin dissociation curve to the right (the Haldane effect), thus decreasing

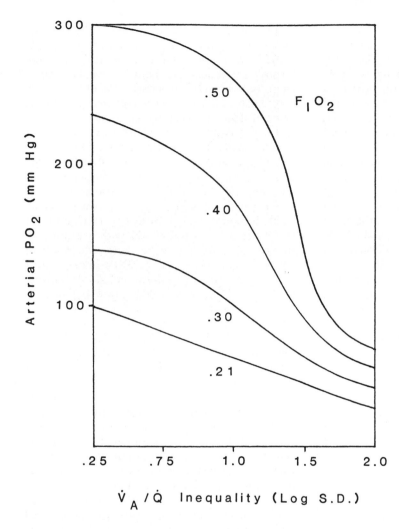

Figure 2–9
The effect of increasing ventilation-perfusion ($\dot{V}_A/\dot{Q}$) inequality on the arterial P_{O_2} at different inspired oxygen fractions ($F_{I_{O_2}}$). In a normal lung, the arterial P_{O_2} increases in a linear fashion with changes in $F_{I_{O_2}}$. As the underlying amount of $\dot{V}_A/\dot{Q}$ inequality increases, the Pa_{O_2} becomes more resistant to changes in $F_{I_{O_2}}$, although at $F_{I_{O_2}}$ of 1.0 the arterial P_{O_2} for any degree of $\dot{V}_A/\dot{Q}$ inequality converges.

its affinity for CO_2. Some increase in Pa_{CO_2} should probably be expected in all hypoxemic, hypercapnic patients who are given supplemental O_2 and should not be seen as a contraindication to O_2 therapy, because the amount of rise is most often limited and is not clinically important. In most patients with chronic respiratory failure due to chronic obstructive pulmonary disease (COPD), arterial Pa_{CO_2} increases by less than 5 to 10 mm Hg with minimal decreases in pH and no evidence of decreased mental function. In these patients, O_2 therapy should be continued. In those few patients in whom a necessary increase in $F_{I_{O_2}}$ leads to progressive hypercapnia and to the onset of CO_2 narcosis, mechanical ventilation should be instituted to ensure adequate oxygenation without acidosis.

SHUNT

Under certain circumstances, venous blood returning from the systemic circulation passes through to the arterial side without exposure to alveolar gas. This finding occurs routinely in the bronchial and thebesian circulations and accounts for the 2 to 3% shunt found in normal subjects. Increased amounts of shunt may develop through anatomic channels, such as atrial or ventricular septal defects, patent ductus arteriosus, or arteriovenous connection within the lung. More commonly, a shunt results from blood passing through pulmonary capillaries within the walls of alveoli that are atelectatic or filled with fluid or inflammatory exudate and are thus unventilated.

A shunt may be viewed as merely one end of the spectrum of $\dot{V}_A/\dot{Q}$ inequality ($\dot{V}_A/\dot{Q} = 0$). This is discussed as a separate entity, however, because the presence of a shunt infers a different spectrum of disorders and its physiologic behavior requires a different approach to therapy. Shunting is the mechanism of hypoxemia in pulmonary edema of both cardiac and noncardiac origin and is the major abnormality in pneumonia and atelectasis (Dantzker et al, 1979; Light et al, 1981; Staub, 1974).

Even small amounts of shunting cause significant hypoxemia because of the marked desaturation of the admixing venous blood (Fig. 2–10). Hypercapnia is a rare feature as long as $\dot{V}E$ remains unchanged and is found only when the shunt is very large (>50%). Even at these high levels of shunt, the $PaCO_2$ is usually low because the combined effects of hypoxemia and the underlying lung pathology stimulate hyperventilation. The hypoxemia of shunt is resistant to correction by increasing the FIO_2, and this feature is often used clinically to differentiate a shunt from $\dot{V}A/\dot{Q}$ inequality. When the shunt is small, a rise in the FIO_2 increases the PaO_2; however, as the shunt increases, the response to supplemental O_2 decreases. With large shunts, even 100% oxygen makes only a small impact on the PaO_2 (unlike even the most severe degree of $\dot{V}A/\dot{Q}$ inequality) (Fig. 2–11A). Because of the shape of the oxyhemoglobin dissociation curve, however, even these small increases in PaO_2 lead to significant increases in oxygen content, which is a major determinant of oxygen delivery to the peripheral tissues (see Fig. 2–11B). Because of the poor response to high concentrations of supplemental oxygen, as well as the potential pulmonary toxic-

ity of a high FIO_2, patients in whom the underlying disease cannot be reversed quickly are usually treated with some form of positive pressure breathing to reduce the shunt by alveolar recruitment (Clark and Lambertsen, 1971). However, considerable controversy currently exists as to the proper balance between increased airway pressure and increased FIO_2 in the ventilatory strategies of the hypoxemic patient (see Chapter 11).

The level of shunt has been shown to vary directly with changes in cardiac output in both animal models of diffuse lung disease as well as in patients with pulmonary edema (Dantzker et al, 1980; Lemaire et al, 1976). The mechanism of this relationship is not known with certainty, although it is thought to be partly the result of concomitant changes in the $P\bar{V}O_2$ and its effect on vascular tone (Sandoval et al, 1983). Although the predominant stimulus to hypoxic vasoconstriction is the alveolar PO_2, the $P\bar{V}O_2$ also affects blood flow distribution (Fishman, 1976). As a result of this interaction, changes in shunt following therapeutic maneuvers that may affect cardiac output must be interpreted in the light of these changes.

A shunt can also be created by breathing enriched O_2 mixtures. Dantzker and associates (1975) demonstrated that as the FIO_2 increases, a point may be reached at which the gas in the alveolus is taken up by the capillary blood faster than it is replaced from the environment, and the lung unit may collapse. The lower the $\dot{V}A/\dot{Q}$ of the lung unit, the lower the FIO_2 required to reach this critical point. Although O_2-induced atelectasis does undoubtedly occur, it is probably of minor clinical importance due to the ability of lung units with low $\dot{V}A/\dot{Q}$ to increase ventilation from adjacent lung units through collateral ventilation.

NONPULMONARY FACTORS

With all other factors remaining constant, the end-capillary PO_2 of any lung unit is affected by a change in the $P\bar{V}O_2$. The degree to which $P\bar{V}O_2$ alters end-capillary PO_2 depends on the $\dot{V}A/\dot{Q}$ of the unit (West, 1977). This concept is most easily understood in the case of a shunt in which the arterial desaturation is caused by the direct admixture of venous blood. For ventilated lung units, the influence of the $P\bar{V}O_2$ is greatest in units in which the $\dot{V}A/\dot{Q}$ is less than 1.0 and is negligible for units with a $\dot{V}A/\dot{Q}$ above 10.0. The resultant effect on the PaO_2 depends on the overall $\dot{V}A/\dot{Q}$ distribution and is greatest in the presence of significant $\dot{V}A/\dot{Q}$ inequality and shunt (Fig. 2–

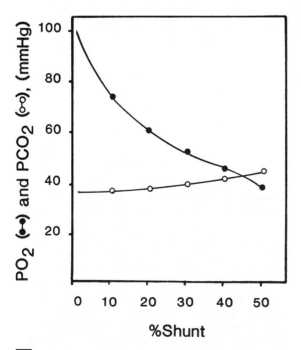

Figure 2–10
The effect of increasing shunt on the arterial PO_2 and PCO_2. The PCO_2 falls precipitously, whereas the PCO_2 is virtually unaffected. (From Dantzker DR: Chronic Obstructive Pulmonary Disease. New York, Churchill Livingstone, 1983. With permission.)

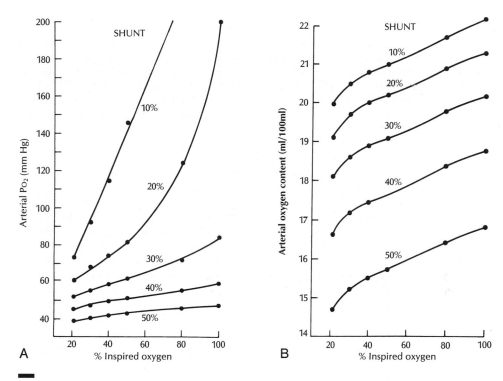

Figure 2–11
(A) The effect of changing the inspired oxygen concentration on arterial P_{O_2} and O_2 content for lungs shunts of 10 to 50%. The increase in P_{O_2} with increasing inspired oxygen is small for lungs with large shunts. (B) However, because of the shape of the hemoglobin dissociation curve, the increase in O_2 content is considerable. (From Dantzker DR: Adult respiratory distress syndrome. Clin Chest Med 3:37, 1982. With permission.)

12A). Factors causing a low $P\bar{v}_{O_2}$ are those that cause a disparity between O_2 requirements and O_2 delivery and include a low cardiac output, low O_2 content, and low hemoglobin concentration, and an increased $\dot{V}_{O_2}$. In a normal lung, the effect of a low $P\bar{v}_{O_2}$ can be overcome by hyperventilation with a subsequent increase in the $\dot{V}_A/\dot{Q}$ of most of the lung units. In the presence of disease, however, this response is less effective because the increased ventilation has minimal impact on the $\dot{V}_A/\dot{Q}$ of poorly ventilated units and has no impact on the shunt (see Fig. 2–12B).

A fall in $P\bar{v}_{O_2}$ is a normal occurrence during exercise, when greater O_2 extraction is used, in addition to an increase in O_2 transfer, to meet the greater metabolic O_2 demands. A highly conditioned athlete can achieve a $P\bar{v}_{O_2}$ as low as 20 mm Hg at peak levels of exercise. What prevents this from being translated into a significant fall in Pa_{O_2} is a shift in the overall distribution of ventilation and blood flow to a higher $\dot{V}_A/\dot{Q}$. Although cardiac output may increase four or even five times during exercise, ventilation increases 15 times or more at peak exercise (see Fig. 2–12).

The importance of alterations in the $P\bar{v}_{O_2}$ to the development or exaggeration of hypoxemia in disease states has been well documented (Dantzker et al, 1984; Dantzker and D'Alonzo, 1986; Huet et al, 1985; Manier et al, 1985). The coexistence of anemia or low cardiac output in the setting of chronic pulmonary disease markedly worsens the hypoxemia present for any degree of underlying lung pathology. The normal decrease in $P\bar{v}_{O_2}$ (already described during exercise) cannot be compensated for in the setting of significant $\dot{V}_A/\dot{Q}$ inequality or shunting because most of the increased ventilation is distributed to the already well-ventilated lung units and thus has little or no impact on the units that are the source of the hypoxemia (see Fig. 2–12). This is the major etiology of exercise-induced hypoxemia. Low cardiac output is the predominant cause of hypoxemia in pulmonary hypertension (Dantzker et al, 1984) and a major contributor to the low Pa_{O_2} found after acute pulmonary embolic disease (Manier et al, 1985). In the acutely ill patient in the intensive care unit in whom the predominant abnormality of pulmonary gas exchange is shunt, alterations in hemoglobin concentration or car-

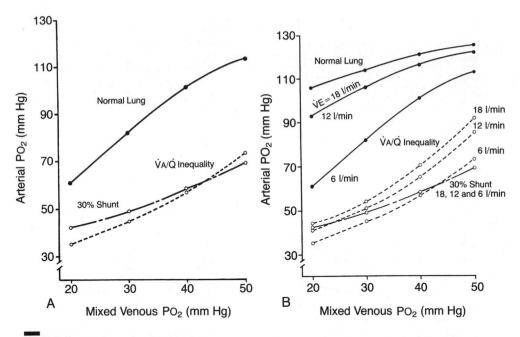

Figure 2–12

(A) The effect of a change of mixed-venous PO_2 on the arterial PO_2 in a theoretical lung with a normal $\dot{V}A/\dot{Q}$ distribution (*solid line*), significant $\dot{V}A/\dot{Q}$ inequality (*dashed line*), and a 30% shunt. The cardiac output and minute ventilation have been held constant, and the mixed venous PO_2 has been allowed to fall by increasing the assumed value of O_2 consumption. (B) The effect of increasing minute ventilation on the relationship between mixed venous PO_2 and arterial PO_2. The conditions are the same as those in A. Increasing minute ventilation is quite effective in preventing the development of hypoxemia in normal lungs but is much less effective when significant ventilation-perfusion inequality or a shunt is also present. (From Dantzker DR: Cardiovascular pulmonary interaction and diseased lung. Clin Chest Med 4:149, 1983. With permission.)

diac output may cause significant changes in PaO_2 (Dantzker et al, 1979). Clearly, a change in $P\overline{v}O_2$ should always be considered as a possible cause of changing PaO_2. One should not merely assume that any change seen must be the result of an alteration in the degree of lung pathology.

MONITORING THE EFFICACY OF GAS EXCHANGE

As with all physiologic functions, the adequate monitoring of gas exchange requires parameters that are sensitive to small changes in lung function and yet are specific enough to separate the various abnormal mechanisms to facilitate the initiation of the correct intervention (Table 2–1). In addition, these parameters should be easily obtainable to allow repeated measurements with sufficient frequency to permit their use in the longitudinal monitoring of critically ill patients.

Continuous measurement would seem to be optimal. However, this is far from clear. Acute changes in metabolic demands, as seen with agitation or fever, or movement can lead to a sharp, transient drop in PaO_2 in the absence of any alteration in lung function. Hence, arterial blood gas values should be accurately interpreted only during relatively steady-state conditions (Young and Woolcock, 1978). Clinicians should refrain from reacting to transient changes in gas exchange not associated with a change in steady-state conditions.

The arterial blood gases are the most commonly used measurements of pulmonary gas exchange efficiency. Ideally, their measurement should be noninvasive. Pulse oximetry can partially accomplish this (Severinghaus and Kelleher, 1992). Oximetry measures the oxygen saturation by light transmission through arterialized blood in the pinna of the ear or in the fingertip. Because pulse oximetry measures saturation rather than partial pressure, its useful range is limited to the steep portion of the oxyhemoglobin dissociation curve. At saturations below 80%, however, the readings are falsely high. In addition, the ability

Table 2–1
Indices of Pulmonary Gas Exchange Efficiency

Variable	Normal Range or Regression Equation
Arterial P_{O_2} (mm Hg)	$104.2 - 0.27 \times$ age (yr)*
Arterial P_{CO_2} (mm Hg)	36–44
pH	7.35–7.45
O_2 saturation (%)	>95
Alveolar arterial O_2 difference (mm Hg)	$2.5 + 0.21 \times$ age (yr)*
Dead space (VD/VT)	$24.6 + 0.17 \times$ age (yr)*
Shunt: Room air	5%*
100% O_2	3%*

*From Mellengaard K: The alveolar-arterial oxygen difference: Its size and components in normal man. Acta Physiol Scand 67:10–20, 1966.

to accurately reflect arterial saturation is critically dependent on adequate blood flow through the skin. The readings are also artificially high when carboxyhemoglobin levels exceed 3% (Chaudhary and Burki, 1978; Vegfors and Lennmarker, 1992).

Devices to measure transcutaneous blood gas tensions have also been developed (Schoemaker and Vidyasagar, 1981). These devices depend on increasing the blood flow through the epidermal capillary loop (usually accomplished by heating the skin) so that the gas diffusing through the skin reflects arterial partial pressures rather than venous blood. Although transcutaneous P_{O_2} (tcP_{O_2}) has proved useful in neonatal units, in critically ill adults it appears to be too dependent on regional blood flow to be useful. Transcutaneous P_{CO_2} (tcP_{CO_2}) is a more accurate reflection of the arterial value, although a significant tc-arterial P_{CO_2} difference exists, and this difference changes with alterations in cardiac output and regional blood flow distribution. Therefore, repeated biologic calibrations, with an actual measurement of the tc-arterial difference, are necessary in the unstable patient.

Continuous monitoring of inspired and expired gases is now both technically and economically practical. However, its usefulness as an index of arterial P_{O_2} and P_{CO_2} is restricted to patients with relatively normal lungs. In the presence of lung disease, a significant difference between the arterial and end-tidal value develops and varies as the degree of lung disease varies.

The direct sampling of arterial blood is still the most accurate and commonly used technique available to evaluate the arterial blood gases. The blood may be obtained from intermittent arterial puncture or from an indwelling arterial cannula.

Although intermittent sampling is accurate, if a large number of samples are required (>5 samples/day), it is preferable to use a cannula to eliminate repeated trauma to the artery. A small chance exists for thrombosis of the artery because of the indwelling line, but this risk is rare when a small-bore catheter is placed (Davis and Stewart, 1980). To maximize both convenience and safety, the order of preference for both puncture and cannulation should be the radial, brachial, femoral, axillary, and ulnar arteries. Advances allow continuous intra-arterial blood gas monitoring. However, the clinical utility of this monitoring remains to be demonstrated (Mahutte, 1991).

As with noninvasive techniques, one must be aware of the potential sources of error that interfere with the accuracy of the measurement. Technical errors, particularly in the calibration of the analytic equipment, are the most common source of problems. Excessive amounts of heparin in the syringe cause a low pH and P_{CO_2}, whereas allowing the blood to remain at room temperature for too long causes the P_{O_2} to fall owing to continued O_2 utilization by the white blood cells and platelets (Cline, 1975; Hansen and Simmons, 1977). This problem is magnified in the presence of marked leukocytosis or thrombocytosis, in which factitious hypoxemia may be seen in even a properly handled specimen (Hess et al, 1979).

Although arterial blood gases are invaluable in the clinical management of patients with lung disease, they are often difficult to use as indices of either an improvement or a progression of the underlying lung disease, especially when patients are breathing enriched O_2 mixtures. When they are breathing room air, there is an almost linear decrease in the Pa_{O_2} as the degree of $\dot{V}A/\dot{Q}$ inequality increases (Fig. 2–13). As the F_{IO_2} increases, the relationship is no longer linear. The same increase in $\dot{V}A/\dot{Q}$ inequality may be associated with a markedly different absolute change in the Pa_{O_2}, depending on the F_{IO_2} level and on how abnormal the lung disease is.

When shunt is the underlying mechanism of disordered gas exchange, changes in the Pa_{O_2} are more sensitive markers of change, at all levels of F_{IO_2}, when lesser amounts of shunt are present. Changes in Pa_{O_2} are less sensitive to changes when the shunt exceeds 30% (Fig. 2–14). With disorders characterized by combinations of these mechanisms of abnormal gas exchange, the relationships are even more complex. The Pa_{CO_2} is so sensitive to changes in $\dot{V}E$ that it is rarely a good index of the efficiency of pulmonary gas exchange.

The alveolar-to-arterial gradient for oxygen ($PA_{O_2} - Pa_{O_2}$) is an index of how much the

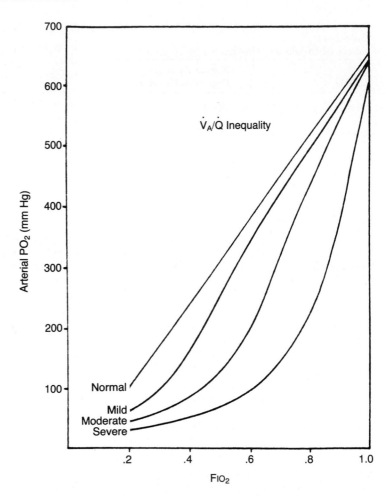

Figure 2–13
The effect of increasing the fractional concentration of inspired O_2 (FIO_2) on the arterial PO_2 in patients with different degrees of ventilation-perfusion ($\dot{V}A/\dot{Q}$) inequality. The degree of ventilation perfusion inequality is quantified by the log SD with 0.25 representing a normal lung and 2.0 severe $\dot{V}A/\dot{Q}$ inequality. When breathing room air, the arterial PO_2 is linearly reduced as the lung becomes more abnormal. However, at a higher FIO_2 the relationship becomes more complex, and thus changes in the degree of abnormality are more difficult to assess.

arterial PO_2 differs from that which would be present if the lung were to be the simple homogeneous model shown in Figure 2–1. The gradient is derived by subtracting the ideal alveolar PO_2 obtained from the alveolar gas equation from the PaO_2. Abnormalities of ventilation and blood flow matching ($\dot{V}A/\dot{Q}$ inequality and shunt) and abnormal diffusion are reflected in a widening of the $PAO_2 - PaO_2$. The $PAO_2 - PaO_2$ has the advantage of being insensitive to changes in the $\dot{V}E$. Thus, patients who are hypoxemic only because of hypoventilation have a normal $PAO_2 - PaO_2$ and can be distinguished from patients who have an underlying lung pathology.

The $PAO_2 - PaO_2$ does not circumvent many of the problems associated with the use of the arterial blood gases. Alterations in the $P\bar{v}O_2$ affect the $PAO_2 - PaO_2$ similar to its effect on the PaO_2. When the FIO_2 is changed, the calculated $PAO_2 - PaO_2$ changes, even though no true alteration in gas exchange efficiency has occurred. When a shunt is the underlying abnormality, the $PAO_2 - PaO_2$ increases progressively as the FIO_2 is

increased (Fig. 2–15). Because of the nonlinear relationship between FIO_2 and PaO_2 in patients with $\dot{V}A/\dot{Q}$ inequality, the relationship between $PAO_2 - PaO_2$ and FIO_2 is also more complex (Fig. 2–16). Because of these complexities, the $PAO_2 - PaO_2$ must be measured at the same FIO_2 each time if it is to meaningfully reflect changes in a patient's lung function.

Even at the same FIO_2, it should be clear from a careful study of Figures 2–14 and 2–15 that, similar to arterial blood gases, the amount of change in the $PAO_2 - PaO_2$ that occurs for any increase in $\dot{V}A/\dot{Q}$ inequality or shunt differs from one FIO_2 to another and depends on the initial degree of abnormality. For example, there are larger increases in $PAO_2 - PaO_2$ for the same increase in shunt when the patient is breathing 100% O_2 than when breathing room air. The changes are also greater when the shunt changes from 10 to 20% than when a similar degree of increase occurs from 40 to 50%. Similar, although even more complex, problems exist when $\dot{V}A/\dot{Q}$ inequality is the major abnormality. Other manip-

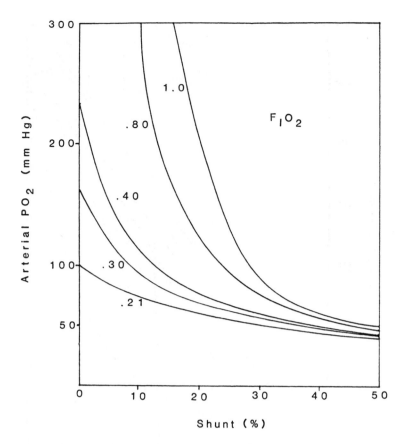

Figure 2–14
The effect of an increasing degree of shunt on the arterial PO_2 at different inspired oxygen fractions (FIO_2). The degree of change in the PaO_2 as the amount of shunt increases and decreases varies widely, depending on the FIO_2.

ulations of these variables have been tried to minimize the difficulties enumerated earlier. Both the PaO_2/PAO_2 and PaO_2/FIO_2 have been suggested as alternatives to the $PAO_2 - PaO_2$ (Gilbert et al, 1979); Modell et al, 1976). Not surprisingly, because they are only further manipulations of the same primary data, they have many of the same limitations. For example, in the setting of both shunt and $\dot{V}A/\dot{Q}$ inequality, an increase in the FIO_2 results in a decrease in both ratios with no change in the underlying lung pathology.

It is often considered more useful to calculate the venous admixture ($\dot{Q}_s/\dot{Q}_t$). This estimation of abnormal gas exchange treats the lung as if it consists of two compartments—an ideal alveolar compartment and a shunt. Increasing hypoxemia is represented as resulting from an increase in the blood flow to the shunt compartment. The $\dot{Q}_s/\dot{Q}_t$ can be quantitated from a simple mixing equation that assumes that the total amount of O_2 in the arterial blood, the product of the cardiac output and the arterial O_2 content ($\dot{Q}_t \times CaO_2$), is equal to the amount coming from the shunt ($\dot{Q}_s \times C\bar{v}O_2$) and the amount in the blood leaving the ideal compartment ($(\dot{Q}_t - \dot{Q}_s) \times CcO_2$):

$$\dot{Q}_t \times CaO_2 = (\dot{Q}_t - \dot{Q}_s) \times CcO_2 + \dot{Q}_s \times C\bar{v}O_2$$

and

$$\dot{Q}_s/\dot{Q}_t = CcO_2 - CaO_2/CcO_2 - C\bar{v}O_2$$

The arterial and venous O_2 contents are obtained directly from the arterial and mixed venous blood gas measurements and the hemoglobin concentration:

$$O_2 \text{ content} = (\text{hemoglobin} \times 1.34) \times \% \text{ saturation} + PO_2 \times 0.003$$

The CcO_2 cannot be measured directly because the end-capillary blood of the ideal alveolus is merely a theoretical construct. The ideal PO_2 is assumed to be the same as that calculated from the alveolar gas equation, and the saturation can be assumed to be 100% if the ideal PO_2 is greater than 150 mm Hg. If it is less, which it often is in patients breathing less than 30% O_2, the saturation must be calculated from the oxyhemoglobin dissociation curve.

There is often no access to mixed venous blood, and one of the many suggested modifications of the standard shunt equation are commonly used. In general, these modified shunt equations assume both an arbitrary a-$\bar{v}O_2$ difference and that both the ideal PO_2 and PaO_2 are

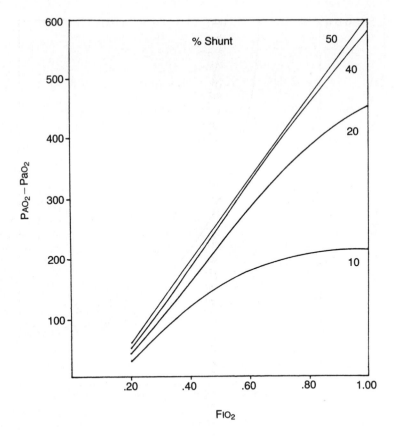

Figure 2–15
The effect of increasing the inspired oxygen fraction (FIO_2) on the calculated alveolar-arterial O_2 gradient ($PAO_2 - PaO_2$) for different amounts of shunt. The alveolar-arterial O_2 gradient appears to increase as the FIO_2 is increased, despite the fact that there is no change in the amount of shunt.

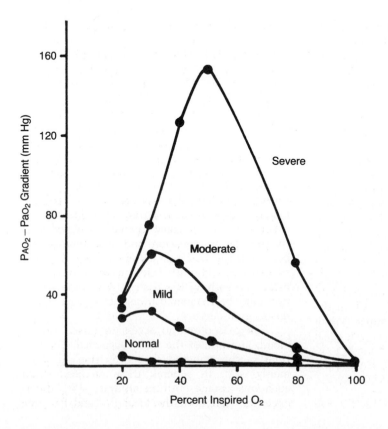

Figure 2–16
The effect of changing the inspired O_2 percentage on the alveolar-arterial gradient for O_2, or $PA - aO_2$, in a normal lung and in one with mild, moderate, and severe ventilation-perfusion inequality. At every level of $\dot{V}A/\dot{Q}$ inequality, the alveolar-arterial gradient varies in a complex manner as the FIO_2 is changed. (From Dantzker DR: Critical Care: A Comprehensive Approach. Park Ridge, IL, American College of Chest Physicians, 1984. With permission.)

high enough to fully saturate the blood (Pontop-pidian et al, 1970). Because the latter assumption is rarely true in critically ill patients and the a-$\bar{V}O_2$ difference is neither predictable nor stable in this population, these simplifications lose more in accuracy and sensitivity than they gain in ease of calculation and should be avoided.

When patients breathe room air, the calculated venous admixture is made up of contributions from both true right-to-left shunt and the shunt-like effect of $\dot{V}A/\dot{Q}$ inequality. As the FIO_2 is increased, the degree to which lung units with low $\dot{V}A/\dot{Q}$ ratios contribute to abnormal gas exchange decreases and, as such, so does their contribution to the venous admixture. When breathing 100% O_2, the venous admixture represents only the amount of true shunt (Fig. 2–17). Thus, in patients in whom $\dot{V}A/\dot{Q}$ inequality is the major physiologic abnormality, $\dot{Q}s/\dot{Q}t$ must be measured at the same FIO_2 for it to be comparable from one point in time to another as with the PaO_2 —

PaO_2. In patients in whom the hypoxemia is predominantly caused by a shunt, however, it makes little difference what FIO_2 is used, as long as the possible influence of a high FIO_2 on the creation of shunt is not thought to be important.

Just as the $\dot{Q}s/\dot{Q}t$ treats the lung as if it contained two lung units, a shunt (made up of true shunt and low $\dot{V}A/\dot{Q}$, depending on the FIO_2) and an ideal lung unit, the dead space, as measured by the Bohr equation:

$$VD/VT = \frac{PaCO_2 - PECO_2}{PaCO_2}$$

looks at the ventilation as being distributed to either an ideal compartment or to dead space (Krogh and Lindhard, 1917). Any difference between $PaCO_2$ and $PECO_2$ is seen as the result of the presence of non-CO_2–containing expired air coming from the unperfused dead space. This dead space is mainly anatomic dead space in normal subjects. However, the expired gas also is diluted, when compared with the $PaCO_2$, by gas coming from overventilated lung units (physiologic dead space). Because the $PaCO_2$ is influenced more by low $\dot{V}A/\dot{Q}$ units (with high alveolar and end-capillary PCO_2) and the $PECO_2$ is influenced more by high $\dot{V}A/\dot{Q}$ units (with low alveolar and end-capillary PCO_2), the greater the $\dot{V}A/\dot{Q}$ inequality, the larger the measured VD/VT. Thus, the dead space is merely another index of the degree of $\dot{V}A/\dot{Q}$ inequality. The VD/VT may be influenced significantly by changes in overall cardiac output and minute ventilation as well as by changes in the degree of $\dot{V}A/\dot{Q}$ inequality.

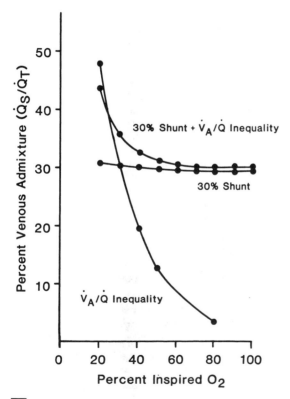

Figure 2–17
The effect of changing the inspired O_2 percentage on the calculated venous admixture for three clinical situations. When only shunt is present, it does not matter at what percentage of inspired O_2 the shunt is measured. (From Dantzker DR: Critical Care: A Comprehensive Approach. Park Ridge, IL, American College of Chest Physicians, 1984. With permission.)

REFERENCES

Anthonisen NR and Cherniack RM: Ventilatory control. In Hornbein T (ed): Lung Disease: Regulation of Breathing. New York, Marcel Dekker, 1981, pp 965–987.

Askanazi J, Rosenbaum SH, Hyman AL, et al: Respiratory changes induced by the large glucose loads of total parenteral nutrition. JAMA 234:1444–1447, 1980.

Aubier M, Marviano D, Milic-Emili J, et al: Effects of the administration of O_2 on ventilation and blood gases in patients with chronic obstructive pulmonary disease during acute respiratory failure. Am Rev Respir Dis 122:747–754, 1980.

Barer GR, Howard P, and Shaw TW: Stimulus-response curves for the pulmonary vascular bed to hypoxia and hypercapnia. J Physiol (Lond) 211:139–155, 1970.

Bergofsky EH: Acute control of the normal pulmonary circulation. In Moser KM (ed): Pulmonary Vascular Disease. New York, Marcel Dekker, 1979, pp 223–278.

Burrows B, Kettel LJ, Niden AT, et al: Patterns of cardiovascular dysfunction in chronic obstructive lung disease. N Engl J Med 286:912–918, 1972.

Chaudhary BA and Burki NK: Ear oximetry in clinical practice. Am Rev Respir Dis 111:173–175, 1978.

Clark JM, and Lambersten CJ: Pulmonary oxygen toxicity: A review. Pharmacol Rev 23:37–133, 1971.

Cline MJ: The White Cell. Cambridge, MA, Harvard University Press, 1975.

Dantzker DR, Brook CH, DeHart P, et al: Gas exchange in adult respiratory distress syndrome and the effects of positive end-expiratory pressure. Am Rev Respir Dis 120:1039–1052, 1979.

Dantzker DR and D'Alonzo GE: The effect of exercise on pulmonary gas exchange in patients with severe chronic obstructive pulmonary disease. Am Rev Respir Dis 134:1135–1139, 1986.

Dantzker DR, D'Alonzo GE, Bower JS, et al: Pulmonary gas exchange during exercise in patients with chronic obliterative pulmonary hypertension. Am Rev Respir Dis 130:412–416, 1984.

Dantzker DR, Lynch P, and Weg JG: Depression of cardiac output is a mechanism of shunt reduction in the therapy of acute respiratory failure. Chest 77:636–642, 1980.

Dantzker DR, Wagner PD, Tornabene VW, et al: Gas exchange after pulmonary thromboembolization in dogs. Circ Res 42:92–103, 1978.

Dantzker DR, Wagner PD, and West JB: Instability of lung units with low $\dot{V}A/\dot{Q}$ ratios during O_2 breathing. J Appl Physiol 38:886–895, 1975.

Davis FM and Stewart JM: Radial artery cannulation: A prospective study in patients undergoing cardiothoracic surgery. Br J Anaesth 52:41–46, 1980.

Fishman AP: Hypoxia on the pulmonary circulation. Circ Res 38:221–231, 1976.

Fishman AP: Vasomotor regulation of the pulmonary circulation. Ann Rev Physiol 42:211–220, 1980.

Gilbert R, Auchincloss JH, Kuppinger M, et al: Stability of the arterial/alveolar oxygen partial pressure rate. Crit Care Med 7:267–272, 1979.

Grant BJB: Effect of the local pulmonary blood flow control on gas exchange. J Appl Physiol 53:1100–1109, 1982.

Greenberg HE, Tarasiuk A, Rao RS, et al: Effect of chronic resistive loading on ventilatory control in a rat model. Am J Resp Crit Care Med 152:666–676, 1995.

Grover RF, Hyers TM, McMurtry IF, et al: High altitude pulmonary edema. In Fishman AP and Renkin EM (eds): Pulmonary Edema. Bethesda, MD, American Physiological Society, 1979.

Hansen JE and Simmons DH: A systematic error in the determination of blood P_{CO_2}. Am Rev Respir Dis 115:1061–1063, 1977.

Hess CE, Nichols AB, Hunt WB, et al: Pseudohypoxemia secondary to leukemia and thrombocytosis. N Engl J Med 301:361–363, 1979.

Huet Y, Lemaire F, Brun-Buisson C, et al: Hypoxemia in acute pulmonary embolism. Chest 88:829–836, 1985.

Hurtado A, Mernio G, and Delgado E: Influence of anoxemia on the hematopoietic activity. Arch Intern Med 75:284–326, 1945.

Kappogoda CJ, Stoker JB, and Linden RJ: A method for continuous measurement of oxygen consumption. J Appl Physiol 37:604–606, 1974.

Krogh A and Lindhard J: The volume of the dead space in breathing and the mixing of gases in the lungs of man. J Physiol (Lond) 51:59–90, 1917.

Lemaire F, Jardin F, Harari A, et al: Assessment of gas exchange during venoarterial bypass using the membrane lung. In Zapol WM and Quist J (eds): Artificial Lungs for Acute Respiratory Failure. New York, Academic Press, 1976.

Light RB, Mink WN, and Wood LDH: Pathophysiology of gas exchange and pulmonary perfusion in pneumococcal lobar pneumonia in dogs. J Appl Physiol 50:524–530, 1981.

Luft U: Aviation physiology—the effects of altitude. In Fenn WD and Rahn H (eds): Respiration. Bethesda, MD, American Physiological Society, 1965, pp 1099–1145.

Lyons HA and Huang CT: Therapeutic use of progesterone in alveolar hypoventilation associated with obesity. Am J Med 44:881–888, 1968.

Mahutte CK: On-line blood gas monitoring. In Tobin MJ (ed): Contemporary Management in Critical Care: Respiratory Monitoring. New York, Churchill Livingstone, 1991, pp 27–49.

Manier G, Castaing Y, and Guenard H: Determinants of hypoxemia during the acute phase of pulmonary embolism in humans. Am Rev Respir Dis 132:332–338, 1985.

Modell JH, Graves SA, and Ketouer A: Clinical course of 91 consecutive near-drowning victims. Chest 70:231–234, 1976.

Moser KM, Luchsinger PC, Adamson JS, et al: Respiratory stimulation with intravenous doxapram in respiratory failure. N Engl J Med 288:427–431, 1973.

Naeij R, Melot C, Mols P, et al: Effects of almitrine in decompensated chronic respiratory insufficiency. Bull Eur Physiopathol Respir 17:153–161, 1981.

Pontoppidan H, Laver ME, and Geffin B: Acute respiratory failure in the surgical patient. Adv Surg 4:163–254, 1970.

Rossaint R, Falke KJ, Lopez F, et al: Inhaled nitric oxide for the adult respiratory distress syndrome. N Engl J Med 328:399–405, 1993.

Roughton FJW and Forster RE: Relative importance of diffusion and chemical reaction rates in the human lung, with special reference to true diffusing capacity of pulmonary membrane and volume of blood in the lung capillaries. J Appl Physiol 11:290–302, 1957.

Sandoval J, Long GR, Skoog C, et al: Independent influence of blood flow rate and mixed venous

PO$_2$ on shunt fraction. J Appl Physiol 55:1128–1133, 1983.

Schoemaker WC and Vidyasagar D (eds): Transcutaneous O$_2$ and CO$_2$ monitoring of the adult and neonate. Crit Care Med 9:689–760, 1981.

Severinghaus JW and Kelleher JF: Recent developments in pulse oximetry. Anesthesiology 76:1018–1038, 1992.

Smithies MN, Royston B, Makita K, et al: Comparison of oxygen consumption measurements: Indirect calorimetry versus the reversed Fick method. Crit Care Med 19:1401-1406, 1991.

Staub N: Pulmonary edema. Physiol Rev 54:678–811, 1974.

Stroud MW, Lambertsen CJ, Ewing R, et al: Effects of aminophylline and meperidine alone and in combination on the respiratory response to carbon dioxide inhalation. J Pharmacol Exp Ther 114:461–469, 1955.

Swensen EW, Finley TN, and Guzman SV: Unilateral hypoventilation in man during temporary occlusion of one pulmonary artery. J Clin Invest 40:828–835, 1961.

Sylvester JT, Harabin AL, Peake MD, et al: Vasodilatory and vasoconstriction responses to hypoxia in isolated pig lungs. J Appl Physiol 49:820–825, 1980.

Vegfors M, Lennmarker C: Carboxyhemoglobinemia and pulse oximetry. Br J Anaesth 77:594–596, 1992.

Wagner PD: Diffusion and chemical reaction in pulmonary gas exchange. Physiol Rev 57:257–312, 1977.

Wagner P, Dantzker D, Dueck D, et al: Ventilation-perfusion inequality in chronic obstructive pulmonary disease. J Clin Invest 59:203–216, 1977.

Wagner PD, Laravuso RB, Uhl RR, et al: Continuous distributions of ventilation-perfusion ratios in normal subjects breathing air and 100% O$_2$. J Clin Invest 54:45–68, 1974.

West JB: Ventilation-perfusion inequality and overall gas exchange in computer models of the lung. Respir Physiol 7:88–110, 1969.

West JB: Ventilation-perfusion relationships. Am Rev Respir Dis 116:919–943, 1977.

Winslow RM, Samaja M, and West JB: Red cell function at extreme altitude on Mount Everest. J Appl Physiol 56:109–116, 1984.

Young IH and Woolcock AJ: Changes in arterial blood gas tensions during unsteady-state exercise. J Appl Physiol 44:93–96, 1978.

CHAPTER

Pathophysiology of the Pulmonary Vascular Bed

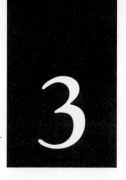

3

Séan P. Gaine, M.B., B.Ch.

Roy G. Brower, M.D., and

Charles M. Wiener, M.D.

The pulmonary vascular bed provides a low-resistance conduit for the movement of venous blood from the right to left heart and a large surface area for intimate contact between blood and alveolar gas. This large surface area also facilitates the production and removal of numerous vasoactive mediators. Pulmonary vascular resistance is modulated both by passive factors, such as lung volume, and active factors, such as alveolar oxygen concentration. Disorders of the pulmonary vasculature are manifested by elevations of pulmonary vasculature resistance and subsequent development of right heart failure. The aim of this chapter is to discuss the unique morphology, physiology, and pathophysiology of the pulmonary vascular bed and to describe the methods to evaluate its function in clinical practice. Disorders of the pulmonary vasculature resulting from or leading to acute lung injury and pulmonary edema are discussed in Chapter 18.

MORPHOLOGY

RIGHT HEART

The morphology of the right heart is determined by its work. *In utero*, when pulmonary vascular resistance is high, the right and left ventricular walls are essentially of similar thickness. As pulmonary vascular resistance falls after birth, however, the relative size of the right ventricle regresses slowly. The adult right ventricle is one-third the thickness of the left ventricle. The output of the adult right ventricle is normally slightly less than that of the left ventricle due to the drainage of bronchial and thebesian veins that bypass the right ventricle. The adult right ventricle is also more compliant than the left ventricle and has a lower resting end-diastolic pressure. As a result, the right heart can tolerate acute increases in volume better than acute increases in pressure (Permutt et al, 1985; Semmens and Reid, 1974). Chronic or insidious elevation in pulmonary pressure or resistance, as discussed later, leads initially to right ventricular hypertrophy, followed by dilation and right heart failure.

PULMONARY VESSELS

The pulmonary artery develops from the sixth branchial arch, which appears *in utero* at about 32 days, and extends branches to the already forming lung buds. By 37 days the proximal ventral aorta is divided so that only blood from the right ventricle goes to the lungs. At this time also the sixth arch on the right thins as the left arch becomes the main pulmonary trunk. The left sixth arch remains attached to the aorta as the ductus arteriosus. The adult pattern of blood supply is complete by 50 days, although there is some ongoing development of the intra-acinar vessels until 18 months, and the "supernumerary" arteries until age 8 years (Hislop and Reid, 1973; Thurlbeck, 1975; Weibel, 1973) (Fig. 3–1).

In the adult, the pulmonary trunk originates from the base of the right ventricle and extends 4 to 5 cm before dividing into the right and left main *pulmonary arteries*. The left pulmonary artery arches over the left main bronchus at the hilum and divides into lobar branches. The right pulmonary artery continues posterior to both the aorta and superior vena cava and anterior to the right main bronchus. The pulmonary arterial system invariably follows the bronchial tree and divides with it. In addition to this conventional dichotomous branching, however, many "supernumerary" or accessory branches arise at points other than the corresponding bronchial divisions and increase in number more distally. As a result, there are more arteries than airways in the lung.

To maintain low vascular resistance, pulmonary blood vessels differ significantly from systemic vessels. Histologically, precapillary vessels are divided into three morphologic types: elastic, muscular, and arteriolar. *Elastic arteries* include the main pulmonary artery and its lobar, segmental, and subsegmental branches, extending to arteries 1 mm in diameter, roughly at the junction of the bronchi and bronchioles. Despite their name, these arteries contain smooth muscle and are capable of vasoconstriction. Elastic arteries provide a distensible elastic reservoir for right ventricular output. Most of the intra-arterial blood volume is contained in the large central elastic arteries as the cross-sectional area of the pulmonary vasculature decreases, moving from the hilus to the periphery (Singhal et al, 1973).

The transition from elastic to *muscular arteries* occurs in vessels from 1 to 0.5 mm in diameter. Pulmonary muscular arteries have internal and external elastic laminae with an intervening layer of smooth muscle cells and have an external diameter of approximately 500 μm down to 70 μm. This is in contrast to systemic muscular arteries

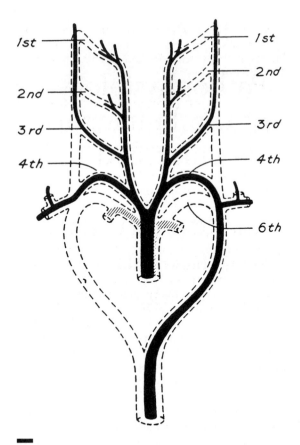

Figure 3–1
Schematic representation of the aortic arches of the embryo. The dashed lines depict the original embryonic arches. The solid black lines are the adult vessels and the shaded lines the adult pulmonary arteries. The left sixth arch maintains communication between the systemic and pulmonary circulations *in utero* as the ductus arteriosus. (From Comroe JH: Physiology of Respiration, 2nd ed. St. Louis, Year Book Medical Publishers, 1974, p 37. With permission.)

in which the external elastic laminae are usually absent or incomplete. The acinar and most supernumerary arteries are muscular. During alveolar hypoxia, the increase in pulmonary vascular resistance comes predominantly from these precapillary muscular arteries (Rock et al, 1985; Weibel, 1973).

Arteries smaller than approximately 70 μm gradually lose their medial smooth muscle to become *arterioles*. These vessels have a thin intima and a single elastic lamina. Within the acinus, arterioles continue to divide and accompany their respective branches of the respiratory tree, along with many accessory branches, and terminate at the alveolar capillary network. Although most of the drop in pressure in the systemic circulation occurs at the precapillary level, the major pressure drop in pulmonary circulation occurs at the capillaries (Bhattacharya and Staub, 1980; Brody et al, 1968; Weibel, 1973).

Each capillary segment has a diameter of about 10 μm, just sufficient to allow a red blood cell through (Weibel, 1963). The *capillary network* is uniquely divided into alveolar and extra-alveolar vessels. Alveolar vessels are in intimate contact with the air-filled alveoli and are exposed to alveolar pressure. Their diameter varies *inversely* with transpulmonary pressure and lung volume. There are approximately 1800 to 2000 capillary segments surrounding each alveolus (Weibel, 1973). The thickness of the blood-gas barrier at the alveolus is approximately 0.5 μm, comprising the alveolar epithelial cell, vascular endothelium, and connective tissue. In the normal adult lung, total capillary surface area has been calculated to be 126 ± 12 m², with a blood volume of approximately 75 ml (Gehr et al, 1978). Under normal resting conditions, each red blood cell moves through the alveolus in 0.75 sec, which is more than adequate for the partial pressures of oxygen (O_2) and carbon dioxide (CO_2) to come into equilibrium across the alveolar membrane (<0.25 sec for equilibration). Extra-alveolar vessels are not exposed to alveolar pressure and are thought to traverse the corner regions between alveolar units. Although these vessels can also exchange gas and filter fluid, their diameter varies *directly* with transpulmonary pressure and lung volume.

From the alveolar network, *pulmonary veins* run separate from the bronchioarterial pathways and return oxygenated blood to the left atrium. There are usually two superior veins draining the middle and upper lobe on the right and upper lobe on the left, and two inferior main pulmonary veins draining both lower lobes (Horsfield and Gordon, 1981). Some return of deoxygenated blood occurs from anastomoses with the venous drainage of the pleura and bronchial circulation. Pulmonary veins are richly innervated and contain vascular receptors similar to pulmonary arteries (Amenta et al 1983; Braun and Stern, 1967; Burch, 1980; Fisher, 1965; Hyman and Kadowitz, 1985; Johnson et al, 1980; Schellenberg and Foster, 1984).

BRONCHIAL VESSELS

The lung has a dual blood supply. The bronchial circulation, which receives approximately 1% of the systemic cardiac output, usually arises from the third intercostal artery on the right and from two arteries directly from the ventral surface of the descending aorta on the left. The arteries enter the hilum to supply the trachea, bronchi, and bronchioli, as well as the vasovasorum of pulmonary vessels. They also perfuse the visceral pleurae, interlobular septal supporting tissues, and middle one-third of the esophagus (Deffebach et al, 1987). Venous drainage from this circulation returns either by bronchial veins to the right heart via the azygos and hemizygous systems or by extensive anastomoses with the pulmonary circulation at the precapillary, capillary, and post-capillary levels, returning to the left heart. This left-sided drainage carries a small (~1%) shunt of mixed venous blood to the systemic circulation. Unlike the pulmonary circulation, the bronchial circulation is angiogenic in adult life. Thus, scars and tumors are supplied by bronchial vessels. Most causes of significant hemoptysis originate from bronchial arteries that are accessible for embolization via the systemic circulation (Deffebach et al, 1987).

PULMONARY ENDOTHELIUM

The *endothelium* is the most common cell type in the lung and lines the entire vascular bed. The endothelium performs a number of important functions. In addition to modulating vascular smooth muscle tone (see later), it has important metabolic activity. The endothelium also maintains vascular integrity and functions as a facilitator of inflammatory responses in the lung.

Endothelial cells release a number of relaxing and contracting mediators, with the balance in favor of relaxation under normal conditions. Under certain conditions and disease states, however, the balance shifts in favor of contraction and smooth muscle proliferation. The metabolic function of the pulmonary endothelium includes the activation and deactivation of a number of circulating mediators. Endothelial cells express angiotensin converting enzyme (ACE) on their surface. The enzyme is responsible for the conversion of angiotensin I to the active vasoconstrictor angiotensin II and for the deactivation of the peptide bradykinin (Ryan et al, 1976).

Endothelial cells also contain adhesion molecules, which are involved in the interaction between blood cells and vessel wall. Circulating leukocytes bind to selectins expressed by both the leukocytes and activated endothelial cells of the pulmonary venules. Leukocytes decelerate by rolling on the endothelium and become activated by local chemoattractants, inducing them to squeeze between endothelial cells and migrate to sites of inflammation. There are three known selectin genes, which are termed *L, E,* and *P.* Disruption of endothelial integrity exposes the subendothelial matrix, stimulating neighboring endothelial cells to express their P-selectin. Platelets also decelerate by rolling, using the endothelial P-selectin, facilitating the recruitment of platelets to the damaged vessel (Frenette and Wagner, 1996; Springer, 1995).

PHYSIOLOGY OF THE PULMONARY CIRCULATION

The pulmonary circulation provides both a low-pressure conduit for the movement of blood from the right to left heart and a large surface area between blood and alveoli for efficient gas exchange. The pulmonary vascular bed is regulated by both passive and active mechanisms that alter vascular resistance.

PULMONARY VASCULAR RESISTANCE

Assuming that the relationship of pressure to flow is linear, we can generate an equation governing resistance in the pulmonary vascular bed derived from Ohm's law.

$$R_{ds} = (P_{pa} - P_{la})/Q_t$$

in which R_{ds} is the resistance downstream from the pulmonary artery, P_{pa} the mean pulmonary artery pressure, P_{la} the mean left atrial pressure, $(P_{pa} - P_{la})$ the pressure gradient for flow, and Q_t the blood flow through the pulmonary vascular bed. Units for resistance can be expressed as either millimeters of mercury per minute per liter or by multiplying by 80, converted to dynes per second per cm^5. Although the pressure gradient for flow through the systemic circulation is approximately 100 mm Hg (upstream minus downstream pressure), the gradient for the normal pulmonary circulation is only about 10 mm Hg. Because flow is similar in the pulmonary and systemic circulations, pulmonary vascular resistance is approximately 10% that of the systemic circulation.

A better understanding of pulmonary hemodynamics is derived by generating pulmonary vascular pressure-flow curves. In a rigid tube with an outflow pressure of zero, the resistance as defined by Ohm's law ($\Delta P/\Delta Q$) is constant and equal to the slope of a straight line through the origin. The normal pulmonary vasculature, however, does not behave like a rigid tube, and resistance is not constant over the physiologic range of pressure and flow. Because pulmonary vessels are distensible, their diameter and resistance vary with pressure, resulting in a curvilinear relationship between pressure and flow in the pulmonary circu-

lation (Roos et al, 1961). The pressure-flow curve is concave to the flow axis, with resistance defined as the instantaneous slope of this relationship. By contrast, pulmonary vascular resistance (PVR) is the slope of a line drawn from any particular point on the pressure flow relation to the origin, or ($P_{pa} - P_{la}/Q_t$). Changes in vascular tone result in shifts of the pressure-flow relationship. Changes in pulmonary vascular resistance, however, can result from alterations in tone or from movement along a nonlinear portion of the pressure-flow relationship (Fig. 3–2). Failure to understand this characteristic of the pulmonary circulation may lead to erroneous conclusions from a single measurement of PVR following a pharmacologic intervention. For example, were cardiac output (flow) to increase following administration of a vasoactive drug (owing to systemic vasodilation without an effect on the pulmonary vasculature), the calculated resistance could decrease without a shift in the pressure-flow relationship. The decrease in calculated resistance can be misinterpreted as pulmonary vasodilation, when in fact it is due to the distensibility of the pulmonary circulation. Indeed, if a pharmacologic intervention did cause pulmonary vasodilation and cardiac output increase, the pressure-flow could shift such that there would be no change in the calculated resistance (Mitzner and Huang, 1987; Mitzner and Wagner, 1989). By taking a number of measurements and plotting pulmonary vascular pressure-flow relationship, the true resistance can be derived, rather than calculating the potentially erroneous PVR.

Passive Regulation of Pulmonary Vascular Resistance

Recruitment and Distensibility in the Pulmonary Vascular Bed

There is considerable reserve in the pulmonary vascular bed. Not only is it a low-pressure high-flow system at rest, but it can accommodate increases in cardiac output of up to three to four times resting values (for example, during exercise) with only a small rise in the inflow pressure. This ability to tolerate increased flow with small changes in pressure occurs by the process of recruitment and distention. When P_{pa} (pulmonary artery pressure) is low, many of the pulmonary capillaries are collapsed without flow. Those that are open are relatively narrow and, therefore, their resistance is relatively high. As P_{pa} and flow increase, however, capillaries open that were previously closed (recruitment), and vessels that were open widen (distention) (Fig. 3–3). By decreasing

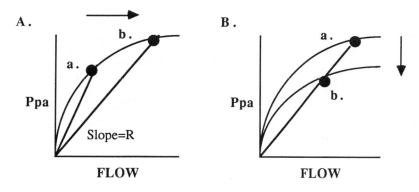

Figure 3-2
Pressure-volume curves depicting two different responses to pharmacologic intervention with a vasodilator. *(A)* Following administration of the vasodilator, the calculated resistance fell, as indicated by the decrease in the slope from point a to point b. The curve did not change, however, because the primary effect of the drug was to increase cardiac output rather than cause a direct response on the true pulmonary vascular resistance. *(B)* In this example the vasodilator caused direct pulmonary vascular vasodilation and shifted the pressure-volume curve downward. The calculated resistance (P_{pa}/flow), as indicated by the slope of the line through point a and point b, however, is unchanged despite the beneficial effect of the drug.

PVR as pressure increases, recruitment and distention of capillaries contribute to the curvilinear shape of the pressure-flow relationship (Glazier et al, 1969). It appears that recruitment is the main mechanism at lower pressure, whereas distention plays a greater role at higher pressure.

Effect of Lung Volume on Resistance

Because the pulmonary circulation has a relatively small amount of vascular smooth muscle, low intravascular pressure, and high distensibility, passive factors such as lung volume and respiration have a large effect on pulmonary resistance.

Resistance varies during respiration because changes in lung inflation affect the diameter of extra-alveolar vessels and alveolar vessels differently (Fig. 3-4). The extra-alveolar compartment comprises arteries, arterioles, veins, and venules, in which "extraluminal" pressure consists of pleural and/or interstitial pressure. During lung inflation, these vessels are pulled open by traction of the surrounding elastic lung parenchyma. During lung deflation, these vessels are squeezed and their diameter decreases (Gil, 1980; Lai-Fook, 1982).

In contrast, alveolar vessels are exposed to alveolar pressure. The diameter of these vessels varies indirectly with transpulmonary pressure (al-

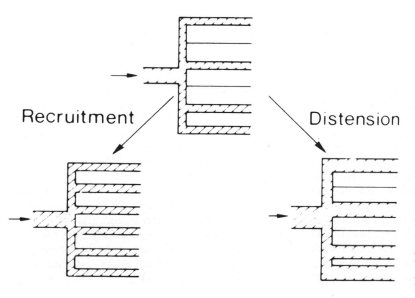

Figure 3-3
Two mechanisms that reduce pulmonary vascular resistance as pulmonary pressures are raised. Recruitment involves opening previously closed vessels, and distention is the expansion of vessels already open. (From West JB: Respiratory Physiology—The Essentials, 4th ed. Baltimore, Williams & Wilkins, 1990, p 37. With permission.)

Figure 3–4
Alveolar vessels are thin-walled and collapsible and are exposed to alveolar pressure. Extra-alveolar vessels are exposed to pleural pressure and are generally thicker walled and resist collapse. (Adapted from Hughes JM, Glazier JB, Maloney JE, et al: Effect of lung volume on the distribution of pulmonary blood flow in man. Respir Physiol 4:58–72, 1968. With kind permission from Elsevier Science–NL, Sara Burgerhartstraat 25, 1055 KV Amsterdam, The Netherlands.)

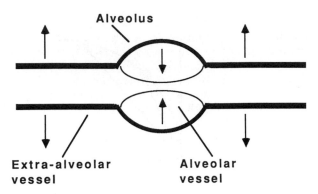

veolar pressure minus pleural pressure) and with lung volume. Factors that increase lung volume, such as positive end-expiratory pressure (PEEP) or air trapping during asthma, compress alveolar vessels and increase resistance. Alveolar corner vessels are functionally extra-alveolar and therefore do not respond to alveolar pressure, except at high lung volumes when they probably become incorporated into the alveolus (Benjamin et al, 1974; Howell et al, 1961).

Effect of Vessel Position on Blood Flow

Regional distribution of pulmonary perfusion is affected by the level of pulmonary artery pressure in relation to the total vertical dimensions of the lung (Dock, 1946; West et al, 1964). West described a three-zone model of pulmonary perfusion in which the relationship between pulmonary arterial pressure (P_{pa}), pulmonary venous pressure (P_{pv}), and alveolar pressure (P_{alv}) governs the regional distribution of blood flow in the lungs. Subsequently, a fourth zone was described to further refine the model (Hughes et al, 1968) (Fig. 3–5).

Zone I conditions are described at the lung apex where flow is obstructed because P_{alv} exceeds both P_{pa} and P_{pv}. This zone probably does not occur in the normal lung (except perhaps briefly in late diastole), but may occur when P_{pa} is decreased significantly, such as in severe hemorrhage or in septic shock, or when P_{alv} increases during the administration of PEEP or continuous positive airway pressure (CPAP), or during air trapping in the course of a severe asthma attack (Culver and Butler, 1980). Zone I conditions result in increased alveolar dead space (V_D) and therefore decreased effective gas exchange.

In zone II, P_{pa} is greater than both P_{alv} and P_{pv}, thereby permitting blood flow. Because P_{alv} remains higher than P_{pv} in zone II, however, changes in P_{pv} do not have an effect on flow or on upstream pressures. This relation between P_{alv}

and P_{pv} produces the characteristics of the so-called waterfall effect or Starling resistor. Zone II is limited to the upper third of the lung because left atrial pressure is normally well above alveolar pressure (Banister and Torrance, 1960; Permutt et al, 1962; Permutt and Riley, 1963).

In zone III, any influence of P_{alv} is removed because the pulmonary veins are below the right atrium and therefore P_{pv} is greater than P_{alv}. In zone III, changes in P_{pv} affect flow and have an effect on upstream pressures. During exercise pulmonary blood flow increases, and inflow (P_{pa}) and outflow (P_{pv}) pressures rise, thus converting

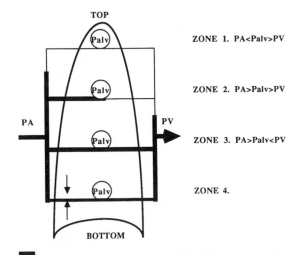

Figure 3–5
The four zones in the lung in which different hemodynamic conditions affect blood flow. The heights of the black lines represent pulmonary arterial (PA) and venous (PV) pressures. Alveolar pressure (P_{alv}) is assumed to be zero. (Adapted from Hughes JM, Glazier JB, Maloney JE, et al: Effect of lung volume on the distribution of pulmonary blood flow in man. Respir Physiol 4:58–72, 1968. With kind permission from Elsevier Science–NL, Sara Burgerhartstraat 25, 1055 KV Amsterdam, The Netherlands.)

all regions to zone III (Levett et al, 1979). Because arterial and venous pressures are increased equally, the driving pressure ($P_{pa} - P_{la}$) across each level of lung remains constant. Zone IV conditions are described at the lung base where the observed decrease in blood flow is postulated to result from increased interstitial pressure (Hughes et al, 1968).

Active Regulation of Pulmonary Vascular Resistance

Pulmonary vascular tone is regulated by a number of active mechanisms, including alveolar oxygen tension, autonomic innervation, circulating vasoactive mediators, and endothelial–smooth muscle interaction.

Effect of Hypoxia

Acute reduction in alveolar O_2 tension (P_aO_2) causes pulmonary vasoconstriction within minutes. On a local level, hypoxic pulmonary vasoconstriction diverts blood to better ventilated regions, thereby reducing shunt and maintaining efficient ventilation-to-perfusion matching. Increased hydrogen ion (H^+) concentration resulting from hypercarbia or metabolic acidosis also cause pulmonary vasoconstriction and augment hypoxic vasoconstriction (Bergofsky et al, 1962). The acute vasoconstrictor response to hypoxia is seen in isolated perfused lungs and in excised pulmonary arterial rings, suggesting local regulation rather than involvement of neural reflexes or systemically released mediators (Kovitz et al, 1996; Wiener et al, 1991). Globally, hypoxic pulmonary vasoconstriction is not beneficial and can lead to smooth muscle hypertrophy and fixed pulmonary vascular disease.

Alveolar hypoxia stimulates the precapillary arteries, which are the predominant site of the observed increased vascular resistance (Isawa et al, 1978; Jamieson, 1964; Marshall and Marshall, 1983; Staub, 1961). Pulmonary venous constriction has also been observed in isolated lung models. The mechanism of hypoxic pulmonary vasoconstriction remains elusive despite years of directed research. The search for a locally produced acute hypoxic mediator has not proved fruitful. Investigators have been led to explore intrinsic responses unique to pulmonary smooth muscle. Study results have demonstrated that some potassium channels in pulmonary vascular smooth muscle are inactivated or inhibited by hypoxia. Inhibition of potassium channels in response to hypoxia results in membrane depolarization, influx of calcium, and cell shortening (Post

et al, 1992). Further evidence that a potassium channel is responsible for hypoxic vasoconstriction derives from the demonstration of a hypoxia-sensing potassium channel in the carotid body. Hypoxic inactivation of these channels may be the mechanism of the acute vasoconstrictor response to hypoxia. It remains to be determined if the endothelium plays a role in augmenting, facilitating, or inhibiting the vascular smooth muscle response (Kovitz et al, 1996).

The mechanism for the elevated PVR and smooth muscle hypertrophy in chronic alveolar hypoxia is either different from or at least more complex than acute hypoxic vasoconstriction. The chronic changes may be explained in part by the peptide endothelin. Studies have demonstrated increases in endothelin gene expression and plasma endothelin levels in response to chronic hypoxia, and the administration of endothelin receptor antagonists attenuated the pulmonary vascular changes associated with chronic hypoxia (DiCarlo et al, 1995; Kourembanas et al, 1991). In addition to endothelin, vascular endothelial growth factor (VEGF) and heme oxygenase gene expression are induced by hypoxia (Kourembanas et al, 1996). These genes and their products may also be involved in the vascular changes induced by chronic hypoxia. Although the cellular sensor for chronic hypoxia is not known, it is interesting that a novel transcription factor, hypoxia inducible factor 1 (HIF-1), which regulates the increased hypoxic expression of endothelin, VEGF, and heme oxygenase, increases in the lung in response to hypoxia (Wang and Semenza, 1996; Wiener et al, 1996). It is unlikely that HIF-1 or any of its gene products mediate acute hypoxic vasoconstriction, but these factors may play an important role in the pulmonary vascular response to chronic hypoxia.

Autonomic Nervous System

The pulmonary circulation is richly innervated by the autonomic nervous system, which includes adrenergic, cholinergic, and nonadrenergic noncholinergic (NANC) systems (Barnes, 1984; Dowing and Lee, 1980). The direct role it plays in the control of the pulmonary circulation appears relatively minor, however (Widdicombe and Sterling, 1970). The indirect effects of the autonomic nervous system in improving cardiac output or increasing venous return are perhaps more significant. Autonomic innervation of the pulmonary vasculature is greatest in the proximal elastic arteries and decreases toward the periphery, suggesting that these nerves modulate pulmonary vascular compliance rather than resistance (Dowing and Lee, 1980). Numerous peptides have been identified in vascular nerve endings in the lung, including vasoactive intestinal peptide (VIP) and bombesin, but their role in regulation of pulmonary vascular tone remains unclear.

Circulating Factors

A number of circulating factors have effects on vasomotor tone in the pulmonary circulation (Bergofsky, 1980). Catecholamine-induced vasoconstriction is mediated via smooth muscle $alpha_1$ and $alpha_2$ receptors, whereas vasodilation is mediated by smooth muscle and endothelial $beta_1$ receptors and endothelial $alpha_2$ receptors. Both serotonin (5-HT), produced locally by circulating platelets, and histamine, stored in basophils or lung mast cells, mediate vasoconstriction in the pulmonary circulation. The lung is a significant site for metabolism of serotonin via the monoamine oxidase (MAO) pathway. Although no defined role has yet been discovered for serotonin in the lung, evidence of increased plasma and decreased platelet serotonin concentrations in patients with primary pulmonary hypertension (PPH), and the persistence of the finding following lung transplantation, are provocative. The same study demonstrated that levels of serotonin released during *in vitro* platelet aggregation were higher in patients than in controls (Herve et al, 1995). Serotonin uptake inhibitors, used as diet suppressant pills, have been associated with the development of primary pulmonary hypertension (Abenhaim et al, 1996; Pouwels et al, 1990; Prime, 1969; Thomas et al, 1995). These observations suggest that serotonin may be involved in the pathogenesis of at least a subset of cases of idiopathic pulmonary hypertension.

Angiotensin II is a potent pulmonary vascular constrictor. When administered to isolated or intact lung preparations it causes rapid-onset nonsustained vasoconstriction alone and potentiates the magnitude of hypoxic vasoconstriction (McMurtry, 1984). The decapeptide angiotensin I is converted to the active angiotensin II by angiotensin converting enzyme, which is located on pulmonary vascular endothelium. Angiotensin receptor antagonists attenuate the increase in pulmonary artery pressure in humans exposed to hypoxia and occasionally decrease pulmonary artery pressure in patients with primary pulmonary hypertension (Kiely et al, 1996). No evidence suggests that elevated levels of angiotensin II are involved in the pathogenesis of primary or hypoxic pulmonary hypertension.

A number of vasodilator peptides have been shown to be active in the pulmonary circulation,

including bradykinin, calcitonin gene-related peptide, and substance P, but their roles remain undefined.

Endothelium-derived Vasoactive Agents

Maintaining low pulmonary vascular tone involves complex interaction between endothelium and smooth muscle. Endothelial cells are capable of releasing various relaxing and constricting factors, in response to hormonal and physical stimuli, that act on vascular smooth muscle cells to modulate vasomotor tone (Furchgott et al, 1989). Under normal physiologic conditions endothelial cells release predominately relaxing or vasodilator mediators; however, under certain physiologic and pathophysiologic conditions the balance may shift toward release of constricting mediators (Fig. 3–6).

ENDOTHELIUM-DERIVED RELAXING FACTORS

The primary endothelium-derived relaxing factors (EDRFs) that are released by the pulmonary endothelium are nitric oxide (NO) and prostacyclin (PGI_2). NO is produced by the enzyme nitric oxide synthase by the conversion of arginine to citrulline. NO activates soluble guanylate cyclase in vascular smooth muscle to produce cyclic GMP–mediated relaxation (Dinerman et al, 1993; Ignarro, 1991).

In experimental preparations, inhibition of NO or NO synthase causes a small increase in pulmonary artery pressure or in vascular resistance. These results suggest that tonic release of NO by the pulmonary endothelium accounts for a small portion of the low pulmonary vascular tone. Inhibition of NO synthase also potentiates the vasomotor response to hypoxia, suggesting that NO modulates hypoxic vasoconstriction. In animals and humans, inhaled NO causes vasodilation in conditions of high pulmonary vascular tone such as chronic hypoxia or primary pulmonary hypertension. Inhaled NO has also been shown to reduce pulmonary artery pressure and reduce shunt in patients with adult respiratory distress syndrome (ARDS). This improvement may be due to increased perfusion of better ventilated lung regions because inhaled NO exerts a preferential effect in ventilated regions (Krafft et al, 1996; Mizutani and Layton, 1996).

It has been generally assumed that any NO released by the pulmonary endothelium that diffused to the intraluminal side of the endothelial cell was scavenged by circulating hemoglobin and had no effect on the systemic circulation. It was demonstrated recently, however, that NO produced in the lung is bound to circulating hemo-

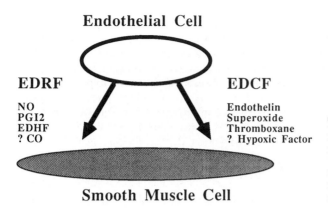

Endothelial Cell

EDRF

NO
PGI2
EDHF
? CO

EDCF

Endothelin
Superoxide
Thromboxane
? Hypoxic Factor

Smooth Muscle Cell

Figure 3–6
Endothelial smooth muscle interaction involves balance between endothelium-derived relaxing factor (EDRF) and contracting factor (EDCF). In normal circumstances, the balance is tipped in favor of relaxing factors.

globin at cysteine residues, rather than to the heme ring, permitting release in the systemic circulation (Jia et al, 1996). This discovery suggests that NO produced in the pulmonary circulation may modulate systemic as well as pulmonary vascular tone. The magnitude of this effect is not clear, however, because studies of inhaled NO do not demonstrate a significant systemic vasodilator effect (Cornfield and Abman, 1996; Lunn, 1995).

Prostacyclin (PGI_2) produced by the cyclooygenase enzyme in endothelial cells is a potent pulmonary vasodilator. Prostacyclin causes relaxation of smooth muscle by increasing cyclic AMP (Vanhoutte, 1993). There does not seem to be much tonic release of PGI_2 from the pulmonary endothelium during normal conditions because inhibition of cyclooxygenase does not cause an increase in vascular resistance. During conditions of high tone, however, such as during hypoxia, inhibition of cyclooxygenase potentiates vasoconstriction, suggesting that PGI_2 modulates these responses. Infusion of PGI_2 into the lung in ARDS causes diffuse vasodilation; it can worsen ventilation-perfusion ($\dot{V}/\dot{Q}$) matching because PGI_2 causes vasodilation in poorly ventilated regions (increasing shunt) as well as in well ventilated regions (Rossart et al, 1993). Inhaled prostacyclin holds promise in ARDS, however, by dilating well ventilated regions, which is similar to the response to inhaled NO (Rossart et al, 1993; Walmrath et al, 1996). A study in patients with primary and secondary pulmonary hypertension demonstrated an increase in the release of the vasoconstrictor thromboxane A_2 and reduced release of prostacyclin, suggesting that reduced endothelial production of PGI_2 may contribute to or promote progression of pulmonary hypertension (Christman et al, 1992).

Other potential endothelial-derived relaxing factors include endothelium-derived hyperpolarizing factor (EDHF) and carbon monoxide. EDHF appears to cause vasodilation by activating a sub-set of potassium channels in vascular smooth muscle and causing hyperpolarization (Nagao and Vanhoutte, 1993). The physiologic role of EDHF is not known. Evidence suggests a role for carbon monoxide in the distal porcine pulmonary circulation in mediating endothelium-dependent relaxation (Zakhary et al, 1996). Carbon monoxide is produced as a byproduct of heme degradation by the enzyme heme oxygenase and stimulates guanylyl cyclase producing cyclic GMP, which is similar to the action of NO. It is not known if endogenous carbon monoxide has a physiologic or pathophysiologic role in humans.

ENDOTHELIUM-DERIVED CONTRACTING FACTORS
The endothelium can also produce constricting factors (EDCFs), which include endothelin; superoxide anion; and the cyclooxygenase-dependent mediators, thromboxane and prostaglandin H_2 (Yanagisawa et al, 1988; Katusic and Vanhoutte, 1989). Endothelin-1 is a 21-amino acid peptide that is a potent constrictor of pulmonary vessels mediated by at least two receptor subtypes (Barnes, 1994). ET-A receptors are found on vascular smooth muscle and mediate constriction. ET-B receptors present on vascular smooth muscle and endothelial cells mediate contraction and release of EDRF-NO, respectively (Hay et al, 1993; Sumner et al, 1992). Thus, endothelin can cause vasoconstriction or vasodilation depending on the level of vascular tone. Hypoxia increases secretion of ET-1 from cultured human endothelial cells (Kourembanas et al, 1991). Administration of ET-A receptor antagonists to rats during chronic (2 weeks) hypoxia reduced right ventricular hypertrophy and pulmonary vascular resistance, suggesting a role for endothelin in mediating or modulating the effects of chronic hypoxia on pulmonary resistance (DiCarlo et al, 1995).

Superoxide anion produced by the endothelium mediates smooth muscle contraction directly. Although it was originally proposed that superoxide was generated by cyclooxygenase in endothelial cells, there are a number of mechanisms capable of producing reactive oxygen species, including nitric oxide synthetase (NOS), xanthine oxidase and NADH oxidoreductase (Katusic and Vanhoutte, 1989; Mohazzab et al, 1994; Pou et al, 1992; Terada et al, 1991). Superoxide can inactivate NO by reacting to form the toxic radical peroxynitrite, which also causes smooth muscle contraction (Squadrito and Prior, 1995). Despite theoretical concern for an increase of peroxynitrite production in response to inhaled NO, however, deleterious effects have not materialized. The cyclooxygenase products thromboxane and PGH_2 mediated smooth muscle contraction. Thromboxane levels are increased initially in venous thromboembolism and following pulmonary embolism, and this effect may explain in part the elevated pulmonary vascular resistance in patients with acute thromboembolism (Klotz et al, 1984; Reeves et al, 1983; Tod et al, 1986). Endoperoxide prostaglandin H_2 is an important intermediate in prostaglandin biosynthesis and can directly mediate platelet aggregation and vascular smooth muscle contraction *in vitro*. It can cause increases in pulmonary arterial pressure *in vivo* (Tod et al, 1986).

PATHOPHYSIOLOGY

DISORDERS OF INCREASED PVR OR PULMONARY HYPERTENSION

The pressure in a blood vessel is determined by the flow through the vessel, resistance downstream from the point of pressure measurement, and pressure at the downstream end of the vessel. For the pulmonary artery

$$P_{pa} = Q_t * R_{ds} + P_{la}$$

in which P_{pa} is mean pulmonary artery pressure, Q_t is cardiac output, R_{ds} is resistance downstream from the pulmonary artery, and P_{la} is mean left atrial pressure or back pressure. Each term in the equation is associated with pathophysiologic states that may result in an elevation of P_{pa}. Not all elevations of P_{pa} are associated with elevations of PVR. For example, in isolated left atrial hypertension due to mitral stenosis or acute left ventricular failure, P_{pa} may be elevated by the rise in back pressure, but the resistance to flow across the lung circuit may not be elevated. In this situation there will be a small gradient (<5 mm Hg) between pulmonary artery diastolic pressure and left atrial pressure. In contrast, pulmonary artery pressure may not be increased substantially despite an elevated PVR if cardiac output is extremely low.

The causes of pulmonary hypertension or increased PVR can be classified by anatomic location (precapillary vs. postcapillary) or by mechanism (active vs. passive). Another logical way to distinguish causes of pulmonary hypertension or elevated PVR is to associate pathophysiologic states with components of the equation that determines P_{pa}. Thus, causes can be grouped by whether they alter P_{la}, R_{ds}, or Q_t.

Elevated Left Atrial Pressure

Elevations of left ventricular end-diastolic pressure or left atrial pressure raise pulmonary artery diastolic pressure via an effect on back pressure. Left ventricular end-diastolic pressure may be elevated in left ventricular failure owing to acute myocardial infarction, aortic valvular disease, or cardiomyopathy. With a patent mitral valve, these elevated pressures are transmitted to the left atrium and may lead to pulmonary hypertension. Elevations of left atrial pressure due to mitral valve disease, left atrial myxoma, or left atrial thrombosis may also cause pulmonary hypertension (Borst et al, 1956; Wagenvoort and Wagenvoort, 1977). This type of pulmonary hypertension which is due to an increase in back pressure, may not result in elevated PVR if the lungs are normal and cardiac output is preserved. Therefore, the gradient between pulmonary artery diastolic pressure and left atrial pressure is normal.

Severe or prolonged elevation of left atrial pressure may cause pulmonary vascular remodeling, which adds to pulmonary hypertension by increasing resistance. In chronic mitral stenosis, there is remodeling of pulmonary veins and arteries. In pulmonary venules there is muscularization of the loosely organized smooth muscle layer (arterialization). Development of a muscular coat also occurs. In small pulmonary arteries there is predominately hypertrophy of the media without onion skin–like intimal hyperplasia or plexiform lesions. In these cases, there is an elevated gradient between pulmonary artery diastolic pressure and left atrial pressure, reflecting the increase in resistance (Wagenvoort and Wagenvoort, 1970, 1977).

Disease of the large pulmonary veins in close proximity to the left atrium can cause pulmonary hypertension in a similar fashion to left atrial hypertension. Sclerosing or fibrosing mediastinitis, which may result from infection with histoplasmosis or tuberculosis, can involve the pulmonary veins close to the left atrium and can create chronic pulmonary hypertension that behaves clinically like mitral stenosis. In these cases, the measured pulmonary capillary wedge pressure may be elevated despite a normal left atrial pressure because measurement of wedge pressure assumes minimal pressure gradient between pulmonary vein and left atrium (Dye et al, 1977). The gradient between pulmonary artery diastolic pressure and measured pulmonary capillary wedge pressure may be normal until there is vascular remodeling.

Elevated Resistance

Pulmonary Veins

Disease of the pulmonary veins can elevate PVR and cause pulmonary hypertension by increasing resistance. Pulmonary venular resistance is elevated in pulmonary veno-occlusive disease. This unusual form of pulmonary hypertension is characterized by intimal proliferation in venules and veins leading to occlusion. Often there is histologic suggestion of fresh or organizing thrombus and evidence of recanalization. There may also be arterialization or muscularization of small pulmonary veins. Patients with this disease are mostly young adults who present with insidious worsening dyspnea on exertion and shortness of breath. No sex prevalence exists. There are usually clinical and radiographic signs of pulmonary interstitial edema because of the elevation of pulmonary capillary pressure. Etiologic associations with viral infections, bleomycin therapies, and connective tissue diseases have been reported. Most patients with pulmonary veno-occlusive disease survive less than 3 years, and to date there is no proven effective therapy (Dail et al, 1978; Horsfield and Gordon, 1981; Wagenvoort and Wagenvoort, 1970).

PULMONARY PARENCHYMA

Vascular resistance in the lung may be increased by passive or active mechanisms. Resistance is elevated passively by processes that significantly reduce the functional cross-sectional area of the pulmonary capillaries or that increase lung volume above functional residual capacity (FRC). This reduction may be due to loss of capillary units, as in emphysema, to parenchymal lung disease that distorts or obstructs capillaries as in pulmonary fibrosis, or to the effect of an increase in transpulmonary pressure on cross-sectional area of alveolar vessels as in the administration of PEEP during mechanical ventilation. Actively, vascular resistance may be increased by alveolar hypoxia causing hypoxic pulmonary vasoconstriction or by circulating vasoactive mediators. These active forms of vasoconstriction may also be modulated by endothelial derived vasoactive factors, CO_2 tension, and pH (Bergofsky, 1979).

Because of the lung's capacity to recruit and distend vasculature, it takes destruction more than 60% of normal lung to increase PVR. Thus, resection of one normal lung should not increase PVR. When cardiac output is increased, however, as with exercise, patients with unilateral lung resections may show pulmonary hypertension. Similarly, in the presence of diffuse lung diseases, resection of less than 60% of lung volume may increase PVR.

Parenchymal lung diseases that cause destruction, distortion, or compression of blood vessels may elevate PVR and cause pulmonary hypertension. Interstitial lung diseases, such as idiopathic pulmonary fibrosis (IPF), progressive systemic sclerosis (PSS), and sarcoidosis, may elevate PVR by distorting or compressing arterioles or capillaries (Fig. 3–7). Obstructive lung diseases, such as emphysema, bronchiectasis, or cystic fibrosis, may elevate PVR by destroying alveolar units and capillaries. Because of the limited distensibility and recruitability of blood vessels in these interstitial and airway diseases, pulmonary hypertension may be present only when cardiac output is elevated, such as during exercise. With severe pulmonary parenchymal disease there may be hemodynamically significant pulmonary hypertension and cor pulmonale. Pulmonary hypertension is common in ARDS and is due to destruction of the capillary network. Early in ARDS, interstitial edema and thrombi are present, increasing resistance. Late in the proliferative and fibrotic stages of ARDS there

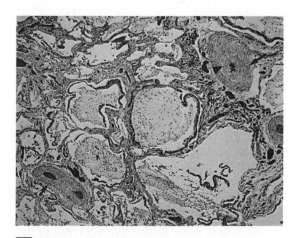

Figure 3–7
Pulmonary hypertension in fibrotic lung disease. There is gross distortion of the alveolar spaces with loss of cross-sectional vascular area. Pulmonary arteries show intimal fibrosis (*arrowhead*) and smooth muscle hyperplasia (*arrows*). (Courtesy of Frederic Askin, M.D.)

may be fibrous obliteration of arterioles and capillaries. (See Chapter 18 for more details.)

As discussed later, alveolar hypoxia superimposed on any parenchymal process exacerbates the elevation of PVR by active mechanisms. Generally, there is no effective treatment for the pulmonary hypertension associated with parenchymal lung disease other than treatment of the underlying condition when possible and administration of O_2 to correct alveolar hypoxia (Culver and Butler, 1980; Cutaia and Round, 1990; Edwards, 1957; Heath et al, 1968; Nocturnal Oxygen Therapy Trial Group, 1980; Smith et al, 1992; Tomashefski et al, 1983; Wright et al, 1992).

Alveolar hypoxia is an important cause of increased PVR or pulmonary hypertension. In systemic arteries and arterioles hypoxia causes vasodilation, presumably to maximize O_2 delivery during this systemic stress. In the pulmonary circulation, however, hypoxia causes vasoconstriction predominantly in small pulmonary arteries or arterioles. Hypoxic vasoconstriction has also been demonstrated in pulmonary veins *in vitro* (Fishman, 1976; Leach and Treacher, 1995; Zhao et al, 1993). Hypoxic pulmonary vasoconstriction is an important mechanism that improves $\dot{V}/\dot{Q}$ matching and decreases shunt during regional hypoxia by diverting blood flow away from poorly ventilated lung regions. This local vasoconstriction should not cause a significant elevation of pulmonary artery pressure because the remainder of the vasculature can recruit and distend. During global hypoxia, however, hypoxic pulmonary vasoconstriction can be deleterious if it causes diffuse vasoconstriction and increases pulmonary artery pressure. Regional hypoxia may also cause pulmonary hypertension in situations such as a reduction in the ability of the pulmonary vasculature to recruit or distend (e.g., interstitial lung disease, obstructive lung disease, or after lung resection). If there is concomitant chronic respiratory failure with these disorders, the elevated CO_2 tension potentiates hypoxic vasoconstriction and worsens pulmonary hypertension (Cutaia and Round, 1990; Fishman, 1976; Harvey et al, 1967; Horsfield and Gordon, 1981; Leach and Treacher, 1995; Marshall and Marshall, 1983; Nocturnal Oxygen Therapy Trial [NOTT] Group, 1981; Rudolph and Yuan, 1966).

For many years the mechanism of hypoxic pulmonary vasoconstriction was unknown. Diffusible vasoactive agents such as prostaglandins or leukotrienes do not mediate hypoxic vasoconstriction, although these agents can potentiate the response. Data suggest that the hypoxia may cause contraction of pulmonary vascular smooth muscle via inhibition of an oxygen-sensitive potassium

channel. Inhibition of this channel depolarizes the cell and leads to external calcium-dependent vasoconstriction. *In vitro* data also suggest that the endothelium may modulate hypoxic vasoconstriction, particularly in small or distal pulmonary arteries (Bergofsky, 1980; Cutaia and Round, 1990; Ganfornina and Lopez-Barneo, 1992; Post et al, 1992). The pulmonary hypertension induced by chronic alveolar hypoxia is likely to be reversible in its early stages if alveolar O_2 tension can be increased. In these cases, administration of supplemental O_2 decreases pulmonary artery pressure. After prolonged hypoxia and sustained pulmonary vasoconstriction, however, the pulmonary vasculature may remodel and develop fixed pulmonary artery hypertension that is not reversed with O_2. This remodeling has a characteristic pathology that is distinct from plexogenic arteriopathy. It is characterized by smooth muscle proliferation in arteries and veins. There is muscularization of pulmonary arterioles smaller than 80 μm and development of longitudinally arranged smooth muscle in the intima of small arteries (Abenhaim et al, 1996; Ashutosh et al, 1983; Leach and Treacher, 1995; Rudolph and Yuan, 1966; Wilkinson et al, 1988) (Fig. 3–8).

The most common cause of pulmonary hypertension that is related to alveolar hypoxia is chronic obstructive pulmonary disease (COPD). Although the pulmonary hypertension of COPD may be related to loss of capillaries, increased blood viscosity, and increased lung volume due to air trapping, much evidence exists to support the conclusion that pulmonary hypertension in COPD

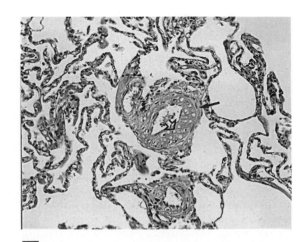

Figure 3–8
Pulmonary hypertension due to chronic hypoxia. There is attenuation of the original media (*closed arrow*) and longitudinal smooth muscle bundles in the intima (*open arrow*). (Courtesy of Frederic Askin, M.D.)

is related to alveolar hypoxia and hypercarbia from $\dot{V}/\dot{Q}$ mismatch. In patients with COPD, deterioration in O_2 and CO_2 tension was associated with increasing pulmonary hypertension. Oxygen therapy has been shown to prolongsurvival in patients with COPD and hypoxemia. Although not proven definitively, it is likely that at least some of this benefit is derived by an effect of O_2 on PVR, although other mechanisms such as increased tissue oxygenation and decreased blood viscosity may also contribute (Ashutosh et al, 1983; Medical Research Council [MRC], 1981; NOTT Group, 1981).

Sources of global hypoxia that may cause pulmonary hypertension include high altitude, central hypoventilation, and obesity hypoventilation syndrome. People living at altitudes higher than approximately 10,000 feet (about where alveolar O_2 tension generally falls below 60–70 mm Hg) may have pulmonary hypertension that is mild at rest but can become pronounced with exercise. Long-term exposure to altitude causes pulmonary vascular remodeling, which increases resistance. The hypertension and remodeling may resolve at lower altitude, but the process can take years. It is also possible that certain populations have adapted to altitude in a fashion that protects the pulmonary vasculature. Two studies of Himalayan residents demonstrated less pulmonary vascular remodeling than had been demonstrated in residents of the Andes.

High-altitude pulmonary edema (HAPE) (see Chapter 27) is an acute fulminant disease that typically occurs in young fit climbers who ascend quickly to more than 2500 meters. Early symptoms include decreased exercise tolerance, fatigue, weakness, cough, and acute mountain sickness. Once fully established there is cyanosis, hypoxemia, and pulmonary edema. HAPE is thought to have a vascular pathophysiology. Studies at altitude demonstrated that patients with HAPE had elevated pulmonary artery pressure and normal pulmonary artery wedge pressure. The condition responds to increasing alveolar O_2 tension with O_2 administration and descent. The calcium channel blocking vasodilator nifedipine, which can inhibit hypoxic pulmonary vasoconstriction, can provide therapeutic and prophylactic benefit (Barst et al, 1996; Bartsch et al, 1991; Schoene et al, 1988).

Patients with primary alveolar hypoventilation (Ondine's curse), secondary alveolar hypoventilation (neurologic disease or drugs), obesity hypoventilation syndrome, or obstructive sleep apnea may have pulmonary hypertension because of alveolar hypoxia. The associated respiratory acidosis potentiates any degree of hypoxic vaso-

constriction. In these cases, increasing ventilation and correcting hypoxia can reverse the pulmonary hypertension if treated early. Once vascular remodeling has been established, O_2 therapy may take years to reverse these changes, if at all (Goerre et al, 1995; Grover et al, 1996; Hackett et al, 1992; Wilkinson et al, 1988).

PULMONARY ARTERIES

Disorders that primarily affect the pulmonary arteries and arterioles may cause pulmonary hypertension or elevated PVR, resulting in obliteration or occlusion of vascular channels. Patients with these disorders often seek medical attention after the pulmonary hypertension is severe with signs of right heart failure. They usually complain of dyspnea on exertion and have little radiographic evidence of parenchymal lung disease (Leach and Treacher 1995; Weir et al, 1989).

Acute pulmonary thromboembolism (see Chapter 22 for more details) may cause pulmonary hypertension and right heart dysfunction. In these instances, the hypertension is predominantly due to pulmonary vascular occlusion resulting in the reduction of the cross-sectional area of the pulmonary arterial system (Fig. 3–9). There may also be a component of active pulmonary vasoconstriction due to release of vasoactive mediators (serotonin and thromboxane) from platelets adherent to the thromboembolus. The severity of pulmonary hypertension after thromboembolism is related to the size of the obstruction, degree of active vasoconstriction, and amount of preexisting vascular disease (Gurewich et al, 1968; Hyland et al, 1963; McIntyre and Sasahara, 1971; Thomas et al, 1966).

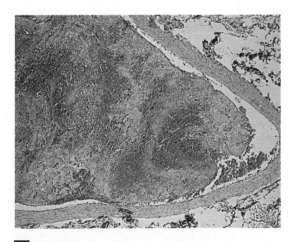

Figure 3–9
Pulmonary thromboembolus. A large thromboembolus is occluding a medium to large pulmonary artery. (Courtesy of Frederic Askin, M.D.)

If there is pulmonary hypertension after acute thromboembolism, the pulmonary hypertension should improve once the clot begins to dissolve via activation of the fibrinolytic system and organization. Serial imaging of the pulmonary vasculature has demonstrated substantial resolution of the perfusion defects over weeks after acute thromboembolism. Thrombolytics cause more rapid resolution of perfusion defects, hemodynamic abnormalities, and echocardiographic demonstration of right ventricular contraction abnormalities than heparin alone. These agents may be useful to reduce life-threatening pulmonary hypertension and right heart failure acutely. There is no difference, however, in the amount of improvement in perfusion defects at 1 to 2 weeks between patients treated with thrombolytics plus heparin and those with heparin alone. Most patients diagnosed with acute pulmonary thromboembolism and treated with anticoagulants do not develop persistent pulmonary hypertension (Dalen et al, 1969; Levine et al, 1990; Tow and Wagner, 1967).

Although the majority of patients with pulmonary thromboembolism do not develop pulmonary hypertension, some with recurrent thromboemboli that do not resolve adequately may develop pulmonary hypertension due to progressive occlusion of the vasculature. Moser and colleagues have described a syndrome of pulmonary hypertension caused by chronic thrombotic occlusion of proximal pulmonary arteries. These patients have symptoms and signs of pulmonary hypertension, including dyspnea on exertion and peripheral edema. Diagnostic evaluation reveals abnormal perfusion scans and angiographically or angioscopically demonstrated thrombi in the main and lobar pulmonary arteries. To date, no systematic defect in fibrinolysis has been identified in these patients. Chronic thromboembolic pulmonary hypotension is important to diagnose because surgical thrombectomy may be curative (D'Alonzo et al, 1984; Moser et al, 1987, 1990; Moser and Bloor, 1993; Rich et al, 1988).

In addition to thrombi, the pulmonary vasculature may be obstructed or occluded by air, fat, amniotic fluid, tumor, or foreign body emboli (Fig. 3–10). Central nervous system (CNS) symptoms predominate in air emboli owing to transpulmonary or transcardiac embolization to the brain. Fat emboli, which occur most frequently after trauma or long bone fracture, cause occlusion of small pulmonary arteries. Patients present with respiratory failure, CNS signs, and petechiae. These findings are thought to be due to the combination of vessel occlusion and inflammatory changes induced by free fatty acids. Amniotic fluid emboli do not occlude the vasculature, but

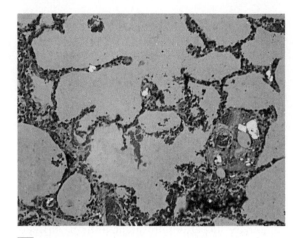

Figure 3–10
Pulmonary hypertension in an injection drug user. Multiple small vessel microemboli with microcrystalline cellulose (*bright white*) demonstrated by polarized light microscopy. (Courtesy of Frederic Askin, M.D.)

instead cause diffuse activation of the coagulation cascade with subsequent respiratory failure and cardiovascular collapse. Tumor emboli, which are most commonly a consequence of lung or breast carcinomas, may cause a presentation of pulmonary hypertension resulting from occlusion of vasculature. In most cases, there is histologic or radiographic evidence of coexisting lymphangitic spread of tumor (Coosling and Pelligrini, 1982; Morgan, 1979).

Inflammatory or collagen vascular diseases may cause pulmonary hypertension. Rheumatoid arthritis, polymyositis, or systemic lupus erythematosus (SLE) may be associated with pulmonary hypertension in the absence of severe parenchymal lung disease. In these cases, there is fibrinoid necrosis with chronic vasculitis, intimal fibrosis, vascular lumen and obliteration. Collagen vascular diseases may also cause pulmonary hypertension due to fibrosis of the vascular adventitia and intima, with medial thickening and no inflammation in muscular pulmonary arteries. This form of pulmonary hypertension is most common in the CREST variant of scleroderma, but may also be seen in SLE and in overlap syndromes (especially with scleroderma features) (Derderian et al, 1985; Hunninghake and Fauci, 1979; Kay and Banik, 1977; Lupi-Herrera and Sanchez-Torres, 1975; Simonson et al, 1989; Stupi et al, 1986). Granulomatous or necrotizing vasculitis of the media or intima may be seen, for example, in disseminated temporal arteritis or Takayasu's arteritis.

Primary pulmonary hypertension is a syndrome characterized by a vasculopathy in the absence of underlying pulmonary parenchymal or cardiac disease. This disorder occurs more frequently in women in their 20s to 40s who typically present to a physician with symptoms of dyspnea on exertion and fatigue that have been present for 1 to 2 years and pulmonary artery pressures that are elevated substantially at the time of diagnosis. A familial form of primary pulmonary hypertension has been described with autosomal dominant inheritance and features of genetic anticipation, in which the disease occurs at a younger age and with greater severity in subsequent generations (Lloyd et al, 1984; Rich et al, 1987; Thompson and McRae, 1970).

Although small pulmonary thromboemboli have been found histologically, the syndrome is thought to be a vasculopathy of muscular pulmonary arteries. Histologically, primary pulmonary hypertension can be graded using the Heath-Edwards Classification of plexogenic pulmonary arteriopathy. The progression from muscularization of arteries (Fig. 3–11) (grade 1), through deposition of collagen and elastin in the intima (grade 3), to development of plexiform lesions (Fig. 3–12) (grades 4–5), and finally to necrotizing arteritis (Fig. 3–13) (grade 6) all contribute to the increased vascular resistance typical of the syndrome (Heath and Edwards, 1958; Palevsky et al, 1989; and Wagenvoort and Wagenvoort, 1970, 1977).

The pathophysiology of primary pulmonary hypertension may be related to dysfunctional endothelium. It is speculated that a dysfunctional endothelium creates an initially reversible increase in vasomotor tone. Chronically, an irreversible state of elevated resistance results from vascular remodeling. In addition to chronic vasoconstriction, the increased presence of prothrom-

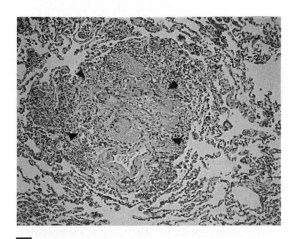

Figure 3–12
Pulmonary hypertension with plexiform lesion. The plexiform lesion (*arrowheads*) has obliterated the lumen of an artery. An intact artery is visible nearby (*open arrow*). (Courtesy of Frederic Askin, M.D.)

botic mediators or decreased presence of antithrombotic mediators promotes platelet aggregation and release of platelet-derived vasoactive mediators (e.g., serotonin), which further raises vascular resistance (Christman et al, 1992; Loscalzo, 1992; Rich et al, 1987). Studies using inhaled NO and prostacyclin as "selective" pulmonary vasodilators demonstrated reductions in pulmonary artery pressure, supporting the hypothesis that early on in the disease, patients with primary pulmonary hypertension have reversible vasoconstriction. Patients without a response to vasodilators may

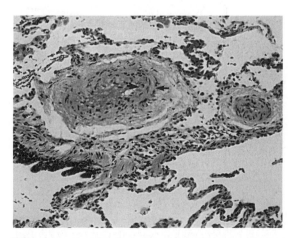

Figure 3–11
Smooth muscle hypertrophy in pulmonary hypertension. There is extensive smooth muscle hyperplasia (*between arrows*). (Courtesy of Frederic Askin, M.D.)

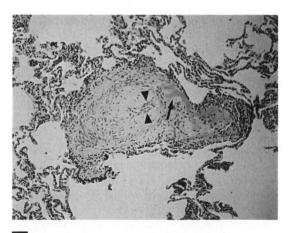

Figure 3–13
Pulmonary hypertension with fibrinoid necrosis. Necrotizing vasculitis (*arrow*) in artery with marked reduction in diameter of the original vessel lumen (*arrowheads*). There is also medial hypertrophy and intimal fibrosis. (Courtesy of Frederic Askin, M.D.)

have already developed irreversible vascular remodeling. Results of retrospective studies have also suggested that anticoagulation with coumadin improves survival in patients with primary pulmonary hypertension, suggesting that *in situ* thrombosis or thromboembolism was important in the pathogenesis of this disorder. These results further support the hypothesis that primary pulmonary hypertension develops in patients with an imbalance between the "good" and the "bad" products of endothelial metabolism (Barst et al, 1994; Palevsky et al, 1989; Pepke-Zaba et al, 1991; Rich et al, 1985).

Although most cases of primary pulmonary hypertension have no identifiable precipitating event, there have been epidemiologic associations with administration of anorexic agents, contaminated rapeseed oil, contaminated L-tryptophan, liver cirrhosis, and infection with human immunodeficiency virus (HIV). Only a minority of those exposed to these agents, however, develop pulmonary hypertension, suggesting that there must be a genetic or environmental predisposition in conjunction with the inciting agent (Abenhaim et al, 1996; Cacoub et al, 1995; Garcia-Dorado et al, 1983; Mette et al, 1992; Nall, 1991).

Increased Pulmonary Blood Flow

Pulmonary hypertension can also develop as a result of an increase in blood flow. As predicted by the equation that determines pulmonary artery pressure, a rise in cardiac output increases pulmonary artery pressure. In the normal lung, this increase is minimal because of the lung's ability to recruit and distend blood vessels. Pulmonary artery pressure rises slightly during exercise. This increase, however, is most notable either in the presence of reduced cross-sectional area of the lung (due to disease or resection) or elevated pulmonary vascular tone due to other factors, such as hypoxia at altitude or chronic lung disease. Increased flow through the lung in a chronic state causes a plexogenic pulmonary arteriopathy, which is histologically indistinguishable from primary pulmonary hypertension. The pathogenesis of this response is not known; it may be related to increased flow and/or to increased pressure. Clinically, this form of pulmonary hypertension is most commonly associated with congenital heart diseases that increase pulmonary blood flow, such as ventricular septal defects, patent ductus arteriosus, persistent truncus arteriosus, atrial septal defects, and anomalous pulmonary venous return. Congenital cardiac defects that do not increase flow do not cause this form of pulmonary hypertension. Correction of the shunt may stop progression or may cause reversal of the arteriopathy before it has reached an advanced stage. Chronically increased flow through small arterial-venous malformations may also explain the pulmonary hypertension of liver cirrhosis (Borst et al, 1956; Heath and Edwards, 1958; Ruttner et al, 1980; Wagenvoort and Wagenvoort, 1977).

CONSEQUENCES OF INCREASED PVR

Increased PVR results in a vicious cycle of secondary vascular remodeling and further elevation in pressure. The matching of pulmonary vascular structure to function leads to a progression of changes in the vessel wall when the wall is exposed to a chronic increase in pressure (Heath and Edwards, 1958). Initial changes, which are thought to be reversible, include medial thickening with smooth muscle hypertrophy. The hypertrophy, however, is followed by irreversible intimal fibrosis and progressive decline in the cross-sectional area of the pulmonary vascular bed. These histologic changes mirror the findings in patients in whom, early in the course of pulmonary hypertension, the elevated PVR responds to pharmacologic agents, but the proportion of patients not responding increases with progression of disease (Fig. 3–14).

Cor pulmonale is defined as the change in right ventricular structure or function due to pulmonary hypertension in which the etiology is disease of the lung or its vasculature. Primary disease of the left heart or congenital heart defects are therefore excluded. Acute cor pulmonale is relatively uncommon, occurring for example in

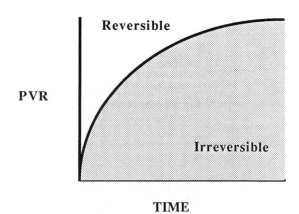

Figure 3–14
Schematic representation of the increase in pulmonary vascular resistance over time in pulmonary hypertension. With the progression of disease and vascular remodeling, the elevated pulmonary resistance becomes irreversible (*shaded area*) and less responsive to pharmacologic intervention.

Table 3–1
Electrocardiographic Criteria of Right Ventricular Hypertrophy

Adult Criterion	% Sensitivity True Positive	% Missed Diagnosis	% Specificity True Negative	% False Positive
QRS axis in frontal plane ≥110°	19	81	96	4
04 sec duration R wave in V_1 > 5 mm	2	98	99	1
R/S ratio in V_1 > 1	6	94	98	2
R/S ratio in V_6 < 1	16	84	93	7
S_1, S_2, S_3 pattern	24	76	87	13
In presence of right bundle branch block:				
a. Axis of early (unblocked) forces > +110°				
b. R' wave in V_1 > 15 mm				

Adapted from Weir KE and Reeves JT: Pulmonary Hypertension. Armonk, NY, Futura Publishing Company, p 11, 1984. With permission.

The above criteria can be applied only in the absence of left ventricular posterior hemiblock and "true" posterior infarction.

the setting of a massive pulmonary embolism. The process usually develops more slowly. Pulmonary artery pressure does not increase significantly until more than 50% of the pulmonary vascular tree is obstructed or obliterated. The right ventricle tolerates elevated pressure (P_{pa}) poorly and compensates by hypertrophy initially, followed by dilation and subsequent heart failure. This condition results in the clinical picture of secondary venous congestion, hepatomegaly, and edema. Edema also accumulates in response to hypoxia-induced renal dysfunction by enhancing salt reabsorption. The most common cause of chronic cor pulmonale is chronic obstructive airways disease due to chronic bronchitis or emphysema; the condition is associated with a poor prognosis (MRC, 1981; NOTT Group, 1981).

The causes of elevated pulmonary pressures in COPD are multiple, although hypoxia is the major factor, and therapy with O_2 improves prognosis. The improved survival is associated with a halt in the progression of pulmonary hypertension, rather than reduced vascular resistance. Other factors, such as the elevated red blood cell mass, are also improved with O_2 therapy and probably contribute to the improved outcome.

The clinical features of cor pulmonale include elevation in the jugular venous pressure, with prominent a waves initially, due to the effects of the hypertrophied atrium and increasingly less complaint ventricular wall. With progressive dilation of the ventricle, tricuspid regurgitation and prominent v waves may be seen. Palpation of the precordium may reveal a right ventricular heave. Auscultation is frequently difficult in patients with emphysema and hyperinflation, but it may reveal a loud P_2 often with abnormal or fixed splitting. Other audible sounds may include a right ventricular gallop, which is often best heard in the epigastrium. Murmurs described include a systolic pulmonic flow murmur, pansystolic murmur of tricuspid regurgitation, or diastolic murmur of pulmonic regurgitation. Hepatomegaly, which is frequently pulsatile from tricuspid regurgitation, and peripheral edema are common as right heart failure progresses.

Electrocardiography is relatively specific, but it is insensitive for diagnosis of right ventricular enlargement. A number of criteria have been developed and are outlined in Table 3–1.

EVALUATING THE PULMONARY VASCULAR BED

NONINVASIVE METHODS

Echocardiography provides a noninvasive method of evaluating right heart size and of estimating pulmonary artery pressure using Doppler technique. Its use is limited, however, by poor sound penetration in many elderly and obese patients or in those with emphysema.

Three types of studies may be performed using echocardiography. *M-mode echocardiography* provides temporal resolution in one dimension and may show changes suggestive of increased pulmonary vascular pressures, such as right ventricular wall thickening and delayed opening and early closure of the pulmonic valve. *Two-dimensional echocardiography* provides spatial resolution, allowing analysis of structural movement in real time, providing information on right ventricular wall thickness and septal wall motion abnormalities indicative of elevated pulmonary vascular pressures. Perhaps the most valuable technique, however, in the evaluation of the pulmonary vascular bed is *Doppler echocardiography,* which detects blood flow velocity and turbulence. When the transmitted sound wave encounters moving red blood cells, the frequency of its reflected signal is altered, allowing calculation of the blood velocity.

Because in the absence of right ventricular outflow tract obstruction, pulmonary artery and right ventricular systolic pressures are almost equal, the pulmonary artery systolic pressure can be estimated from measurements of right ventricular systolic pressure. The most frequently used method measures the flow velocity in a tricuspid regurgitant jet, which is common in patients with elevated pulmonary vascular pressures, to estimate the right ventricular to right atrial pressure gradient.

Pressure gradients can be calculated by using a modified Bernoulli equation. When blood flows through a stenotic segment blood velocity is accelerated. The Bernoulli equation relates the resultant decrease in pressure across the segment to the velocity of the blood flow

$$\Delta P = 4V^2$$

in which ΔP is the pressure gradient in millimeters of mercury Hg and V the velocity in meters per second. Once the transvalvular gradient (ΔP) is determined, using the estimated or measured right atrial pressure during systole, estimated right ventricular systolic pressure is possible. Combined Doppler and imaging techniques permit the calculation of cardiac output by estimating the stroke volume of the ventricle.

INVASIVE METHODS

Right heart catheterization remains the standard method for evaluating pulmonary vascular hemodynamics. Swan and Ganz introduced the balloon-tipped flow-directed pulmonary artery (PA) catheter in 1970 (Swan et al, 1970). Although questions have been asked about its effectiveness in routine clinical practice, the catheter can help to provide important information about pulmonary and cardiovascular hemodynamics (Matthay and Chatterjee, 1988).

The standard flow-directed catheter in current use has three lumens. The proximal lumen is located 30 cm from the tip and allows measurement of right atrial pressure. The distal lumen allows measurement of the pulmonary artery pressure. Inflation of the distal balloon via the third lumen permits wedging of the catheter in a peripheral artery and measurement of the downstream pressure. A thermistor located 4 cm from the tip of the catheter allows measurement of temperature for estimation of cardiac output with the thermodilution method. To minimize the influence of intrathoracic pressure, the pressure is measured at end expiration, which is the point in the respiratory cycle when pleural pressure is closest to zero.

The indications for placement of a PA catheter are varied, but include discrimination between the cardiac and noncardiac causes of acute pulmonary infiltrates, determination of the etiology of hypotension, titration of fluid therapy to avoid pulmonary edema, and evaluation of pharmacologic interventions in pulmonary hypertension.

Balloon inflation isolates the distal tip of the catheter from upstream pulmonary arterial pressure, thus creating a static, nonflowing column of blood distal to the balloon. Without flow there is no pressure drop along this column of fluid, and therefore the pressure at the catheter tip measures pressure in the pulmonary vein (pulmonary capillary wedge pressure [PCW]). Because there is normally minimal resistance in the pulmonary veins, it is assumed that the pressure measured approximates the pressure in the left atrium (P_{la}) (Hellems et al, 1949). Therefore, in the absence of mitral valve disease, P_{la} approximates left ventricular end diastolic pressure (LVEDP). Confirmation that the balloon is indeed wedged can be achieved by gas analysis of left ventricular end-diastolic pressure blood from the distal lumen, in which the values should approximate those of systemic arterial blood rather than mixed venous blood.

To obtain reliable values, proper technique is essential. The transducer must be zeroed and balanced correctly. If the transducer is below the zero position, intravascular pressures are overestimated, and they are underestimated if the transducer is above the zero position. Calibration is best accomplished periodically with a mercury manometer. Excessive damping due to too-long or too-compliant tubing or to air bubbles can lead to erroneous mean values. Data from a digital readout may be misleading, and a correctly calibrated analogue pressure tracing is essential.

It may be difficult to interpret pressure readings from patients on mechanical ventilation with applied PEEP, or from patients with severe airway obstruction who may have significant auto-PEEP. Positive end-expiratory pressure may convert zone III areas in the lung to zone I or II areas. Therefore, PCW no longer reflects P_{la}, because downstream pressure is then alveolar pressure. It is not recommended that PEEP be removed to measure the PCW, because doing so may alter oxygenation and produce hemodynamic changes. Usually less than half of the applied PEEP contributes to the measured PCW when lung compliance is reduced. In conditions in which lung compliance is increased, however, such as in emphysema, the effect of applied PEEP may be greater.

CONCLUSIONS

The pulmonary vascular bed provides a low-pressure conduit for blood flow to the left heart and for efficient exchange of gases. There are a number of passive and active mechanisms that regulate pulmonary blood flow. Only through advances in our understanding of the normal physiology can we make progress into our understanding and treatment of pulmonary vascular disease.

REFERENCES

Nocturnal Oxygen Therapy Trial Group: Continuous or nocturnal oxygen therapy in hypoxemic chronic obstructive lung disease: A clinical trial. Ann Intern Med 263:2347–2353, 1980.

Medical Research Council: Long term domiciliary oxygen therapy in chronic hypoxaemic cor pulmonale complicating chronic bronchitis and emphysema. Lancet 1:681–686, 1981.

Abenhaim L, Moride Y, Brenot F, et al: Appetite-suppressant drugs and the risk of primary pulmonary hypertension. International Primary Pulmonary Hypertension Study Group. N Engl J Med 335:609–616, 1996.

Amenta F, Cavallotti C, Ferrante F, et al: Cholinergic innervation of the human pulmonary circulation. Acta Anat 117:58–64, 1983.

Ashutosh K, Mead G, and Dunksy M: Early effects of oxygen administration and prognosis in chronic obstructive pulmonary disease and cor pulmonale. Am Rev Respir Dir 127:399–404, 1983.

Banister J and Torrance RW: The effects of the tracheal pressure upon flow: Pressure relations in the vascular bed of isolated lungs. Q J Exp Physiol 45:352–367, 1960.

Barnes PJ: The third nervous system in the lung: Physiology and clinical perspective. Thorax 39:561, 1984.

Barnes PJ: Endothelins and pulmonary disease. J Appl Physiol 77:1051, 1994.

Barst RJ, Rubin LJ, Long WA, et al: A comparison of continuous intravenous epoprostenal

(prostacyclin) with conventional therapy for primary pulmonary hypertension: The Primary Pulmonary Hypertension Study Group. N Engl J Med 334:296–302, 1996.

Barst, RJ, Rubin LJ, McGoon MD, et al: Survival in primary pulmonary hypertension with long-term continuous intravenous prostacyclin. Ann Intern Med 121:409–415, 1994.

Bartsch P, Maggiorini M, Ritter M, et al: Prevention of high-altitude pulmonary edema by nifedipine. N Engl J Med 325:1284–1289, 1991.

Benjamin JJ, Murtagh PS, Proctor DF, et al: Pulmonary vascular interdependence in excised dog lobes. J Appl Physiol 37:887–894, 1974.

Bergofsky EH: Pulmonary Vascular Disease: Active control of the normal pulmonary circulation. New York, Marcel Dekker, 1979.

Bergofsky EH: Humoral control of the pulmonary circulation. Annu Rev Physiol 42:221–223, 1980.

Bergofsky EH, Lehr DE, and Fishman AP: The effect of changes in hydrogen ion concentration on the pulmonary circulation. J Clin Invest 41:1492, 1962.

Bhattacharya J and Staub NC: Direct measurements of microvascular pressures in the isolated perfused dog lung. Science 210:327–328, 1980.

Borst HG, McGregor M, Whittenberger JL, et al: Influence of pulmonary arterial and left atrial pressures on pulmonary vascular resistance. Circ Res 4:393–399, 1956.

Braun K and Stern S: Functional significance of the pulmonary venous system. Am J Cardiol 20:56–65, 1967.

Brody JS, Stemmeler EJ, and DuBois AB: Longitudinal distribution of vascular resistance in the pulmonary arteries, capillaries, and veins. J Clin Invest 47:483–499, 1968.

Burch GE: Of pulmonary venous receptors. Am Heart J 99:814, 1980.

Cacoub P, Dorent R, Nataf P, et al: Pulmonary hypertension and dexfenfluramine. Eur J Clin Pharmacol 48:81–83, 1995.

Christman BW, McPherson CD, and Newman JH: An imbalance between the excretion of thromboxane and prostacyclin metabolites in pulmonary hypertension. N Engl J Med 327:70–75, 1992.

Coosling H and Pelligrini V: Fat embolism syndrome. Clin Orthop 165:68–92, 1982.

Cornfield DN and Abman SH: Inhalational nitric oxide in pulmonary parenchymal and vascular disease. J Lab Clin Med 127:530–539, 1996.

Culver BH and Butler J: Mechanical influences on the pulmonary circulation. Annu Rev Physiol 42:187–198, 1980.

Cutaia M and Round S: Hypoxic pulmonary vasoconstriction: Physiologic significance, mechanism, and clinical relevance. Chest 97:706–718, 1990.

D'Alonzo GE, Barst RJ, and Ayres SM: Survival in patients with primary pulmonary hypertension. Results from a national prospective registry. Ann Intern Med 115:343–349, 1991.

D'Alonzo GE, Bower JS, and Dantzker DR:

Differentiation of patients with primary thromboembolic pulmonary hypertension. Chest 85:457–461, 1984.

Dail DH, Liebow AA, Gmelich J, et al: A study of 43 cases of pulmonary veno-occlusive disease. Lab Invest 38:340–350, 1978.

Dalen JE, Banas JS, and Brooks HL: Resolution rate of acute pulmonary embolism in man. N Engl J Med 280:1194–1199, 1969.

Deffebach ME, Charan NB, Lakshminarayan S, and Butler J: The bronchial circulation. Small, but a vital attribute of the lung. Am Rev Respir Dis 135:463–481, 1987.

Derderian SS, Tellis CJ, Abbrecht PH, et al: Pulmonary involvement in mixed connective tissue disease. Chest 88:45–48, 1985.

DiCarlo VS, Chen SJ, Meng QC, et al: ETA-receptor antagonist prevents and reverses chronic hypoxia-induced pulmonary hypertension in rats. Am J Physiol 269:L690–L697, 1995.

Dinerman JL, Lowenstein CJ, and Snyder SH: Molecular mechanisms of nitric oxide regulation. Circ Res 72:217–222, 1993.

Dinh-Xuan AT: Endothelial modulation of pulmonary vascular tone. Eur Resp J 5:757–762, 1992.

Dock W: Apical localization of phthisis. Its significance in treatment by prolonged rest in bed. Am Rev Tuberc 53:297–305, 1946.

Dowing SE and Lee JC: Nervous control of the pulmonary circulation. Annu Rev Physiol 42:199–210, 1980.

Dye TE, Saab SB, Almond CH, et al: Sclerosing mediastinitis with occlusion of pulmonary veins. Manifestations and management. Thorac Cardiovasc Surg 74:137–141, 1977.

Edwards JE: Functional pathology of the pulmonary vascular tree in congenital cardiac disease. Circulation 15:164–196, 1957.

Fisher AW: The intrinsic innervation of the pulmonary vessels. Acta Anat 60:481–496, 1965.

Fishman AP: Hypoxia and the pulmonary circulation. Circ Res 38:221–231, 1976.

Frenette PS and Wagner DD: Adhesion molecules. Part II: Blood vessels and blood cells. N Engl J Med 335:43–45, 1996.

Furchgott RR and Vanhoutte PM: Endothelium-derived relaxing and contracting factors. FASEB J 3:2007–2018, 1989.

Ganfornina MD and Lopez-Barneo J: Gating of O_2-sensitive K+ channels of arterial chemoreceptor cells and kinetic modifications induced by low PO_2. J Gen Physiol 100:427–455, 1992.

Garcia-Dorado D, Miller DD, Garcia EJ, et al: An epidemic of pulmonary hypertension after toxic rapeseed oil ingestion in Spain. J Am Coll Cardiol 5:1216–1222, 1983.

Gehr P, Bachofen M, and Weibel ER: The normal human lung: Ultrastructure and morphometric estimation of diffusing capacity. Respir Physiol 32:121–140, 1978.

Gil J: Organization of microcirculation of the lung. Annu Rev Physiol 42:177–186, 1980.

Glazier JB, Hughes JMB, Maloney JE, et al: Measurements of capillary dimensions and blood volume in rapidly frozen lungs. J Appl Physiol 26:65–76, 1969.

Goerre S, Wenk M, Bartsch P, et al: Endothelin-1 in pulmonary hypertension associated with high-altitude exposure. Circulation 31:359–364, 1995.

Grover RF, Vogel JHK, Voight CK, et al: Reversal of high altitude pulmonary hypertension. Am J Cardiol 18:928–932, 1996.

Gurewich V, Cohen ML, and Thomas DP: Humoral factors in massive pulmonary embolism: An experimental study. Am Heart J 76:784–794, 1968.

Hackett PH, Roach RC, Hartig GS, et al: The effect of vasodilators on pulmonary hemodynamics in high altitude pulmonary edema: A comparison. Int J Sports Med 13:S68–S71, 1992.

Harvey RM, Enson Y, Betti R, et al: Further observations on the effect of hydrogen ion on the pulmonary circulation. Circulation 35:1019–1027, 1967.

Hay DWP, Luttman MA, Hubbard WC, et al: Endothelin receptor subtypes in human and guinea-pig pulmonary arteries. Br J Pharmacol 110:1175–1183, 1993.

Heath D, Gillund TD, Kay JM, et al: Pulmonary vascular disease in honeycomb lung. J Pathol Bacteriol 95:423–430, 1968.

Heath DI and Edwards JE: The pathology of hypertensive pulmonary vascular disease: A description of six grades of structural changes in the pulmonary arteries with special reference to congenital cardiac septal defect. Circulation 18:533–547, 1958.

Hellems HK, Haynes FW, and Dexter L: Pulmonary "capillary" pressure in man. J Appl Physiol 2:24–29, 1949.

Herve P, Launay JM, Scrobohaci ML, et al: Increased plasma serotonin in primary pulmonary hypertension. Am J Med 99:249–254, 1995.

Hislop A and Reid L: Pulmonary arterial development during childhood: Branching pattern and structure. Thorax 28:129, 1973.

Horsfield K and Gordon WL: Morphometry of pulmonary veins in man. Lung 159:211–218, 1981.

Howell JBL, Permutt S, Proctor DF, et al: Effect of inflation of the lung on different parts of pulmonary vascular bed. J Appl Physiol 16:71–76, 1961.

Hughes JMB, Glazier JB, Maloney JE, et al: Effect of lung volume on the distribution of pulmonary blood flow in man. Respir Physiol 4:58–72, 1968.

Hunninghake GW and Fauci AS: Pulmonary involvement in the collagen vascular diseases. Am Rev Respir Dis 119:471–503, 1979.

Hyland JW, Smith GT, McGuire LB, et al: Effect of selective embolization of various sized pulmonary arteries in the dog. Am J Physiol 204:619–625, 1963.

Hyman AL and Kadowitz PJ: Evidence for existence of postjunctional alpha 1- and alpha 2-

adrenoceptors in cat pulmonary vascular bed. Am J Physiol 249:H891–H898, 1985.

Ignarro LJ: Heme-dependent activation of guanylate cyclase by nitric oxide: A novel signal transduction mechanism. Blood Vessels 28:67–73, 1991.

Isawa T, Teshima T, Hirano T, et al: Regulation of regional perfusion distribution in the lungs: Effect of regional oxygen concentration. Am Rev Respir Dis 118:55, 1978.

Jamieson AG: Gaseous diffusion from alveoli into pulmonary arteries. J Appl Physiol 19:448–452, 1964.

Jia L, Bonaventura C, Bonaventura J, et al: S-nitrosohaemoglobin: A dynamic activity of blood involved in vascular control. Nature 380:221–226, 1996.

Johnson AR, Schulz WW, Noguiera LA, et al: Kinins and angiotensins. Angiotensin I converting enzyme (kininase II) in endothelial cells cultured from human pulmonary arteries and veins. Clin Exp Hypertens 2:659–674, 1980.

Katusic ZS and Vanhoutte PM: Superoxide anion is an endothelium-derived contracting factor. Am J Physiol 257:H33–H37, 1989.

Kay JM and Banik S: Unexplained pulmonary hypertension with pulmonary arteritis in rheumatoid disease. Br J Dis Chest 71:53–59, 1977.

Kiely DG, Cargill RI, and Lipworth BJ: Angiotensin II receptor blockade and effects on pulmonary hemodynamics and hypoxic pulmonary vasoconstriction in humans. Chest 110:698–703, 1996.

Klotz TA, Cohn LS, and Zipser RD: Urinary excretion of thromboxane B2 in patients with venous thromboembolic disease. Chest 85:329–335, 1984.

Kourembanas S, Marsden PA, McQuillan LP, et al: Hypoxia induces endothelin gene expression and secretion in cultured human endothelium. J Clin Invest 88(3):1054–1057, 1996.

Kovitz KL, Aleskowitch TD, Sylvester JT, et al: Endothelium-derived contracting and relaxing factors contribute to hypoxic responses of pulmonary arteries. Am J Physiol 256:H139–H148, 1996.

Krafft P, Fridrich P, Fitzgerald RD, et al: Effectiveness of nitric oxide inhalation in septic ARDS. Chest 109:486–493, 1996.

Lai-Fook SJ: Perivascular interstitial fluid pressure measured by miropipettes in isolated dog lung. J Appl Physiol 52:9–15, 1982.

Leach RM and Treacher DF: Physiological Society Symposium: Control of the pulmonary circulation: Clinical aspects of hypoxic pulmonary vasoconstriction. Exp Physiol 80:865–875, 1995.

Levett JM and Replogle RL: Thermodilution cardiac output: A critical analysis and review of the literature. J Surg Res 27:392–404, 1979.

Levine M, Hirsh J, Weitz J, et al: A randomized trial of a single bolus dosage regimen of recombinant tissue plasminogen activator in patients with acute pulmonary embolism. Chest 98:1473–1479, 1990.

Lloyd JE, Primm RK, and Newman JH: Familial primary pulmonary hypertension: Clinical patterns. Am Rev Respir Dis 129:194–197, 1984.

Loscalzo J: Endothelial dysfunction in pulmonary hypertension. N Engl J Med 327:117–119, 1992.

Lunn RJ: Inhaled nitric oxide therapy. Mayo Clin Proc 70:247–255, 1995.

Lupi-Herrera E, Sanchez-Torres G, and Horwitz S: Pulmonary artery involvement in Takayasu's arteritis. Chest 67:69–74, 1975.

McIntyre KM and Sasahara AA: The hemodynamic response to pulmonary embolism in patients without prior cardiopulmonary disease. Am J Cardiol 28:288–294, 1971.

McMurtry IF: Angiotensin is not required for hypoxic construction in salt solution–perfused rat lungs. J Appl Physiol 56:375–380, 1984.

Marshall C and Marshall B: Site and sensitivity for stimulation of hypoxic pulmonary vasoconstriction. J Appl Physiol 55:711, 1983.

Matthay MA and Chatterjee K: Bedside pulmonary artery catheterization: Risks versus benefits. Ann Intern Med 109:826–834, 1988.

Mette SA, Palevsky HI, Pietra GG, et al: Primary pulmonary hypertension in association with human immunodeficiency virus infection. Am Rev Respir Dis 145:1196–1200, 1992.

Mitzner W and Huang I: Interpretation of pressure-flow curve in the pulmonary vascular bed. In Will JA (ed): The Pulmonary Circulation in Health and Disease. Orlando, Academic Press, 1987, pp 215–230.

Mitzner W and Wagner E: Pulmonary and bronchial vascular resistance. In Scharf SM, Cassidy SS (eds): Heart-Lung Interactions in Health and Disease. New York, Marcel Dekker, 1989, pp 45–73.

Mizutani T and Layon AJ: Clinical applications of nitric oxide. Chest 110:506–524, 1996.

Mohazzab KM, Kaminski PM, and Wolin MS: NADH oxidoreductase is a major source of superoxide anion in bovine coronary artery endothelium. Am J Physiol 266:H2568–H2572, 1994.

Morgan M: Amniotic fluid embolism: A review. Anesthesiology 34:20–31, 1979.

Moser KM, Auger WR, and Fedullo PF: Chronic major vessel thromboembolic pulmonary hypertension. Circulation 81:1735–1743, 1990.

Moser KM and Bloor CM: Pulmonary vascular lesions occurring in patients with chronic major vessel thromboembolic pulmonary hypertension. Chest 103:685–692, 1993.

Moser KM, Daily PO, and Peterson K: Thromboendarterectomy for chronic, major vessel thromboembolic pulmonary hypertension: Immediate and long-term results in 42 patients. Ann Intern Med 107:560–565, 1987.

Nagao T and Vanhoutte PM: Endothelium-derived hyperpolarizing factor and endothelium-dependent relaxations. Am J Respir Cell Mol Biol 8:1–6, 1993.

Nall KC, Rubin LJ, and Lipskind S: Reversible pulmonary hypertension associated with anorexigen use. Am J Med 91:97–99, 1991.

Palevsky HI, Schloo BL, Pietra GG, et al: Primary pulmonary hypertension: Vascular structure, morphometry, and responsiveness to vasodilator agents. Circulation 80:1207–1221, 1989.

Pepke-Zaba J, Higgenbottam TW, Dinh-Xuan AT, et al: Inhaled nitric oxide as a cause of selective pulmonary vasodilatation in pulmonary hypertension. Lancet 338:1173–1174, 1991.

Permutt S, Bromberger-Barnea B, and Bane HN: Alveolar pressure, pulmonary venous pressure, and the vascular waterfall. Med Thorac 19:239–260, 1962.

Permutt S and Riley RL: Hemodynamics of collapsible vessels with tone: The vascular waterfall. J Appl Physiol 18:924–932, 1963.

Permutt S, Wise RA, and Sylvester JT: Interaction between the circulatory and ventilatory pumps. In Roussos C, and Macklem PT (eds): Thorax: Lung Biology in Health and Disease. New York, Marcel Dekker, 1985, pp 701–735.

Post JM, Hume JR, Archer SL, et al: Direct role of potassium channel inhibition in hypoxic pulmonary vasoconstriction. Am J Physiol 262:C882–C890, 1992.

Pou S, Pou WS, Bredt DS, et al: Generation of superoxide by purified brain nitric oxide synthase. J Biol Chem 267:24173–24176, 1992.

Pouwels HM, Smeets JL, Cheriex EC, et al: Pulmonary hypertension and fenfluramine. Eur Respir J 3:606–607, 1990.

Prime FJ: Dangers of certain appetite suppressants. Br Med J 3:177, 1969.

Reeves WC, Demers LM, Wood MA, et al: The release of thromboxane A2 and prostacyclin following experimental acute pulmonary embolism. Prostaglandins Leukot Med 11:1–10, 1983.

Rich S, Brundage BH, and Levy PS: The effect of vasodilator therapy on the clinical outcome of patients with primary pulmonary hypertension. Circulation 71:1191–1196, 1985.

Rich S, Dantzker DR, Ayres SM, et al: Primary pulmonary hypertension. Ann Intern Med 107:216–223, 1987.

Rich S, Kaufman E, and Levy PS: The effect of high doses of calcium-channel blockers on survival in primary pulmonary hypertension. N Engl J Med 327:76–81, 1992.

Rich S, Levitsky S, and Brundage BH: Pulmonary hypertension from chronic pulmonary thromboembolism. Ann Intern Med 108:425–434, 1988.

Rock P, Patterson GA, Permutt S, et al: Nature and distribution of vascular resistance in hypoxic pig lungs. J Appl Physiol Respir Environ Exercise Physiol 59:1891–1901, 1985.

Roos A, Thomas LJ Jr, Nagel EL, et al: Pulmonary vascular resistance as determined by lung inflation and vascular pressures. J Appl Physiol 16:77–84, 1961.

Rossart R, Falke KJ, Lopez F, et al: Inhaled NO for the ARDS. N Engl J Med 328:399–405, 1993.

Rubin LJ, Mendoza J, and Hood M: Treatment of primary pulmonary hypertension with continuous intravenous prostacyclin (epoprostenol). Ann Intern Med 112:485–491, 1990.

Rudolph AM and Yuan S: Response of the pulmonary vasculature to hypoxia and H^+ ion concentration changes. J Clin Invest 45:399–411, 1966.

Ruttner JR, Bartschi J-P, Niedermann R, et al: Plexogenic pulmonary arteriopathy and liver cirrhosis. Thorax 35:133–136, 1980.

Ryan US, Ryan JW, Whitaker C, et al: Localization of angiotensin-converting enzyme (kininase II). II. Immunocytochemistry and immunofluorescence. Tissue Cell 8:125, 1976.

Schellenberg RR and Foster A: Differential activity of leukotrienes upon human pulmonary vein and artery. Prostaglandins 27:475–482, 1984.

Schoene RB, Swenson ER, Pizzo CJ, et al: The lung at high altitude: Bronchoalveolar lavage in acute mountain sickness and pulmonary edema. J Appl Physiol 64:2605–2613, 1988.

Semmens M and Reid L: Pulmonary arterial muscularity and right ventricular hypertrophy in chronic bronchitis and emphysema. Br J Dis Chest 68:253–263, 1974.

Simonson JS, Schiller NB, Petri M, et al: Pulmonary hypertension in systemic lupus erythematosus. J Rheumatol 16:918–925, 1989.

Singhal S, Henderson R, Horsfield K, et al: Morphometry of the human pulmonary arterial tree. Circ Res 33:190–194, 1973.

Smith P, Rodgers B, Heath D, et al: The ultrastructure of pulmonary arteries and arterioles in emphysema. J Pathol 167:69–75, 1992.

Springer TA: Traffic signals on endothelium for lymphocyte recirculation and leukocyte emigration. Annu Rev Physiol 57:827–872, 1995.

Squadrito GL and Pryor WA: The formation of peroxynitrite in vivo from nitric oxide and superoxide. Chem Biol Interact 96:203–206, 1995.

Staub N: Gas exchange vessels in the cat lung. Fed Proc 20:107–109, 1961.

Stupi AM, Steen VD, Owens GR, et al: Pulmonary hypertension in the CREST Syndrome variant of systemic sclerosis. Arth Rheum 29:515–524, 1986.

Summer MJ, Cannon TR, Mundin JW, et al: Endothelin ETA and ETB receptors mediate vascular smooth muscle contraction. Br J Pharm 107:858–860, 1992.

Swan HJ, Ganz W, Forrester J, et al: Catheterizaion of the heart in man with use of a flow-directed balloon-tipped catheter. N Engl J Med 283:447–451, 1970.

Terada LS, Willingham IR, Rosandich ME, et al: Generation of superoxide anion by brain endothelial cell xanthine oxidase. J Cell Physiol 148:191–196, 1991.

Thomas DP, Gurewich V, and Ashford TP: Platelet adherence to thromboemboli in relation to the pathogenesis and treatment of pulmonary embolism. N Engl J Med 274:953–956, 1966.

Thompson P and McRae C: Familial pulmonary hypertension: Evidence of autosomal dominant inheritance. Br Heart J 32:758–760, 1970.

Thomas SH, Butt AY, Corris PA, et al: Appetite suppressants and primary pulmonary hypertension in the United Kingdom. Br Heart J 74:660–663, 1995.

Thurlbeck WM: Postnatal growth and development of the lung. Am Rev Respir Dis 111:803, 1975.

Tod ML, Cassin S, McNamara DB, et al: Effects of prostaglandin H2 on perinatal pulmonary circulation. Pediatr Res 20:565–569, 1986.

Tomashefski JF Jr, Davies P, Boggis L, et al: The pulmonary vascular lesions of the adult respiratory distress syndrome. Am J Pathol 112:112–126, 1983.

Tow DE and Wagner HN Jr: Recovery of pulmonary arterial blood flow in patients with pulmonary embolism. N Engl J Med 276:1053–1059, 1967.

Vanhoutte PM: Other endothelium-derived vasoactive factors. Circulation 87:V9–V17, 1993.

Wagenvoort CA and Wagenvoort N: Primary pulmonary hypertension: A pathologic study of the lung vessels in 156 clinically diagnosed cases. Circulation 42:1163–1184, 1970.

Wagenvoort CA and Wagenvoort N: Pathology of Pulmonary Hypertension. New York, John Wiley & Sons, 1977.

Walmrath D, Schneider T, Schermuly R, et al: Direct comparison of inhaled nitric oxide and aerosolized prostacyclin in acute respiratory distress syndrome. Am J Respir Crit Care Med 153:991–996, 1996.

Wang GL and Semenza GL: Oxygen sensing and response to hypoxia by mammalian cells. Redox Report 2:89–96, 1996.

Weibel ER: Morphometry of the Human Lung. New York, Academic Press, 1963.

Weibel ER: Morphological basis of alveolar-capillary gas exchange. Physiol Rev 53:419–495, 1973.

Weir EK, Rubin LJ, Ayres SM, et al: The acute administration of vasodilators in primary pulmonary hypertension. Am Rev Respir Dis 140:1623–1630, 1989.

West JB, Dollery CT, and Naimark A: Distribution of blood flow in isolated lung: Relation to vascular and alveolar pressures. J Appl Physiol 19:713–724, 1964.

Widdicombe JG and Sterling GM: The autonomic nervous system and breathing. Arch Intern Med 126:311–329, 1970.

Wiener CM, Dunn A, and Sylvester JT: ATP-dependent K^+ channels modulate vasoconstrictor responses to severe hypoxia in isolated ferret lungs. J Clin Invest 88:500–504, 1991.

Wiener CM, Booth G, Semenza GL: In vivo expression of mRNAs encoding HIF–1. Biochem Biophys Res Comm 225:485–488, 1996.

Wilkinson M, Langhorne CA, Heath D, et al: A pathophysiological study of 10 cases of hypoxic cor pulmonale. Q J Med 66:65–85, 1988.

Wright JL, Petty T, and Thurlbeck WM: Analysis of the structure of the muscular pulmonary arteries in patients with pulmonary hypertension and COPD: National Institutes of Health nocturnal oxygen therapy trial. Lung 170:109–124, 1992.

Yanagisawa M, Kurihara H, Kimura S, et al: A novel potent vasoconstrictor peptide produced by vascular endothelial cells. Nature 332:411–415, 1988.

Zakhary R, Gaine SP, Dinerman JL, et al: Heme oxygenase-2: Endothelial and neuronal localization and role in endothelium-derived relaxation. Proc Natl Acad Sci U S A 93:795–798, 1996.

Zhao Y, Packer CS, and Rhoades RA: Pulmonary vein contracts in response to hypoxia. Am J Physiol 265:L87–L92, 1993.

C H A P T E R

Mechanical Cardiopulmonary Interactions in Critical Care

Steven M Scharf, M.D., Ph.D.

The primary function of the cardiovascular system is to transport oxygen (O_2) and carbon dioxide (CO_2) between the lungs and peripheral tissues. As such, cardiac output needs to be tuned to the metabolic demands of the body. Furthermore, the linkage between the cardiovascular and pulmonary systems, important for the normal functioning of both systems, occurs on a number of different levels including humoral, neurologic, and mechanical. There are also numerous circulatory adjustments engendered by abnormal arterial blood gas tensions associated with respiratory failure. However, in this chapter, we concentrate on the mechanical circulatory-respiratory interactions important in critical care. The reader is referred to any of a number of excellent reviews for material related to the other aspects of cardio-circulatory interactions (De Burgh Daly, 1986; Hoffman and Cassidy, 1989; Heistad and Abboud, 1980). We review some of the basic principles governing the mechanical interactions of the cardiovascular and respiratory systems. In particular, we make use of circulatory models to understand the interaction between these systems.

In general, the circulatory effects of the normally functioning respiratory system are small. However, drastic changes in respiratory function can result in substantial changes in lung volume, pulmonary vascular resistance, and intrathoracic pressure. All of these can have profound effects on normal and abnormal circulatory function. This is true whether the patient is in respiratory distress and is generating large negative swings in intrathoracic pressure as in airway obstruction or if the patient is sedated and paralyzed and is being ventilated with positive-pressure ventilation. The physiologic changes caused by altered respiration can either hinder or enhance circulatory function. To begin, we review some of the aspects of the control of the circulation that are affected by respiration.

A MODEL FOR THE CONTROL OF CARDIAC OUTPUT

The reader is referred to the next chapter for a review of aspects of venous return from specific organ beds, especially the abdomen, and for changes in venous return with endotoxic shock. A model such as that shown in Figure 4–1 yields an analysis of the circulation similar to that used by Guyton and colleagues (1973) and has formed the basis for numerous analyses of the effects of abnormal respiration on the circulation (Sylvester et al, 1983; Nanas and Magder, 1992; Fessler et al, 1992; Tarasiuk and Scharf 1993; Scharf, 1992, to name but a few). This model consists of a number of elements that work together to regulate cardiac output. There is a reservoir, representing the lumped compliance of the circuit. Volume into the reservoir is divided into two compartments. That below the dotted line is referred to as *unstressed volume*. It is called that because it does not generate any pressure within the reservoir. In the model, the pressure at the inflow end of the veins, represented by P_s, does not begin to rise until the volume in the reservoir rises above the unstressed volume, V_0. The *stressed volume* is the difference between total volume, V, and stressed volume. In this model, venous return, VR, is equal to:

$$VR = \frac{P_s - P_{ra}}{R_v} \qquad [1]$$

where P_s is the mean circulatory pressure, P_{ra} is the pressure in the right atrium, and R_v is the resistance to venous return. The pressure gradient driving venous return is therefore $P_s - P_{ra}$. One can also express P_s in terms of the stressed volume in the reservoir and its compliance and rewrite equation 1 as:

$$VR = \frac{\frac{(V - V_0)}{C_s} - P_{ra}}{R_v} = \frac{(V - V_0) - C_s P_{ra}}{R_v C_s} \qquad [2]$$

where $V - V_0$ is the stressed volume of the reservoir and C_s is its compliance. The product $R_v C_s$ is called the *time constant* of the reservoir. It can be shown that if the reservoir drains a total amount of volume V, the time it takes to drain to 1/e of this volume is equal to the product $R_v C_s$. The shorter the time constant, the faster blood drains from the reservoir into the right atrium.

The venous circuit also contains a collapsible segment, shown in the figure as the portion of this circuit just below the label P_{pl}. This collapsible segment is acted upon by forces external to the segment. In this case, an intrathoracic collapsible segment is shown being acted upon by pleural pressure (P_{pl}). However, collapsible segments in the great veins also exist outside the chest and are acted upon by the appropriate external pressure, abdominal pressure for the inferior vena cava (IVC), and atmospheric (or subcutaneous) pressure for the superior vena cava (SVC).

Figure 4–2 shows venous return and cardiac function curves. In the circuit shown in the previous figure, and according to equations 1 and 2, P_{ra} is the back pressure to venous return. Thus, as P_{ra} increases, venous return decreases. Venous return becomes zero when P_{ra} is equal to P_s, which is the mean circulatory pressure. The downward slope of the VR curve is $-1/R_v$. The value for mean circulatory pressure is shown here as approximately 7 mm Hg, which is that found in anesthetized dogs undergoing right heart bypass (Guyton et al, 1973). Studies in closed-chest animals yield estimates somewhat greater (Nanas and Magder, 1992; Fessler et al, 1992; Tarasiuk and Scharf, 1993). Mean circulatory pressure has been measured in anesthetized humans (Beloucif et al, 1995) and is in the range of 10 to 12 mm Hg.

As P_{ra} decreases, venous return increases until

Figure 4–1
A good working model of the circulation. In this model, the periphery is depicted as a reservoir with both unstressed (V_0) and stressed volume ($V - V_0$). The reservoir drains through a resistance, called *the resistance to venous return*, and a collapsible section into the right heart. The heart is shown as a bilge pump that alternately fills and empties through a system of one-way valves. Blood volume in the heart and lungs is ignored. (See the text for development of the model.)

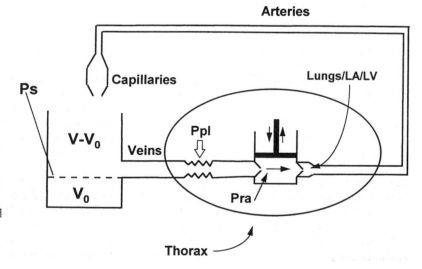

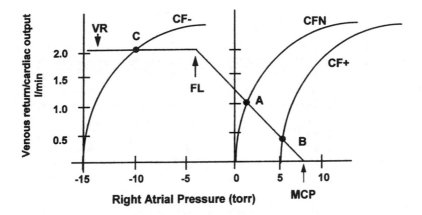

Figure 4–2

Graphic analysis of the circulation of a normal dog based on the model in Figure 4–1.
VR = venous return curve; CFN = cardiac function curve in the "normal" state; CF+ = cardiac
function curve when intrathoracic pressure is increased by 5 mm Hg; CF− = cardiac function
curve when intrathoracic pressure is decreased by 15 mm Hg; FL = point of flow limitation;
MCP = mean circulatory pressure.

a point when further decreases in P_{ra} fail to elicit increases in flow. This *flow limiting point* (FL) is related to the collapse of the great veins, which is approximately −4 mm Hg in the studies of Guyton and colleagues (1973). However, respiratory maneuvers that change the critical closing pressure around the great veins may also change the point of flow limitation.

The figure also shows cardiac function curves, depicted as classic Frank-Starling curves. Because in the steady state venous return and cardiac output must be equal, the system exists at the point where cardiac function and venous return curves intersect. For the normal situation, CFN is the normal cardiac function curve, and the system exists at point A.

Because the right atrium and its overlying pericardium are compliant structures, as a first approximation they transmit changes in intrathoracic pressure. In this model, an increase in intrathoracic pressure of 5 mm Hg displaces the cardiac function curve by +5 torr (CF+ in Figure 4–2). This results in a shift of the point of intersection to point B, at which P_{ra} is increased, but flow is decreased. Conversely, if intrathoracic pressure decreases, it is transmitted to the right atrium and cardiac structures. A decrease in intrathoracic pressure of 15 mm Hg is shown in Figure 4–2. This decrease results in a displacement of the cardiac function curve by −15 mm Hg (CF−) and a change in the point of intersection to point C, at which cardiac output is increased and P_{ra} is decreased. However, because of flow limitation (FL), the degree to which venous return and

hence cardiac output increase with decreases in intrathoracic pressure is limited.

We have shown the cardiac function curves in Figure 4–2 as if they were merely displaced by changes in intrathoracic pressure with no change in shape. This supposes that transmission of intrathoracic pressure to the cardiac surface is perfect, and that there is no change in the slope of the cardiac function curve with changes in intrathoracic pressure. Furthermore, it presupposes that the venous return curve remains unchanged with alterations in respiratory mechanics. The system is more complicated than this, and these points are considered later.

MULTIPLE VENOUS RESERVOIRS — A BETTER MODEL

Although the circuit shown in Figure 4–1 is useful for understanding many of the main principles governing the control of venous return and cardiac output from the periphery, it is an oversimplification and does not take into account the fact that there are multiple circuits in the vascular system that may be affected differently by respiratory maneuvers. Figure 4–3 shows a multiple-circuit model in which the vascular compartment is subdivided into nonsplanchnic, thoracic, and abdominal components, each with its reservoir consisting of stressed and unstressed volume (the latter is the greatest in the abdominal compartment). For simplicity we have ignored the legs. However, the reader may wish to consider the legs

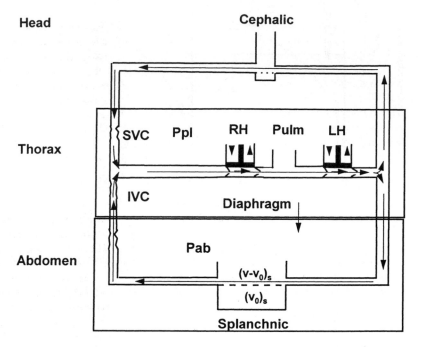

Figure 4-3
A better model of the circulatory system dividing the circulation into different beds. Three different compartments are shown here, the nonsplanchnic "cephalic" reservoir shown as exposed to atmospheric pressure (an oversimplification); a thoracic compartment; and an abdominal compartment, which is exposed to abdominal pressure (Pab). The thoracic compartment is shown with the right and left hearts (RH and LH, respectively) exposed to pleural pressure and the pulmonary blood volume reservoir (Pulm) exposed to alveolar pressure. The splanchnic compartment (including intestines, liver, and spleen), exposed to abdominal pressure, is the largest reservoir and has the largest unstressed volume compartment. A segment of the intra-abdominal IVC is shown as collapsible as well. (See the text for discussion.)

as belonging to the nonsplanchnic or "cephalic" compartment. The proportion of blood flow between the reservoirs is determined by the fractional arterial resistance to each compartment. Each reservoir has its own compliance. Total systemic vascular compliance is:

$$C = C_{ns} + C_s + C_p + C_{r+1} \qquad [3]$$

where C_{ns} is nonsplanchnic compliance, C_s is splanchnic compliance, C_p is pulmonary compliance, and C_{r+1} is the combined compliance of right and left heart. Mean systemic pressure is determined not only by stressed and unstressed volume but also by pressures in the relevant compartments.

$$P_s = \frac{V - V_0}{C} + P_{abd}\left(\frac{C_s}{C}\right) + P_{alv}\left(\frac{C_p}{C}\right) + P_{pl}\left(\frac{C_{r+1}}{C}\right) \qquad [4]$$

Changes in pressure in one compartment relative to another can shift volume from one to another.

For example, positive airway pressure increases both P_{alv} and P_{pl}. This acts to shift volume from intrathoracic (pulmonary and cardiac) reservoirs to extrapulmonary reservoirs. Because splanchnic compliance is far greater than nonsplanchnic compliance, most of this shifted volume is found in the splanchnic compartment. In the multiple-circuit model it can be shown that the resistance to venous return (the R_v component of equations 1 and 2) is equal to

$$R_v = F_s\left(\frac{C_s}{C}\right)R_{vs} + F_{ns}\left(\frac{C_{ns}}{C}\right)R_{vns} + \left(\frac{C_p}{C}\right)R_{vp} \qquad [5]$$

where F_s and F_{ns} are the fractional distribution of flow to splanchnic and nonsplanchnic compartments, and R_{vs}, R_{vns}, and R_p are the resistance to venous return from the individual splanchnic, nonsplanchnic, and pulmonary reservoirs, respectively (see Caldini et al, 1974). Because the time constant for drainage (T) is equal to RC, equation 5 becomes:

$$R_v = \frac{F_sT_s + F_{ns}T_{ns} + T_p}{C} \qquad [6]$$

Now, if the time constants of the splanchnic and nonsplanchnic compartments are different enough—in general the time constant of the splanchnic is longer than that of the nonsplanchnic compartment—a shift in blood flow between compartments owing to changes in the distribution of arterial resistance can affect the resistance to venous return and, hence, venous return according to equations 1 and 2. To put it simply, a shift in arterial flow toward venous drainage beds with short time constants (well-draining beds) increases venous return, and a shift in arterial flow toward venous drainage beds with long time constants decreases venous return.

To summarize, the multiple-compartment model means that changes in overall venous return can be caused by changes in overall stressed blood volume, relationships between pressures in the various compartments (affecting mean systemic pressure), and distribution of arterial blood flow between the compartments (affecting the resistance to venous return). All of these components can be affected by respiratory maneuvers.

TRANSMURAL PRESSURE AND MECHANICAL HEART-LUNG INTERACTIONS

Critically ill patients frequently require monitoring of intravascular pressure. Intravascular pressure especially is used for measuring the preload of any given cardiac chamber: P_{ra} or central venous pressure for the right ventricle (RV) and pulmonary artery occlusion or "wedge" pressure for the left ventricle (LV). If intravascular pressure is referenced to atmospheric pressure, as is usual for most critical care units and cardiac catheterization laboratories, changes in intrathoracic pressure that are transmitted to the heart are also measured. In normal subjects at rest, this approach leads to only small errors. But with respiratory distress, when intrathoracic pressure decreases substantially during inspiration, or with positive pressure ventilation with high levels of positive end-expiratory pressure (PEEP), this error can be large. The state of "filling" of a cardiac structure is best reflected by referencing the intracardiac pressure to the pressure on the cardiac surface. This *transmural* pressure reflects the stress across the wall of the chamber (Robotham and Scharf, 1983) during both systole and diastole.

Many studies of cardiac function during respiratory failure attempt to estimate transmural right and left ventricular filling (end-diastolic) and end-systolic pressures. Often esophageal pressure is used as the referent for intracardiac pressure. Although changes in body position and the weight of mediastinal contents on the esophagus can alter baseline esophageal pressure (Marini et al, 1982), it is assumed that changes in cardiac surface pressure with respiration are adequately represented by changes in esophageal pressure. Unfortunately, this assumption is not always valid.

Figure 4–4 shows a diagram of a cross section of the heart and lungs. The heart is located within the pericardial sac and this in turn is located within a space between the lungs called the *pericardial fossa*. As lung volume increases, there are mechanical interactions between the heart and lungs that are not adequately reflected by esophageal pressure. Thus, at large lung volumes, the heart is in effect mechanically compressed by the expanding lung (Wallis, et al, 1983; Cassidy and Ramanathan, 1984; Marini et al, 1981; Bell et al, 1987; Scharf et al, 1989; Smiseth et al, 1994). This effect increases cardiac fossa and cardiac surface (pericardial) pressure to a degree greater than that measured in the esophagus. Thus, with large increases in lung volume (above the normal tidal range), esophageal pressure *underestimates* the degree to which cardiac surface pressure increases. In fact, in patients with hyperinflated lungs due to emphysema, gas trapping in the lower lobes associated with exercise leads to a rise in pressure in the cardiac fossa. This in turn leads to increases in pulmonary artery occlusion (wedge) pressure with exercise, which is frequently observed in these patients (Butler et al, 1988). Thus, increased pulmonary artery occlusion pressure does not necessarily reflect increased "filling" (i.e., transmural) pressure of the LV but may reflect increased cardiac surface pressure associated with expanding lungs.

A second factor influencing cardiac surface pressure not reflected in esophageal pressure is related to the elasticity of the pericardium. Although the pericardium is normally thought of as a relaxed membrane transmitting all pressure changes, the pericardium normally limits cardiac expansion, even at physiologic cardiac volumes (Glantz et al, 1978). This finding suggests that external forces constrain cardiac filling over the physiologic range of cardiac volumes. This concept has been shown to apply to humans as well as experimental animals (Dauterman et al, 1995). In terms of its elasticity, pericardial volume is normally above the unstressed level. Thus, pericardial pressure is equal to the arithmetic sum of

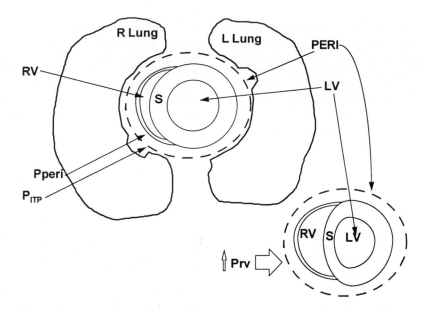

Figure 4–4
Diagram of the anatomic relationships between heart and lungs. The lung is peeled away from the pericardium to allow a potential space between lung and pericardium—the pericardial fossa. The pericardium is set back from the heart. Normally the surface of the heart, pericardium, and lungs are contiguous structures. RV = right ventricle; LV = left ventricle; S = septum; Pperi = pericardial (or cardiac surface) pressure; P_{ITP} = intrathoracic (or pericardial fossa) pressure; PERI = pericardium. The inset shows the effects of increased RV pressure (Prv) and RV dilation on the LV. Note flattening of the septum with decreased LV septal–free wall dimension.

two pressures, cardiac fossa (intrathoracic) pressure and transpericardial pressure:

$$P_{cs} = P_{itp} + P_{tp} \qquad [7]$$

where P_{cs} = cardiac surface (often called pericardial) pressure, P_{itp} = intrathoracic or cardiac fossa pressure, and P_{tp} = transpericardial or cardiac elastic recoil pressure. At low cardiac volumes, P_{tp} is small and the pericardial contribution to cardiac surface pressure is small. However, at elevated cardiac volumes, this component of cardiac surface pressure is large (Takata and Robotham, 1991).

Thus, the balance of the determinants of cardiac surface pressure changes as heart size increases from primarily cardiac fossa pressure to primarily pericardial elastic pressure. At large cardiac volumes, by not taking into account the transpericardial component of cardiac surface pressure, changes in esophageal pressure actually *overestimate* changes in cardiac surface pressure during large negative swings in intrathoracic pressure (Scharf et al, 1989). As the heart contracts, during ventricular ejection, regional pericardial pressure over the LV decreases (Scharf et al, 1989; Scharf et al, 1992). This change in pressure is not measured in the esophagus. Calculations of end-

systolic LV transmural pressure using esophageal pressure therefore do not reflect the true value of end-systolic wall stress.

From the earlier discussion it can be seen that estimates of changes in "preload" made from estimates of "filling pressure" can be difficult to interpret, which is true even if esophageal pressure is used as the referent for intracavitary pressure. However, a sophisticated knowledge of the relevant conditions allows the clinician to interpret the readings obtained in the light of the physiologic and clinical circumstances. If right atrial and ventricular compliance is high, and the pericardium relatively relaxed (Pinsky et al, 1992), swings in central venous (right atrial) pressure during respiration become a reasonable estimate for changes in intrathoracic (cardiac surface) pressure with respiratory maneuvers.

An alternative measurement, which has been suggested for use in patients ventilated with mechanical ventilation and PEEP, is the use of the "nadir" pulmonary arterial occlusion (wedge) pressure. To estimate the degree to which the inflated lungs lead to increased pulmonary arterial occlusion pressure during PEEP via mechanical interactions, one can briefly discontinue the PEEP. Pressure measured by the wedged pulmonary arterial catheter drops immediately by the amount that the PEEP increased cardiac surface pressure. After a few more seconds the pulmonary arterial occlusion pressure begins to increase again as venous return increases. However, the nadir value for the wedge pressure can be used to predict LV end-diastolic filling pressure; the difference between pulmonary arterial wedge pressure and the nadir pressure equals the amount by which cardiac surface pressure is influenced by the PEEP (Pinsky et al, 1991).

EFFECTS OF LUNG VOLUME

Many diseases relevant to the critical care setting are associated with increased lung volume. These include asthma, emphysema, and ventilation with high airway pressures. We have discussed the mechanical effects of increasing lung volume on cardiac filling and function. A number of investigators have noted a biphasic relationship between lung volume and pulmonary vascular resistance and capacitance (Howell et al, 1961; Permutt et al, 1961; Whittenberger et al, 1960). In the normal lung, as lung volume increases from residual volume to functional residual capacity (FRC), pulmonary vascular resistance decreases and vascular capacitance increases. Then as lung volume increases from FRC to total lung capacity, pulmonary vascular resistance increases and capacitance decreases. Thus, increases in lung volume above FRC lead to increased pulmonary vascular resistance and decreased capacitance. Thus, at constant pulmonary vascular pressures, this increased lung volume above FRC leads to decreased blood flow and pulmonary vascular volume.

The biphasic behavior of pulmonary vasculature with increasing lung volume is explained by postulating at least two kinds of pulmonary vessels. Microvasculature located within interalveolar septa are exposed to alveolar pressure and are constricted or shut off when lung volume increases. These vessels are called *intra-alveolar* vessels because they are physiologically influenced by alveolar pressure. Vessels located in the corners where alveoli join or within peribronchial spaces are exposed to expanding forces as lung volume increases. These are called *extra-alveolar* vessels; they tend to dilate or open with increases in lung volume. The overall effect on pulmonary vascular resistance is the arithmetic sum of the effects on these two types of vessels, which are in series. Thus, as lung volume increases from residual volume to FRC, effects on extra-alveolar vessels predominate and pulmonary vascular resistance decreases. As lung volume increases from FRC to total lung capacity, the effects on intra-alveolar vessels predominate and pulmonary vascular resistance increases. Lung volume–related increases in pulmonary vascular resistance are compounded by the presence of edematous fluid around pulmonary microvasculature, hypoxia, and acidosis-mediated vasoconstriction and thrombi/emboli within the pulmonary vasculature. All of these conditions are associated with respiratory failure in patients in the critical care unit.

RV afterload is partly related to RV wall stress, which in turn is a function of RV end-systolic pressure and volume (reviewed in Maughan, 1987). Clearly, the more lung volume is above FRC, the greater the afterload placed on the RV. This tendency is exaggerated the more that cardiac output is maintained at high lung volumes with fluids and pressors. The effects can be hemodynamically significant when lung volume is increased with high levels of positive end-expiratory pressure; venous return is preserved or increased; and concomitant pulmonary edema, vasoconstriction, LV failure, or thromboembolic disease is present. In patients with adult respiratory distress syndrome, this combination of events can lead to RV failure (Dhainaut et al, 1989). In contrast, with increased airway pressure, as venous return decreases, the hemodynamic effects on the RV are usually dominated by preload (venous return) rather than by afterload effects.

VENTRICULAR INTERACTION

The ventricles are connected in series through the pulmonary circulation. Diminution of the output from the RV leads to decreased preload and output from the LV. The *series interaction* is familiar to most readers. However, the ventricles also share common fiber bundles and septum and coexist within the same pericardial sac. These features are responsible for *parallel interactions* between the ventricles. If the diastolic volume of one ventricle increases, the diastolic compliance of the other decreases (Janicki et al, 1989). One of the more familiar interactions in critical care units is the effect of RV diastolic overload on the LV (see Fig. 4-4). This leads to increased RV end-diastolic volume. The interventricular septum flattens, and there is a decrease in the septum-LV free wall dimension, sometimes called *leftward septal shift*. With no change in LV end-diastolic volume, there is an increase in LV end-diastolic filling pressure. With no change in LV end-diastolic filling pressure, there is a decrease in LV end-diastolic volume (i.e., LV preload).

The degree of interdependence between the

chambers is influenced by a number of factors. Septal compliance is an important determinant of interdependence; the stiffer the septum, the less the interaction. The pericardium is an important amplifier of interdependence. Interdependence can be expressed as the *gain* between the ventricles. In 1987, Maughan and colleagues presented a relatively simple model to explain the interdependence between the ventricles. Although this model was specifically designed to explain systolic interactions, most of the features are pertinent for diastolic interactions as well. This simple model views the heart as a three-compartment structure with three relevant volume elastances belonging to the RV and LV free walls and the septum, respectively. At constant volume, when pressure is changed in one chamber, there is a concomitant change in pressure in the other. The cross-talk gain is defined as the ratio of the resultant change in pressure in the second chamber to the change in pressure in the primary chamber. For example, when volume is held constant in the LV, for a primary change in pressure in the RV, the cross-talk gain (G_{RL}) is:

$$G_{RL} = \frac{\Delta LVP}{\Delta RVP} \qquad [8]$$

[In terms of the elastances of the free walls and septum, right-left gain is expressed as:

$$G_{RL} = \frac{E_{LF}}{E_S + E_{LF}} \qquad [9]$$

[where E_{LF} = LV free wall elastance and E_S = septal (and common fiber) elastance. The effect of perturbations in one ventricle depend on the elastance of the free wall of the opposite ventricle. The stiffer the LV free wall (and the less stiff the septum), the greater the effect of perturbations of RV end-diastolic pressure and volume on the LV.

For respiratory maneuvers, the most important diastolic interactions are those resulting from increased RV volume and pressure. This interaction occurs during spontaneous inspiration when, according to the principles governing venous return, decreased intrathoracic pressure leads to increased venous return during inspiration. These effects are magnified with airways obstruction when the negative inspiratory swings in intrathoracic pressure are exaggerated (Scharf, 1991). As reviewed later, at least part of the inspiratory fall in stroke volume associated with airway obstruction (pulsus paradoxus) is likely to be due to decreased LV preload associated with interdependence effects. Interdependence effects also are seen when there is a large increase in RV afterload, as with pulmonary hypertension,

associated with the primary disease process or with large increases in lung volume (high levels of PEEP), especially when venous return is preserved (Jardin et al, 1981). These effects are exaggerated when RV dysfunction leads to increased RV dilation in response to elevated RV afterload with high levels of PEEP (Schulman et al, 1990).

EFFECTS OF INTRATHORACIC PRESSURE ON CARDIAC FUNCTION

The term *intrathoracic pressure* does not always signify a single pressure within the chest. One must specify which intrathoracic pressure one is dealing with—esophageal, pleural, pericardial fossa, or cardiac surface (pericardial) pressure. Because these pressures are subject to different mechanical forces, they may change differently with varying respiratory maneuvers. The difference between esophageal and cardiac surface pressure and the influence of the surrounding lungs and pericardium have been reviewed. However, it is helpful in some circumstances to continue to use the term in an unspecified way when discussing the general principle of the effects of respiratory maneuvers on cardiac function.

In 1853, the physiologist Donders recognized that just as decreasing intrathoracic pressure encouraged the influx of blood *into* the thorax from the periphery, the same phenomenon also hindered the egress of blood *from* the thorax to the periphery. This concept was once again brought to scientific consideration by the classic studies of Charlier (1967). In modern terminology, decreasing intrathoracic pressure—really cardiac surface pressure—acts to impede the ejection of blood from the LV, and increasing intrathoracic pressure acts to aid the ejection of blood from the LV. In other words, decreasing intrathoracic pressure acts as an increase in LV afterload and vice versa.

Figure 4–5 illustrates the principles involved. The left ventricle is shown as a one-way plunger-type pump that needs to overcome the pressure drop between left atrial and arterial pressure. Panel A illustrates the normal situation. In panel B, the level of arterial pressure has been increased relative to the level of the pump outflow and the left atrium. This is easily recognizable as analogous to increasing arterial pressure with a pressor. Obviously LV work has to increase. Panel C illustrates the effect of maintaining the relationship between LV outflow and arterial pressure constant but lowering left atrial pressure. This could occur if decreases in intrathoracic pressure are transmitted to the left atrium with relatively little change

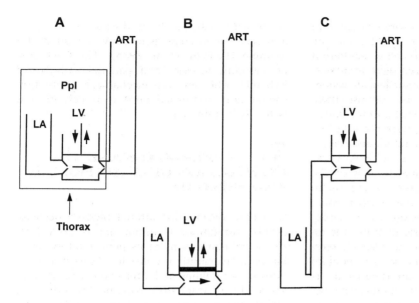

Figure 4–5
Illustration of the effects of decreased intrathoracic pressure on LV function. ART = arterial pressure level; LA = left atrial pressure level; LV = left ventricle; Ppl = pleural pressure. (See the text for explanation.)

in arterial pressure. In this case, the pressure gradient between arterial and left atrial pressure is increased and LV work is increased. From the point of the LV, the response would be the same as in panel B.

Returning to Panel A, the left atrium and LV are shown encased in the pleural space. If pleural pressure decreases here, the response of the LV is equivalent to that shown in Panel C. The LV "sees" this as an increase in LV afterload. If one measured LV end-systolic pressure relative to atmospheric pressure, it would not necessarily change much or might even decrease with a

decrease in pleural pressure. However, if LV transmural pressure were measured (LV relative to intrathoracic pressure), it would clearly be shown to increase. LV end-systolic transmural pressure is one measure of LV wall stress, which thus increases with decreases in intrathoracic pressure.

The effects of sustained decreases in intrathoracic pressure (Mueller maneuver) on the mechanics of venous return are shown in Figure 4–6. The normal venous return and cardiac function curves (VR and CF Normal, respectively) intersect at point A. If there were no effect on cardiac function, during a Mueller maneuver the cardiac

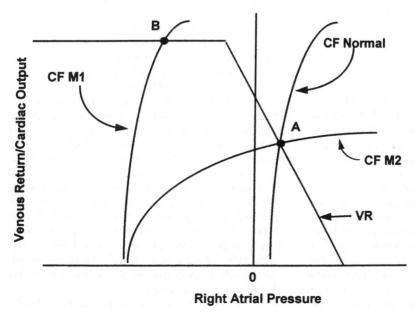

Figure 4–6
Illustration of the effects of sustained decreases in intrathoracic pressure (Mueller maneuver) on the venous return–cardiac function system. VR = venous return curve; CF Normal = normal cardiac function curve; CF M1 = cardiac function curve during the Mueller maneuver as if there were no change in cardiac function; CF M2 = a more realistic cardiac function curve during the Mueller maneuver, which acts to increase LV afterload. (See the text for explanation.)

function curve would shift in a parallel fashion to the left (CF M1). This shift would move the intersection of cardiac function and venous return curves to point B (i.e., decreased right atrial pressure and increased cardiac output [equals venous return in the steady state]). In contrast, there could be no change in right atrial pressure during the Mueller maneuver. If this were the case, the point of intersection of venous return and cardiac function curves would remain at point A. However, the cardiac function curve itself would be vastly altered to show the effects of the increase in afterload. In fact, right atrial transmural pressure would have increased unit for unit with the decrease in intrathoracic pressure. In truth, the effects of sustained decreases in intrathoracic pressure are usually not as dramatic so as to produce no change in ventricular pressure (relative to atmosphere), but are somewhat intermediate between the two cardiac function curves.

There is ample experimental verification of the effects of the Mueller maneuver on ventricular function and the demonstration that there are substantial increases in transmural filling pressures and/or end-systolic and end-diastolic ventricular volumes (Buda et al, 1979; Scharf et al, 1979c, 1981, 1987; Brinker et al, 1980; Magder et al, 1983). In fact, in patients with ischemic heart disease, regional LV wall akinesis may appear during the Mueller maneuver because of the degree of increased afterload (Scharf et al, 1981, 1987).

In general, when patients are removed from mechanical ventilators there is a small increase in cardiac output, which is probably related to greater metabolic demands and decreases in mean intrathoracic pressure. Beach and colleagues (1973) reported that cardiac output decreased in 18 of 37 patients with ischemic heart disease during weaning from mechanical ventilation. Other investigators have demonstrated evidence of subclinical congestive heart failure (Lemaire et al, 1988) and/or the onset of cardiac ischemia (Räsänen et al, 1984; Hurford et al, 1991) during weaning from mechanical ventilation in patients with ischemic heart disease. Although changes in autonomic tone and metabolic demands may well contribute to these changes, the decreases in mean intrathoracic pressure occurring on removal of positive-pressure ventilation may also be a major contributing factor. Decreased intrathoracic pressure allows for increased venous return and ventricular preload and increased LV afterload, both of which increase myocardial oxygen demand.

Because these effects may retard the weaning process, thought should be given to this factor when encountering difficulties in weaning patients with ischemic heart disease. Appropriate anti-ischemic therapy may allow for successful weaning (Lemaire et al, 1988). The same line of reasoning suggests that patients with active ischemia who are on mechanical ventilation should not be weaned until it is certain that ischemia is stabilized.

PULSUS PARADOXUS AND THE INTERACTION OF LV AFTERLOAD AND PRELOAD

LV stroke volume and arterial pressure decrease during inspiration. If inspiration is prolonged, stroke volume returns to its preinspiratory level. Furthermore, during the first few beats of expiration, stroke volume and arterial pressure increase above the preinspiratory baseline (Scharf et al, 1979a; Scharf, 1991; Scharf et al, 1992). The difference between maximum and minimum systolic arterial pressure is normally not more that 10 mm Hg. When the inspiratory-arterial pressure difference is greater than 10 mm Hg, the phenomenon is called *pulsus paradoxus*. The term was first coined by Kussmaul (1873). He observed that in patients with fibrosing mediastinitis and pericarditis, the peripheral pulse disappeared during inspiration, whereas heart sounds continued to be heard. This was the "paradox" giving rise to the name. Dornhorst (reviewed in Dornhorst, 1952) later described this in patients with severe airway obstruction. Pulsus paradoxus is a good indicator of the severity of airway obstruction (Knowles and Clark, 1973; Rebuck and Pengelly, 1973).

Many mechanisms have been proposed to explain pulsus paradoxus. These include pooling of blood in the lungs during inspiration, phase lag between RV and LV output, and reflex myocardial depression. However, the interaction between LV preload and afterload during inspiration appears to be largely responsible with some modulation by direct transmission of intrathoracic pressure to the arterial system. (For a thorough review of the topic see Scharf, 1991.) As intrathoracic pressure decreases, RV filling increases, which, via the mechanisms of diastolic interaction, leads to a decrease in LV preload. Numerous studies have demonstrated increased RV end-diastolic volume and decreased LV end-systolic volume during normal and obstructed inspiration in animals as well as in humans (Scharf, 1991; Scharf et al, 1979; Blaustein et al, 1986; Friedman et al, 1980; Jardin et al, 1982; Wayne et al, 1984). Thus, decreased LV preload plays a role in decreasing LV stroke output during inspiration.

This mechanism is illustrated in Figure 4–7,

Spontaneous Ventilation

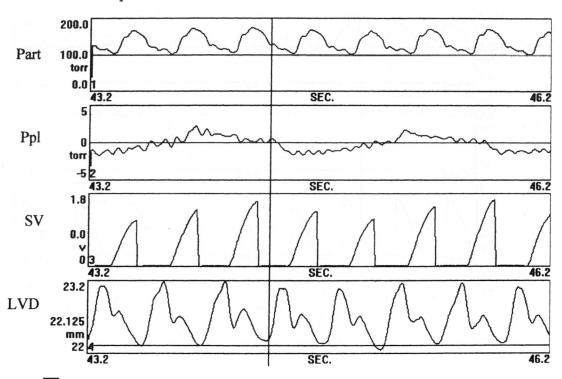

Figure 4–7
An illustration of the hemodynamic effects of normal inspiration in a sedated pig. Part = arterial pressure; Ppl = pleural pressure (esophageal balloon); SV = stroke volume (integrated aortic flow from the electromagnetic flow probe); LVD = anteroposterolateral LV dimension. Note that during inspiration there is a decrease on LV diastolic dimension corresponding to a decrease in LV stroke volume. The vertical line represents the start of an inspiration.

showing spontaneous respiration in a long-term instrumented, sedated pig. Note that during inspiration there is a decrease in LV stroke volume corresponding to decreased LV end-diastolic dimension. Furthermore, there is a decrease in end-systolic dimension during inspiration, indicating a decrease in LV afterload probably resulting from decreased aortic pressure during inspiration (hard to see in the figure owing to the compressed scale). Increased LV end-diastolic transmural pressure during inspiration, at the time when LV end-diastolic size is decreasing, is consistent with LV stiffening as expected from the effects of interventricular interdependence reviewed earlier (Scharf et al, 1979a; Scharf et al, 1992; Khilnani et al, 1992).

With increasing respiratory distress, inspiratory swings in intrathoracic pressure become more negative. This response would lead to greater effects on LV afterload. Figure 4–8 shows results in the same animal illustrated in Figure 4–7. How-

ever, this time the animal has been breathing against an obstructed airway for approximately 30 sec. Arterial Po_2 has been maintained by having the animal breathing 100% O_2. Note the large inspiratory decrease in pleural pressure. As stroke volume decreases during inspiration, LV end-systolic and end-diastolic dimension increases. Thus, as inspiratory efforts become greater, LV afterload effects become more important in the genesis of pulsus paradoxus.

The interaction between preload (interdependence) and afterload (intrathoracic pressure) effects during inspiration was illustrated by the work of Peters and colleagues (1988a, b), who timed decreases in intrathoracic pressure to ventricular systole and diastole. These investigators demonstrated decreases in LV preload when intrathoracic pressure dropped during LV diastole and increases in LV preload when intrathoracic pressure dropped during LV systole. Thus, there is an interaction between venous return–related de-

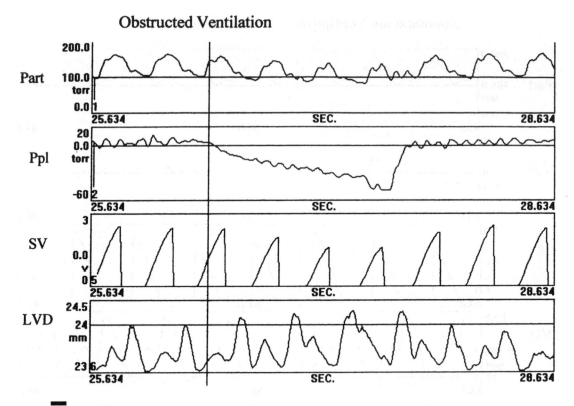

Figure 4–8
Results in the same animal illustrated in Figure 4–7. This time the animal has been breathing against an obstructed airway (obstructed apnea) for 30 sec. Arterial Po_2 is greater than 100 because the animal has been breathing from a 100% O_2 source.

creases in LV preload (via ventricular interdependence) and inspiratory increases in LV afterload, which produce the pulsus paradoxus observed in patients with airway obstructions.

EFFECTS OF PEEP ON VENOUS RETURN

For the final section of this chapter, we review some of the modern ideas concerning the effects of PEEP on venous return an cardiac output. A complete review of all the cardiovascular effects of PEEP is beyond the scope of this chapter, and the reader is referred elsewhere for aspects not covered here (Scharf, 1992; Chapter 5). Positive airway pressure has been used to oxygenate blood in patients with respiratory problems for at least 100 years. It has also been known from the late 1940s (Cournand et al, 1948) that cardiac output decreases as airway pressure decreases. Many studies have confirmed that increasing PEEP is associated with decreasing cardiac output (reviewed in Scharf, 1992). Contrary to some early reports

(Manny et al, 1979) that PEEP may be associated with humorally mediated ventricular depression, cardiac function has generally been observed to be normal with PEEP (Scharf et al, 1977, 1979b, 1992; Berglund et al, 1993, 1994). Thus, decreased cardiac output with PEEP appears to be due to a decrease in venous return. Administration of fluids or sympathomimetics is usually sufficient to overcome a decrease and restore cardiac output in clinical situations (see Hemmer, 1987).

At first approximation, the explanation for decreased venous return with PEEP is relatively simple. As lung volume increases with PEEP, intrathoracic pressure increases by an amount determined by chest wall compliance and the rise in lung volume. This effect is transmitted to the right atrium, which then decreases venous return. This situation is illustrated in Figure 4–2. As intrathoracic pressure increases, the point of intersection of venous return and cardiac function curve should "slide down" the venous return curve from point A to point B in Figure 4–2. In their initial studies, Scharf and colleagues (1977) plotted venous return as a function of right atrial pressure with increasing PEEP and concluded that the decreases in venous return seen with PEEP were far less than would be expected if all that was happening with PEEP was a slide down the venous return curve. They predicted that there must have been an increase in the mean circulatory pressure that buffered the decrease in output caused by rising airway pressure. One mechanism for increasing mean circulatory pressure is to transfer volume from intrathoracic to extrathoracic reservoirs (Fenn et al, 1947; Versprille et al, 1990). Applying enough PEEP to decrease cardiac output by 65% leads to the translocation of 7.2 ml/kg blood from central to peripheral compartments. Indeed, increased blood volume in splanchnic compartments has been observed during PEEP ventilation (Risoe et al, 1991; Manyari et al, 1993; Peters et al, 1993). To the extent that this transfer results in an increase in the upstream pressure for venous return, it buffers the decrease in cardiac output associated with PEEP.

Another mechanism for increased mean circulatory pressure is a sympathoadrenal response to decreased cardiac output. Scharf and Ingram (1977) and later Fessler and colleagues (1991) demonstrated that there was a sympathoadrenal response to PEEP. This response acts to increase mean circulatory pressure (Fessler et al, 1991; Nanas and Magder, 1992). However, both Fessler and colleagues (1991) and Nanas and Magder (1992) concluded that even though mean circula-

tory pressure increases with PEEP, there was no change in the gradient for venous return. There is, therefore, an increase in the resistance to venous return with PEEP. This increased resistance may be due to mechanical compression and narrowing of the great veins and/or to shunting of blood from well draining to poorly draining vascular beds.

Actually, the situation is even more complex. As demonstrated in preliminary studies on cardiopulmonary interactions (Robotham and Scharf, 1983; Sylvester et al, 1983) and in a study by Fessler and colleagues (1992), there is a shift rightward (increase) in mean circulatory pressure and in the point of flow limitation. The effects of PEEP on the venous return scheme developed in the earlier discussion are thus illustrated in Figure 4–9. Note that there is an increase in the point of flow limitation in the venous return curve (the inflection in the curve) with PEEP. This increase has the effect of limiting maximal venous return. As PEEP increases from 0 to 20, there is a progressive rightward shift in the cardiac function curves. The point of intersection between cardiac function and venous return curves shifts from A to B to C. Point D is a theoretical point of intersection between the original venous return curve and the cardiac function curve on PEEP 10, which would have been the situation had mean circulatory pressure not increased with PEEP. Thus, increased mean circulatory pressure buffered the effects of increased PEEP on cardiac output and venous

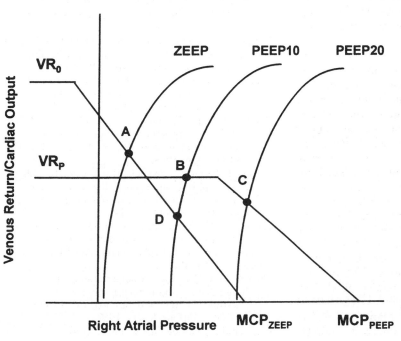

Figure 4–9
Effects of PEEP on the determinants of venous return. VR_0 = venous return curve with no end-expiratory pressure; VR_P = venous return curve with PEEP; ZEEP = cardiac function curve with zero end-expiratory pressure; PEEP 10 = cardiac function curve with PEEP 10; PEEP20 = cardiac function curve with PEEP 20; MCP_{ZEEP} = mean circulatory pressure with zero end-expiratory pressure; MCP_{PEEP} = mean circulatory pressure with PEEP. (See the text for discussion.)

return. The figure also shows a decrease in the downward slope of the venous return curve with PEEP. This finding corresponds to the findings of Fessler and colleagues (1992) and suggests an increase in the resistance to venous return as well.

What causes the point of flow limitation to increase with PEEP? In their follow-up study, Fessler and colleagues (1993) demonstrated sudden pressure increases in the inferior vena cava of dogs as a catheter was moved from the abdomen to the right atrium when the animals were in the supine position. This finding suggested the presence of a vascular waterfall in the inferior vena cava associated with mechanical compression of the lower lobes of the right lung on the inferior vena cava. This vascular waterfall causes flow limitation in this vessel, which carries approximately three times the flow as the superior vena cava. Flow limitation was not observed in the superior vena cava.

Direct mechanical effects of PEEP on the inferior vena cava may explain some of the differential effects of single-lung PEEP. Studies have shown that cardiac output (venous return) is decreased the most by bilaterally applied PEEP compared with PEEP applied to a single lung. However, PEEP applied to the right lung alone limits cardiac output substantially more than PEEP applied to the left lung alone (Veddeng et al, 1992). This effect may be explained on the basis of direct mechanical compression by the inflating lung on the right ventricle and right atrium with greater increases in right atrial pressure and hence greater decreases in venous return. However, these findings may be equally well explained by the advent of a critical closure pressure on the intrathoracic portion of the inferior vena cava.

Thus, the effects of PEEP on venous return are the result of a complicated interaction between increases in intrathoracic pressure, mechanical compression of the inflating lungs on the heart, mechanical compression of the inflating right lung on the inferior vena cava, and effects on right ventricular function (see earlier). The effects are modified by factors, primarily sympathoadrenal, that buffer the effects of increasing airway pressure on venous return. Although this discussion specifically applies to PEEP, the same principles also apply to newer modes of positive-pressure ventilation, such as inverse ratio ventilation either pressure- or volume-controlled. Because of the extended inspiratory time, inverse ratio ventilation may have greater detrimental effects on venous return than standard mode ventilation with increased airway pressure (Ludwigs et al, 1994; Mancebo et al, 1994; Mang et al, 1995).

In this chapter we have discussed a number of mechanical factors that interact in critically ill patients to produce resultant cardiovascular changes and that may limit peripheral O_2 delivery. The clinician should be familiar with these factors as he or she begins to determine the causes of changes noted in a patient's cardiocirculatory function.

REFERENCES

Beach T, Millen E, and Genvik A: Hemodynamic response to discontinuance of mechanical ventilation. Crit Care Med 1:85–92, 1973.

Bell RC, Robotham JL, Badke RR, et al: Left ventricular geometry during intermittent positive pressure ventilation in dogs. J Crit Care 2:230–244, 1987.

Beloucif S, Bizot J, Leenhardt A, and Paten D: PEEP increases mean systemic pressure in humans (abstr). Am J Resp Crit Care Med 151: A708, 1995.

Berglund JE, Haldén E, Jakobson S, and Svensson J: PEEP ventilation does not cause humorally mediated cardiac output depression in pigs. Intensive Care Med 20:360–364, 1994.

Berglund JE, Haldén E, and Jakobson S: The effect of PEEP-ventilation on cardiac function in closed chest pigs. Ups J Med Sci 99:167–178, 1994.

Blaustein A, Risser RA, Weiss JW, et al: Mechanisms of pulsus paradoxus during resistive respiratory loading and asthma. J Am Coll Cardiol 8:529–536, 1986.

Braunwald E, Binion J, Morgan W, et al: Alterations in central blood volume and cardiac output induced by positive pressure breathing and counteracted by metaraminal (Aramine). Circ Res 5:670–675, 1957.

Brinker JA, Weiss JL, Lappe DL, et al: Leftward septal displacement during right ventricular loading in man. Circulation 61:626–633, 1980.

Buda AJ, Pinsky MR, Ingels NB, et al: Effect of intrathoracic pressure on left ventricular performance. N Engl J Med 301:453–459, 1979.

Butler J, Schrijen F, Henriquez A, et al: Cause of the raised wedge pressure on exercise in chronic obstructive pulmonary disease. Am Rev Resp Dis 138:350–354, 1988.

Caldini P, Permutt S, Wadell JP, and Riley RL: Effect of epinephrine on pressure, flow and volume relationships in the systemic circulation of dogs. Circ Res 34:606–623, 1974.

Cassidy SS and Ramanathan M: Dimensional analysis of the left ventricle during PEEP: Relative septal and lateral wall displacements. Am J Physiol 246:H792–H805, 1984.

Charlier AA: Beat to beat hemodynamic effects of lung inflation and normal respiration in anesthetized and conscious dogs (monograph). Brussels, Editions Arscia, 1967.

Cournand A, Motley HL, Werko L, et al:

Physiological studies of the effects of intermittent positive pressure breathing on cardiac output in man. Am J Physiol 152:162–174, 1948.

Dauterman K, Pak PH, Maughan WL, et al: Contribution of external forces to left ventricular diastolic pressure: Implications for the clinical use of the Starling Law. Ann Intern Med 122:737–742, 1995.

De Burgh Daly M: Interactions between respiration and circulation. In Cherniack N and Fishman AP (eds): Handbook of Physiology, vol 2, pt 2. Baltimore, MD, Williams & Wilkins, 1986, pp 529–594.

Dhainaut JF, Aouate P, and Brunet FP. Circulatory effects of positive end-expiratory pressure in patients with acute lung injury. In Scharf SM and Cassidy SS (eds): Heart-Lung Interactions in Health and Disease. New York, Marcel Dekker, 1989, pp 809–838.

Donders FC: Contribution to the mechanism of respiration and circulation in health and disease. In West JB (ed): Translations in respiratory physiology. Stroudsburg, PA, Dowden, Hutchinson and Ross, 1853, pp 529–594.

Dornhorst AC, Howard P, and Lethar GL: Pulsus paradoxus. Lancet 1:746–748, 1952.

Fenn W, Otis A, Rahn H, et al: Displacement of blood from the lungs by pressure breathing. Am J Physiol 151:258–269, 1947.

Fessler HE, Brower RG, Shapiro EP, and Permutt S: Effects of positive end-expiratory pressure and body position on pressure in the thoracic great veins. Am Rev Resp Dis 148:1657–1664, 1993.

Fessler HE, Brower RG, Wise RA, et al: Effects of positive end-expiratory pressure on the gradient for venous return. Am Rev Resp Dis 143:19–24, 1991.

Fessler HE, Brower RG, Wise RA, and Permutt S: Effects of positive end-expiratory pressure on the canine venous return curve. Am Rev Resp Dis 146:4–10, 1992.

Friedman HS, Sakurai H, Sakurai H, et al: Pulsus paradoxus: A manifestation of a marked reduction of left ventricular end-diastolic volume in cardiac tamponade. J Thorac Cardiovasc Surg 79:74–82, 1980.

Glantz SA, Misbach GA, Moores WY, et al: The pericardium substantially affects the left ventricular diastolic pressure-volume relationship in the dog. Circ Res 42:433–441, 1978.

Guyton AC and Adkins LH: Quantitative aspects of the collapse factor in relation to venous return. Am J Physiol 177:523–527, 1954.

Guyton AC, Jones CE, and Coleman TG: Circulatory Physiology: Cardiac Output and its Regulation. Philadelphia, WB Saunders, 1973.

Heistad DD and Abboud FM: Circulatory adjustments to hypoxia. Circulation 61:463–473, 1980.

Hemmer M: Cardiovascular support during mechanical ventilation with PEEP. In Vincent JL and Suter PM (eds): Cardiopulmonary Interaction in Acute Respiratory Failure. Berlin, Springer-Verlag, 1987, pp 239–249.

Hoffman MP and Cassidy SS: Reflex effects of lung inflation and other stimuli on the heart and circulation. In Scharf SM and Cassidy SS (eds): Heart-Lung Interactions in Health and Disease. New York, Marcel Dekker, Inc. 1989, pp 339–364.

Howell JBL, Permutt S, Proctor D, and Riley RL: Effect of inflation of the lung on different parts of the pulmonary bed. J Appl Physiol 16:71–76, 1961.

Hurford WE, Lynch KE, Strauss HW, et al: Myocardial perfusion as assessed by thallium-201 scintigraphy during the discontinuation of mechanical ventilation in ventilatory-dependent patients. Anesthesiology 174:1007–1012, 1991.

Janicki JS, Shroff SG, and Weber KT: Ventricular interdependence. In Scharf SM and Cassidy SS (eds): Heart-Lung Interactions in Health and Disease. New York, Marcel Dekker, 1989, pp 285–308.

Jardin F, Farcot JC, Boisante L, et al: Influence of positive end-expiratory pressure on left ventricular performance. N Engl J Med 304:387–392, 1981.

Jardin F, Farcot JC, Boisante L, et al: Mechanism of paradoxic pulse in bronchial asthma. Circulation 66:887–892, 1982.

Khilnani S, Graver LM, Balaban K, and Scharf SM: Effects of inspiratory loading on left ventricular myocardial blood flow and metabolism. J Appl Physiol 72:1488–1492, 1992.

Knowles GK and Clark TJH: Pulsus paradoxus as a valuable sign indicating severity of asthma. Lancet 2:1356–1359, 1973.

Kussmaul A: Weber schwielige Mediastino-pericarditides und den paradoxen puls. Klin Wochenschr 10:433, 1873. Translated in Shapir E and Salick AL: A clarification of the paradoxic pulse. Am J Cardiol 16:426–431, 1965.

Lemaire F, Teboul JC, Cinotti L, et al: Acute left ventricular dysfunction during unsuccessful weaning from mechanical ventilation. Anesthesiology 69:171–176, 1988.

Ludwigs U, Klingstedt C, Baehrendtz S, et al: A functional and morphologic analysis of pressure controlled inverse ratio ventilation in oleic acid induced lung injury. Chest 106:925–931, 1994.

Magder SA, Lichtenstein S, and Adelman AG: Effects of negative pleural pressure on left ventricular hemodynamics. Am J Cardiol 52:588–593, 1983.

Mancebo J, Vallverdu I, Bak E, et al: Volume-controlled ventilation and pressure controlled inverse ratio ventilation: A comparison of their effects in ARDS patients. Monaldi Arch Chest Dis 49:201–207, 1994.

Mang H, Kacmarek RM, Ritz R, et al: Cardiorespiratory effects of volume and pressure controlled ventilation at various I/E ratio in an acute lung injury model. Am J Respir Crit Care Med 151:731–736, 1995.

Manny J, Patten MT, Liebman PR, et al: The association of lung distension, PEEP, and biventricular failure. Ann Surg 187:151–159, 1979.

Manyari DE, Wang Z, Cohen J and Tyberg JV: Assessment of the human splanchnic venous volume-pressure relation using radionuclide plethysmography. Effect of nitroglycerin. Circulation 87:1142–1151, 1993.

Marini JJ, Culver BH, and Butler J: Mechanical effect of lung distension with positive pressure on cardiac function. Am Rev Respir Dis 124:382–386, 1981.

Marini JJ, O'Quinn R, Culver BH, and Butler J: Estimation of transmural cardiac pressures during ventilation with PEEP. J Appl Physiol 53:384–391, 1982

Maughan WL: Right ventricular function. In Scharf SM and Cassidy SS (eds): Heart-Lung Interactions in Health and Disease. New York, Marcel Dekker, 1989, pp 179–220.

Maughan WL, Sunagawa K, and Sagawa K: Ventricular systolic interdependence: Volume elastance model in isolated canine hearts. Am J Physiol 253 (Heart Circ Physiol 22):H1381–H1390, 1987.

Nanas S and Magder S: Adaptations of the peripheral circulation to PEEP. Am Rev Respir Dis 146:688–693, 1992.

Permutt S, Howell JBL, Proctor D, and Riley RL: Effects of lung inflation on static pressure-volume characteristics of pulmonary vessels. J Appl Physiol 16:64–70, 1961.

Peters J, Hecker B, Neuser D, et al: Regional blood volume distribution during positive and negative airway pressure in supine humans. J Appl Physiol 75:1740–1747, 1993.

Peters J, Kindred MK, and Robotham JL: Transient analysis of cardiopulmonary interactions I. Diastolic events. J Appl Physiol 64:1506–1517, 1988a.

Peters J, Kindred MK, and Robotham JL: Transient analysis of cardiopulmonary interactions II. Systolic events. J Appl Physiol 64:1518–1526, 1988b.

Pinsky MR, Desmet JM, and Vincent JL: Effect of positive end-expiratory pressure on right ventricular function in humans. Am Rev Resp Dis 146:681–687, 1992.

Pinsky M, Vincent JL, and De Smet JM: Estimating left ventricular filling pressure during positive end-expiratory pressure in humans. Am Rev Resp Dis 143:25–31, 1991.

Räsänen J, Nikki P, and Heikkilä J: Acute myocardial infarction complicated by respiratory failure. The effects of mechanical ventilation. Chest 85:21–29, 1984.

Rebuck AS and Pengelly LD: Development of pulsus paradoxus in the presence of airway obstruction. N Engl J Med 288:66–76, 1973.

Risoe C, Hall C, and Smiseth OA: Splanchnic vascular capacitance and positive end-expiratory pressure in dogs. J Appl Physiol 70:818–824, 1991.

Robotham J and Scharf SM: The effects of positive and negative pressure ventilation on cardiac performance. Clin Chest Med 4:161–167, 1983.

Scharf SM: Cardiovascular effects of airways obstruction. Lung 169:1–23, 1991.

Scharf SM: Cardiovascular effects of positive pressure ventilation. J Crit Care 7:268–279, 1992.

Scharf SM, Bianco JA, Town DE, and Brown R: The effects of large negative intrathoracic pressure on left ventricular function in patients with coronary artery disease. Circulation 63:871–876, 1981.

Scharf SM, Brown R, Saunders N, and Green LH: Effects of normal and loaded spontaneous inspiration on cardiovascular function. J Appl Physiol 47:582–590, 1979a.

Scharf SM, Brown R, Saunders N, and Green LH: Changes in canine left ventricular size and configuration with positive end-expiratory pressure. Circ Res 44:672–678, 1979b.

Scharf SM, Brown R, Tow DE, and Parisi AF: Cardiac effects of increased lung volume and decreased pleural pressure. J Appl Physiol 47:257–262, 1979c.

Scharf SM, Brown R, Warner KG, and Khuri S: Intrathoracic pressures and left ventricular configuration with respiratory maneuvers. J Appl Physiol 66:481–491, 1989.

Scharf SM, Caldini P, and Ingram RH Jr: Cardiovascular effects of increasing airway pressure in the dog. Am J Physiol 232:H35–H43, 1977.

Scharf SM, Graver LM, Khilnani S, and Balaban K: Respiratory phasic effects of inspiratory loading in left ventricular hemodynamics in vagotomized dogs. J Appl Physiol 73:995–1003, 1992.

Scharf SM and Ingram RH: Influence of abdominal pressure and sympathetic vasoconstriction on the cardiovascular response to PEEP. Am Rev Resp Dis 116:661–670, 1977.

Scharf SM, Woods B O'B, Brown R, et al: Effects of the Mueller maneuver on global and regional left ventricular function in angina pectoris with or without previous myocardial infarction. Am J Cardiol 59:1305–1309, 1987.

Schulman DS, Biondi JW, Aoghi S, et al: Left ventricular diastolic function during positive end-expiratory pressure. Am Rev Resp Dis 145:515–522, 1990.

Smiseth OA, Thompson, CR, Ling H, et al: Juxtacardiac pleural pressure during positive end-expiratory pressure ventilation: An intraoperative study in patients with open pericardium. J Am Coll Cardiol 23:753–758, 1994.

Sylvester JT, Goldberg HS, and Permutt S: The role of the vasculature in the regulation of cardiac output. Clin Chest Med 4:111–126, 1983.

Takata M and Robotham JL: Ventricular external constraint by the lung and pericardium during positive end-expiratory pressure. Am Rev Resp Dis 143:872–875, 1991.

Tarasiuk A and Scharf SM: Venous return in obstructive apneas. Am Rev Resp Dis 148:323–329, 1993.

Veddeng OJ, Myhre ES, Risow C, and Smiseth OA:

Selective positive end-expiratory pressure and intracardiac dimensions in dogs. J Appl Physiol 73:2016–2020, 1992.

Versprille A, Jansen J, Frietman R, et al: Negative effect of insufflation on cardiac output and pulmonary blood volume. Acta Anaesth Scand 34:607–615, 1990.

Wallis TW, Robotham JL, Compear R, et al: Mechanical heart-lung interactions with positive end-expiratory pressure. J Appl Physiol 54:1039–1047, 1983.

Wayne VS, Bishop RL, and Spodick DH: Dynamic effects of pericardial effusion without tamponade. Br Heart J 51:202–204, 1984.

Whittenberger JL, McGregor M, Berglund E, et al: Influence of state of inflation of the lung on pulmonary vascular resistance. J Appl Physiol 15:878–882, 1960.

Peripheral Control of Venous Return in Critical Illness: Role of the Splanchnic Vascular Compartment

Nicola Brienza, M.D.

Takao Ayuse, D.D.S., Ph.D.

Jean-Pierre Revelly, M.D.

James L. Robotham, M.D.

The heart and the peripheral circulation are linked to each other, and cardiac output depends on their interaction. An efficient heart pumps all the blood returning to it, and, under steady-state conditions, venous return (VR) (flow coming into the heart) equals cardiac output (flow coming out of the heart). If the heart is replaced by a mechanical pump with unlimited capacity to increase flow maintaining right atrial pressure near zero, the limits of cardiac output are exclusively determined by the peripheral factors affecting venous return (Permutt and Caldini, 1978). Venous return depends on the drainage of blood from the capacitance regions of the peripheral circulation to the heart. Venous return is proportional to the pressure gradient between the average pressure in the circulation (i.e., mean systemic vascular pressure [P_{ms}]), and the right atrial pressure (P_{ra}) and is inversely related to the resistance to venous return (R_{vr}):

$$VR = (P_{ms} - P_{ra})/R_{vr} \qquad [1]$$

Therefore, all the parameters affecting venous return are peripheral, except for right atrial pressure. However, it should be pointed out that under many physiologic and pathologic conditions the downstream pressure for either regional or total venous return does not correspond to right atrial pressure because of the presence of venous vascular waterfalls (critical closing pressures) that effectively disconnect the peripheral compartments from the central compartment.

VENOUS RETURN

THE VENOUS RETURN CURVE

The reader is referred to the previous chapter for a detailed review of the venous return–cardiac output relationship.

Analysis of venous flow at different right atrial pressures classically defines the venous return curve (Guyton et al, 1957). This curve is a plot of blood flow to the right atrium (venous return) on the y axis, versus right atrial pressure on the x axis (Fig. 5–1). According to this curve, the intercept on the right atrial pressure axis

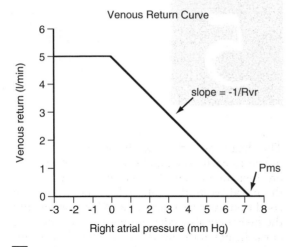

Figure 5–1
The venous return curve is a plot of blood flow to the right atrium (venous return) versus right atrial pressure. The intercept on the right atrial pressure axis is the pressure at which venous return is zero and corresponds to the mean systemic vascular pressure (P_{ms}). The slope of the relationship corresponds to -1/resistance to venous return (R_{vr}). At right atrial pressure below zero, venous return reaches its maximal value and plateaus, owing to the collapse of the large intrathoracic veins at the entry of the chest. In the plateau region, venous return is equal to P_{ms}/R_{vr}.

represents the pressure at which venous return is zero and corresponds to the mean systemic vascular pressure. Below this value, as right atrial pressure decreases, venous return increases, as defined by equation 1. The slope of this relationship is $-1/R_{vr}$. At a right atrial pressure below zero, venous return reaches its maximal value and plateaus, owing to the collapse of the large intrathoracic veins at their entry to the chest (Guyton and Adkins, 1954). In the plateau region, VR = P_{ms}/R_{vr}.

VENOUS VASCULAR WATERFALLS

The analysis of the venous return curve shows that when right atrial pressure is below zero, it does not correspond to the effective downstream pressure determining venous return. Venous beds are subjected not only to the effect of vascular smooth muscle tone, but also to the effect of surrounding pressure (Permutt and Riley, 1963) (Fig. 5–2). The venous system travels through different chambers characterized by different surrounding pressures (e.g., the intrathoracic pressure for the thoracic veins, the intra-abdominal pressure for the veins between diaphragm and pelvis, the tissue-surrounding pressure for the veins in

the limbs [Moreno et al, 1969], and intracranial pressure for the cerebral veins). In such vessels, when the surrounding pressure is higher than downstream pressure, the flow becomes proportional to the difference between inflow pressure and surrounding pressure. The downstream pressure, as long as it remains lower than surrounding pressure, is effectively disconnected from the upstream system. This concept has been classically applied in defining pulmonary vascular zones (West et al, 1964) and in characterizing the relationship between alveolar (P_{alv}) and left atrial (P_{la}) pressures. In the lung, when P_{alv} is higher than P_{la}, the downstream P_{la} is disconnected from the right ventricle, which is analogous to the way the river bed below a waterfall has no effect on the flow over the waterfall (Permutt et al, 1962; Permutt and Riley, 1963; Brower et al, 1990). When the P_{la} is greater than P_{alv}, the downstream river bed rises "above" the waterfall, and the flow is determined by the difference between upstream and downstream vascular pressures.

The plateau of the venous return curve is one

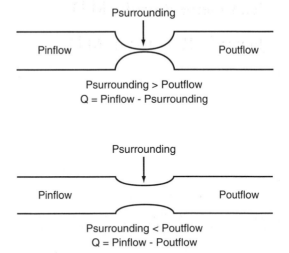

Figure 5–2
When the surrounding pressure is higher than outflow pressure, the downstream bed is disconnected from the upstream bed, and, analogous to the way the river bed below a waterfall has no effect on the flow over the waterfall, flow ($\dot{Q}$) is determined by the pressure gradient between inflow pressure and surrounding pressure. When outflow pressure is greater than surrounding pressure, the downstream river bed rises "above" the waterfall, and the flow is determined by the difference between inflow and outflow vascular pressures.

of the conditions in which right atrial pressure does not affect venous return. As expected from the venous return equation, for constant P_{ms} and resistance to venous return, venous return should increase with inspiration because of the decrease in intrathoracic and right atrial pressures. Although some studies have shown a phasic increase in the inferior vena cava (IVC) blood flow during spontaneous inspiration (Lloyd, 1983; Smith et al, 1985), using both model and experimental systems, Holt reported that an inspiratory decrease in right atrial pressure did not cause a further increase in flow (Holt, 1941; 1942). A decrease in IVC flow observed during inspiration (Wexler et al, 1968; Smith et al, 1985) has been associated with the collapse of the IVC (Smith et al, 1985). Duomarco and Rimini (1954) suggested that this venous collapse is the hydrostatic analogy of a waterfall. The waterfall concept can be applied to the thoracic veins to explain how the inspiratory fall in right atrial pressure may produce a collapse of the veins near their point of entrance into the thoracic cavity (Duomarco and Rimini, 1954).

Another situation in which venous return can be affected independently from any change in right atrial pressures occurs with an increase in lung volume (Willeput et al, 1984). Fessler and colleagues have shown that lung inflation can directly compress the thoracic vena cava affecting venous return independently from the effect on pleural pressure (Fessler et al, 1993). This situation is typically reproduced in chronic obstructive pulmonary disease (COPD) in which the increase in end-expiratory lung volume from the static elastic equilibrium volume (or relaxation volume) of the respiratory system is a cardinal feature of the underlying pathophysiology (Kimball et al, 1982).

A fall in IVC blood flow associated with an inspiratory increase in femoral venous pressure has been reported in 6 of 15 patients with emphysema and lung hyperinflation (Nakhjavan et al, 1966). The fall in the IVC flow, with the increase in peripheral venous pressure, has been related to a direct mechanical compressive effect of the lung or the contracting diaphragm on the vena cava that creates a vascular waterfall, disconnecting the peripheral from the central compartment (Nakhjavan et al, 1966). An inspiratory blood flow limitation at the thoracic inlet of the abdominal IVC has been reported also in acute asthma (Jardin et al, 1982). Willeput and colleagues observed that if abdominal pressure increased due to diaphragmatic descent during inspiration, venous return from the legs decreased (Willeput et al, 1984).

Another clinical condition in which the development of a venous vascular waterfall has been postulated occurs during application of positive end-expiratory pressure (PEEP) (Fessler et al, 1992). Fessler and colleagues have observed that application of PEEP increases the effective downstream pressure for venous return in both the superior and inferior vena caval compartments. This increase was independent of any change in right atrial pressure that in the experimental conditions was kept constant. Therefore, during the application of PEEP, the driving pressure for venous return was not represented by the difference between ($P_{ms} - P_{ra}$), but rather the venous return equation should be rewritten as

$$VR = (P_{ms} - P_{crit})/R_{vr} \qquad [2]$$

where P_{crit} is the new effective downstream critical closing pressure for venous return, which by definition is higher than right atrial pressure. The site of development of a new effective downstream pressure is difficult to locate. However, on the basis of a nonuniform increase in regional pleural pressures with lung inflation (Brookhart and Boyd, 1947; Marini et al, 1981), the authors postulated that the development of the vascular waterfalls is related to the presence of high surrounding pressure around the vena cava and/or to an active reflex increasing the tone of small muscular veins (Fessler et al, 1992).

The concept of vascular waterfalls and critical closing pressures has been applied not only to defining how venous return may be affected by respiratory-induced variations in lung volume and intrathoracic or abdominal pressures (Takata et al, 1990; 1992; Takata and Robotham, 1992), but also in defining regional venous return from single vascular beds or compartments. In the splanchnic compartment, a vascular waterfall has been used to explain the relationship between right atrial and upstream venous pressures. The splanchnic compartment has a blood reservoir function with a vascular compliance nearly double the compliance of the remaining vasculature (Mitzner and Goldberg, 1975). This specific characteristic makes control of the splanchnic compartment's venous pressure a critical function for the maintenance of hemodynamic homeostasis. In anesthetized dogs, Green (1977) observed an effective downstream pressure upstream from the right atrium, which regulated venous return from the splanchnic compartment. Bennett and Rothe (1981) raised hepatic venous pressure while keeping portal flow constant, and reported a "threshold" pressure of about 3.5 mm Hg, below which any increase in outflow pressure was not transmitted to the portal vein pressure (P_{pv}). A critical pressure, higher than the outflow venous pressure, has been defined in the portal-sinusoidal bed (Mitzner, 1974b; Brienza et al, 1995a). The portal-sinusoidal critical pressure mimics the behavior of a classic vascular waterfall (Brienza et al, 1995a) in that when P_{ra} is less than P_{crit}, portal flow (Qpv) is determined by

$$Qpv = (P_{pv} - P_{crit})/Rpv' \qquad [3]$$

whereas, when P_{ra} is greater than P_{crit}, flow is determined by

$$Qpv = (P_{pv} - P_{ra})/Rpv'' \qquad [4]$$

where Rpv is the portal vein resistance, which is also affected by the relationship between P_{ra} and P_{crit} (*vide infra*). The portal P_{crit} value is in the range of 1 to 3 mm Hg (Mitzner, 1974b; Brienza et al, 1995a), small as an absolute value, but, nevertheless, representing a substantial percentage (20–25%) of the upstream portal vein driving pressure. The portal vascular waterfall can be affected by drug administration or pathologic states. Green and colleagues (Green 1975; 1977; Green et al, 1978) observed that the portal waterfall is sensitive to the level of anesthesia and to the administration of morphine (most likely due to the release of endogenous histamine) (Robotham et al, 1984). More recent work confirms that endotoxemia increases the portal venous critical pressure (Ayuse et al, 1995b; Brienza et al, 1995b).

When right atrial pressure rises above the critical pressure that defines the waterfall, another mechanism acts to stabilize portal pressure, minimizing fluctuations in the splanchnic blood volume. Consistent with its unique position in the venous system, the liver shares the high capacitance–low pressure properties of veins and can be conceptualized as a single vessel composed of sinusoids. Any increase in right atrial pressure above the portal vein waterfall causes an increase in both the transmural distending pressure and the cross-sectional area of the portal-sinusoidal bed, thus lowering resistance to venous flow across the liver (Brienza et al, 1995a). This is why two values of Rpv are presented in equations 3 and 4, with Rpv'' less than Rpv' because of the decrease in portal resistance occurring when P_{ra} is greater than portal P_{crit} (Fig. 5–3). This portal vascular distention accounts for the minimal changes in portal pressure when right atrial pressure increases (Lautt et al, 1991; Lautt and Legare, 1992; Brienza et al, 1995a). Therefore, the association of *both* vascular waterfall and distensibility characteristics within the portal sinusoidal bed allows effective isolation of the splanchnic compartment from large negative-pressure decreases and moderate positive-pressure increases in central venous pressure. This stability of the portal vein pressure despite substantial swings in right atrial pressure is a crucial homeostatic mechanism maintaining both splanchnic venous return and splanchnic blood volume relatively constant. This explains why, in the presence of right-sided congestion with an increase in right atrial pressure, splanchnic venous return is constant, maintaining the same upstream driving pressure, whereas in the superior vena caval compartment, the upstream driving pressure increases (Engler et al, 1983). This implies an independent modulation of these regional beds as a mechanism of circulatory regulation (Engler et al, 1983).

EFFECT OF ABDOMINAL PRESSURE ON VENOUS RETURN

The mechanical properties of abdominal blood vessels make them especially sensitive to changes in the pressure on their outer surface (Sylvester et al, 1983). Because the abdominal vascular compartment has a large capacity and is directly upstream from the intrathoracic vascular compartment, changes in abdominal pressure can influence systemic venous return (Takata et al, 1990). The effects of abdominal pressure on venous return are complex, because abdominal pressure can affect both mean systemic vascular pressure and resistance to venous return, producing opposing effects on venous return. An increase in mean systemic vascular pressure, the driving pressure for venous return caused by the increase in pressure surrounding the capacitance compartments, augments venous return, whereas an increase in resistance caused by the compression of the inferior vena cava decreases venous return (Doppman et al, 1966). The predominance of either effect can explain why an increase in abdominal pressure can cause an increase (Kelman et al, 1972; Ivankovich et al, 1975), no change (Richardson and Trinkle, 1976), or a decrease (Masey et al, 1985) in venous return and thus cardiac output. A potential explanation for these conflicting results has been provided by Kashtan and colleagues (1981), who generated venous return curves for abdominal pressure from 0 to 40 mm Hg. They observed that an increase in abdominal pressure at low right atrial pressures depresses venous return, whereas at high right atrial pressures, venous return is augmented.

Takata and colleagues (1990) presented the concept of an abdominal vascular zone, which provides a theoretical framework for a coherent interpretation of these apparently conflicting results based on the relationships between right

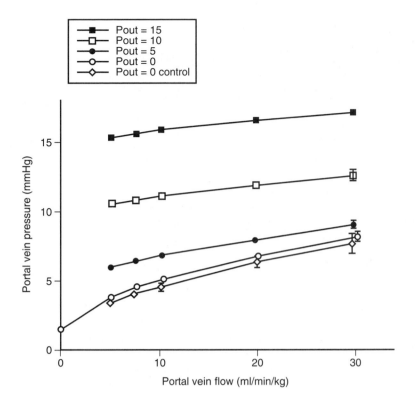

Figure 5–3
Portal vein pressure-flow relationships at liver outflow pressure (P_{out}) of 0, 5, 10, 15, and 0 (control) mm Hg. The data points are mean ± SE of pressure and flow, and the pressure measured at zero portal flow at P_{out} of 0 mm Hg is also shown. Note that at P_{out} of 0 mm Hg, a critical closing pressure higher than outflow pressure is present in the portal vein. When this zero flow pressure is overcome by outflow pressure, the slope of the pressure-flow relationships decrease, consistent with distention of the system above the waterfall. (From Brienza N, Ayuse T, O'Donnell C, et al: Regional control of venous return: Liver blood flow. Am J Resp Crit Care Med 152:511–518, 1995a. With permission.)

atrial and abdominal pressures. The concept of abdominal vascular zone conditions is analogous to the pulmonary vascular zone conditions described by West and colleagues (1964). According to this analysis, the abdominal vascular compartment can function either as a capacitor or as a collapsible Starling resistor (i.e., a vascular waterfall), depending on whether the transmural inferior vena cava pressure where it leaves the abdomen at the level of the diaphragm is above or below its critical closing transmural pressure.

The simple model of the inferior vena cava circulation developed by Takata and colleagues (1990) is shown in Figure 5–4. The model includes an upstream extra-abdominal compartment surrounded by atmospheric pressure and consisting of the compliant vessels of the legs and abdominal wall, and a downstream abdominal compartment surrounded by abdominal pressure (P_{abd}). Both compartments are connected in series and empty into the thoracic IVC (Takata et al, 1990). The relationship between right atrial and abdominal pressures accounts for the dual nature of the abdominal vascular bed and for increases or decreases in IVC flow. A steady-state elevation in abdominal pressure occurring when the abdomen is in zone III (the inferior vena cava pressure, $P_{ivc} > P_{abd}$, as in pulmonary zone III where left atrial pressure, $P_{la} > P_{alv}$, alveolar pressure) decreases the effective compliance of the abdominal

venous compartment and thus increases venous return. In this situation, the pressure in the thoracic inferior vena cava acts as the downstream pressure for venous return from the abdominal vena cava. In contrast, a steady-state elevation in abdominal pressure when the abdomen is in zone II ($P_{ivc} < P_{abd}$, as in pulmonary zone II, $P_{la} < P_{alv}$) would increase the back pressure to flow within the abdominal vena cava at the level of the diaphragm, impeding venous return. Under the latter condition, the downstream pressure to venous return is represented by the vascular waterfall developed upstream from the right atrium at the site where the vena cava exits from the abdominal compartment. Thus, the relationships among the downstream right atrial pressure, abdominal pressure, and upstream femoral venous pressure define the behavior of venous return through the inferior vena cava with an increase in abdominal pressure. The blood volume status of the subject, right heart performance, and resistance and compliance of the component venous beds all contribute to determining those key parameters of pressure that regulate venous return through the abdomen.

The role of the abdominal vascular compartment may be important during the weaning from ventilator support of patients with COPD. During the weaning of patients with severe COPD and pre-existing heart disease, a marked increase in transmural left ventricular filling pressure, with

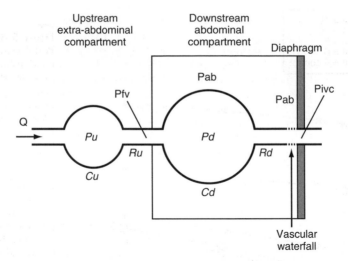

Figure 5–4

The simple model of the inferior vena cava circulation developed by Takata and coworkers is represented. The model includes an upstream extra-abdominal compartment surrounded by atmospheric pressure and consisting of the compliant vessels of the legs and abdominal wall, and a downstream abdominal compartment surrounded by abdominal pressure (P_{ab}). Both the compartments are connected in series and empty into the thoracic inferior vena cava. The relationship between right atrial and abdominal pressures accounts for the dual nature of the abdominal vascular bed and for increases or decreases in inferior vena cava flow. A steady-state elevation in abdominal pressure occurring when the abdomen is in zone III (the inferior vena cava pressure—$P_{ivc}>P_{ab}$) decreases the effective compliance of the abdominal venous compartment (Cd) and increases venous return. A steady-state elevation in abdominal pressure when the abdomen is in zone II ($P_{ivc}<P_{ab}$) increases the back pressure to flow at the diaphragm, impeding venous return. $\dot{Q}$ = flow; P_u and P_d = pressures in the upstream extra-abdominal and downstream abdominal compartments; P_{fv} = femoral venous pressure; C_u and C_d = the compliances of the upstream extra-abdominal and downstream abdominal compartments; R_u and R_d are the resistances between upstream extra-abdominal and downstream abdominal compartments, and between downstream abdominal compartment and thorax, respectively. (From Takata M, Wise RA, and Robotham JL: Effects of abdominal pressure on venous return: Abdominal vascular zone conditions. J Appl Physiol 69:1961–1972, 1990. With permission.)

consequent weaning failure, has been observed (Lemaire et al, 1988). Subsequent weaning was successful when the patients who failed the first weaning trial underwent diuretic therapy. Translocation of blood from the peripheral to the central circulation has been proposed as the cause of the initial failure to wean (Permutt, 1988). During spontaneous inspiration, the active descent of the diaphragm with contraction produces a fall in pleural pressure and an increase in abdominal pressure, with the resultant increase in transdiaphragmatic pressure. If the abdominal viscera are congested with a reduced compliance of the abdominal cavity, the increase in transdiaphragmatic pressure enhances venous return to the heart and lungs, shifting blood volume from the abdominal compartment to the thoracic compartment (Permutt, 1988). The increase in both pulmonary and cardiac transmural pressures may be expected to adversely affect any attempts to wean

a patient with left ventricular dysfunction from ventilatory support. Reducing the circulating blood volume can minimize translocation of blood into the thoracic compartment. At the opposite extreme, increasing transdiaphragmatic pressure during a relative hypovolemic state may reduce venous return (Takata et al, 1990).

Changes in abdominal pressure are often considered to be the same throughout the whole abdominal cavity. For example, a change in gastric pressure is considered to reflect a change in the whole abdominal pressure. However, in the absence of ascites, abdominal pressure changes are inhomogeneous throughout the abdominal compartment. The pressure swings in the abdomen are greater where the force is applied than in sites distant from the application (Decramer et al, 1984). Thus, the abdomen does not behave as a classic liquid-filled container, where pressure swings, equilibrating at the speed of sound, are the same all over the abdomen (Agostoni and Rahn, 1960).

The inhomogeneity of the abdominal pressure is important in understanding how the same increase in abdominal pressure may hypothetically produce different responses during respiration. Depending on the different contributions of the intercostal and accessory muscles, diaphragm, and abdominal muscles to the breathing pattern, differences in regional abdominal pressure occur (Decramer et al, 1984). Recruitment of abdominal muscle has been reported in COPD patients quietly breathing (Ninane et al, 1992) or during an unsuccessful weaning trial (Tobin et al, 1986). Expiratory contraction of the abdominal muscles is considered a physiologic response to increased ventilation or mechanical loading (Younes, 1992). Patients with COPD show a phasic activation of expiratory muscles, specifically the musculus transversus abdominis, when breathing at rest (Ninane et al, 1992). Under these circumstances, the pressure generated by the abdominal muscles should be greater on the outer surface of the splanchnic vasculature than on the inferior vena cava at the thoracic inlet. Moreover, in most acutely ill patients with COPD, there is little change in gastric pressure during spontaneous respiration (Murciano et al, 1982), and the diaphragm is reported to act as a fixator during inspiration (Derenne et al, 1988). Under these conditions (i.e., increased abdominal pressure on the outer surface of the capacity compartment with little change in the pressure in the diaphragmatic region and with $P_{ra} > P_{abd}$ at the IVC level), the abdominal vascular compartment should behave as an abdominal zone III, with the abdominal breathing thus enhancing venous return.

With a predominant pattern of diaphragmatic breathing, the diaphragmatic descent produces a mechanical compressive force on the liver, independent from any effect on the generalized abdominal pressure, because it occurs even with the abdomen widely opened (Moreno et al, 1967; Takata and Robotham, 1992). Alexander (1951) observed a reduction in portal flow with an increase in portal pressure during tetanic stimulation of the diaphragm. A mechanical focal compression on the liver has been reported to cause a phasic inspiratory reduction in hepatic outflow (Moreno and Burchell, 1982). The inspiratory arrest of splanchnic outflow was shown to be related to the anatomic location of the liver below and in intimate contact with the diaphragm (Moreno et al, 1969). Compression on the liver surface from the downward displacement of the diaphragm could reduce the diameter and the number of the perfused sinusoidal channels, producing a decrease in liver venous flow. As suggested by Brauer (1963), the main reduction in the liver vasculature should occur at the site of least resistance, potentially represented by the hepatic venules, which are devoid of connective tissue support. A prolonged diaphragmatic descent, with an increase in end-expiratory lung volume, as produced by PEEP application, produces a similar compression, increasing portal venous resistance, decreasing splanchnic venous return (Brienza et al, 1995c), and thus simulating an abdominal zone II condition. Although increased pressure over the liver surface may increase resistance, reducing outflow, a surface pressure applied over the liver with a replete capacity, analogous to an abdominal zone III, increases liver outflow (Takata and Robotham, 1992).

Thus, the effects of abdominal pressure on venous return are complex and depend on many factors. However, application of the concept of abdominal vascular zone conditions to both splanchnic and nonsplanchnic venous return from the abdomen provides a theoretical framework to examine the variables in a consistent and logical manner.

REGIONAL VENOUS RETURN

In Guyton's original description, the venous return curve was characterized by the presence of gradual upper and lower inflections at the transition from the plateau to the slope and near the intercept on right atrial pressure axis, respectively (Guyton et al, 1957). This latter inflection has been interpreted to be the consequence of the interaction of venous return from multiple beds (Engler et al, 1983). The venous return curve of the entire circulation is a composite of venous return curves from several compartments, with significant differences between the splanchnic and nonsplanchnic compartments (Caldini et al, 1974; Takata et al, 1992; Takata and Robotham, 1992). When measured separately, upstream driving pressures and resistances to venous return are different in the splanchnic and nonsplanchnic systemic beds (Engler et al, 1983). By analogy, a change in the downstream right atrial pressure may differentially affect venous return from individual venous compartments because of differences in blood volume shifts among the beds (Engler et al, 1983). Moreover, the presence of regional venous beds with different drainage characteristics (i.e., different time constants, the product of resistance multiplied by compliance) explains why alterations of the distribution of the cardiac output are able to affect total venous return (Krogh, 1912; Caldini et al, 1974). The time constant of the splanchnic bed is nearly double that of either the nonsplanchnic IVC or SVC regions (Mitzner and Goldberg, 1975). Decreasing the fractional flow to the splanchnic region, by increasing the fractional flow to faster time constant regions, leads to an increase in steady-state venous return and cardiac output.

Such analyses become extremely interesting as therapeutic measures are directed toward pharmacologic manipulation of the arterial distribution of blood flow. For example, Caldini and colleagues (1974) have postulated that the main mechanism underlying the increase in cardiac output with epinephrine is the redistribution of flow from slow to fast time constant regions with a consequent shift in blood volume. Although this explanation has been challenged (Mitzner and Goldberg, 1975; Deschamps and Magder, 1992) because of the concomitant effects of epinephrine on not only arterial flow distribution but also venous tone and baroreceptor reflexes, the key role of the arterial flow distribution to compartments with different time constants has been clearly shown in many physiologic and pathologic conditions (Guyton and Sagawa, 1961; Mitzner and Goldberg, 1975; Malo et al, 1984; Deschamps and Magder, 1992).

POSITIVE END-EXPIRATORY PRESSURE AND VENOUS RETURN FROM THE ABDOMEN

The previous chapter reviews some of the pertinent aspects of the effects of PEEP on venous return.

Measurements of "resistance" and "capacity" are often used to describe the mechanical properties that determine venous return. However, the presence of critical closing pressures is often not accounted for in the calculations of "resistance" of a peripheral vascular bed or, for that matter, for the entire circulation. Similarly, the presence of unstressed volume needs to be accounted for in the calculation of "compliance" or, to be exact, the "capacity" of a particular vascular bed.

Two parameters are necessary to define the resistive properties of a vascular bed: the zero flow pressure and the slope of the pressure-flow (P-Q) relationship. The zero flow pressure can be estimated from the extrapolation of a P-Q curve and is considered as the effective back pressure, or critical closing pressure, of the vascular bed (Mitzner, 1974b). The slope of the P-Q relationship describes the ratio of a change in pressure to a change in flow (i.e., incremental resistance).

During flow conditions, the vascular pressure is determined by a flow-dependent resistive component, described by the slope of the relationship (Δpressure/Δflow), and by a flow-independent pressure, described by the zero flow intercept. Pressure rises by increasing flow (no change in the slope and intercept), increasing the slope (higher resistance), and/or increasing the zero flow intercept (Fig. 5–5A–C). If the presence of the zero flow intercept, often the critical closing pressure of the vascular bed, is not accounted for, erroneous conclusions regarding changes in the components of the resistive load will be drawn.

The same concepts apply to systemic vascular pressures, with the difference that instead of a pressure-flow relationship, one must deal with a pressure-volume relationship. Two parameters are necessary to determine mean systemic pressure, the compliance of the vasculature (slope of the pressure-volume relationship) and the volume contained at zero transmural pressure, which is the unstressed volume. Thus, pressure can increase in the system by either a rise in the stressed volume, possibly by transfer of unstressed volume to stressed compartments), or by a rise in the pressure volume slope (decreased compliance, increased elastance). These concepts apply well to the determination of mean systemic pressure, which is the upstream pressure for venous return (Fig. 5–6A–C). Although both of these mechanisms can be caused by venoconstriction, there are important differences. For example, venoconstriction is an adaptive response to hemorrhage. If venoconstriction increases P_{ms} by decreasing vascular compliance, the blood volume mobilized would be progressively smaller as intravascular pressure decreases (Rothe and Drees, 1976). By contrast, increasing P_{ms} by decreasing the unstressed volume allows for pressure-independent mobilization of blood, which is more efficient and offers survival advantage. When Nanas and Magder (1992) studied the changes in P_{ms} with PEEP, they observed a leftward parallel shift in the pressure-volume curve. This suggests that P_{ms} increases with positive end-expiratory pressure by shifting volume from unstressed to stressed compartments with no change in compliance or overall blood volume (Fig. 5–7).

In addition to translocation of blood from intrathoracic to extrathoracic compartments and neurovascular reflexes, a third potential mechanism of the increase in P_{ms} with PEEP would be an increase in abdominal pressure induced by downward displacement of the diaphragm. The increase in the abdominal pressure would augment the pressure surrounding splanchnic vessels, and thus P_{ms}. However, no significant role has been

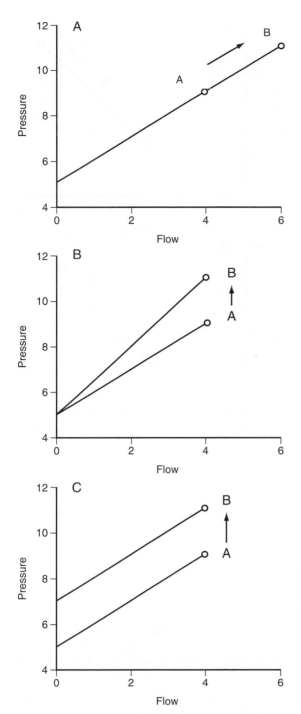

Figure 5–5
Pressure-flow relationships describe the critical closing pressure (zero flow pressure intercept) and the ratio of a change in pressure to a change in flow (i.e., incremental resistance). Pressure increases from A to B by increasing flow (A, no change in the slope and intercept), by increasing the slope of the relationship (B, with no change in flow and intercept), or by increasing the zero flow pressure (C, with no change in flow and slope).

confirmed for this factor in determining the rise in P_{ms} with PEEP (Fessler et al, 1991). An equal percentage decrease in cardiac output has been observed when PEEP was applied when the abdomen was intact, open, or bound (Scharf and Ingram, 1977). Therefore, abdominal pressure seems to exert a minimal role in the effects of PEEP on venous hemodynamics. However, it seems possible

that the local mechanical force applied over the liver during diaphragmatic descent, independent of the generalized abdominal pressure, may contribute significantly to peripheral venous response to PEEP (Brienza et al, 1995c).

We have seen that even though PEEP increases P_{ra}, it also increases P_{ms} by a similar amount (Fessler et al, 1991; Nanas and Magder,

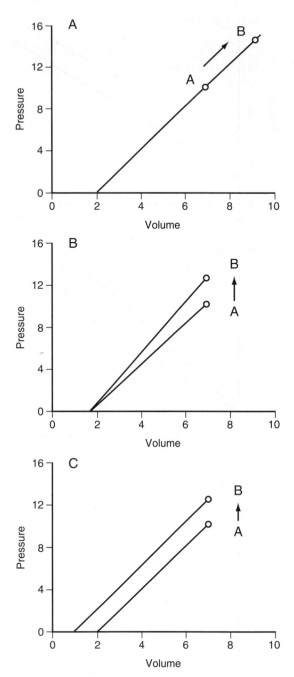

Figure 5–6
Volume-pressure relationships describe the compliance of the vasculature (i.e., the slope of the pressure-volume relationship), and the volume contained in the vasculature at zero pressure (i.e., the unstressed volume). Mean systemic vascular pressure may raise from A to B by increasing the total amount of volume inside the circulation (A, with no change in slope of the pressure-volume relationship and in unstressed volume); by decreasing the compliance of the circulation (i.e., decreasing the slope of the pressure-volume relationship) (B, with no change in either unstressed volume or total volume); or by decreasing unstressed volume (C, with no change in total volume or in the slope of the pressure-volume relationship).

1992). Therefore, the pressure gradient for venous return does not change. This implies that the decrease in cardiac output with PEEP must be caused by other factors. Two mechanisms have been proposed. On one hand, PEEP could raise the effective back pressure to venous return above the level of P_{ra} by causing upstream venous collapse, leading to the development of a vascular waterfall upstream from the right atrium (Fessler et al, 1992) in the superior and inferior vena cava.

PEEP may increase the tissue pressure surrounding vessels in the liver or other abdominal organs directly, and may increase the pressure surrounding intracranial vessels by raising cerebrospinal fluid pressure.

On the other hand, a second mechanism that may underlie the decrease in venous return with PEEP is an increase in resistance to systemic venous return (Fessler et al, 1992; Nanas and Magder, 1992). As with the development of vas-

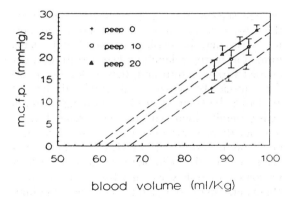

Figure 5-7
Volume-pressure relationships of the systemic circulation during application of PEEP. P_{ms} corresponds to the mean circulatory filling pressure$_{ms}$ (i.e., the driving pressure for venous return). P_{ms} increases with PEEP. The increase is due to a parallel leftward shift of the volume-pressure relationships, which is caused by a decrease in the unstressed volume (the zero pressure intercept on the x-axis), with no change in total blood volume or compliance of the vasculature. (From Nanas S and Magder S: Adaptations of the peripheral circulation to PEEP. Am Rev Respir Dis 146:688–693, 1992. With permission.)

cular waterfalls, an increase in resistance to venous return with PEEP may be due to reflex constriction or mechanical compression on the venous system.

SPLANCHNIC VENOUS RETURN AND PEEP

Both the development of vascular waterfalls and an increase in resistance to venous return with PEEP have been observed in experimental conditions in which it was not possible to investigate the relative contribution of regional venous returns. As described earlier, total venous return is a composite of regional venous returns, and the splanchnic venous return represents the single most important regional venous return. PEEP reduces splanchnic venous return (Brienza et al, 1995c). This reduction is associated with an increase in both the back pressure and resistance to flow through the liver venous system (Fig. 5–8). This behavior is similar to that of systemic venous return with PEEP (Fessler et al, 1992; Nanas and Magder, 1992). The increase in back pressure to splanchnic flow with PEEP is directly related to an increase in right atrial pressure. The rise in intrathoracic pressure with PEEP causes a parallel

increase in right atrial pressure and portal venous back pressure to flow (Brienza et al, 1995c).

The increase in venous resistance to splanchnic outflow results in sequestration of blood volume in the upstream prehepatic splanchnic bed (Manyari et al, 1993; Peters et al, 1993). Potential causes of the increase in splanchnic venous resistance include the increase in right atrial pressure, a baroreceptor-mediated reflex, and the increase in generalized or regional abdominal pressures. If the effects of PEEP on portal venous hemodynamics were uniquely the result of passive distention resulting from the increase in right atrial pressure (Risoe et al, 1991), a decrease, and not an increase, in portal resistance would have been expected. This implies that an increase in right atrial pressure due to rises in the central blood volume (heart failure, pulmonary hypertension, hypervolemia) has different effects on the splanchnic venous system than does an increase in P_{ra} caused by an increase in intrathoracic pressure during mechanical ventilation and PEEP.

A PEEP-induced baroreceptor-mediated decrease in unstressed volume (Nanas and Magder, 1992) in the splanchnic bed cannot be the dominant factor because splanchnic volume increases (Manyari et al, 1993; Peters et al, 1993). The contribution of regional compartments to the pe-

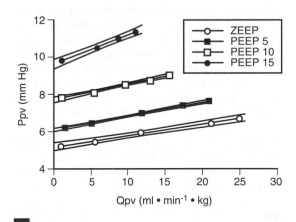

Figure 5-8
Portal vein pressure–flow relationships generated at different levels of PEEP (95% confidence intervals of the linear regressions are also shown). The increase in the zero flow pressure intercept of the relationships is due to the increase in downstream right atrial pressure with PEEP. However, independent from the increase in right atrial pressure, PEEP causes a significant increase in the slope of the pressure-flow relationships (i.e., portal vein incremental resistance increases). (From Brienza N, Revelly J, Ayuse T, et al: Effects of PEEP on liver arterial and venous blood flows. Am J Respir Crit Care Med 152:504–510, 1995a. With permission.)

ripheral response of the baroreceptor reflex has been investigated, with specific focus on the splanchnic compartment (Deschamps and Magder, 1992). Deschamps and Magder (1992) observed that hypotension elicits the expected decrease in unstressed volume, increasing P_{ms} and venous return, but with a 56% decrease in splanchnic venous resistance. Consistent with this finding, decreasing carotid sinus pressure shifts volume out of the splanchnic bed (Brunner et al, 1981). Therefore, the increase in splanchnic venous resistance with PEEP is the opposite of what is expected with a baroreceptor-mediated reflex. Furthermore, a reduction in carotid sinus pressure by as much as 100 mm Hg produces only a minimal change in portal venous resistance (Carneiro and Donald, 1977). The most likely explanation of the increase in splanchnic venous resistance with PEEP is the increase in abdominal pressure and, more specifically, the increase in local pressure over the liver surface produced by diaphragmatic descent, as previously suggested by other authors (Alexander, 1951; Moreno et al, 1967).

What are the clinical implications of this increase in splanchnic venous resistance with PEEP? Although splanchnic venous resistance can be decreased by beta-agonists (Green, 1977), their use to counteract the PEEP-induced decrease in splanchnic venous return is not useful if the decrease is related to mechanical compression on the liver. However, if volume expansion is performed during PEEP, splanchnic venous flow returns to its pre-PEEP values (Brienza et al, 1995c) not only through the expected rise in upstream venous driving pressure, P_{ms}, but also through a reduction in splanchnic venous resistance. This effect seems dependent on the increase in transmural distending pressure across the portal system (Brienza et al, 1995a; 1995c) that is able to counteract the PEEP-induced mechanically mediated increase in resistance.

SEPSIS AND PERIPHERAL VENOUS BEDS

The peripheral vascular response to sepsis is characterized by hypotension and inadequate tissue perfusion associated with alterations in vascular reactivity, which is typified by the arterial vasodilation (Sibbald and Martin, 1991; Szabo et al, 1993). There is substantially less known about the hemodynamics of the venous compartment during sepsis, which, if altered, may profoundly affect venous return (Magder and Quinn, 1991). Clinical experience and laboratory studies strongly suggest that a major factor in propagating the acute relative "hypovolemic" shock state during sepsis may be pooling of blood and edema formation in the splanchnic bed, resulting in decreased venous return and, hence, decreased cardiac output (Brockman et al, 1967; Hinshaw et al, 1970; Teule et al, 1984). Although arterial beds generally dilate with the sepsis-related hypotension, there is evidence of increased resistance and acute hypertension in beds with venous characteristics. In the pulmonary circulation (a low-resistance, high-flow vascular bed, with "venous" characteristics) endotoxemia causes acute pulmonary hypertension. The pulmonary hypertension is related to increases in both the slope of the P-Q relationship, presumptively because of vessel narrowing, and to increases in the back pressure to flow because of vessel obstruction and derecruitment (D'Orio et al, 1992). Moreover, increased P_{ms} and resistance to the total systemic venous return have been reported during sepsis (Bressack et al, 1987), in contrast to the vasodilation observed on the arterial side of the circulation.

Because of the in-series arrangement between the splanchnic organs and liver, all the flow perfusing the gut, spleen, stomach, and other organs must pass through the liver portal-sinusoidal pathway before returning to the right heart. This flow accounts for 30 to 40% of total venous return (Mitzner and Goldberg, 1975; Engler et al, 1983) and almost two-thirds of the inferior vena caval flow. The unique characteristics of the liver, which is perfused by both an arterial and a venous bed, allow independent determination of each inflow bed but, more importantly, provide the opportunity to directly measure the upstream driving pressure in a systemic venous bed. The physiologic meaning of portal pressure may be far more than a regional venous pressure. As stated by Rothe (1993): "The mean systemic vascular pressure, which can be estimated by the mean circulatory filling pressure, is less than capillary pressure, [and] is closely similar to the portal venous pressure and the venule pressure of most tissues. . . ." Thus, the study of regional portal system during sepsis may represent a window of exploration for organ-specific venous bed events and may offer important insights into the behavior of the systemic venous vascular bed.

Conflicting results have been reported on the behavior of the splanchnic venous compartment during sepsis. In a canine model of endotoxemia, no change in splanchnic venous resistance was observed (Magder and Quinn, 1991). However, in other studies, an increase in portal pressure (Kuida et al, 1961; Nolan and O'Connell, 1965;

Brockman et al, 1967; Ayuse et al, 1995b; Brienza et al, 1995b) is a common finding. This increase is consistent with the observation that P_{ms} is also increased with sepsis. Although the administration of endotoxin is not the same as sepsis, the combined effects of administering endotoxin and supportive fluid therapy in pigs seem to reproduce the hemodynamic pattern of septic shock observed in humans (Breslow et al, 1987; Fink and Heard, 1990). The similarities between pigs and humans with regard to the cardiovascular and liver systems (Dodds, 1982), particularly with increasing interest in the possibility of the porcine liver being used for "bridging" to transplantation or permanent direct xenotransplantation in humans, strengthens the rationale for using a porcine model in the study of liver hemodynamics (Cattral and Levy, 1994; Lu et al, 1994).

EFFECTS OF ENDOTOXIN ON PORTAL VEIN P-Q RELATIONSHIP

How an increase in portal pressure during endotoxemia is partitioned between increases in back pressure and incremental resistance has been examined in a porcine model of endotoxic shock. Although reproducing a typical global pattern of hyperdynamic septic shock, increases in portal vein pressure in endotoxic shock result from both an upward shift of the portal vein P-Q relationships over the whole range of flow analyzed compared with P-Q relationships obtained under control conditions resulting from an increase in both the slope and the pressure intercept of the P-Q relationships (Ayuse et al, 1995b; Brienza et al, 1995b).

The endotoxin-induced increase in portal closing pressure averaged 2 mm Hg, which is a substantial percentage of the total portal pressure. This increase has been observed in both a vascularly isolated liver preparation (Brienza et al, 1995b) (Fig. 5–9) and the intact anesthetized pig, in which during endotoxemia, portal back pressure progressively increases over time (Ayuse et al, 1995b). A reduction in the cross-sectional area because of portal-sinusoidal constriction can explain the increase in the slope of the P-Q relationship, and complete obstruction of sinusoids with derecruitment may explain the increase in critical closing pressure.

Whether other venous beds, in addition to the liver and lung venous beds, exhibit an increase in pressure during sepsis is experimentally difficult to define because these are the only two organs with separate arterial (bronchial and hepatic arterial) and venous (pulmonary artery and portal vein) inflows allowing independent evalua-

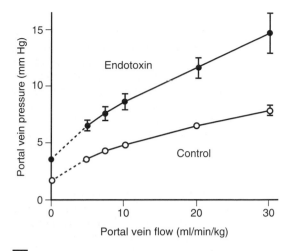

Figure 5–9
Mean ($\pm$SE) values of pressure and flow in the portal vein for control and endotoxin conditions. Note that endotoxin causes an upward shift of the pressure-flow relationships due to an increase in both zero flow pressure and slope. (From Brienza N, Ayuse T, Revelly J-P, et al: Effects of endotoxin on the isolated porcine liver: Pressure-flow analysis. J Appl Physiol 78:784–792, 1995b. With permission.)

tion of the arterial and venous input hemodynamic characteristics. However, despite differences in the microvascular anatomic structure between liver and lung (sinusoids and alveoli), the remarkable similarity in findings strongly suggests that this may be a common finding in multiple organs. It further suggests that hemodynamic differences between the systemic arterial and pulmonary vascular beds conventionally ascribed to systemic-pulmonary vascular bed differences may, in reality, reflect differences between arterial beds and microvascular/venous beds that are normally not "seen" because of the presence of upstream arterial critical closing pressures.

Whereas the increased portal closing pressure results in a constant, flow-independent, increase in portal pressure, the increase in incremental resistance results in flow-proportional increases in portal pressure. These phenomena can cause critical alterations in the upstream splanchnic compartment. One-half of the splanchnic blood is in the intestinal circulation (Morse and Rutlen, 1994), accounting for about 25% (Rothe, 1983) of total blood volume. Splanchnic blood pooling occurs during experimental endotoxemia (Chien et al, 1966), and this may contribute to reduced cardiac preload, edema formation, and third space loss, which are all prominent features of septic shock with its associated increased vascular permeability (Parrillo, 1993). Any increase in the portal vein critical closing pressure contributes to sequestration of vascular volume in the upstream splanchnic compartment, independently from any change in portal flow. An isolated increase in the critical closing pressure of the portal vein also decreases venous return for a constant total blood volume, as occurs after morphine administration (Green et al, 1978). Furthermore, during endotoxemia, a concurrent increase in incremental resistance when the critical closing pressure is raised results in higher portal and upstream splanchnic pressures for any given level of splanchnic flow.

Sepsis-induced increases in mean circulatory filling pressure are associated with the formation of edema in the splanchnic organs as a result of an increase in capillary hydrostatic pressure (Bressack et al, 1987). The well-recognized increase in vascular permeability in sepsis (Esbenshade et al, 1982) further increases edema formation and third space loss. These factors when taken together may explain why the gut is considered the most susceptible organ to edema during experimental septic shock (Bressack et al, 1987). The increases in splanchnic venous pressures result in pooling of blood, increased edema formation, and third space loss that leads to the decrease in effective circulating blood volume and to the self-propagating cycle of acute "hypovolemic" shock observed in sepsis (Reilly and Bulkey, 1993; Revelly et al, 1995).

Endotoxemia causes not only quantitative but also qualitative changes in the portal back pressure. Indeed, the waterfall behavior of the portal vein is substantially modified after endotoxin administration in that a constant positive difference (approximately 2–3 mm Hg) between back pressure and outflow pressure is always present, independent from the outflow pressure value (Brienza et al, 1995b). This is in contrast to the normal condition in which, once hepatic venous outflow pressure exceeds 3 mm Hg, the waterfall/critical closing pressure can no longer be found. There is a reasonable likelihood that endotoxin causes the development of active tone in the sinusoidal cells, creating a critical pressure that acts in addition to P_{out}. Thus, the quantitative and qualitative changes in the portal vein waterfall occurring after endotoxin administration appear to be the result of active contraction with an increase in back pressure to flow. When outflow pressure rises, the portal vein waterfall is not overcome, but portal resistance is reduced to a degree by distention of the portal system. This distention must occur in a portion of the vasculature proximal to the site of the increase in back pressure (i.e., in upstream sinusoids and/or portal vein branches) (Fig. 5–10). Thus, analysis of portal vein P-Q relationships enables differentiation of mechanically reversible (resistance-related) and mechani-

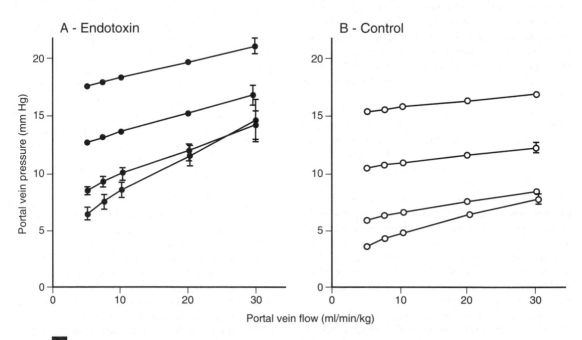

Figure 5–10
Mean (±SE) values of pressure and flow in portal vein for (B) control and (A) endotoxin conditions at multiple levels of outflow pressure (0, 5, 10, and 15 mm Hg from bottom to top). (From Brienza N, Ayuse T, Revelly J-P, et al: Effects of endotoxin on the isolated porcine liver: Pressure-flow analysis. J Appl Physiol 78:784–792, 1995b. With permission.)

cally irreversible (back pressure-related) increases in portal pressure, hence partitioning of the behavior of upstream and downstream compartments within the liver's venous vascular bed.

Dominant changes in the portal hemodynamics during inflammatory states, such as endotoxemia, are the result of sinusoidal alterations, including cell swelling, hemorrhage, congestion, and extravasation outside the sinusoidal endothelial barrier (McCuskey et al, 1987; Ayuse et al, 1995b). Moreover, vasoconstrictive mediators are reported to increase with endotoxemia and may contribute to the development of active tone inside the sinusoidal pathway. Both the lung and the liver are considered to be organs with a high density of endothelin receptors. In the pulmonary circulation, human idiopathic pulmonary hypertension is associated with elevated plasma endothelin levels (Giaid et al, 1993), and experimental chronic hypoxic pulmonary hypertension in the rat can be prevented by an endothelin receptor antagonist (Eddahibi et al, 1995).

In the liver, pathologic states may activate Kupffer and Ito cells (Housset et al, 1993). After activation, Kupffer cells swell, partially obstructing sinusoidal lumena (McCuskey et al, 1983). Ito cells, which functionally act as sinusoidal sphincters, are regulated by endothelin (Bauer et al, 1994) whose circulating levels are elevated during endotoxemia (Voerman et al, 1992). When administered directly in the portal vein, endothelin is able to reproduce the increases in both portal vein back pressure and resistance, which are observed after endotoxemia, and to cause a decrease in both portal vein flow and venous return to the right heart (Fig. 5–11). Studies suggest that both endothelins and cyclooxygenase products are the vasoactive agents responsible for the increases in incremental resistance and critical closing pressure in the portal system (Yamamoto et al, 1996; Pannen et al, 1996a). Following endotoxin exposure, the responsiveness of the portal bed to endothelin increases, thus further enhancing both presinusoidal and sinusoidal resistances for a given endothelin level (Pannen et al, 1996b).

Under normal conditions, because arterial resistances are normally much higher than venous resistances, it is the regional upstream arterial resistances that determine the regional distribution of blood flow. If arterial resistances decrease while venous resistances markedly increase, a highly unusual condition is produced in which venous parameters increasingly determine regional blood and total cardiac output (Permutt and Wise, 1987). This condition may apply to the splanchnic-liver regional compartment during

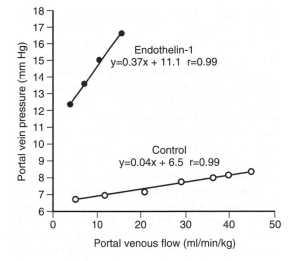

Figure 5–11
Effects of endothelin-1 on the portal vein pressure-flow relationship in the intact liver. Endothelin-1 at the dose of 1 μg/min was infused in the portal vein, and pressure-flow relationships were then generated. Note that endothelin-1 caused a marked increase in both portal vein back pressure and slope, as evidenced by the equations of the least square regression lines. These increases were associated with a decrease in venous return to the right heart.

sepsis, in that while inflow arterial resistance decreases, outflow venous resistance increases. This implies that therapeutic strategies must include consideration of the influence of an intervention on both the arterial and venous beds.

THERAPEUTIC OPTIONS

Under experimental shock conditions, at the macrocirculatory level, vigorous volume resuscitation is required to maintain venous return and cardiac output (Breslow et al, 1987; Fink and Heard, 1990). The increase in systemic venous resistance described during sepsis (Bressack et al, 1987) can be overcome by volume resuscitation. Similarly, in the splanchnic compartment, volume resuscitation may increase the P_{ms}, replace third space loss, and increase central venous pressure. This decreases portal venous resistance and enhances splanchnic venous return despite the increase in the portal critical closing pressure (Brienza et al, 1995b). This may explain why volume resuscitation may be a therapeutic option in raising venous return during sepsis. However, consistent with clinical and laboratory experience, the maintenance or increase in venous return may be obtained only at the expense of further progressive blood pooling and third space loss in the abdominal compartment.

A more interesting option is to change the flow distribution. Under physiologic conditions, arterial inflow resistance in a regional vascular bed increases with rising venous outflow pressure. This phenomenon has been observed in the canine hindlimb (Haddy and Gilbert, 1956), in the liver (Hinshaw et al, 1965), and in the intestine (Selkurt and Johnson, 1958; Johnson, 1959; Mitzner, 1974a; Revelly et al, 1995), where it has been called the venoarterial response. The venoarterial response provides a homeostatic regional mechanism to preserve the effective circulating blood volume by limiting arterial inflow and, hence, blood pooling in the splanchnic circulation (Mitzner, 1974a). An increase in portal pressure, while causing blood pooling, induces an increase in superior mesenteric arterial resistance and a decrease in its fractional flow (Revelly et al, 1995). This decrease in the mesenteric fractional flow limits blood pooling in the splanchnic vascular bed and causes an increase in fractional flow to other regions with faster time constants, thus minimizing the decrease in venous return (Caldini et al, 1974).

Does this mechanism operate during sepsis? Although endotoxin increases portal pressure, it also decreases superior mesenteric arterial resistance, consistent with the global sepsis-induced systemic arterial dilation. Under these endotoxic conditions, if portal pressure is further increased as a result of increased central venous pressure, portal venous resistance and/or a portal venous critical closing pressure, mesenteric arterial resistance, rather than rising as normally, is found to decrease without a change in fractional flow (Fig. 5–12). Thus, with endotoxemia, the normal redistribution of arterial flow away from the splanchnic circulation does not occur, and, as a result, splanchnic blood pooling continues unabated (Revelly et al, 1995). The loss of the venoarterial response during endotoxic shock appears to remove a key mechanism protecting the gut and whole organism hemodynamic homeostasis when portal pressure increases.

A therapeutic strategy may therefore include altering the capacity and resistive properties of regional vascular compartments. As suggested by Magder (1993), the use of norepinephrine is a potential means to increase venous return during sepsis through an increase in stressed volume and a decrease in unstressed volume (Appleton et al, 1985). This effect is the result of the venoconstriction of the capacity vessels through alpha-adrenergic receptors. The concomitant effect of norepinephrine on the predominant beta-adrener-

gic receptors of the large veins and of hepatic sphincters (Green, 1975) also contributes to reduced splanchnic venous resistance, thus fostering the drainage of the abdominal compartment.

Another potential strategy to avoid splanchnic pooling and enhance venous return is to act on flow redistribution, for example, to shift arterial flow from slow to fast time constant regions. However, the therapeutic advantages of redistributing arterial flow by constricting arterial vessels (e.g., the splanchnic arteries) could be negated by the consequent reduction in flow. Although during human septic shock vasoconstrictors do not decrease renal blood flow (Desjars et al, 1989), this could occur in the gut. Even though a reduction in flow to the splanchnic bed reduces blood pooling, reduction in flow in the gut-liver axis may also aggravate cellular ischemia. During sepsis in humans, the liver seems to be characterized by a state of relative ischemia, in that the increased metabolic requirements are not matched by an increased blood flow (Dahn et al, 1987). Thus, maneuvers decreasing gut-liver blood flow should be evaluated carefully.

Nitric oxide (NO) has been shown to account for the systemic arterial hypotension and vascular hyporeactivity observed during septic shock (Wright et al, 1992; Szabo et al, 1993) and to attenuate vascular response to multiple vasoconstricting substances, including endothelin (Filep et al, 1993). Inhibition of NO synthase has been used to reverse systemic hypotension in a clinical setting (Petros et al, 1991), but detailed studies on the venous hemodynamics during NO inhibition are few. Under controlled conditions, NO does not regulate the portal venous bed (Ayuse et al, 1995a). However, following endotoxin administration, NO dramatically ameliorates the adverse effects produced by endotoxin in the portal bed (Ayuse et al, 1995a). Although inhibition of nitric oxide synthase (NOS) does not modify portal vein P-Q relationships under control conditions, a marked increase in both back pressure and resistance is observed when NO is inhibited after endotoxemia is induced (Ayuse et al, 1995a) (Fig. 5–13). These alterations following NOS inhibition during endotoxic shock in a porcine model are associated with an increase in arterial systemic pressure, but also with marked decreases in both cardiac output and portal venous flow. This implies that, during sepsis, NO is important in the maintenance of the hepatic sinusoidal microcirculation. NO acts in minimizing hepatic damage either by preventing platelet aggregation and thrombosis or by attenuating the increase in vascular tone induced by vasoconstricting substances. Studies in a rat liver preparation confirm

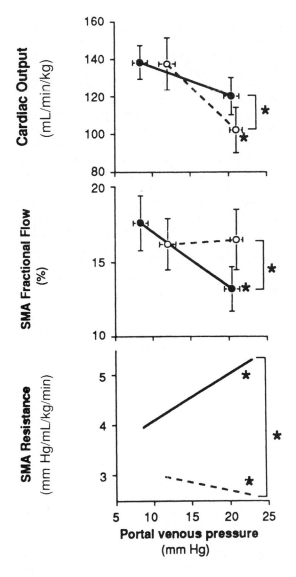

Figure 5–12
Effects of endotoxin on the relationships between portal pressure and systemic and superior mesenteric artery hemodynamics. *(Top)* Effects of endotoxin on the relationship between cardiac output and portal pressure. Under control conditions *(solid circles)*, the increase in portal pressure does not decrease cardiac output; whereas, after endotoxemia *(open circles)*, the same increase in portal pressure significantly decreased cardiac output. *(Middle)* Effects of endotoxin on the relationship between superior mesenteric artery (SMA) fractional flow and portal pressure. Under control conditions *(solid circles)*, the increase in portal pressure causes a selective decrease of the SMA fractional flow; whereas, after endotoxemia *(open circles)*, the same increase in portal pressure does not affect SMA fractional flow. *(Bottom)* Effects of endotoxin on the relationship between SMA resistance and portal pressure. Under control conditions *(solid circles)*, the increase in portal pressure increases SMA resistance (venoarterial response); whereas, after endotoxemia *(open circles)*, the same increase in portal pressure significantly decreases SMA resistance, to signify that the venoarterial response is dysregulated (* = $p<0.05$). (From Revelly J, Ayuse T, Brienza N, et al: Dysregulation of the veno-arterial response in the superior mesenteric artery during endotoxic shock. Crit Care Med 23:1519–1527, 1995. With permission.)

the role of endogenous NO in ameliorating the constrictive effects of endogenous endothelin on the sinusoid microcirculatory bed following endotoxin administration (Pannen et al, 1996b).

The role of NO in the liver circulation under normal and endotoxemic conditions is remarkably similar to the role played by NO in the lung circulation under the same conditions. The pulmonary bed is minimally regulated under basal conditions by NO, whereas, after endotoxin, the presence of NO is critical in attenuating the increase in pulmonary vascular resistance (Cobb et al, 1992; Ayuse et al, 1995a). Therefore, in the two critically important venous beds that allow measurement of inflow pressures following endotoxin exposure, rapidly occurring enhanced NO release acts to counteract the effects of vasoconstricting mediators activated by endotoxemia.

Thus, clinical strategies to inhibit NO, particularly in the presence of intractable arterial hypotension, require very careful titration and monitoring to produce benefit without harm. Adverse effects that can be anticipated appear to include diminished regional flow to the liver and gut (Gardiner et al, 1990; Wright et al, 1992; Ayuse et al, 1995a). The potential for acute disastrous consequences by inhibiting NO synthase during sepsis may be ascribed to increased resistance to venous return across the pulmonary and portal vascular beds (Ayuse et al, 1995a).

CONCLUSIONS

In past years, hemodynamic treatment of critical care patients has progressively changed its targets.

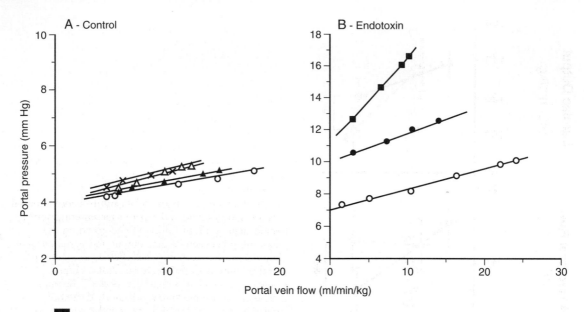

Figure 5–13
Effects of NO-inhibition by nitro-L-arginine methyl ester (L-NAME) on portal vein pressure-flow (P-Q̇) relationships under control and endotoxin conditions. *(A)* L-NAME was administered at incremental doses *(empty circles,* control; *full triangles,* 2.5 mg/kg of L-NAME; *empty triangles,* 7.5 mg/kg of L-NAME; *crosses,* 25 mg/kg of L-NAME). No change was observed in portal vein P-Q̇ relationships. *(B)* L-NAME at the dose of 2.5 mg/kg was administered after infusion of endotoxin *(empty circles,* control; *full circles,* endotoxin; *full squares,* endotoxin + L-NAME). Note the increase in back pressure after endotoxin, and the further marked increase in back pressure and slope of the P-Q̇ relationships when L-NAME was administered after endotoxin. (Modified from Ayuse T, Brienza N, Revelly J, et al: Role of nitric oxide in porcine liver circulation under normal and endotoxemic conditions. J Appl Physiol 78:1319–1329, 1995a.)

From the simple monitoring and treatment of the systemic arterial pressure, the hemodynamic target has moved toward obtaining supranormal values of cardiac output (Shoemaker et al, 1982; 1988) or normal values of mixed venous oxygen saturation, even though recent data suggest that "... hemodynamic therapy aimed at achieving supranormal values for the cardiac index or normal values for mixed venous oxygen saturation does not reduce morbidity and mortality among critically ill patients" (Gattinoni et al, 1995). In recent years, regional and single organ perfusion has become the focus of many clinicians and researchers. The use of more "organ-specific" drugs (e.g., dopamine for the kidney, dopexamine for the splanchnic organs) to improve regional flow has increased. Liver failure, a critical determinant of adult respiratory distress syndrome/multiorgan failure/sepsis (Schwartz et al, 1989) is initiated and propagated by hemodynamic alterations associated with cellular dysfunction (Machiedo et al, 1988). Liver hemodynamic alterations are detrimental not only for the liver in itself, but also for overall peripheral O₂ delivery as determined by venous return/cardiac output. Moreover, the response of the liver double (arterial and venous) inflow to pathologic stresses may represent a generalizable model for the vascular abnormalities occurring in multiple organs. Consistent with this possibility, most of the alterations observed in the portal venous bed in experimental endotoxic shock resemble those observed in the pulmonary arterial bed, which is a vascular compartment more easily accessible for hemodynamic evaluation in the clinical setting. Whether these findings can be generalized to microvascular/venous beds in other organs and whether therapeutic strategies directed at hemodynamic events alter outcome remain to be investigated.

ACKNOWLEDGMENTS

Appreciation is extended to Mr. Hillary Burman for performing the studies and Ms. Alice Trawinski for editing and organizing this paper.

REFERENCES

Agostoni E and Rahn H: Abdominal and thoracic pressures at different lung volumes. J Appl Physiol 15:1087–1092, 1960.

Alexander RS: Influence of the diaphragm upon portal blood flow and venous return. Am J Physiol 167:738–748, 1951.

Appleton C, Olajos M, Morkin E, et al: Alpha-1 adrenergic control of the venous circulation in intact dogs. J Pharmacol Exp Ther 233:729–734, 1985.

Ayuse T, Brienza N, Revelly J, et al: Role of nitric oxide in porcine liver circulation under normal and endotoxemic conditions. J Appl Physiol 78:1319–1329, 1995a.

Ayuse T, Brienza N, Revelly J, et al: Alterations in liver hemodynamics in an intact porcine model of endotoxin shock. Am J Physiol 268:H1106–H1114, 1995b.

Bauer M, Zhang JX, Bauer I, et al: Endothelin-1–induced alterations of hepatic microcirculation: Sinusoidal and extrasinusoidal sites of action. Am J Physiol 267:G143–G149, 1994.

Bennett TD and Rothe CF: Hepatic capacitance responses to changes in flow and hepatic venous pressure in dogs. Am J Physiol 240:H18–H28, 1981.

Brauer R: Liver circulation and function. Physiol Rev 43:115–213, 1963.

Breslow MJ, Miller CF, Parker SD, et al: Effect of vasopressors on organ blood flow during endotoxin shock in pigs. Am J Physiol 252:H291–H300, 1987.

Bressack MA, Morton NS, Hortrup J: Group B streptococcal sepsis in the piglet: Effects of fluid therapy on venous return, organ edema and organ blood flow. Circ Res 61:659–669, 1987.

Brienza N, Ayuse T, O'Donnell C, et al: Regional control of venous return: Liver blood flow. Am J Respir Crit Care Med 152:511–518, 1995a.

Brienza N, Ayuse T, Revelly J-P, et al: Effects of endotoxin on the isolated porcine liver: Pressure-flow analysis. J Appl Physiol 78:784–792, 1995b.

Brienza N, Revelly J, Ayuse T, et al: Effects of PEEP on liver arterial and venous blood flows. Am J Respir Crit Care Med 152:504–510, 1995c.

Brockman SK, Thomas CS, and Vasko JS: The effect of escherichia coli endotoxin on the circulation. Surg Gynecol Obstet 125:763–774, 1967.

Brookhart J and Boyd T: Local differences in intrathoracic pressure and their relation to cardiac filling pressure. Am J Physiol 148:434–444, 1947.

Brower R, Sylvester J, and Permutt S: Flow-volume characteristics in the pulmonary circulation. J Appl Physiol 69:1746–1753, 1990.

Brunner M, Shoukas A, and MacAnespie C: The effect of carotid sinus baroreceptor reflex on blood flow and volume redistribution in the total systemic vascular bed of the dog. Circ Res 48:274–285, 1981.

Caldini P, Permutt S, Waddell J, et al: Effect of epinephrine on pressure, flow, and volume relationship in the systemic circulation in dogs. Circ Res 34:606–623, 1974.

Carneiro J and Donald D: Change in liver blood flow and blood content in dogs during direct and reflex alteration of hepatic sympathetic nerve activity. Circ Res 40:150–158, 1977.

Cattral MS and Levy GA: Artificial liver support—pipe dream or reality? N Engl J Med 331:268–269, 1994.

Chien S, Dellenback R, Usami S, et al: Blood volume and its distribution in endotoxin shock. Am J Physiol 210:1411–1418, 1966.

Cobb J, Natanson C, Hoffman W, et al: Nω-amino-L-arginine, an inhibitor of nitric oxide synthase, raises vascular resistance but increases mortality rates in awake canines challenged with endotoxin. J Exp Med 176:1175–1182, 1992.

D'Orio V, Fatemi M, Marnette J, et al: Pressure-flow relationships of the pulmonary circulation during endotoxin infusion in intact dogs. Crit Care Med 20:1005–1013, 1992.

Dahn M, Lange P, Lobdell K, et al: Splanchnic and total body oxygen consumption differences in septic and injured patients. Surgery 101:69–80, 1987.

Decramer M, De Troyer A, Kelly S, et al: Regional differences in abdominal pressure swings in dogs. J Appl Physiol 57:1682–1687, 1984.

Derenne J, Fleury B, and Pariente R: Acute respiratory failure of chronic obstructive pulmonary disease. Am Rev Respir Dis 138:1006–1033, 1988.

Deschamps A, and Magder S: Baroreflex control of regional capacitance and blood flow distribution with or without α-adrenergic blockade. Am J Physiol 263:H1755–H1763, 1992.

Desjars P, Pinaud M, Bugnon D, et al: Norepinephrine therapy has no deleterious renal effects in human septic shock. Crit Care Med 17:426, 1989.

Dodds WJ: The pig model for biomedical research. Fed Proc 41:247–256, 1982.

Doppman J, Robinson R, Rockoff S, et al: Mechanism of obstruction on the infradiaphragmatic portion of the inferior vena cava in the presence of increased intra-abdominal pressure. Invest Radiol 1:37–53, 1966.

Duomarco J, Rimini R: Energy and hydraulic gradient along systemic veins. Am J Physiol 178:215, 1954.

Eddahibi S, Raffestin B, Clozel M, et al: Protection

from pulmonary hypertension with an orally active endothelin receptor antagonist in hypoxic rats. Am J Physiol 268:H828–835, 1995.

Engler R, Freeman G, and Covell J: Regional venous return: Nitroprusside effect in normal and chronically congested dogs. Am J Physiol 245:H814–H823, 1983.

Esbenshade A, Newman J, Lams P, et al: Respiratory failure after endotoxin infusion in sheep: Lung mechanics and lung fluid balance. J Appl Physiol 53:967–976, 1982.

Fessler H, Brower R, Shapiro E, et al: Effects of positive end-expiratory pressure and body position on pressure in the thoracic great veins. Am Rev Respir Dis 148:1657–1664, 1993.

Fessler HE, Brower RG, Wise R, et al: Effects of positive end-expiratory pressure on the gradient for venous return. Am Rev Respir Dis 143:19–24, 1991.

Fessler HE, Brower RG, Wise RA, et al: Effects of positive end-expiratory pressure on the canine venous return curve. Am Rev Respir Dis 146:4–10, 1992.

Filep J, Földes-Filep E, Rousseau A, et al: Vascular responses to endothelin-1 following inhibition of nitric oxide synthesis in the conscious rat. Br J Pharmacol 110:1213–1221, 1993.

Fink MP and Heard SO: Laboratory models of sepsis and septic shock. J Surg Res 49:186–196, 1990.

Gardiner S, Compton A, Kemp P, et al: Regional and cardiac hemodynamic effects of NG-nitro-L-arginine methyl ester in conscious, Long Evans rats. Br J Pharmacol 101:625–631, 1990.

Gattinoni L, Brazzi L, Pelosi P, et al: A trial of goal-oriented hemodynamic therapy in critically ill patients. SvO2 Collaborative Group. N Engl J Med 333:1025–1032, 1995.

Giaid A, Yanagisawa M, Langleben D, et al: Expression of endothelin-1 in the lungs of patients with pulmonary hypertension. N Engl J Med 328:1732–1739, 1993.

Green J: Pressure-flow and volume-flow relationships of the systemic circulation of the dog. Am J Physiol 229:761–769, 1975.

Green J: Mechanism of action of isoproterenol on venous return. Am J Physiol 232:H152–H156, 1977.

Green JF, Jackman AP, and Parsons G: The effects of morphine on the mechanical properties of the systemic circulation in the dog. Circ Res 42:474–478, 1978.

Guyton A and Adkins L: Quantitative aspects of the collapse factor in relation to venous return. Am J Physiol 177:523–527, 1954.

Guyton AC, Lindsey AW, Abernathy B, et al: Venous return at various right atrial pressures and the normal venous return curve. Am J Physiol 189:609–615, 1957.

Guyton A and Sagawa K: Compensations of cardiac output and other circulatory functions in areflexic dogs with large a-v fistulae. Am J Physiol 200:1157–1165, 1961.

Haddy F and Gilbert R: The relation of a venous-

arteriolar reflex to transmural pressure and resistance in small and large systemic vessels. Circ Res 4:25–32, 1956.

Hinshaw LB, Shanbour LL, Greenfield LJ, et al: Mechanism of decreased venous return. Arch Surg 100:600–606, 1970.

Hinshaw LB, Reins DA, Wittmers R, et al: Venous-arteriolar response in the canine liver. Proc Soc Exp Biol Med 118:979–982, 1965.

Holt J: The collapse factor in the measurement of venous pressure: The flow of fluid through collapsible tubes. Am J Physiol 134:292–299, 1941.

Holt J: The effect of positive and negative intrathoracic pressure on cardiac output and venous pressure in dogs. Am J Physiol 135:594–603, 1942.

Housset C, Rockey D, and Bissell D: Endothelin receptors in rat liver: Lipocytes as a contractile target for endothelin-1. Proc Natl Acad Sci USA 90:9266–9270, 1993.

Ivankovich A, Miletich D, Albrecht R, et al: Cardiovascular effects of intraperitoneal insufflation with carbon dioxide and nitrous oxide in dogs. Anesthesiology 42:281–287, 1975.

Jardin F, Farcot J, Boisante L, et al: Mechanism of paradoxic pulse in bronchial asthma. Circulation 66:887–894, 1982.

Johnson P: Myogenic nature of increase in intestinal vascular resistance with venous pressure elevation. Circ Res 7:992–998, 1959.

Kashtan J, Green JF, Parsons EQ, et al: Hemodynamic effects of increased abdominal pressure. J Surg Res 30:249–255, 1981.

Kelman G, Swapp G, Smith I, et al: Cardiac output and arterial blood–gas tension during laparoscopy. Br J Anaesth 44:1155–1161, 1972.

Kimball W, Leith D, and Robins A: Dynamic hyperinflation and ventilatory dependence in chronic obstructive pulmonary disease. Am Rev Respir Dis 126:991–995, 1982.

Krogh A: The regulation of the supply of blood to the right heart (with a description of a new circulation model). Scand Arch Physiol 27:227–248, 1912.

Kuida H, Gilbert RP, Hinshaw LB, et al: Species differences in effect of gram-negative endotoxin in circulation. Am J Physiol 200(6):1197–1202, 1961.

Lautt W, Greenway C, and Legare D: Index of contractility: Quantitative analysis of hepatic venous distensibility. Am J Physiol 260:G325–G332, 1991.

Lautt W and Legare D: Passive autoregulation of portal venous pressure: Distensible hepatic resistance. Am J Physiol 263:G702–G708, 1992.

Lemaire F, Teboul J, Cinotti L, et al: Acute left ventricular dysfunction during unsuccessful weaning from mechanical ventilation. Anesthesiology 69:171–179, 1988.

Lloyd T: Effect of inspiration on inferior vena caval blood flow in dogs. J Appl Physiol 55:1701–1706, 1983.

Lu CY, Khair-El-Din TA, Dawidson IA, et al: Xenotransplantation. FASEB J 8:1122–1130, 1994.

Machiedo GW, Hurd T, Rush BF, et al: Temporal relationship of hepatocellular dysfunction and ischemia in sepsis. Arch Surg 123:424–427, 1988.

Magder S: Shock Physiology. In Pinsky M, Dhainaut J-F (eds): Pathophysiologic Foundations of Critical Care. Baltimore, Williams & Wilkins, 1993, pp 140–160.

Magder S and Quinn R: Endotoxin and the mechanical properties of the canine peripheral circulation. J Crit Care 6(2):81–88, 1991.

Malo J, Goldberg H, Graham R, et al: Effect of hypoxic hypoxia on systemic vasculature. J Appl Physiol 56:1403–1410, 1984.

Manyari DE, Wang Z, Cohen J, et al: Assessment of the human splanchnic venous volume-pressure relation using radionuclide plethysmography. Effect of nitroglycerin. Circulation 87:1142–1151, 1993.

Marini J, Culver B, and Butler J: Mechanical effect of lung distention with positive pressure on cardiac function. Am Rev Respir Dis 124:382–386, 1981.

Masey S, Koehler R, Rock J, et al: Effect of abdominal distention on central and regional hemodynamics in neonatal lmb. Pediatr Res 19:1244–1249, 1985.

McCuskey R, Urbaschek R, McCuskey P, et al: In vivo microscopic observations of the responses of Kupffer cells and the hepatic microcirculation to mycobacterium bovis BCG alone and in combination with endotoxin studies of the responses of the liver to endotoxin. Infect Immun 42:362–367, 1983.

McCuskey RS, McCuskey PA, Urbaschek R, et al: Kupffer cell function in host defense. Rev Infect Dis 9:S616–S619, 1987.

Mitzner W: Effect of portal venous pressure on portal venous inflow and splanchnic resistance. J Appl Physiol 37:706–711, 1974a.

Mitzner W: Hepatic outflow resistance, sinusoid pressure, and the vascular waterfall. Am J Physiol 227:513–519, 1974b.

Mitzner W and Goldberg H: Effects of epinephrine on resistive and compliant properties of the canine vasculature. J Appl Physiol 39:272–280, 1975.

Moreno A, Burchell A, Van Der Woude R, et al: Respiratory regulation of splanchnic and systemic venous return. Am J Physiol 213(2):455–465, 1967.

Moreno A, Katz A, and Gold L: An integrated approach to the study of venous system with steps toward a detailed model of the dynamic of venous return to the right heart. IEEE Trans 16:308–324, 1969.

Moreno AH and Burchell AR: Respiratory regulation of splanchnic and systemic venous return in normal subjects and in patients with hepatic cirrhosis. Surg Gynecol Obstet 154:257–267, 1982.

Morse M and Rutlen D: Influence of nitroglycerine on splanchnic capacity and splanchnic capacity-cardiac output relationship. J Appl Physiol 76:112–119, 1994.

Murciano D, Aubier M, Bussi S, et al: Comparison of esophageal, tracheal and mouth occlusion pressure in patients with chronic obstructive pulmonary disease during acute respiratory failure. Am Rev Respir Dis 126:837–841, 1982.

Nakhjavan F, Palmer W, and McGregor M: Influence of respiration on venous return in pulmonary emphysema. Circulation 33:8–16, 1966.

Nanas S and Magder S: Adaptations of the peripheral circulation to PEEP. Am Rev Respir Dis 146:688–693, 1992.

Ninane V, Rypens F, Yernault J, et al: Abdominal muscle use during breathing in patients with chronic airflow obstruction. Am Rev Respir Dis 146:16–21, 1992.

Nolan JP and O'Connell C: Vascular response in the isolated rat liver. I. Endotoxin, direct effect. J Exp Med 122:1063–1073, 1965.

Pannen BHJ, Bauer M, Zhang JX, et al: Endotoxin pretreatment enhances the portal venous contractile response to endothelin-1. Am J Physiol 270:H7–H15, 1996a.

Pannen BHJ, Bauer M, Zhang JX, et al: A time-dependent balance between endothelins and nitric oxide regulating portal resistance after endotoxin pretreatment. Am J Physiol 271:H1953–H1961, 1996b (Heart Circ Physiol 40).

Parrillo J: Pathogenic mechanisms of septic shock. N Engl J Med 328:1471–1477, 1993.

Permutt S: Circulatory effects of weaning from mechanical ventilation: The importance of transdiaphragmatic pressure. Anesthesiology 69:157–160, 1988.

Permutt S, Bromberger-Barnea B, and Bane H: Alveolar pressure, pulmonary venous pressure, and the vascular waterfall. Med Thorac 19:239–260, 1962.

Permutt S and Caldini P: Regulation of cardiac output by the circuit: Venous return. In Baan J, Noordegraff A, Raines J (eds): Cardiovascular System Dynamics, Cambridge, MA, MIT Press, 1978, pp 465–479.

Permutt S and Riley RL: Hemodynamics of collapsible vessels with tone: The vascular waterfall. J Appl Physiol 18:924–932, 1963.

Permutt S and Wise R: The control of cardiac output through coupling of heart and blood vessels. In Yin F (ed): Ventricular/Vascular Coupling. Clinical, Physiological, and Engineering Aspects. New York, Springer-Verlag, 1987, pp 159–179.

Peters J, Hecker B, Neuser D, et al: Regional blood volume distribution during positive and negative airway pressure breathing in supine humans. J Appl Physiol 75:1740–1747, 1993.

Petros A, Bennett D, and Valance P: Effect of nitric oxide synthase inhibitors on hypotension in patients with septic shock. Lancet 338:1557–1558, 1991.

Reilly P and Bulkey G: Vasoactive mediators and

splanchnic perfusion. Crit Care Med 21:S55–S68, 1993.

Revelly J, Ayuse T, Brienza N, et al: Dysregulation of the veno-arterial response in the superior mesenteric artery during endotoxic shock. Crit Care Med 23:1519–1527, 1995.

Richardson J and Trinkle J: Hemodynamic and respiratory alterations with increased intra-abdominal pressure. J Surg Res 20:401–404, 1976.

Risoe C, Hall C, and Smiseth OA: Splanchnic vascular capacitance and positive end-expiratory pressure in dogs. J Appl Physiol 70:818–824, 1991.

Robotham JL, Doherty KC, and Lange DG: A comparison of the hemodynamic effects of fentanyl and morphine in right heart bypassed dogs. Anesthesiology 61:A76, 1984.

Rothe C and Drees J: Vascular capacitance and fluid shifts in dog during prolonged hemorrhagic hypotension. Circ Res 38:347–356, 1976.

Rothe CF: Venous system: Physiology of the capacitance vessels. In Shepherd JT and Abboud FM (eds): Handbook of Physiology. The Cardiovascular System. Peripheral Circulation and Organ Blood Flow. Vol. III. Bethesda, MD, American Physiological Society, 1983, pp 397–452.

Rothe CF: Mean circulatory filling pressure: Its meaning and measurements. J Appl Physiol 74:499–509, 1993.

Scharf SM and Ingram RH: Influence of abdominal pressure and sympathetic vasoconstriction on the cardiovascular response to positive end-expiratory pressure. Am Rev Respir Dis 116:661–670, 1977.

Schwartz DB, Bone RC, Balk RA, et al: Hepatic dysfunction in the adult respiratory distress syndrome. Chest 95:871–875, 1989.

Selkurt E and Johnson P: Effect of acute elevation of portal venous pressure on mesenteric blood volume, interstitial fluid volume and hemodynamics. Circ Res 6:592–599, 1958.

Shoemaker WC, Appel PL, Kram HB, et al: Prospective trial of supranormal values of survivors as therapeutic goals in high-risk surgical patients. Chest 94:1176–1186, 1988.

Shoemaker WC, Appel PL, Waxman K, et al: Clinical trials of survivors' cardiorespiratory patterns as therapeutic goals in critically ill postoperative patients. Crit Care Med 10:398–403, 1982.

Sibbald W and Martin C: Abnormalities of vascular reactivity in the sepsis syndrome. Chest 100:S155–S159, 1991.

Smith H, Grottum P, and Simonsen S: Ultrasonic assessment of abdominal venous return. I. Effect of cardiac action and respiration on mean velocity pattern, cross-sectional area and flow in the inferior vena cava and portal vein. Acta Radiol Diagn 26:581–588, 1985.

Sylvester JT, Goldberg HS, and Permutt S: The role of the vasculature in the regulation of cardiac output. Clin Chest Med 4:111–126, 1983.

Szabo C, Mitchell J, and Thiemermann C, et al: Nitric oxide–mediated hyporeactivity to noradrenaline precedes the induction of nitric oxide synthase in endotoxin shock. Br J Pharmacol 108:786–792, 1993.

Takata M, Beloucif S, Shimada M, et al: Superior and inferior vena caval flows during respiration: Pathogenesis of Kussmaul's sign. Am J Physiol 262:H763–H770, 1992.

Takata M and Robotham J: Effects of inspiratory diaphragmatic descent on inferior vena caval venous return. J Appl Physiol 72:597–607, 1992.

Takata M, Wise RA, and Robotham JL: Effects of abdominal pressure on venous return: Abdominal vascular zone conditions. J Appl Physiol 69:1961–1972, 1990.

Teule GJ, von Lingen A, Verwey von Vught MA, et al: Role of peripheral pooling in porcine escherichia coli sepsis. Circ Shock 12:115–123, 1984.

Tobin M, Perez W, and Guenther S: The pattern of breathing during successful and unsuccessful trials of weaning from mechanical ventilation. Am Rev Respir Dis 134:1111–1118, 1986.

Voerman HJ, Stehouwer CDA, van Kamp GJ, et al: Plasma endothelin levels are increased during septic shock. Crit Care Med 20:1097–1101, 1992.

West J, Dollery C, and Naimark A: Distribution of blood flow in isolated lung: Relation to vascular and alveolar pressures. J Appl Physiol 19:713–724, 1964.

Wexler L, Bergel D, and Gabe I, et al: Velocity of blood flow in normal human venae cavae. Circ Res 23:349–359, 1968.

Willeput R, Rondeux C, and DeTroyer A: Breathing affects venous return from legs in humans. J Appl Physiol 57:971–976, 1984.

Wright C, Rees D, and Moncada S: Protective and pathological roles of nitric oxide in endotoxin shock. Cardiovasc Res 26:48–57, 1992.

Yamamoto S, Burman H, O'Donnell CP, et al: Endothelin causes portal and pulmonary hypertension in porcine endotoxemia. Am J Physiol 272 (Heart Circ Physiol 41). In press.

Younes M: Determinants of thoracic excursions during exercise. In Whipp B and Wassermann K (eds): Exercise. Pulmonary Physiology and Pathophysiology. New York, Marcel Dekker, 1992, pp 1–65.

The Muscles of Respiration

Steven G. Kelsen, M.D.

Bernard R. Borbely, M.D.

The respiratory skeletal muscles apply force to the rigid structures of the rib cage, spine, and pectoral and pelvic girdles, thereby deforming the chest wall away from its relaxed configuration. The magnitude of the negative swings in intrathoracic pressure generated by the inspiratory muscles determines the rate of inspiratory airflow and tidal volume. Moreover, the act of sighing by the inspiratory muscles (i.e., inflation to total lung capacity) minimizes lung compliance by redistributing alveolar surfactant.

The expiratory muscles, on the other hand, compress the thorax and generate positive swings in intrathoracic pressure, which accelerate expiratory airflow and facilitate increases in ventilation. Exaggerated positive swings in intrathoracic pressure during coughing compress the intrathoracic airways, thereby clearing secretions and minimizing airflow resistance. Impairments in the ability of the inspiratory and expiratory muscles to generate appropriate swings in intrathoracic pressure, therefore, quickly lead to atelectasis, retained secretions, and, ultimately, hypercapnic respiratory failure. Proper functioning of the inspiratory and expiratory muscles is required to preserve the normal mechanical properties of the lungs and airways and to generate a level of ventilation appropriate to the needs of body metabolism. The respiratory striated muscles, therefore, are a vital thoracic pump like the heart.

Intense investigation within the past decade indicates that the respiratory skeletal muscles are highly plastic and capable of adaptive changes in structure, biochemical properties, and contractile function in response to altered patterns of use (Leith et al, 1976). However, respiratory muscle function deteriorates slowly with aging and senescence; and muscle function deteriorates quickly during highly intense contractions (i.e., fatigue) and when blood chemistry is abnormal (Tolep et al, 1995; Aubier et al, 1985a; Juan et al, 1984).

MECHANICAL ACTION

Conceptually, the ventilatory pump may be viewed as consisting of two compartments: the rib cage and abdomen, separated by the diaphragm

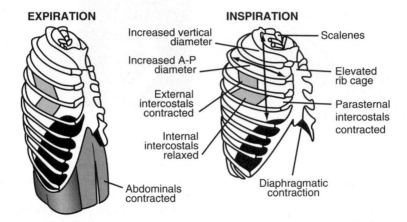

Figure 6–1
The muscles of respiration. Primary muscles of inspiration: diaphragm, parasternal intercartilaginous, external intercostal, and scalenus muscles. Accessory muscles of inspiration: sternocleidomastoid muscles. Muscles of exhalation: abdominal muscles (rectus abdominis, internal and external oblique, transversus abdominis), internal intercostals (excluding parasternals). Arrows indicate vector forces applied by the muscle. (Adapted from Luce JM, and Culver BH: Critical review. Respiratory muscle function in health and disease. Chest 81:82, 1982. With permission.)

(Macklem et al, 1983) (Figs. 6–1 and 6–2). The rib cage is composed of the sternum, ribs, thoracic vertebrae, and costal cartilage. Contraction of the inspiratory or expiratory muscles, which displaces the ribs in an anterior (pump-handle) or a lateral (bucket-handle) direction, changes intrathoracic and abdominal pressure. Moreover, because the costal and crural regions of the diaphragm are in apposition to the inner aspect of the lower rib cage, the lower four to six ribs (laterally and posteriorly) function as part of the abdominal wall. The portion of the diaphragm that abuts the inside of the rib cage occupies slightly more than one-fourth of the internal surface of the thorax. Accordingly, changes in abdominal pressure are transmitted to the lower rib cage via the zone of apposition; conversely, expansion or compression of the lower rib cage alters abdominal pressure.

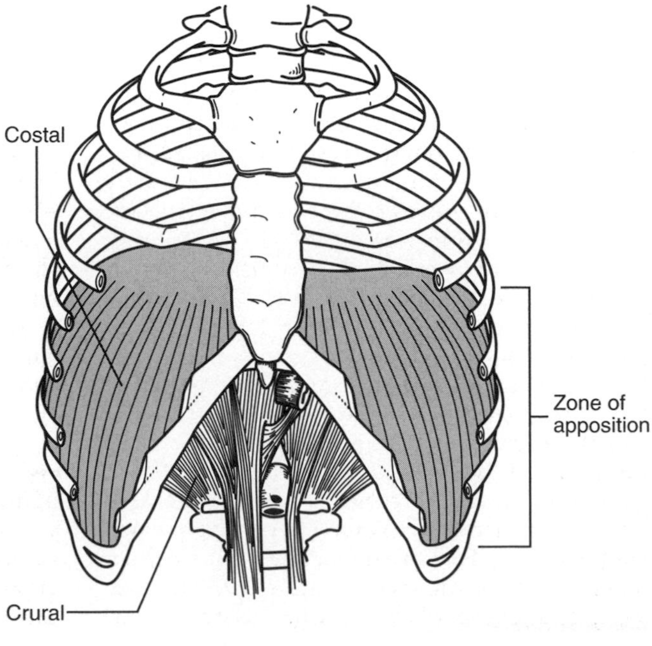

Figure 6–2
The human diaphragm. The crural diaphragm is posterior and caudal and attaches to the vertebrae. The costal diaphragm arises from the lower six ribs. The costal and crural diaphragms abut the lower ribs in the region of the zone of apposition. (Redrawn from Rochester DF: The diaphragm: Contractile properties and fatigue. J Clin Invest 75:1397–1402, 1985. With permission.)

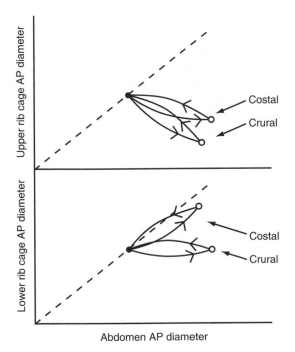

Figure 6–3
Konno-Mead diagram of the relationship between the abdomen and rib cage during isolated contraction of the costal and crural diaphragm. Without contribution from the chest wall and neck muscles the diaphragm primarily produces a paradoxical expiratory action on the upper rib cage during inspiration. The crural diaphragm has little effect on the lower rib cage during inspiration while the costal diaphragm expands this part of the thorax.

The abdominal contents are essentially incompressible, and most of the structures surrounding the abdominal cavity are rigid (e.g., pelvis, dorsal spine, iliac crests, rib cage). Therefore, an increase in abdominal pressure generated by descent of the diaphragm can be dissipated only by moving the ventral abdominal wall outward. Conversely, an increase in abdominal pressure generated by contraction of the abdominal or rib cage expiratory muscles can be dissipated only by displacing the diaphragm cranially. This relationship allows the diaphragm and lower rib cage muscles to affect abdominal pressure and the abdominal muscles to affect intrathoracic pressure.

The mechanical action of the respiratory muscles is reflected in the volume changes of the rib cage and abdomen during breathing and their pattern of movement relative to each other. Rib cage and abdominal volume changes (expansion and deflation) have been assessed from their anteroposterior or transverse dimensions. The temporal relationship of their change relative to one another is generally assessed by displaying rib cage and abdominal dimensions on an x-y plot, which has been termed a Konno-Mead diagram after the investigators who originated it (Figs. 6–3 and 6–4).

MUSCLES OF INSPIRATION

Diaphragm

In normal subjects, contraction of the diaphragm, the primary muscle of ventilation, accounts for the largest portion of the change in intrathoracic pressure. Normally, the diaphragm has an ellip-

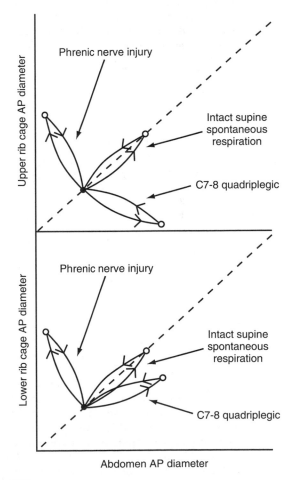

Figure 6–4
Konno-Mead diagram of the relationship between the abdomen and rib cage in patients with neurologic injury. The C7 to C8 quadriplegic patient selectively uses the diaphragm and the sternocleidomastoid muscles for respiration. The patient with phrenic nerve injury (i.e., phrenic nerve frostbite post-CABG) primarily uses the chest wall and neck muscles to generate negative intrathoracic pressure.

tical and cylindrical shape. The diaphragm has several hiatal openings and triangular spaces (foramina of Morgagni and Bochdalek), which may transmit gas or fluid, thereby affecting the pressure difference between the abdomen and rib cage.

The diaphragm anatomically and functionally may be considered as two distinct muscles (Macklem et al, 1983; De Troyer et al, 1981). Costosternal fibers (costal diaphragm) originating from the xiphoid process of the sternum and the upper margins of the lower six ribs insert on the central tendon. Vertebral muscle fibers (crural diaphragm), arising from the ventrolateral aspect of the first three lumbar vertebrae and the aponeurotic ligaments, also insert on the central tendon.

Normally, at end expiration the costal and crural diaphragm muscle fibers are oriented in a direction parallel to and abutting the inner surface of the rib cage. This zone of apposition allows the lower ribs (laterally and posteriorly) to function as part of the abdominal wall because the wall is acted on by abdominal pressure.

Contraction of the costal diaphragm applies an inspiratory action on the lower rib cage in two ways. Abdominal pressure generated by caudal movement of the diaphragm is transmitted across the zone of apposition and expands the lower rib cage (Urmey et al, 1988). This positive pressure in the lower pleural space during inspiration is known as the appositional force and is proportional to the area of the zone of apposition and the total abdominal pressure. Second, the contraction force applied directly by the costal diaphragm fibers on insertional sites on the lower six ribs generates an inspiratory pump and buckethandle motion. The inspiratory action of the costal diaphragm is the sum of the appositional and insertional forces. In contrast, the inspiratory action of the crural diaphragm is based solely on the appositional force. There is no insertion of the crural diaphragm on the ribs and hence no direct insertional action. The crural diaphragm thus contributes to a lesser degree to the inspiratory action of the diaphragm (see Fig. 6–3). Injury or dysfunction of the costal diaphragm, therefore, causes more impairment than that of the crural diaphragm (see Fig. 6–3).

In contrast to their effects on the lower rib cage, contraction of the costal and crural diaphragm produces an expiratory action on the upper rib cage by decreasing pleural pressure. This expiratory effect is illustrated by collapse of the upper rib cage during inspiration in patients with lower cervical cord transection in whom the diaphragm contracts in isolation (Mortola et al, 1978; Mead et al, 1984) (see Fig. 6–4). Expansion of the upper rib cage during inspiration, therefore,

requires contraction of the scalene and parasternal intercostal muscles.

Lung volume has important mechanical effects on the diaphragm. As lung volume increases, caudal movement of the diaphragm, which appears to descend in piston-like fashion, decreases the area of the zone of apposition and the appositonal force (Loring et al, 1982; 1985). Moreover, hyperinflation, which is induced by obstructive lung diseases such as chronic obstructive pulmonary disease (COPD) and asthma, alters diaphragm shape. As lung volume approaches total lung capacity, the diaphragm becomes flattened and the insertional force may be directed medially, causing a decrease in lower rib cage volume during inspiration. Accordingly, with marked hyperinflation, as in patients with emphysema, the costal and crural diaphragm may exert an expiratory action on the lower rib cage. The clinical sign of inward (expiratory) movement of the lower rib cage during inspiration is called *Hoover's sign* and is frequently seen in patients with marked hyperinflation. On the other hand, as lung volume decreases, the area of the zone of apposition and the appositonal force increase. Reductions in lung volume augment the mechanical advantage of the costal and crural diaphragm.

The inspiratory action of the diaphragm is also dependent on the compliance of the abdominal cavity (Druz et al, 1981). The lower the abdominal compliance (i.e., the stiffer the abdominal wall), the greater the increase in abdominal pressure for a given diaphragmatic descent. Decreases in the abdominal compliance also facilitate lower rib cage expansion by allowing greater force to be applied insertionally. Conditions associated with decreased abdominal compliance include ascites, obesity, abdominal bandages, ileus, supine posture, and hyperinflation. Increases in abdominal compliance (i.e., from open abdominal wounds or evisceration) produce the opposite effect and impair diaphragmatic efficiency.

The costal diaphragm is innervated by branches of the phrenic nerve, which arise from the third and fourth cervical nerves. The crural diaphragm is innervated by branches of the fourth and fifth cervical nerves. Injury of the cervical cord in the C3 to C5 region, therefore, denervates the diaphragm. However, the topographic innervation of the diaphragm in a rostral-caudal direction allows function of the costal diaphragm to be preserved in subjects injured below the C3-C4 segment. In the thorax, the phrenic nerves travel between the parietal pleura and the pericardium until they enter the diaphragm lateral to the heart and anterior to the central tendon. This position of the phrenic nerves makes them extremely vulnerable to surgical procedures that involve the pericardium (e.g., cardiac cooling). Phrenic nerve injury is associated with a paradoxical inward movement of the anterior abdominal wall during inspiration as the abdominal wall becomes subatmospheric and the flaccid diaphragm moves cranially into the thorax in response to the negative intrathoracic pressure swing (see Fig. 6–4).

Intercostal Muscles

Three groups of intercostal muscles show phasic inspiratory electrical activity during eupneic breathing in man and hence may be considered primary inspiratory muscles: the parasternal intercostals, upper external intercostals, and levator costae. Contraction of these muscles causes cranial (inspiratory) displacement of the upper and lower ribs and offsets the deflationary action of negative pleural pressure on the upper rib cage. These muscles receive their sensory and motor innervation from the first to twelfth thoracic nerves.

The parasternal muscles are located ventrally between the costochondral junctions and the sternum (see Fig. 6–1). The parasternal muscles arise from the inner portion of the superior rib and insert on the rostral portion of the next lower rib. The fibers run in a caudal and lateral direction. During eupneic breathing, inspiratory activity is more concentrated in the rostral interspaces. When the scalenes are voluntarily inhibited, parasternal muscle activity increases.

The external intercostals arise from the tubercles of the superior ribs and insert on the inferior costal cartilage medially. Contraction of the external intercostals causes a pump-handle, cranial elevation of the ribs about the dorsal spinal articulation. During eupneic breathing, the external intercostals are primarily active in the rostral interspaces posteriorly where they have greatest inspiratory mechanical advantage. They appear to be less active and involve fewer motor units than the parasternal muscles during inspiration (De Troyer, 1991).

The levator costae arise from the transverse processes of the seventh cervical and eleven upper dorsal thoracic vertebrae and insert on the inferior rib caudally and laterally. The levator costae contribute to the pump-handle and bucket-handle motion of the ribs.

Scalene Muscles

The scalene muscles (anterior, medial, and posterior) originate from the transverse processes of all the cervical vertebrae and insert on the superior surface of the first and second ribs. The scalenes elevate the first and second ribs during inspiration. A significant contribution to inspiration during normal breathing is suggested for the scalenes because they are electrically active during eupneic breathing. The scalenes are innervated by branches of the fourth to seventh cervical nerves and so may be denervated in high cervical cord injury.

Sternocleidomastoid Muscle

The sternocleidomastoid has two heads that arise from the manubrium of the sternum and the medial clavicle and insert on the ipsilateral mastoid process of the temporal bone. This muscle is inactive during eupneic breathing but can be recruited during forceful, large inspirations. The sternocleidomastoid muscle displaces the sternum cranially and enlarges the upper rib cage in an anteroposterior direction (Danon et al, 1979). In normal humans, the sternocleidomastoid is recruited during hyperventilation, increased ventilatory load (e.g., increased airway resistance, decreased lung compliance), or inspiration to total lung capacity. This muscle is innervated by the eleventh cranial nerve and the second cervical nerve. Accordingly, sternocleidomastoid function is preserved in patients with high cervical cord injury.

MUSCLES OF EXPIRATION

Intercostal Muscles

The interosseous, internal intercostal muscles (excludes parasternal intercostal muscles) produce a deflationary pump-handle motion of the ribs. During eupneic breathing, activity of the internal intercostals is confined to the caudal interspaces, where they have the greatest mechanical advantage.

Abdominal Muscles

The abdominal muscles include the external and internal oblique, rectus abdominis, and transversus abdominis. The abdominal muscles are innervated by the seventh to eleventh intercostal, iliohypogastric, and ilioinguinal nerves.

The abdominal muscles are inactive during normal breathing in the supine position. However, they are recruited under conditions of increased ventilatory demand caused by exercise, hypercapnia, and increased ventilatory loads and when assuming the upright posture. Their tonic activity in the upright position may improve the mechanical action of the diaphragm by minimizing diaphragm descent when assuming the upright posture and during inspiration. The transverse abdominis is usually recruited before the rectus abdominis or external oblique (De Troyer et al, 1990).

When active, these muscles decrease abdominal anteroposterior and lateral diameter and abdominal compliance; they increase intra-abdominal pressure (Mier et al, 1985). By virtue of their insertions on the ribs, they pull the lower ribs caudally and decrease rib cage volume and increase pleural pressure. Pleural pressure is also increased by displacing the diaphragm cranially. In part, the deflationary action of the abdominal muscles on the lower rib cage is offset by the insertional forces of the diaphragm, which are increased as the diaphragm is displaced cranially.

The abdominal muscles contracting against a closed glottis create forces required for a normal cough. Impairment of abdominal muscle function by laparotomy or neuromuscular disease, therefore, impairs the clearance of airway secretions. Abdominal muscle contraction is also necessary for phonation, micturition, and parturition.

Triangularis Sterni

The triangularis sterni is a thin muscle located on the inner side of the anterior chest wall, deep to the sternum and parasternal muscles. Its fibers arise from the lower part of the posterior sternum and course superiorly and laterally to insert on the lower inner borders of the third to seventh ribs. It is innervated by the intercostal nerves. When active, it decreases rib cage volume by displacing the ribs caudally and the sternum cranially. The triangularis sterni, therefore, has an opposite effect to that of the parasternal intercostal muscles on the rib cage but may have an agonistic effect by increasing parasternal intercostal precontractile length (De Troyer et al, 1987). This muscle is not electrically active in normal humans in the supine position but is recruited during hyperventilation.

RESPIRATORY MUSCLE CONTRACTILE PROPERTIES

Respiratory muscle force depends on (1) fiber composition and fiber mass; (2) intensity of central nervous system motor outflow as reflected in the force-frequency relationship and pattern of motor unit recruitment; (3) fiber length; (4) velocity of fiber shortening; and (5) fatigability.

MUSCLE FIBER COMPOSITION

The respiratory skeletal musculature represents a mix of slow and fast twitch fiber types (Akabas et al, 1989; Kelsen et al, 1993; Reid W et al, 1992). The precise mix varies considerably from muscle to muscle and even regionally within a given muscle. Differences in muscle fiber type account, in a large part, for the considerable differences that exist between the several respiratory muscles in force generation, velocity of shortening, and susceptibility to fatigue.

Slow oxidative (type I) and fast oxidative (type IIa) fibers are highly fatigue-resistant. In contrast, fast glycolytic fibers (type IIb) are highly susceptible to fatigue. Fast fibers have larger cross-sectional area and hence generate greater force as well as shorten considerably faster than slow fibers. In addition, the size of fast motor units (i.e., the number of muscle fibers innervated by a single alpha motor neuron) is 5 to 20 times greater than the size of slow motor units (Fournier et al, 1988). Accordingly, activation of fast motor units represents a "force reserve," which permits strenuous respiratory efforts but only for brief periods before fatigue ensues.

Fiber composition is dynamic and changes throughout neonatal and adult life (Maxwell et al, 1983; Sieck et al, 1991; Kelly et al, 1991). The respiratory muscles of adults tend to have a higher percentage of slow fatigue-resistant fibers than the same muscles in the newborn. The adult human diaphragm consists of approximately 50% slow oxidative fibers, 25% fast oxidative fibers, and 25% fast glycolytic fibers (Lieberman et al, 1973; Keens et al, 1978). However, considerable interindividual differences in diaphragm muscle fiber composition contribute to important differences in muscle strength and endurance (Laporta et al, 1985). Moreover, fiber cross-sectional area is highly plastic and is affected by activity, nutritional status, and hormonal milieu. For example, inspiratory resistive load training increases diaphragm fiber size and aerobic capacity (Akabas et al, 1989). Conversely, chronic protein-calorie undernutrition (Kelsen et al, 1985), cachexia resulting from uncontrolled infection and carcinoma (Arora and Rochester, 1982a, b), and chronic corticosteroid excess (Ferguson et al, 1990; Dekhuijzen et al, 1995) cause diaphragm fiber atrophy, with greater effects on fast- than slow-twitch fibers.

Muscle mass is the product of average muscle fiber diameter and the number of fibers present. Normative data for respiratory muscle mass is largely unavailable. However, it is clear that diaphragm muscle mass varies considerably between individuals (Rochester et al, 1985). Differences in diaphragm mass probably reflect body habitus, hormonal and nutritional factors, and, perhaps most importantly, differences in the level of muscle activity. For example, diaphragm thickness and weight are greater in men than women and greater in manual laborers than sedentary adults.

CENTRAL NERVOUS SYSTEM OUTPUT

Force-frequency Relationship

Application of a single supramaximal threshold depolarizing stimulus (i.e., 1.2 to 1.5 times the voltage that generates a maximal compound action potential) to an axon innervating a respiratory muscle motor unit (or muscle sarcolemma) initiates the bell-shaped tension wave form shown in Figure 6–5 (i.e., a twitch). The time from tension development to its peak (i.e., the contraction time) is generally shorter than the time from peak back to baseline (i.e., the relaxation time).

In contrast to a twitch, the force-frequency curve is generated by applying a train of stimuli for approximately 1 to 2 seconds (see Fig. 6–5). At stimulus frequencies in excess of 50 Hz, a fully fused tetanic contraction is developed and motor

unit force output is maximal. For the diaphragm, axonal firing rates of 50 to 75 depolarizations/sec develop maximal force output. Accordingly, the force output of individual respiratory muscles can be increased by moving each motor unit up its force-frequency relationship toward the plateau. It is estimated that during eupneic breathing the firing rate of phrenic motor neurons is approximately 15/sec (Iscoe et al, 1976). During high levels of activation, such as during a cough or sneeze, phrenic firing rates may exceed of 200/sec.

The shape of the force-frequency relationship varies for slow- and fast-twitch fibers. Slow fibers that generate and dissipate tension more slowly achieve maximal force at lower stimulus frequencies than fast-twitch muscle fibers. As a result, the axonal firing frequency required to fully activate a fast motor unit is greater than that required to maximally activate a slow-twitch motor unit.

In man, quasi-isometric contractions have been accomplished for the diaphragm by occluding the airway at end expiration while the cervical phrenic nerves are stimulated electrically using transcutaneous or percutaneous electrodes. (Aubier et al, 1981a, 1985a; Bellemare et al, 1984, 1986). In this method, a single supramaximal pulse of 0.1 ms is applied to the phrenic nerves

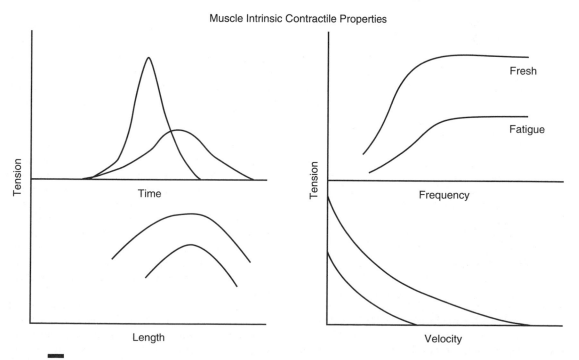

Muscle Intrinsic Contractile Properties

Figure 6–5
The twitch-tension wave form (*left upper panel*), the length-tension relationship (*left lower panel*), the force-frequency relationship (*right upper panel*), and the isotonic force-velocity relationship (*right lower panel*). Responses of fatigued muscle are indicated by the lower tracing in each panel.

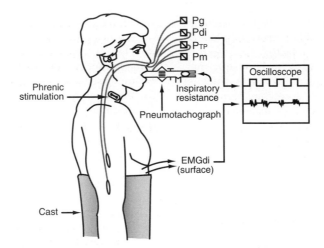

Figure 6–6

Schematic representation of the experimental approach used to assess diaphragm strength and endurance in man. Transdiaphragmatic pressure (P_{di}) is measured by catheters in the esophagus (P_{es}) and stomach (P_g) and displayed on an oscilloscope for visual feedback to the subject. The diaphragm EMG is recorded with the surface electrode on the lower rib cage. Phrenic nerves may be stimulated in the neck transcutaneously. Constancy of lung volume and thoracoabdominal configuration is achieved by monitoring end-expiratory transpulmonary pressure (P_{TP}) and by placing a cast around the abdomen and lower 1/4 of the rib cage. To assess diaphragm endurance, subjects inspire against ventilatory loads of varying severity to produce target levels of P_{di}. (Redrawn from Aubier M, Farkas A, DeTroyer RM, et al: Detection of diaphragmatic fatigue in man by phrenic stimulation. J Appl Physiol 50(3):538–544, 1981a. With permission.)

bilaterally during breath-holding at end expiration. The force output of the diaphragm is assessed from the transdiaphragmatic pressure (P_{di}) (Fig. 6–6). Transdiaphragmatic pressure is measured as the difference in abdominal and esophageal pressure ($P_{di} = P_{abd} - [-P_{es}]$). Because esophageal pressure is opposite in sign to abdominal pressure, P_{di} during inspiration may be taken as the sum of the absolute values of P_{abd} and P_{es}. The evoked diaphragmatic muscle compound action potential is recorded from surface electrodes on the anterior rib cage at the sixth or seventh intercostal space in the midclavicular line or endoesophageally to ensure that supramaximal conditions of current or voltage are achieved.

The diaphragm may shorten considerably despite airway occlusion because of collapse of the rib cage. To counteract this effect, the abdomen may be casted at functional residual capacity to prevent outward movement of the anterior abdominal wall and hence descent of the diaphragm. In the case of the sternocleidomastoid muscle, the head and neck are immobilized in a rigid frame and the airway remains open.

Motor Unit Recruitment

When the respiratory muscles are activated endogenously during volitional or reflexly driven contractions, motor unit recruitment follows a stereotypic hierarchy (Fournier et al, 1988). During eupneic breathing, only motor units made up of slow-twitch, fatigue-resistant (i.e., type I) muscle fibers are activated. While efforts of greater magnitude are made, as occurs during hypercapnea, hypoxia, bronchoconstriction, and other effects, populations of fast-twitch, oxidative (i.e., type IIa) fibers are recruited, followed ultimately by recruitment of fast-twitch, glycolytic fibers (i.e., type IIb) (Kelsen et al, 1977; Oliven et al, 1989). As mentioned, the susceptibility to fatigue of the three fiber types demonstrates the following rank order: IIb greater than IIa greater than I (Sieck et al, 1991). Accordingly, eupneic breathing is accomplished by highly fatigue-resistant type I fibers, whereas strenuous efforts approaching maximum involve more easily fatigued types IIa and IIb fibers.

The force output of a contracting skeletal muscle can be increased, therefore, by recruitment of inactive motor units. Because motor unit size is smallest for slow oxidative fibers, intermediate for fast oxidative fibers, and greatest for fast glycolytic motor units, recruitment of progressively larger fast-twitch motor units allows disproportionate rises in force to be generated.

The rank order of motor unit recruitment

most likely accounts for the fact that the diaphragm contracts rhythmically, 24 hours a day, for a lifetime and does not fatigue. In contrast, progressively more strenuous inspiratory efforts approaching the maximum may be required when ventilatory drive is high (e.g., during severe hypoxia, acidosis, hypercapnia) or when the mechanics of breathing are markedly deranged (as with pulmonary edema or asthma). However, such intense efforts are difficult to maintain for prolonged periods and predispose to muscle fatigue (see later).

LENGTH-TENSION RELATIONSHIP

Active isometric force of the respiratory muscles is a function of the extent of actin-myosin contractile filament overlap as reflected in muscle fiber length (i.e., the active length-tension relationship). For any given motor unit firing rate, active tension increases progressively as fiber length is increased. However, at some muscle fiber length overlap of actin and myosin filaments is optimal and active tension is maximal (L_0). On the other hand, passive tension depends on muscle elasticity and increases progressively in curvilinear fashion as length increases. The total force output of a respiratory muscle at any length is the sum of the active and passive tension.

In the body, respiratory muscle fiber length depends primarily upon lung volume, and to a lesser extent on thoracoabdominal configuration (Hubmayr et al, 1989; Grassino et al, 1978). Progressive increases in lung volume shorten the inspiratory muscles and lengthen the expiratory muscles. At functional residual capacity (FRC), the diaphragm is close to L_0 while the parasternal intercostals, sternocleidomastoid, and scalene muscles are shorter than L_0 (Farkas et al, 1985). Increases in lung volume, therefore, decrease the mechanical advantage of the diaphragm. Expanding lung volume increases the mechanical advantage of the parasternal and neck inspiratory muscles. In contrast, the expiratory muscles of the abdominal wall appear to be below L_0 and approach L_0 as lung volume increases. The fact that individual respiratory muscles "sit" at different positions on the length-tension curve at any given lung volume allows the aggregate pressure-generating ability of the respiratory muscles to be well maintained over a wide range of lung volume.

The effect of lung volume on the force output of the human inspiratory and expiratory muscles in aggregate is reflected in the maximal active pressure-volume diagram of the respiratory system (Fig. 6–7). To construct this relationship, subjects make maximal inspiratory or expiratory efforts against an occluded airway while muscle mechanical output is assessed from the maximal static pressure generated at the mouth. However, the recoil pressure of the relaxed respiratory system contributes to airway pressure at all lung volumes except functional residual capacity (where it is zero). The pressure generated by the actively contracting muscles, P_{mus}, is calculated by subtracting recoil pressure from maximal static inspiratory and

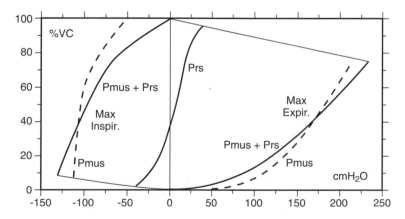

Figure 6–7
The active pressure-volume relationship of the respiratory system. Maximum static inspiratory (PI_{max}) and expiratory (PE_{max}) pressures are measured at the airway opening during a maximal voluntary effort. The pressure generated by the actively contracting muscles (P_{mus}) represents the difference between PI_{max} or PE_{max} and respiratory system passive recoil pressure (P_{rs} is represented by the solid line). Note that P_{mus} of the inspiratory muscles decreases with increasing lung volume while expiratory P_{mus} increases. (Redrawn from Roussos C [ed]: The Thorax, 2nd ed, Vol 85, 1995, p 480. With permission of Marcel Dekker, Inc.)

expiratory pressure. As can be seen, P_{mus} for the inspiratory muscles is greatest at lung volumes ranging from residual volume (RV) to FRC and progressively decreases thereafter. P_{mus} for the inspiratory muscles reaches minimal values (30 cm H_2O) at full lung inflation (i.e., at total lung capacity [TLC]). In fact, the lung volume at TLC is that lung volume at which P_{mus} is equal and opposite to respiratory system recoil pressure. In contrast, P_{mus} for the expiratory muscles is greatest at TLC and least at RV. In fact, RV is the lung volume at which expiratory P_{mus} is equal and opposite to respiratory system recoil.

The expiratory muscles are considerably stronger (about 250 cm H_2O) than the inspiratory muscles (about 150 cm H_2O). The important nonrespiratory tasks performed by these muscles that require marked increases in intra-abdominal pressure include defecation, micturition, parturition, and weight-bearing. In normal subjects, P_{mus} generated by the inspiratory muscles even during strenuous hyperventilation rarely exceeds 30 to 40 cm H_2O. Therefore, both the inspiratory and expiratory muscles have a vast reserve of pressure over that required to maintain ventilation. This considerable reserve of the respiratory muscles is essential in patients with lung or chest wall diseases in whom the mechanics of breathing are markedly deranged. PI_{max} is lower in women than men, and in men PI_{max} and P_{di} decrease with aging (Black et al, 1969; Tolep et al, 1995) (Fig. 6–8).

It is apparent from the earlier discussion that hyperinflation in the setting of obstructive lung disease represents a marked mechanical disadvantage to the inspiratory muscles but a mechanical advantage to the action of the expiratory muscles. Maximal static inspiratory pressure in subjects with COPD may be reduced to as little as approximately one-third of the values obtained in age-matched normal adults (Sharp et al, 1968) (Fig. 6–9).

Changes in thoracoabdominal configuration achieved by changes in body posture also alter fiber length and configuration of the respiratory muscles at a given lung volume (Grassino et al, 1978; Hubmayr et al, 1989). For example, at a given lung volume, P_{di} is greater when abdominal volume is decreased and rib cage volume is increased. Presumably, this chest wall configuration diminishes the radius curvature of the diaphragm (R) and results in greater pressure for the same tension (T) in accordance with the LaPlace relationship (i.e., $P_{di} = 2 \, T/R$). The supine posture (typical of bedridden critically ill patients) reduces abdominal volume and increases rib cage volume and, everything else being equal, augments the mechanical action of the diaphragm.

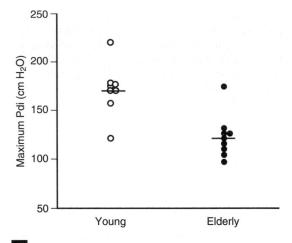

Figure 6–8
The effect of aging on maximal static transdiaphragmatic pressure (Pdi_{max}) in normal young and elderly men. Pdi_{max} measured during the performance of an expulsive Mueller maneuver with visual feedback of the P_{di} signal. Note that Pdi_{max} is about 25% lower in the healthy elderly group. (Redrawn from Tolep K, Higgins N, Muza S, et al: Comparison of diaphragm strength between healthy adult elderly and young men. Am J Crit Care Med 152:677–682, 1995. With permission.)

Conversely, the flattened diaphragm in patients who are hyperinflated with severe COPD or asthma has a greater radius of curvature, and hence converts tension into pressure less effectively than when the curvature is normal. Of interest, severely ill patients with COPD spontaneously adopt body postures that favorably affect the mechanical action of the inspiratory muscles. For example, patients with severe obstructive lung disease flex the trunk, compress the abdomen, and hyperextend the head. This posture improves the mechanical advantage of the diaphragm and neck inspiratory muscles (Druz et al, 1982). It is important to note, however, that chronic alterations in lung volume and thoracoabdominal configuration induce adaptive changes in the length-tension characteristics of the diaphragm. For example, in experimental animals, chronic hyperinflation causes a leftward shift of the length-tension characteristic of the costal regimen of the diaphragm (Supinski et al, 1982; Farkas et al, 1982) (Fig. 6–10). In patients with chronic hyperinflation, this alteration could help to restore the mechanical advantage of the diaphragm toward normal (Oliven et al, 1986; Similowski et al, 1991). Length-tension adaptations, however, do not overcome the deleterious effects of diaphragm flattening, which act through the LaPlace relationship.

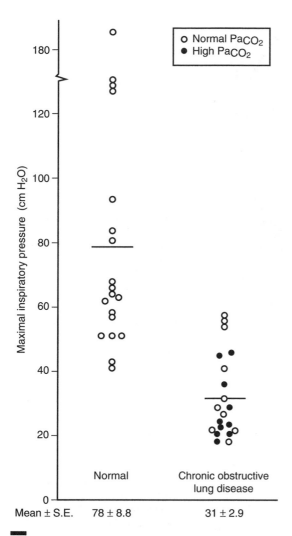

Figure 6–9
Maximum static inspiratory pressure (PI_{max}) measured in stable outpatients with COPD and age-matched normal subjects. COPD subjects demonstrate significantly lower PI_{max} than normals because of hyperinflation and muscle wasting. Hypercapnic COPD subjects *(solid symbols)* generated lower PI_{max} than eucapnic subjects *(open symbols)*. (Redrawn from Sharp JT, van Lith P, Nuchprayoon C, et al: The thorax in chronic obstructive lung disease. Am J Med 44:39–46, 1968. With permission.)

FORCE-VELOCITY RELATIONSHIP

The respiratory muscles do not contract isometrically but rather shorten against a load. Application of loads diminishes the velocity of shortening and converts the energy of crossbridge cycling into force (i.e., the isotonic force-velocity relationship) (see Fig. 6–5). The force developed by contracting respiratory muscles is inversely related to the velocity of shortening. *In vivo*, the inspiratory muscles contract against a load (i.e., the inspiratory impedance), which increases throughout inspiration as the muscle shortens. Inspiratory impedance is a function of respiratory resistance and compliance. (The resistive load progressively decreases while the elastic load increases.) The analogue of the isotonic force-velocity relationship in intact man is the maximal inspiratory pressure-flow curve. This relationship is nearly linear rather than hyperbolic (Agostoni et al, 1960; McCool et al, 1986) (Fig. 6–11).

An important consequence of the force-velocity relationship is that it provides an intrinsic muscle mechanism to augment force output when the load on the contracting respiratory muscles is increased. Derangements in the mechanical properties of the lungs and airways that increase inspiratory impedance reduce muscle shortening velocity and, hence, increase force generation.

Another implication of the force-velocity relationship is that assessment of inspiratory muscle strength in patients must be performed when the airway is occluded so as to minimize muscle shortening. (Some degree of inspiratory muscle shortening occurs despite airway occlusion because of thoracic gas decompression and paradoxical movement of the abdomen and rib cage.)

FATIGABILITY

Respiratory muscle fatigue has been defined as a loss in the capacity to develop force and/or shorten resulting from muscle fiber activity under load that was reversible by rest (Respiratory Muscle Fatigue Workshop, 1990). The important operational components of the definition of fatigue involve impaired mechanical output of the muscle and its reversibility with rest. In addition, fatigue-induced mechanical impairment of muscle function is viewed as developing when the muscle is highly active and generating appreciable levels of force. Recovery from fatigue is generally observed over a short time scale (i.e., minutes to hours). A commonly accepted classification of fatigue based on presumed sites of impaired function within the neuromuscular system is given in Table 6–1.

In contrast to fatigue, respiratory muscle weakness has been defined as impairment in the capacity of a fully rested muscle to generate force. Muscle weakness is commonly caused by muscle fiber atrophy, metabolic derangements that impair the ability of crossbridges to generate force (e.g., acidosis or electrolyte abnormalities that affect intracellular calcium flux), or chronic reductions in muscle precontraction length that impose a

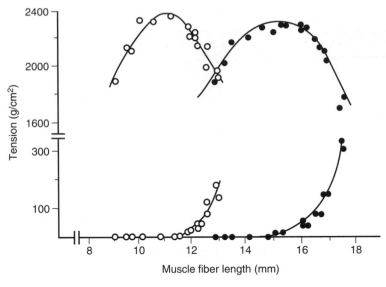

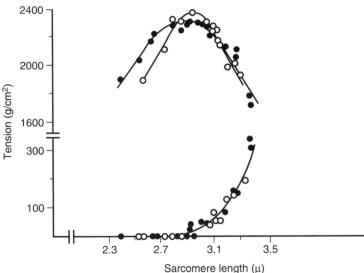

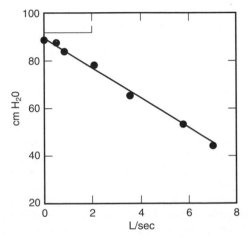

Figure 6–10
Active *(upper panel)* and passive *(lower panel)* length-tension relationship of the costal diaphragm of emphysematous *(open circles)* and normal hamsters *(solid circles)*. The apex of the active length-tension curve represents Lo. Note that in emphysematous animals, the length-tension curve is displaced toward shorter fiber lengths. This adaptive change allows the diaphragm to generate maximal tension (force) at shorter fiber lengths and helps preserve the contractile performance in the face of considerable hyperinflation. (Redrawn from Supinski GS and Kelsen SC: Effect of elastase-induced emphysema on the force-generating ability of the diaphragm. J Clin Invest 70:978–988, 1982. With permission.)

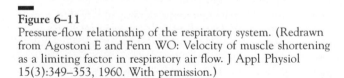

Figure 6–11
Pressure-flow relationship of the respiratory system. (Redrawn from Agostoni E and Fenn WO: Velocity of muscle shortening as a limiting factor in respiratory air flow. J Appl Physiol 15(3):349–353, 1960. With permission.)

Table 6–1
Classification of Respiratory Muscle Fatigue

Central: decreases in phrenic motor output mediated by spinal or supraspinal mechanisms

Peripheral: fatigue occurring at the level of the muscle itself
Transmission—failure of mechanisms involved in muscle excitation (i.e., high-frequency fatigue)
Contractile—failure of mechanisms involved in excitation-contraction coupling or contractile protein function (i.e., low-frequency fatigue)

mechanical disadvantage (e.g., hyperinflation of the thorax and its effects on the inspiratory muscles). Implied in the definition of weakness is the idea that alterations in muscle function are the consequence of alterations in muscle structure or lung volume, and hence they induce changes that are more slowly reversible than fatigue (e.g., days to weeks).

In the clinical setting, the distinction between muscle weakness and fatigue is difficult and is not easily accomplished. Moreover, as will become apparent in the remainder of this chapter, a close association exists between respiratory muscle weakness and respiratory muscle fatigue. In fact, weak muscles are predisposed to fatigue (see later).

The changes in muscle contractile properties produced when the respiratory muscles fatigue are shown in Figure 6–5 and have been studied extensively (Aubier et al, 1981a, b, c; Aubier et al, 1985a; Kelsen et al, 1982; Road et al, 1987; Enoka and Stewart, 1992).

Fatigue prolongs contraction and relaxation time. Slowing of the tension wave form is thought to result from impaired calcium release from storage sites in the sarcoplasmic reticulum and in its rate of reuptake (Fitts, 1994). Fatigue also depresses the force generated at a given frequency and displaces the isometric length-tension relationship downward so that at a given fiber length, tension is diminished. Fatigue also diminishes the velocity of muscle fiber shortening against a given load. These changes indicate that fatigue not only diminishes the load-bearing capacity of the respiratory muscles (i.e., maximal force output) but also slows the velocity of shortening at a given force or load.

Depending upon the nature of the fatigue-inducing regimen, depression of force output can occur at primarily subtetanizing frequencies (e.g., <15–20 Hz), which is a condition called low-frequency fatigue, or at frequencies greater than

50 Hz, which is a condition called high-frequency fatigue (Aubier et al, 1981a) (see Table 6–1). The biochemical and biophysical processes that underlie low-frequency and high-frequency fatigue differ. Muscle force responses to tetanizing frequencies of stimulation (i.e., >50 Hz) are primarily determined by the processes of neuromuscular transmission (Metzger et al, 1986). High-frequency fatigue reflects impairment in muscle excitation at the level of neurotransmitter release at the neuromuscular junction, sarcolemma propagation of an action potential, or charge transfer within the T tubular system.

At subtetanizing frequencies (i.e., generally <15–20 Hz) muscle mechanical output is primarily determined by the processes of excitation-contraction coupling (e.g., calcium release from the sarcoplasmic reticulum, calcium-troponin interactions). Low-frequency fatigue appears to reflect impairments in the dihydropyridine-sensitive charge sensor in the T tubular system, the ryanodine-sensitive calcium channel in the sarcoplasmic reticulum, or the binding affinity of activator calcium to tropomyosin (Fitts, 1994). Low-frequency fatigue may be caused in part by oxygen free radical–induced injury (Reid M et al, 1992; Nashawati et al, 1993; Anzueto et al, 1994). Low- and high-frequency fatigue reflect impairments occurring at the level of the muscle and hence have been termed *peripheral fatigue*. Of interest, recovery from high-frequency fatigue is more rapid (i.e., minutes) than recovery from low-frequency fatigue (i.e., hours) (Aubier et al, 1981a; Laghi et al, 1995). Moreover, the two forms of fatigue have different physiologic consequences. High-frequency fatigue impairs muscle force output under conditions in which the muscle is maximally driven by the central nervous system (CNS) (i.e., when muscle strength is being evaluated). Low-frequency fatigue, on the other hand, impairs force generation during eupneic breathing when phrenic motor unit discharge rates are typically approximately 15 Hz (Iscoe et al, 1976).

Low-frequency fatigue may preferentially affect the tension developed at shorter fiber lengths when the activation process in general appears to be submaximal. Slowing of the twitch contraction wave form in the fatigued muscle, especially the prolonged rate of muscle relaxation, may displace the force-frequency curve leftward. That is, the stimulation frequency required to achieve a fully fused contraction may be lower following fatigue if relaxation time is markedly prolonged. Changes in the rate of relaxation of fatigued muscle seem to be sensed by the CNS and elicit a slowing in neuronal firing rates in limb muscles during maximal isometric voluntary contractions.

Fatigue during performance of ventilatory tasks requiring intense efforts may also be associated with a reduction in central motor output and failure of the CNS to fully activate the respiratory muscles (Bazzy and Haddad, 1984; Scardella et al, 1986; Bellemare and Bigland-Ritchie, 1987; Petrozzino et al, 1990). That is, conditions in which the mechanics of breathing are markedly abnormal may be associated with a reduction in diaphragm electromyogram (EMG) or phrenic neural activity. This failure of CNS mechanisms to fully activate the muscle has been termed *central fatigue*.

The mechanisms underlying central fatigue are poorly understood. It is not clear whether central fatigue represents a behavioral response elicited by the unpleasant sensations present during ventilatory loading (see dyspnea, later) or is mediated reflexly. Of interest, afferent information arising in diaphragm golgi tendon organs and type III and type IV endings and spindle organs in the intercostal muscles reflexly modify the intensity and timing of phrenic motor activity in deeply anesthetized animals (Bolser et al, 1987; Frazier et al, 1991). Central fatigue may be mediated by changes in brain endorphin levels; it can be partially reversed by intravenous administration of the opiate antagonist naloxone (Scardella et al, 1986).

Fatigue also alters the power spectral content of the raw EMG of the respiratory muscles (Bigland-Ritchie et al, 1981; Moxham et al, 1982; Aldrich et al, 1983; Hägg et al, 1992). The EMG power spectral content can be analyzed by fast Fourier transform to generate the curvilinear relationship shown in Figure 6–12. In the fresh diaphragm, the power (or voltage) contained in the EMG wave form reaches a maximum between approximately 85 to 105 Hz, and thereafter declines. Maximal power in the EMG of the diaphragm, parasternal intercostal, and sternocleidomastoid muscles occurs at somewhat different frequencies, however. Fatigue-inducing contractions cause a leftward shift of the power spectral density of respiratory muscle such that more of the power in the EMG is contained in a lower frequency domain. Of note, the power spectral density of the contracting diaphragm changes almost immediately in the setting of fatiguing contractions and considerably before the mechanical output of the muscle fails (Bellemare and Grassino, 1982a, b). The EMG power spectrum has been taken as a useful indicator of the presence of muscle fatigue because it is minimally invasive and requires no cooperation from the subject. Accordingly, the EMG power spectrum has proved to be a useful tool to study the patho-

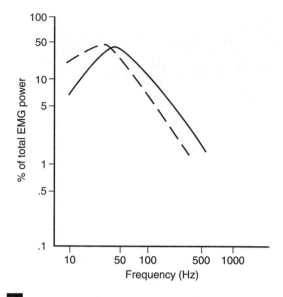

Figure 6–12
Schematic representation of the power spectral density of a respiratory muscle EMG determined by fast fourier transform. Note the concave appearance of the relationship. Note that fatigue decreases and increases power in the high- and low-frequency domains, respectively, thereby shifting the relationship toward the left. (Redrawn from Moxham J, Edwards RHT, Aubier M, et al: Changes in EMG power spectrum (high-to-low ration) with force fatigue in humans. J Appl Physiol 53(5):1094–1099, 1982. With permission.)

physiologic mechanisms of human respiratory muscle fatigue.

The physiologic basis for shifts in the power spectral density of the muscle is not well understood (Hägg et al, 1992). Possibilities include slowing in action potential conduction velocity along the sarcolemma membrane; reduction in the activity of upper and/or lower respiratory motor neurons with consequent reductions in motor unit firing rate; and greater synchronization of firing of activated motor units. There is strong evidence that the EMG power spectrum depends primarily on the firing pattern of the bulbospinal respiratory motor neurons in the medulla, which project to the spinal phrenic motor neuron pool. In fact, the power spectrum may change when central respiratory motor output is heightened even in the absence of fatigue (e.g., hypercapnia in the absence of load) (Sieck et al, 1985). Moreover, the power spectrum of the diaphragm may increase in response to centrally acting drugs (e.g., the endogenous opiate antagonist naloxone) even when the muscle is fatigued by severe inspiratory ventilatory loads (Scardella et al, 1986).

In humans, studies examining the pathogenesis of respiratory muscle fatigue have largely been performed in a laboratory setting on highly motivated subjects performing intense volitional contractions (Roussos and Macklem, 1977; Bellemare and Grassino, 1982a, b; Clanton et al, 1985; Pardy et al, 1985). Experiments have involved severe ventilatory loads to the point of exhaustion and have focused on the diaphragm because of its importance in respiration and its accessibility to measurement. The endpoint of these fatigue trials has been taken as the point at which target P_{di} could not be maintained (Loke et al, 1982; Levine et al, 1988; Murciano et al, 1988) Mador et al, 1993; Johnson et al, 1993) (Figs. 6–13 to 6–15).

However, diaphragm fatigue also occurs in normal subjects during the performance of maximal exercise, and in mechanically ventilated patients with severe cardiopulmonary disease.

Laboratory studies have demonstrated that susceptibility of the diaphragm to fatigue depends on: (1) the pattern of muscle use; (2) muscle strength; and (3) muscle blood flow. However, the most important determinant of fatigue is the intensity and timing of diaphragm contractile activity (Bellemare and Grassino, 1982a; Clanton et al, 1985, 1990). The fatigability of the diaphragm can be quantitated in terms of the ratio between peak P_{di} generated during contraction to the maximal possible P_{di} ($P_{di}/P_{di_{max}}$). Figure 6–14

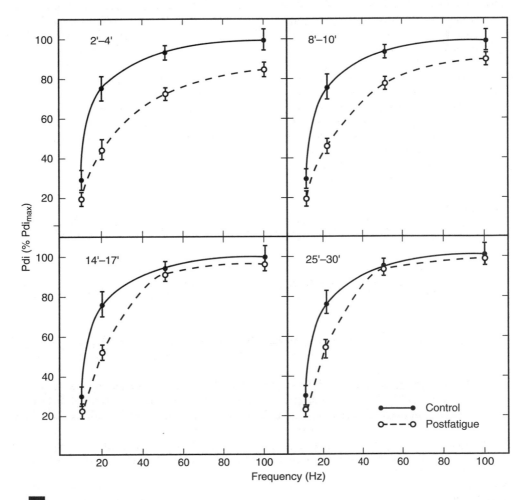

Figure 6–13
Force-frequency relationship of the human diaphragm showing the rate of recovery from high- and low-frequency fatigue. Data obtained in a single subject before and after a period of inspiratory resistive loading to t_{lim} (time to fatigue). Note the presence of both high- and low-frequency fatigue immediately after loading. Note also that high-frequency fatigue disappears within 10 to 14 minutes but low-frequency fatigue persists for the duration of the study. (Redrawn from Aubier M, Farkas A, DeTroyer RM, et al: Detection of diaphragmatic fatigue in man by phrenic stimulation. J Appl Physiol 50(3):538–544, 1981a. With permission.)

Figure 6–14

Effect of increasing P_{di}/Pdi_{max} (i.e., the ratio of peak inspiratory P_{di} during resistance breathing over maximal static P_{di} (*ordinate*) on the time of onset of mechanical failure of the diaphragm, t_{lim} (*abscissa*). Data are from three normal subjects (*shown as separate symbols*). Note that progressive increases in P_{di}/Pdi_{max} are associated with more rapid onset of diaphragm fatigue. Note also the curvilinear nature of the relationship with apparent asymptote between 40 and 50% P_{di}/Pdi_{max}, which represents a fatigue threshold. (Redrawn from Roussos CS and Macklem PT: Diaphragmatic fatigue in man. J Appl Physiol 43(2):189–197, 1977. With permission.)

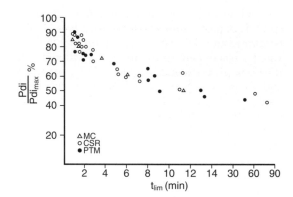

demonstrates the effect of increasing P_{di}/Pdi_{max} on the time to fatigue (t_{lim}). With very high values of P_{di}/Pdi_{max}, time to fatigue is short but increases rapidly as P_{di}/Pdi_{max} decreases.

Because the diaphragm contracts rhythmically, its activity is reflected not only in the peak inspiratory P_{di}, but as well in the duration of inspiration (Ti) and can be quantitated as the area under a curve of tension versus time. This parameter has been termed the tension-time index (TTI) and is the product of peak P_{di}/Pdi_{max} multiplied by Ti over the duration of the total respiratory cycle (i.e., Ti/Ttot). Mathematically, the TTI = $P_{di}/Pdi_{max} \times$ Ti/Ttot. (The Ti/Ttot ratio has been termed the *duty cycle of breathing* and represents the portion of the respiratory cycle during which the diaphragm is active.) When the diaphragm TTI exceeds approximately 15 to 20% of maximum, fatigue occurs (Bellemare and Grassino, 1982a, b; Bellemare and Grassino, 1983b) (Figs. 6–16 and 6–17). Thus, the fatigue threshold can be reached by increasing P_{di} or Ti/Ttot or decreasing Pdi_{max}.

Increases in P_{di} occur when minute ventila-

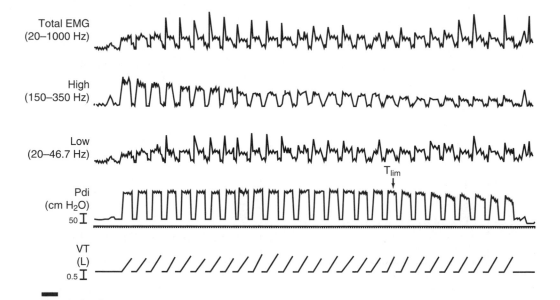

Figure 6–15

Polygraph record of a fatigue run at 75% Pdi_{max} and a t_i/t_{tot} of 60% produced during inspiratory resistive ventilatory loading. Total integrated diaphragm EMG signal in bandwidth is between 20 and 1000 Hz; high integrated EMG signal is in bandwidth 150 to 350 Hz; low integrated EMG signal is in the bandwidth 20 to 46.7 Hz. Time markers on the x axis are 1 sec; t_{lim} indicates the time that the breathing effort could be sustained. Note that the EMG power in the high- and low-frequency domain change on the first several breaths well before t_{lim} occurs. (Redrawn from Bellemare F and Grassino A: Evaluation of human diaphragm fatigue. J Appl Physiol 53(5):1196–1206, 1982b. With permission.)

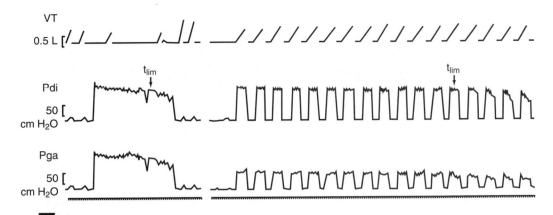

Figure 6–16

Polygraph record effect of the breathing duty cycle, t_i/t_{tot}, on the time of mechanical failure of the diaphragm, t_{lim}. Subject is generating the same level of peak P_{di} (75%) but two different values of t_i/t_{tot}. Note that the continuous effort, a t_i/t_{tot} of 100%, is associated with more rapid onset of diaphragm fatigue. (Redrawn from Bellemare F and Grassino A: Effect of pressure and timing of contraction on human diaphragm fatigue. J Appl Physiol 53(5):1190–1195, 1982a. With permission.)

tion increases (i.e., inspiratory airflow or the tidal volume increase); when airway resistance is increased by bronchoconstriction or retained secretions; or when lung or chest wall compliance is

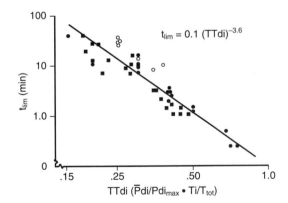

Figure 6–17

Relationship of the time of mechanical failure of the diaphragm, t_{lim}, and TT_{di}, the diaphragm pressure-time index (i.e., the product of $P_{di}/Pdi_{max} \times t_i/t_{tot}$). Data were obtained in normal subjects during strenuous volitional contractions performed in the setting of inspiratory resistive ventilatory loading. The two scales are logarithmic. Note that above approximately 15% TT_{di}, t_{lim} decreases progressively with increasing TT_{di}. These data indicate that the effects of the magnitude and timing of diaphragm contractions on diaphragm endurance collapse into the primary factor, the TT_{di}. (Redrawn from Bellemare F and Grassino A: Effect of pressure and timing of contraction on human diaphragm fatigue. J Appl Physiol 53(5):1190–1195, 1982a. With permission.)

decreased by lung edema, atelectasis, or pneumonia. In addition, tachypnea decreases the duration of expiration (Te) out of proportion to the duration of inspiration (Ti), thereby increasing the Ti/Ttot ratio and the TTI. Diaphragm contractions above approximately 50 to 60% of maximum predispose to fatigue since the Ti/Ttot usually ranges between 33 and 40%.

Alternatively, the TTI can be increased by factors that impair diaphragm strength (i.e., decreased Pdi_{max}). Decreases in Pdi_{max} increase the TTI for a given set of lung mechanical properties and minute ventilation. Reductions in Pdi_{max} occur with aging hyperinflation, muscle atrophy (e.g., prolonged undernutrition or cachexia), or derangements in blood chemistry (e.g., hypercapnia, profound hypoxia, hypocalcemia, hypokalemia, hypomagnesemia).

The clinical conditions that predispose to inspiratory muscle fatigue are listed in Table 6–2.

RESPIRATORY MUSCLE BLOOD FLOW

The long-term maintenance of respiratory muscle function depends upon the balance between the rate at which adenosine triphosphate (ATP) supplies are generated and broken down. Respiratory muscle blood flow is the major mechanism by which these processes are maintained in equilibrium and fatigue prevented. In turn, respiratory muscle blood flow, like blood flow in other skeletal muscles, depends on neural, humoral, mechan-

Table 6–2

Clinical Conditions Predisposing to Respiratory Muscle Fatigue

1. Abnormal lung or chest wall mechanics—hyperinflation, increased airway resistance, decreased compliance (e.g., COPD, asthma, interstitial pulmonary fibrosis, kyphoscoliosis, ARDS)
2. Increased ventilatory drive—hypoxemia, hypercapnia, fever, acidosis, lung injury inflammation (e.g., sepsis, ARDS, pneumonia, pulmonary embolus, post-thoracotomy)
3. Low cardiac output state—cardiogenic, hypovolemic or septic shock; congestive heart failure
4. Metabolic abnormalities—hypercapnia, metabolic acidosis, hypoxemia, electrolyte disturbances
5. Nutritional depletion—chronic protein-calories malnutrition, hypoglycemia, starvation
6. Aging

ical (intramuscular pressure), and circulatory factors (e.g., arterial profusion pressure, blood volume, and cardiac output).

Most information on respiratory muscle blood flow has been accumulated from studies on the diaphragmatic vascular bed. The diaphragm blood flow has several sources of inflow and extensive collateralization (Comtois et al, 1987) (Fig. 6–18). In the human diaphragm, the intercostal, *ipsilateral* inferior phrenic and internal mammary arteries anastomose head-to-head to form costo-

phrenic arcades. The venous drainage exhibits a similar configuration. The high degree of collateral flow through these several arterial inputs allows diaphragm contractile activity to be unaffected by ligation of the inferior phrenic arteries even in the face of highly intense contractions.

The level of respiratory muscle contractile activity is the most important determinant of respiratory muscle blood flow. Respiratory muscle blood flow rises with increases in minute ventilation achieved by physical exertion, hypercapnia, or hypoxia. Nonetheless, the largest increases in diaphragm blood flow occur during inspiratory resistive-loaded breathing or phrenic nerve pacing, with values approximating 210 to 265 ml/min per 100 g of tissue. Cardiac muscle is the only organ with higher blood flow (approximately 600 ml/min per 100 g of tissue). It seems likely that the substantial rise in respiratory muscle blood flow in response to increased muscle metabolic demand is achieved by release of endothelium–derived relaxing factor identified pharmacologically as nitric oxide (NO) and other known mediators of exercised-induced hyperemia (e.g., adenosine, ATP, lactate, inorganic phosphate, and potassium).

Although increasing contractile activity heightens muscle blood flow, sufficiently intense contractions can actually interrupt blood flow (Bellemare et al, 1983a; Bark et al, 1987) (Fig. 6–19). The effect of contraction on diaphragm blood flow is achieved by increases in intramuscular pressure compressing the intramuscular blood vessels. Diaphragm blood flow in the dog is com-

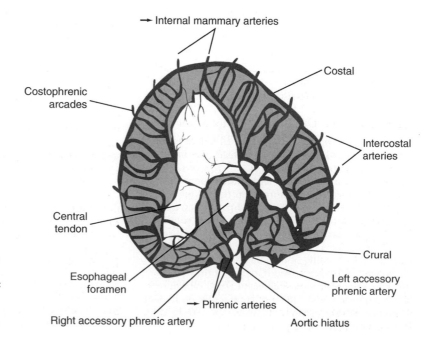

Figure 6–18

Anatomy of the arterial supply of the dog diaphragm. (Redrawn from Roussos C [ed]: The Thorax, 2nd ed, Vol 85, 1995, p 638. With permission of Marcel Dekker, Inc.)

Internal mammary arteries

Costal

Costophrenic arcades

Intercostal arteries

Central tendon

Crural

Esophageal foramen

Left accessory phrenic artery

Phrenic arteries

Right accessory phrenic artery

Aortic hiatus

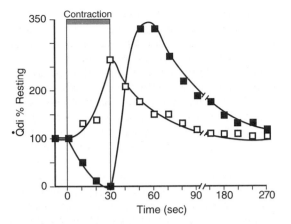

Figure 6–19

Effect of a single sustained contraction (30 seconds) on diaphragm muscle blood flow in the anesthetized dog. Blood flow ($\dot{Q}_{di}$) to the perfused costal diaphragm muscle strip preparation was measured by collecting the phrenic venous effluent. Muscle contraction was induced by electrical stimulation of the phrenic neve. The contraction period is followed by 4 minutes of rest. (*Open squares*) Tension = 10% of maximum; (*closed squares*) tension = 80% of maximum. Note that 80% contraction mechanically impedes blood flow during the period of contraction and elicits a post-contraction hyperemia lasting several minutes. (Redrawn from Bark H and Supinski G: Relationship of changes in diaphragmatic muscle blood flow to muscle contractile activity. J Appl Physiol 62(1):291–299, 1987. With permission.)

pletely abolished when P_{di} is equal to or greater than 80% of maximum. In fact, contractions above 30 to 40% of Pdi_{max} impede blood flow, and blood flow largely occurs during expiration. Progressive increases in Ti/Ttot, at a given P_{di}/Pdi_{max}, therefore, further compromise blood flow. Accordingly, diaphragm blood flow is a function of the TTI. Diaphragmatic perfusion, therefore, appears to be similar to that of perfusion through the myocardium. Diaphragmatic blood flow is reduced or interrupted during inspiration (systole), and is re-established during expiration (diastole).

The relationship between TTI and blood flow in the dog diaphragm is shown in Figures 6–19 and 6–20 (Bellemare et al, 1983a; Bark et al, 1987). Blood flow increases as TTI increases to approximately 20%. At TTI above 20%, diaphragm blood flow falls, however. Therefore, increases in muscle contractile activity up to a TTI of approximately 20% are associated with increases in muscle energy supply. Contractions above TTI of 20% predispose to fatigue by decreasing blood supply while at the same time increasing muscle energy consumption.

The pattern of pleural and abdominal pressure changes also influences diaphragm blood flow at a given TTI. High positive abdominal pressures tend to decrease diaphragm blood flow, presumably by reducing venous return to the right heart. Moreover, increases in diaphragm length decrease muscle blood flow, presumably by passive increases in intramuscular pressure. A salient feature of diaphragmatic blood flow is its ability to autoregulate in response to changes in arterial pressure, which is a feature of blood flow regulation in many organs (Hussain et al, 1988). For example, in the dog, blood flow appears to be largely unchanged over a range of mean arterial pressure from approximately 70 to 120 mm Hg (Fig. 6–21). Below this range, diaphragm blood flow decreases in proportion to reductions in arterial pressure. Therefore, the dog diaphragm compensates effectively for sudden changes in arterial pressure or

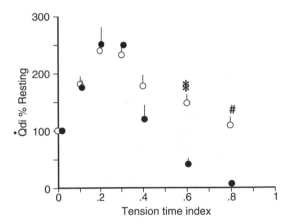

Figure 6–20

The relationship of diaphragm blood flow to diaphragm contractile activity as reflected in the tension time index of the electrically stimulated, rhythmically contracting dog diaphragm (same preparation as in Fig. 6–19). Note the curvilinear relationship of blood flow and contractile activity during 30 seconds of contraction. (*Closed circles*) T_i/t_{tot} of 100%; (*open circles*) tension 100% of maximum. Blood flow reaches a maximum at a tension time index of approximately 20% of maximum and thereafter falls progressively with increasing activity. Note, however, that above the critical tension time index of 20%, duty cycle of 100% produces greater reductions in blood flow than tension of 100%. These data indicate that the level of diaphragm activity reflected in the TTI determines its blood flow and that the pattern of contractions has important effects. (Redrawn from Bark H and Supeniski G: Relationship of changes in diaphragmatic muscle blood flow to muscle contractile activity. J Appl Physiol 62(1):291–299, 1987. With permission.)

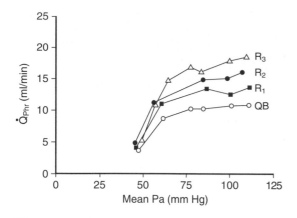

Figure 6–21
Effect of changes in arterial blood pressure on diaphragm blood flow in the dog. Note that blood flow is relatively constant over a wide range of blood pressure (autoregulation). However, below a critical level of hypotension, blood flow falls. (Redrawn from Roussos C [ed]: The Thorax, 2nd ed, Vol 85, 1995, p 654. With permission.)

cardiac output over a modest range. Assuming that a similar operating range applies to the human diaphragm, reduction in mean arterial pressure to less than 60 mm Hg will reduce diaphragm blood flow and predispose to fatigue. Accordingly, patients with hypotension are likely to experience a reduction in diaphragm blood flow. Unfortunately, hypotension and sepsis also heighten ventilatory demand, thus increasing the TTI of the diaphragm and its metabolic activity. Sepsis also impedes oxygen extraction and reduces the arteriovenous oxygen content difference. In animal models, sepsis increases lactate production by the diaphragm.

Hypotension and sepsis, therefore, are likely to severely stress the relationship between diaphragm metabolic demand and the ability of the diaphragm circulation to deliver vital substrates. The development of respiratory failure in the hypotensive or septic patient may be a consequence of a reduction in diaphragm blood flow or impaired oxygen uptake.

BEDSIDE ASSESSMENT OF RESPIRATORY MUSCLE FUNCTION

SYMPTOMS

Dyspnea

The precise mechanisms that underlie the sensation of dyspnea are unclear and probably multifac-

torial (Manning et al, 1995). However, dyspnea occurs commonly in the setting of inspiratory muscle weakness and/or fatigue. In fact, an important determinant of the sense of dyspnea is the magnitude of the CNS motor command to the inspiratory muscles (Killian et al, 1985; Manning et al, 1995). Inspiratory muscle weakness or fatigue requires an increase in neuronal firing rate and/or motor unit recruitment to preserve inspiratory pressure. Increased dyspnea in the setting of inspiratory muscle fatigue probably reflects the greater motor command required to generate a given level of muscle force. In fact, the factors that contribute to respiratory muscle dysfunction, that is, the TTI, also underlie the sensation of respiratory effort or dyspnea. In particular, the magnitude of the sense of dyspnea depends on: (1) inspiratory pressure swings as a percent of maximum, (i.e., P/P_{max}); (2) duration of inspiration, Ti; and (3) the respiratory rate (i.e., 60/Ttot) (Killian et al, 1985). The sensation of dyspnea can be expressed quantitatively by each of these parameters raised to a power:

$$\text{Dyspnea} = P^{1.3} \times Ti/Ttot^{1.14} \times freq^{-0.97}.$$

Given the greater exponential value for P than for the timing variables, it can be seen that the magnitude of the swing in inspiratory pressure is the predominant factor. In contrast, respiratory muscle fatigue does not appear to depend upon the manner in which a TTI is arrived at, whereas dyspnea does. That is, whether a given TTI is arrived at by a higher P/P_{max} or a higher Ti/Ttot is irrelevant in the development of fatigue but is important in the generation of respiratory sensations.

Of interest, the diaphragm appears to be relatively insensate, and it may be possible to selectively fatigue the diaphragm without generating a sense of dyspnea (Bradley et al, 1986; Ward et al, 1988). This procedure is likely to be rare clinically and is confined to patients with cervical spine injury. Dyspnea may be related to the level of activity of neck and rib cage accessory inspiratory muscles. Because recruitment of the neck and rib cage inspiratory muscles occurs when ventilatory demand is increased or the mechanics of breathing are deranged, the sense of dyspnea may reflect a condition in which reserve inspiratory muscles are recruited to cope with ventilatory stress.

PHYSICAL SIGNS OF RESPIRATORY MUSCLE DYSFUNCTION

Physical signs of respiratory muscle dysfunction revolve around (1) evidence of accessory respiratory muscle recruitment; (2) abnormal thoracoabdominal movement; and (3) tachypnea.

Use of Accessory Muscles

Intense respiratory efforts are associated with visible activation of the neck accessory muscles, interosseous intercostals, abdominal expiratory muscles, and flaring of the nostrils via the alae nasi muscles. These signs can be detected by inspection and palpation.

Abnormal Thoracoabdominal Movement

Normally in the supine posture, the anterior abdominal wall displays a prominent outward movement during inspiration. With impaired diaphragm function, as occurs in the setting of diaphragm paralysis (e.g., "phrenic frostbite" following cold cardioplegia) or fatigue, the abdominal wall may move inward on inspiration (so-called abdominal paradox [see Fig. 6–4]). Abdominal paradox reflects cephalad movement of the contracting diaphragm in response to the negative intrathoracic pressure generated by the inspiratory action of the neck and intercostal muscles. Abdominal paradox may also be present in patients with marked derangements in lung mechanics in whom inspiratory intrathoracic pressure swings exceed 30% of maximum (Tobin et al, 1987). Abdominal paradox, therefore, is not specific for diaphragm weakness or fatigue.

Abdominal paradox resulting from ineffectual contractions of the diaphragm should be distinguished from "pseudo-abdominal paradox" resulting from strong contractions of the expiratory muscles during expiration with rapid relaxation during early inspiration, as is seen in some patients with COPD. For example, intense contraction of the transverse abdominis muscles causes inward movement of the lateral abdominal wall and outward movement of the anterior abdominal wall during expiration. Subsequent relaxation of the abdominal muscles with the onset of inspiration causes outward movement of the lateral abdominal wall and inward movement of the anterior abdominal wall. Tenseness of the lateral abdominal wall during expiration easily distinguishes pseudo-abdominal paradox from true abdominal paradox.

In addition, inward movement of the anterior abdominal wall because of transient reduction in abdominal pressure is not maintained throughout inspiration. Descent of the diaphragm later in inspiration subsequently increases abdominal pressure and causes outward movement of the abdominal wall. Measurement of swings in gastric pressure during inspiration can help distinguish true paradox ($P_{gastric}$ decreases) from pseudoparadox ($P_{gastric}$ increases). This can be accomplished by placing a gastric balloon. In patients with nasogastric tubes, the direction of change of a water column in the tube may provide the same information.

Tachypnea

Conscious humans fatigued by inspiratory resistive loads in the laboratory adopt a shallow, rapid pattern of breathing after fatigue. Patients with acute exacerbations of COPD in hypercapnic respiratory failure demonstrate a similar pattern of breathing, which tends to disappear as patients improve clinically (Sorli et al, 1978; Aubier et al, 1980). Rapid, shallow breathing is accomplished by reductions in the duration of Ti and the duration of expiration, Te. However, reductions in Ti are disproportionately greater than reductions in Te. Accordingly, the Ti/Ttot ratio is decreased. A rapid shallow breathing pattern minimizes the TTI of the inspiratory muscles and, therefore, represents a mechanism to reduce their activity level. However, reductions in tidal volume tend to increase the dead space/tidal volume ratio and predispose to hypercapnea. A rapid shallow breathing pattern, therefore, tends to increase $PaCO_2$.

The pattern of breathing has been quantitated in adults receiving ventilatory support for acute respiratory failure from the ratio of respiratory rate (breaths/min) divided by tidal volume (liters) (Yang et al, 1991). This parameter has been termed the rapid shallow breathing index (RSBI) and has proved to be an extremely powerful way of assessing weanability from respirators in adults with a variety of medical and surgical conditions. The greater the value, the more rapid and shallow the pattern of breathing. Values for the RSBI exceeding 100 are associated with a high probability (~80%) of failure to wean from mechanical ventilation.

In animal models, tidal volume is decreased with fatigue because of reductions in Ti and peak diaphragm and external intercostal electrical activity (Oliven et al, 1988). In addition, tidal volume is decreased because the pressure generated for a given level of muscle excitation (i.e., diaphragm EMG activity) is decreased.

The neurophysiologic mechanisms driving the altered pattern of breathing are unclear. Moreover, whether changes in breathing pattern are reflexly induced or whether they reflect changes in brain neurotransmitter levels (e.g., endorphins) is unclear. In addition, behavioral mechanisms activated when breathing efforts are increased may be operating in an attempt to minimize the sensation of dyspnea. The intensity of dyspnea is minimized at a given level of ventilation by breathing shallowly and rapidly because dyspnea is chiefly a function of peak inspiratory intrathoracic pressure. Increases in the frequency of breathing have quantitatively trivial effects on the sense of dyspnea. In fact, those subjects with COPD and with the greatest sensory acuity for changes in inspiratory pressure show the greatest reductions in tidal volume while breathing against severe inspiratory flow resistive loads (Oliven et al, 1985). Further work is required to determine the neurophysiologic mechanisms that alter breathing pattern and the acute situations in which these defense mechanisms are insufficient to prevent fatigue from ensuing.

The sensitivity and specificity of the symptoms and physical signs associated with diaphragm dysfunction have not been studied systematically, and their positive and negative predictive value as indicators of respiratory muscle dysfunction is unknown. However, they are useful when present.

MAXIMUM STATIC INSPIRATORY PRESSURE (PI_{max})

Perhaps the most practical bedside method of assessing the function of the inspiratory muscles contracting in aggregate is from the pressure generated during maximal volitional contractions against an occluded airway at functional residual capacity.

Reductions in PI_{max} indicate inspiratory muscle weakness or high-frequency fatigue. Improvements in maximal static inspiratory pressure occurring over several hours to several days in the patient with obstructive lung disease suggest that lung volume is improving toward normal and the mechanical disadvantage imposed on the inspiratory muscles is disappearing. More rapid improvements occurring over hours may indicate resolution of high-frequency fatigue or elimination of the metabolic disturbances (e.g., hypercapnia, hypophosphatemia) that depress inspiratory muscle function. Of note, the PI_{max} does not detect low-frequency fatigue.

Maximal static inspiratory pressure (PI_{max}) is critically dependent on patient cooperation and motivation. This often limits its use in critical care situations. However, with training, many patients can provide reproducible values. Performance of the maneuver at end-expiratory lung volume at FRC is preferred because this is the lung volume at which respiratory system recoil is zero. That is, at FRC, changes in airway pressure during inspiratory efforts equal inspiratory P_{mus}. Interpretation of changes in PI_{max} must, therefore, take into account changes in FRC with time. For example, FRC decreases with therapy in patients with asthma, which in itself increases PI_{max}.

Investigators have suggested that use of a one-way valve in which subjects exhale freely to atmosphere while the airway is occluded during inspiration for 20 to 30 seconds yields values for PI_{max} that are more reproducible than those obtained by other methods. Maintained occlusion of the airway presumably provides an asphyxia stimulus that stimulates greater inspiratory efforts. [Reproducibility is not the same as accuracy, and the use of PI_{max} to determine weaning ability and to assess inspiratory muscle function is highly controversial.]

Maximal static expiratory pressure (PE_{max}) has been used in the laboratory setting to assess the endurance properties of the expiratory muscles. However, the measurement has not been used much at the bedside because of the perception that it is more difficult to obtain consistent values of PE_{max} than of PI_{max} in breathless people.

DETECTION OF RESPIRATORY MUSCLE FATIGUE

Diaphragm muscle fatigue has been diagnosed in intact man from changes in the: (1) response of the muscle to electrical stimulation; (2) power spectral content of the EMG; and (3) PI_{max}. As will be seen, the force-frequency relationship and EMG power spectrum analyses are complex and require sophisticated electronics and instrumentation. Consequently, their use has been confined to the research laboratory. On the other hand, the PI_{max} is convenient and easily performed at the bedside but suffers from relative nonspecificity.

Electrical Stimulation

The force-frequency relationship represents a way of assessing muscle mechanical output over a wide range of stimulus intensities. Because fatigue shifts the force-frequency downward (and possibly to the left), the magnitude of the shift in the force-frequency relationship can be used to assess the severity of low- and high-frequency fatigue and the time course of recovery.

Electrical stimulation of the muscle of interest has several advantages. It allows the muscle to be activated in response to a standard stimulus without the cooperation of the subject. Hence, neurologic deficits, decreased effort, or central fatigue, which may diminish muscle activation, are circumvented and peripheral fatigue can be detected. Unfortunately, tetanizing stimuli are painful, making this an unpalatable option in unanesthetized subjects. Moreover, current spread of the stimulus activates adjacent muscles in the neck and shoulder girdle and may lead to unpleasant or dangerous side effects. Activation of other respiratory muscles that insert on the chest wall may change chest wall compliance, or the activity of agonist and/or antagonist muscles capable of changing intrathoracic pressure.

A development that shows considerable promise is electrophrenic twitch stimulation of the diaphragm (Aubier et al, 1981a, 1985a; Bellemare and Bigland-Ritchie, 1984; Gandevia et al, 1985). This approach is well tolerated. In addition, electrophrenic twitch stimulation can detect the presence of low-frequency fatigue. As is the case with skeletal muscles, prior contraction of the diaphragm to greater than 33% of maximal P_{di} elicits contraction intensity, after contraction "twitch potentiation" (i.e., 16–70% augmentation of peak twitch height). Twitch potentiation is relatively short-lived, however, and generally dissipates within 3 minutes.

By combining twitch contraction during breath-holding at end expiration with superimposed twitches applied during the performance of graded inspiratory efforts, which is the twitch occlusion technique, Pdi_{max} can be calculated. The rationale behind the twitch occlusion pressure is as follows. As a muscle is activated to a progressively greater extent, progressively more motor units are recruited. Individual motor units move up their force-frequency curve toward the plateau. Consequently, the magnitude of the superimposed twitch is inversely proportional to the extent of muscle activation (Fig. 6–22). When the muscle is maximally activated (that is, all motor units are recruited and on the flat portion of their force-frequency curve), the superimposed twitch is undetectable or zero. The twitch-occlusion technique is analyzed quantitatively by plotting the magnitude of the volitional contraction on the x axis against the magnitude of the superimposed twitch on the y axis (see Fig. 6–22). The relationship is inversely linear. When extrapolated to the x axis (that is, to zero superimposed twitch), the maximal pressure output of the muscle is determined. The twitch-occlusion technique therefore allows detection of high-frequency fatigue as well as low-frequency fatigue.

The twitch-occlusion technique has been used to assess diaphragm function in stable outpatients with COPD (Similowski et al, 1991) and to assess mechanisms of fatigue in normal subjects during volitional contractions against large external inspiratory resistive loads to exhaustion

(Bellemare et al, 1987). The twitch-occlusion method demonstrates that the fresh diaphragm can be maximally activated volitionally. However, task performance during prolonged ventilatory loading to exhaustion (that is, the ability to generate a targeted P_{di}) is in part limited by central fatigue (Bellemare and Bigland-Ritchie, 1987).

EMG Power Spectrum

The diaphragmatic EMG power spectrum can be obtained from the raw EMG of the muscle recorded from surface electrodes on the chest wall or within the esophagus. It is, therefore, relatively noninvasive and well tolerated. Moreover, the EMG power spectrum, unlike maximal static pressure, can be measured continuously (i.e., breath-by-breath) and does not require subject cooperation.

The effect of fatigue on the spectral content of the respiratory muscles has been assessed in several ways. Initial studies assessed leftward shifts in the power spectrum using band pass filters to partition the raw signal into high-frequency (>125–150 Hz) and low-frequency domains (<50 Hz) (Bellemare and Bigland-Ritchie, 1986). The integrated activity in the high- and low-frequency domains was taken as a reflection of the position of the spectrum. Leftward shifts in the spectrum induced by fatigue decrease the EMG power in a high-frequency domain (i.e., >150 Hz) and increase the power in a low-frequency domain (i.e., <50 Hz). The ratio of activity in the greater than 150-Hz range over activity in the less than 50-Hz range was taken as a reflection of this leftward shift of the EMG power spectrum and, therefore, is termed the *high/low ratio*. Twenty to thirty percent reductions in the high/low ratio have been taken as evidence of fatigue. This method obviates the need for fast Fourier analysis and, hence, sophisticated computational analysis of the EMG wave form. It can also be assessed in real time with relatively inexpensive equipment.

Another method of assessing the spectral content of an EMG signal is via the centroid (or median) frequency (i.e., the frequency at which the power below and above are equal). The centroid frequency requires sophisticated computational analysis to construct the fast Fourier transform and at present cannot be performed real time. The centroid frequency, unlike the high/low ratio, is a concept based on sound principles of signal analysis. It has a lower signal-to-noise ratio and is more stable than the high/low ratio. A significant caveat in the use of the power spectrum is the suggestion that it may be unable to

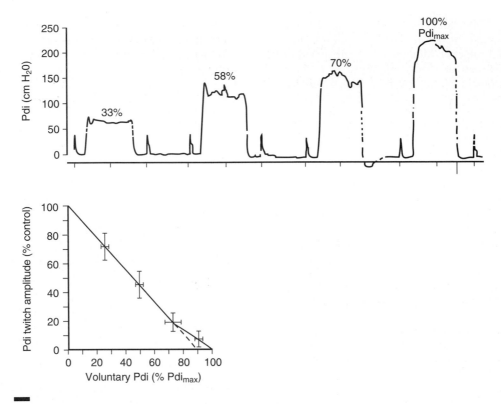

Figure 6–22

Effect of diaphragm contraction intensity as reflected in the transdiaphragmatic pressure (P_{di}) on the magnitude of the superimposed twitch contraction *(bottom panel)* and the diaphragm EMG *(top panel)*. The subject is performing progressively more intense diaphragm contractions. Vertical dotted lines in top and bottom panels mark the time at which electrical stimulus is applied to the phrenic nerves. Note that the superimposed twitch P_{di} is greatest when the diaphragm is relaxed at FRC and decreases progressively with increasingly intense volitional efforts from 33% to 100% of maximum. *(Lower panel)* Relationship between the amplitude of the voluntary P_{di} and the superimposed twitch contraction. Voluntary P_{di} and twitch P_{di} are normalized as percentages of Pdi_{max}. Note the inverse linear relationship. Maximum static P_{di} is reflected in the **x** intercept. (Redrawn from Bellemare F and Bigland-Ritchie B: Assessment of human diaphragm strength and activation using phrenic nerve stimulation. Resp Physiol 58:263–267, 1984. With permission of Elsevier Science—NL, Sara Burgerhartstraat 25, 1055 KV Amsterdam, The Netherlands.)

detect low-frequency fatigue (Moxham et al, 1982).

TREATMENT

RESPIRATORY MUSCLE WEAKNESS

The treatment of respiratory muscle weakness depends upon the pathogenic mechanisms operating. For example, inspiratory muscle weakness related to the hyperinflation of obstructive lung disease is best treated by aggressively improving airway function (e.g., β-adrenergic agonist and anticholinergic bronchodilators and corticosteroids). On the other hand, decreases in muscle strength caused by electrolyte abnormalities (e.g., hypophosphatemia) or protein calorie malnutrition are best dealt with by repleting the deficits.

The time course of recovery of muscle function is likely to depend on whether the weakness is due to an abnormality in blood chemistry or to reductions in muscle mass. For example, hypophosphatemia-induced diaphragm weakness can be corrected within hours (Aubier et al, 1985b). On the other hand, weakness related to undernutrition or prolonged corticosteroid use most likely requires days to weeks to accomplish (Rogers et al, 1992).

Inotropic agents have been used investigationally to provide long-term improvement in inspiratory muscle strength in normal subjects and outpatients with stable COPD (Murciano et al, 1989). Theophylline in doses that achieve therapeutic blood levels (i.e., 10–15 µg/ml) produces modest (i.e., ~10–20%) improvements in diaphragm contractile function in this population (Aubier at al, 1981c). However, theophylline has not been used in critically ill patients in an intensive care unit setting and it is doubtful that this class of drugs has important beneficial effects on respiratory muscle strength given its rather unfavorable therapeutic-to-toxic ratio. It seems advisable to limit the use of theophylline to its recognized role as a bronchodilator in patients with obstructive lung disease.

RESPIRATORY MUSCLE FATIGUE

The treatment of diaphragm respiratory muscle fatigue has not been systematically studied. However, several approaches based on theoretical considerations appear to be applicable (Tables 6–3 and 6–4). It is clear that diaphragm fatigue is a result of muscle overactivity (i.e., a TTI >20%). In turn, diaphragm overactivity is usually a consequent of derangements in lung mechanics (e.g., increases in airway resistance or decreases in longer chest wall compliance); increases in ventilatory drive (e.g., hypoxia, pulmonary interstitial lung disease, fever); or, most commonly, a combination of both factors. Accordingly, attempts should be made to decrease the TTI of the inspiratory muscles to values below the fatigue thresh-

Table 6–3
Principles of Therapy of Respiratory Muscle Fatigue

Decrease Inspiratory Swings in Transdiaphragmatic Pressure (P_{di})

Improve the mechanics of breathing (e.g., decrease airway resistance, improve thoracic compliance and static lung volume)

Decrease ventilatory drive (e.g., relieve hypoxemia, hypercapnia, metabolic acidosis, fever, pulmonary congestion/inflammation, ARDS)

Increase P_{dimax}

Correct hyperinflation

Correct muscle atrophy induced by protein-calorie deficiency

Correct electrolyte and blood gas abnormalities (e.g., hypoxemia, hypercapnia, hypophosphatemia, hypokalemia, hypocalcemia, hypomagnesemia)

Optimize Muscle Blood Flow and Substrate Availability

Correct low cardiac output state (e.g., cardiogenic shock, hypovolemic shock)

Correct hypoxemia, anemia, hypoglycemia

Table 6–4
Overview of Therapeutic Approaches to the Treatment of Respiratory Muscle Fatigue

Well Accepted	Experimental
Decrease pressure-time index	Vasoactive drugs (e.g., dopamine)
Optimize muscle blood flow	Antioxidants (e.g., glutathione, vitamin E, N-acetylcysteine)
Training	Muscle inotropic agents (e.g., digitalis, methylxanthines, β-adrenergic agonists)

old by addressing these two factors. For example, improvements in lung mechanics or reduction of ventilatory drive decrease the phasic swings in inspiratory pressure. In patients with abnormalities in airway resistance and hyperinflation resulting from severe obstructive lung disease, this can best be accomplished with anticholinergic and β_2-adrenergic agonist bronchodilators and corticosteroids. Reductions in ventilatory drive in hypoxic or febrile patients can be accomplished by administration of oxygen and/or antipyretics.

Studies in animal models suggest that diaphragm fatigue can be partially reversed by increasing diaphragmatic blood flow. In part, increases in blood flow may prevent or reverse fatigue by washing out toxic metabolites (e.g., H^+, lactate) (Metzger et al, 1987; Ward et al, 1992). Although mechanically produced increases in diaphragm blood flow postpone fatigue in animal models, the role of pharmacologically induced increases in diaphragm blood flow in humans is unclear. In fact, administration of the potent NO-liberating vasodilator nitroprusside fails to increase diaphragmatic blood flow during fatigue induced by electrical stimulation in experimental preparations. These data indicate a lack of a vasodilator reserve in the intensely activated fatiguing diaphragm.

In theory, diaphragm blood flow may be increased by raising arterial pressure with vasoconstrictors. The precise role of vasoconstrictors such as norepinephrine or dopamine on human respiratory muscle blood flow remain to be determined. An interesting study, however, suggests that augmenting diaphragm blood flow with dopamine (8 µg/kg per min) acutely increases P_{di} by approximately 30% in COPD subjects in acute hypercapnic respiratory failure (Aubier et al, 1983) (Fig. 6–23). The number of subjects in this study was small and the results have not as yet been confirmed, making the approach provocative but not yet advisable.

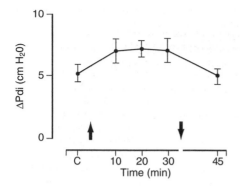

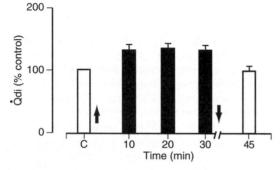

Figure 6–23
Time course of changes in twitch P_{di} during electrophrenic stimulation (*top panel*) and diaphragm blood flow ($\dot{Q}_{di}$, *bottom panel*) in eight COPD subjects in acute respiratory failure. Arrows indicate the point at which dopamine infusion (8 µg/min/kg) started and stopped. Note that dopamine infusion increased P_{di} and diaphragm blood flow. (Redrawn from Aubier M, Muriano D, Lecocquic Y, et al: Bilateral phrenic stimulation: A simple technique to assess diaphragmatic fatigue in humans. J Appl Physiol 58(1):58–64, 1985a. With permission.)

Although the role of vasoconstrictors and cardiac inotropic agents in the prevention and treatment of respiratory failure in patients with normal cardiovascular function is unclear, hypotensive patients with respiratory muscle fatigue should be treated with volume resuscitation to restore intravascular volume and vasoconstrictors as appropriate. Attempts should be made to maintain mean arterial pressure greater than 70 mm Hg. Low cardiac output states that compromise respiratory muscle blood flow (e.g., cardiogenic shock) should be treated with cardiac inotropic agents. A point that is also of importance in the setting of septic or cardiogenic shock, the respiratory muscles may be a major source of lactic acidosis and may divert blood flow from important viscera like the brain, heart, and kidney (Aubier et al, 1981b, 1982; Hussain et al, 1985; Magder et al, 1985). Accordingly, reductions in respiratory

muscle contractile activity, which decrease the demand of the respiratory muscles for blood flow, may improve visceral blood flow and blood pH. Resting the respiratory muscles during shock is thus often indicated even in the absence of overt respiratory failure until hemodynamic resuscitation is achieved.

Studies in animal models suggest that diaphragm fatigue can be partially reversed by administering free-radical scavenging, antioxidant agents such as *N*-acetylcysteine, glutathione, or vitamin E (Shindoh et al, 1990; Anzueto et al, 1994; Supinski et al, 1995). The role of these agents in the treatment of human respiratory muscle fatigue is at present investigational and awaits further study.

Unloading the inspiratory muscles by reducing the TTI may be sufficient to prevent or reverse fatigue and allow the muscle to recover. However, in some cases, respiratory muscle fatigue may be sufficiently advanced so that the muscle must be placed at complete rest. Mechanical ventilation and ventilatory muscle rest are certainly indicated when the pH is less than 7.25 or the patient appears unable to maintain ventilation and blood gas tensions.

The precise duration of mechanical ventilation to rest the inspiratory muscles in patients with respiratory muscle fatigue is unclear. However, no attempts at weaning should be made until the conditions that initiated fatigue are reversed. That is, lung mechanics, ventilatory drive, and respiratory muscle blood flow should have been corrected toward normal. Because low-frequency fatigue persists for 24 hours or more (Laghi et al, 1995), it may not be advisable to wean patients from mechanical ventilation in the setting of respiratory muscle fatigue for at least 24 hours, even if the factors that caused fatigue have been corrected.

REFERENCES

Agostoni E and Fenn WO: Velocity of muscle shortening as a limiting factor in respiratory air flow. J Appl Physiol 15(3):349–353, 1960.

Akabas SR, Bazzy AR, DiMaurio S, et al: Metabolic and functional adaptation of the diaphragm to training with resistive loads. J Appl Physiol 66(2):529–535, 1989.

Aldrich TK, Adams JM, Arora NS, et al: Power spectral analysis of the diaphragm electromyogram. J Appl Physiol 54(6): 1579–1584, 1983.

Anzueto A, Supinski GS, Levine SM, et al: Mechanisms of disease: Are oxygen derived free radicals involved in diaphragmatic dysfunction?

Am J Respir Crit Care Med 149:1048–1052, 1994.

Arora NS and Rochester DF: Respiratory muscle strength and maximal voluntary ventilation in undernourished patients. Am Rev Respir Dis 126:5 8, 1982a.

Arora NS and Rochester DF: Effect of body weight and muscularity on human diaphragm muscle mass, thickness, and area. J Appl Physiol 52(1):64–70, 1982b.

Aubier M, Murciano D, Rournier M, et al: Central respiratory drive in acute respiratory failure of patients with chronic obstructive pulmonary disease. Am Rev Respir Dis 122:191–200, 1980.

Aubier M, Farkas A, DeTroyer AM, et al: Detection of diaphragmatic fatigue in man by phrenic stimulation. J Appl Physiol 50(3):538–544, 1981a.

Aubier M, Trippenbach T, and Roussos C: Respiratory muscle fatigue during cardiogenic shock. J Appl Physiol 51(2):499–508, 1981b.

Aubier M, DeTroyer A, Sampson M, et al: Aminophylline improves diaphragmatic contractility. N Engl J Med 305:249–252, 1981c.

Aubier M, Murciano D, Lecocguic Y, et al: Bilateral phrenic stimulation: a simple technique to assess diaphragmatic fatigue in humans. J Appl Physiol 58(1):58–64,1985a.

Aubier M, Murciano D, Lecocguic Y, et al: Effect of hypophosphatemia on diaphragmatic contractility in patients with acute respiratory failure. N Engl J Med 313:420–424, 1985b.

Aubier M, Murciano D, Menu Y, et al: Dopamine effects on diaphragmatic strength during acute respiratory failure in chronic obstructive pulmonary disease. Ann Intern Med 110:17–23, 1983.

Aubier M, Viires N, Syllie G, et al: Respiratory muscle contribution to lactic acidosis in low cardiac output. Am Rev Respir Dis 126:648–652, 1982.

Bark H and Supinski G: Relationship of changes in diaphragmatic muscle blood flow to muscle contractile activity. J Appl Physiol 62(1):291–299, 1987.

Bazzy AR and Haddad GG: Diaphragmatic fatigue in unanesthetized adult sheep. J Appl Physiol 57(1):182–190, 1984.

Bellemare F and Grassino A: Effect of pressure and timing of contraction on human diaphragm fatigue. J Appl Physiol 53(5):1190–1195, 1982a.

Bellemare F and Grassino A: Evaluation of human diaphragm fatigue. J Appl Physiol 53(5):1196–1206, 1982b.

Bellemare F, Wight CM, Lavigne CM, et al: Effect of tension and timing of contraction on the blood flow of the diaphragm. J Appl Physiol 54(6):1597–1606, 1983a.

Bellemare F and Grassino A: Force reserve of the diaphragm in patients with chronic obstructive pulmonary disease. J Appl Physiol 55(1): 8–15, 1983b.

Bellemare F and Bigland-Ritchie B: Assessment of human diaphragm strength and activation using phrenic nerve stimulation. Resp Physiol 58:263–277, 1984.

Bellemare F and Bigland-Ritchie B: Central components of diaphragmatic fatigue assessed by phrenic nerve stimulation. J Appl Physiol 62(3):1307–1316, 1987.

Bellemare F, Bigland-Ritchie B, and Woods JJ: Contractile properties of the human diaphragm in vivo. J Appl Physiol 61(3):1153–1161, 1986.

Bigland-Ritchie B, Donovan EF, and Roussos CS: Conduction velocity and EMG power spectrum changes in fatigue of sustained maximal efforts. J Appl Physiol 51(5):1300–1305, 1981.

Black LF and Hyatt R: Maximal respiratory pressures: Normal values and relationship to age and sex. Am Rev Respir Dis 99:696–702, 1969.

Bolser DC, Linsey BG, and Shannon R: Medullary inspiratory activity: Influence of intercostal tendon organs and muscle spindle endings. J Appl Physiol 62(3):1046–1056, 1987.

Bradley TD, Chartrand D, Fitting JW, et al: The relation of inspiratory effort sensation to fatiguing patterns of the diaphragm. Am Rev Respir Dis 134:1119–1124, 1986.

Clanton TL, Ameredes BT, Thomson DB, et al: Sustainable inspiratory pressures over varying flows, volumes, and duty cycles. J Appl Physiol 69(5):1875–1882, 1990.

Clanton TL, Dixon GF, Drake J, et al: Effects of breathing pattern on inspiratory muscle endurance in humans. J Appl Physiol 59(6):1834–1841, 1985.

Comtois A, Gorczyca W, and Grassino A: Anatomy of diaphragm circulation. J Appl Physiol 62:238–244, 1987.

Danon J, Druz WS, Goldberg NB, et al: Function of the isolated paced diaphragm and the cervical accessory muscles in C1 quadriplegics. Am Rev Respir Dis 111:909–919, 1979.

Dekhuijzen PNR, Gayan-Ramirez G, Bisschop A, et al: Corticosteroid treatment and nutritional deprivation cause a different pattern of atrophy in rat diaphragm. J Appl Physiol 78(2):629–637, 1995.

De Troyer A: Inspiratory elevation of the ribs in the dog: Primary role of the parasternals. J Appl Physiol 70(4):1447–1455, 1991.

De Troyer A, Estenne M, Ninane V, et al: Transversus abdominis muscle function in humans. J Appl Physiol 68(3):1010–1016, 1990.

De Troyer A, Ninane V, Gilmartin JJ, et al: Triangularis sterni muscle use in supine humans. J Appl Physiol 62(3):919–925, 1987.

De Troyer A, Sampson M, Sigrist S, et al: The diaphragm: Two muscles. Science 213: 237–238, 1981.

Divertie MB and Brass A (eds): The Ciba Collection of Medical Illustrations, Vol 7. West Caldwell, NJ, Ciba, 1980, p 47.

Druz WS and Sharp JT: Activity of respiratory muscles in upright and recumbent humans. J Appl Physiol 51(6):1552–1561, 1981.

Druz WS and Sharp JT: Electrical and mechanical activity of the diaphragm accompanying body position in severe chronic obstructive pulmonary disease. Am Rev Respir Dis 125:275–280, 1982.

Enoka RM and Stuart DG: Neurobiology of muscle fatigue. J Appl Physiol 72(5):1631–1648, 1992.

Farkas GA and Roussos C: Adaptability of the hamster diaphragm to exercise and/or emphysema. J Appl Physiol 53(5):1263–1272, 1982.

Farkas GA, Decramer M, Rochester DF, et al: Contractile properties of intercostal muscles and their functional significance. J Appl Physiol 59(2):528–535, 1985.

Ferguson GT, Irvin CG, Cherniack RM: Effect of corticosteroids on respiratory muscle histopathology. Am Rev Respir Dis 142:1047–1052, 1990.

Fitts RH: Cellular mechanisms of muscle fatigue. Physiol Rev 74(1):49–74, 1994.

Fournier M and Sieck GC: Mechanical properties of motor units in the cat diaphragm. J Neurophysiol 59(3):1055–1065, 1988.

Frazier DT and Revelette WR: Role of phrenic nerve afferents in the control of breathing. J Appl Physiol 70(2):491–496, 1991.

Gandevia SC and McKenzie DK: Activation of the human diaphragm during maximal static efforts. J Physiol 367:45–56, 1985.

Grassino A, Goldman MD, Mead J, et al: Mechanics of the human diaphragm during voluntary contraction: Statics. J Appl Physiol 44(6):829–839, 1978.

Hägg GM: Interpretation of EMG spectral alterations at sustained contraction. J Appl Physiol 73(4):1211–1217, 1992.

Hubmayr RD, Litchy WJ, Gay PC, et al: Transdiaphragmatic twitch pressure. Am Rev Respir Dis 193:547–652, 1989.

Hussain SNA and Roussos C: Distribution of respiratory muscle and organ blood flow during endotoxic shock in dogs. J Appl Physiol 59(6):1802–1808, 1985.

Hussain SNA, Roussos C, and Magder S: Autoregulation of diaphragmatic blood flow in dogs. J Appl Physiol 64(1):329–336, 1988.

Hussain SNA, Roussos C, and Magder S: Effects of tension, duty cycle, and arterial pressure on diaphragmatic blood flow in dogs. J Appl Physiol 66(2):968–976, 1989.

Iscoe S, Dankoff J, Migicovsky R, et al: Recruitment and discharge frequency of phrenic motoneurons during inspiration. Respir Physiol 26:113–128, 1976.

Johnson BD, Babcock MA, and Suman OE: Exercise-induced diaphragmatic fatigue in healthy humans. J Physiol 460:385–405, 1993.

Juan DA, Calverley P, Talamo C, et al: Effect of carbon dioxide on diaphragmatic function in human beings. N Engl J Med 310:874–879, 1984.

Keens TG, Bryan AC, Levison H, et al: Developmental pattern of muscle fiber types in human ventilatory muscles. J Appl Physiol 44(6):909–913, 1978.

Kelly AM, Rosser BWC, Hoffman R, et al: Metabolic and contractile protein expression in developing rat diaphragm muscle. J Neurosci 11(5):1231–1242, 1991.

Kelsen SG, Altose MD, and Cherniack NS: Interaction of lung volume and chemical drive on respiratory muscle EMG and respiratory timing. J Appl Physiol 42(2):287–294, 1977.

Kelsen SG, Bao S, Thomas AJ, et al: Structure of parasternal intercostal muscles in the adult hamster: Topographic effects. J Appl Physiol 75(3):1150–1154, 1993.

Kelsen SG, Ference M, and Kapoor S: Effects of prolonged undernutrition on structure and function of the diaphragm. J Appl Physiol 58(4):1354–1359, 1985.

Kelsen SG and Nochomovitz ML: Fatigue of the mammalian diaphragm in vitro. J Appl Physiol 53(2):440–447, 1982.

Killian KJ, Summers E, Basalygo M, et al: Effect of frequency on perceived magnitude of added loads to breathing. J Appl Physiol 58(5):1616–1621, 1985.

Laghi F, D'Alfonso N, and Tobin MJ: Pattern of recovery from diaphragmatic fatigue over 24 hours. J Appl Physiol 79(2):539–546, 1995.

Laporta D and Grassino A: Assessment of transdiaphragmatic pressure in humans. J Appl Physiol 58(5):1469–1476, 1985.

Leith DE and Bradley M: Ventilatory muscle strength and endurance training. J Appl Physiol 41(4):508–516, 1976.

Levine S and Henson D: Low-frequency diaphragmatic fatigue in spontaneously breathing humans. J Appl Physiol 64(2):672–680, 1988.

Lieberman DA, Faulkner JA, Craig AB, et al: Performance and histochemical composition of guinea pig and human diaphragm. J Appl Physiol 34(2):233–237, 1973.

Loke J, Mahler DA, and Virgulto JA: Respiratory muscle fatigue after marathon running. J Appl Physiol 52(4):821–824, 1982.

Loring SH and Mead J: Action of the diaphragm on the rib cage inferred from a force-balance analysis. J Appl Physiol 53(3):756–760, 1982.

Loring SH, Mead J, and Griscom NT: Dependence of diaphragmatic length on lung volume and thoracoabdominal configuration. J Appl Physiol 59(6):1961–1970, 1985.

McCool FD, McCann DR, Leith DE, et al: Pressure-flow effects on endurance of inspiratory muscles. J Appl Physiol 60(1):299–303, 1986.

Macklem PT and DeTroyer A: A model of inspiratory muscle mechanics. J Appl Physiol 55(2):547–557, 1983.

Mador MJ, Magalang UJ, Rodis A, et al: Diaphragmatic fatigue after exercise in healthy human subjects. Am Rev Respir Dis 148:1571–1575, 1993.

Magder S, Lockhat D, Luo BJ, et al: Respiratory muscle and organ blood flow with inspiratory elastic loading and shock. J Appl Physiol 58(4):1148–1156, 1985.

Manning HL and Schwartzstein RM: Pathophysiology of dyspnea. N Engl J Med 333(23):1547–1553, 1995.

Maxwell LC, McCarter JM, Kuehl TJ, et al: Development of histochemical and functional properties of baboon respiratory muscles. J Appl Physiol 54(2):551–561, 1983.

Mead J, Banzett RB, Lehr J, et al: Effect of posture on upper and lower rib cage motion and tidal volume during diaphragm pacing. Am Rev Resp Dis 130:320–321, 1984.

Metzger JM and Fitts RH: Fatigue from high- and low-frequency muscle stimulation: Role of sarcolemma action potentials. Exp Neurol 93:320–333, 1986.

Metzger JM and Fitts RH: Role of intracellular pH in muscle fatigue. J Appl Physiol 62(4):1392–1397, 1987.

Mier A, Brophy C, Estenne M, et al: Action of abdominal muscles on rib cage in humans. J Appl Physiol 58(5):1438–1443, 1985.

Mortola JP and Sant'Ambrogio G: Motion of the rib cage and the abdomen in tetraplegic patients. Clin Sci Mol Med 54:25–32, 1978.

Moxham J, Edwards RHT, Aubier M, et al: Changes in EMG power spectrum (high-to-low ration) with force fatigue in humans. J Appl Physiol 53(5):1094–1099, 1982.

Murciano D, Auclair M, Pariente R, et al: A randomized controlled trial of theophylline in patients with severe chronic obstructive pulmonary disease. N Engl J Med 320:1521–1525, 1989.

Murciano D, Boczkowski J, Lecocguic Y, et al: Tracheal occlusion pressure: A simple index to monitor respiratory muscle fatigue during acute respiratory failure in patients with chronic obstructive pulmonary disease. Ann Intern Med 108:800–805, 1988.

Nashawati E, Dimarco A, and Supinski G: Effects produced by infusion of a free radical generating solution into the diaphragm. Am Rev Respir Dis 147:60–65, 1993.

Oliven A and Kelsen SG: Effect of hypercapnia and PEEP on expiratory muscle EMG and shortening. J Appl Physiol 66(3):1408–1413, 1989.

Oliven A, Kelsen SG, Deal EC, et al: Respiratory pressure sensation. Am Rev Respir Dis 132:1214–1218, 1985.

Oliven A, Lohda S, Adams ME, et al: Effect of fatiguing resistive loads on the level and pattern of respiratory activity in awake goats. Resp Physiol 73:311–324, 1988.

Oliven A, Supinski GS, Kelsen SG: Functional adaptation of diaphragm to chronic hyperinflation in emphysematous hamsters. J Appl Physiol 60(1):225–231, 1986.

Pardy RL and Bye PT: Diaphragmatic fatigue in normoxia and hyperoxia. J Appl Physiol 58(3):738–742, 1985.

Petrozzino JJ, Scardella AT, and Li JKJ: Effect of

naloxone on spectral shifts of the diaphragm EMG during inspiratory loading. J Appl Physiol 68(4):1376–1385, 1990.

Reid MB, Haack KE, Francik KM, et al: Reactive oxygen in skeletal muscle. I. Intracellular oxidant kinetics and fatigue in vitro. J Appl Physiol 73:1797–1804, 1992.

Reid WD, Wiggs BR, Paré PD, et al: Fiber type and regional differences in oxidative capacity and glycogen content in the hamster diaphragm. Am Rev Respir Dis 146(5):1266–1271, 1992.

Respiratory Muscle Fatigue Workshop Group: Respiratory muscle fatigue. Am Rev Respir Dis 142:474–480, 1990.

Road J, Vahi R, Rio PD, et al: In vivo contractile properties of fatigued diaphragm. J Appl Physiol 63(2):471–478, 1987.

Rochester DF: The diaphragm: Contractile properties and fatigue. J Clin Invest 75:1397–1402, 1985.

Rogers RM, Donahoe M, and Costantino J: Physiologic effects of oral supplemental feeding in malnourished patients with chronic obstructive pulmonary disease. Am Rev Respir Dis 146:1511–1517, 1992.

Roussos CS and Macklem PT: Diaphragmatic fatigue in man. J Appl Physiol 43(2):189–197, 1977.

Scardella AT, Parisi RA, Phair DK, et al: The role of endogenous opioids in the ventilatory response to acute flow resistive loads. Am Rev Respir Dis 133:26–31, 1986.

Sharp JT, van Lith P, Nuchprayoon C, et al: The thorax in chronic obstructive lung disease. Am J Med 44:39–46, 1968.

Shindoh C, DiMarco A, Thomas A, et al: Effect of N-acetylcysteine on diaphragm fatigue. J Appl Physiol 68(5):2107–2113, 1990.

Sieck GC, Fournier M, and Blanco CE: Diaphragm muscle fatigue resistance during postnatal development. J Appl Physiol 71(2):458–464, 1991.

Sieck GC, Mazer A, and Belman MJ: Changes in diaphragmatic EMG spectra during hyperpneic loads. Respir Physiol 61:137–152, 1985.

Similowski T, Yan S, and Gauthier AP: Contractile properties of the human diaphragm during chronic hyperinflation. N Engl J Med 325:917–923, 1991.

Sorli J, Grassino A, Lorange A, et al: Control of breathing in patients with chronic obstructive lung disease. Clin Sci Mol Med 54:295–304, 1978.

Supinski GS, Kelsen SC: Effect of elastase-induced emphysema on the force-generating ability of the diaphragm. J Clin Invest 70:978–988, 1982.

Supinski GS, Stofan D, Ciufo SR, et al: N-acetylcysteine administration and loaded breathing. J Appl Physiol 79(1):340–347, 1995.

Tobin MJ, Perez W, Guenther SM, et al: Does rib cage-abdominal paradox signify respiratory muscle fatigue? J Appl Physiol 63(2):851–860, 1987.

Tolep K, Higgins N, Muza S, et al: Comparison of diaphragm strength between healthy adult elderly

and young men. Am J Crit Care Med
152:677–682, 1995.

Urmey WF, De Troyer A, Kelley KB, et al: Pleural
pressure increases during inspiration in the zone
of apposition of diaphragm to rib cage. J Appl
Physiol 65(5):2207–2212, 1988.

Ward ME, Eidelman D, Stubbing DG, et al:
Respiratory sensation and pattern of respiratory
muscle activation during diaphragm fatigue. J
Appl Physiol 65(5):2181–2189, 1988.

Ward ME, Magder SA, and Hussain SNA: Oxygen
delivery independent effect of blood flow on
diaphragm fatigue. Am Rev Respir Dis
145:1058–1063, 1992.

Yang KL and Tobin MJ: A prospective study of
indexes predicting the outcome of trials of
weaning from mechanical ventilation. N Engl J
Med 324(21):1445–1450, 1991.

CHAPTER 7

Cardiac Function

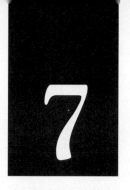

Obi N. Nwasokwa, M.D., Ph.D

The cardiac chamber is a mechanical pump made of myocardium. Therefore cardiac chamber pump function depends to a large extent on the mechanical behavior of its constituent myocardium. Thus, there are two broad frames of reference in the context of which cardiac function has been studied and analyzed: myocardial function and cardiac chamber pump function. This chapter therefore is a discussion of cardiac function from these dual perspectives of muscle and pump. The left ventricle (LV) is the most important and best studied of the cardiac chambers. Therefore, virtually all the discussion of cardiac chamber function is about left ventricular function. However, this discussion applies to other chambers as well, because LV behavior typifies the mechanical behavior of other chambers.

Cardiac mechanical function has yet another duality. It is more than simply the pumping of blood around the body during systole. To function properly, the heart must first fill with blood at low pressures during diastole. This filling function is just as important as the pumping function. Therefore there are two sides to the coin of cardiac mechanics: (a) pumping or systolic function and (b) filling or diastolic function. This duality applies to both muscle and pump function.

MYOCARDIAL MECHANICS

MYOCARDIAL SYSTOLIC FUNCTION

There are four levels of structural organization relevant to myocardial mechanical function. From the lowest to the highest levels, these are the crossbridge, the sarcomere, the myofibril, and the bulk myocardium.

Biochemistry of Cardiac Muscle Contraction

Cardiac muscle, like all striated muscle, is made principally of myofilaments whose interaction causes contraction. There are two types of myofilaments: the thick and the thin. Each thick filament consists of a bundle of 300 longitudinal myosin molecules. Each molecule has a long rod-like tail and a bilobed globular head. The heads occur in sets of three so that each half of the myosin filament has 50 such triplets. These myosin heads are the crossbridges that interact with actin sites to generate force and shortening.

The thin filament is a complex of the contractile protein actin and the regulatory proteins tropomyosin and troponin. Tropomyosin blocks the active sites of actin and thus ordinarily prevents the interaction of actin and myosin. Troponin has three components. Troponin T binds troponin to actin and tropomyosin; troponin C triggers contraction when it binds calcium; and troponin I also inhibits the interaction of actin and myosin.

Crossbridge Function as the Fundamental Activity Responsible for Systole

The myocardial crossbridge is the smallest unit of myocardial ultrastructure associated with the smallest identifiable mechanical event responsible for systolic activity. This event is the crossbridge cycle. The cyclical interaction of the crossbridge with the adjacent actin filament is responsible for myocardial mechanical activity. This interaction is triggered by calcium when it binds to troponin C and thereby removes the inhibitory effect of troponin I and causes a conformational change in tropomyosin. This conformational change unmasks active sites on actin, permitting it to bind to the myosin crossbridge in the presence of adenosine triphosphate (ATP). Subsequent hydrolysis of ATP by myosin, which also has enzymatic activity, releases the energy that enables the myosin head to move or flex and to tense up. Depending on the resistance encountered by the myosin filament, this motion and tension may result in the longitudinal translocation of the actin filament to cause shortening or in the generation of force or both. When summed over an ensemble of crossbridges, these unitary activities account for myocardial shortening and force generation on a macroscopic scale.

The Sarcomere as the Unit of Myocardial Function

The next unit of myocardial structure and function is the sarcomere. Each sarcomere is delimited longitudinally by a specific invagination of the sarcolemma, the Z-line. The sarcomere contains actin and myosin filaments. The actin filaments are in two groups associated with each half of the sarcomere; each group emanates from the opposite Z-line and there is a gap between both groups at the midsection of the sarcomere. Each myosin or

thick filament is located in the central part of the sarcomere where it straddles the gap between the contralateral actin groups. Thus each myosin filament is between and interdigitates with adjacent actin filaments (Fig. 7–1) and is studded with crossbridges that are therefore well positioned to interact with the neighboring actin filament. The midsegment of the myosin filament lacks crossbridges; it faces the gap between contralateral actin filaments. The myosin filament has polarity such that crossbridges in opposite halves of a myosin filament pull the actin filament in opposite directions.

Functionally, each sarcomere may be viewed as an ensemble of crossbridges and actin sites that generate force or shortening when they interact. When the crossbridge interacts with actin sites, the thin filament slides past the thick without change in the length of either filament, to produce shortening (see Fig. 7–1). The filaments also tense up to different extents to generate force. The overall activities of these crossbridges are coordinated to produce the total force output and/or shortening of the sarcomere. Indeed, the sarcomere is the smallest unit of myocardial structural and functional organization that manifests the bulk mechanical behavior of the myocardium in miniature. Such behavior includes the dependence of force output on sarcomere length, which undergirds the dependence of myocardial force on fiber length.

The myofibril consists of sarcomeres stacked end to end with the stacks in turn bundled side to side in such a way that adjacent sarcomeres that are side by side have their myofilaments in register, giving the muscle its striated appearance. Several myofibrils side by side form a strip of myocardium. Thus, any strip of myocardium can ultimately be considered an ensemble of sarcomeres whose individual activities summate to produce the total mechanical activity of the myocardium.

Determinants of Myocardial Systolic Performance

There are two broad general categories of factors that control myocardial systolic performance. The first comprises physical factors intrinsic to the myocardium, namely the length of the myocardial fiber and the force experienced by the myocardium. The second involves extrinsic control through changes in contractility.

Length Dependence of Myocardial Force Output: Starling's Law

Stretch-induced increase in the length of the myocardial fiber causes an increase in the force

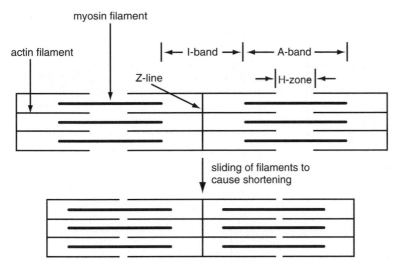

actin filament

myosin filament

Z-line

|← I-band →|← A-band →|

→|H-zone|←

sliding of filaments to cause shortening

Figure 7–1
Structure of the sarcomere under light microscopy. Actin and myosin filaments interdigitate and produce a pattern of bands including the A and I bands and the H zone. Shortening occurs when the myofilaments slide past each other following interaction of myosin crossbridges and actin sites in the presence of ATP.

output of the muscle (Fig. 7–2). This is Starling's law of the heart. Starling and his coworkers expressed this law this way (Patterson et al, 1914):

> ... the mechanical energy set free on passage from the resting to the contracted state depends on the area of "chemically active surfaces" i.e. on the length of the muscle fibers.

This statement is remarkable because it foreshadows the later discovery of the role of crossbridges in myocardial force generation and in the mechanism of Starling's law.

The force required to stretch the muscle to a particular length before it becomes active is the preload. Thus, in general, an increase in preload results in an increase in force output.

However, although increase in length results in increase in force output, the relationship between myocardial fiber length and force output is not monotonic. At a certain length called L_{max}, the force output peaks (see Fig. 7–2). Beyond L_{max}, the force output either stays constant or decreases slightly. Starling's law is also manifested as a higher absolute value of instantaneous derivative (dF/dt) of isometric force at longer muscle lengths up to L_{max} (see Fig. 7–2).

Putative Ultrastructural Basis of Starling's Law

Much recent research has addressed the mechanism of Starling's law. Because the sarcomere is the fundamental unit that exhibits the bulk mechanical behavior of the myocardium, the mechanism of Starling's law must reside in the mechanical behavior of the sarcomere (Gordon et al, 1966).

An attractive hypothesis shown to be true in skeletal muscle was that the degree of overlap of actin and myosin filaments accounts for Starling's law (Fig. 7–3). Thus, below L_{max}, stretch-induced increase in the length of the muscle fiber and sarcomere led to an increase in the number of crossbridges that were in register with actin sites to generate force. At short lengths below 1.6 μm, which is the length of the myosin filament, the deformation of the myosin filament at both ends and the double overlap of actin filaments from opposite ends of the sarcomere undermine force development (see Fig. 7–3). Because the negative effect of these factors on force development diminishes with increase in muscle length, sarcomere force output increases as the muscle is stretched at these short lengths towards 1.6 μm. The length of two actin filaments end to end is 2.0 μm. Below this sarcomere length, actin filaments from opposite ends of the sarcomere overlap each other and interfere with force generation. As sarcomere length increases from 1.6 toward 2.0 μm, the degree of double overlap of actin filaments from opposite halves of the sarcomere decreases and force output increases. At a sarcomere length of 2.05 to 2.2 μm, the degree of overlap of actin and myosin filaments is optimal and the number of crossbridges in register with actin sites is maximal and the sarcomere force output is maximal. This sarcomere length corresponds to L_{max}. Above a length of 2.2 μm, the degree of overlap of actin and myosin filaments and the number of crossbridges in register with actin sites diminish progressively, resulting in the decline of sarcomere force output beyond L_{max} (see Fig. 7–3).

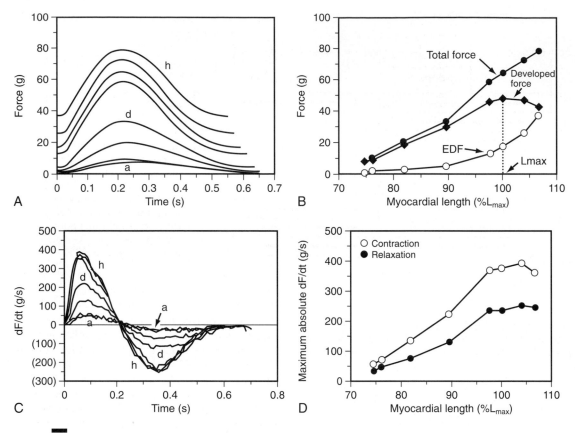

Figure 7–2
Starling's law in the *in situ* canine papillary muscle preparation studied under isometric conditions by the author. *(A)* Curves of the time course of myocardial isometric force as muscle length was increasing from curve a to curve h. Panel *(B)* Plot of total force, developed force, and end-diastolic force against myocardial length expressed as a percentage of L_{max}, the length at which developed force is a maximum. *(C)* Curves of the time course of the derivatives (dF/dt) of the isometric force curves in A showing progressive increase in instantaneous and peak values of dF/dt as muscle length increases. *(D)* Plots of the peak dF/dt during contraction and relaxation against myocardial length expressed as a percentage of L_{max}.

Sarcomere Length Dependence of Calcium Activation as the Mechanism of Starling's Law of the Heart

The above mechanism seems plausible for skeletal muscle, which operates over a wide range of sarcomere lengths. In contrast, the myocardial sarcomere length versus force relationship is rather steep. The myocardium operates within a narrow range of sarcomere lengths. In the unloaded myocardium, sarcomere length is 1.8 to 1.9 μm but not shorter. Moreover, the myocardium is stiffer than skeletal muscle such that stretch of the myocardium to increase sarcomere length beyond 2.2 μm damages the muscle. Thus, the operational range of sarcomere length in the myocardium is from 1.9 to 2.2 μm. Investigators believe that within this short operational range of sarcomere

lengths, change in degree of myofilament overlap alone cannot account for change in muscle force.

If the degree of myofilament overlap cannot account for the myocardial force-length relationship, what does? It is now established that an increase in sarcomere and myocardial fiber length also increases both the sensitivity of troponin C to calcium as well as the amount of calcium available to trigger the interaction of myofilaments to generate force and shortening (Allen et al, 1974; Fabiato and Fabiato, 1975; Gordon and Pollack, 1980; Allen and Kurihara, 1982; Kentish et al, 1986; Hofmann and Fuchs, 1987; Lakatta, 1987b; Babu et al, 1988; Stefanon et al, 1990; Gamble et al, 1992). Thus, the mechanism of Starling's law depends on the availability of calcium. It is therefore not realistic to make a sharp distinction between inotropic mechanism and

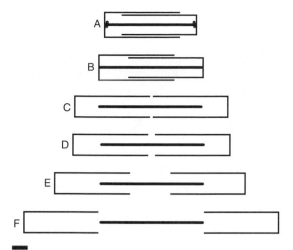

Figure 7–3
Change in sarcomere length may change the degree of myofilament overlap and thereby the force output of the sarcomere. *(A)* At very short lengths (i.e., below 1.6 μm, the length of a myosin filament), the ends of the myosin filament are squeezed against the Z-line and deformed. There is also double overlap of actin filaments. Both effects interfere with force generation and decrease sarcomere force output. *(B)* At 1.6 μm, the myosin filaments are no longer deformed. *(C)* At a sarcomere length of 2.0 μm, the length of two actin filaments end-to-end, degree of overlap of filaments is first optimal and force output peaks. *(D)* At a sarcomere length of 2.2 μm, the degree of overlap is still optimal. *(E)* Between a sarcomere length of 2.2 μm and 3.6 μm, the degree of overlap diminishes progressively and the sarcomere force output diminishes commensurately. *(F)* At a sarcomere length of 3.6 μm and above, there is no overlap and zero force output.

length-dependence of myocardial performance because both depend on changes in the availability of calcium.

Myocardial Force (Afterload)

Myocardial force output and shortening are two sides of the coin of myocardial mechanical activity and represent two reciprocal manifestations of myocardial power output. Therefore, the greater the force the myocardium has to generate to overcome the prevailing load, the less it shortens (Fig. 7–4). This inverse relationship between the force output of the myocardium and its shortening is called the *force-velocity relationship*. The greater the force generated to overcome the prevailing load, the lower the shortening velocity. Afterload may thus be defined as the force on the muscle when it shortens. This force opposes shortening, and so both the extent and the velocity of short-

ening have an inverse relationship to myocardial afterload (see Fig. 7–4).

Short and Long-term "Memory" of Myocardial Force and Length Changes

Although myocardial length determines its force output and myocardial force determines the amount of shortening, the relationship between myocardial length and force output on the one hand and myocardial force and shortening on the other, at any given instant in the contraction cycle, depends to some extent on the mechanical events that occurred before that instant. These antecedent events constitute the mechanical history before the instant in question. Many studies (Nwasokwa et al, 1984) have shown that events that occurred both in previous beats (long-term history) and within the same beat (short-term history) alter the instantaneous myocardial length-force output and force-shortening relationship.

Thus, antecedent shortening within the same beat results in decreased force output at any instant following the shortening, whereas a history of force development may have the opposite effect (Nwasokwa et al, 1984). Small amounts of shortening actually potentiate rather than impair subsequent instantaneous force output (Nwasokwa et al, 1984). To the extent that instantaneous myocardial mechanical response depends on its previous experience within the same twitch (short-term history), the myocardium is said to have short-term memory (Nwasokwa et al, 1984). Myocardial short-term memory is therefore the dependence of instantaneous active force-length relationship on antecedent mechanical events (force and length history) within the same twitch or contraction cycle.

Other studies (Kaufman et al, 1972; Parmley and Chuck, 1973; Jewell and Rovell, 1973) have shown that force and length changes in previous beats and the manner in which such changes came about alter instantaneous force-length relationships. An increase in length in a previous beat produces not only an instantaneous increase in force output but a progressive increase in force output in subsequent beats and vice versa. This is an example of what may be called long-term memory because the instantaneous force-length relationship of muscle is altered by mechanical history within a previous twitch.

Myocardial Contractility

Contractility or inotropic state is that aspect of myocardial performance that reflects the intrinsic ability of the myocardium to generate force and

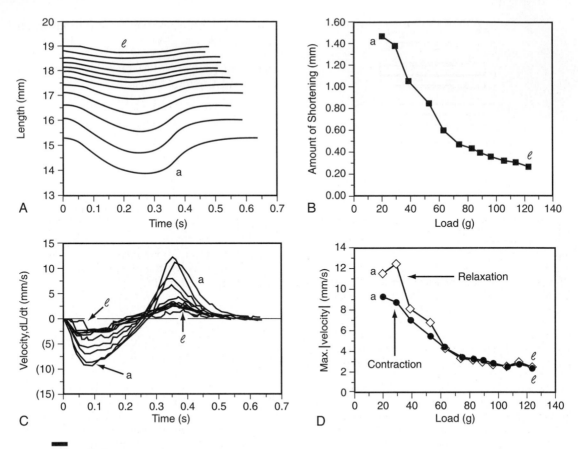

Figure 7–4

Effect of load on myocardial shortening in the *in situ* canine papillary muscle studied under isotonic conditions by the author. (A) Curves of the time course of myocardial isotonic shortening at progressively increasing loads from twitch a to twitch l. (B) Plot of the amount of shortening versus load showing the inverse relationship between both variables. (C) Curves of the time course of isotonic shortening velocity (derivatives of the curves in A) as the load increases progressively from a to l. (D) Plot of the peak velocity of isotonic shortening during contraction and relaxation versus the load or force on the muscle during shortening. The inverse relation between shortening velocity and load is the force-velocity relation.

shorten. It is therefore traditionally viewed as independent of the prevailing preload and afterload. Inotropic state is thought to be dependent on the amount of calcium available to trigger the interaction of myofilaments. Indeed, interventions that enhance myocardial contractility such as the catecholamines and dobutamine (Fig. 7–5), invariably do so by increasing the amount of calcium that triggers myofilament interaction. However, changes in myocardial performance traditionally not considered inotropic changes have been shown to involve, at least in part, a change in calcium availability. Thus, change in myocardial fiber length is now thought to change force output partly by altering the amount of calcium available for myofilament interaction and partly by altering the sensitivity of the myofilaments to

calcium (Allen et al, 1974; Fabiato and Fabiato, 1975; Gordon and Pollack, 1980; Allen and Kurihara, 1982; Kentish et al, 1986; Hofmann and Fuchs, 1987; Babu et al, 1988; Lakatta, 1987b; Stefanon et al, 1990; Gamble et al, 1992) leading to the view that one must not draw too sharp a contrast between load-dependent and contractility-dependent alterations in cardiac function. Notwithstanding, many students of cardiac mechanics still consider it useful to make a distinction between changes in performance related to load changes and those related to contractility.

The Ionic Basis of Myocardial Contractility: Excitation-contraction Coupling

Excitation-contraction (E-C) coupling is the process whereby electrical depolarization of cardiac

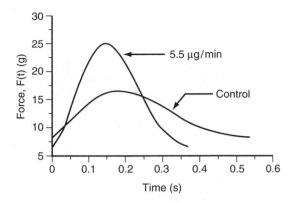

Figure 7–5
Effect of dobutamine on myocardial contractility in the *in situ* canine papillary muscle. Note the increase in both peak and developed force, the decrease in end-diastolic force, and the decrease in both time to peak force and total twitch duration.

muscle causes the release of calcium, which then triggers the interaction of actin and myosin filaments to produce mechanical contraction. This is a membrane process. The membrane structures responsible include the sarcolemma, the transverse or T-tubules, and the sarcoplasmic reticulum (SR) (Fig. 7–6). These structures are anatomically and functionally specialized to bring about E-C coupling.

The sarcolemma is rich in fast sodium channels whose activity maintains and propagates the action potential. The T-tubules are invaginations of the sarcolemma that abut on the junctional SR or terminal cistern and thereby provide a mechanism for the action potential to reach the calcium release channels of the SR (see Fig. 7–6). The T-tubules have sodium channels but are also

rich in L-type calcium channels. The SR has two distinct sites. The junctional SR (JSR) (see Fig. 7–6) is specialized to release calcium. Toward this end, it has a high density of calcium-release channels, which on electron microscopy appear as projections or "foot" processes that span the space between the JSR and the adjacent T-tubule (see Fig. 7–6). The other site, the longitudinal SR (LSR) is specialized for the reuptake or sequestration of calcium to produce relaxation after myofilament interaction. It therefore has a calcium pump, calcium ATPase, that, for each ATP molecule hydrolyzed, transports two calcium ions across the LSR membrane against a concentration gradient (see Fig. 7–6). To fine-tune control of calcium sequestration, the LSR contains phospholambam, a membrane protein that is an allosteric regulator of the calcium ATPase enzyme. When phosphorylated by a cAMP-dependent protein kinase, phospholambam increases the ATPase enzyme's affinity for calcium, thereby enhancing calcium transport. When dephosphorylated, it impairs calcium uptake (Tada and Katz, 1982; Katz et al, 1986).

E-C coupling occurs in the following stages. Sodium entry through the SL fast sodium channels depolarizes the SL to produce an action potential and propagates this depolarization. The T-tubules, which are invaginations of the sarcolemma that abut on the sarcoplasmic reticulum, are critical to excitation-contraction coupling because they conduct the action potential to the vicinity of the junctional sarcoplasmic reticulum, which is the calcium release site. Depolarization of the T-tubule at this site causes voltage-dependent L-type calcium channels to open, thereby allowing calcium to enter the sarcoplasm. This calcium current is not large enough to trigger the

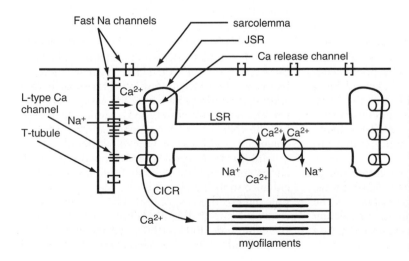

Figure 7–6
Ionic basis of myocardial inotropy. This diagram depicts the principal membrane-related structures involved in excitation-contraction coupling and modulation of inotropy. JSR = junctional sarcoplasmic reticulum; LSR = longitudinal sarcoplasmic reticulum; CICR = calcium-induced calcium release.

interaction of myofilaments but goes to the "foot" processes to cause the junctional sarcoplasmic reticulum to release an avalanche of calcium by a process of calcium-induced calcium release (CICR) (Fabiato, 1983). This latter calcium current is released in multiple quentized units called *calcium sparks*. Each spark is the response to a unitary event involving the interaction of trans-sarcolemmal calcium ion and the junctional sarcoplasmic reticulum. All the calcium sparks provide sufficient calcium to trigger the interaction of the myofilaments (see Fig. 7–6).

Modulation of E-C Coupling and Inotropic State: Effect of Drugs and Other Interventions

The structures for E-C coupling provide the myocardium with a mechanism that can be manipulated by extrinsic interventions to change myocardial contractility and, thereby, myocardial performance. Such interventions alter or modulate sarcolemmal ion currents by altering the function of various sarcolemmal ion pumps and channels. Although the final common pathway involves a change in calcium ion flux, the ion transport initially altered by an intervention need not be calcium itself.

Various mechanisms for control of sarcolemmal ion channel and pump function include alteration of the state of phosphorylation of various proteins relevant to pump or channel function; direct agonism of a channel; blockade of a channel; and inhibition of pump function. Interventions such as beta-agonists and cAMP phosphodiesterase inhibitors increase the level of cAMP. This in turn activates a cAMP-dependent protein kinase, which then phophorylates various proteins. When phosphorylated, a protein that is resident within the sarcolemmal L-type calcium channel facilitates calcium entry through the channel. The entry of calcium through the L-type calcium channel may then cause CICR at the JSR and thereby enhance contractility by increasing the availability of calcium for myofilament interaction. Phosphorylation of phospholambam facilitates calcium sequestration (Tada and Katz, 1982) making it keep pace with the increased release of calcium in the same circumstances. Phosphorylation of troponin I, on the other hand, results in decreased sensitivity of troponin C to calcium (Zhang et al, 1995).

Beta-blockers are competitive inhibitors of beta-receptors and thus decrease cAMP levels, resulting eventually in less phosphorylation of the slow calcium channel protein, decreased calcium entry, decreased CICR, and decreased contractility.

There are several other substances that affect channel and pump function. Angiotensin increases contractility through an agonist effect on the L-type calcium channel. Potassium channel agonists such as adenosine decrease contractility because they facilitate repolarization. This shortens the action potential duration and the duration of phase 2 of the action potential. Because phase 2 is the time during which calcium enters through the calcium channel, shortening of this phase decreases calcium availability and has a negative inotropic effect.

Sarcolemmal ion channel antagonism is another way to control contractility. Calcium channel blockers block sarcolemmal L-type calcium channels, thereby decreasing calcium entry, CICR, and calcium availability for myofilament interaction. The effect of sodium channel blockers is more complicated because they do not alter calcium fluxes directly. Rather, these agents block the fast sodium channel and thereby decrease sodium entry (Fig. 7–7).

How does this effect alter calcium flux? Decrease of sodium entry reduces the concentration of sodium within the restricted subsarcolemmal space, the so-called *fuzzy space* (Leblanc and Hume, 1990; Lederer et al, 1990; Sham et al, 1992; Carmeliet, 1992; Levesque et al, 1994; Kohmoto et al, 1994) (see Fig. 7–7). This space does not permit free diffusion of sodium to the rest of the sarcoplasm. Local sodium concentration therefore may change considerably within the fuzzy space relative to the rest of the sarcoplasm. Decrease of sodium concentration within the fuzzy space activates the sodium-calcium pump, causing it to pump calcium out in exchange for sodium, thereby decreasing CICR and the amount of calcium available for myofilament interaction (Leblanc and Hume, 1990; Lederer et al, 1990; Sham et al, 1992; Levesque et al, 1994; Carmeliet, 1992; Kohmoto et al, 1994) (see Fig. 7–7). The movement of sodium down its concentration gradient probably provides the energy for the movement of calcium. Potassium channel blockade causes a positive inotropic effect by delaying repolarization, thereby maintaining the voltage higher and longer during phase 2 of the action potential (Singh and Nademanee, 1985). More calcium enters the cell through L-type channels, resulting in enhanced CICR and enhanced contractility.

Inhibition of certain sarcolemmal ion pumps affects inotropy. For example, digitalis glycosides enhance inotropy by inhibiting the sodium/potassium pump, thereby presumably causing sodium to accumulate in the subsarcolemmal fuzzy space (Leblanc and Hume, 1990; Lederer et al, 1990; Sham et al, 1992; Carmeliet, 1992; Levesque et

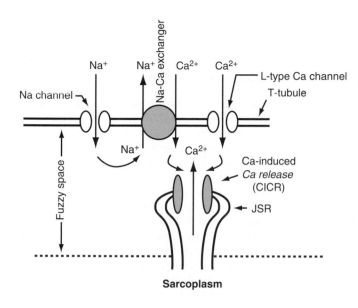

Figure 7–7
How modulation of a sarcolemmal ion current other than calcium may alter contractility by altering the amount of calcium released to the myofilaments. The subsarcolemmal "fuzzy" space is thought to be a restricted space from which sodium does not diffuse freely to the rest of the sarcoplasm.

al, 1994; Kohmoto et al, 1994). This activates the sodium/calcium pump and makes it operate in reverse mode, pumping calcium into, and sodium out of, the cell. The trans-sarcolemmal inward calcium transport stimulates CICR at the JSR and thereby enhances inotropy.

Increase in heart rate has an effect equivalent to that of an agonist on the fast sodium channel, causing increased sodium transport into the cell and thereby raising sodium concentration within the fuzzy space (Leblanc and Hume, 1990; Lederer et al, 1990; Sham et al, 1992; Carmeliet, 1992; Kohmoto et al, 1994; Levesque et al, 1994; Nwa-sokwa, 1994). This again stimulates the sodium/calcium pump, resulting in increased entry of calcium and eventually enhanced inotropy. Decrease in heart rate has the opposite effect.

Alteration of Myofilament Sensitivity to Calcium

Another way to alter myocardial contractility does not involve change in calcium availability but instead entails altering the sensitivity of the myofilaments to calcium (Blinks and Endoh, 1986). Thus, agents like sulmazole and Bay K 8644 increase contractility partly by increasing the sensitivity of myofilaments to calcium.

MYOCARDIAL DIASTOLIC FUNCTION

As with systolic function, ventricular diastolic function is determined to a great extent by myocardial diastolic function. There are two main components to myocardial diastolic function: myocardial relaxation, an active process, and the passive elastic properties of the myocardium—compliance and stiffness.

Myocardial Relaxation

Myocardial relaxation occurs as a result of the sequestration of calcium by the longitudinal SR (Katz, 1989). This transport of calcium from the sarcoplasm into the LSR (see Fig. 7–6) is necessarily an active process because the concentration of calcium within the SR is as high as 10^{-2} molar whereas its concentration in the sarcoplasm at the end of myofilament interaction is no more than 10^{-5} molar. At end-diastole following calcium sequestration, sarcoplasmic calcium is 10^{-7} molar. A calcium-stimulated magnesium (Mg)-ATPase is responsible for this and transports two calcium ions for each ATP molecule hydrolyzed. This process is modulated by the membrane protein, phospholambam, which is resident in the LSR, such that when phospholambam is phosphorylated by a cAMP-dependent protein kinase, sequestration of calcium is greatly facilitated (Katz et al, 1986). Interventions that increase cAMP levels therefore enhance calcium sequestration and myocardial relaxation and are said to be positively lusitropic. Such interventions include catecholamines and cAMP phosphodiesterase inhibitors.

Passive Elastic Properties

Myocardial stiffness is the property that makes the myocardium resist passive stretch. It may be defined as the force required to produce unit change in myocardial length or the rate of change of passive myocardial force relative to its length, dF/dL (Fig. 7–8). A stiffer or less compliant myocardium requires more passive force to stretch it by a given amount. Because the ventricle is made

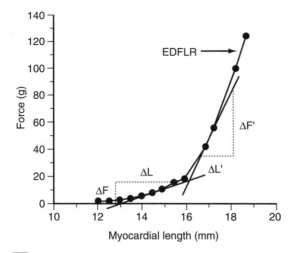

Figure 7–8
Myocardial end-diastolic force-length relation and stiffness. Stiffness is the slope, dF/dL, of the end-diastolic force-length relation and may change in two ways: Muscle operates over a different range of the same curve or over a different curve (*not shown*). dF/dL is approximated by ΔF/ΔL where ΔF and ΔL are small changes in force and length, respectively, along the end-diastolic force-length curve.

of myocardium, the passive elastic properties of the myocardium are largely, although not exclusively, responsible for the passive elastic properties of the ventricle.

What confers these passive elastic properties on the myocardium? At the ultrastructural level, in addition to myofibrils and other organelles such as mitochondria and SR, the myocardium also contains a matrix of connective tissue including collagen fibers, fine microfibrils, and elastin. These give the myocardium its tensile strength and other passive elastic properties. They also impose a limit on how much the myocardium can stretch.

VENTRICULAR PUMP FUNCTION

CARDIAC CHAMBER MECHANICAL CYCLE IN THE TIME DOMAIN

The two fundamental variables of ventricular pump function are pressure and volume. Their change during mechanical activity constitutes the events of the cardiac cycle. These events may be described in the time domain by looking at changes in pressure and volume separately as a function of time. Alternatively it is also useful to examine change in pressure as a function of change in volume in the pressure-volume plane

during the cardiac cycle. The latter approach gives pressure-volume (P-V) loops.

Ventricular Contraction

Cardiac chamber function during systole and diastole may be characterized by the time course of intracavitary pressure and volume (Fig. 7–9). Changes in pressure and volume are interdependent. Volume changes only in response to a favorable pressure gradient between a proximal and a downstream site. At the onset of systole, left ventricular pressure is less than aortic pressure and the aortic valve is closed. The mitral valve had also closed at the end of diastole as soon as LV pressure exceeded left atrial pressure. Thus, in the earliest phase of systole, the mitral and aortic valves are closed. Left ventricular volume is therefore constant in this isovolumic phase of contraction to ensure that pressure rise is rapid (see Fig. 7–9). When LV pressure exceeds aortic pressure, the aortic valve opens and the gradient of pressure between the LV and aorta drives the blood from the LV to the aorta. During this phase of rapid ejection, LV cavity volume decreases rapidly, and the rate of rise of pressure is not as rapid as in the phase of isovolumic contraction (see Fig. 7–9). Subsequently, LV pressure peaks and begins to decline slowly, causing ejection to be slower and ventricular volume to decline less steeply.

Ventricular Filling Dynamics

Ventricular diastole has several phases, namely isovolumic relaxation, rapid filling phase, diastasis, and atrial systole.

Isovolumic Relaxation

As soon as LV pressure drops below aortic pressure, the aortic valve closes and ejection stops. The closure of the aortic valve is marked by a slight transient increase in aortic pressure, which is the dicrotic notch. With aortic valve closure, systole ends and diastole begins with the relaxation phase. Initially, after closure of the aortic valve, ventricular relaxation is isovolumic because the mitral valve is still closed and blood cannot enter or leave the LV. This phase of isovolumic relaxation is brief, being marked by a precipitous decline in LV pressure (see Fig. 7–9). This rapid decay of LV pressure is necessary because the maintenance of a high pressure in diastole is counterproductive. During systole, rapid pressure rise is necessary to quickly overcome the impedance to ejection. But at the completion of ejection, a high premium is placed on the dissipa-

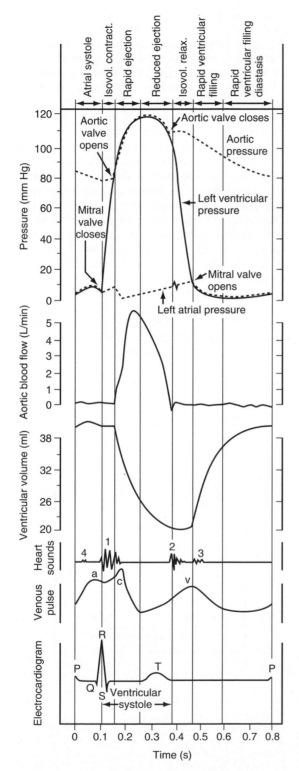

Figure 7–9
The cardiac cycle. Time course of ventricular pressure, volume, and aortic flow. The various phases of the cardiac cycle are shown. (From Berne RM and Levy MN: Physiology, 3rd ed. St Louis, CV Mosby, 1993 with permission.)

tion of this pressure. For ventricular filling to occur, LV pressure has to drop below LA pressure. The faster the LV pressure falls, the earlier the mitral valve can open so that filling can begin.

Rapid Early Filling Phase

For most of early diastole, LV filling is entirely "passive." Under normal conditions this phase of filling accounts for close to 70% of total ventricular filling. The pressure gradient between the LA and the LV is the motive force for the flow of blood from the LA into the LV (Thomas et al, 1991; Thomas and Weyman, 1991). The amount of filling depends on this gradient. Factors that alter this gradient alter the extent of diastolic filling in this early passive filling phase. There are three principal determinants of ventricular filling during early passive filling.

The first determinant is atrial pressure. The higher the atrial pressure, the greater the pressure gradient. However, under normal circumstances atrial pressure is maintained at low levels; raising the atrial pressure is not usually a means to increase diastolic filling. However, in various heart disease states, LA pressure may be high. This has the effect of maintaining LV diastolic filling especially in the face of increased LV diastolic pressure.

Important determinants of atrial pressure are atrial stiffness, atrial contractility, and the extent of atrial emptying in the previous atrial systole. An increase in atrial stiffness increases left atrial pressure for the same amount of atrial filling and thus tends to increase the atrioventricular pressure gradient. Left atrial contractility determines how strong atrial systole is in completing ventricular filling toward end-diastole. If the atrium is hypocontractile or not contracting as in atrial fibrillation, this late boost to ventricular filling is weak or lost, respectively. The extent of atrial emptying in the previous systole is important because the less complete the previous atrial systole, the more blood remains in the atrium; the more distended the atrium and the greater the atrial pressure and the atrioventricular pressure gradient; and the greater the filling of the ventricle, both as a result of the enhanced passive filling and of the more forceful atrial systole as a result of Starling's law.

The second determinant of passive ventricular filling is ventricular relaxation and the associated elastic recoil and diastolic suction. Even after the mitral valve opens and ventricular filling commences, the ventricular pressure continues to drop because the ventricle continues to relax. The fact that ventricular pressure is dropping even as its volume is increasing as it fills has given rise to the concept of diastolic ventricular suction and relaxation filling (Sabbah and Stein, 1981; Ishida et al, 1986; Cheng et al, 1990) (Fig. 7–10). Thus, during its filling, the role of the ventricle is more than simply that of a passive recipient of blood. By continuing to relax as it fills, the ventricle actively "sucks" blood in. The faster and more complete the ventricular relaxation, the better maintained the pressure gradient for filling and the greater the amount of ventricular filling.

The third determinant of passive filling of the ventricle is ventricular compliance and the passive elastic properties of the ventricle in diastole. These determine how much ventricular pressure rises for each unit of volume it fills and therefore how quickly the pressure gradient for filling is dissipated. The more compliant the ventricle, the less its pressure rises as it fills, the less the pressure gradient is dissipated, and the greater the extent of filling. Ventricular chamber compliance depends directly on myocardial compliance, ventricular wall thickness, and size of the ventricular cavity. It is also affected indirectly by ventricular interaction with the other ventricle, pericardial pressure, and lung inflation.

Diastasis

The early passive filling phase ends when the pressure gradient is dissipated largely because of a

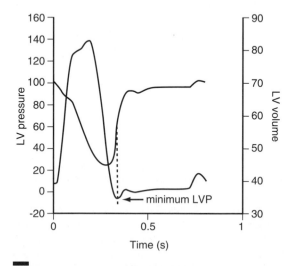

Figure 7–10
Relaxation filling. Time course of ventricular pressure and volume showing an increase in volume and filling even as ventricular pressure continues to fall. (From Cheng C-P, Freeman GL, Santamore WP, et al: Effects of loading conditions, contractile state and heart rate on early diastolic left ventricular filling in conscious dogs. Circ Res 66:814–823, 1990. With permission of the American Heart Association.)

rise in diastolic LV pressure to equal LA pressure. The next phase of diastole is marked by virtual cessation of LV filling and very little change in LV volume. This phase is called *diastasis*.

Atrial Contraction

The final phase of diastole is atrial systole. The atrium contracts and completes ventricular filling. The importance of atrial filling to overall ventricular filling depends on how well the ventricle filled during the passive filling phase. If early ventricular filling was deficient because the magnitude of the determining factors discussed earlier was unfavorable, and the pressure gradient for filling was not properly maintained, the contribution of atrial contraction to ventricular filling is commensurately higher. This higher atrial contribution to ventricular filling is partly as a result of the fact that the less early filling there was, the more blood remains in the atrium, stretching the atrium. Starling's law therefore results in a more forceful atrial contraction. Thus, for instance, a ventricle that is stiff or one that relaxes poorly relies more on atrial systole and less on early passive filling for its filling function. The presence of a fourth heart sound or S_4 is the hallmark of such situations. Moreover, atrial fibrillation is poorly tolerated in such situations because it robs the ventricle of the crucial atrial contribution (atrial "kick") to its filling.

CARDIAC CYCLE IN THE PRESSURE-VOLUME PLANE: PRESSURE-VOLUME LOOPS

The P-V loop (Fig. 7–11) is another description of events in the cardiac cycle. It is a plot of left ventricular pressure against left ventricular volume throughout the cardiac cycle. This plot forms a closed loop with four sides, representing the four major phases of the cardiac cycle. The extreme right and vertical part of the loop in which pressure is increasing at constant volume represents isovolumic contraction (see Fig. 7–11). This is followed by the ejection phase, in which volume decreases at variable pressure. The next phase is the phase of isovolumic relaxation, during which pressure drops at constant volume. Finally, there is a ventricular filling phase, during which ventricular pressure and volume increase together as dictated by the passive elastic properties of the left ventricle (see Fig. 7–11). Although the idealized P-V loop is usually depicted as four-sided, in practice, the sides are not straight lines. For instance, the transition from isovolumic relaxation to ventricular filling governed by passive

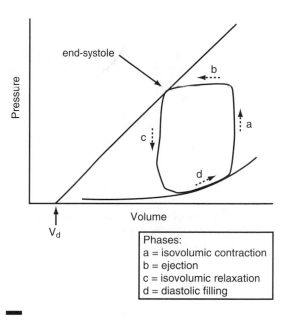

Figure 7–11
The left ventricular pressure-volume loop and the phases of ventricular mechanical activity.

elastic ventricular properties is curvilinear (see Fig. 7–11) because of relaxation filling, a mini-phase, in which filling is occurring and LV volume is increasing even as LV pressure continues to fall by relaxation.

VENTRICULAR SYSTOLIC FUNCTION

Pressure generation and ejection of blood volume are the two systolic activities of the ventricular pump and are analogous to, and indeed depend on, force generation and shortening of the component myocardium. Not surprisingly, as in the myocardium, ventricular systolic function depends both on factors more or less intrinsic to the ventricle—preload and afterload—and on influences extrinsic to the ventricle through change in contractility.

Determinants of Ventricular Systolic Performance

Ventricular End-diastolic Volume, Preload, and the Frank-Starling Law

By enhanced filling during diastole, an increase in left ventricular end-diastolic volume usually results in an increase in ventricular performance in the next systole, as evidenced by enhanced pressure generation and/or ejection (Patterson et al, 1914; Frank, 1895). This property of the ventricle is the Frank-Starling law of the ventricle

(Patterson et al, 1914; Frank, 1895) and depends on the force output versus length relationship of the active myocardium (see Fig. 7–2). Increased filling of the ventricle stretches the constituent myocardium to accommodate the increased diastolic volume, causing the myocardium to generate more force (Fig. 7–12). Enhanced force generation by the myocardium accounts for the more forceful ventricular contraction. This phenomenon is autoregulatory because it ensures that if ventricular filling increases, the ventricle contracts more forcefully to eject the larger quantity of blood that entered it during diastole.

Preload can be a confusing term. It was borrowed from the protocol of early cardiac muscle experiments that used an isotonic lever and a stop

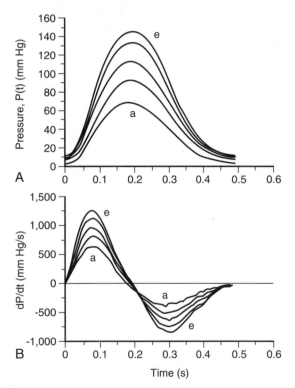

Figure 7–12
Starling's law in the isovolumic left ventricle of the Suga-Sagawa cross-circulated canine heart preparation studied by the author. (A) Curves of the time course of left ventricular pressure in entirely isovolumic (nonejecting) beats at progressively larger end-diastolic volumes from beat a to beat e. Note the progressive increase in peak pressure and developed pressure with little or no increase in time to peak pressure. (B) Curves of the time course of the derivative of pressure, dP/dt, obtained from the curves in A. Note the progressive increase in instantaneous dP/dt, and maximal dP/dt during both contraction and relaxation.

to make the muscle experience various loads at various times before and after it became active (Braunwald et al, 1976). In those experiments, preload was the force or load that stretched the muscle *before* (hence pre-load) it was stimulated and generated force or shortening actively. This muscle preload is therefore analogous to the diastolic filling pressure or wall stress of the ventricle, because the latter stretches the ventricle before systole. However, the variable that determined myocardial force in those early experiments was actually the length of the myocardial fiber. The preload was only an indirect determinant because it stretched the fiber. If the investigator applied a preload insufficient to stretch the muscle fiber, this preload force had no effect whatever on myocardial force or shortening.

In the ventricle, the equivalent of myocardial preload is often said to be ventricular filling pressure or diastolic wall stress. This, however, is able to alter the force of ventricular contraction and ventricular performance in general only if it is associated with increase in ventricular diastolic volume. Indeed, ventricular filling pressure generally increases in lockstep with ventricular diastolic volume, provided that ventricular compliance is unchanged. If ventricular compliance changes or if ventricular stiffness is high, ventricular filling pressure becomes an unreliable indicator of ventricular volume. Frank (1895) recognized this relationship when he wrote:

> Tension rises as filling increases . . . [and] would furnish a measure of filling if one knew the distensibility curve of resting heart muscle. The determination of this relationship would be helpful in connection with many problems of cardiac filling . . . Initial tension could be used to deduce the volume of the heart in relaxation.

Confusion arises if the term *preload* is equated to myocardial fiber length and ventricular diastolic volume and is thus assumed to be the proximate variable that is linked to myocardial and ventricular performance. One must emphasize that although preload is the force or pressure that tends to stretch the myocardium, it is important to remember that the proximate influence on cardiac performance as defined by Starling's law is myocardial fiber length, not diastolic pressure or wall stress. Indeed, Starling addressed this issue and cited an experiment that enabled him to say that increased "tension" or pressure was not the variable responsible for the increase in performance: it is possible to increase volume substantially with little or no increase in muscle tension or force and yet see substantial increase in pressure generation in the next systole (Starling, 1897).

Determinants of Preload and Ventricular End-diastolic Volume

The two major determinants of preload are venous return and atrial contraction.

Venous Return

An increase in venous return raises preload. Venous return depends on several factors, including gravity and posture, compression of lower extremities, intrathoracic pressure, venous tone, ventricular relaxation, and the passive pressure-volume relationships of the ventricle. Chapters 4 and 5 review the determinants of venous return in detail.

Because of gravity, an upright posture causes pooling of blood in the lower extremities and thereby impairs venous return, whereas a supine posture or leg elevation causes less pooling of blood in the lower extremities. With exercise involving lower extremity muscles, the compression effect of the muscles on lower extremity veins propels blood toward the heart, enhancing venous return. Inflation of a positive pressure suit has a similar effect. An increase in intrathoracic pressure such as occurs with positive pressure respiration or a pneumothorax compresses the great veins of the thorax and thereby decreases venous return. Inspiration, on the other hand, causes a negative intrathoracic pressure, opening up the thoracic veins and increasing venous return. Venoconstriction, such as that occurring during exercise and anxiety and in response to sympathomimetics, decreases venous capacitance and propels venous blood back to the heart. Venodilation, such as that which occurs in response to vasodilator drugs, decreases preload by increasing venous capacitance, thereby sequestering blood that should have returned to the heart in the venous system.

The faster the ventricle relaxes in early diastole, the lower its pressure and the greater the pressure gradient from the atrium to the ventricle and the greater ventricular filling.

The passive diastolic pressure-volume relationships of the ventricle determine how much its pressure rises as it fills with blood. The stiffer or less compliant or distensible the ventricle is, the more its pressure rises in response to the same amount of filling and therefore the faster the atrioventricular pressure gradient that drives ventricular filling is dissipated. Thus, a stiff ventricle

is associated with deficient ventricular filling, whereas a compliant one has the opposite effect.

Atrial Contraction

Atrial systole occurs towards the end of diastole and augments ventricular filling. Normally it accounts for about 20 to 30% of ventricular filling. The atrial contribution to ventricular filling is greater and is particularly important if passive filling in early diastole is impaired either because of relatively slow ventricular relaxation or increased ventricular stiffness such as that which occurs in the setting of left ventricular hypertrophy.

To be useful, atrial contraction has to be synchronized with ventricular contraction. For instance, with atrioventricular dissociation and junctional rhythm, atrial systole is improperly timed relative to ventricular contraction (i.e., it does not precede ventricular systole and occurs either simultaneous with or after ventricular systole). Such asynchrony means that the ventricle is unable to make use of the atrial contribution to its filling. Finally, with atrial fibrillation, there is no effective atrial contraction, and the atrial contribution to ventricular filling is lost completely. This could become disastrous if the ventricle relies heavily on the atrial contribution to its filling to maintain an adequate stroke volume.

Measures of Preload

The ideal variable related to preload that directly determines myocardial and ventricular performance is the average sarcomere length within the ventricle during diastole. It is, however, impractical to measure this variable so that some variable that increases *pari passu* with sarcomere length is a good substitute. Because sarcomere length increases as the ventricle is distended and the myocardium stretched, the end-diastolic volume of the ventricle is a more practical measure of the configuration of myocardial sarcomeres. However, in clinical situations this variable is often not easily measured. Therefore, a variable that increases with the degree of filling is often used. This variable is end-diastolic pressure. Because it is much easier to measure pressure than volume, pressure measurement is widely used even in clinical situations when the balloon-tipped catheter readily provides fairly reliable measurements of pulmonary occlusion ("wedge") pressure, which is very similar to mean left atrial and left ventricular end-diastolic pressures. In addition to left ventricular end-diastolic pressure, LV diastolic wall stress has also been used as a measure of preload, the force stretching the ventricular myocardium (see later for the formula for wall stress).

Preload Reserve

When myocardial fiber length is lower than L_{max}, further stretch of the myocardium during diastole results in more forceful contraction because increased sarcomere length toward the optimum for contraction (L_{max}) results in increased release of calcium as well as increased sensitivity of the myofilaments to calcium. This ability to stretch the myocardium further is the mobilization of preload reserve to improve systolic function. Preload reserve is therefore the amount of unused "useful and usable" myocardial fiber length to which the myocardium may be stretched to optimize or improve its systolic performance at a given time. It depends on sarcomere length.

Sarcomere length is longest in the mid-wall. At this site it is about 1.9 μm when the ventricle is empty and increases with ventricular filling, reaching the optimal value 2.2 μm at a left ventricular end-diastolic pressure of 10 to 12 mm Hg (Ross et al, 1967; Sonnenblick et al, 1967). At these pressures, sarcomere lengths at other locations across the ventricular wall are shorter than optimal. As filling pressure increases further, the mid-wall sarcomeres cease to elongate, whereas the shorter sarcomeres at other sites become longer and thereby account for further rise in force of contraction. Such recruitment of suboptimally stretched sarcomeres is one way to mobilize preload reserve.

In the intact heart the ability to mobilize preload reserve is limited if the myocardium is stiff because a stiff myocardium exacts a price in the form of increased pressure when it is stretched to mobilize its heterometric or preload reserve. How much the pressure rises depends on the diastolic elastic properties of the myocardium and ventricular chamber. In a stiff ventricle, the pressure tends to rise excessively for the same amount of filling. Moreover, it is important to remember that pericardial pressure, lung inflation, and RV-LV interdependence and interaction can alter the apparent ventricular chamber stiffness.

During diastole, the mitral valve is open. The LV is therefore in communication with the pulmonary circulation so that LV diastolic filling pressure tends to equilibrate with pulmonary pressure. This hydrostatic coupling of the heart to the lungs makes it necessary that LV diastolic filling occur at low pressures. It therefore imposes limits on how much the myocardium may be stretched because the lung is unable to tolerate the high pressures necessary to stretch the myocardium to

the upper limits of its preload reserve. Such high pressures cause interstitial and alveolar pulmonary edema and impair gas exchange severely. The stiffer the myocardium the greater the penalty exacted in terms of high diastolic pressures and risk of pulmonary congestion by any attempt to mobilize the upper reaches of preload reserve.

Ventricular Contractility

Ventricular contractility, like myocardial contractility, is an attribute that, independent of prevailing loading conditions, reflects the intrinsic capacity of the ventricular pump to generate pressure and/or eject volume. Thus, contractility measures how good the ventricle is as a pump independent of its loading conditions.

Causes of Change in Ventricular Contractility

A change in contractility is usually the result of a change in the amount of calcium available to trigger the interaction of myofilaments. This is illustrated by the LV response to the infusion of dobutamine (Fig. 7–13). Less commonly, contractility is related to an increase in calcium sensitivity of the myofilaments. Various interventions that may cause a change in calcium availability were discussed earlier in relation to the ionic basis of myocardial contractility and do so by altering or modulating myocardial ion transport by blocking or potentiating various ion channel and pump functions.

Measures of Ventricular Contractility

Several measures of ventricular contractility have been proposed. These have included ejection fraction, stroke work, stroke power, peak rate of pressure rise during isometric contraction, dP/dt, dP/dt/P (i.e., the peak rate of isometric pressure generation normalized to the peak isometric pressure), preload recruitable stroke work, and end-systolic pressure-volume relation. None of them is perfect.

Ejection phase indices such as ejection fraction and mean velocity of circumferential fiber shortening, V_{cf}, are quite sensitive to contractility. Although moderate alterations of preload have little effect, these indices are exquisitely sensitive to afterload which has an inverse relation with them. If afterload is kept nearly constant, these variables can reflect contractility. If both preload and afterload are held constant, ejection fraction, V_{cf}, stroke volume, cardiac output, stroke work, and stroke power may all be used as measures of contractility. Stroke power is defined as the prod-

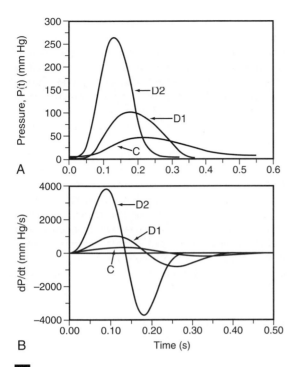

Figure 7–13
Effect of dobutamine on left ventricular contractility studied in the Suga-Sagawa cross-circulated canine heart. (A) Curves of the time course of canine left ventricular pressure in entirely isovolumic contractions under control conditions (C) and at two different doses of dobutamine, D1 (5.73 μg/min) and D2 (11.46 μg/min). (B) The time derivative (dP/dt) of the curves in (A) are shown. Note the increase in peak dP/dt with dobutamine. Dobutamine was infused into the coronary circulation.

uct of ventricular pressure and the rate of change of ventricular volume.

The isovolumic phase indices, dP/dt and dP/dt/DP40, are sensitive to afterload and preload, respectively, but if these types of load are held constant, these indices reflect inotropic state. dP/dt/DP40 is the dP/dt at developed pressure of 40 mm Hg (Quinones et al, 1976).

END-SYSTOLIC PRESSURE-VOLUME RELATIONSHIP (ESPVR) I The ESPVR is the most widely accepted measure of ventricular contractility and the one that comes closest to conforming to the requirement of load insensitivity. To obtain this relationship, several pressure-volume loops are constructed under different levels of preload and afterload. The end-systolic point for each loop is identified and all the end-systolic points are then joined. These points tend to lie on a straight line (Fig. 7–14). The slope of this line is an index of

ventricular contractility. This slope is virtually equal to end-systolic elastance, (E_{es}), or maximal elastance E_{max} (Suga et al, 1973; Suga and Sagawa, 1974; Sagawa, 1978). Elastance is defined as the slope of isochronal pressure volume lines (Suga et al, 1973; Suga and Sagawa, 1974). A rise in contractility causes the slope of the ESPVR line to increase (see Fig. 7–14), whereas negative inotropic interventions decrease this slope (Suga et al, 1973; Suga and Sagawa, 1974; Sagawa, 1978). In the LV, the volume intercept of the isochronal lines is constant throughout the cardiac cycle (Suga et al, 1973; Suga and Sagawa, 1974; Sagawa, 1978).

Although ESPVR has been studied best in the left ventricle, similar relationships apply to the right ventricle (Maughan et al, 1979) and the right atrium (Lau et al, 1979). However, there are some differences. E_{es} is more sensitive to loading conditions in the RV than in the LV (Maughan et al, 1979). In addition, the volume intercept, V_d, of isochronal lines on the x-axis changes throughout the cardiac cycle in the RV (Maughan et al, 1979). In the left atrium, E_{es} is load invariant as in the LV (Suga and Sagawa, 1974), but unlike the LV, and more like the RV, V_d changes

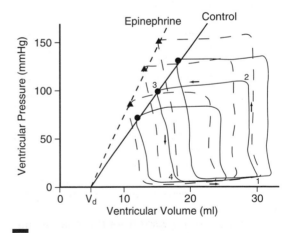

Figure 7–14
Pressure volume loops showing the effect of contractility on the end-systolic pressure-volume relationship. The effect of contractility is in contrast to the lack of effect of afterload represented by mean arterial pressure that was fixed at three different levels while cardiac output was clamped at a constant value during both the control (solid lines) and the enhanced (2 μg/kg/min epinephrine infusion) (broken lines) contractile states. (From Suga H, Sagawa K, and Shoukas AA: Load independence of the instantaneous pressure-volume ratio of the canine left ventricle and the effects of epinephrine and heart rate on the ratio. Circ Res 32:314–322, 1973. With permission of the American Heart Association.)

with time during the cardiac cycle in the left atrium (Alexander et al, 1987).

The ESPVR is not a flawless measure of contractility. Several studies have shown that the ESPVR is not strictly load-independent even in the LV. Thus, ejecting beats tend to fall short of the ESPVR line of the isovolumic (nonejecting) beats if ejection is substantial but go beyond it if ejection is small (Suga and Yamakoshi, 1977; Sigiura et al, 1989; Hunter, 1989). In addition, over a wide range of contractility, the ESPVR is curvilinear rather than a straight line over a wide enough range of volume (Burkhoff et al, 1987; Kass et al, 1989). Although it is less load-sensitive, the ESPVR is not as sensitive to contractility as the ejection and isovolumic phase indices (Kass et al, 1987).

DIFFICULTIES ENCOUNTERED IN THE CLINICAL USE OF THE END-SYSTOLIC PRESSURE-VOLUME RELATION I Although it is widely used in investigations, there are difficulties with clinical use of ESPVR as an index of contractility. There is no universally accepted definition of end-systole. It is therefore often difficult to identify end-systole from P-V loops obtained in patients. It is tempting to equate end-systole with end-ejection but in some hemodynamic lesions such as mitral regurgitation, this is wrong because end-ejection or the moment of the smallest ventricular volume tends to occur in the relaxation phase (Iizuka, 1978). Suga has defined end-systole as "the moment at which the contraction becomes maximal and the relaxation starts" (Suga, 1979), but concedes that identification may be very difficult if the left upper corner of the P-V loop is rounded.

To obtain end-systolic points, it is necessary to alter both preload and afterload. The patient may not tolerate such changes in loading conditions. Moreover, a reflex response to altered load may change contractility and heart rate (Carabello and Spann, 1984; Sagawa, 1984). Volume measurement in the clinical setting is usually imprecise. Ventricular volume but not pressure depends on the size of the human subject, so that small hearts tend to have higher end-systolic elastance even when contractility is normal (Carabello and Spann, 1984; Suga et al, 1984). In the setting of ventricular hemodynamic overload, end-systolic elastance may be unreliable as a measure of contractility. For instance, in pressure overload, regardless of contractility, pressure is high while ventricular volume is low, resulting in spuriously high end-systolic elastance. In volume overload, ventricular volume is high, resulting in spuriously low end-systolic elastance. It has been proposed that substitution of stress for pressure in

pressure overload corrects for the effect of low volume in pressure overload. However, use of the end-systolic stress-volume relationship has its limitations because a change in contractility may produce a parallel shift (i.e., change in the x-axis intercept) in the end-systolic stress-volume relationship line instead of a change in its slope (Grossman et al, 1977; Carabello and Spann, 1984).

E_{max} and E_{es} are based on total pressure rather than developed pressure. Therefore, if end-diastolic pressure is increased enough, it is possible for developed pressure to decrease without much change in total pressure. In the presence of diastolic dysfunction such as that which occurs with ischemia-reperfusion and hypertrophy, E_{max} may not change even though contractility has changed, as evidenced by a lower developed isovolumic pressure (Zile et al, 1991).

History Dependence of Ventricular Contractility and Effect of Short- and Long-term Memory for Previous Mechanical Conditions

Just as a history of shortening within the same twitch results in deficient myocardial performance, a history of ejection results in a decrease in ventricular end-systolic pressure. Pressure generation, as typified by a completely isovolumic contraction, results in apparent enhancement of inotropic state because the ESPVR line is such that end-systolic elastance is greater than is the case if ejection were allowed to occur (Suga and Yamakoshi, 1977). This echoes the effect of force generation in the myocardium. Moreover, small amounts of ejection, as is the case with small amounts of myocardial shortening, cause the greatest apparent enhancement of contractility (Sigiura et al, 1989; Hunter, 1989). Furthermore, events in previous beats such as a sudden change in volume alter contractility by changing P-V relations in subsequent beats (Lew, 1988). Similarly, a sudden increase in afterload also enhances contractility in subsequent beats. This phenomenon is called *homeometric autoregulation* (Von Anrep, 1912; Sarnoff et al, 1960).

Impedance to Ventricular Ejection (Afterload)

Left ventricular afterload may be defined as the aggregate of the external forces that oppose the shortening of myocardial fibers and therefore ventricular ejection. Afterload is usually computed clinically as systemic vascular resistance. This definition is not strictly accurate because the variables flow and pressure, from which systemic vascular resistance is calculated, are changing constantly throughout the cardiac cycle. Moreover, both resistance and compliance should be taken into consideration (Milnor, 1975). Afterload may therefore be better measured as aortic input impedance. This is frequency-dependent and is therefore measured as an impedance spectrum. To measure vascular impedance spectrum, the time course of pressure P(t) and flow F(t) are decomposed into sinusoidal waves of different frequencies by Fourier analysis. At any particular frequency, the ratio of pressure amplitude to the flow amplitude is an impedance at that frequency. The impedance spectrum is therefore a plot of impedance versus frequency, and this spectrum constitutes the afterload. For complete representation of the impedance spectrum and, therefore, the afterload, one should also include a plot of the phase angle versus the frequency. The two major components of afterload are arterial compliance, which is analogous to electrical capacitance, and arterial resistance. The former is a property of the large arteries, whereas the latter is a property of the arterioles. For practical clinical purposes, only arterial resistance is measured.

Although ventricular impedance is probably the most rigorous measure of afterload, in practice numerous variables have been used to represent afterload. These have included ventricular systolic wall stress, systemic vascular resistance alone, and aortic pressure. Systemic vascular resistance is computed as the ratio of mean pressure gradient to the mean flow (i.e., [mean aortic pressure − mean RAP/cardiac output]) where RAP is right atrial pressure. To obtain ventricular wall stress, investigators have assumed various models of the left ventricle. The simplest of these is the spherical model. The Laplace relationship gives the wall stress in a spherical ventricle as follows:

$$\sigma = Pa/2h$$

where σ is average wall stress; a is radius at the endocardial surface; P is intraventricular pressure; and h is wall thickness.

The more rigorous and more commonly adopted model for the ventricle is the ellipsoid. For an ellipsoidal ventricle, the circumferential wall stress is given by the formula:

$$\sigma = (Pb/h)\cdot(1 - b^2/2a^2 - h/2b + h^2/8a^2)$$

where σ is mean circumferential wall stress; P is instantaneous intraventricular pressure; a is mid-wall semi-major axis; and b is mid-wall semi-minor axis (Mirsky 1979; Yin, 1981).

Ventricular afterload closely parallels ventricular pressure during ejection, and the latter may suffice as a simple and practical measure of afterload.

Afterload is an important determinant of ventricular performance. Increase in afterload impairs ventricular ejection performance, whereas a reduction in afterload improves ventricular ejection (Fig. 7–15). In heart failure, neuroendocrine activation increases the levels of many vasoconstrictors including norepinephrine, angiotensin II, arginine vasopressin, and endothelin. These changes in the ambient biochemical milieu of systolic heart failure cause a preponderance of vasoconstriction over vasodilation. This further increases afterload and makes afterload reduction an important means to improve ventricular performance in heart failure.

The Coupling of the Ventricular Pump to the Arterial Load: Impedance Matching

In general, power generators transfer power to a load in which the power is utilized. A general principle of operation of power sources is that they optimize power transfer to the load. This is done by matching the impedance of the source to the impedance of the load.

The left ventricle is the power source for the circulation. It transfers this power to its arterial load in the form of stroke volume under an arterial pressure. There is an infinite number of possible pairs of values of stroke volume and arterial pressure obtainable as a manifestation of the transfer of a given amount of stroke power from the ventricular pump to the arterial load. Yet, various studies (Sunagawa et al, 1985; Van den

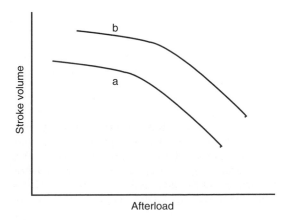

Figure 7–15
Effect of afterload on systolic performance as measured by the stroke volume. In general, increase in afterload causes a decrease in performance to produce one plot (a) of stroke volume versus afterload under control inotropic conditions. With enhanced contractility, the curve is higher but has the same shape and therefore shows the same relationship.

Horn et al, 1985; Myhre et al, 1988) show that the ventricle chooses to partition its power output between stroke volume and arterial pressure such that the stroke work is at a maximum. This condition is invariably achieved by matching the source impedance of the ventricular pump to the input impedance of the arterial load. In various studies the variables used to represent ventricular source impedance and arterial input impedance have varied somewhat.

Sunagawa and coworkers (1985) used ventricular elastance to represent the relevant operational variable of the ventricle and the arterial effective elastance as the input impedance of the arterial load property. Arterial effective elastance was defined as the slope of the end-systolic pressure-stroke volume relationship. They showed that under different values of afterload, contractility, and heart rate, they could maximize the stroke work only if the effective arterial elastance was equal to the ventricular elastance (Sunagawa et al, 1985).

In another study of ventriculoarterial interaction or coupling, Van den Horn et al (1985) showed that for a given preload, contractility, and heart rate, at the "working point" of the ventricle (i.e., the prevailing pressure and flow at which the ventricle operates) the power output is maximal and source resistance of the ventricle is matched (i.e., equal) to the peripheral resistance of the arteries. Source resistance was defined as the difference between actual and maximal mean left ventricular pressure divided by the mean outflow. The arterial resistance was the ratio of mean aortic pressure to mean flow.

More recently, Myhre et al (1988) showed that the mutual optimization of the ventricle and its arterial load is achieved at normal contractility but breaks down after an acute depression of ventricular contractility.

Definitive studies of the clinical relevance of impedance matching are lacking. However, the functional state of the ventricle, its performance, and indeed its fate and the fate of the patient may be influenced by the proper match of the ventricular source impedance to the arterial load in various pathologic cardiac conditions. This is well illustrated by dilated cardiomyopathy and some valve lesions.

In dilated cardiomyopathy, ventricular contractility is impaired. Therefore, ventricular elastance, a representation of its source impedance, is low. The large volume of the dilated heart is one reason why the ventricular elastance is low. Such ventricles tolerate a high afterload poorly because a high afterload is associated with a high effective arterial elastance, which is the input impedance.

Thus, if afterload is high, there is impedance mismatch, which causes further impairment of ventricular performance. Afterload reduction is therefore necessary to ensure impedance match and optimize ventricular performance. Experience in 1996 suggests that LV volume reduction surgery may improve ventricular performance and clinical outcome (Altman, 1996). If more studies confirm this early experience, it would not be surprising because reducing LV volume tends to increase ventricular elastance, provided that the smaller ventricle can generate pressures comparable to values before volume reduction. This increase in ventricular elastance would make for better impedance match.

In chronic severe mitral regurgitation, the ventricle adapts to the low-input impedance it encounters by having a low source impedance. The latter is accomplished by remodeling of the ventricular chamber such that sarcomeres are laid down in series to produce a dilated left ventricle with relatively thin wall, compared with its cavity diameter (i.e., relatively low ratio of wall thickness to cavity radius) (Grossman et al, 1975). The increased radius of the dilated ventricle ensures that ventricular elastance, and therefore source impedance, are low, and match the low-input impedance engendered by ejection into the left atrium. After mitral valve replacement, the low-input impedance is suddenly removed by preventing ejection into the left atrium so that the ventricle is now forced to eject not mainly into the low-impedance left atrium but entirely into the higher impedance aorta, without allowing time for proper remodeling of the ventricle to achieve impedance match at the new input impedance. Thus, initially following mitral valve replacement, left ventricular failure may occur because of impedance mismatch. It seems logical to propose that impedance match following mitral valve replacement or repair for mitral regurgitation may be improved by LV volume reduction during the operation.

The situation in pure critical aortic stenosis is the opposite of that in chronic mitral regurgitation. Here, as before, the ventricle adapts by matching its source impedance to its outflow input impedance. The source impedance is high to match the abnormally high outflow input impedance. Adaptation is accomplished by laying down sarcomeres in parallel to produce concentric hypertrophy and a high ratio of wall thickness to cavity radius (Grossman et al, 1975). After aortic valve replacement, the outflow input impedance is markedly decreased, whereas the ventricular source impedance remains high initially. An impedance mismatch exists, but this time the mismatch is skewed in favor of the ventricle, which tends to handle its arterial load remarkably well. As a result, left ventricular performance shows considerable improvement following aortic valve replacement for aortic stenosis.

Characterization of Ventricular Systolic Performance

Ventricular performance represents the extent of ventricular contraction under the prevailing conditions of preload, afterload, and contractility. Clinicians and investigators have characterized ventricular performance within different reference frames including P-V loops; and in relation to preload (Starling curves), and in relation to afterload or some measure of the impedance to ejection. Because the function of the heart is to pump blood, some measure of ejection performance such as stroke volume or cardiac output is usually the dependent variable in ventricular function curves.

Effect of Isolated Changes in Preload, Afterload, and Contractility on Ventricular Performance in the P-V Reference Frame

In this P-V reference frame, the end-systolic P-V relationship line (ESPVRL) and the end-diastolic pressure volume curve (EDPVC) define the limits of the contraction space of the ventricle. Within this space, the trajectories of particular P-V loops may be plotted to illustrate the effect of preload, afterload, and contractility subject to the following constraints: (1) ventricular volume either remains constant or decreases but does not increase during systole; (2) during diastole, ventricular volume may not decrease: it may remain constant or increase; (3) at a given level of ventricular contractility, end-systolic pressure volume coordinates must fall on the ESPVR line; pressure and volume never drop below the EDPVC. The amount of ejection (stroke volume) is measured by the decrease in volume and the amount of pressure generation by the increase in pressure. The pressure generated before the aortic valve is opened is regarded as a measure of the afterload, whereas the end-diastolic pressure is regarded as a measure of preload.

Increase in preload at constant afterload and contractility results in an increase in stroke volume (Fig. 7–16). A decrease in preload has the opposite effect. On the other hand, increase in afterload at constant preload causes a decrease in stroke volume, and vice versa (Fig. 7–17). Enhancement of inotropic state rotates the ESPVR line counterclockwise, resulting in higher

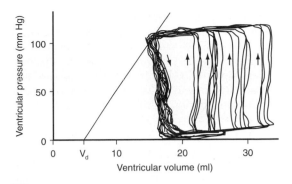

Figure 7–16
Pressure-volume loops showing the relative lack of effect of preload on the end-systolic point given the same afterload (mean arterial pressure) and contractile state. However, note that stroke volume increases as preload increases. This is a manifestation of Starling's law. (From Suga H, Sagawa K, and Shoukas AA: Load independence of the instantaneous pressure-volume ratio of the canine left ventricle and the effects of epinephrine and heart rate on the ratio. Circ Res 32:314–322, 1973. With permission of the American Heart Association.)

stroke volumes at the same preload and afterload (see Figs. 7–14 and 7–17).

Stroke Volume Versus End-diastolic Volume: Effect of Preload (Starling Curves)

If afterload, contractility, and compliance are held constant, an increase in end-diastolic volume re-

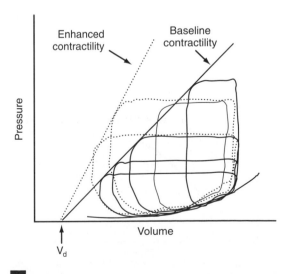

Figure 7–17
Pressure-volume loops showing the effect of afterload and contractility on ventricular performance at constant preload.

flects an increase in preload and causes the stroke volume to increase (Fig. 7–18). The stroke volume versus EDV curve represents one cardiac function curve. An increase in contractility or a decrease in afterload shifts this curve upward and to the left, whereas a decrease in contractility or increase in afterload shifts it downward and to the right (see Fig. 7–18).

Stroke Volume Versus Afterload: Effect of Afterload

Stroke volume or another measure of ejection performance such as cardiac output may be plotted against afterload, as measured by systemic vascular resistance or wall stress in systole, with contractility and preload held constant, to give an inverse relation between both variables. Thus, as afterload increases, ejection performance decreases (see Fig. 7–15). An increase in contractility or preload shifts this curve upward, whereas a decrease has the opposite effect (see Fig. 7–15).

VENTRICULAR DIASTOLIC FUNCTION

Diastolic function is normal if the cardiac chamber fills adequately at low pressures.

Determinants of Diastolic Performance

The determinants of diastolic ventricular performance were discussed earlier and include relaxation, ventricular stiffness, heart rate, atrioventricular pressure gradient, atrial stiffness, atrial contractility, and the extent of emptying in the previous diastole.

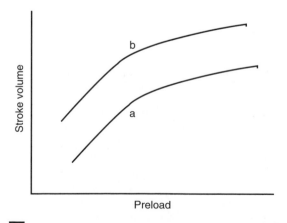

Figure 7–18
Effect of preload on ventricular performance as measured by the stroke volume at two different levels of contractility.

Measures of Ventricular Diastolic Function

Because diastolic function has many facets, no one index suffices to measure it. Therefore, different measures and indices based on different methodologies and technologies have been proposed for different aspects of diastolic performance.

Radionuclide Indices of Diastolic Performance

The radionuclide method of measuring diastolic function uses technetium 99, which is injected intravenously (Spirito et al, 1986). Time-activity curves are then plotted. This is done by plotting the ventricular radioactivity in successive frames several milliseconds apart. Instantaneous radioactivity counts are proportional to ventricular volume and independent of geometry but do not give absolute volume. These counts are normalized to counts at end-diastole. The ventricular time-activity curves represent the time course of LV volume normalized to end-diastolic volume during the course of the cardiac cycle.

Various attributes of the time-activity curve have been proposed as measures of diastolic performance. These include the peak ventricular filling rate, time to peak ventricular filling rate, and first third filling fraction (i.e., the proportion of LV filling that occurs during the first third of diastole) (Spirito et al, 1986).

Doppler Echocardiographic Indices

The Doppler echocardiographic indices of LV filling dynamics and diastolic function and dysfunction are based on monitoring the pattern of flow from the LA across the mitral valve into the LV by recording the spectral pattern of flow velocity across the mitral valve (Spirito and Maron, 1988; Labovitz and Pearson, 1987; Nishimura et al, 1989a; 1989b). Prominent aspects of such a recording include an E-wave, representing the flow velocity profile during the rapid filling phase of early diastole, and the A-wave, which is the velocity profile during atrial systole. The initial slope of the E-wave is the acceleration of flow, whereas the final slope represents deceleration of flow. The measures of diastolic performance include the E-wave amplitude, the A-wave amplitude, the acceleration half time and the deceleration half time, and the E/A ratio (i.e., the ratio of the amplitudes of the E and A waves) (Labovitz and Pearson, 1987; Spirito and Maron, 1988; Nishimura et al, 1989a; 1989b) (Fig. 7–19). E/A ratio reflects the extent to which diastolic filling occurred in early relative to late diastole. Because it is noninvasive and easily derived, the E/A ratio is commonly

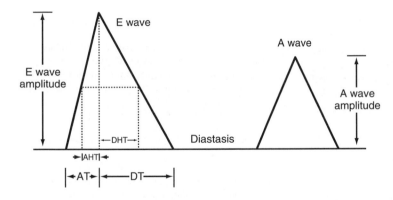

Figure 7–19
Assessment of global left ventricular diastolic function with Doppler echocardiography. The diagram shows transmitral diastolic flow velocity spectrum (inflow pattern into the LV) and relevant intervals and amplitudes. AT = acceleration time; DT = deceleration time; AHT = acceleration half time; DHT = deceleration half time.

used as a measure of diastolic performance. The normal ratio is greater than 1.0, and because diastolic function is progressively impaired with advancing age, the E/A ratio decreases with age (Bryg et al, 1987b).

Although the E/A ratio may reflect various aspects of diastolic function including ventricular relaxation and stiffness, one important drawback is that it lacks specificity for disturbances of diastolic function. Thus, although diastolic dysfunction usually causes a decrease in E/A ratio, a decrease unrelated to diastolic dysfunction may also be seen with rapid heart rate (Harrison et al, 1991) and decreased preload, as occurs with nitroglycerin administration. Increased E/A, which may mask diastolic dysfunction, is seen with increased preload such as with restrictive cardiomyopathy, mitral regurgitation, overt congestive heart failure, and volume overload. At heart rates greater than 90 beats per minute, the E and A waves tend to merge, making it more difficult to determine indices of diastolic function.

Time Constant of Isovolumic Relaxation, τ

Isovolumic relaxation from the time of peak negative (minimum) dP/dt to mitral valve opening has been modeled mathematically as a simple exponential function:

$$P(t) = P_0 \exp(-t/\tau) + P_B$$

where P(t) is instantaneous pressure at time t between the time of peak negative (minimum) dP/dt to mitral valve opening; P_0 is magnitude of pressure at peak negative dP/dt; P_B is the baseline pressure toward which the exponential decays; and τ (pronounced "tau") is time constant of isovolumic pressure fall (i.e., time it takes for pressure to fall to 1/e [37%] of its amplitude at peak negative dP/dt).

Tau measures the rapidity of relaxation. The drawbacks of τ as a measure of relaxation include the fact that it represents a small fraction of

diastole and does not even represent the whole of isovolumic relaxation, because the period of isovolumic relaxation from aortic valve closure to peak negative dP/dt is not represented. Moreover, relaxation usually continues after mitral valve opening, and this period is not addressed by τ.

Isovolumic Relaxation Time (IVRT)

The total duration of isovolumic relaxation has been used as a measure of the adequacy of relaxation. This is the period from aortic valve closure to mitral valve opening. It is identified on the M-mode echocardiogram and measured. Impaired relaxation such as that which occurs with ventricular hypertrophy results in prolongation of isovolumic relaxation time. Enhanced relaxation has the opposite effect. One disadvantage of the IVRT is that the effect of heart rate is not addressed. At slower heart rates, isovolumic relaxation time will tend to be higher. Moreover, at high left atrial pressures, the mitral valve opens sooner and this shortens the IVRT spuriously.

Causes of Diastolic Dysfunction

The three major disorders that cause diastolic dysfunction are hypertrophy (Malhotra et al, 1981; Colan et al, 1985; Topol et al, 1985; Pearson et al, 1986; Lorell and Grossman, 1987; Bryg et al, 1987a; Diver et al, 1988; Pearson et al, 1988; Shepherd et al, 1989; Takamoto et al, 1990), ischemic heart disease, infiltrative processes that alter ventricular stiffness, and, finally, aging.

Left ventricular hypertrophy occurs most commonly because of pressure overload due to hypertension and causes diastolic dysfunction (Shepherd et al, 1989). Other causes of hypertrophy and diastolic dysfunction include valvular heart disease, notably aortic stenosis (Diver et al, 1988) and aortic regurgitation, hypertrophic cardiomyopathy (Bryg et al, 1987a), and hypertensive hypertrophic cardiomyopathy of the elderly (Topol et al, 1985; Pearson et al, 1988). Hypertrophic cardiomyopathy is a unique disease in which the hemodynamic disturbance is exclusively diastolic dysfunction caused by extreme and apparently gratuitous hypertrophy of the LV. Not only does this increase myocardial and LV chamber stiffness and impair relaxation, but it also causes myocardial ischemia, which further impairs diastolic performance. Cardiac chamber hypertrophy may also occur in athletes, but this does not usually cause diastolic dysfunction (Colan et al, 1985; Pearson et al, 1986; Takamoto et al, 1990), probably because exercise improves ventricular lusitropic performance partly by enhancing reuptake of calcium by the sarcoplasmic reticulum (Malhotra et al, 1981).

Various manifestations of ischemic heart disease including chronic asymptomatic coronary artery disease (Carroll et al, 1985; Lawson et al, 1988; Inoue et al, 1992), myocardial ischemia (Labovitz et al, 1987; Wind et al, 1987), and myocardial infarction (Joseph et al, 1990; Chenzbraun et al, 1992; Nonogi et al, 1994; Algom and Schlesinger, 1995; Persson et al, 1995) have all been shown to impair diastolic function by increasing myocardial and ventricular stiffness and impairing relaxation.

Diastolic dysfunction worsens with aging (Miyatake et al, 1984; Miller et al, 1986; Arora et al, 1987; Bonow et al, 1988; Wong et al, 1989; Bryg et al, 1987b); the myocardium becomes stiffer (Gerstenblith et al, 1977; Spurgeon et al, 1977; Templeton et al, 1979) and ventricular relaxation is slower (Lakatta, 1987a). Reasons for the increase in stiffness include an increase in left ventricular wall thickness with age (Gerstenblith et al, 1977), partly as a result of progressive increase in blood pressure with age and partly independently of blood pressure. The poor relaxation is related to impairment of calcium reuptake by the LSR with age (Lakatta et al, 1987b). Moreover diastolic dysfunction is generally more prevalent with aging because other disorders that cause it increase in prevalence with age.

There are some pathologic conditions, which, although they do not affect the myocardium *per se*, nonetheless lead to impairment of ventricular filling. These include pericardial diseases causing pericardial effusion, pericardial tamponade and pericardial constriction, and hyperinflation of the lungs (see Chapter 4).

REFERENCES

Alexander J Jr, Sunagawa K, Chang N, and Sagawa K: Instantaneous pressure-volume relation of the ejecting canine left atrium. Circ Res 61:209–219, 1987.

Algom M and Schlesinger Z: Serial changes in left ventricular diastolic indexes derived from Doppler echocardiography after anterior wall acute myocardial infarction. Am J Cardiol 75:1272–1273, 1995.

Allen DG, Jewell BR, and Murray JW: The contribution of activation processes to the length-tension relation of cardiac muscle. Nature 248:606–607, 1974.

Allen DG and Kurihara S: The effects of muscle length on intracellular calcium transients in mammalian cardiac muscle. J Physiol 327:79–94, 1982.

Altman LK: Brazil surgeon develops a bold, promising operation for patients with heart failure. New York Times, June 14, 1996, p A16.

Arora RR, Machac J, Goldman ME, et al: Atrial kinetics and left ventricular diastolic filling in the healthy elderly. J Am Coll Cardiol 9:1255–1260, 1987.

Babu A, Sonnenblick E, and Gulati J: Molecular basis for the influence of muscle length on myocardial performance. Science 240:74–76, 1988.

Blinks JR and Endoh M: Modification of myofibrillar responsiveness to Ca^{2+} as an inotropic mechanism. Circulation 73 [suppl III]:85–98, 1986.

Bonow RO, Vitale DF, Bacharach SL, et al: Effects of aging on asynchronous left ventricular regional function and global ventricular filling in normal human subjects. J Am Coll Cardiol 11:50–58, 1988.

Braunwald E, Ross J, and Sonnenblick EH: Mechanisms of Contraction of the Normal and Failing Heart, 2nd ed. Boston, Little, Brown, 1976.

Bryg RJ, Pearson AC, Williams GA, and Labovitz AJ: Left ventricular systolic and diastolic flow abnormalities determined by Doppler echocardiography in obstructive hypertrophic cardiomyopathy. Am J Cardiol 59:925–931, 1987a.

Bryg RJ, Williams GA, and Labovitz AJ: Effect of aging on left ventricular diastolic filling in normal subjects. Am J Cardiol 59:971–974, 1987b.

Burkhoff D, Sugiura S, Yue DT, and Sagawa K: Contractility-dependent curvilinearity of end-systolic pressure-volume relations. Am J Physiol 252:H1218–H1227, 1987.

Carabello BA and Spann JF: The uses and limitations of end-systolic indexes of left ventricular function. Circulation 69:1058–1064, 1984.

Carmeliet E: A fuzzy subsarcolemmal space for intracellular Na^+ in cardiac cells? Cardiovasc Res 26:433–442, 1992.

Carroll JD, Hess OM, Hirzel HO, et al: Left ventricular systolic and diastolic function in coronary artery disease: Effects of revascularization on exercise-induced ischemia. Circulation 72:119–129, 1985.

Cheng C-P, Freeman GL, Santamore WP, et al: Effects of loading conditions, contractile state and heart rate on early diastolic left ventricular filling in conscious dogs. Circ Res 66:814–823, 1990.

Chenzbraun A, Keren A, and Stern S: Doppler echocardiographic patterns of left ventricular filling in patients early after acute myocardial infarction. Am J Cardiol 70:711–714, 1992.

Colan SD, Sanders SP, MacPherson D, and Borrow KM: Left ventricular diastolic function in elite athletes with physiologic cardiac hypertrophy. J Am Coll Cardiol 6:545–549, 1985.

Diver DJ, Royal HD, Aroesty JM, et al: Diastolic function in patients with aortic stenosis: Influence of left ventricular load reduction. J Am Coll Cardiol 12:642–648, 1988.

Fabiato A: Calcium-induced release of calcium from the cardiac sarcoplasmic reticulum. Am J Physiol 245:C1–C14, 1983.

Fabiato A and Fabiato F: Dependence of the contractile activation of skinned cardiac cells on the sarcomere length. Nature 256:54–56, 1975.

Frank O: On the dynamics of cardiac muscle. Translated by Chapman CB and Wasserman E. Am Heart J 58:282–317, 1959, and Am Heart J 58:467–477, 1959.

Gamble J, Taylor PB, and Kenno KA: Myocardial stretch alters twitch characteristics and Ca^{2+} loading of sarcoplasmic reticulum in rat ventricular muscle. Cardiovasc Res 26:865–870, 1992.

Gerstenblith G, Frederiksen J, Yin FCP, et al: Echocardiographic assessment of a normal adult aging population. Circulation 56:273–278, 1977.

Gordon AM, Huxley AF, and Julian FJ. The variation in isometric tension with sarcomere length in vertebrate muscle fibres. J Physiol (London) 184:170–192, 1966.

Gordon AM and Pollack GH: Effects of calcium on the sarcomere length-tension relation in rat cardiac muscle. Implications for the Frank-Starling mechanism. Circ Res 47:610–619, 1980.

Grossman W, Braunwald E, Mann T, et al: Contractile state of the left ventricle in man evaluated from end-systolic pressure-volume relations. Circulation 56:845–852, 1977.

Grossman W, Jones D, and McLaurin LP: Wall stress and patterns of hypertrophy in the human left ventricle. J Clin Invest 56: 56–64, 1975.

Harrison MR, Clifton GD, Pennell AT, and DeMaria AN: Effect of heart rate on left ventricular diastolic transmitral flow velocity patterns assessed by Doppler echocardiography in normal subjects. Am J Cardiol 67:622–627, 1991.

Hofmann PA and Fuchs F: Effect of length and cross-bridge attachment on Ca^{2+} binding to cardiac troponin C. Am J Physiol 253:C90–C96, 1987.

Hofmann PA and Fuchs F: Bound calcium and force development in skinned cardiac muscle bundles: Effect of sarcomere length. J Mol Cell Cardiol 20:667–677, 1988.

Hunter WC: End-systolic pressure as a balance between opposing effects of ejection. Circ Res 64:265–275, 1989.

Iizuka M: End-systolic pressure-volume relations. Circulation 58:379, 1978.

Inoue T, Morooka S, Hayashi T, et al: Left ventricular diastolic dysfunction in coronary artery disease: Effects of coronary revascularization. Clin Cardiol 15:577–581, 1992.

Ishida Y, Meisner JS, Tsujiokak S, et al: Left ventricular filling dynamics: Influence of left ventricular relaxation and left atrial pressure. Circulation 74:187–196, 1986.

Jewell BR and Rovell JM: Influence of previous mechanical events on the contractility of cat papillary muscle. J Physiol (London) 235:725–740, 1973.

Joseph G and Jose VJ. Right ventricular filling abnormalities in acute inferior wall myocardial infarction—a pulsed Doppler study. Indian Heart J 42:437–440, 1990.

Kass DA, Beyar R, Lankford E, et al: Influence of contractile state on curvilinearity of in situ end-systolic pressure-volume relations. Circulation 79:167–178, 1989.

Kass DA, Maughan WL, Guo ZM, et al: Comparative influence of load versus inotropic states on indexes of inotropic state: Experimental and theoretical analysis based on pressure-volume relationships. Circulation 76:1422–1436, 1987.

Katz AM: Sarcoplasmic reticular control of cardiac contraction and relaxation. In Grossman W and Lorell BH (eds): Diastolic Relaxation of the Heart. Basic Research and Current Applications for Clinical Cardiology. Boston, Martinus Nijhoff, 1989, pp 11–15.

Katz AM, Takenaka H, and Watras J: The sarcoplasmic reticulum. In Fozzard HA, Haber E, Jennings RB, et al (eds): The Heart and Cardiovascular System. Scientific Foundations. New York, Raven Press, 1986, pp 731–746.

Kaufman RL, Bayer RM, and Harnasch C: Autoregulation of contractility in the myocardial cell. Displacement as a controlling parameter. Pflugers Arch 332:96–116, 1972.

Kentish JC, ter Keurs HEDJ, Ricciardi L, et al: Comparison between the sarcomere length-force relations of intact and skinned trabeculae from rat right ventricle. Circ Res 58:755–768, 1986.

Kohmoto O, Levi AJ, and Bridge JHB: Relation between reverse sodium-calcium exchange and sarcoplasmic reticulum calcium release in guinea pig ventricular cells. Circ Res 74:550–554, 1994.

Labovitz AJ, Lewen MK, Kern M, et al: Evaluation of left ventricular systolic and diastolic dysfunction during transient myocardial ischemia produced by angioplasty. J Am Coll Cardiol 10:748–755, 1987.

Labovitz AJ and Pearson AC: Evaluation of left ventricular diastolic function: Clinical relevance and recent Doppler echocardiographic insights. Am Heart J 114:836–851, 1987.

Lakatta EG: Cardiac muscle changes in senescence. Ann Rev Physiol 49:519–531, 1987a.

Lakatta EG: Starling's Law of the heart is explained by an intimate interaction of muscle length and myofilament calcium activation. J Am Coll Cardiol 10:1157–1164, 1987b.

Lau VK, Sagawa K, and Suga H: Instantaneous pressure-volume relationship of right atrium during isovolumic contraction in canine heart. Am J Physiol 236:H672–H679, 1979.

Lawson WE, Seifert F, Anagnostopoulos C, et al: Effect of coronary artery bypass grafting on left ventricular diastolic function. Am J Cardiol 61:283–287, 1988.

Leblanc N and Hume JR: Sodium current-induced release of calcium from cardiac sarcoplasmic reticulum. Science 248:372–376, 1990.

Lederer JW, Niggli E, and Hadley RW: Sodium-calcium exchange in excitable cells: Fuzzy space. Science 248:283, 1990.

Levesque PC, Leblance N, and Hume JR: Release of calcium from guinea pig cardiac sarcoplasmic reticulum induced by sodium-calcium exchange. Cardiovasc Res 28:370–378, 1994.

Lew WYW: Time-dependent increase in left ventricular contractility following acute volume loading in the dog. Circ Res 63:635–647, 1988.

Lorell BH and Grossman W: Cardiac hypertrophy: The consequences for diastole. J Am Coll Cardiol 9:1189–1193, 1987.

Malhotra A, Penpargkul S, Schaible T, and Scheuer J: Contractile proteins and sarcoplasmic reticulum in physiologic cardiac hypertrophy. Am J Physiol 241:H263–H267, 1981.

Maughan WL, Shoukas AA, Sagawa K, and Weisfeldt ML: Instantaneous pressure-volume relationship of the canine right ventricle. Circ Res 44:309–315, 1979.

Miller TR, Grossman SJ, Schectman KB, et al: Left ventricular diastolic filling and its association with age. Am J Cardiol 58:531–535, 1986.

Milnor WR: Arterial impedance as ventricular afterload. Circ Res 36:565–570, 1975.

Mirsky I: Elastic properties of the myocardium: A quantitative approach with physiological and clinical applications. In Berne RM (ed): Handbook of Physiology, Vol 1, Section 2, The Cardiovascular System. Heart. Bethesda, MD, American Physiological Society, 1979, pp 501–527.

Miyatake K, Okamoto M, Kinoshita N, et al: Augmentation of atrial contribution to left ventricular inflow with aging as assessed by intracardiac Doppler flowmetry. Am J Cardiol 53:586–589, 1984.

Myhre ESP, Johansen A, and Piene H: Optimal matching between canine left ventricle and afterload. Am J Physiol 254:H1051–H1058, 1988.

Nishimura RA, Housmans PR, Hatle LK, and Tajik AJ: Assessment of diastolic function of the heart: Background and current applications of Doppler echocardiography. Part I. Physiologic and pathophysiologic features. Mayo Clin Proc 64:71–81, 1989a.

Nishimura RA, Housmans PR, Hatle LK, and Tajik AJ: Assessment of diastolic function of the heart: Background and current applications of Doppler echocardiography. Part II. Clinical studies. Mayo Clin Proc 64:181–204, 1989b.

Nonogi H, Kawase Y, Miyazaki S, et al: Assessment of left ventricular filling dynamics utilizing Doppler echocardiography in acute coronary syndrome. Jpn Heart J 35:163–173, 1994.

Nwasokwa O, Sagawa K, and Suga H: Short-term memory in the in situ canine myocardium. Am J Physiol 247:H8–H16, 1984.

Nwasokwa ON: Effect of heart rate on myocardial relaxation in isometric twitches. Cardiovasc Res 28:92–99, 1994.

Parmley WW and Chuck L: Length-dependent changes in myocardial contractile state. Am J Physiol 224:1195–199, 1973.

Patterson SW, Piper H, and Starling EH: The regulation of the heart beat. J Physiol (London) 48:475–513, 1914.

Pearson AC, Gudipati CV, and Labovitz AJ: Systolic and diastolic flow abnormalities in elderly patients with hypertensive hypertrophic cardiomyopathy. J Am Coll Cardiol 12:989–995, 1988.

Pearson AC, Schiff M, Mrosek D, et al: Left ventricular diastolic function in weight lifters. Am J Cardiol 58:1254–1259, 1986.

Persson H, Linder-Klingsell E, Eriksson SV, and Erhardt L: Heart failure after myocardial infarction: The importance of diastolic dysfunction. A prospective clinical and echocardiographic study. Eur Heart J 16:496–505, 1995.

Quinones MA, Gaasch WH, and Alexander JK: Influence of acute changes in preload, afterload and contractile state and heart rate on ejection and isovolumic indices of myocardial contractility in man. Circulation 53:293–302, 1976.

Ross J, Sonnenblick EH, Covell JW, et al: Architecture of the heart in systole and diastole: Technique of rapid fixation and analysis of left ventricular geometry. Circ Res 21:409–421, 1967.

Sabbah HN and Stein PD: Pressure-diameter relations during early diastole in dogs. Circ Res 45:357–365, 1981.

Sagawa K: The ventricular pressure-volume diagram revisited (brief review). Circ Res 43:677–687, 1978.

Sagawa K: End-systolic pressure-volume relations in retrospect and prospect. Introduction. Fed Proc 43:2399–2401, 1984.

Sarnoff SJ, Mitchell JH, Gilmore JP, et al: Homeometric autoregulation of the heart. Circ Res 8:1077–1091, 1960.

Sham JSK, Cleemann L, and Morad M: Gating of the cardiac Ca^{2+} release channel: The role of Na^+ current and Na^+-Ca^{2+} exchange. Science 255:850–853, 1992.

Shepherd RFJ, Zachariah PK, and Shub C: Hypertension and left ventricular diastolic function. Mayo Clin Proc 64:1521–1532, 1989.

Sigiura S, Hunter WC, and Sagawa K: Long-term

versus intrabeat history of ejection as determinants of canine ventricular end-systolic pressure. Circ Res 64:255–264, 1989.

Singh BN and Nademanee K: Control of cardiac arrhythmias by selective lengthening of repolarization: Theoretic considerations and clinical observations. Am Heart J 109:421–430, 1985.

Sonnenblick EH, Ross J, Covell JW, et al: Ultrastructure of the heart in systole and diastole. Changes in sarcomere length. Circ Res 21:423–431, 1967.

Spirito P and Maron BJ: Doppler echocardiography for assessing left ventricular diastolic function. Ann Intern Med 109:122–126, 1988.

Spirito P, Maron BJ, and Bonow RO: Noninvasive assessment of left ventricular diastolic function: Comparative analysis of Doppler echocardiographic and radionuclide angiographic techniques. J Am Coll Cardiol 7:518–526, 1986.

Spurgeon HA, Thorne PR, Yin FCP, et al: Increased dynamic stiffness of trabeculae carneae from senescent rats. Am J Physiol 232:H373–H380, 1977.

Starling EH: The Arris and Gale lectures on some points in the pathology of heart disease. Lecture 1. The compensating mechanism of the heart. Lancet 1:569–572, 1897.

Stefanon I, Vassallo DV, and Mill JG: Left ventricular length dependent activation in the isovolumetric rat heart. Cardiovasc Res 24:254–256, 1990.

Suga H: End-systolic pressure-volume relations. Circulation 59:419–420, 1979.

Suga H, Hisano R, Goto Y, and Yamada O: Normalization of end-systolic pressure-volume relation and E_{max} of different sized hearts. Jpn Circ J 48:136–143, 1984.

Suga H and Sagawa K: Instantaneous pressure-volume relationships and their ratio in the excised, supported canine left ventricle. Circ Res 35:117–126, 1974.

Suga H, Sagawa K, and Shoukas AA: Load independence of the instantaneous pressure-volume ratio of the canine left ventricle and the effects of epinephrine and heart rate on the ratio. Circ Res 32:314–322, 1973.

Suga H and Yamakoshi K: Effects of stroke volume and velocity of ejection on end-systolic pressure of canine left ventricle. End-systolic volume clamping. Circ Res 40:445–450, 1977.

Sunagawa K, Maughan WL, and Sagawa K: Optimal arterial resistance for the maximal stroke work studied in isolated canine left ventricle. Circ Res 56:586–595, 1985.

Tada M and Katz AM: Phosphorylation of the sarcoplasmic reticulum and sarcolemma. Ann Rev Physiol 44:401–423, 1982.

Takamoto KA, Marshak D, Lopez JF, et al: Exercise training diminishes the left ventricular diastolic filling abnormalities associated with aging. J Am Coll Cardiol 15:163A, 1990.

Templeton GH, Platt MR, Willerson JT, and Weisfeldt ML: Influence of aging on left ventricular hemodynamics and stiffness in beagles. Circ Res 44:189–194, 1979.

Thomas JD, Newell JB, Choog CY, and Weyman AE: Physical and physiological determinants of transmitral velocity. Am J Physiol 260:H1718–H1731, 1991.

Thomas JD and Weyman AE: Echocardiographic Doppler evaluation of left ventricular diastolic function. Circulation 84:977–990, 1991.

Topol EJ, Traill TA, and Fortuin NJ: Hypertensive hypertrophic cardiomyopathy of the elderly. N Engl J Med 312:277–283, 1985.

Van den Horn GJ, Westerhof N, and Elzinga G: Optimal power generation by the left ventricle. A study in the anesthetized open thorax cat. Circ Res 56:252–261, 1985.

Von Anrep G: On the part played by the suprarenals in the normal vascular reactions of the body. J Physiol (London) 45:307–330, 1912.

Wind BE, Snider R, Bufs SJ, et al: Pulsed Doppler assessment of left ventricular diastolic filling in coronary artery disease before and immediately after coronary angioplasty. Am J Cardiol 59:1041–1046, 1987.

Wong WF, Gold S, Fukuyama O, and Blanchette P: Diastolic dysfunction in elderly patients with congestive heart failure. Am J Cardiol 63:1526–1528, 1989.

Yin FCP: Ventricular wall stress. Circ Res 49:829–842, 1981.

Zhang R, Zhao J, and Mandveno A: Cardiac troponin I phosphorylation increases the rate of cardiac muscle relaxation. Circ Res 76:1028–1035, 1995.

Zile MR, Izzi G, and Gaasch WH: Left ventricular diastolic dysfunction limits use of maximum systolic elastance as an index of contractile function. Circulation 83:674–680, 1991.

Oxygen Transport and Utilization

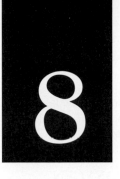

8

Guillermo Gutierrez, M.D., Ph.D.

Qamar U. Arfeen, M.D.

Critical illness often results from diseases that affect one or several components of the oxygen (O_2) transport process. For example, during acute lung injury O_2 fails to diffuse from alveoli into pulmonary capillary blood, whereas the flow of oxygenated blood from the lungs to the tissues decreases during heart failure. Other pathologic conditions, such as sepsis, are known to adversely affect microvascular control (Drazenovic, 1992) and perhaps may even interfere with the biochemical reactions of cellular energy metabolism (Vary, 1986).

Sustained decreases in cellular O_2 delivery result in irreversible cellular damage, especially in organs with high metabolic requirements, such as the heart and brain. A survival strategy used by most vertebrates to prevent tissue hypoxia is to increase systemic O_2 transport, which is a goal usually attained by a faster heart rate. This is the case during exercise, as blood flow to contracting muscles increases to meet the higher metabolic demands for O_2. The exercise paradigm has led to the hypothesis that increasing systemic O_2 delivery should prevent cellular hypoxia. However, several studies designed to test this hypothesis in critically ill patients have yielded disappointing results, and at least one study reported greater mortality in patients subjected to increased O_2 transport (Hayes et al, 1994). The failure of these therapeutic trials suggests that the maintenance of adequate energy supply to the cells during critical illness is not a simple function of systemic O_2 transport and tissue oxygenation. Rather, cellular energy balance depends on complex mechanisms of mass transport, microvascular control, and cellular bioenergetic metabolism.

The extreme pathologic conditions that characterize critical illness sometimes interfere with the adequate O_2 supply to all cells. To achieve this goal in most patients requires a clear understanding of the physiologic determinants of systemic O_2 transport as it relates to capillary O_2 delivery and tissue oxygenation, mitochondrial O_2 utilization, and cellular aerobic energy production. This chapter offers an overview of the physiology of

Supported in part by an American Lung Association Career Investigator Award.

the O_2 transport process and of the biochemical reactions involved in the production of cellular energy. Furthermore, the clinical application of these principles and the practical use of monitors of tissue oxygenation are discussed.

EVOLUTION OF AN OXYGEN TRANSPORT SYSTEM

Simple aerobic organisms appeared in the earth's oceans toward the end of the Archean era, approximately 1500 million years ago. The earth's atmosphere at that time contained less than 1% oxygen (Orgel, 1973). Primordial prokaryotic organisms lacked specialized respiratory mechanisms; instead, passive diffusion of O_2 and carbon dioxide (CO_2) across the cell membrane was sufficient to provide these organisms with the required flux of O_2. At some point in the evolutionary scale there appeared cells with chloroplast, an organelle capable of employing the energy from sunlight. The propagation of photosynthetic organisms was accompanied by an increase in atmospheric O_2, because these cells consumed CO_2 and produced O_2 as a waste product. Greater O_2 concentrations in air led to the development of cells capable of using O_2 as the final acceptor in a chain of organic electron donors, the cytochromes, located in the inner surface of the mitochondrion. The latter is a remarkable organelle capable of generating large quantities of energy in the form of adenosine triphosphate (ATP). It is unknown whether primitive organisms developed mitochondria or if these organelles evolved as separate entities that were later incorporated into aerobic cells. Whatever was the case, the increase in cellular energy resulting from aerobic metabolism made possible the emergence of complex multicellular life forms. The evolution of multicellular organisms in turn led to the development of efficient gas exchange mechanisms for the delivery of O_2 and for the removal of CO_2 from the innermost cells in the tissues.

In land-dwelling vertebrates, the delivery of O_2 to the tissues is accomplished by the combined action of the lungs, cardiovascular system, and blood (Wood and Lenfant, 1979). Atmospheric O_2 is brought into intimate contact with blood in the pulmonary capillaries, and O_2 diffuses across the alveolocapillary membrane into the erythrocytes, where it binds to hemoglobin. The pumping action of the heart carries blood to the tissue capillaries. There, O_2 dissociates from hemoglobin and diffuses into the cells by passive diffusion (Weibel et al, 1981).

As shown in Figure 8–1, the transport of O_2 from the atmosphere to the mitochondria occurs along a wide P_{O_2} gradient that, at sea level, ranges from 150 mm Hg to less than 0.1 mm Hg. This transport process can be broadly divided into convection, chemical reaction, and tissue diffusion. Each of these subprocesses may be affected by critical illness.

TRANSPORT OF OXYGEN TO THE PERIPHERAL CAPILLARIES

Alveolar O_2 diffuses into pulmonary capillary blood. The amount of O_2 transferred from alveoli to pulmonary blood depends mainly on the ventilation-perfusion relationship of the lungs and on the inspired O_2 concentration, F_{IO_2}. Other important factors that determine pulmonary O_2 exchange are the diffusion characteristics of the alveolocapillary membrane, hemoglobin concentration in blood, and affinity of hemoglobin for O_2.

The O_2 concentration in plasma is a function of the atmospheric pressure, proportion of O_2 in air, and solubility coefficient of plasma for O_2. This relationship, also known as Henry's law, states that:

$$\text{Dissolved } O_2 = c \times P_{O_2}/P_{atm} \quad [1]$$

The term c represents the solubility coefficient of O_2 in blood, 0.023 ml O_2/ml of blood at 38°C (Roughton, 1964), P_{atm} is the atmospheric pressure, and P_{O_2} is the partial pressure of O_2 in blood. Expressing dissolved O_2 in terms of milliliters of O_2/100 ml of blood (STPD) or, as it is commonly known, milliliters of O_2/vol %:

$$\text{Dissolved } O_2 = \frac{100 \times 0.023}{P_{atm} - 47} \times P_{O_2} \approx 0.0031 \times P_{O_2} \quad [2]$$

Under normal physiologic conditions, the concentration of O_2 dissolved in plasma is not sufficient to meet the metabolic requirements of the tissues. Instead, the bulk of O_2 in blood is carried by hemoproteins that bind molecular O_2 in the peripheral gas exchange organs and release it in the tissue capillaries. Among these hemoproteins are the hemocyanins of invertebrates and the hemoglobins of vertebrates.

PROPERTIES OF HEMOGLOBIN

Hemoglobin is a complex protein composed of four individual peptide chains bound to a heme residue by a noncovalent linkage. Two of the peptide chains, the α chains, have 141 amino acids. The remaining two chains, the β chains,

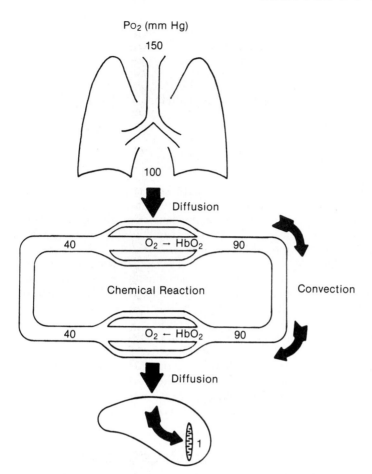

Figure 8–1
The oxygen transport system from atmosphere to mitochondria. The numbers represent the partial pressures of oxygen in millimeters of mercury (mm Hg). By the processes of diffusion, convection, and chemical reaction, oxygen moves down a gradient of 150 mm Hg in sea level air to 1 mm Hg or less in the mitochondria.

contain 146 amino acids. Each heme residue contains an iron atom capable of binding reversibly with O_2. This iron atom does not change valence as O_2 is bound to or released by hemoglobin, but remains in the Fe^{2+} (ferrous) state. The addition of ferricyanide to hemoglobin changes the iron atom to the Fe^{3+} (ferric) state. This produces methemoglobin, a molecule that binds O_2 irreversibly (Antonini and Brunori, 1971).

The binding of O_2 to hemoglobin exhibits the characteristics of a homotropic enzyme system (Antonini, 1979), where the substrate (O_2) also serves as a modulator of catalytic activity. This behavior results in the sigmoid-shaped oxyhemoglobin dissociation curve (ODC) shown in Figure 8–2. The ODC depicts the O_2 saturation of hemoglobin (S_{O_2}) as a function of plasma P_{O_2}.

The cooperative binding of O_2 to hemoglobin is the result of mechanical interaction among the heme residues. Hemoglobin behaves functionally as if composed by two separate subunits, instead of a tetramer. Each subunit contains an α chain tightly bound to a β chain (Antonini and Brunori, 1971). When a molecule of O_2 binds to the

heme group of an α chain, it also changes its conformation. This transformation is mechanically transmitted to the β chain of the α-β subunit, enhancing its affinity for O_2 and promoting the binding of a second O_2 molecule. This produces further spatial rearrangements of the α-β subunit, causing the adjacent α-β subunit to assume a higher O_2 affinity. These changes ultimately result in the complete saturation of the hemoglobin molecule.

The ability of hemoglobin to change its affinity for O_2 makes it an ideal O_2 carrier. In the pulmonary capillaries the binding to hemoglobin is facilitated, whereas in the tissue capillaries the dissociation of O_2 is promoted. The main factors that determine the degree of capillary O_2 uptake and release are the concentration of hemoglobin (Hb) and the kinetics of the O_2-Hb reaction.

KINETICS OF THE O_2-HEMOGLOBIN REACTION

The kinetics of the reaction between O_2 and Hb were described originally by Hufner (1890) as a unimolecular, first-order system of the form:

$$[Hb] + [O_2] \overset{k'}{\underset{k}{\leftrightarrow}} [HbO_2] \qquad [3]$$

A mathematical expression of this stoichiometric equation is:

$$\frac{d[HbO_2]}{dt} = k'\,[O_2]\,[Hb] - k\,[HbO_2] \qquad [4]$$

In this equation the parameters k and k' are the forward and backward reaction-velocity coefficients, respectively. Hufner's model did not account for the homotropic effect of O_2 binding to Hb. At equilibrium, which is defined mathematically by the condition in which $d[HbO_2]/dt = 0$, this model describes a rectangular hyperbola instead of the sigmoid-shaped ODC determined experimentally (Bohr et al, 1904). Because of its simplicity, however, equation 4 has been used widely in many first-order models of capillary O_2 exchange (Fletcher, 1978; Kety, 1957; Roughton et al, 1957). A better model was proposed by Hill (1910; 1921) who assumed that n mole of O_2 bind to hemoglobin, thus converting Hufner's model into an nth order reaction,

$$[Hb]_n + n\,[O_2] \overset{k'}{\underset{k}{\leftrightarrow}} [HbO_2]_n \qquad [5]$$

At equilibrium, this equation becomes:

$$So_2 = (Po_2)/(Po_2^n + k/k') \qquad [6]$$

The aforementioned equation yields an accurate mathematical description of the ODC for values of n between 2.5 and 2.7. However, the discovery that 4 mole of O_2 bind to 1 mole of Hb (instead of approximately 2.5 mole) deprived Hill's equation of its physicochemical significance (Barcroft and Hill, 1910). Hill's equation has a rightful place as an empirical expression of the ODC because of its simplicity. In this equation a single number, the Hill coefficient n, characterizes the region of physiologic interest of the ODC. For that reason, Hill's equation is widely used as a descriptor of hemoglobin kinetics in several time-dependent mathematical models of capillary O_2 exchange (Homer et al, 1981; Popel, 1989).

A physicochemically accurate model was suggested by Adair (1925), in what was defined as the intermediate compound hypothesis. Adair described the O_2-Hb reaction by a series of four steps, each having different association and dissociation velocity constants.

$$[Hb_4] + [O_2] \overset{k_1'}{\underset{k_1}{\leftrightarrow}} [Hb_4O_2] \qquad [7a]$$

$$[Hb_4] + [O_2] \overset{k_2'}{\underset{k_2}{\leftrightarrow}} [Hb_4O_4] \qquad [7b]$$

$$[Hb_4] + [O_2] \overset{k_3'}{\underset{k_3}{\leftrightarrow}} [Hb_4O_6] \qquad [7c]$$

$$[Hb_4] + [O_2] \overset{k_4'}{\underset{k_4}{\leftrightarrow}} [Hb_4O_8] \qquad [7d]$$

Because of its complexity, and because numerous undetermined velocity constants are needed to describe the intermediate steps, the use of Adair's model to describe capillary O_2 exchange has proved impractical.

When blood is saturated with oxygen and cellular energy requirements are low, the time needed by the red blood cells (RBCs) to release the O_2 required by the tissues is much shorter than the capillary transit time. Under those conditions, the effect that changes in O_2 dissociation kinetics have on tissue oxygenation is negligible. However, during maximal exercise or when O_2 supply is decreased, the kinetics of RBC deoxygenation may become the rate-limiting step in the O_2 delivery process (Gayeski and Honig, 1986; Gutierrez, 1986).

OXYHEMOGLOBIN DISSOCIATION CURVE

The equilibrium relationship of O_2 and human hemoglobin, at 37° C temperature and pH 7.40, is described by the sigmoid-shaped ODC in Figure 8–2 (Severinghaus, 1979). In the absence of carbon monoxide (CO) or methemoglobin, the ODC of human blood is 97.5% saturated at Po_2 of 100 mm Hg (Roughton and Severinghaus, 1973). Decreases in Po_2 to 60 mm Hg result in relatively small decreases in So_2 to 90.9%. However, below this Po_2 level lies the steep portion of the ODC, where further reductions in Po_2 are accompanied by large decreases in So_2. The sigmoidicity of hemoglobin, a consequence of its homotropic properties, makes hemoglobin an excellent O_2 carrier, one that binds O_2 in the O_2-rich pulmonary capillaries and releases it in the tissue capillaries, where Po_2 is low (Antonini and Brunori, 1971; Haldane and Smith, 1896).

POSITION OF THE OXYHEMOBLOGIN DISSOCIATION CURVE

The position of the ODC varies with changes in the association and dissociation velocity coefficients. For example, when the association reac-

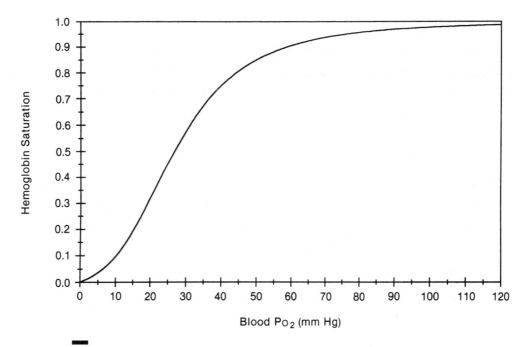

Figure 8–2
The standard oxyhemoglobin dissociation curve at pH 7.40 and temperature 37°C.

tion coefficient (k′) is greater than the dissociation coefficient (k), the affinity of hemoglobin for O_2 increases. This increase in affinity is manifested by a shift to the left in the position of the ODC. Likewise, increases in the dissociation coefficient shift the ODC to the right, resulting in greater amounts of O_2 released at a lower P_{O_2} (Malmberg et al, 1979). The position of the ODC is characterized by its P_{50}, defined as the P_{O_2} corresponding to 50% O_2 saturation of hemoglobin. Under standard conditions, the P_{50} of human blood is 26.7 mm Hg (Aberman et al, 1975; Severinghaus, 1979).

CHANGES IN P_{50}

Changes in the affinity of hemoglobin are the result of conformational changes in the α-β subunits produced by hydrogen ions ([H^+]), 2,3-diphosphoglycerate (2,3-DPG), and CO (Antonini and Brunori, 1971; Shappell and Lenfant, 1972). The influence of these ligands on the position of the ODC depends on temperature and on each other. Changes in temperature can shift the ODC by changing the quaternary structure of hemoglobin and the binding of 2,3-DPG. Shifts in P_{50} also occur with hemoglobinopathies, such as sickle cell disease (Bromberg and Jensen, 1967) or with chronic hypoxemic states (Fairweather et al, 1974; Neilan et al, 1980; Ross and Hlastala, 1981) (Table 8–1).

BOHR EFFECT

Shifts in P_{50} produced by varying the concentration of [H^+] in blood were described originally by Bohr and associates (1904). They noted that the addition of CO_2 to oxygenated blood displaced O_2 from hemoglobin. This is known as the CO_2 Bohr effect. A few years later, Margaria and Green (1933) made the observation that CO_2 has a dual influence on the position of the ODC. The main effect of CO_2 on the ODC occurs from the hydration of CO_2 into carbonic acid with the production of [H^+] (the fixed acid Bohr effect). Acidosis shifts the P_{50} to the right, promoting the release of O_2 to the tissues, whereas alkalosis has the opposite effect. Increases in CO_2 also shift the ODC independently of the acid-base status of blood by forming carbamino compounds that attach to the N-terminal amino acids of the hemoglobin chains (the direct CO_2 effect). The direct effect of CO_2 is relatively minor when compared with the shifts produced by changes in [H^+] (Hlastala, 1979).

The CO_2 Bohr effect is the sum of the fixed acid effect and the direct CO_2 effect. The magnitude of the CO_2 Bohr effect is a function of the O_2 saturation of hemoglobin and of the 2,3-DPG concentration (Hlastala and Woodson, 1975). The CO_2 Bohr effect is magnified by low levels of S_{O_2} and of 2,3-DPG concentration. This is an important property of hemoglobin, because it pro-

Table 8–1
Factors Associated With Changes in Hemoglobin-oxygen Affinity

Increased Affinity (Left Shift)	Decreased Affinity (Right Shift)
Increased pH	Decreased pH
Decreased Pco_2	Increased PCO_2
Decreased temperature	Increased temperature
Decreased 2,3-DPG	Increased 2,3-DPG
Stored blood	Hypoxemia
Phosphate depletion	Anemia
RBC pyruvate kinase excess	Hyperphosphatemia
RBC hexokinase deficiency	RBC pyruvate kinase deficiency
Abnormal hemoglobins	Abnormal hemoglobins
Hereditary	Hereditary (sickle cell disease)
Acquired (carboxyhemoglobin, methemoglobin)	

motes the release of O_2 in the tissues, where O_2 concentration is low but CO_2 is high (Bellingham et al, 1971; Hill, 1910; Nakamura and Staub, 1964). The CO_2 Bohr effect at a given pH and Pco_2 can be calculated using the following empirical expression (Severinghaus, 1979):

$$\Delta \ln Po_2 = (7.4 - pH) [(Po_2/P_{50})\ 0.184 + 0.003\ BE - 2.2] \quad [8]$$

in which $\ln Po_2$ represents the difference in Po_2 at the measured blood pH and at pH 7.4:

$$\Delta \ln Po_2 = (\ln Po_2)_{7.4} - (\ln Po_2)_{pH} \quad [9]$$

In the aforementioned equations BE represents the base excess, ln is the natural logarithm, and the term $\ln(Po_2)_{7.4}$ is the natural logarithm of Po_2 corrected to a standard pH of 7.4. BE accounts for the independent effect of CO_2 on the ODC.

TEMPERATURE

Warmer temperatures shift the ODC to the right. The opposite effect occurs when blood cools (Reeves, 1980). The effect of temperature does not depend on the O_2 saturation (Zwart et al, 1984b). The temperature coefficient of Po_2 is:

$$(\ln Po_2/(T) = 0.058\ [(0.243 \times Po_2/100)\ 3.88 + 1]^{-1} + 0.013 \quad [10]$$

where T = (blood temperature in °C − 37°C).

Temperature alters Pco_2 in the following manner (Nunn et al, 1965):

$$(\log \Delta Pco_2)/(\Delta T) = 0.019 \quad [11]$$

in which log ΔPco_2 is the base 10 logarithm of the Pco_2 at body temperature minus the Pco_2 measured at 37°C.

The effect of temperature on pH at a constant CO_2 content is

$$(\Delta pH)/(\Delta T) = -0.017 \quad [12]$$

in which ΔpH is the pH at body temperature minus the pH measured at 37°C (Rahn et al, 1975; White, 1981).

ORGANIC PHOSPHATES

Erythrocytes are ideal O_2 carriers, because they do not generate ATP aerobically. Instead, these cells use an alternate anaerobic pathway, the hexose-monophosphate shunt, to ferment glucose into pyruvate and lactate. The use of this pathway results in the accumulation of 2,3-DPG. The average 2,3-DPG concentration in human erythrocytes is 4.5 mmol. An increase in the concentration of 2,3-DPG produces a shift to the right of the ODC (Benesch and Benesch, 1967; Chanutin and Curnish, 1967). This effect is related to the binding of 2,3-DPG by deoxyhemoglobin. 2,3-DPG also acts on the ODC by altering the Gibbs-Donnan equilibrium in the cell and lowering intracellular pH (Bauer et al, 1973). The effect of 2,3-DPG on the position of the ODC also depends on temperature and O_2 saturation. Decreases in blood 2,3-DPG concentration are produced by acidosis, blood storage, and a reduction in inorganic phosphate. Hypoxia and altitude increase the 2,3-DPG concentration (Weiskopf and Severinghaus, 1972; Winslow et al, 1981, 1984).

The effect of changes in blood pH and temperature on the position of the ODC takes place rapidly, but alterations in P_{50} resulting from changes in 2,3-DPG require a longer time. The rate of accumulation of 2,3-DPG is a function of RBC glycolysis, and measurable changes in the position of the ODC require 4 to 24 hours to occur (Klocke, 1972). The Bohr effect regulates the position of the ODC in response to sudden changes in blood pH, whereas the function of 2,3-

DPG is to maintain a normal P_{50} during chronic acid-base disturbance (Fairweather et al, 1974). Figure 8–3 shows in graphic form the combined effect of the various parameters discussed on the P_{50} of the human ODC (Woodson, 1977). The interaction of temperature [H^+], CO_2, and 2,3-DPG, as well as their effects on the affinity of hemoglobin for O_2 are also shown in Figure 8–3 (Hlastala and Woodson, 1975). The solid lines represent a positive effect of these variables on hemoglobin affinity and on each other, whereas the broken lines denote a negative or inhibitory effect. For example, a rise in temperature directly decreases hemoglobin affinity, while promoting the effects of decreases in pH or a rise in 2,3-DPG concentration. Conversely, a rise in temperature increases hemoglobin affinity and enhances the inhibitory influence of CO_2. The influence of SO_2 on these variables is not included in Figure 8–3.

CARBON MONOXIDE

Hemoglobin binds reversibly to CO with great tenacity, with approximately 230 times the avidity for O_2 (Collier, 1976). The binding of CO by hemoglobin decreases the sites available for the transport of O_2 and shifts the ODC to the left (Coburn, 1979; Douglas et al, 1912; Forster et al, 1957; Hlastala et al, 1976; Ledwith, 1978). The effect that different concentrations of carboxyhemoglobin have on the ODC is shown in Figure 8–4. The following relationship describes the equilibrium condition between P_{O_2} and P_{CO} in plasma and their respective hemoglobin saturations (Coburn et al, 1965; Haldane, 1895; Roughton, 1964).

$$S_{CO}/S_{O_2} = (M \times P_{CO})/P_{O_2} \qquad [13]$$

In the equation, M is Haldane's constant and has an approximate value of 230. The effect of CO on the position of the ODC has been described by Zwart and associates (1984a) as:

$$P_{50} = -0.28 \times S_{CO}\% + 26.8 \qquad [14]$$

MATHEMATICAL MODEL OF THE OXYHEMOGLOBIN-DISSOCIATION CURVE

A number of mathematical expressions have been developed to describe the ODC (Aberman et al, 1973; Kelman, 1965; Neilan et al, 1980; Nordby

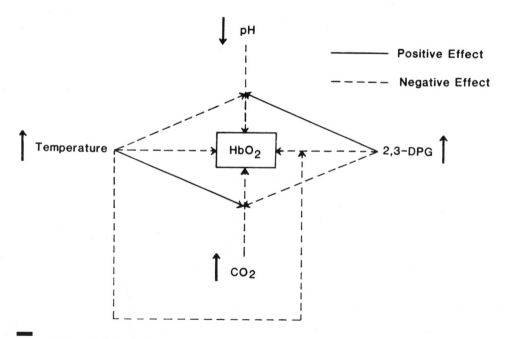

Figure 8–3
Interaction of temperature, CO_2, pH, and 2,3-DPG and their effects on the affinity of hemoglobin for oxygen. HbO_2 represents the affinity of hemoglobin for oxygen. The effect of these variables on hemoglobin affinity and on each other is shown by solid lines (a positive effect) and by broken lines (a negative effect). (From Hlastala MP: Physiological significance of the interaction of oxygen and carbon dioxide in blood. Crit Care Med 7:374–379, 1979. © by Williams & Wilkins.)

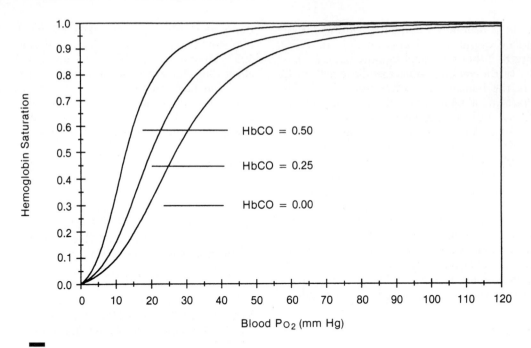

Figure 8–4
Carbon monoxide shifts the oxyhemoglobin dissociation curve to the left. Shown here is the effect of increasing concentrations of HbCO from 0.00 to 0.50 on the position of the oxyhemoglobin dissociation curve.

and Ellis, 1981; Tien and Gabel, 1977). The following equation, proposed by Severinghaus (1979), is simple to use, and it has a mean absolute error of 0.26% for any value of SO_2.

$$SO_2 = \{[(PO_2{}^3 + 150\, PO_2)^{-1} \times 23,400] + 1\}^{-1} \quad [15]$$

The inverse of the aforementioned equation can be used to obtain the standard PO_2 (pH = 7.4; T = 37°C) from a known saturation fraction SO_2:

$$PO_2 = \exp\{0.385\ln [SO_2{}^{-1} - 1]^{-1} + 3.32 - [72SO_2]^{-1} - [SO_2)^6/6]\} \quad [16]$$

The P_{50} of blood can be calculated from a sample of SO_2 and PO_2, measured at 37°C, by the following method (Severinghaus, 1979): (1) compute the standard PO_2 from equation 16 (Bauer et al, 1973); (2) correct the observed PO_2 for the patient's pH and temperature by using equations 8 and 10, respectively; (3) enter these values in the following expression:

$$P_{50} = 26.7 \times (PO_2)_{obs}/(PO_2)_{std} \quad [17]$$

OXYGEN CONTENT OF BLOOD

The total concentration, or content, of O_2 in blood is the sum of dissolved plasma O_2 and O_2 bound to hemoglobin. As shown by equation 2,

the O_2 content of plasma equals 0.0031 × PO_2 ml per 100 ml of blood. The O_2 bound to hemoglobin can be calculated by noting that 4 moles of O_2 bind to 1 mole of hemoglobin. Because each mole of O_2 is equivalent to 22,400 ml, and the molecular weight of hemoglobin is approximately 64,500 (Lehninger, 1975), the O_2 content of saturated hemoglobin is:

$$\left(4 \times \frac{22,400}{64,500}\right) = 1.39\, \text{ml}\, O_2 \quad [18]$$

This number varies from 1.34 to 1.39, depending on the value used for the molecular weight of hemoglobin. In addition, small quantities of methemoglobin can result in an underestimation of the aforementioned number when direct measurements of the O_2-carrying capacity of blood are performed.

The amount of O_2 carried by hemoglobin depends on its degree of O_2 saturation. The total O_2-carrying capacity of blood is lowered by the presence of other ligands, such as CO, or nonfunctional hemoglobins in the form of methemoglobin. The O_2 content of blood, expressed in milliliters of O_2 per liter of blood, is:

$$O_2\ \text{content} = 1.39 \times SO_2 \times [\text{Hb}]_{total} + 0.0031 \times PO_2 \times 10 \quad [19]$$

Figure 8–5 shows the O_2 content curve of

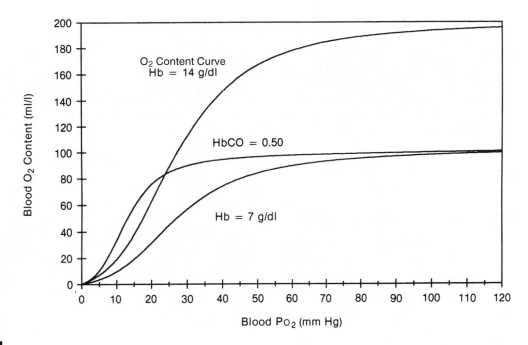

Figure 8–5
The standard calculated blood oxygen content curve based on a hemoglobin concentration of 14 g/dl. Shown also are effects of 50% reduction in hemoglobin concentration (7 g/dl) and 50% increase in carboxyhemoglobin. At high P_{O_2} values, both conditions decrease the O_2 content by 50%, but the left shift of the ODC produced by carbon monoxide results in lower venous P_{O_2} values for a given O_2 content.

blood with a normal $[Hb]_{total}$ of 14 g/dl. Also shown are the effects of anemia with $[Hb]_{total} = 7$ g/dl and that of CO, $S_{CO} = 0.50$. Both abnormal conditions reduce the maximal attainable O_2 content by 50%. Shifts in the position of the ODC have a significant effect on venous P_{O_2}. For example CO and anemia depress the O_2 content curve, but CO also shifts the curve to the left, resulting in a lower venous P_{O_2} for a given arterovenous O_2 difference. This may explain why severe anemia is better tolerated than similar reductions in O_2 content produced by CO (Coburn et al, 1965).

PHYSIOLOGIC DETERMINANT OF SYSTEMIC OXYGEN TRANSPORT AND OXYGEN CONSUMPTION

The transport of O_2 to the tissues, $\dot{T}_{O_2}$, is the product of the cardiac output ($\dot{Q}$), expressed in liters per minute, and the arterial O_2 content, Ca_{O_2}:

$$\dot{T}_{O_2} = \dot{Q} \times Ca_{O_2}\,\text{ml } O_2/\text{min} \qquad [20]$$

It is evident that an adequate cardiac output is very important in the transport of O_2 to the tissues. Although individual decreases in $[Hb]_{total}$, Sa_{O_2}, or $\dot{Q}$ result in similar decreases in $\dot{T}_{O_2}$, the capacity of the cardiac output to increase

in response to a fall in S_{O_2} or in hemoglobin concentration provides an immediate compensatory mechanism. Conversely, compensatory responses to decreases in cardiac output do not occur rapidly or to a significant degree, owing to the slow process of hemoglobin generation and to the flattened shape of the ODC at normal P_{O_2} levels (60 to 100 mm Hg). Furthermore, in the clinical setting, anemia or hypoxemia sometimes are easier to correct than improving the pumping capacity of a failing left ventricle.

O_2 consumption by the tissues ($\dot{V}_{O_2}$) is determined by Fick's equation:

$$\dot{V}_{O_2} = \dot{Q} \times (Ca_{O_2} - C\bar{v}_{O_2})\,\text{ml } O_2/\text{min} \qquad [21]$$

in which the mixed venous content, $C\bar{v}_{O_2}$, is calculated from the $P\bar{v}_{O_2}$ and $S\bar{v}_{O_2}$ of pulmonary artery blood. The term $(Ca_{O_2} - C\bar{v}_{O_2})$ is the arterovenous content difference.

A useful physiologic parameter to describe the ability of the tissues to remove O_2 from blood is the extraction ratio (ER_{O_2}), defined as $ER_{O_2} = \dot{V}_{O_2}/\dot{T}_{O_2}$, or its reciprocal, the coefficient of oxygen delivery (COD) (Tenney and Mithoefer, 1982).

Another method to calculate systemic $\dot{V}_{O_2}$ relies on measurements of minute ventilation ($\dot{V}_E$), the fractions of O_2 in the inspired and expired gases (F_{IO_2} and F_{EO_2}), and the expired gas CO_2 fraction (F_{ECO_2}) (Otis, 1964). The error in this calculation of $\dot{V}_{O_2}$ increases in direct proportion to the F_{IO_2}, and it becomes unreliable when the inspired O_2 fraction is greater than 0.60. Some clinical studies suggest that this method of calculating $\dot{V}_{O_2}$ in critically ill patients may be preferable to using Fick's equation.

OXYGEN UTILIZATION BY THE TISSUES

REDISTRIBUTION OF CARDIAC OUTPUT

The level of perfusion of different tissue beds is accomplished by the combined action of arterioles and the microcirculation. Moderate hypoxemia results in increases in cardiac output and decreases in peripheral vascular resistance (Adachi et al, 1976; Malo et al, 1984; Sylvester et al, 1979). There is a preferential increase in flow to the coronary, cerebral, adrenal, and skeletal muscle circulations (Nesarajah et al, 1983). Flow to the kidneys and abdominal viscera remains unchanged or decreases (Heistad and Abboud, 1980), which may explain the propensity of these organs to early ischemic injury. Changes in cardiac output and peripheral resistance are associated with increases in plasma catecholamines and renin activity, which in turn may regulate the angiotensin II level to produce optimal vasomotor control during hypoxia (Davidson and Stalcup, 1984).

CHANGES IN HEMOGLOBIN AFFINITY

Changes in hemoglobin affinity reflect alterations in the kinetics of RBC deoxygenation in the capillaries. Shifts in the position of the ODC have a significant impact on tissue oxygenation because they affect the O_2 content of arterial blood (Riggs et al, 1973; Ross and Hlastala, 1981; Wagner, 1974; Winslow et al, 1981; Woodson, 1977, 1979). The relationship between arterial O_2 content and P_{50} is discussed in the preceding sections of this chapter. The possible effects that changes in P_{50} may have on tissue oxygenation are more difficult to define. A right-sided shift of the ODC improves tissue oxygenation under most circumstances, except when alveolar hypoxia is present, such as may occur at high altitude. In that case, hemoglobin in the pulmonary capillaries is not fully saturated and arterial blood content is decreased (Bencowitz et al, 1982; Willford et al, 1982).

Although it is commonly accepted that decreases in hemoglobin affinity promote the release of O_2 in the tissue capillaries, there is considerable debate over the effect that a curve with a shift to the left has on O_2 delivery. Barcroft (1925) speculated that an increase in affinity plays a role in acclimatization to high altitude because as it maintains adequate arterial hemoglobin saturation with lowered alveolar P_{O_2}. Subsequent measurements demonstrated a rise in 2,3-DPG, usually accompanied by chronic hyperventilation and respiratory alkalosis (Hurtado, 1964). The net effect of these opposing factors on the ODC is either no change in P_{50} or a slight increase in affinity (Weiskopf and Severinghaus, 1972). Measurements obtained at the summit of Mt. Everest showed a shift in arterial blood P_{50} to 19.4 mm Hg when Pa_{O_2} decreased to 28 mm Hg, suggesting that under conditions of extreme hypoxemia a shift to the left of the ODC may improve tissue oxygenation (Winslow et al, 1984). On the other hand, Gutierrez and Andry (1989a) measured changes in rabbit skeletal muscle $\dot{V}_{O_2}$ and phosphocreatine levels using magnetic resonance spectroscopy (MRS) and found that a left-shifted ODC does not improve $\dot{V}_{O_2}$ during hypoxemia. The reason was a proportional decrease in tissue ERO_2 as hemoglobin affinity increased. In other words, higher affinity hemoglobin binds more oxygen in the lungs at a given alveolar P_{O_2}, but has difficulty releasing it to the tissues. It is possible that with maximal exercise, hemoglobin shifts to the left in the pulmonary capillaries, the result of hyperventilation-induced alkalemia, and then shifts to the right in the capillaries of working muscles where pH is decreased. This phasic adjustments in P_{50} provide the optimal conditions for O_2 transfer from the lungs to the tissues. The role that a left-shifted ODC has in the management of critically ill patients with severe hypoxemia remains to be determined.

MICROCIRCULATION

The microcirculation is the largest and least understood portion of the O_2 transport system. It consists of the terminal arterioles, capillaries, and postcapillary venules. The capillaries consist of a single layer of endothelial cells that allow the free exchange of water, solutes, and gases, but retain large-sized molecules such as albumin. The average diameter of a capillary is 3.5 μm, which is approximately the same diameter as an RBC. As the RBCs traverse the capillaries, O_2 dissociates from oxyhemoglobin and diffuses into the tissues, obeying Fick's law of passive diffusion:

$$\dot{V}_{O_2} = D_t \times (P_{cap}O_2 - P_{mit}O_2) \qquad [22]$$

in which D_t is the Krogh O_2 diffusion coefficient (Krogh, 1919b), $P_{cap}O_2$ is the capillary plasma PO_2, and $P_{mit}O_2$ is the mitochondrial PO_2. Transport of O_2 from the capillaries to the cells is a direct function of the O_2 needs of the tissues and the diffusion distance for O_2 (Cole et al, 1982; Ellsworth and Pittman, 1984). The diffusion distance in turn depends on the number of perfused capillaries and their arrangement within the tissue. The range of diffusion distances from the capillary to the mitochondria varies from 50 μm in resting muscle to less than 10 μm in contracting muscle (Hansson-Mild and Linderholm, 1984).

DISTRIBUTION OF BLOOD FLOW AMONG ORGANS

MICROVASCULAR CONTROL MECHANISMS

The distribution of oxygen in the tissues is determined by local microvascular control mechanisms that regulate total RBC flow, capillary transit time, and capillary recruitment. The arteriolar sphincters react to signals from the autonomic nervous system (neurogenic control) and to local vasoactive substances and pH (metabolic control). Increases in PO_2 cause constriction of the arterioles, whereas hypoxemia produces arteriolar vasodilation (Crystal and Weiss, 1980). The control mechanisms that determine the number of opened capillaries in tissue appear to be mediated by tissue adenosine released in response to hypoxia (Honig and Frierson, 1980; Schantz, 1983). Propranolol and epinephrine also appear to increase the density of tissue capillaries (Vetterlein and Schmidt, 1984). The effect that these and other vasoactive drugs (e.g., dopamine) have on tissue oxygenation is not well understood.

Systemic Regulation

The efficiency of O_2 extraction by the tissues depends on the degree of microcirculatory regulation provided by systemic and local vascular control mechanisms. At the systemic level, increases in O_2 extraction ratio are produced by redistributing cardiac output to organs vital to the survival of the organism (i.e. the heart, brain, skeletal muscle, and adrenal glands). At the individual organ level, ERO_2 is maximized by increasing the number of perfused capillaries for a given volume of tissue. Capillary recruitment is a defense mechanism well suited to organs capable of large increases in capillarity, such as skeletal muscle and, to a lesser extent, the myocardium. Organs with

poor capillary reserve are at a disadvantage during hypoxia, especially those with countercurrent microvascular arrangements (i.e., the intestinal villi and the kidney medulla).

Regional vascular resistance determines the distribution of the cardiac output among the various organs. Regional vascular resistance is a function of humoral and neurogenic control mechanisms that regulate arteriolar constriction, and of local mechanisms of vascular control that determine microflow. Neurogenic control is mediated primarily by vasomotor fibers, which include sympathetic adrenergic and cholinergic fibers as well as parasympathetic cholinergic fibers. Arterioles and venules have sympathetic adrenergic nerves whose stimulation leads to smooth muscle contraction and vasoconstriction. This action is mediated by the transmitter norepinephrine acting on α-receptors of vascular smooth muscle. Most organs also have tonic adrenergic activity that can be nullified by denervation or by blockade of α-receptors, resulting in vasodilation. The overall effect of sympathetic adrenergic enervation is to increase vascular resistance and reduce blood volume and flow.

Sympathetic adrenergic activity also mediates a vasodilator reaction through the stimulation of β-receptors, but this response is usually masked by adrenergic vasoconstriction. There are some microvascular beds, such as the skin, that are enervated by nerves with neurotransmitters other than norepinephrine and acetylcholine. These transmitters include histamine, ATP, and peptides. The action of these nerves on the microvasculature is unknown.

Local Regulation

Local regulatory mechanisms are responsible for microvascular autoregulation. Changes in intraluminal pressure result in arteriolar dilation or constriction (Borgstrom and Gestrelius, 1987). This action serves to prevent alterations in flow produced by rapid changes in arterial pressure. The endothelium also responds to the shear stresses produced by increases in flow. This type of autoregulation appears to be mediated by the release of endothelium-derived relaxing factor (EDRF). This substance has been identified as nitric oxide produced by the endothelial cells from the amino acid L-arginine (Moncada and Higgs, 1993).

Endothelium-derived nitric oxide appears to be important in regulating vascular reactivity during hypoxia and sepsis, by activating soluble guanylate cyclase into guanosine 3',5'-cyclic monophosphate (Lamas et al, 1991), a potent intracellular mediator of vasodilation (Murad, 1986; Julou-Schaeffer et al, 1990). Pohl and Busse (1989) found increases in EDRF release in rabbit femoral artery strips during hypoxia, when luminal PO_2 values was 24 mm Hg. The adventitial side of these preparations were maintained at high PO_2 (~300 mm Hg), which complicates the interpretation of these data. Conversely, Vallet and coworkers (1994) concluded that the inhibition of NO does not affect hypoxic vasodilation or increases in O_2 extraction in canine skeletal muscle. They inhibited NO production with N^{ω}-nitro-L-arginine methyl ester (L-NAME) in an isolated dog hindlimb preparation exposed to hypoxia (PO_2 ~ 28 mm Hg) and compared results with a control group. There were no differences in hindlimb vascular resistance, O_2 extraction, or O_2 consumption between the groups, suggesting that a vascular mediator other than NO is responsible for hypoxic vasodilation.

Inhibition of endothelial NO synthesis may play an important role in reversing the vasodilation associated with NO overproduction by the inducible pathway, as might occur during septic states. Kilbourn and coworkers (1990a) infused N^G-methyl-L-arginine, an inhibitor of NO synthesis, to hypotensive dogs following the administration of either *Escherichia coli* endotoxin, tumor necrosis factor-α (TNF-α) (Kilbourn et al, 1990b), and interleukin-2 (Kilbourn et al, 1994). In each case they noted the reversal of the hypotensive response to these cytokines. Their findings have been confirmed by Baudry and Vicaut (1993), who examined changes in second- third-, and fourth-order arterioles and noted an acute vasodilator effect of TNF-α that was mediated by both prostaglandins and NO, because it was prevented by the simultaneous infusion of inhibitors of cyclooxygenase and NO synthetase. Meyer and coworkers (1992) found that the intravenous administration of L-NAME to septic ewes increased mean arterial pressure and decreased the pulmonary shunt fraction. It appears that NO also may decrease myocardial contractility in sepsis, as shown by Brady and coworkers (1992) in isolated ventricular myocytes from septic guinea pigs, which is a phenomenon reversed by N^G-methyl-L-arginine.

Improved mortality or a reduction in organ system failure, by the infusion of NO synthesis inhibitors in sepsis, has not been demonstrated in animals or humans. The synthesis of inducible NO probably plays an important role in mediating the systemic vasodilation of sepsis. Because vasodilation may represent a beneficial cellular response to sepsis-related cytokines, blocking this response may have deleterious consequences to tissue perfusion. Inhibition of NO synthesis is associated with decreased cardiac output (Lorente et al, 1993), suggesting that increases in blood pressure by nonselective systemic vasoconstriction may occur at the expense of nutritive flow to individual tissues. More experimental and clinical data are needed before endorsing the use of NO synthesis inhibitors in patients with septic shock.

CAPILLARY TRANSIT TIME

The rate of RBC deoxygenation in relation to the time spent by the RBC in the capillaries appears to be an important parameter of tissue oxygenation (Gutierrez, 1986; Honig et al, 1983). A slow rate of O_2 release in relation to capillary transit time results in the development of a significant PO_2 gradient from the RBC to the surrounding plasma. The decrease in capillary PO_2 may result in a reduction in $\dot{V}O_2$ as the O_2 driving pressure into the tissues falls (Lawson and Forster, 1967). Capillary transit time depends on the number of open capillaries, the length of the capillaries, and the RBC velocity. Transit times may vary from 2.0 to 0.9 sec at rest and decrease to 0.2 sec during exercise (Honig et al, 1982; Sarelius and Duling, 1982). Under conditions of reduced O_2 supply, the RBCs may not have sufficient time to release the O_2 required by the tissues. This situation creates the equivalent of a diffusion block to O_2 delivery. Likewise, when the vascular control of the microcirculation is deranged, which may occur during septic shock, an increase in cardiac output may result in a very short capillary transit time. Under these conditions, the RBC velocity may be too fast to allow the complete release of O_2 to the tissues. As a result, venous blood has a high O_2 saturation, although the tissues may be starving for O_2, which is a condition akin to a functional peripheral O_2 shunt.

MICROCIRCULATORY HEMATOCRIT

A major determinant of O_2 delivery is the hemoglobin concentration. A cursory examination of the factors that determine arterial O_2 content (see equation 18) may give the impression that tissue O_2 delivery is a linear function of hemoglobin concentration. That is, the greater the hemoglobin concentration, the more oxygen is delivered to the tissues. However, capillary hematocrit and the spacing of the RBCs also affect the flux of O_2 into the tissues (Homer et al, 1981; Klitzman and Duling, 1979; Restorff et al, 1975; Robertson et al, 1982; Woodson and Auerbach, 1982). As the result of a slow-moving plasma layer next to the endothelium, RBCs travel across the capillaries faster than the surrounding plasma (the Fahraeus-Lindqvist effect). This phenomenon results in capillary hematocrit values on the order of 50 to 25% those of arterial blood (Klitzman and Duling, 1979).

Changes in hematocrit have variable effects on tissue oxygenation. Decreases in hematocrit tend to decrease blood viscosity and promote tissue perfusion (Messmer et al, 1973), whereas an abnormally high hematocrit increases blood viscosity, resulting in clumping and aggregation of RBCs, capillary occlusion, and regional redistribution of the circulation. There is no evidence to support the idea that high hemoglobin concentration is beneficial in hypoxic patients, and the doping of blood (i.e., increasing hematocrit to supernormal levels) is not indicated. Owing to its carrying capacity, however, hemoglobin concentration in these patients should be maintained at levels greater than 10 g/dl.

CAPILLARY RECRUITMENT

A major regulatory control of the microcirculation depends on its ability to recruit additional capillaries to promote O_2 delivery to the tissues. The number of open capillaries determines the functional intercapillary distance and the diffusion distance for O_2. At rest, only a few of the capillaries are opened to accommodate RBCs, whereas the remaining capillaries only allow the passage of plasma. During the transition from rest to exercise, skeletal muscle increases mean capillary density 1.5- to 3-fold, resulting in a 7-fold increase in flow (Duling, 1980; Federspiel and Sarelius, 1984; Sarelius and Duling, 1982). The myocardium does not have the same capacity as skeletal muscle to recruit capillaries; instead, the heart increases blood flow to compensate for tissue hypoxia (Bourdeau-Martin et al, 1974; Grunewald and Sowa, 1978).

PERIPHERAL VASCULAR SHUNTS

The presence of peripheral vascular shunts has been invoked as explanation for the elevated venous O_2 values measured in septic shock. However, anatomic vascular shunts have not been found in skeletal muscle (Hammersen, 1970) or in the coronary circulation (Feldstein et al, 1978). The lack of anatomic evidence for peripheral shunting does not preclude the existence of functional shunts (Honig et al, 1983). As an example, decreases in the rate of O_2 release from the erythrocytes, in relation to the time spent by the RBC in the capillaries, may have a significant impact on diffusion of O_2 into the tissues. A slower rate

of O_2 release by the erythrocyte, or conversely, a very fast capillary transit time, may result in significant O_2 remaining inside the RBCs as they exit the capillaries (Heidelberger and Reeves, 1990a). Insufficient time in the capillary for RBC O_2 release is the equivalent of a diffusion block to cellular O_2 delivery, resulting in tissue PO_2 lower than venous PO_2. The time spent by the red cells in the capillaries is a complex function of RBC velocity, number of open capillaries, and length of the capillaries. Transit times vary from 0.2 sec during maximal exercise to 2.0 sec at rest (Honig et al, 1980; Hester and Duling, 1988)

The kinetics of erythrocyte O_2 release constitutes another important factor affecting the rate of O_2 transfer in the capillaries. The half-time values for erythrocyte O_2 uptake range from 10 to 15 ms, whereas the half-time for O_2 release is longer, from 21 to 91 ms (Heidelberger and Reeves, 1990b). The clinical importance of this time-related phenomenon has not been established. However, mathematic models of the microcirculation suggest that, under extreme conditions of hypoxia or anemia, the kinetics of erythrocyte O_2 release may play a significant role in determining capillary O_2 transfer (Gutierrez, 1986). Measurements of skeletal muscle PO_2 with surface Clark-type microelectrodes show that muscle PO_2 is less than effluent venous PO_2 during hypoxemia, anemia, and sepsis (Gutierrez et al, 1989, 1990, 1991).

Another model capable of explaining the differences noted between venous and tissue PO_2 is the one proposed by Piiper and coworkers (1975). This model proposes that O_2 diffuses directly from the arterioles into the adjacent venules, forming a gas exchange countercurrent system. The predictions of this model are supported by the findings of Stein and coworkers (1993), who evaluated the relationship between systemic venous PO_2 and end-capillary PO_2 in hamster skeletal muscle using *in vivo* video microscopy and O_2 microelectrodes. They found greater venous PO_2 than end-capillary PO_2 and concluded that there is a significant rate of O_2 diffusion from arteriole to venule in muscle.

METABOLIC CONSIDERATIONS

CELLULAR RESPIRATION

Cellular respiration is defined as the orderly transfer of electron metabolic pathways from organic compounds to O_2. This process produces high-energy phosphates in the form of ATP to provide the free energy needed by the tissue cells. Figure

8–6 shows the metabolic pathways responsible for the generation of ATP. The oxidation of carbohydrates, amino acids, and fatty acids results in the production of acetylcoenzyme A (acetyl-CoA). This molecule enters the tricarboxylic acid cycle (TCA), yielding CO_2 and four pairs of electrons. Nicotinamide dinucleotide (NAD^+) and flavine adenine dinucleotide (FAD^+) serve as electron acceptors and transport the electron pairs to the cytochrome system in the mitochondria. In the inner mitochondrial membrane, the electron pairs move down a series of oxidation-reduction reactions in the cytochrome system. Each oxidation-reduction reaction is associated with progressively lower energy levels until the final cytochrome reduces molecular O_2. ATP is generated in large quantities during this process, which is called *oxidative phosphorylation* and is a feature of all aerobic cells. ATP is hydrolized by the ATPases to provide the energy for the various cellular functions and to preserve cellular membrane permeability (Harold, 1986). The hydrolysis of ATP results in the production of ADP, inorganic phosphate (P_i), and hydrogen ions (Gevers, 1977):

$$ATP + H_2O \rightarrow ADP + P_i + H^+ \qquad [23]$$
$$ATPase$$

When the supply of O_2 is adequate, ADP, P_i, and H^+ are recycled in the mitochondria to produce ATP by oxidative phosphorylation. In this manner, the cytosolic concentrations of ADP, P_i, and H^+ are maintained within a narrow range. The phosphorylation potential (PP), defined as:

$$PP = \frac{[ATP]}{[ADP]\,[P_i]} \qquad [24]$$

appears to provide the control signal for oxidative phosphorylation (Wilson et al, 1977, 1979) and

for the consumption of O_2. Aerobic metabolism is depressed when PP is elevated, and it is stimulated with decreases in PP. The former occurs when O_2 transport is adequate and the cellular concentration of ATP is high. Conversely, with accelerated hydrolysis of ATP, such as occurs during exercise, there are increases in [ADP] and [P_i], resulting in decreases in PP. These changes are accompanied by elevations in tissue blood flow and O_2 consumption (Nuutinen et al, 1982). [ADP] and [P_i] also increase during hypoxia, but given the limited O_2 supplies, O_2 consumption does not increase. O_2 consumption decreases as O_2 deprivation increases.

Another important determinant of ATP production is the adenine nucleotide content (ATP + ADP + AMP) in the mitochondria (Hochachka and Guppy, 1987). As ADP and P_i accumulate in the cytosol, they are transported back into the mitochondria by the ADP/ATP translocases, the P_i/OH^- carrier, and the ATP/P_i carrier (Aprille, 1988). These transport mechanisms regulate the respective size of the adenine nucleotide pool in the cytosol and in mitochondria. Under normoxic conditions the steady-state distribution of the adenine nucleotide pools in the cytosol and in the mitochondria are balanced.

$$[ATP]+[ADP]+[AMP] \leftrightarrow [ATP]+[ADP]+[AMP] \qquad [25]$$
$$cytosol \qquad\qquad\qquad mitochondria$$

Hypoxia shifts the distribution of the adenine nucleotides toward an increase in the cytosolic pool. This process may be hastened by a decrease in pH, because the ATP/P_i carrier is pH-dependent and is pH-dependent, favoring the net loss of ATP from the mitochondria with increasing acidity of the cytosol. As the adenine nucleotide pool of the mitochondria diminishes, so does the

---

Figure 8–6

During aerobic metabolism, glucose, free fatty acids, and, under conditions of starvation, proteins, enter the Krebs', or tricarboxylic acid, cycle by their conversion to acetyl CoA. The electron pairs produced in the Krebs' cycle are transported by NADH to the cytochrome system where ATP is produced with the consumption of oxygen. ATP is transported to the cytosol where it is hydrolyzed to release the energy stored in its high-energy phosphate bonds. The products of ATP hydrolysis are recycled in the mitochondria during normoxia but accumulate in the cytosol during hypoxia, resulting in cellular acidosis.

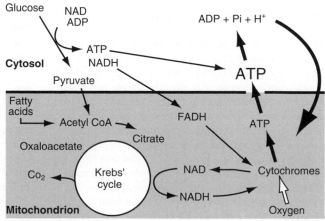

rate of oxidative phosphorylation. The mitochondrial adenylate pool eventually becomes so small that ATP production ceases. After a net loss of adenine nucleotides, the mitochondria may not be capable of renewing aerobic ATP production when O_2 supply returns to normal.

When the production of ATP by oxidative phosphorylation is insufficient to satisfy cellular energy needs, anaerobic sources of energy are used. These are glycolysis, the creatine kinase reaction, and the adenylate kinase reaction.

During the hypoxia, the production of [ATP] lags behind cellular energy needs, and cytosolic [AMP] accumulates. This in turn stimulates glycolysis, with the production of lactate and the generation of ATP (Harris et al, 1986).

$$Glucose + 2\ P_i + 2\ ADP \rightarrow 2\ lactate^- \atop + 2\ ATP + 2\ H_2O \qquad [26]$$

The increase in glycolytic rate with hypoxia has been called the *Pasteur effect*. Glucose is used preferentially during hypoxia, because the P:O ratio (i.e., the ratio of moles of ATP produced per mole of O_2 consumed) is higher with glucose than with any other metabolic fuel. Therefore, glucose consumption maximizes the utilization of available O_2. On the other hand, the ATP yield of anaerobic glycolysis, 2 mole ATP/mole glucose, is small in comparison with oxidative phosphorylation, 36 mole ATP/mole glucose. Glycolysis has the additional disadvantage of increasing cytosolic lactate concentration.

Another source of ATP is the creatine kinase reaction, in which phosphocreatine (PCr) is used to phosphorylate ADP (Chance et al, 1985a). This reaction is present in skeletal muscle, heart, and brain:

$$[PCr] + [ADP] + [H^+] \leftrightarrow [ATP] \atop + [creatine] \qquad [27]$$

The advantages of this reaction are numerous. In addition to providing a ready source of ATP, it also ameliorates the cytosolic accumulation of [ADP] and [H⁺]. However, this reaction has limited benefit during hypoxia because of the small tissue concentrations of PCr.

In a persistent state of cellular hypoxia, ADP accumulates in the cytosol and stimulates the adenylate kinase reaction (Meyer et al, 1980):

$$[ADP] + [ADP] \leftrightarrow [ATP] + [AMP] \qquad [28]$$

The adenylate kinase reaction helps to keep the [ATP]/[ADP] ratio constant, but it also results in accumulation of [AMP].

The buildup of cytosolic AMP may be a key event in the development of organ failure. AMP can be deaminated to inosine monophosphate (IMP), with the production of ammonia (Dudley and Terjung, 1985; Manfredi and Holmes, 1984; Meyer et al, 1980; Terjung et al, 1985), or converted to adenosine by 5'-nucleotidase (Van Belle et al, 1987). Adenosine diffuses out of the cell into the microvasculature, where it is a potent vasodilator because it binds to receptors in blood vessels (Berne, 1986). This provides the tissues with a metabolic feedback mechanism to control capillary blood flow as a function of the cellular energy balance. Deamination of AMP with the formation of IMP may lead to the formation of inosine or hypoxanthine and to the production of O_2 free radicals in the xanthine oxidase reaction (Bontemps et al, 1986; Franco and Canela, 1984; Granger et al, 1986). O_2 free radicals may result in cellular membrane damage (Kim and Akera, 1987; Takeda et al, 1986) and in the activation of the arachidonic acid cascade by the action of the phospholipases. The lipooxygenase and cyclooxygenase pathways of arachidonic acid degradation produce powerful metabolites, which can also exert a strong influence in microvascular regulation.

RELATIONSHIP OF OXYGEN TRANSPORT TO OXYGEN CONSUMPTION

The consumption of O_2 by the tissues is slightly greater than aerobic ATP production. The lack of a one-to-one correspondence between $\dot{V}O_2$ and mitochondrial ATP production is related to the utilization of O_2 by other cellular oxidative processes (estimated to be 2% of $\dot{V}O_2$), as it occurs during the generation of reactive O_2 metabolites, such as superoxide, hydrogen peroxide, and hydroxyl radicals (Grisham and McCord, 1986). Another factor that determines the number of ATP molecules produced per molecule of O_2 consumed is the substrate used by the tissues, the P:O ratio. As mentioned previously, glycolysis increases during hypoxia because glucose metabolism has a higher P:O ratio (3:1) than either fat or protein. This property makes glucose consumption the most effective means to produce energy from the scarce cellular O_2. For the purposes of this discussion, and for most clinical or physiologic considerations, one may assume that $\dot{V}O_2$ represents the aerobic production of ATP.

The relationship of $\dot{T}O_2$ to $\dot{V}O_2$ was initially described by Stainsby and Otis (1964), who found that $\dot{V}O_2$ in isolated dog skeletal muscle responds in a nonlinear or biphasic manner to the progressive reductions in $\dot{T}O_2$. This is shown schematically in Figure 8–7, in which $\dot{V}O_2$ is shown as a

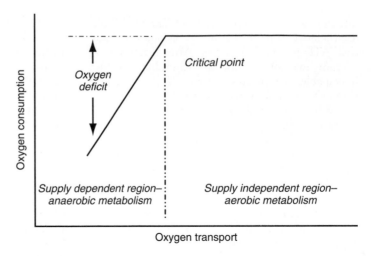

Figure 8–7
Schematic representation of the relationship between O_2 transport and O_2 consumption as determined from animal experiments. The supply-independent (aerobic metabolism) and supply-dependent regions (anaerobic metabolism) are separated by a sharply demarcated critical point.

function of $\dot{T}O_2$. As $\dot{T}O_2$ decreases, $\dot{V}O_2$ remains more or less unchanged. The constancy of the $\dot{V}O_2$ is the result of microvascular adaptations resulting in increases in ERO_2. Further declines in $\dot{T}O_2$ can overwhelm these microvascular adaptations, and aerobic ATP production falls below the level required by cellular metabolism. At that level of $\dot{T}O_2$, also called the "critical" $\dot{T}O_2$ ($\dot{T}O_{2crit}$), anaerobic sources of energy are recruited to supplement ATP production. This response to decreases in $\dot{T}O_2$ has been described as O_2 regulation (Hochachka, 1986).

The nonlinear nature of the $\dot{T}O_2$-$\dot{V}O_2$ relationship has been confirmed in numerous animal experiments, including studies in which $\dot{V}O_2$ was measured independent of the cardiac output by using the gas-exchange method (Pepe and Culver, 1985). These studies also found a $\dot{T}O_{2crit}$ of approximately 10 ml/min per kilogram, supporting the theory that $\dot{T}O_{2crit}$ is a fixed quantity that may be useful as an index of O_2 transport system failure. However, hypothermic dogs have been shown to have significantly lower levels of $\dot{T}O_{2crit}$ when compared with normothermic controls (Gutierrez et al, 1986b). As previously mentioned, increasing hemoglobin O_2 affinity decreases tissue O_2 extraction and increases the $\dot{T}O_{2crit}$ (Gutierrez and Andry, 1989a). Increases in $\dot{T}O_{2crit}$ have also been shown in hypoxemic dogs fed sodium cyanate, with a resultant shift of the ODC to the left (Warley and Gutierrez, 1988). These results indicate that the $\dot{T}O_{2crit}$ is not a fixed quantity, but that it varies with the metabolic needs for O_2 and with factors that affect the O_2 transport system.

Results from clinical studies show a different type of $\dot{T}O_2$-$\dot{V}O_2$ relationship. With the exception of the work of Shibutani and associates (1983), who found a nonlinear $\dot{T}O_2$-$\dot{V}O_2$ relationship with a clearly defined critical point in 58 patients un-

dergoing cardiac surgery, all the published clinical studies show a linear relationship between $\dot{T}O_2$ and $\dot{V}O_2$. Among the earliest clinical studies on the $\dot{T}O_2$-$\dot{V}O_2$ relationship are those of Lutch and Murray (1972) and of McMahon and associates (1973). These investigators found no changes in systemic $\dot{V}O_2$ when small decreases in $\dot{T}O_2$ were produced by the application of positive end-expiratory pressure (PEEP) in mechanically ventilated patients. Conversely, Powers and associates (1973) noted linear decreases in $\dot{V}O_2$ in 33 patients with ARDS when declines in cardiac output were produced by PEEP. This finding was supported by the study of Rhodes and associates (1978), who measured the effect of increasing $\dot{T}O_2$ by intravenous infusions of mannitol and noted proportional increases in $\dot{V}O_2$.

The proportional relationship of $\dot{V}O_2$ to decreases in $\dot{T}O_2$ was firmly established in the clinical literature by the now classic work of Danek and associates (1980), who measured $\dot{T}O_2$, $\dot{V}O_2$, and mixed venous PO_2 in 20 patients with adult respiratory distress syndrome (ARDS) and in 12 patients with various diseases. In all except one of the patients, the $\dot{T}O_2$-$\dot{V}O_2$ relationship was linear, even in regions in which the $\dot{T}O_2$ rose to approximately 50 ml/min per kilogram, three times that of normal subjects at rest (Fig. 8–8). In the patients without ARDS, the $\dot{V}O_2$ appeared to be unrelated to the $\dot{T}O_2$. This finding was confirmed by Mohsenifar and associates (1983) and by Nishimura (1984). The latter concluded that patients behave as O_2 conformers, increasing their $\dot{V}O_2$ in response to an increment in $\dot{T}O_2$.

Kaufman and coworkers (1984) found that increases in $\dot{T}O_2$ in patients with septic shock and hypovolemia result in proportional increases in $\dot{V}O_2$ for both conditions. Dorinsky and coworkers (1988) compared the $\dot{T}O_2$-$\dot{V}O_2$ relationship from

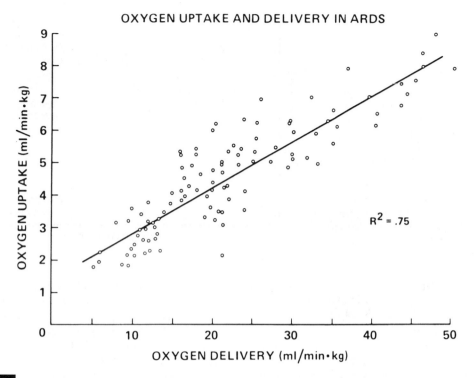

Figure 8–8
The relationship between O_2 transport and O_2 consumption obtained from clinical studies is a linear function, as shown by the data from patients with ARDS. (From Danek SJ, Lynch JP, Weg JG, et al: The dependence of oxygen uptake on oxygen delivery in the adult respiratory distress syndrome. Am Rev Respir Dis 122:387–395, 1980. With permission.)

10 patients with non-ARDS respiratory failure who were treated with volume infusions to that obtained from six patients with ARDS who were subjected to increases in PEEP. They found $\dot{V}O_2$ dependency on $\dot{T}O_2$ for both groups. Measurements of venous samples from the jugular and brachial veins showed marked differences in regional values, which they interpreted as variations in regional adaptation to tissue hypoxia. They concluded that a linear relationship is not unique to patients with ARDS and may not predict regional response to critical reductions in $\dot{T}O_2$.

Gutierrez and Pohil (1986) measured changes in $\dot{T}O_2$ and $\dot{V}O_2$ in 30 critically ill patients who had at least eight serial measures obtained at 6-hour intervals. They noted that patients could be segregated according to their ability to increase O_2 extraction in response to decreases in $\dot{T}O_2$. The group unable to increase ERO_2 was composed mostly of patients with sepsis, ARDS, and acute gastrointestinal bleeding (80%). This group showed marked $\dot{V}O_2$ dependency on $\dot{T}O_2$ and had a mortality rate of 70%. The group able to increase ERO_2, and in which $\dot{V}O_2$ was independent of $\dot{T}O_2$, had a significantly lower mortality rate

(30%). The latter group also had fewer patients with sepsis or ARDS (30%) and required significantly lesser use of vasopressor agents. These data suggest that diseases that affect the microcirculation, such as sepsis, are characterized by a loss of O_2 extraction capacity, resulting in O_2 supply dependency.

Cain (1984) proposed the phrase *pathologic O_2 supply dependency* to explain the finding of a linear $\dot{T}O_2$-$\dot{V}O_2$ function in patients with sepsis or ARDS, as opposed to the nonlinear $\dot{T}O_2$-$\dot{V}O_2$ curve observed in animal studies (Fig. 8–9). According to this concept, critically ill patients have greater energy needs for O_2, perhaps as a consequence of inflammation or hypermetabolism, resulting in a higher $\dot{V}O_2$ plateau. Their microvascular control also may be affected, impairing their ability to increase ERO_2. The combination of a higher $\dot{V}O_2$ plateau and impaired O_2 extracting mechanisms results in a greater critical $\dot{T}O_2$. A reasonable corollary to this hypothesis is that patients with pathologic O_2 supply dependency reach supply independency when subjected to pharmacologic increases in $\dot{T}O_2$ (Edwards and Clarke, 1991).

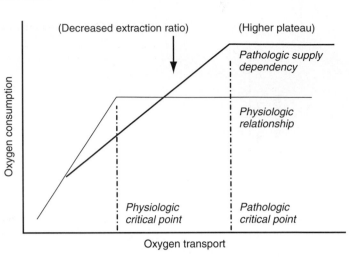

Figure 8–9
The concept of pathologic O_2 supply dependence assumes that basal energy requirements (the plateau of the curve) are higher in patients with sepsis and ARDS, perhaps because of the action of inflammatory agents. In addition, microcirculatory derangements may interfere with the efficient extraction of O_2 from the capillaries, resulting in a shallower slope in the O_2 supply-dependent region, and consequently a greater critical O_2 transport point.

OXYGEN SUPPLY DEPENDENCY AS A PATHOLOGIC CONDITION, AN ONGOING DEBATE

Several clinical studies dispute the existence of "pathologic supply dependency." These studies have as a common denominator the measurement of $\dot{V}O_2$ by analysis of the expired gases. This eliminates mathematic coupling of data as being the cause of the linear $\dot{T}O_2$-$\dot{V}O_2$ function observed in clinical studies. Because both $\dot{T}O_2$ and $\dot{V}O_2$ are calculated from common variables, CaO_2 and cardiac output, random errors in the measurement of these variables may result in a factitious spread of values for $\dot{T}O_2$ and $\dot{V}O_2$ along a straight line. This problem was analyzed mathematically by Moreno and coworkers (1986), who concluded that mathematic coupling, although present when determinations of $\dot{T}O_2$ and $\dot{V}O_2$ share a common variable, probably plays a minor role in the genesis of the linear $\dot{T}O_2$-$\dot{V}O_2$ function, as long as changes in $\dot{T}O_2$ are sufficiently large. Although pooled data from several patients may show large variations in $\dot{T}O_2$, these variations may still be small for a given patient. In that case, measuring $\dot{V}O_2$ independently of $\dot{T}O_2$ using the expired gases method may avoid the possibility of mathematic coupling (Stratton et al, 1987).

Annat and coworkers (1986) measured $\dot{V}O_2$ in eight mechanically ventilated patients with ARDS using the expired gas method. They decreased $\dot{T}O_2$ by applying PEEP and found no change in $\dot{V}O_2$ or increases in blood lactate, implying that these patients could increase O_2 extraction to meet cellular O_2 requirements. Furthermore, they also found no differences in basal $\dot{V}O_2$ between the patients with ARDS and other ventilated patients without ARDS. When $\dot{V}O_2$

was measured by the expired gases method in patients with ARDS in whom $\dot{T}O_2$ was increased by blood transfusion, there were no changes in $\dot{V}O_2$, even in patients with initial elevations in plasma lactate (Ronco et al, 1991). Conversely, $\dot{V}O_2$ increased if calculated using Fick's equation, suggesting that O_2 supply dependency may be the result of a methodologic error involving shared variables. In a similar study, Hanique and coworkers (1994a, 1994b) made simultaneous measures of $\dot{V}O_2$ using the expired gases method and Fick's principle in 32 patients subjected to increases in $\dot{T}O_2$ by colloid infusion. O_2 supply dependency was present when $\dot{V}O_2$ was calculated by Fick's principle, whereas directly measured $\dot{V}O_2$ did not change with changes in $\dot{T}O_2$. Furthermore, an elevated arterial lactate level failed to identify O_2 supply dependency in these patients. Other studies in which $\dot{V}O_2$ consumption was measured from the expired gases by indirect calorimetry also have failed to show sepsis-associated "pathologic O_2 supply dependency" (Manthous et al, 1993; Ronco et al, 1993a, 1993b).

It is also possible that the $\dot{T}O_2$-$\dot{V}O_2$ relationship in patients may represent the normal physiologic response of the system, instead of an abnormal manifestation of impaired oxygen extraction. As mentioned previously, animal experiments usually consist of a healthy animal preparation exposed for a relatively short time to reductions in $\dot{T}O_2$. Under these conditions, $\dot{V}O_2$ is clearly the dependent variable, whereas $\dot{T}O_2$ is the manipulated variable. This is not the case in the clinical setting, where variations in $\dot{T}O_2$ occur spontaneously in response to changes in the patient's metabolic rate. Perhaps a linear $\dot{T}O_2$-$\dot{V}O_2$ relationship is the manifestation of temporal changes in O_2 demand. That is, increases $\dot{V}O_2$ in response to agitation, fever, work of breathing and other factors result in appropriate increases in $\dot{T}O_2$. This physiologic response of $\dot{T}O_2$ to increases in $\dot{V}O_2$ is akin to that of exercise. One must consider that organs such as the liver, kidney, or heart can alter their O_2 demand in response to changes in blood flow (Schlichtig, 1991), which is a condition called O_2 conformity. A proportional $\dot{T}O_2$-$\dot{V}O_2$ relationship resulting from this adaptive response does not represent tissue hypoxia or O_2 supply dependency. On the contrary, it represents the dependency of O_2 supply on O_2 demand, which is a normal physiologic state.

Dantzker and coworkers (1991) noted that increases in energy requirements during exercise result in proportional increases in cardiac output and $\dot{T}O_2$. During strenuous exercise, anaerobic metabolism helps supplement aerobic energy production when O_2 supply is unable to satisfy cellular energy requirements. This condition has been defined as the lactate threshold (Whipp, 1994), which is a condition analogous to the critical $\dot{T}O_2$ during conditions of decreased O_2 supply. Whereas ERO_2 at the anaerobic threshold is approximately 0.60, the critical ERO_2 for patients under conditions of decreased O_2 supply is much lower, in the range of 0.30 to 0.40. Increases in ERO_2 during exercise occur as blood flow is directed toward contracting skeletal muscle, which is an organ capable of autoregulating blood flow according to energy requirements by substantial increases in capillary recruitment. Similarly, blood flow during severe hypoxia is also preferentially redistributed to skeletal muscle, except that now skeletal muscle is at rest and uses but a fraction of the delivered O_2; its regional ERO_2 will be low. Because of this preferential muscle perfusion, blood flow to other organs, such as the gut and kidneys, may be reduced to the point where they cannot maintain adequate aerobic energy production. These underperfused organs will have high ERO_2 values. Because of this heterogeneous perfusion pattern, large quantities of venous blood from overperfused organs mix with lesser amounts of blood from underperfused tissues, resulting in a low systemic ERO_{2crit}. Patients experiencing this condition may not be able to increase ERO_2 in the gut and in the kidneys. This results in decreases in aerobic energy production in these organs, which in turn may lead to their dysfunction and ultimately to death.

INCREASED $\dot{V}O_2$ AS A MARKER OF TISSUE HYPOXIA

Several investigators have attempted to combine information derived from the $\dot{T}O_2$-$\dot{V}O_2$ relationship and elevations in blood lactate levels to test for the existence of covert tissue hypoxia in critically ill patients. Haupt and coworkers (1985) noted that the infusion of colloidal fluids increased $\dot{V}O_2$ in septic patients with concurrent lactic acidosis. In a subsequent study (Gilbert et al, 1986), these investigators found that the infusion of fluids or blood increased $\dot{V}O_2$ in patients with sepsis who also had blood lactate levels greater than 2.2 mM. In contrast, dobutamine raised $\dot{V}O_2$ in septic patients with or without lactic acidosis. They concluded that fluid or blood infusion could be used to predict the presence of anaerobic metabolism in sepsis, whereas dobutamine was not as useful, because this catecholamine appeared to exert a direct positive effect on metabolic rate. These findings have been supported by studies using fluids (Wolf et al, 1987) and RBC transfusions (Lucking et al, 1990) to increase $\dot{T}O_2$.

The results from a study by Bihari and coworkers (1987) also support the notion that many critically ill patients suffer from inadequate tissue oxygenation. They increased $\dot{T}O_2$ in critically ill patients by infusing prostacyclin, which is a potent vasodilator. $\dot{V}O_2$ increased with prostaglandin in a group of patients that uniformly died. In another group who survived their stay in the intensive care unit (ICU), prostaglandin administration increased $\dot{T}O_2$ but $\dot{V}O_2$ remained constant. Bihari and coworkers concluded that patients who had increases in $\dot{V}O_2$ had a substantial oxygen deficit. The results of this study may have criticized by the finding that these patients were relatively hypovolemic. A subsequent study by De Backer and coworkers (1993) failed to show a difference in the response to prostacyclin in survivors and nonsurvivors in 17 patients with sepsis. Furthermore, when $\dot{V}O_2$ was measured from the expired gases in 15 patients with postoperative septic shock (Hannemann et al, 1994) the infusion of prostacyclin did not produce an increase in $\dot{V}O_2$, although $\dot{T}O_2$ rose 14%.

Vincent and coworkers (1990) proposed a short-term trial of dobutamine to disclose an O_2 uptake/supply dependency condition in sepsis. They found increased $\dot{V}O_2$ in response to a dobutamine infusion of 5 μg/kg per minute in a septic group of patients with lactic acidosis. There were no increases in $\dot{V}O_2$ in another group of septic patients with normal lactate levels. Based on these results, these investigators concluded that, at the dose used, dobutamine does not increase $\dot{V}O_2$ in critically ill patients, unless there is coexisting tissue hypoxia evidenced by lactic acidosis.

The prognostic value of the dobutamine test was tested by Vallet and coworkers (1993) in

50 patients with sepsis syndrome. They excluded patients in shock and those with lactate concentrations greater than 2.0 mM. They found 23 responders in whom $\dot{T}O_2$ increased on the average 39% and $\dot{V}O_2$ 41%. The mortality rate was significantly greater in the nonresponders (44% vs. 9%). The authors concluded that increases in $\dot{V}O_2$ in the responders were related to the calorigenic effect of dobutamine, given that these were patients without shock or hyperlactatemia. They also proposed that failure to respond to dobutamine, and worse prognosis, may be related to β-adrenoreceptor dysfunction.

INCREASES IN OXYGEN TRANSPORT AND OXYGEN CONSUMPTION IN CRITICALLY ILL PATIENTS

It is not clear whether pharmacologic increases in $\dot{V}O_2$ affect the survival of critically ill patients. However, if the concept of pathologic supply dependency is correct, it would be reasonable to increase $\dot{T}O_2$ to a level compatible with the patient's O_2 requirements. Russell and coworkers (1990) studied 29 patients with ARDS and found that survivors (n = 13) had greater $\dot{T}O_2$ and $\dot{V}O_2$ within the first 24 hours of onset of ARDS. No effort was made in this study to increase $\dot{T}O_2$ to supernormal levels. Conversely, Gutierrez and coworkers (1992a) found lower $\dot{T}O_2$ and $\dot{V}O_2$ in survivors of a heterogeneous group of critically ill patients monitored longitudinally during their stay in the ICU. They associated greater $\dot{V}O_2$ with increased tissue inflammation and greater metabolic requirements in these patients.

The notion that increasing $\dot{T}O_2$ to supernormal values in critically ill patients improves survival is based on the work of Shoemaker and coworkers (1988). These investigators found better postoperative survival rates in nonseptic patients in whom pulmonary artery catheters (PA) were used to help maximize cardiac output, $\dot{V}O_2$, and $\dot{T}O_2$. This prospective, randomized study compared three groups: one treated according to the information derived from central venous lines (CVP-control), another using pulmonary artery catheters to achieve normal values of oxygenation parameters as therapeutic goals (PA-control), and a protocol group, wherein patients with PA catheters were treated with fluids and catecholamines (mainly dobutamine) in efforts to reach supernormal levels of $\dot{V}O_2$ and $\dot{T}O_2$ as therapeutic end points (PA-protocol). Hospital mortality rates

were 38%, 23%, and 4% for the CVP-control, PA-control, and PA-protocol groups, respectively, suggesting that prevention of an O_2 debt improved mortality in this group of patients.

The results of the 1988 study were confirmed by Boyd and coworkers (1993) in a prospective, randomized trial testing the effect of deliberate increases in $\dot{T}O_2$ during the perioperative period on morbidity and mortality. A control group of patients classified as high-risk (n = 38) received standard perioperative care, and the results were compared with those of a protocol group (n = 43) in whom $\dot{T}O_2$ was maintained at 600 ml/min/m² or more during surgery and postoperatively until arterial lactate concentration was less than 1.5 mM. Dopexamine hydrochloride was used to augment cardiac output in the protocol group. The protocol group achieved higher $\dot{T}O_2$ than the control group, but significantly, there were no differences in $\dot{V}O_2$. The 28-day mortality in the protocol group was significantly lower than that for the control group (7.0% vs. 23.7%; p = 0.04).

The studies of Shoemaker and coworkers (1988) and Boyd and coworkers (1993) suggest that maintenance of adequate O_2 transport during the perioperative period improves survival. However, their results should be interpreted in the context of patients who presumably have intact microvascular control and whose tissues are adequately oxygenated before sustaining the insult of surgery. Preventing tissue hypoxia under those conditions appears to be a beneficial therapeutic intervention. Conversely, the application of the supernormal $\dot{T}O_2$ concept to a heterogeneous population of critically ill patients, many of whom have already sustained irreversible cellular damage, has met with little success. The few studies in the literature in which a consistent effort has been applied to maintain greater-than-normal values of $\dot{T}O_2$ in critically ill patients show disappointing results. In a randomized, double-blind trial for treatment of ARDS (Bone et al, 1989; Silverman et al, 1990) a study group (n = 50) was randomized to receive prostaglandin E_1 (PGE₁) for seven days. Results in this group were compared with those of an equal number of patients given placebo. An unexpected finding of the trial was a significantly greater $\dot{T}O_2$ and $\dot{V}O_2$ for the study group, which was probably related to the vasodilator effect of PGE₁. Survival, however, was similar for both groups (60% for the PGE₁ vs. 48% for placebo). Tuchschmidt and coworkers (1989) studied a group of patients with septic shock (n = 26) in whom cardiac index was increased to 6.0 l/min/m² for 72 hours using dobutamine. Results in this group were compared with those in a normal treatment control with cardiac indices averaging 3.6 l/min/m². They found no difference in mortality between the groups (p<0.14), although their sample may not have had sufficient power to detect a significant difference.

A study by Hayes and coworkers (1994) showed increased mortality when dobutamine was used to raise $\dot{T}O_2$ in a group of critically ill patients. This was a randomized, prospective study in which a treatment group (n=50) was given dobutamine until the following goals were achieved simultaneously: cardiac index higher than 4.5 l/min/m², $\dot{T}O_2$ values higher than 600 ml/kg/m², and $\dot{V}O_2$ higher than 170 ml/kg/m². A control group (n=50) was given dobutamine only if the cardiac index was below 2.8 l/min/m². ICU mortality rates were 50% for the treatment group and 30% for the control group (p=0.04). It is not clear why the treatment group had greater mortality, although the very high doses of dobutamine used (up to 200 μg/kg per minute) may have been responsible for the worse outcome. As acknowledged by the investigators, perhaps the larger doses of dobutamine exacerbated the poor distribution of blood flow in the microcirculation, resulting in impaired perfusion of vital organs, such as the gastrointestinal tract.

For all practical purposes, the calculation of systemic O_2 transport and consumption add little to the knowledge gained from measures of arterial O_2 content and cardiac output. Although the interpretation of arterial O_2 content is relatively straightforward, alterations in cardiac output are more difficult to understand in the context of its effect on tissue oxygenation. Sometimes it is difficult to establish the optimal cardiac output in a given patient, in particular those with hemodynamic sepsis and hyperlactatemia. To best manage these patients, we require an accurate assessment of regional blood flow distribution and tissue energy requirements, because systemic measures of O_2 transport offer little information regarding the distribution of O_2 supply to individual organs and the effectiveness of their gas exchange (Fiddian-Green et al, 1993). Improved clinical means are needed to quantify the distribution of blood flow to individual organs and to determine cellular energy balance in all organs. This knowledge is of particular importance in organs with insufficient capillary reserve, such as the gut and the kidneys. They are the so-called sentinel organs, because they manifest alterations produced by decreases in O_2 supply earlier than organs with greater microvascular control, including the heart, brain, and skeletal muscle. The gut has been called "the canary of the body" (Dantzker, 1993), in reference to the heightened sensitivity of canaries to CO and their role as CO monitors for miners.

MONITORING THE ADEQUACY OF TISSUE OXYGENATION IN THE INTENSIVE CARE UNIT

ARTERIAL AND MIXED VENOUS BLOOD GASES

At the present time, arterial and mixed venous blood gases are the mainstay of tissue oxygenation assessment in the ICU. Arterial blood gases can be drawn from the radial, brachial, or femoral artery into a heparinized syringe with a small-gauge needle. The skin over the puncture site should be cleansed thoroughly with povidone-iodine or a similar agent, and sterile techniques should be used. The blood sample must be processed immediately or put in an iced container to prevent artifactual changes in the composition of the blood gases.

Significant decreases in PO_2 have been reported in patients with a high leukocyte count, because these cells consume the available O_2. The PO_2 of the sample is measured by polarographic techniques with a PO_2 electrode, usually at a temperature of 37°C. The PCO_2 and the pH are measured with pH electrodes. The oxyhemoglobin saturation is measured in a CO-Oximeter by spectrophotometry (de la Huerga and Sherrick, 1971). This instrument also measures the carboxyhemoglobin and methemoglobin levels in the same blood sample. Some laboratories do not have a CO-Oximeter, and the oxyhemoglobin saturation is calculated from the measured PO_2. If this is the case, care must be taken when significant fractions of methemoglobin or CO are present, because the O_2 content may be decreased despite a normal or high PO_2.

Mixed venous PO_2 is a nonspecific marker of global tissue oxygenation, because it represents the combined effluent concentration of O_2 from all tissues. Kety (1957) and later Tenney (1974) used the cylindrical tissue-capillary model of Krogh (1919b), using different capillary PO_2 profiles (Krogh, 1919a, b). In this manner, tissue PO_2 distribution could be calculated. Results from this model identify a portion of the tissue corresponding with the venous end that is exposed to the lowest capillary O_2 concentration (Fig. 8–10). This region of tissue presumably is the first to experience the effects of hypoxia, and it is called the *lethal corner*. Assuming that PO_2 at the end of the capillary is equal to the $P\bar{v}O_2$, a simple mathematic analysis reveals a close relationship

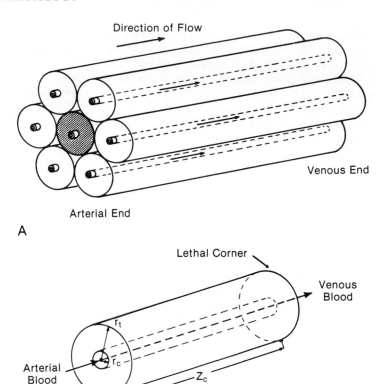

Figure 8–10
The concept of concentric, parallel capillaries as proposed by Krogh (1919). Each cylinder has a central capillary that supplies a cylindrical volume around it. The region corresponding to the lowest tissue P_{O_2} values is the lethal corner, which is located at the venous end of the capillary. (From Fletcher JE: Mathematical modeling of the microcirculation. Math Biosci 38:159–202, 1978. With permission.)

between an idealized mean tissue P_{O_2} and $P\bar{v}_{O_2}$ (Tenney, 1974). This relationship has been used to suggest that $P\bar{v}_{O_2}$ is a valid index of tissue oxygenation.

Mixed venous blood gases are obtained from the distal port of a flow-directed pulmonary artery catheter. Care must be taken not to draw the blood sample too fast or with the balloon inflated. Such practices increase the P_{O_2} of the sample, because oxygenated blood from the pulmonary capillaries may be pulled back into the catheter. The significance of the mixed-venous P_{O_2} or saturation has been discussed earlier, and it should be reiterated that this variable has been overrated as a measure of tissue oxygenation. Absolute values of $P\bar{v}_{O_2}$ or $S\bar{v}_{O_2}$ may not accurately reflect the true state of tissue oxygenation as a result of functional peripheral shunting or mixing of the effluents from the capillary beds of various organs. However, knowledge of the mixed venous blood O_2 content is important because it allows the computation of the total O_2 consumption and the extraction ratio.

CONTINUOUS $S\bar{v}_{O_2}$ MEASUREMENT

The serial or continuous measurement of the $S\bar{v}_{O_2}$ is valuable in certain conditions of decreased O_2

supply, especially in states of low-cardiac output. Measurement can be performed on a continuous basis with a flow-directed oximetry catheter. This catheter transmits light of a certain wavelength into the pulmonary artery, where it is reflected by the RBCs. The oxyhemoglobin saturation is computed by spectrographic analysis with a microprocessor. This technique may produce erroneous results in severe anemia, because there are fewer cells to reflect the emitted light. Thus, clinical data show a good correlation between the results of this method and *in vitro* oximetry.

The advantage of continuous $S\bar{v}_{O_2}$ monitoring lies on the trending aspect of this technique. A serial assessment of the ability of the tissues to utilize the O_2 delivered can be helpful, especially when sudden changes from a stable baseline are detected. Used in this manner, continuous measurement of the $S\bar{v}_{O_2}$ appear to be a valuable tool. However, one should keep in mind when judging the adequacy of O_2 delivery that $S\bar{v}_{O_2}$ also depends on O_2 uptake and on the ability of the tissues to extract O_2 from the blood. Monitoring transient changes in oxygenation, which may occur during suctioning of the endotracheal tube, has been advocated as an indication for the use of these catheters. The clinical significance of these changes has not been established (Schweiss, 1983).

INDWELLING Po_2 ELECTRODES

Indwelling Po_2 catheters have been developed to continuously monitor the arterial O_2 tension. These catheters contain a Clark-type electrode, which is an electrochemical cell that uses a polarographic technique to measure Po_2. Intravascular Po_2 electrodes appear to be reasonably accurate when tested in experimental and clinical studies (Green et al, 1987; Shapiro et al, 1989). However, they have not been widely accepted because of a tendency for electrode drift and the need for frequent calibration. In addition, the Clark electrode consumes O_2, yielding false readings in low-flow states, and offers the risk of vessel thrombosis at the site of insertion.

Optical fluorescence systems for the continuous intra-arterial measurement of pH, Po_2, and Pco_2 have been developed. The term *optode* was given to describe these optical electrodes. Subsequent development has led to an intra-arterial blood-gas system consisting of three optical fibers that can be inserted through a 20-gauge catheter (Tremper and Barker, 1989). Shapiro and associates (1989) evaluated this technique in dogs and in a group of critically ill patients. They found excellent agreement with independently measured pHa and $Paco_2$ but not with Pao_2.

TRANSCUTANEOUS AND CONJUNCTIVAL Po_2

Transcutaneous Po_2 electrodes provide a reasonable estimate of arterial Po_2, especially in neonates and in adults under anesthesia (Severinghaus, 1982). O_2 diffuses from the cutaneous capillaries across the dermal and epidermal layers and into the electrode positions over the skin. This diffusion cascade reduces the Po_2 measured by the electrode to a fraction of the arterial Po_2. The ratio of measured-to-arterial Po_2 is called the Pto_2 index and is approximately 70%. Factors that affect the Pto_2 are the choice of skin site and skin preparation. Preferred sites are the chest, lateral abdomen, and buttocks. The extremities should be avoided because these electrodes are very sensitive to cutaneous blood flow, and erroneous measurements are obtained with vasoconstriction.

A Po_2 electrode attached to a scleral contact lens can provide a continuously measure of conjunctival Po_2. An advantage of this technique is the elimination of the heating artifact associated with transcutaneous $Ptco_2$ measurements. Another advantage is the evaluation of cerebral oxygenation, because the conjunctiva is supplied by the ophthalmic branch of the internal carotid artery. However, studies in healthy volunteer subjects revealed a wide variation between conjunctival Po_2 and Pao_2 among subjects (Chapman et al, 1986). Neither transcutaneous nor conjunctival Po_2 are used in clinical practice to determine tissue oxygenation.

Po_2 MICROELECTRODES

Po_2 microelectrodes fall into two categories, needle Po_2 electrodes (Whalen et al, 1967) and surface microelectrodes. Needle microelectrodes have been developed to a very small size. The major problem with these electrodes is the damage caused as they penetrate the tissues, which may result in false-high readings if bleeding occurs. Surface Po_2 microelectrodes provide a histogram view of the Po_2 distribution within 40 to 50 μm from the organ surface (Kessler et al, 1976). Changes in Po_2 distribution also provide a measure of microcirculatory changes (Gutierrez and Andry, 1989b). Attaching both the needle and surface Po_2 electrodes is an invasive procedure and their use in the clinical setting has been relegated to research studies.

PULSE OXIMETRY

Pulse oximetry relies on the principle that oxyhemoglobin and reduced hemoglobin have different light absorbance characteristics evident by their difference in color. The oximeter determines the percentage of hemoglobin saturation by measuring the absorbance of two wavelengths of light detected through a vascular bed. Ear oximetry was first tested by Comroe and Botelho (1947) in a group of volunteers whose hemoglobin saturation was changed by breathing different concentrations of O_2. They concluded that clinical signs were unreliable for detecting cyanosis until Sao_2 was less than or equal to 80%.

The development of pulse oximetry is attributed to the work of Aoyagi and associates (1971), who realized that the pulsatile signal in the earlobe was related to the saturation of arterial blood. Among the clinical conditions that may interfere with the correct measurement of arterial O_2 saturation by pulse oximetry are elevated levels of carboxyhemoglobin and methemoglobin (Douglas et al, 1979). Other conditions that interfere with the accuracy of pulse oximetry include jaundice (Chaudary and Burki, 1978); skin pigmentation (Ries et al, 1989); nail polish (Cote et al, 1988); shock states (Lawson et al, 1982); and severe hypoxic states. Intense light also can interfere with the oximeter signal and, therefore, it is helpful to cover the sensor whenever it appears to be giving erroneous data (Tremper, 1989).

CARDIAC OUTPUT

An accurate assessment of cardiac function is important in the management of critically ill patients. Invasive measurements of cardiac output include the Fick equation and the indicator dilution method modified for thermodilution (TD). Three noninvasive techniques are available to measure cardiac output: Doppler velocimetry combined with ultrasonic echo imaging of the ascending aorta; thoracic electrical bioimpedance (TEB); and the partial CO_2 rebreathing technique.

The computation of cardiac output by the reverse Fick's equation requires the simultaneous measurement of arterial and mixed venous blood gases, as well as the collection of expired gases to measure $\dot{V}O_2$ (Otis, 1964). With recent technical advances in flowmeter and expired-gas analyzers, this method is becoming increasingly popular.

Indicator dye–dilution methods have been superseded by the TD method (Khalil et al, 1966; Wiedemann et al, 1984), in which a bolus of saline at a known temperature is injected through the proximal port of a pulmonary artery catheter located in the right atrium. The change in temperature in the blood leaving the right ventricle is detected by a thermistor located near the end of the catheter. The recorded signal is a simple exponential decay, and the cardiac output is inversely proportional to the area under the curve. Most cardiac output computers use a modification of the Stewart-Hamilton equation:

$$\text{Cardiac output} = K \times (T_B - T_i)/A \quad [29]$$

in which A is the area under the temperature curve, K is a computation constant, and T_B and T_i are the temperature of the blood and the injectate, respectively. Normal saline or dextrose solutions can serve as the injectate. The use of an iced-fluid bolus increases the signal-to-noise ratio. However, clinical trials have not shown a significant loss of accuracy when the injectate is at room temperature, even in hypothermic patients (Merrick et al, 1980; Shellock et al, 1983).

Cardiac output varies with the ventilatory cycle, and its measurement should be performed at the end of expiration (Stevens et al, 1985). Preferably, the mean of three consecutive determinations should be recorded. A possible source of error is the procedure used to inject the fluid bolus, which should be performed at a constant rate of infusion for 3 to 5 sec, depending on the volume injected. A strip-chart recording of the temperature curve provides an easy check on the adequacy of the injecting technique.

Although TD is the technique most used in measuring cardiac output in critically ill patients, this technique has certain drawbacks. It is expensive and invasive, because it requires a pulmonary artery catheter insertion, with its potential complications. Furthermore, acquisition of data is intermittent. Cardiac output measurements by TD correlate well with those made using the Fick principle (Davies et al, 1986) or dye-dilution techniques (Sorenson et al, 1976).

Another noninvasive method to measure cardiac output is by impedance plethysmography. The electrical impedance of the thoracic cavity changes with blood flow, which is the result of changes in the size of the arteries and in blood viscosity with pulsations. These changes increase the electrical conductance of the cavity and cause a bioimpedance wave form. An estimate of SV can be determined from the impedance wave form. Changes in thoracic electrical impedance were first used to calculate cardiac output by Nyboer (1959). Subsequently, Kubicek and associates (1970) developed an equation that visualized the thorax as a truncated cone and yielded good results in healthy individuals. However, the correlation between cardiac output measured by TEB and by other methods was poor when a more heterogeneous group of patients with various illnesses and body habitus was tested (Keim et al, 1976). A new set of equations has been suggested by Sramek (1981) and by Bernstein (1986), and a commercial TEB device has been developed. Animal (Tremper et al, 1986) and clinical studies have shown an acceptable correlation with invasive reference flow standards (Spinale et al, 1987). However, this method yields poor results in patients with dysrhythmias, aortic regurgitation, ventricular septal defects, sepsis, metal in the chest or chest wall, and possibly hypertension (Appel et al, 1986).

The partial CO_2 rebreathing technique (Capek and Roy, 1988) is based on Fick's equation for CO_2 balance in the lungs:

$$\dot{Q} = \frac{\dot{V}CO_2}{C\bar{v}CO_2 - CaCO_2} \quad [30]$$

Because $C\bar{v}CO_2$ and $CaCO_2$ require sampling of arterial and mixed venous blood, a differential form of the aforementioned equation was developed that uses the PCO_2 at the end of expiration (end-tidal) as an estimate of arterial $PaCO_2$. An estimate of mixed venous PCO_2 is obtained from partial rebreathing for 30 seconds. The procedure is fully automated and provides estimates of cardiac output every few minutes. Animal studies show a correlation coefficient of 0.91 when compared with the TD technique (Capek and Roy, 1988). The clinical usefulness of this technique has not been established.

EXTRACTION RATIO

The extraction ratio ($\dot{V}O_2/\dot{T}O_2$) includes measures of O_2 supply and tissue O_2 demand in a single measurement. Under normal conditions of O_2 supply, the extraction ratio is 15 to 20%. As the supply of O_2 is reduced, the extraction ratio may rise to levels reaching 40 to 50%. Animal experiments show that the extraction ratio may reach levels of 70 to 80% before death. As with the other variables of tissue oxygenation, the ERO_2 is not always an accurate indicator of tissue hypoxia. Capillary recruitment, capillary transit time, changes in the O_2 tissue diffusion, and alterations in microvascular control can reduce the amount of O_2 extracted from blood, which can result in low extraction ratios, although the tissue metabolic needs remain unaltered. It remains to be determined if serial measurements of ERO_2 can be useful in assessing changes in tissue oxygenation.

MAGNETIC RESONANCE SPECTROSCOPY

High levels of exercise or hypoxia result in the accumulation of ADP, P_i, and lactate as well as in decreases in PCr and pH_i. The decrease in PCr and the concomitant increase in P_i provide a convenient index of cellular energy state (i.e., the PCr/P_i ratio). This index has been used to characterize the state of cell bioenergetics in skeletal muscle, heart, and brain (Chance et al, 1980). It appears that the PCr/P_i ratio may be equivalent to the parameter associated most closely with the control of mitochondrial respiration, the phosphate potential (Gyulai et al, 1985).

In the past, measurements of the phosphate potential or the PCr/P_i ratio could be obtained only by destructive tissue biopsy procedures. This has changed with the introduction of ^{31}P-magnetic resonance spectroscopy (MRS), a technique that makes it possible to sequentially monitor changes in PCr, P_i, and ATP during hypoxia in an accurate and noninvasive manner.

A magnetic resonance spectrometer consists of a radio transmitter capable of directing high-frequency radio waves into a tissue sample placed inside a strong, homogeneous, magnetic field. These radio frequency waves are absorbed by certain atomic nuclei in the magnetic field, altering their spatial orientation. Maximal energy is transferred to these isotopes at their resonant frequency. Achieving resonance depends on matching the rotation or spin frequency of the isotope nuclei with the radio-pulse frequency. As the radio pulse fades, these nuclei return to their original position but in the process generate electrical signals that are used to develop a frequency spectrum.

The resonant frequency of the isotope nuclei under study is also affected by its associated molecule. Therefore, the MRS spectrum contains several peaks, each corresponding with a different molecule that contains the isotope nuclei. Because the peak area is the total of the resonating nuclei, this area can be used to quantify the concentration of the compound under investigation.

Proton, or H^-, which is an abundant isotope present in fat and water, has been used to obtain tomographic images (magnetic resonance imaging [MRI]). Given the close association of phosphorus with the various bioenergetic phenomena, ^{31}P spectroscopy has been very useful in characterizing metabolic changes. The reader is referred to a review by Gutierrez and Andry (1989b).

Figure 8–11 shows a ^{31}P-MRS spectrum obtained from skeletal muscle. ^{31}P is a naturally occurring isotope that forms part of several important molecules that participate in the transfer of energy within the cell. These peaks correspond to the resonance of P_i, PCr, and the three phosphate bonds of ATP, γ, α, and β. Because the resonance of ADP also contributes to the γ and α peaks, the concentration of ATP is determined from the area under the β peak. Intracellular pH can be accurately measured from the separation between the P_i and PCr peaks, the so-called chemical shift (Moon and Richards, 1973). Changes in the peak areas and in the chemical shift can be used as noninvasive measures of changes in cellular energy metabolism.

MRS has certain limitations that must be kept in mind when interpreting the spectra. The signals derived from an MRS experiment represent a spatial and temporal average, and, therefore, the technique is inherently poor in spatial localization (Chance et al, 1985b). The sensitivity of the MRS measurement depends greatly on the concentration of the nuclei under study and on the length of time during which the spectra are accumulated. MRS can detect metabolites found in concentrations of approximately 1 mM, but it cannot measure those present in smaller or trace amounts. The latter include many biologically important molecules, including hormones and drugs.

INCREASES IN TISSUE P_{CO_2}—GASTRIC TONOMETRY

Increases in cellular H^+ concentration occur during hypoxia as anaerobically generated ATP un-

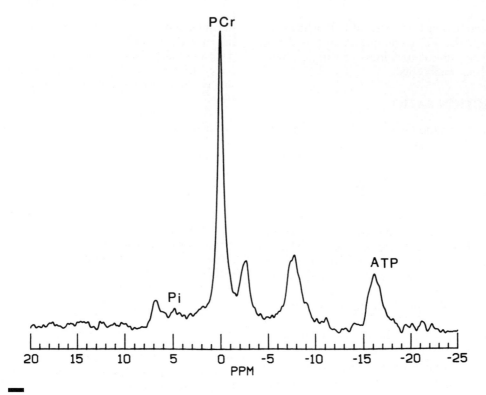

Figure 8–11

A typical skeletal muscle ^{31}P spectrum. The areas under the peaks for inorganic phosphate (Pi), phosphocreatine (PCr), and ATP are proportional to their concentration in tissue. The intracellular pH can be estimated from the separation of the frequencies for Pi and PCr.

dergoes hydrolysis. This is accompanied by increased tissue production of CO_2 by the buffering action of bicarbonate on hydrogen ions:

$$H^+ + HCO^-_3 \leftrightarrow H_2O + CO_2 \qquad [31]$$

Measuring increases in tissue P_{CO_2} by a tonometric method has emerged as a potentially useful monitoring modality in the ICU (Gutierrez and Brown, 1995; Clark and Gutierrez, 1992; Fiddian-Green, 1991). Tonometry is a relative noninvasive technique that measures either gastric or intestinal mucosal P_{CO_2} by allowing the equilibration of CO_2 pressures between a fluid-filled balloon and the interstitial fluid of the mucosa (Fig. 8–12). The tissues normally generate CO_2 during the metabolism of O_2 at a rate determined by the cellular respiratory quotient. With hypoxia, there is excess production of CO_2 as hydrogen ions resulting from anaerobic metabolism accumulate in the cytosol and are buffered by tissue bicarbonate. Therefore, the basis of tonometry as a monitor of cellular energy balance is that increases in tissue CO_2 occur during cellular hypoxia.

An important characteristic of the intestinal and gastric mucosa is their vulnerability to de-

creases in oxygenation. This phenomenon is partly related to the countercurrent microcirculation found in the gastric and intestinal mucosa, in which diffusion of O_2 from the arterioles to the adjacent venules occurs. As a result of this capillary diffusional shunt, the cells located at the tip of the intestinal villus have a lower P_{O_2} than those located at the base. Countercurrent vascular systems are characteristic of the' renal and splanchnic microcirculation. These systems are well suited for the absorption of solutes but fare poorly with hypoxia. This property has earned the gut and the kidney the sobriquet of "sentinel" organs (Dantzker, 1993), because they manifest early the harmful effects of decreases in cardiac output in shock, or the release of potent vasoactive substances during sepsis.

Tonometry provides the indirect assessment of gut mucosal pH (Fiddian-Green et al, 1982). This concept is based on the assumptions that (1) CO_2 diffuses freely in tissue; (2) P_{CO_2} in the luminal fluid is in equilibrium with the mucosal P_{CO_2}; (3) arterial bicarbonate concentration ([HCO^-_3]) equals intestinal mucosa bicarbonate. The application of the Henderson-Hasselbalch

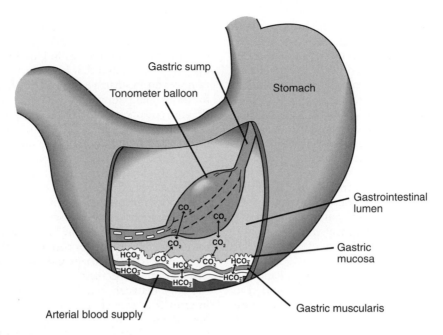

Figure 8–12

A gastric tonometer consists of a fluid-filled balloon inserted in the lumen of the stomach. The mucosal layers and the fluid CO_2 concentrations equilibrate, providing an indirect measurement of changes in tissue CO_2 concentration. (From Clark CH and Gutierrez G: Gastric intramucosal pH: A noninvasive method for the indirect measurement of tissue oxygenation. Am J Crit Care 1:53–60, 1992. With permission.)

equation to these assumptions variables allows the calculation of the intra-mucosal pH (pHi):

$$pH_i = 6.1 + \log \frac{HCO_3^-}{\alpha \cdot \text{tonometer } P_{CO_2}} \quad [32]$$

where α represents the solubility of CO_2 in plasma ($\alpha = 0.03$).

There is an association between decreases in gastric pH_i and greater patient mortality. Gys and associates (1988) measured gastric pH_i by gastric fluid aspiration in 59 postsurgical subjects upon admission to the ICU. Patients with admission pH_i levels less than 7.32 had a 37% short-term mortality rate (defined as death within 72 hours of ICU admission) compared with 0% in those with pH_i levels of 7.32 or greater. They also found that 90% of patients with sepsis had pH_i levels less than 7.32. They found no correlation between gastric pH_i measured on ICU admission and hospital mortality.

The prognostic characteristics of pH_i were further established by Doglio and coworkers (1991), who measured gastric pH_i with a tonometer in a heterogeneous group of 80 patients at the time of admission to the ICU and again 12 hours later. A pH_i of 7.35 was used as the lower range of normal. The group admitted with low pH_i had

greater ICU mortality (65% vs. 44%; p<0.04). Furthermore, patients with persistently low pH_i 12 hours after ICU admission had the highest mortality rate (87%), compared with a mortality rate of only 27% for the group with normal pH_i since admission. The prevalence of sepsis was greater in the low pH_i group (59% vs. 26%; p<0.01). This study was repeated by Maynard and colleagues (1993), who found a remarkably concordance in the data from both studies. They compared the predictive ability of pH_i to that of lactate concentration, D_{O_2}, and $\dot{V}_{O_2}$, among others, and found that gastric pH_i had a very high sensitivity (88%) and the highest likelihood ratio of the variables tested. Further analysis of the data using a step-down logistic regression analysis showed that pH_i at 24 hours was the only independent predictor of mortality.

In a prospective study comparing measures of gastric pH_i to standard measures of oxygen transport and consumption in a group of 22 patients, Gutierrez and coworkers (1992a) found that only gastric pH_i mixed venous pH measurements differentiated survivors from nonsurvivors. Marik (1993) obtained similar results in a study of 30 ICU patients, in whom gastric pH_i and mixed venous pH were lower in those who developed multiple systems organ failure or in those who died. He concluded that indices of oxygenation, including pH_i and arterial lactate, are superior to hemodynamic or oxygen-derived variables as predictors of outcome in patients with sepsis.

Changes in pH_i have been used to guide therapy in critically ill patients. Mythen and Webb (1995) used volume expansion to maintain pH_i levels higher than 7.32 during elective cardiac surgery in 60 patients. The incidence of mucosal hypoperfusion ($pH_i < 7.32$) was only 7% in the protocol group compared with 56% in the control group. A lower pH_i was associated with significantly greater incidence of major complications (6 vs. 0), greater ICU length of stay (1.7 vs. 1.0 days), and greater hospital length of stay (10.1 vs. 6.4 days).

In a more ambitious study, Gutierrez and colleagues (1992b) studied 260 patients admitted to the ICU of eight participating hospitals with Acute Physiology and Chronic Health Evaluation (APACHE) II scores of 15 to 25. After insertion of a gastric tonometer, each patient was randomized to a control or protocol group within an admission category (normal ≥ 7.35; low < 7.35). The control groups were treated according to standard ICU practices, whereas the protocol group received, in addition, treatment to increase systemic DO_2 whenever pH_i level fell below 7.35, or by more than 0.10 units from the previous measurements. The intervention protocol consisted of standard treatment of hypotension, hypoxia, anemia, fever, and other factors , if present, followed by the infusion of fluids and the inotrope dobutamine. The protocol was used in all patients admitted with low pH_i and, because pH_i fell at some time during their ICU stay, in 85% of those admitted with normal pH_i. They found that for patients admitted with pH_i level lower than 7.35, survival was similar in the protocol and control groups (37% vs. 36%) whereas for those admitted with normal pH_i, survival was significantly greater in the protocol treated group (58% vs. 42%; $p < 0.01$). The authors concluded that pH_i-guided resuscitation may improve outcome in the subpopulation of patients admitted to the ICU with normal pH_i, perhaps by preventing splanchnic ischemia and the development of a systemic oxygen deficit.

BLOOD LACTATE CONCENTRATION

The interpretation of blood lactate concentration as a marker of tissue hypoxia may be complicated by the profound pathologic conditions encountered in critically ill patients. In a retrospective analysis of 24 patients (8 with ARDS), Rashkin

and coworkers (1985) identified a critical O_2 transport threshold of 8 ml/kg per minute, corresponding to rapid increases in blood lactate. However, they also noted that blood lactate concentration was an insensitive measure of changes in TO_2 for individual patients. In a subsequent study, Astiz and coworkers (1988) monitored changes in 50 patients with sepsis and 50 patients with acute myocardial infarction and were unable to identify a threshold value for TO_2 corresponding to increases in blood lactate in either group.

An elevated arterial lactate concentration in a hemodynamically stable patient should be interpreted as a marker of disease, one that portends a bad outcome. Increases in blood lactate concentration in these patients correlate with the severity of illness and perhaps indicate severe cellular dysfunction in specific tissues. On the other hand, causality between cellular hypoxia and increases in arterial or mixed venous blood lactate has not been demonstrated (Connet et al, 1984). Therefore, the presence of lactic acidosis should not be taken as proof of an oxygen debt requiring increases in systemic O_2 transport to supernormal values. Furthermore, the treatment of lactic acidosis with sodium bicarbonate or with dichloroacetate is not supported by clinical studies (Graf et al, 1985; Benjamin et al, 1994; Stacpoole et al, 1992).

INDIVIDUAL ORGAN FUNCTION

Assessment of the adequacy of tissue oxygenation by the response of organ function to hypoxia is an insensitive technique and is one that defeats the purpose of optimizing O_2 delivery and utilization.

The response of an individual organ to a reduction on O_2 delivery depends on the ability of that organ to increase its ERO_2 and on systemic vasoregulatory mechanisms. Changes in the function of an organ or even an organ system, therefore, do not provide sufficient information to ascertain the regional or generalized causes for the reduction in O_2 delivery. As mentioned earlier, hypoxemia produces a redistribution of the cardiac output to the brain and heart. These are high-extraction organs that do not demonstrate the effects of hypoxia until exposed to extremely severe reductions in O_2 delivery. Once the compensatory mechanisms are overwhelmed, further increases in hypoxia produce dramatic abnormalities. Other organs, such as the gut and kidneys, are more sensitive indicators of hypoxia, because they are affected early in the process of O_2 reduction. Severe peripheral vasoconstriction and a reduction in urine output should alert the physician to disturbances in the O_2 transport system.

From the aforementioned discussion, it is clear that no single measurement of tissue oxygenation provides a complete picture of the adequacy of cellular respiration. Instead, a critical evaluation should be made, and the information provided by these variables should be integrated to gain an accurate picture of the state of tissue oxygenation.

OPTIMIZATION OF TISSUE OXYGENATION IN THE CRITICALLY ILL PATIENT

The successful treatment of patients suffering from derangement in tissue gas exchange is a formidable task. It is nearly impossible to devise a detailed therapeutic algorithm for the treatment of this condition, given the multiplicity of diseases associated with regional dysoxia, as well as the heterogeneity of the patient population. Therefore, treatment should be guided by broad guidelines revolving around the principle of adequate regional tissue oxygenation (Bone et al, 1992; Fiddian-Green et al, 1993).

It is important to ensure adequate ventilation of the lungs by establishing a patent airway. Given the hemodynamic instability of these patients, as well as the frequency with which respiratory failure is associated with critical illness, many of these patients require mechanical ventilation. The smooth coupling of the patient's respiratory efforts to ventilator driven breaths cannot be overemphasized, because coupling minimizes the work of breathing, allowing blood flow to be diverted to and from the respiratory muscles to organs that may be hypoperfused (Mohsenifar et al, 1993).

The uppermost therapeutic goal in the treatment of critically ill patients is the maintenance of adequate cellular oxygenation in all organs. Loss of microvascular control results in the unregulated opening of capillary beds, decreases in peripheral vascular resistance, cardiac output maldistribution, and overperfusion of some organs while others are underperfused. Hemodynamic and oxygenation parameters should be monitored regularly, at least every 6 hours in acutely ill patients. The adequacy of systemic O_2 transport may be assessed using pulmonary artery catheters to determine cardiac output, pulse oximetry to measure arterial blood oxygenation, and gastric tonometry to assess the adequacy of tissue oxygenation in a sentinel organ. The placement of an arterial line should be considered, because it allows continuous monitoring of systemic blood pressure and serves to sample arterial blood for blood gases. Serial measurements of $\dot{T}O_2$, $\dot{V}O_2$, ERO_2, and gastric mucosal pH provide valuable information regarding the oxygenation-metabolic state of the patient. Alterations in regional tissue oxygenation and metabolism usually do not result in hemodynamic alterations or in end-organ function for several hours. This provides the clinician with an early warning period that should be used judiciously if organ failure is to be avoided. Important questions that must be answered during that time are: what are the causes of inadequate oxygenation? Are the data correct? Is it a local or a global phenomenon? Is the cardiac output adequate? Is the patient bleeding? Is there a continuing source of cytokine release, such as an abscess, resulting in impaired microvascular control?

Unless new studies prove otherwise, increases in $\dot{T}O_2$ to supernormal levels should not be attempted in every patient. Provided that control of the microvasculature is not impaired, many patients have perfectly adequate tissue perfusion at relatively low levels of $\dot{T}O_2$. The infusion of dobutamine or other catecholamines in that case may be deleterious because it may provoke a loss of microvascular autoregulation. On the other hand, increasing systemic $\dot{T}O_2$ in patients with signs of regional underperfusion may be beneficial, but the aim of this therapy should be to achieve a systemic $\dot{T}O_2$ high enough to satisfy the O_2 requirements of all organs, no more, no less. Only in response to rapid increases in arterial lactate concentration, decreases in pH_i to values less than 7.25 in patients without arterial acidosis, or changes in organ function, such as rapidly deteriorating renal or hepatic function, should one attempt to increase $\dot{T}O_2$. Increasing $\dot{T}O_2$ accomplished by infusing fluids or blood products, or by the infusion of dobutamine. Usually a rate of 5 to 10 μg/kg per minute of dobutamine is sufficient to reverse a low pH_i, although greater concentrations may be required in individual cases (Silverman and Tuma, 1992).

It is obvious that increasing systemic $\dot{T}O_2$ is a grossly inefficient method to assure adequate oxygenation to all tissues. However, we lack selective vasoactive agents capable of redirecting cardiac output to those tissues where the need for O_2 is greatest. Dopexamine hydrochloride, a potent β_2-adrenergic and dopaminergic agonist, may be useful in this respect (Bredle and Cain, 1991; Colardyn et al, 1989) Cain and Curtis (1992) treated dogs with a combination of dextran and dopexamine following the infusion of *E. coli* endotoxin and found greater intestinal $\dot{V}O_2$ and decreased gut lactate efflux in that group when compared with those in a control group treated with dextran only. Clinical experience on the use of dopexamine to improve splanchnic perfusion is encouraging. Smithies and coworkers (1994) infused dopexamine to a maximum dose of 6 μg/kg per minute for 1 hour in 10 patients with sepsis and acute respiratory failure. Cardiac index increased from 4.0 to 4.8 l/min/m² with dopexamine but returned to baseline 1 hour after the infusion ceased. Gastric pH_i measured with tonometry also increased from a mean of 7.21 to 7.28. This improvement in pH_i was maintained after the infusion of dopexamine ceased, suggesting that it was an effect independent of dopexamine's systemic action.

Close attention to the patient's nutritional requirements, frequent changes of intravenous and intra-arterial lines, and a high level of nursing care are paramount at improving the patient's chances of survival. These are complex clinical cases and only by the coordinated action of the ICU health care team composed of physicians, nurses, respiratory therapists, dietitians, and others can we improve the odds of survival from a syndrome that has become a major cause of death in our intensive care units.

CONCLUSIONS

Humans have developed an efficient and resilient system to transport O_2 from the atmosphere to every cell in the body. When the delivery of O_2 is reduced by pathologic processes, adaptive mechanisms respond to maintain cellular respiration. The issue confronting physicians caring for critically ill patients is the inability of these adaptive mechanisms to cope with an overwhelming failure in the O_2 delivery system. The advent of sophisticated technology has provided us with a clearer perception of the process of tissue oxygenation and the effect that various therapeutic measures have on this process. Although there are still many unanswered questions with regard to basic physiologic mechanisms in tissue oxygenation, as our knowledge expands and we answer some of these questions, the care of hypoxic patients continues to improve.

REFERENCES

Aberman A, Cavanilles JM, Trotter J, et al: An equation for the oxygen hemoglobin dissociation curve. J Appl Physiol 35:570–571, 1973.

Aberman A, Cavanilles JM, Weil MH, et al: Blood P_{50} calculated from a single measurement of pH, PO_2, and SO_2. J Appl Physiol 38:171–176, 1975.

Adachi H, Strauss HW, Ochi H, et al: The effect of hypoxia on the regional distribution of cardiac output in the dog. Circ Res 39:314–319, 1976.

Adair GS: The hemoglobin system. VI: The oxygen dissociation curve of hemoglobin. J Biol Chem 63:529–545, 1925.

Annat G, Viale J, Pereival C, et al: Oxygen delivery and uptake in the adult respiratory distress syndrome. Am Rev Respir Dis 133:999–1001, 1986.

Antonini E: History and theory of the oxyhemoglobin dissociation curve. Crit Care Med 7:360–367, 1979.

Antonini E and Brunori M: Hemoglobin and Myoglobin in Their Reactions with Ligands. Vol 21: Frontiers of Biology. Amsterdam, North Holland Research Monographs, 1971.

Aoyagi T, Kish M, et al: Improvements of an ear oximeter. Abstracts of the 13th Annual Meeting of the Japanese Society for Medical Electronics and Biological Engineering, 1971, pp 90–91.

Appel DL, Kram HB, Mackabee J, et al: Comparison of measurements of cardiac output by bioimpedance and thermodilution in severely ill surgical patients. Crit Care Med 14:933–935, 1986.

Aprille JR: Regulation of the mitochondrial adenine nucleotide pool size in liver: Mechanism and metabolic role. Fed Am Soc Exper Biol 2:2547–2556, 1988.

Astiz ME, Rackow EC, Kaufman B, et al: Relationship of oxygen delivery and mixed venous oxygenation to lactic acidosis in patients with sepsis and acute myocardial infarction. Crit Care Med 16:655–658, 1988.

Barcroft J: The Respiratory Function of Blood. Part 1: Lessons from High Altitude. London, Cambridge University Press, 1925.

Barcroft MA and Hill AV: The nature of oxyhemoglobin with a note on its molecular weight. J Physiol (Lond) 39:411–428, 1910.

Baudry N and Vicaut E: Role of nitric oxide in effects of tumor necrosis factor-α on microcirculation of rat. J Appl Physiol 75:2392–2399, 1993.

Bauer C, Klocke A, Kamp D, et al: Effect of 2, 3-diphosphoglycerate and H^+ on the reaction of O_2 and hemoglobin. Am J Physiol 224:838–847, 1973.

Bellingham AJ, Detter C, and Lenfant C: Regulatory mechanisms of hemoglobin oxygen affinity in acidosis and alkalosis. J Clin Invest 50:700–706, 1971.

Bencowitz HZ, Wagner PD, and West JB: Effect of change in P_{50} on exercise tolerance at high altitude: A theoretical study. J Appl Physiol 53:1487–1495, 1982.

Benesch R and Benesch RE: Effect of organic phosphates from human erythrocytes on the allosteric properties of haemoglobin. Biochem Biophys Res Commun 26:162–167, 1967.

Benjamin E, Oropello JM, Abalos AM, et al: Effects of acid-base correction on hemodynamics, oxygen dynamics, and resuscitability in severe canine hemorrhagic shock. Crit Care Med 22:1616–1623, 1994.

Berne RM: Adenosine: An important physiological regulation. N Physiol Sci 1:163, 1986.

Bernstein D: A new stroke volume equation for thoracic electrical bioimpedance: Theory and rationale. Crit Care Med 14:904–909, 1986.

Bihari D, Smithies M, Gimson A, and Tinker J: The effects of vasodilation with prostacyclin on oxygen delivery and uptake in critically ill patients. N Engl J Med 317:397–403, 1987.

Bohr C, Hasselbalch K, and Krogh A: Ubereinen biologischer Beziehung wichtigen Einfluss den die Kohlen-saurespannung des Blutes auf dessen Sauerstoffbindung abt. Skand Arch Physiol 16:402–412, 1904.

Bone RC, et al: Definitions for sepsis and organ failure and guidelines for the use of innovative therapies in sepsis. Crit Care Med 20:864–874, 1992.

Bone RC, Slotman G, Maunder RJ, et al: Randomized double-blind, multicenter study of prostaglandin E_1 in patients with the adult respiratory distress syndrome. Chest 96:114–119, 1989.

Bontemps F, Van den Berghe G, and Hers HG: Pathways of adenine nucleotide catabolism in erythrocytes. J Clin Invest 77:824–830, 1986.

Borgstrom P and Gestrelius S: Integrative myogenic and metabolic control of vascular tone in skeletal muscle during autoregulation of blood flow. Microvasc Res 33:353–376, 1987.

Bourdeau-Martin J, Odoroff CL, and Honig CR: Dual effect of oxygen on magnitude and uniformity of coronary intercapillary distance. Am J Physiol 226:800–810, 1974.

Boyd O, Grounds RM, and Bennett ED: A randomized clinical trial of the effect of deliberate perioperative increase of oxygen delivery on mortality in high-risk surgical patients. JAMA 270:2699–2707, 1993.

Brady AJB, Poole-Wilson PA, Harding SE, et al: Nitric oxide production within cardiac myocytes reduces their contractility in endotoxemia. Am J Physiol 263:H1963–H1966, 1992.

Bredle DL and Cain SM: Systemic and muscle oxygen uptake/delivery after dopexamine infusion in endotoxic dogs. Crit Care Med 19:198, 1991.

Bromberg PA and Jensen WN: Blood oxygen dissociation curves in sickle cell disease. J Lab Clin Med 70:480–488, 1967.

Cain SM: Supply dependency of oxygen uptake in ARDS: Myth or reality? Am J Med Sci 288:119–129, 1984.

Cain SM and Curtis SE: Systemic and regional oxygen uptake and lactate flux in endotoxic dogs resuscitated with dextran and dopexamine or dextran alone. Circ Shock 38:173, 1992.

Capek J and Roy R: Noninvasive measurement of cardiac output using partial CO_2 rebreathing.

IEEE Trans Biomed Eng (BME) 35:653–661, 1988.

Chance B: Oxygen transport and oxygen reduction? In Chien H (ed): Electron Transport and Oxygen Utilization. Amsterdam, Elsevier North Holland, 1982, pp 225–266.

Chance B, Eleff S, and Leigh JS: Noninvasive, nondestructive approaches to cell bioenergetics. Proc Natl Acad Sci USA 77:7430–7434, 1980.

Chance B, Leigh JS, Clark BJ, et al: Control of oxidative metabolism and oxygen delivery in human skeletal muscle: A steady-state analysis of the work/energy cost transfer function. Proc Natl Acad Sci USA 82:8384–8488, 1985a.

Chance B, Leigh JS, and Nioka S: Micro-heterogeneity: The Achilles heel of NMR spectroscopy and imaging: Some calculations for brain ischemia and muscle exercise. N Metab Res 2:26–31, 1985b.

Chanutin A and Curnish R: Effect of organic and inorganic phosphates on the oxygen equilibrium of human erythrocytes. Arch Biochem Biophys 121:96–102, 1967.

Chapman K, Liu F, Watson R, et al: Conjunctival oxygen tension and its relationship to arterial oxygen tension. J Clin Monit 2:100–104, 1986.

Chaudary BA and Burki NK: Oximetry in clinical practice. Am Rev Respir Dis 117:173–175, 1978.

Clark CH and Gutierrez G: Gastric intramucosal pH: A noninvasive method for the indirect measurement of tissue oxygenation. Am J Crit Care 1:53–60, 1992.

Coburn RF: Mechanisms of carbon monoxide toxicity. Prev Med 8:310–322, 1979.

Coburn RF, Forster RE, and Kane BP: Considerations of the physiological variables that determine the blood carboxyhemoglobin concentration in man. J Clin Invest 44:1899–1910, 1965.

Colardyn FC, VanDenbogaerde JF, Vogelaers DP, et al: Use of dopexamine hydrochloride in patients with septic shock. Crit Care Med 17:999–1003, 1989.

Cole RP, Sukanek PC, Wittenberg JB, et al: Mitochondrial function in the presence of myoglobin. J Appl Physiol 53:1116–1124, 1982.

Collier CR: Oxygen affinity of human blood in the presence of carbon monoxide. J Appl Physiol 40:487–490, 1976.

Comroe JH and Botelho S: The reliability of cyanosis in the recognition of arterial anoxemia. Am J Med Sci 214:1–6, 1947.

Connett RJ, Gayeski TE, and Honig CR: Lactate accumulation in fully aerobic working dog gracilis muscle. Am J Physiol 246:H120–H128, 1984.

Cote CJ, Goldstein A, Fuchsman WH, et al: The effect of nail polish on pulse oximetry. Anesth Analg 67:683–686, 1988.

Crystal GJ and Weiss HR: V_{O_2} of resting muscle during arterial hypoxia: Role of reflex vasoconstriction. Microvasc Res 20:30–40, 1980.

Danek SJ, Lynch JP, Weg JG, et al: The dependence of oxygen uptake on oxygen delivery in the adult respiratory distress syndrome. Am Rev Respir Dis 122:387–395, 1980.

Dantzker D: Editorial: The gastrointestinal tract: The canary of the body? JAMA 270:1247–1248, 1993.

Dantzker DR, Foresman B, and Gutierrez G: Oxygen supply and utilization relationships: A reevaluation. Am Rev Respir Dis 143:675–679, 1991.

Davidson D and Stalcup SA: Systemic circulatory adjustments to acute hypoxia and reoxygenation in unanesthetized sheep. J Clin Invest 73:317–328, 1984.

Davies GG, Jebson PJR, Glasgow BM, et al: Continuous Fick cardiac output compared to thermodilution cardiac output. Crit Care Med 14:881–885, 1986.

De Backer D, Berre J, Zhang H, et al: Relationship between oxygen uptake and oxygen delivery in septic patients: Effects of prostacyclin versus dobutamine. Crit Care Med 21:1658–1664, 1993.

de la Huerga J and Sherrick JC: Measurement of oxygen saturation of the blood. Ann Clin Lab Sci 1:261–271, 1971.

Doglio GR, Pusajo JF, Egurrola MA, et al: Gastric mucosal pH as a prognostic index of mortality in critically ill patients. Crit Care Med 19:1037–1040, 1991.

Dorinsky PM, Costello JL, and Gadek JE: Relationship of oxygen uptake and oxygen delivery in respiratory failure not due to the adult respiratory distress syndrome. Chest 93:1013–1019, 1988.

Douglas CG, Haldane JS, and Haldane JBS: The laws of combination of hemoglobin with carbon monoxide and oxygen. J Physiol (Lond) 44:275–304, 1912.

Douglas NJ, Brash HM, Wraith PK, et al: Accuracy, sensitivity to carboxyhemoglobin, and speed of response of the Hewlett-Packard 47201 ear oximeter. Am Rev Respir Dis 119:311–313, 1979.

Drazenovic R, Samsel RW, Wylam ME, et al: Regulation of perfused capillary density in canine intestinal mucosa during endotoxemia. J Appl Physiol 72:259–265, 1992.

Dudley GA and Terjung RL: Influence of aerobic metabolism on IMP accumulation in fast-twitch muscle. Am J Physiol 248:C37–C42, 1985.

Duling BR: Local control of microvascular function: Role in tissue oxygen supply. Ann Rev Physiol 42:373–382, 1980.

Edwards JD and Clarke C: Therapeutic implications of oxygen transport in critically ill patients. In Gutierrez G and Vincent JL (eds): Update in Intensive Care and Emergency Medicine. Vol 12. Tissue Oxygen Utilization. New York, Springer-Verlag, 1991, pp 286–299.

Ellsworth ML and Pittman RN: Heterogeneity of oxygen diffusion through hamster striated muscles. Am J Physiol 246:H161–H167, 1984.

Fairweather LJ, Walker J, and Flenley DC: 2,3-Diphosphoglycerate concentrations and the dissociation of oxyhaemoglobin in ventilatory failure. Clin Sci Molec Med 47:577–588, 1974.

Federspiel WJ and Sarelius IH: An examination of the contribution of red cell spacing to the uniformity of oxygen flux at the capillary wall. Microvasc Res 27:273–285, 1984.

Feldstein ML, Henquell L, and Honig CR: Frequency analysis of coronary intercapillary distances: Site of capillary control. Am J Physiol 235:H321–H325, 1978.

Fiddian-Green RG: Editorial: Should measurements of tissue pH and PO_2 be included in the routine monitoring of intensive care unit patients? Crit Care Med 19:141–143, 1991.

Fiddian-Green RG, Haglund U, Gutierrez G, et al. Goals for the resuscitation of shock. Crit Care Med 21:S25, 1993.

Fiddian-Green RG, Pittenger G, and Whitehouse WM: Back-diffusion of CO_2 and its influence on the intramural pH in gastric mucosa. J Surg Res 33:39–48, 1982.

Fisher AB and Dodia C: Lung as a model for evaluation of critical intracellular PO_2 and PCO. Am J Physiol 241:E47–E50, 1981.

Fletcher JE: Mathematical modeling of the microcirculation. Math Biosci 38:159–202, 1978.

Forster RE, Roughton FJW, Kreuzer F, et al: Photocolorimetric determination of rate of uptake of CO and O_2 by reduced human red cell suspensions at 37°C. J Appl Physiol 11:260–268, 1957.

Franco R and Canela EI: Computer simulation of purine metabolism. J Biochem 144:305–315, 1984.

Gayeski TEJ and Honig CR: O_2 gradients from sarcolemma to cell interior in red muscle at maximal V_{O_2}. (Heart Circ Physiol 20) Am J Physiol 251:H789–H799, 1986.

Gayeski TEJ and Honig CR: Intracellular PO_2 in long axis of individual fibers in working dog gracilis muscle. Am J Physiol 254:H1179–H1186, 1988.

Gevers W: Generation of protons by metabolic processes in heart cells. J Mol Cell Cardiol 9:864–874, 1977.

Gilbert E, Haupt M, Mandanas R, et al: The effect of fluid loading, blood transfusion, and catecholamine infusion on oxygen delivery and consumption in patients with sepsis. Am Rev Respir Dis 134:873–878, 1986.

Graf H, Leach W, and Arieff AI: Evidence for a detrimental effect of bicarbonate therapy in lactic acidosis. Science 227:754–756, 1985.

Granger DN, Hollwarth MA, and Parks DA: Ischemia reperfusion injury: Role of oxygen derived free radicals. Acta Physiol Scand 126[Suppl 548]:47–63, 1986.

Green G, Hassell K, and Mahutte C: Comparison of arterial blood gas with continuous intra-arterial and transcutaneous PO_2 sensors in adult critically ill patients. Crit Care Med 15:491–494, 1987.

Grisham MB and McCord JM: Chemistry and cytotoxicity of reactive oxygen metabolites. In Taylor AE, Matalon S, and Ward P (eds): Physiology of Oxygen Radicals. Bethesda, MD, American Physiological Society, 1986, pp 1–18.

Grunewald WA and Sowa W: Distribution of the myocardial tissue Po_2 in the rat and in the inhomogeneity of the coronary bed. Pflugers Arch 374:57–66, 1978.

Gutierrez G: The rate of oxygen release and its effect on capillary O_2 tension: A mathematical analysis. Respir Physiol 63:79–96, 1986.

Gutierrez G and Andry J: Increased hemoglobin O_2 affinity does not improve O_2 consumption in hypoxemia. J Appl Physiol 66:837–843, 1989a.

Gutierrez G and Andry J: Nuclear magnetic resonance measurements: Clinical applications. Crit Care Med 17:73–82, 1989b.

Gutierrez G, Bismar H, Dantzker D, et al: Comparison of gastric intramucosal pH with measures of oxygen transport and consumption in critically ill patients. Crit Care Med 20:451, 1992a.

Gutierrez G and Brown SD: Gastric tonometry: A new monitoring modality in the intensive care unit. J Intensiv Care Med 10:34–44, 1995.

Gutierrez G, Lund N, and Palizas F: Rabbit skeletal muscle Po_2 during hypodynamic sepsis. Chest 99:224–229, 1991.

Gutierrez G, Marini C, Acero A, et al: Skeletal muscle Po_2 during hypoxemia and isovolemic anemia. J Appl Physiol, 68:2047–2053, 1990.

Gutierrez G, Palizas F, Doglio G, et al: Gastric intramucosal pH as a therapeutic index of tissue oxygenation in critically ill patients. Lancet 339:195–199, 1992b.

Gutierrez G and Pohil R: Oxygen consumption is linearly related to O_2 supply in critically ill patients. J Crit Care 1:45–53, 1986.

Gutierrez G, Warley A, and Dantzker D: Oxygen delivery and utilization in hypothermic dogs. J Appl Physiol 60:751–757, 1986.

Gyulai L, Roth Z, Leigh J, et al: Bioenergetic studies of mitochondrial oxidative phosphorylation using 31-phosphorus NMR. J Biol Chem 260:3947–3954, 1985.

Gys T, Hubens A, Neels H, et al: Prognostic value of gastric intramural pH in surgical intensive care patients. Crit Care Med 16:1222–1224, 1988.

Haldane J: The relation of the action of carbonic oxide to oxygen tension. J Physiol (Lond) 18:201–218, 1895.

Haldane J and Smith JL: The oxygen tension of arterial blood. J Physiol (Lond) 20:497–520, 1896.

Hammersen F: The terminal vascular bed in skeletal muscle with special regard to the problem of shunts. In Crone C, and Lassen NA (eds): Capillary Permeability. New York, Academic Press, 1970, pp 351–365.

Hanique G, Dugernier T, Laterre PF, et al: Significance of pathologic oxygen supply dependency in critically ill patients: Comparison between measured and calculated methods. Intensive Care Med 20:12–18, 1994a.

Hanique G, Dugernier T, Laterre PF, et al: Evaluation of oxygen uptake and delivery in critically ill patients: A statistical reappraisal. Intensive Care Med 20:19–26, 1994b.

Hannemann L, Reinhart K, Meier-Hellmann A, et al: Prostacyclin in septic shock. Chest 105:1504–1510, 1994.

Hansson-Mild K and Linderholm H: Some factors of significance for respiratory gas exchange in muscle tissue. Acta Physiol Scand 112:395–404, 1984.

Harold FM: The vital force: A study of bioenergetics. New York, Freeman, 1986, pp 28–56.

Harris K, Walker PM, Mickle DAL, et al: Metabolic response of skeletal muscle to ischemia. Am J Physiol 250:H213–H220, 1986.

Haupt M, Gilbert E, and Carlson R: Fluid loading increases oxygen consumption in septic patients with lactic acidosis. Am Rev Respir Dis 131:912–916, 1985.

Hayes MA, Timmins AC, Yau EHS, et al: Elevation of systemic oxygen delivery in the treatment of critically ill patients. N Engl J Med 330:1717–1722, 1994.

Heidelberger E and Reeves RB: Factors affecting whole blood O_2 transfer kinetics: Implications for $\theta(O_2)$. J Appl Physiol 68:1865–1874, 1990a.

Heidelberger E and Reeves RB: O_2 transfer kinetics in a whole blood unicellular thin layer. J Appl Physiol 68:1854–1864, 1990b.

Heistad DD and Abboud FM: Circulatory adjustments to hypoxia. Circulation 61:463–471, 1980.

Hester RL and Duling BR: Red cell velocity during functional hyperemia: Implications for rheology and oxygen transport. Am J Physiol 255:H236–H244, 1988.

Hill AV: The possible effects of the aggregation of the molecules of haemoglobin on its dissociation curves. J Physiol (Lond) 40:IV–VII, 1910.

Hill AV: LXXI: The combinations of haemoglobin with oxygen and carbon monoxide, and the effects of acid and carbon dioxide. Biochem J 15:577–586, 1921.

Hlastala MP: Physiological significance of the interaction of oxygen and carbon dioxide in blood. Crit Care Med 7:374–379, 1979.

Hlastala MP, McKenna HP, Franada RL, et al: Influence of carbon monoxide on hemoglobin-oxygen binding. J Appl Physiol 41:893–899, 1976.

Hlastala MP and Woodson RD: Saturation dependency of the Bohr effect: Interactions among H^+, CO_2, and DPG. J Appl Physiol 38:1126–1131, 1975.

Hochachka PW: Defense strategies against hypoxia and hypothermia. Science 231:234–241, 1986.

Hochachka PW and Guppy M: Metabolic arrest and the control of biological time. Cambridge, MA, Harvard University Press, 1987, pp 10–35.

Homer LD, Weathersby PK, and Kiesow LA: Oxygen gradients between red blood cells in the microcirculation. Microvasc Res 22:308–323, 1981.

Honig CR and Frierson JL: Role of adenosine in exercise vasodilation in dog gracilis muscle. Am J Physiol 238:H703–H715, 1980.

Honig CR, Gayeski TEJ, Federspiel W, et al: Muscle O_2 gradients from hemoglobin to cytochrome:

New concepts, new complexities. In Lubbers DW, Acker H, Leninger-Follerte A, and Goldsmith TK: Oxygen Transport to Tissue—IV. New York, Plenum Press, 1983, pp 23–38.

Honig CR, Odoroff CL, and Frierson JL: Capillary recruitment in exercise: Rate, extent, uniformity, and relation to blood flow. Am J Physiol 238:H31–H42, 1980.

Honig CR, Odoroff CL, and Frierson JL: Active and passive capillary control in red muscle at rest and in exercise. Am J Physiol 243:H196–H206, 1982.

Hufner GV: Uber das Gesetz der Dissociation des Oxyhaemoglobins und uber einige sich Knupfende wichtige Fragen aus der Biologie. Arch Anat Physiol 1:1–27, 1890.

Hurtado A: Animas in high altitude, resident man. In Handbook of Physiology: Adaptation to Environment. Washington DC, American Physiological Society, 1964, pp 54, 843–860.

Julou-Schaeffer G, Gray G, Fleming I, et al: Loss of vascular responsiveness induced by endotoxin involves L-arginine pathway. Am J Physiol 259:H1038–1042, 1990.

Kaufman BS, Rackow EC, and Falk JL: The relationship between oxygen delivery and consumption during fluid resuscitation of hypovolemic and septic shock. Chest 85:336–340, 1984.

Keim HJ, Wallace JM, Thurston H, et al: Impedance cardiography for determination of stroke index. J Appl Physiol 41:797–799, 1976.

Kelman GR: Digital computer subroutine for the conversion of oxygen tension into saturation. J Appl Physiol 21:1375–1376, 1965.

Kessler M, Hofer J, and Krumme B: Monitoring of tissue perfusion and cellular function. Anesthesiology 45:184–197, 1976.

Kety SS: Determinants of tissue oxygen tension. Fed Proc 16:666–670, 1957.

Khalil HH, Richardson RQ, and Guyton AC: Measurement of cardiac output by thermal-dilution and direct Fick methods in dogs. J Appl Physiol 21:1131–1135, 1966.

Kilbourn RG, Jubran A, Gross SS, et al: Reversal of endotoxin-mediated shock by N^G-methyl-L-arginine, an inhibitor of nitric oxide synthesis. Biochem Biophys Res Com 172:1132–1138, 1990a.

Kilbourn RG, Gross SS, Jubran A, et al: N^G-methyl-L-arginine inhibits tumor necrosis factor-induced hypotension: Implications for the involvement of nitric oxide. Proc Natl Acad Sci, USA, 87:3629–3632, 1990b.

Kilbourn RG, Owen-Schaub LB, Cromeens DM, et al: N^G-methyl-L-arginine, an inhibitor of nitric oxide formation, reverses IL-2 mediated hypotension in dogs. J Appl Physiol 76:1130–1137, 1994.

Kim MS and Akera T: O_2 free radicals: Cause of ischemia: Reperfusion injury to cardiac $Na^+ K^+$-ATPase. Am J Physiol 252:H252–H257, 1987.

Klitzman B and Duling BR: Microvascular hematocrit and red cell flow in resting and contracting striated muscle. Am J Physiol 237:H481–H490, 1979.

Klocke RA: Oxygen transport and 2,3-diphospho-glycerate (DPG). Chest 62[Suppl:79S]:795–855, 1972.

Kreuzer F and Cain S: Regulation of peripheral vasculature and tissue oxygenation in health and disease. Crit Care Clin 1:453–470, 1985.

Krogh A: The number and distribution of capillaries in muscles with calculations of the oxygen pressure head necessary for supplying the tissue. J Physiol (Lond) 52:409–415, 1919a.

Krogh A: The rate of diffusion of gases through animal tissues, with some remarks on the coefficient of invasion. J Physiol (Lond) 52:391–408, 1919b.

Kubicek WG, Frour AHL, Patterson RP, et al: Impedance cardiology as a noninvasive means to monitor cardiac function. J Assoc Adv Med Instrum 4:79–85, 1970.

Kwan M and Fatt I: A noninvasive method of continuous arterial oxygen tension estimation from measured palpebral conjunctival oxygen tension. Anesthesiology 35:309–314, 1971.

Lamas S, Michel T, Brenner BM, et al: Nitric oxide synthesis in endothelial cells: Evidence for a pathway inducible by TNF-α. Am J Physiol 261:C634–C641, 1991.

Lawson WH and Forster RE: Oxygen tension gradients in peripheral capillary blood. J Appl Physiol 22:970–973, 1967.

Lawson D, Norley S, Kochou G, et al: Blood flow limits and pulse oximeter signal detections. Anesthesiology 67:599–603, 1982.

Ledwith JW: Determining P_{50} in the presence of carboxyhemoglobin. J Appl Physiol 44:317–321, 1978.

Lehninger A: Biochemistry: The Molecular Basis of Cell Structure and Function. New York, Worth Publishers, 1975.

Lorente JA, Landin L, De Pable R, et al: L-Arginine pathway in the sepsis syndrome. Crit Care Med 21:1287–1295, 1993.

Lucking SE, Williams TM, Chaten FC, et al: Dependence of oxygen consumption on oxygen delivery in children with hyperdynamic septic shock and low oxygen extraction. Crit Care Med 18:1316–1319, 1990.

Lutch JC and Murray JF: Continuous positive-pressure ventilation: Effects of systemic oxygen transport and tissue oxygenation. Ann Intern Med 76:193–202, 1972.

McMahon SM, Halprin GM, and Sieker HO: Positive end-expiratory airway pressure in severe arterial hypoxemia. Am Rev Respir Dis 108:526–535, 1973.

Malmberg PO, Hlastala MP, and Woodson RD: Effect of increased blood-oxygen affinity on oxygen transport in hemorrhagic shock. J Appl Physiol 47:889–895, 1979.

Malo J, Goldberg H, Graham R, et al: Effect of hypoxic hypoxia on systemic vasculature. J Appl Physiol 56:1403–1410, 1984.

Manfredi JP and Holmes ED: Control of the purine nucleotide cycle in extracts of rat skeletal muscle:

Effects of energy state and concentrations of cycle intermediates. Arch Biochem Biophysiol 233:515–529, 1984.

Manthous CA, Schumacker PT, Pohlman A, et al: Absence of supply dependence of oxygen consumption in patients with septic shock. J Crit Care 8:203–211, 1993.

Margaria R and Green AA: The first dissociation constant, pK_1, of carbonic acid in hemoglobin solutions and its relation to the existence of a combination of hemoglobin with carbon dioxide. J Biol Chem 103:611–634, 1933.

Marik PE: Gastric intramucosal pH: A better predictor of multiorgan dysfunction syndrome and death than oxygen-derived variables in patients with sepsis. Chest 104:225–229, 1993.

Maynard N, Bihari D, Beale R, et al: Assessment of splanchnic oxygenation by gastric tonometry in patients with acute circulatory failure. JAMA 270:1203–1210, 1993.

Merrick SH, Hessel EA, and Dillard DH: Determination of cardiac output by thermodilution during hypothermia. Am J Cardiol 46:419–423, 1980.

Messmer K, Sunder-Plasmann L, Jesch L, et al: Oxygen supply to the tissues during limited normovolemic hemodilution. Respir Exp Med 159:152–166, 1973.

Meyer RA, Dudley GA, and Terjung RL: Ammonia and IMP in different skeletal muscle fibers after exercise in rats. J Appl Physiol 49:1037–1041, 1980.

Meyer J, Traber LD, Nelson S, et al: Reversal of hyperdynamic response to continuous endotoxin administration by inhibition of NO synthesis. J Appl Physiol 73:324–328, 1992.

Mohsenifar A, Goldbach P, Tashkin DP, et al: Relationship between O_2 delivery and O_2 consumption in the adult respiratory distress syndrome. Chest 84:267–271, 1983.

Mohsenifar Z, Hay A, Hay J, et al: Gastric intramural pH as a predictor of success or failure in weaning patients from mechanical ventilation. Ann Intern Med 119:794–798, 1993.

Moncada S and Higgs A: The L-arginine-nitric oxide pathway. N Engl J Med 239:2002–2012, 1993.

Moon R and Richards J: Determination of intracellular pH by ^{31}P magnetic resonance. J Biol Chem 2348:7276–7278, 1973.

Moreno LF, Stratton HH, Newell JC, et al: Mathematical coupling of data: Correction of a common error for linear calculations. J Appl Physiol 60:335, 1986.

Murad F: Cyclic guanosine monophosphate as a mediator of vasodilation. J Clin Invest 78:1–5, 1986.

Mythen MG and Webb AR: Prospective, randomized study in patients undergoing elective cardiac surgery. Arch Surg 130:423–429, 1995.

Nakamura T and Staub NC: Synergism in the kinetic reactions of O_2 and CO_2 with human red blood cells. J Physiol (Lond) 173:161–177, 1964.

Neilan BA, Gunter P, Adams AB, et al: Estimated and determined P_{50} values in erythrocytosis. Chest 77:572–574, 1980.

Nesarajah MS, Matalon S, Krasney JA, et al: Cardiac output and regional oxygen transport in the acutely hypoxic conscious sheep. Respir Physiol 53:161–172, 1983.

Nishimura N: Oxygen conformers in critically ill patients. Resuscitation 12:53–58, 1984.

Nordby GL and Ellis JH: Efficient computer subroutines for interconversion of oxygen tension and saturation. J Appl Physiol 51:1080–1085, 1981.

Nunn JF, Bergman A, Bunatyan A, et al: Temperature coefficients for PCO_2 and PO_2 of blood in vitro. J Appl Physiol 20:23–26, 1965.

Nuutinen EM, Nishiki K, Erecinska M, et al: Role of mitochondrial oxidative phosphorylation in regulation of coronary blood flow. Am J Physiol 243:H159–H169, 1982.

Nyboer J: Electrical Impedance Plethysmography. Springfield, IL, Charles C Thomas, 1959.

Orgel LE: The Origins of Life: Molecules and Natural Selection. New York, John Wiley & Sons, 1973.

Otis AB: Quantitative relationships in steady-state gas exchange. In Handbook of Physiology. Vol 1. Respiration. Washington, American Physiological Society, 1964, pp 681–698.

Pepe PE and Culver CH: Independently measured oxygen consumption during reduction of oxygen delivery by positive end-expiratory pressure. Am Rev Respir Dis 132:788–792, 1985.

Piiper J, Meyer M, and Scheid P: Dual role of diffusion in tissue gas exchange: Blood-tissue equilibration and diffusion shunt. Respir Dis 112:165–172, 1975.

Pohl U and Busse R: Hypoxia stimulates release of endothelium-derived relaxing factor. Am J Physiol 257:H1595–H1600, 1989.

Popel AS: Theory of oxygen transport to tissue. Crit Rev Biomed Eng 17:257–321, 1989.

Powers SR, Mannal R, Neclerio M, et al: Physiological consequences of positive-end expiratory pressure (PEEP) ventilation. Ann Surg 178:265–272, 1973.

Rahn H, Reeves RB, and Howell BJ: Hydrogen ion regulation, temperature, and evolution. Am Rev Respir Dis 112:165–172, 1975.

Rashkin MC, Bosken C, and Baughman RP: Oxygen delivery in critically ill patients. Relationship to blood lactate and survival. Chest 87:580–584, 1985.

Reeves RB: The effect of temperature on the oxygen equilibrium curve of human blood. Respir Physiol 42:317–328, 1980.

Restorff WV, Hofling B, Holtz J, et al: Effect of increased blood fluidity through hemodilution on general circulation at rest and during exercise in dogs. Pflugers Arch 357:25–34, 1975.

Rhodes GR, Newell JC, Shah D, et al: Increased oxygen consumption accompanying increased oxygen delivery with hypertonic mannitol in adult respiratory distress syndrome. Surgery 84:490–497, 1978.

Ries A, Prewitt L, and Johnson J: Skin color and ear oximetry. Chest 96:287–290, 1989.

Riggs TE, Shafter AW, and Guenter CA: Acute changes in oxyhemoglobin affinity, effects on oxygen transport and utilization. J Clin Invest 52:2660–2663, 1973.

Robertson RJ, Gilcher R, Metz KF, et al: Effect of induced erythrocythemia on hypoxia tolerance during physical exercise. J Appl Physiol 53:490–495, 1982.

Ronco JJ, Fenwick JC, Tweeddale MG, et al: Identification of the critical oxygen delivery for anaerobic metabolism in critically ill septic and nonseptic humans. JAMA 270:1724–1730, 1993.

Ronco JJ, Fenwick JC, Wiggs BR, et al: Oxygen consumption is independent of increases in oxygen delivery by dobutamine in septic patients who have normal or increased plasma lactate. Am Rev Respir Dis 147:25, 1993b.

Ronco JJ, Phang PT, and Walley JR: Oxygen consumption is independent of changes in oxygen delivery in severe adult respiratory distress syndrome. Am Rev Respir Dis 143:1267, 1991.

Ross BK and Hlastala MP: Increased hemoglobin-oxygen affinity does not decrease skeletal muscle oxygen consumption. J Appl Physiol 51:864–870, 1981.

Roughton FJW: Transport of oxygen and carbon monoxide. In Handbook of Physiology. Vol 1. Respiration. Washington, DC, American Physiological Society, 1964, pp 767–825.

Roughton FJW, Forster RE, and Cander L: Rate at which carbon monoxide replaces oxygen from combination with human hemoglobin in solution and in the red cell. J Appl Physiol 11:269–281, 1957.

Roughton FJW and Severinghaus JW: Accurate determination of O_2 dissociation curve of human blood above 98.7 percent saturation with data on O_2 solubility in unmodified human blood from 0° to 37°C. J Appl Physiol 35:861–869, 1973.

Russell JA, Ronco JJ, Lockhat D, et al: Oxygen delivery and consumption and ventricular preload are greater in survivors than in nonsurvivors of the adult respiratory distress syndrome. Am Rev Respir Dis 141:659–665, 1990.

Sarelius IH and Duling BR: Direct measurement of microvessel hematocrit, red cell flux, velocity, and transit time. Am J Physiol 243:H1018–H1026, 1982.

Schantz P: Capillary supply in heavy-resistance trained non-postural human skeletal muscle. Acta Physiol Scand 117:153–155, 1983.

Schlichtig R, Kramer DJ, Boston JR, et al: Renal O_2 consumption during progressive hemorrhage. J Appl Physiol 70:1957–1962, 1991.

Schweiss JF (ed): Continuous Measurements of Blood Oxygen Saturation in the High-Risk Patient. California, Beach International, 1983.

Severinghaus JW: Simple, accurate equations for human blood O_2 dissociation computations. J Appl Physiol 46:599–602, 1979.

Severinghaus JW: Transcutaneous blood gas analysis. Respir Care 27:152–159, 1982.

Shapiro B, Cane R, Chomba C, et al: Preliminary evaluation of an intra-arterial blood gas system in dogs and humans. Crit Care Med 17:455–460, 1989.

Shappell SD and Lenfant CJM: Adaptive, genetic, and iatrogenic alterations of the oxyhemoglobin-dissociation curve. Anesthesiology 37:127–139, 1972.

Shellock FG, Riedinger M, Bateman TM, et al: Thermodilution cardiac output determination in hypothermic post cardiac surgery patients. Crit Care Med 11:668–670, 1983.

Shibutani K, Komatsu T, Kubal K, et al: Critical level of oxygen delivery in anesthetized man. Crit Care Med 11:640–643, 1983.

Shoemaker W, Appel P, Kram H, et al: Prospective trial of supranormal O_2 values as therapeutic goals in high risk surgical patients. Chest 94:1176–1186, 1988.

Silverman HJ, Slotman G, Bone RC, et al: Effects of prostaglandin E_1 on oxygen delivery and consumption in patients with the adult respiratory distress syndrome. Chest 98:405–410, 1990.

Silverman HJ and Tuma P: Gastric tonometry in patients with sepsis. Effects of dobutamine infusions and packed red blood cell transfusions. Chest 102:184–188, 1992.

Smithies M, Yee TH, Jackson L, et al: Protecting the gut and the liver in the critically ill: Effects of dopexamine. Crit Care Med 22:789–795, 1994.

Sorenson MB, Bille-Brahe NE, and Engel HC: Cardiac output measurements by thermal dilution: Reproducibility and comparison with dye-dilution technique. Ann Surg 183:67–72, 1976.

Spinale F, Reines HD, and Crawford F: Electrical bioimpedance as a method for continuous noninvasive estimation of cardiac output: Experimental and clinical studies. Crit Care Med 15:364–370, 1987.

Sramek BB: Noninvasive technique for measurement of cardiac output by means of electrical impedance. Proceedings of the Fifth International Conference on Electrical Bioimpedance, Tokyo, Japan, 1981, pp 39–42.

Stacpoole PW, Wright EC, Baumgartner TG, et al: A controlled clinical trial of dichloroacetate for treatment of lactic acidosis in adults. The Dichloroacetate-Lactic Acidosis Study Group. N Engl J Med 327:1564–1569, 1992.

Stainsby WN and Otis AB: Blood flow, oxygen tension, oxygen uptake, and oxygen transport in skeletal muscle. Am J Physiol 206:858–866, 1964.

Stein JC, Ellis CG, and Ellsworth ML: Relationship between capillary and systemic venous PO_2 during nonhypoxic and hypoxic ventilation. Am J Physiol 265:H537–H542, 1993.

Stevens JH, Raffin TA, Mihm FG, et al: Thermodilution cardiac output measurement. JAMA 253:2240–2242, 1985.

Stratton HH, Feustel PJ, and Newells JC: Regression of calculated variables in the presence of shared measurement error. J Appl Physiol 62:2083–2093, 1987.

Sylvester JT, Scharf SM, Fitzgerald GRS, et al: Hypoxic and CO hypoxia in dogs: Hemodynamics, carotid reflexes, and catecholamines. Am J Physiol 236:H22–H28, 1979.

Takeda K, Shimada Y, Okada T, et al: Lipid peroxidation in experimental septic rats. Crit Care Med 14:719–723, 1986.

Tenney SM: A theoretical analysis of the relationship between venous blood and mean tissue oxygen pressures. Respir Physiol 20:283–296, 1974.

Tenney SM and Mithoefer JC: The relationship of mixed venous oxygenation to oxygen transport. Am Rev Respir Dis 125:474–479, 1982.

Terjung R, Dudley GA, and Meyer RA: Metabolic and circulatory limitations to muscular performance at the organ level. J Exper Biol 115:307–318, 1985.

Tien Y-K and Gabel RA: Prediction of PO_2 from SO_2 using the standard oxygen hemoglobin equilibrium curve. J Appl Physiol 42:985–987, 1977.

Tremper K: Pulse oximetry. Chest 95:713–715, 1989.

Tremper K and Barker S: The optode: Next generation in blood gas measurement. Crit Care Med 17:481–482, 1989.

Tremper KK, Hufstedler SM, Barker SJ, et al: Continuous noninvasive estimation of cardiac output by electrical bioimpedance: An experimental study in dogs. Crit Care Med 14:231–233, 1986.

Tuchschmidt J, Fried J, Swinnery R, et al: Early hemodynamic correlates of survival in patients with septic shock. Crit Care Med 17:719–723, 1989.

Vallet B, Chopin C, Curtis SE, et al: Prognostic value of the dobutamine test in patients with sepsis syndrome and normal lactate values: A prospective, multicenter study. Crit Care Med 21:1868–1875, 1993.

Vallet B, Curtis SE, Winn MJ, et al: Hypoxic vasodilation does not require nitric oxide (EDRF/NO) synthesis. J Appl Physiol 76:1256–1261, 1994.

Van Belle H, Goossens F, and Wynanta J: Formation and release of purine catabolites during hypoperfusion, anoxia, and ischemia. Am J Physiol 252:H886–H893, 1987.

Vary TC, Siegel JH, Nakatani T, et al: Effect of sepsis on activity of PDH complex in skeletal muscle and liver. Am J Physiol 250:E634–E640, 1986.

Vetterlein F and Schmidt G: Effects of propranolol and epinephrine on density of capillaries in rat heart. Am J Physiol 246:H189–H196, 1984.

Vincent JL, Roman A, De Backer D, et al: Oxygen uptake/supply dependency. Effect of short-term dobutamine infusion. Am Rev Respir Dis 142:2–7, 1990.

Wagner PD: The oxyhemoglobin dissociation curve and pulmonary gas exchange. Semin Hematol 11:405–421, 1974.

Warley A and Gutierrez G: Chronic administration of sodium cyanate decreases O_2 extraction ratio in dogs. J Appl Physiol 64:1584–1590, 1988.

Weibel ER, Taylor CR, Gehr P, et al: Design of the mammalian respiratory system. IX: Functional and structural limits for oxygen flow. Respir Physiol 44:151–164, 1981.

Weiskopf RB and Severinghaus JW: Lack of effect of high altitude on hemoglobin oxygen affinity. J Appl Physiol 33:276–277, 1972.

Whalen W, Riley J, and Nair P: A microelectrode for measuring intracellular PO_2. J Appl Physiol 23:789–791, 1967.

Whipp BJ: The bioenergetic and gas exchange basis of exercise testing. Clin Chest Med 15:173–192, 1994.

White FN: A comparative physiological approach to hypothermia. J Thorac Cardiovasc Surg 82:821–831, 1981.

Wiedemann HP, Matthay MA, and Matthay RA: Cardiovascular-pulmonary monitoring in the intensive care unit, Part 1. Chest 85:537–549, 1984.

Willford DC, Hill EP, and Moores WY: Theoretical analysis of optimal P_{50}. J Appl Physiol 52:1043–1048, 1982.

Wilson DF, Erecinska M, Drown C, et al: Effect of oxygen tension on cellular energetics. Am J Physiol 233:C135–C140, 1977.

Wilson DF, Erecinska M, Drown C, et al: The oxygen dependency on cellular energy metabolism. Biochem Biophys 195:485–493, 1979.

Winslow RM, Monge CC, Statham NJ, et al: Variability of oxygen affinity of blood: Human subjects native to high altitude. J Appl Physiol 51:1411–1416, 1981.

Winslow RM, Samaja M, and West JB: Red cell function at extreme altitude on Mount Everest. J Appl Physiol 56:109–116, 1984.

Wolf YG, Cotev S, Perel A, et al: Dependence of oxygen consumption on cardiac output in sepsis. Crit Care Med 15:198–203, 1987.

Wood SC and Lenfant C: Oxygen transport and oxygen delivery. In Wood SC and Lenfant C (eds): Evolution of Respiratory Processes. New York, Marcel Dekker, 1979.

Woodson RD: O_2 transport: DPG and P_{50}: Basics of respiratory disease. Am Thorac Soc 5:1–6, 1977.

Woodson RD: Physiological significance of oxygen dissociation curve shifts. Crit Care Med 7:368–373, 1979.

Woodson RD and Auerbach S: Effect of increased oxygen affinity and anemia on cardiac output and its distribution. J Appl Physiol 153:1299–1306, 1982.

Zwart A, Kwant G, Oeseburg B, et al: Human whole-blood oxygen affinity: Effect of carbon monoxide. J Appl Physiol 57:14–20, 1984a.

Zwart A, Kwant G, Oeseburg B, et al: Human whole-blood oxygen affinity: Effect of temperature. J Appl Physiol 57:429–434, 1984b.

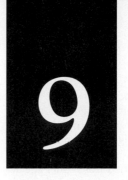

The Microcirculation and Tissue Oxygenation

Heidi V. Connolly, M.D.

Thomas E. J. Gayeski, M.D., Ph.D.

In this chapter we consider the relationship between the microcirculation and tissue oxygenation. Because there are few clinical tools available for making direct observations of microcirculation and tissue oxygenation, most of the discussion is based on basic science literature. Within this literature, the majority of the systematic studies have been in skeletal muscle of animals. Although there are limitations to extrapolating from one organ and species to another, the principles derived from these studies are generally believed to apply to all organs and mammalian species.

APPLICABILITY OF ANIMAL MODELS

Resting whole-body oxygen consumption is remarkably well conserved among species. When oxygen consumption is plotted against weight for mammals ranging in size from a shrew (7 g) to an elephant (800 kg), results fall on a line of a log–log plot (Hoppeler et al, 1981; Schmidt-Nielsen, 1979). In humans, hemodynamic parameters are frequently normalized to body surface area to standardize values among individuals of different sizes.

Only minor differences exist in slope between the relationship of body weight to resting oxygen consumption (0.71) or body surface area (0.67). During maximal exercise, most of the body's oxygen consumption results from skeletal muscle contraction. When average maximal oxygen consumption is plotted against weight, values obtained from 21 different species extending in size from mice to horses also identify a straight line on a log–log plot (Taylor et al, 1981). The slope of this line is 0.81, however, which is too large a difference from the resting relationship to be attributed to experimental error. Although resting oxygen consumption is fixed regardless of size, larger animals are able to achieve a higher maximal oxygen consumption rate during exercise.

Although there is some scatter within the data from skeletal and cardiac muscle, capillary density (the number of capillaries per cross-sectional area of muscle) and mitochondrial density are directly proportional regardless of the animal species studied (Honig and Gayeski, 1993). If capillary density is the limiting factor in the capacity of the microvascular system to deliver oxygen, capillary density is tightly coupled to the capacity of the oxygen consumers, the mitochondria. Hence, principles learned from other species should be applicable to humans, and data obtained from a particular muscle should be applicable to other muscle types, including cardiac muscle.

Extrapolation of microcirculatory data from muscle to other organs is generally believed to be appropriate by investigators studying the microcirculation. Data confirming this belief are limited, however. Mesentery is one organ in which direct observation demonstrates that the capillary module structure is similar to that of muscle (Chambers and Zweifach, 1944). Currently there are no published comparisons of the microcirculation among different organs. Any extrapolation must be considered carefully and should include an analysis of the pattern of oxygen utilization by the organ, biochemical reserves of high-energy phosphate (adenosine triphosphate [ATP] or phosphocreatine), sites of ATP consumption relative to ATP production, and sites of ATP production relative to the capillary structures or oxygen source.

ARTERIOLAR AND VENULAR ANATOMY

The main arterial supply is variably anastomotic on the muscle surface (Stingl, 1969, 1970, 1976). Within the muscle there are two vascular networks—a macromesh, which is a two-dimensional area that is 1 to 2 cm wide and 1 to 5 cm long, and a micromesh, which is 5 to 15 mm wide. The arterial macromesh is formed by the primary and secondary arteries that branch from the supply vessels. These arteries have diameters ranging from 100 to 400 μm in cat. The corresponding diameters of the venular macromesh vessels range from 300 to 700 μm. Often there are two venules for each artery at this level. The secondary arteries generally run parallel to the length of the muscle. We hypothesize that the secondary arteries of the macromesh supply blood to several centimeters along the length of muscle fascicle.

The arterial micromesh covers an area 5 to 15 mm wide and begins with branches from the secondary arteries. Distribution arterioles of the arteriole tree passes between fascicles in the fascial planes. The interconnecting tree structure of arte-

rioles branches into transverse arterioles that are about 1 mm in length (Lubbers and Wodick, 1969). Four or more branches emanate from the transverse arteriole, which end in the terminal arteriole. One to five capillary modules originate from each terminal arteriole (Delashaw and Duling, 1991; Lund et al, 1984). Observations of the microcirculation show that blood flow through branches off the terminal arteriole is not equal (Frame and Sarelius, 1993a, 1993b; Sweeney and Sarelius, 1990). Because a capillary module may supply a length of a fascicle above or below the level of the transverse arteriole, the longitudinal length influenced by such an arteriole is twice that of a single capillary module, or approximately 2000 μm.

CAPILLARY MODULE ANATOMY

The capillary module consists of several interconnected individual capillary flow paths (Berg and Sarelius, 1994; Frame and Sarelius, 1993b; Cain, 1977; Lubbers and Wodick, 1969). The capillary module is a two-dimensional structure with approximate dimensions of 200 μm in width and 1000 mm in length. Capillary modules are composed of a network of capillary segment lengths. Because capillary segments interconnect within a module as well as between modules, red blood cell–flow path lengths may differ from anatomically defined capillary lengths.

Heterogeneity of red blood cell flux among flow paths has been described (Cain, 1977). A capillary segment length is the smallest *microcirculatory oxygen supply unit*. A typical capillary segment length is approximately 300 to 500 μm long (Berg and Sarelius, 1994; Frame and Sarelius, 1993b), and it runs parallel to the longitudinal axis of the myocyte. The total longitudinal length of a capillary module is 700 to 1000 μm. At rest, approximately 50% of the capillary modules are perfused. Within each perfused module only 50% of the capillary segment lengths receive red blood cell flow. Hence, the perfusion and organization of capillary modules should influence myocyte myoglobin PO_2 (PMbO_2).

Longitudinally, a single myocyte is supplied by at least 100 capillary modules along its entire length. Transversely, one capillary module supplies a cluster of myocytes but only for the length of the capillary module. Currently, the number of myocytes in such a cluster must be inferred from two-dimensional muscles such as cheek pouch or cremaster muscle, where a capillary module is 200 to 400 μm in width, or 4 to 8 myocytes. The volume of tissue supplied by a capillary module is dependent on oxygen consumption (V_{O_2}) per myocyte and capillary module density. Using the Krogh cylinder radius to scale the radial dimension of the capillary module and the myoglobin (Mb) diffusion constant of Clark and coworkers (1985), one estimates a Krogh radius of less than a myocyte diameter for maximal V_{O_2} and up to several hundred micrometers for resting V_{O_2}. We estimate the volumes of tissue supplied by a capillary module by multiplying width of a capillary module, as estimated from two-dimensional muscles, by the observed capillary module length times a Krogh cylinder radius (10^8 μm^3 for rest and 10^6 μm^3 for maximal exercise). The spatial resolution of any measuring technique must be smaller than these volumes to determine heterogeneity at these spatial scales.

HETEROGENEITY

Heterogeneity is a hallmark of biologic systems. Heterogeneity may be expressed as diversity of adaptations to the same environment among species or as diversity among members of the same species. Organs respond differently to similar physiologic conditions, indicating heterogeneity within organisms. Heterogeneity within an individual organ or tissue may be a consequence of cells performing different tasks, or heterogeneity may be a consequence of loci of identical cells receiving different blood flow.

In muscle, heterogeneity of blood flow exists over wide ranges of the spatial scale. Macroheterogeneity has been measured among tissue volumes (e.g., 0.75 cm³ within a 100-mg muscle) (Marconi et al, 1988; Piiper et al, 1985, 1989), whereas microheterogeneity exists among volumes of tissue supplied by a single capillary module (e.g., approximately 4×10^{-4} cm³) (Berg and Sarelius, 1995; Delashaw and Duling, 1991; Federspiel and Sarelius, 1984; Frame and Sarelius 1993b; Sarelius, 1990; Sarelius and Duling, 1982; Sweeney and Sarelius, 1990). Heterogeneity of blood flow may lead to heterogeneity of tissue P_{O_2} level. In tissues containing Mb pigment, such as skeletal muscle, measured Mb saturation can be used to calculate myocyte PMb_{O_2} values in segments of individual myocytes (Voter and Gayeski, 1995). The heterogeneity of PMb_{O_2} is important because it may limit organ function or viability.

An example related to the importance of sample volume and heterogeneity is a simple two-compartment model. In the first case, the PMb_{O_2} level is equal in the entire sample and has a value of 1 mm Hg. In the second, the sample has two compartments of equal size. One compartment

has a PMb_{O_2} value of 2 mm Hg, whereas the other compartment has a value of 0 mm Hg, thereby resulting in an average PMb_{O_2} value of 1 mm Hg. Because a P_{O_2} level greater than 0.1 mm Hg is required for mitochondrial cytochrome aa3 to produce ATP to meet myocyte demands (Chance et al, 1973; Starlinger and Lubbers, 1972, 1973), in the first case, oxygen levels are high enough to meet demand. In the second case, however, the same average P_{O_2} value cannot meet mitochondrial demands, and tissue dysoxia occurs. Hence, knowledge of the spatial scale of PMb_{O_2} heterogeneity is important in defining the relationship among myocyte (or any other cell type) P_{O_2} level, cell biochemistry, and muscle function.

The source of oxygen for the myocyte is a capillary module (Berg and Sarelius, 1995; Frame and Sarelius, 1993b; Lund et al, 1987). Because a capillary module is approximately 600 to 1000 μm long (Berg and Sarelius, 1995) and a myocyte in large mammals is several centimeters long, there is not a unique measure of P_{O_2} level that describes the entire myocyte, but rather there is a distribution of P_{O_2} values along the length of a myocyte. Therefore, heterogeneity of myocyte P_{O_2} exists even within a single myocyte. We define PMb_{O_2} as the P_{O_2} level of a myocyte at a particular location along its length. Oxygen flux into a given myocyte occurs along partial pressure gradients both from intravascular supply of oxygen (in association with hemoglobin or dissolved in plasma) and from adjacent myocytes. Thus, PMb_{O_2} distribution is influenced by the perfusion of individual capillary modules along the length of the myocyte as well as by the PMb_{O_2} level of adjacent myocytes. For the population of myocytes in the muscle, there are identical considerations for each.

ANIMAL MODEL

Canine skeletal muscle is selected because myocytes are relatively large (approximately 50 μm in diameter) and contain sufficient myoglobin to determine saturation in subcellular volumes. A dog, weighing approximately 20 kg, is maintained under pentobarbital anesthesia. The gracilis muscle is vascularly and anatomically isolated. This muscle contains both fast and slow oxidative fibers, but glycolytic fibers are absent (unpublished results of Dr. Odile Matthieu-Costello). In all experiments discussed here, the muscle is studied at rest. Freezing of the muscle through surface application of a liquid nitrogen–cooled copper block rapidly stops metabolism and flow, allowing for observation of spatial heterogeneity of *in-situ*

$PMbO_2$ existing at the time of freezing (Voter and Gayeski, 1995). The frozen muscle sample is immersed in liquid nitrogen, divided into blocks of approximately 0.8 cm wide by 1.5 cm long, and stored in liquid nitrogen. Only the first 1 mm of muscle thickness is used for analysis to ensure adequate freezing rates.

Myoglobin saturation in frozen samples (observed at $-110°C$) can be determined utilizing spectrophotometric methods that have five wavelengths (Voter and Gayeski, 1995) and multiple wavelengths (Lubbers, 1972; Lubbers and Wodick, 1969; Voter and Gayeski, 1995; Wodick and Lubbers, 1973) of incident light. The former method involves determining a ratio of reflected light intensities to derive myoglobin saturation, whereas the latter method reconstructs an unknown spectrum from a spectrum of fully saturated and fully desaturated myoglobin. This latter, nonlinear multicomponent analysis developed by Dr. Lubbers (Lubbers and Wodick, 1969; Lubbers, 1972) offers an advantage over the five-wavelength method in that relative concentrations of myoglobin can also be derived. The catchment volume of each individual measurement is a hemisphere with a 60-μm radius, or a radius of approximately $2 \times 10^5 \ \mu m^3$. Although the catchment volume is slightly larger in cross-section than an individual myocyte, signal strength is strongest from the central region. Additionally, the volume of tissue supplied by a capillary module is greater than $4 \times 10^7 \ \mu m^3$ during rest, making the catchment volume of $PMbO_2$ measurements small relative to both the length of myocyte supplied by a capillary module and the total volume supplied by a capillary module.

Myocyte sampling in transverse planes for determining $PMbO_2$ and myoglobin concentration is undertaken in three ways. To describe dispersion and average and median values for whole muscles, myoglobin saturation and concentration are determined from myocytes separated by distances of 500 μm on a transverse surface of each block. This distance is selected to ensure that each sampled myocyte is supplied by a different capillary module. For determining dispersion within a fascicle, measurements are obtained from every other myocyte in a transverse plane in a checkerboard-like pattern. Based on preliminary results, this sampling frequency defines the $PMbO_2$ for the fascicle reproducibly, including the fifth and ninety-fifth percentiles. For determining the impact of blood flow heterogeneity at the level of the capillary module on $PMbO_2$ distributions, groups of contiguous myocytes are sampled, thereby defining the $PMbO_2$ pattern of a cluster of myocytes. With the exception of the whole-muscle sampling protocol, the other methods are new to our laboratory and results are preliminary.

$PMbO_2$ DISTRIBUTION OF WHOLE MUSCLE

Piiper and coworkers (1985), employing microspheres to determine heterogeneity, found a tenfold range of blood flow within muscle. This heterogeneity was found among 0.75-ml volumes and is present for both resting and exercising muscles. To determine if increased flow to resting muscle resulted in increased $PMbO_2$, we infused adenosine and acetylcholine into the circulation of the autoperfused isolated muscle. By infusing locally we minimized the impact on the entire dog. Both drugs resulted in a 25-fold increase in resting blood flow. Resting VO_2 of the muscles was unchanged within the error of the measurement. In both cases the arterial and venous hemoglobin saturations were equal because oxygen extraction relative to blood flow was low.

Figure 9–1 shows the cumulative $PMbO_2$ probability plot for each infusate. The $PMbO_2$ distribution measured during acetylcholine infusion is left-shifted and is more homogeneous than that measured during adenosine infusion. Adenosine infusion increases the perfused surface area of the capillary bed as measured by permeability

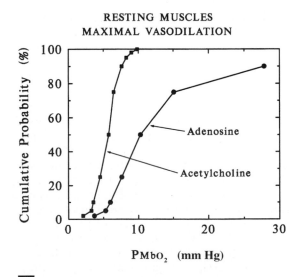

**RESTING MUSCLES
MAXIMAL VASODILATION**

Figure 9–1
The cumulative probability plots of $PMbO_2$ from two resting muscles that had increased blood flow due to infusion of acetylcholine and adenosine. These probability plots represent the highest and lowest values for resting muscles collected under pentobarbital anesthesia.

surface area (PS) product, and acetylcholine decreases that area (Carter et al, 1974; Joyner et al, 1974). This relationship between the changes in PS product and distribution of PMbO$_2$ suggests that resting PMbO$_2$ may be determined by the perfused capillary density.

In addition to the clear left shift of PMbO$_2$ distribution during acetylcholine infusion relative to adenosine infusion, there are three salient points for resting whole-muscle PMbO$_2$ distributions. First, the upper tail of the adenosine distribution is much larger than the acetylcholine one. Hence, the distribution is skewed to the right. Second, a population of 18 resting muscles that were analyzed had PMbO$_2$ distributions that fell between these two ranges. These muscles included those with a blood flow range of 1.5 to 20 ml/ 100 g/min, those that were both innervated and denervated, and those that were not fully isolated to minimize "preparation damage." Third, three of these muscles were analyzed utilizing the nonlinear multicomponent (NLMC) analysis. This subset consisted of innervated muscles only. These muscles had a relatively strong correlation between myoglobin concentration and saturation, as seen in Figure 9–2. This finding suggests that fiber type may influence capillary module perfusion. In addition, neither blood flow nor venous effluent was a good predictor of PMbO$_2$ distribution.

REGIONAL HETEROGENEITY

Piiper and coworkers (1985, 1989) have reported that blood flow is heterogeneously distributed in

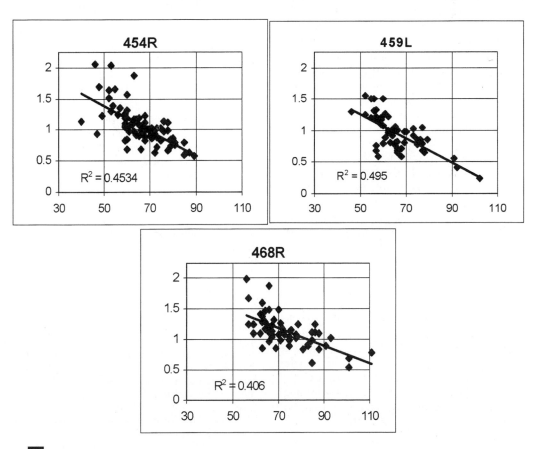

Figure 9–2
The ordinate for each graph is the relative myoglobin concentration, and the abscissa is the percent myoglobin saturation. Each separate graph represents the relationship between these two variables from a different resting muscle. The solid line is the least mean square fit with the R^2 value. Although R^2 is not particularly high, it is noteworthy that this relationship exists at all because the variables were taken from random loci within the muscle and therefore represent myoglobin saturation values from both arterial and venous ends of capillaries. Determining if fiber type plays a role in modules perfused at rest can help elucidate control mechanisms determining perfused capillaries.

muscle during both rest and exercise. Furthermore, there is greater spatial than temporal heterogeneity (Marconi et al, 1988). If spatial heterogeneity of blood flow is important in determining PMbO$_2$, flow heterogeneity can affect the median, the width of the PMbO$_2$ distribution of the whole muscle, or both. Likewise, the shape of the PMbO$_2$ distribution of whole muscle may not be reflective of local patterns of myocyte PO$_2$ distribution. To obtain preliminary results from an innervated resting muscle that had blood flow above average for resting muscles, we collected distributions from transverse sections of four adjacent fascicles (i.e., all fascicles on one block). After determining the distributions for each of the four fascicles in the initial transverse plane, approximately 1000 μm was removed from the length of the block. Measures of PMbO$_2$ were repeated to define the distributions of each of the four fascicles. This process was repeated for four additional transverse planes. The sampled volume of muscle was approximately 8 mm in width, 1 mm in depth, and 5 mm in length. This approach yielded 6 PMbO$_2$ distributions for each of the 4 fascicles, for a total of 24.

To determine if global heterogeneity of PMbO$_2$ exceeds regional heterogeneity, we compared PMbO$_2$ distributions obtained from an autoperfused muscle from an animal that had undergone volume expansion. Figure 9–3A shows the cumulative probability of one randomly selected fascicle compared with the whole muscle, whereas Figure 9–3B shows a comparison of two different fascicles. In a non-parametric test to compare two cumulative distributions (Kolmogorov-Smirnov test), those distributions in Figure 9–3A were statistically different, whereas those in Figure 9–3B were not. Of the 24 distributions from transverse planes of individual fascicles, 85% were statistically indistinguishable from one another, yet 92% were different from that of the whole muscle. From a muscle from an animal that had undergone volume constriction, PMbO$_2$ distributions of five randomly selected and widely spaced fascicles were statistically equal to the distribution of the whole muscle. Hence, based on this early finding, it is likely that sympathetic vasomotor tone influences regional heterogeneity of PMbO$_2$.

RELATIONSHIP BETWEEN MYOCYTE PO$_2$ AND CAPILLARY MODULE

Blood flow through the capillary module is influenced by nitric oxide (Frame and Sarelius, 1995) and prostaglandin (Rivers and Duling, 1992). It is likely that there are other chemical and me-

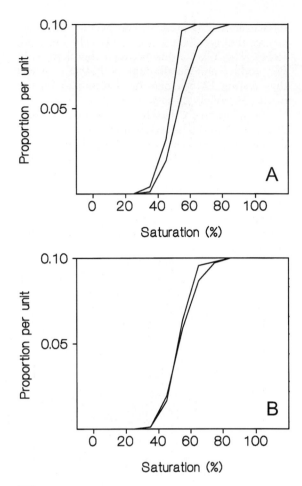

Figure 9–3
(A) The difference between a cumulative probability plot from the whole muscle (*right shifted curve*) and a transverse plane of an individual fascicle. Although these distributions are statistically different, the physiologic importance of the difference in PMbO$_2$ is minimal if any. The steeper slope of the fascicular distribution can represent the effect of local homogeneity of blood flow as compared with its global heterogeneity. (B) The same distributions from two different fascicles within a 5-mm distance of one another. No statistical difference exists between these two distributions. In fact, 85% of fascicular distributions within a 1-mm × 5-mm × 5-mm volume had no statistical difference among them, but 92% were different from the distribution of the whole muscle. Hence, local PMbO$_2$ may be influenced by local blood flow, but the resulting differences in PMbO$_2$ are small.

chanical mechanisms involved as well. These effectors act in a coordinated fashion, as seen through both immediate and conducted responses within arterioles (Frame and Sarelius, 1995; Segal et al, 1989). Application of a drug at one site influences both a concurrent and a later response at another site (Frame and Sarelius, 1995). No unifying model of microvascular coordination exists at the present time. This description of the microcirculation suggests that patterns of PMbO$_2$ should reflect capillary modular organization.

To determine if capillary module organization is reflected in PMbO$_2$ pattern, we collected the Mb saturation for each myocyte in the small fascicle shown in Figure 9–4. Clearly in these preliminary results, this fascicle has clusters of myocytes at high PMbO$_2$, whereas there are many myocytes at lower PMbO$_2$ levels surrounding these clusters. This PMbO$_2$ pattern is consistent with the microcirculatory observations and supports the applica-

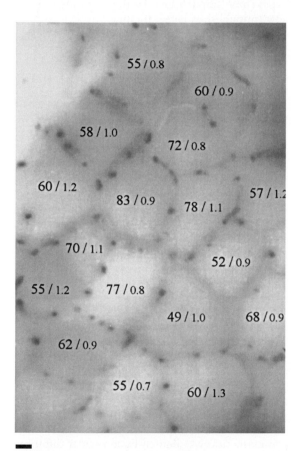

Figure 9–4
Photomicrograph of transverse section of muscle at −210°C. The myocyte outlines are enhanced by the black dots, which are red cells in capillaries. Each myocyte is labeled with two numbers. The numerator is the myoglobin saturation, and the denominator is the relative myoglobin concentration for that myocyte. Note the pattern of a cluster of myocytes with high myoglobin saturation in the center of the figure. This cluster is surrounded by myocytes with a lower myoglobin saturation. This pattern is typical of resting muscle.

tion of findings in thin muscles to thicker ones. These results may also explain how venous effluent PO$_2$ values can be much greater than PMbO$_2$ values. The clustering of perfused capillaries into modules increases the oxygen flux density per capillary flow path. The perfused capillary must supply oxygen to both myocytes adjacent to it as well as to neighboring myocytes that have no other perfused capillaries to supply oxygen.

Consider for a moment the effect of fast and slow transit times on the PMbO$_2$ level within a capillary module. In this *thought* experiment, a short transit time (high red blood cell velocity) results in little extraction per red blood cell. Hence, within the capillary, the PO$_2$ values at the arterial and venous ends are essentially equal. The result would be little change in the PMbO$_2$ pattern from the arterial to the venous end of the capillary module. If this result were true for all capillary modules, it would produce an increased number of myocytes with high PMbO$_2$ and thereby a right skew to the PMbO$_2$ distribution. The resulting cumulative probability plot may be similar to that of the adenosine muscle of Figure 9–1. If transit time is long, producing a low capillary red blood cell velocity, the PO$_2$ along the capillary module decreases along each flow path, and the PMbO$_2$ of the adjacent myocytes also decreases. The long transit time results in a reduction in the PO$_2$ level measured in myocytes residing at the venous end of the capillary module. Fewer myocytes with high PMbO$_2$ levels are present, and the distribution is left-skewed. The distribution for the acetylcholine muscle in Figure 9–1 may be anticipated in this condition.

In the context of this thought experiment, the PMbO$_2$ distributions in Figure 9–1 lead to the conjecture that the apparent blood flow shunts in the adenosine and acetylcholine muscles are different. The acetylcholine muscle has no significant upper tail, and therefore the muscle has few portions of a myocyte with a high PMbO$_2$ value. Hence, the transit times will be long and extraction high. The value of venous PO$_2$ from the organ is much higher than that of PMbO$_2$, however, suggesting that a large non-nutrient shunt exists during infusion of acetylcholine. In contrast, the adenosine muscle has a significant population of myocytes with increased PMbO$_2$ values, suggesting a short transit time. This result suggests that shunting through nutrient channels exists during adenosine infusion.

In addition to the above data and thought experiment, other data suggest that anatomic shunts do exist in skeletal muscle. Using microspheres to detect anatomic shunt, Marconi and coworkers (1988) and Piiper and coworkers

(1985) found only a 3% anatomic shunt in skeletal muscle. Their oxygen extraction ratio for muscle was 33%, however. This is a large extraction ratio for resting skeletal muscle and suggests that the animals may have been volume-contracted as a consequence of the length of the preparation or of hemorrhage during surgery. Yano and Takaori (1994) have reported that the depth of anesthesia influences anatomic blood flow shunt. With use of isoflurane, an inhalational anesthetic that increases muscle blood flow, it was reported (Hartman et al, 1992; Yano and Takaori, 1994) that shunt fraction ranged from 25 to 50% as the depth of anesthesia was increased. Thus, the anatomic and physiologic shunts may be present in skeletal muscle under normal physiologic conditions, following the administration of vasodilating drugs and in pathologic states such as the systemic inflammatory response syndrome (Bone, 1996; Pinsky, 1996). Although there are few data, the same can probably be said for other organs. Shunting may contribute to the multiple organ failure syndrome in sepsis.

SYSTEMIC LIMITATION OF OXYGEN DELIVERY

Limitation of oxygen delivery, which is the product of arterial oxygen content (CaO_2) and blood flow, frequently occurs in clinical medicine. Anemia and hypoxemia both result in the reduction of arterial oxygen content. Cardiovascular collapse can result in the presence of reduced organ blood flow. Frequently, reduction in CaO_2 is compensated for by an increase in blood flow, whereas a reduction in blood flow is compensated for by an increase in oxygen extraction. Compensation may be imperfect, however, leading to inadequate tissue oxygen levels relative to demand, thereby resulting in dysoxia. Dysoxia can result from inadequate intravascular oxygen content at the venous end of capillary modules—a concept described as the "lethal corner" by Krogh (1918). Alternatively, dysoxia can be caused by microvascular maldistribution of oxygen supply resulting in clustered loci of dysoxic myocytes.

The point at which oxygen supply limitation occurs, the critical oxygen delivery, is independent of the means by which supply is reduced. In experiments performed by Cain (1977) and Schumacker and coworkers (1987), the point at which oxygen consumption becomes limited by supply is similar in progressive anemia and hypoxia. Likewise, a similar onset of critical supply limitation occurs during progressive reductions in blood flow. The distribution of myocyte PO_2 during critical supply limitation is unknown. Molecular diffusion of oxygen from the capillary to the mitochondria, however, can be responsible for limiting O_2 uptake, as theorized by Krogh (1918). If true for each capillary module, heterogeneity should then be similar among different regions of the muscle. Dysoxic cells should be clustered around venous ends of the capillary module, and portions of a myocyte residing near the arterial end of capillaries should be adequately oxygenated. Alternatively, if microvascular maldistribution occurs "upstream" from the capillary module, clusters of dysoxic myocytes should be observed. By using spectrophotometry to measure myocyte PO_2 during anemia (Honig and Gayeski, 1993), hypoxemia (unpublished data), and limited blood flow (unpublished data), the myocyte PO_2 pattern during supply limitation has been identified as follows.

ANEMIA

Euvolemic exchange transfusion with hetastarch was employed to hemodilute to an average hemoglobin concentration of 7.5 g/dl. Muscles were analyzed at different VO_2 (18) values, ranging from rest to exercise rates equaling 67% of maximal oxygen consumption (VO_{2max}). Resting $PMbO_2$ distributions were indistinguishable from $PMbO_2$ distributions obtained from control muscles. At 67% of VO_{2max}, however, muscle $PMbO_2$ distributions were left-shifted relative to controls. Percentage of reduction in oxygen consumption and active muscle tension development, as well as the percentage of myocytes measured in the transverse plane with a $PMbO_2$ level indistinguishable from zero, were all equally decreased. Furthermore, the myocyte segments with $PMbO_2$ levels indistinguishable from zero were distributed among all portions of the muscle. Hence, the decreased Hb concentration did not result in regional heterogeneity of $PMbO_2$ ($PMbO_2$ pattern over cm^3 to mm^3), suggesting that oxygen supply was distributed uniformly and that myocyte oxygen extraction was limited by molecular diffusion of oxygen.

HYPOXEMIA

Pentobarbital-anesthetized dogs were mechanically ventilated with hypoxic gas mixtures, resulting in decreased arterial PO_2 levels. Under resting conditions, arterial hemoglobin saturations of 30% and 60% resulted in no change in muscle oxygen consumption and only minor changes in the PMbO$_2$ distribution compared with controls. During exercise, under conditions of 30% arterial hemoglobin saturation, muscle performance was markedly reduced. During exercise (67% of VO$_{2max}$), with an arterial hemoglobin saturation of 60%, the value of VO$_2$ was unchanged, but the PMbO$_2$ distribution was left-shifted. Myocytes measured in the transverse plane with low PMbO$_2$ values were uniformly distributed among all portions of the muscle.

LOW FLOW

Systemic hemorrhage was utilized to decrease muscle blood flow to near the point of critical supply dependency. At rest, muscle oxygen consumption and PMbO$_2$ distribution were unchanged relative to controls. Myocytes with low PMbO$_2$ levels were uniformly distributed within the muscle, as seen in resting conditions during anemia and hypoxemia.

Maginniss and coworkers (1994) have shown that sympathetic tone affects the minimum blood flow at which muscle oxygen consumption decreases. This minimum blood flow is referred to as the *critical point*. When sympathetic tone is high, oxygen consumption is maintained at a blood flow that is approximately 25% less than that observed with low sympathetic tone. One possible explanation for this response is the regional heterogeneity of blood flow leading to regional dysoxia (Connolly et al, 1997). To separate effects of sympathetic tone from bulk blood flow, muscles were pump-perfused at similar flow rates.

Systemic hemorrhage and volume expansion were used to alter sympathetic tone. Figure 9–5 shows a plot of the median values of PMbO$_2$ of each of 10 and 9 blocks for the high and low sympathetic tone muscles, respectively. Although the median values of both muscles were similar, regional heterogeneity was greater during low sympathetic tone. Thus, local dysoxia on the spatial scale of at least cubic millimeters during conditions of low sympathetic tone is a possible mechanism for impaired muscle oxygen extraction during critical supply limitation. Furthermore, under conditions of high sympathetic tone, the absence of regional heterogeneity of PMbO$_2$ suggests that blood flow heterogeneity measured among tissue volumes of 0.75 ml (Piiper et al, 1985) may not correlate with changes in PMbO$_2$.

SUMMARY

Heterogeneity of blood flow can be demonstrated at multiple levels of the microvascular network. Capillary module perfusion measured during two-dimensional videomicroscopy *in vivo* is consistent with PMbO$_2$ patterns measured *in situ* in a thick muscle preparation. By utilizing microspheres to label regional blood flow distribution, heterogeneity is identified but does not predict regional differences in cellular PO$_2$ levels. When oxygen supply is adequate relative to demand, there is little heterogeneity of cellular PO$_2$, and few cells with low PO$_2$ levels are found. When oxygen supply cannot meet demand, the level of sympathetic tone is important in determining microvascular

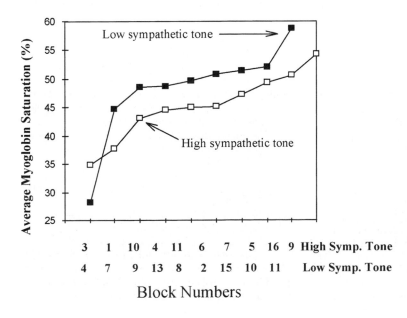

Figure 9–5
Depicted is the average myoglobin saturation for individual blocks from two muscles: one with high and one with low sympathetic tone. The muscle with high sympathetic tone has a narrower range of average myoglobin saturations (17%) compared with those from the muscle with low sympathetic tone (29%). This difference may suggest that blood flow distribution in muscles with low sympathetic tone is less homogeneous and that this inhomogeneity may lead to occult tissue dysoxia.

distribution of oxygen offered. When sympathetic tone is low, maldistribution of oxygen supply relative to demand occurs, thereby resulting in localized regions of tissue dysoxia.

Increases in oxygen offered do not *a priori* augment cellular PO_2 levels. Regional maldistribution of oxygen supply can result in tissue dysoxia despite high levels of global oxygen supply, and occult tissue hypoxia may occur. Oxygen content of venous effluent from a tissue bed represents the flow-weighted average of capillary venous oxygen content. As such, little helpful information regarding cellular oxygenation can be gained by studying venous PO_2. Under all conditions, the value of median myocyte PO_2 is significantly less than the value of venous effluent PO_2. Infusion of vasodilators, inotropes, and vasoconstrictors in the clinical setting have an unknown effect on cellular PO_2 level and microvascular blood flow heterogeneity. Hence, conclusions about tissue oxygenation based on global measures of oxygen offered or venous effluent oxygen content must be interpreted with caution. This principle may explain the difficulty in assessing tissue oxygenation under clinical conditions like sepsis in which regional heterogeneity of microcirculation may contribute to end-organ failure.

REFERENCES

Berg B and Sarelius IH: Architecture and flow properties in capillary networks in striated muscle. Faseb J 7:A885, 1994.

Berg BR and Sarelius IH: Functional capillary organization in striated muscle. Am J Physiol 268:H1215–22, 1995.

Bone RC: Toward a theory regarding the pathogenesis of the systemic inflammatory response syndrome: What we do and do not know about cytokine regulation (review). Crit Care Med 24:163–172, 1996.

Cain SM: Oxygen delivery and uptake in dogs during anemic and hypoxic hypoxia. J Appl Physiol 42:228–234, 1977.

Carter RD, Joyner WL, and Renkin EM: Effects of histamine and some other substances on molecular selectivity of the capillary wall to plasma proteins and dextran. Microvasc Res 7:31–48, 1974.

Chambers R and Zweifach BW: Topography and function of the mesenteric capillary circulation. Am J Anat 75:173–198, 1944.

Chance B, Oshino N, Sugano T, and Mayevsky A: Basic principles of tissue oxygen determination from mitochondrial signals. Adv Exp Med Biol 37A:277–292, 1973.

Clark A Jr, Federspiel WJ, Clark PAA, and Cokelet GR: Oxygen delivery from red cells. Biophys J 47:171–181, 1985.

Connolly HV, Maginniss LA, and Schumacker PT: Transit time heterogeneity in canine small intestine: Significance for oxygen transport. J Clin Invest 99:225–228, 1997.

Delashaw JB and Duling BR: Heterogeneity in conducted arteriolar vasomotor response is agonist dependent. Am J Physiol 260:H1276–H1282, 1991.

Duling BR and Damon DH: An examination of the measurement of flow heterogeneity in striated muscle. Circ Res 60:1–13, 1987.

Federspiel W and Sarelius I. An examination of the contribution of red blood cell spacing to the uniformity of oxygen flux at the capillary wall. Microvasc Res 27:273–285, 1984.

Frame MD and Sarelius IH: Arteriolar bifurcation angles vary with position and when flow is changed. Microvasc Research 46:190–205, 1993a.

Frame MD and Sarelius IH: Regulation of capillary perfusion by small arterioles is spatially organized. Circ Res 73:155–163, 1993b.

Frame MD and Sarelius IH: L-Arginine-induced conducted signals alter upstream arteriolar responsivity to L-arginine. Circ Res 77:695–701, 1995.

Hartman JC, Pagel PS, Proctor LP, et al: Influence of desflurane, isoflurane and halothane on regional tissue perfusion in dogs. Can J Anaesth 39:877–887, 1992.

Honig CR and Gayeski TEJ: Resistance to O_2 diffusion in anemic red muscle: Roles of flux density and cell PO_2. Am J Physiol 265:H868–H875, 1993.

Hoppeler H, Mathieu O, Weibel ER, et al: Design of the mammalian respiratory system. VIII. Capillaries in skeletal muscles. Resp Physiol 44:129–150, 1981.

Joyner WL, Carter RD, Raizes GS, and Renkin EM: Influence of histamine and some other substances on blood-lymph transport of plasma protein and dextran in the dog paw. Microvasc Res 7:19–30, 1974.

Krogh A: The rate of diffusion of gases through animal tissues, with some remarks on the coefficient of invasion. J Physiol (London) 52:391–408, 1918.

Lubbers DW: Spectrophotometric examination of tissue oxygenation. In Bicher HI and Bruley DF (eds): Oxygen Transport to Tissue: Instrumentation, Methods, and Physiology. New York, Plenum Publishing, 1972, pp 45–54.

Lubbers DW and Wodick R: The examination of multicomponent systems in biological materials by means of a rapid scanning photometer. Appl Optics 8:1055–1062, 1969.

Lund N, Damon DH, Damon DN, and Duling BR: Capillary grouping in hamster tibialis anterior muscles: Flow patterns and physiological significance (abstract). Int J Microcirc 5:359–372, 1987.

Lund N, Damon DN, and Duling BR: Functional capillary grouping in striated muscle:

Organization and flow patterns. Microvasc Res 27:254–278, 1984.

Maginniss LA, Connolly H, Samsel RW, and Schumacker PT: Adrenergic vasoconstriction augments tissue O_2 extraction during reductions in O_2 delivery. J Appl Physiol 76:1454 1461, 1994.

Marconi C, Heisler N, Meyer M, et al: Blood flow distribution and its temporal variability in stimulated dog gastrocnemius muscle. Respir Physiol 74:1–13, 1988.

Piiper J, Marconi C, Heisler N, et al: Spatial and temporal variability of blood flow in stimulated dog gastrocnemius muscle. Adv Exp Med Biol 248:719–728, 1989.

Piiper J, Pendergast DR, Marconi C, et al: Blood flow distribution in dog gastrocnemius muscle at rest and during stimulation. J Appl Physiol 58:2068–2074, 1985.

Pinsky MR: Organ-specific therapy in critical illness: Interfacing molecular mechanisms with physiological interventions (review). J Crit Care 11:95–107, 1996.

Rivers RJ and Duling BR: Arteriolar endothelial cell barrier separates two populations of muscarinic receptors. Am J Physiol 262:H1311–H1315, 1992.

Sarelius IH: An analysis of microcirculatory flow heterogeneity using measurements of transit time. Microvasc Res 40:88–98, 1990.

Sarelius IH and Duling BR: Direct measurement of microvessel hematocrit, red blood cell flux, velocity, and transit time. Am J Physiol 243:H1018–H1026, 1982.

Schmidt-Nielsen K: Animal Physiology. Cambridge, Cambridge University Press, 1979.

Schumacker PT, Long GR, and Wood LDH: Tissue oxygen extraction during hypovolemia: Role of hemoglobin P50. J Appl Physiol 62:1801–1807, 1987.

Segal SS, Damon DN, and Duling BR: Propagation of vasomotor responses coordinates arteriolar resistances. Am J Physiol 256:H832–H837, 1989.

Starlinger H and Lubbers DW: [Methodical studies on the polarographic measurement of respiration and "critical oxygen pressure" in mitochondria and isolated cells with membrane-covered platinum electrodes.] [German] Pflug Archiv—Eur J Physiol 337:19–28, 1972.

Starlinger H and Lubbers DW: Polarographic measurements of the oxygen pressure performed simultaneously with optical measurements of the redox state of the respiratory chain in suspensions of mitochondria under steady-state conditions at low oxygen tensions. Pflug Archiv—Eur J Physiol 341:15–22, 1973.

Stingl J: Arrangement of the vascular bed in the skeletal muscles of the rabbit. Folia Morphol (Praha) 17:257–264, 1969.

Stingl J: [The vascular system of the skeletal muscles.] [German] Acta Anat 76:488–504, 1970.

Stingl J: Fine structure of precapillary arterioles of skeletal muscle in the rat. Acta Anat 96:196–205, 1976.

Sweeney TE and Sarelius IH: Spatial heterogeneity in striated muscle arteriolar tone, cell flow, and capillarity. Am J Physiol 259:H124–H136, 1990.

Taylor CR, Maloiy GM, Weibel ER, et al: Design of the mammalian respiratory system. III. Scaling maximum aerobic capacity to body mass: Wild and domestic mammals. Respir Physiol 44:25–37, 1981.

Voter WA and Gayeski TEJ: Determination of myoglobin saturation of frozen specimens using a reflecting cryospectrophotometer. Am J Physiol 269:H1328–1341, 1995.

Wodick R and Lubbers DW: Quantitative Analyse von Reflexionsspektren und anderen Spektren mit Inhomogen Lichtwegen an Mehrkomponentensystemen mit Hilfe der Queranalyse, II. Z Physiol Chem 354:916–922, 1973.

Yano H and Takaori M: The microcirculation during enflurane and isoflurane anaesthesia in dogs. Can J Anaesth 41:149–155, 1994.

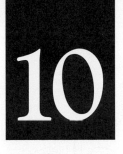

C H A P T E R

Pulmonary Mechanics in Critical Care

John J. Marini, M.D.

BASIC CONCEPTS OF RESPIRATORY MECHANICS

The mechanical properties of the respiratory system are the characteristics that influence the energy cost of breathing. Mechanical properties vary from site to site within the thoracic cavity, especially in the setting of heterogeneous lung disease (Fig. 10–1). Although this regionality of mechanical properties carries profound implications for gas exchange, at present clinicians are able to measure imperfectly only the cumulative properties of the entire lung, entire chest wall, or entire integrated respiratory system.

Because pressure gradients provide the forces driving gas flow and counterbalancing elastic recoil, the assessment of respiratory mechanics involves the measurement of flows, volumes (flow integrated over time), and pressure gradients (Fig. 10–2). Indeed, the simplified inspiratory equation of motion of the respiratory system, an expression of these relationships, can be written (Otis et al, 1950):

$$P = R\dot{V} + \frac{V}{C} + P_{ex}$$

In this equation, P is the pressure applied across the respiratory system, R is inspiratory resistance, C is inspiratory (dynamic) compliance, $\dot{V}$ and V are flow and volume inspired in excess of the end-expiratory value, and P_{ex} is end-expiratory alveolar pressure. Flow, which is the rate of volume change, can be directly measured with a variety of sensing instruments. Alternatively, flow can be determined indirectly by mathematically differentiating spirometric volume. The volumes of interest during routine assessment of respiratory system mechanics are those that exceed the passive equilibrium value. The equilibrium point of the respiratory system is the position at which the system is at rest, with pressure at the alveolar level the same as unchanging pressure at the airway opening. Thus, when positive end-expiratory pressure is applied, the equilibrium position is displaced to that higher volume corresponding to positive end-expiratory pressure [PEEP]. Although regional mechanics are of unquestioned impor-

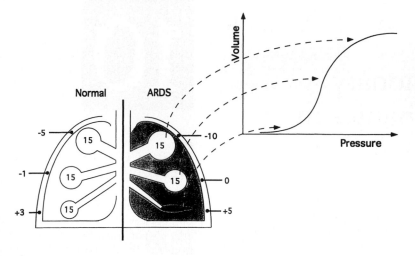

Figure 10–1
Influence of the gravitational gradient of pressure on regional alveolar mechanics. Dependent alveoli at the base of the lung may remain collapsed at airway pressures that threaten to overdistend those in nondependent regions. Regional mechanics are especially heterogeneous in the setting of ARDS. (From Marini JS and Wheeler AP: Critical Care Medicine, The Essentials, 2nd ed. Baltimore, Williams & Wilkins, 1997. With permission.)

tance in determining ventilation and gas exchange, technology available at the bedside currently limits clinical measurement to the global properties of the respiratory system.

Flow is most commonly measured by pneumotachography. Volume changes relative to functional residual capacity (FRC) are tracked by integrating the resulting flow signal. Impedance plethysmography is another alternative (Chadha et al, 1982). Pressure changes relevant to the lungs must be assessed as the difference between the airway pressure (P_{aw}) and the average pleural pressure (P_{pl}) that surrounds them. The esophagus provides a convenient site for estimating changes in intrapleural pressure. With the airway occluded and flow stopped, pressure measured at the airway opening serves also to estimate alveolar pressure. Because the lungs are inherently passive, their mechanical properties can be assessed during any form of spontaneous, pressure-assisted, or controlled ventilation. The mechanical properties of the chest wall, in contrast, can be evaluated only during controlled ventilation. With the chest wall relaxed, the pressure acting to distend that struc-

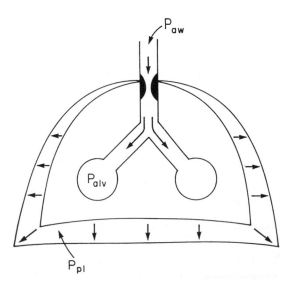

Figure 10–2
The pressure gradient driving gas to the alveolar level against resistive forces is the airway pressure (P_{aw}) minus the alveolar pressure. The pressure gradient expanding the lung is P_{alv} minus pleural pressure (P_{pl}). The pressure gradient tending to expand the relaxed chest wall is reflected by the pleural pressure. The total transpulmonary pressure is indexed by the airway opening pressure.

ture can be directly estimated as the average pleural pressure.

In clinical practice, the monitoring of respiratory mechanics assumes greatest importance for the patient who is intubated and mechanically ventilated with high airway pressures. Patients with severe airflow obstruction and acute respiratory distress syndrome (ARDS) provide common examples. Although readily available, measurements of airway pressure are of limited use unless assessed using passive conditions or supplemented using esophageal pressure (P_{es}). Most clinicians rarely consider measuring esophageal pressure, either because of unfamiliarity with the method or belief that it is neither needed nor well tolerated. In fact, intrapleural pressure estimation can be of great value in decision-making, for both the respiratory and cardiovascular systems. Under conditions of controlled inflation, swings in central venous pressure (CVP) also provide a useful, if somewhat imprecise, indicator of changes in intrathoracic pressure. During vigorous spontaneous efforts, the reliability of the CVP may be somewhat less, but this is relatively unstudied. In the absence of P_{es} or some other estimate of P_{pl}, resistance and compliance, and the mechanics measures on which they are based, cannot be reliably assessed from P_{aw} alone in patients making active efforts. Except as otherwise noted, the remaining discussion of this chapter assumes passive conditions and availability of airway pressure, flow, and spirometric volumes.

MONITORING LUNG AND CHEST WALL MECHANICS

During spontaneous breathing and all conventional forms of mechanical ventilation, gas is driven to and from the alveoli by differences in pressure developed between the airway opening and the alveoli. Under passive conditions, all required power is provided by the mechanical ventilator. The difference between applied airway pressure and atmospheric pressure is the sum of two components: the pressure needed to drive gas between the airway opening and the alveolus, and that required to hold the alveoli expanded against the combined elastic recoil of the lung and chest wall (Otis et al, 1950). In a passively ventilated system, the elastic component is most easily assessed by measuring pressure at the airway opening under stop-flow (static) conditions.

STATIC PRESSURE-VOLUME RELATIONSHIPS

When flow stops at the end of tidal expiration, the difference between pressures at the airway

opening and alveolus disappears, and the system is at equilibrium. The pressure (ΔP_L) required to expand the lung by a certain volume (ΔV) is the corresponding change in transpulmonary pressure (P_L = alveolar pressure, P_{alv}, minus pleural pressure, P_{pl}). Lung compliance ($C_L = \Delta V/\Delta P_L$), the inverse of elastance, indicates the pressure required per unit change in lung volume. Under passive conditions, the pressure needed to simultaneously expand the chest wall by the same ΔV is given by the average change in "intrathoracic" pressure (ΔP_{pl}), which is usually and most conveniently sampled in the esophagus. The distensibility of the relaxed chest wall is characterized by chest wall compliance ($C_W = \Delta V/\Delta P_{pl}$). Thus, the slope of the pressure-volume relationship for the total respiratory system (C_{RS}) is $\Delta V/\Delta P_{alv}$. Because the inspiratory pressure-volume relationship is curvilinear, compliance varies with the imposed volume change. Moreover, compliance varies with the number of lung units available to accept the delivered gas. In ventilator-derived calculations of compliance, ΔV must be measured at the inlet of the endotracheal tube, or total expired volume must be adjusted for the amount of gas stored in compressible circuit elements during (pressurized) inspiration. Most conveniently, tidal (or chord) compliance is computed; ΔV is taken as the tidal volume and ΔP_{alv} is the difference in alveolar pressure at the two extremes of the tidal cycle (the peak static plateau pressure, P_S, minus the sum of PEEP and auto-PEEP).

Compliance measurements may have therapeutic and prognostic value in patients with acute failure to oxygenate the arterial blood. When PEEP is applied incrementally with tidal volume held constant, static compliance tends to reach its highest value coincident with maximal recruitment of lung units, reduction in shunt fraction, and improvement in oxygen delivery (Suter et al, 1975; Blanch et al, 1987). It is a good general principle not to use values of end-expiratory pressure or tidal volume that significantly depress thoracic compliance, unless safe transpulmonary pressures can be obtained and objective evidence exists of improved O_2 delivery (Suter, 1984). Excessive tidal pressures, as a rule those greater than 35 cm H_2O between alveolus and pleural space (*transalveolar pressure*), risk barotrauma and hemodynamic compromise without tangible benefit to gas exchange or oxygen delivery. Because lung units at the ventral surface of the lung are surrounded by lower pleural pressures, a decreasing tangential compliance can be observed at plateau airway pressures that are considerably lower.

Serial changes in the respiratory pressure-volume curve and computed static compliance also tend to reflect the worsening or resolution of acute lung injury (Lamy et al, 1976; Matamis et al, 1984). Maximal depression of lung compliance in ARDS often requires 1 to 2 weeks to develop. Normal compliance of the respiratory system is approximately 80 to 100 ml/cm H_2O. Severe disease is implicated when compliance falls to 30 ml/cm H_2O or less.

Both the number of aerated alveoli and their relative distention influence the compliance value. Therefore, caution must be exercised when attempting to use C_{RS} as an indicator of underlying tissue elastance. Ideally, compliance would be referenced to a measure of absolute lung volume (V_{abs}) (such as FRC or TLC) to produce a "specific compliance" C_{RS}/V_{abs} (Comroe, 1974). For example, identical pressures drive greatly different volumes into the normal lungs of elephants and mice. C_L is influenced by this volume difference; in theory, C_L/V_{abs} is not. Calculated airflow resistance may also be high when there has been a substantial loss of patent air channels, as in ARDS. Even in the same patient, C_{RS} can change greatly near the extremes of the vital capacity range. Thus, most patients with hyperinflated lungs who are ventilated for acute exacerbations of asthma or chronic obstructive pulmonary disease (COPD) have a depressed C_{RS}, despite supernormal tissue distensibility when assessed in a lower volume range. This reduction in compliance is due, in part, to lung overdistention and, in part, to the inward recoil of the chest wall at high thoracic volumes. Furthermore, C_{RS} can be apparently depressed if the pressure component corresponding to dynamic hyperinflation is not considered (Rossi et al, 1985b).

C_{RS} may also be depressed at the lower extremes of lung volume if substantial atelectasis occurs, as during hydrostatic pulmonary edema or ARDS (Suter et al, 1975; Suter, 1984; O'Quin et al, 1985). As the chest expands, the number of recruited alveoli tends to increase, improving C_{RS} toward its normal value. The reverse phenomenon, derecruitment, occurs during tidal lung deflation, producing hysteresis of the static pressure-volume curve. Thus, C_L and C_{RS} may appear to vary with increasing tidal volume, improving until fewer alveolar units open than reach their elastic limit at end-inspiration. During acute respiratory failure, the presence of an inflection point of compliance change (P_{flex}) on the static pressure-volume curve appears to indicate recruitable lung and potential benefit from additional PEEP (Matamis et al, 1984; Benito and LeMaire, 1990). In reality, there is not a single "inflection" point, but a region of transition to best compliance, because basilar lung units are more difficult to recruit

than those less dependent (Marini, 1996). (See Chapter 18 for additional details.)

Although seldom calculated, thoracic elastance (E_{RS}), the reciprocal of C_{RS}, has certain advantages for clinical use (Katz et al, 1981). Unlike the subcomponents of respiratory system compliance, elasticities of the lung (E_L) and chest wall (E_W) add in series:

$$E_{RS} = E_L + E_W$$

In contrast, their respective compliances add in parallel:

$$\frac{1}{C_{RS}} = \frac{1}{C_L} + \frac{1}{C_W}$$

Therefore, even though C_{RS} is often used to assess the elastic properties of the lung, the relationship of C_{RS} to C_L is not entirely straightforward (Fig. 10–3):

$$C_{RS} = \frac{C_L C_W}{(C_W + C_L)}$$

For this reason, the impact of chest wall compliance should be taken into account when attempting to evaluate the lung on the basis of total respiratory system behavior (Chapin et al, 1979). The interpretation of changes in elastance is considerably easier (Fig. 10–4).

Chest wall distensibility is often disturbed by abdominal distention, pleural effusions, increased muscular tone, recent surgery, position changes, soft tissue injury, and many other factors common to the critical care setting. Such changes in chest wall compliance are important to consider, in that they influence the functional residual capacity (Fig. 10–5), work of breathing, efficacy of pulmonary gas exchange, and interpretation of hemodynamic data (for example, the pulmonary artery occlusion or wedge pressure, P_W) as well as calculation of chest mechanics data.

The C_{RS} is the appropriate measure for calculating the effect of PEEP on lung volume. A given peak airway pressure has different hemodynamic and prognostic significance, however, depending on whether the lung or chest wall primarily accounts for that value. The fraction of end-expiratory alveolar pressure (P_{ex}) partitioned to the pleural space depends on the relative compliances of the lungs and chest wall (Katz et al, 1981; O'Quin et al, 1985):

$$\Delta V_L = C_L(\Delta[P_{ex} - P_{pl}])$$
$$\Delta V_W = C_W(\Delta P_{pl})$$

and since $\Delta V_L = \Delta V_W$,

$$\Delta P_{pl} = \Delta P_{ex}\left(\frac{C_L}{(C_L + C_W)}\right)$$

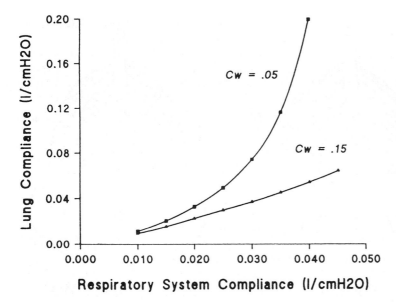

Figure 10–3
Relationship of lung compliance to respiratory system compliance for two different values of chest wall compliance. Note the extreme curvilinearity of this relationship under stiff chest wall conditions. (From Marini JJ: Lung mechanics in the adult respiratory distress syndrome. Recent conceptual advances and implications for management. Clin Chest Med 11(4):673–690, 1990. With permission.)

This equation indicates that the *relative* stiffness of the lungs and chest wall determines the effect of PEEP on hemodynamics and measured P_W. In healthy individuals, C_L approximates C_W over the tidal volume range, so that ΔP_{pl} is approximately $1/2$ ΔP_{ex}. Accordingly, about half a given PEEP (or auto-PEEP) increment is normally reflected in the pleural pressure. With stiff lungs this "transmission" fraction falls to a lower value, and with a stiff chest wall (e.g., with obesity) it rises to a higher value (see Fig. 10–5).

USE OF THE AIRWAY PRESSURE TRACING TO CALCULATE EFFECTIVE COMPLIANCE AND RESISTANCE OF THE RESPIRATORY SYSTEM

Inspiratory Resistance and Thoracic Compliance

Digital technology has greatly expanded monitoring capability, especially during mechanical ventilation. During passive inflation, some systems now

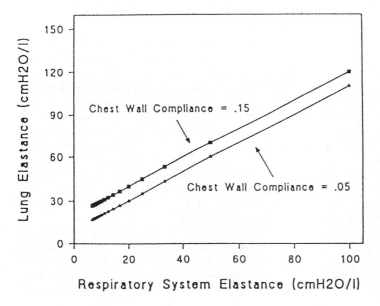

Figure 10–4
Relationship of lung elastance to respiratory system elastance for the same data depicted in Figure 10–3. (From Marini JJ: Lung mechanics in the adult respiratory distress syndrome. Recent conceptual advances and implications for management. Clin Chest Med 11(4):673–690, 1990. With permission.)

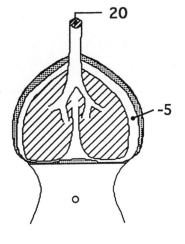
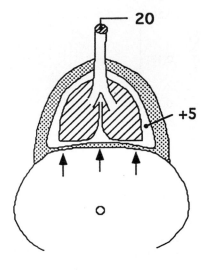

Figure 10–5
Effect of chest wall compliance on lung volume. The effect of positive airway pressure (here, 20 cm H_2O) on lung volume is influenced by the compliance of the chest wall. In this example, the distending force across the lung is 25 cm H_2O when the chest wall is normal, but only 15 cm H_2O when the chest wall is stiff. A patient with a stiff chest wall requires a higher PEEP to achieve the same physiologic effect. (From Marini JS and Wheeler AP: Critical Care Medicine, The Essentials, 2nd ed. Baltimore, Williams & Wilkins, 1997. With permission.)

Normal   **Stiff Chest Wall**

provide breath-to-breath estimates of R and C_{RS} as well as tracings of flow and airway pressure. All ventilators monitor pressure in the external airway. When a mechanical ventilator expands the chest of a passive subject using constant flow, calculations of total system compliance and resistance can be made from airway pressure alone. During active efforts, P_{aw} must be supplemented by esophageal pressure to make the relevant calculations for the lung.

Airway pressure must overcome the frictional and elastic forces opposing ventilation. The pressures required for these tasks are characterized by resistance (the pressure cost per unit of flow) and compliance (the inverse of the pressure cost per unit volume) (Otis et al, 1950; Marini et al, 1986c). These system characteristics can be gauged in several ways. When flow is transiently stopped at end-inspiration, P_{aw} falls rapidly toward a stable level, which represents an average of the peak alveolar pressure existing in regions with both higher and lower values. The difference between this end-inspiratory "stop flow," "plateau," or "peak static" (P_S) pressure and end-expiratory alveolar pressure (P_{ex}, the sum of PEEP and auto-PEEP) determines the component of end-inspiratory inflation pressure needed to overcome the elastic forces of tidal inflation (Fig. 10–6). When tidal volume (adjusted for gas compression) is divided by ($P_S - P_{ex}$), static effective compliance (C_{eff}) can be computed (Capps and Hicks, 1987):

$$C_{eff} = \frac{V_t - [(P_S - PEEP)(\text{circuit compression factor})]}{(P_S - P_{ex})}$$

During dynamic cycling, P_D should be substituted for P_S in this equation to obtain the appropriate tidal volume correction for *dynamic* conditions. In clinical practice it is wise to determine the relationship of C_{eff} to tidal volume to avoid over-distention. At a minimum, the inspiratory dynamic airway pressure tracing obtained during constant flow under passive conditions should be carefully inspected for signs indicating overdistention. During constant flow, time is a direct analogue of delivered volume, so that the slope of the airway pressure tracing reflects dynamic elastance ($1/C_{RS}$) (see Fig. 10–6). Unfortunately, even under constant flow conditions, it is not always possible to draw a single tangent to the P_{aw} inflation curve that characterizes the entire inspiratory period.

When a flow signal is not available, the mechanics of the system can still be readily assessed if either flow or inspiratory airway pressure is known to be constant. Other wave forms (decelerating flow, sinusoidal flow, and so forth) are more difficult to use. Constant-flow volume-cycled ventilation is perhaps the most widely employed mode in current practice, and a monitored flow signal is not often readily available. If the ventilator's performance characteristics are good and the flow values actually delivered are nominal, estimates of R and C acceptable for clinical purposes can be made.

Under conditions of constant flow, the pressure achieved just before the cessation of gas delivery, the peak dynamic pressure (P_D), is the total pressure needed to drive gas to the alveolar level at the set flow rate and to expand the lungs and

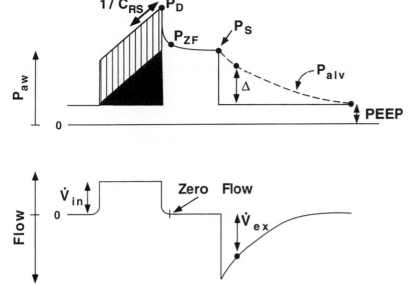

Figure 10–6
Computation of the compliance and resistance of the respiratory system under passive conditions during constant inspiratory flow (V_{in}). An end-inspiratory pause allows the identification of peak dynamic (P_D), peak static (P_S), and zero-flow pressures needed to compute airway resistance and respiratory system compliance.

chest wall by the full tidal volume. The difference between P_D and P_S approximates the gradient of pressure driving end-inspiratory gas flow and varies with the resistance of the lungs, chest wall, and endotracheal tube. The term *resistance* usually refers to the ratio between the pressure necessary to drive flow (P_R) and flow itself. P_R is usually a nonlinear function of flow, however, so that R does not remain constant across all flow rates: P_R is approximately $k\dot{V}^\epsilon (1 \leq \epsilon \leq 2)$. Thus, for unchanging geometry, computed resistance usually increases as flow increases, especially if flow is highly turbulent.

The ratio of delivered tidal volume (compression-corrected) to the ($P_D - PEEP$) difference, the "dynamic characteristic" (Bone, 1983), provides an index of the overall difficulty of chest expansion, provided that tidal volume and inspiratory flow rate stay unchanged and that inflation occurs passively. (Note that this is not a true dynamic compliance value, due to the kinetic nature of the measurement.) Because P_D is influenced by both the frictional and elastic properties of the respiratory system, it may be a simple yet valuable indicator of bronchodilator response (Gay et al, 1987). Here, P_D reflects not only the decline in frictional work during effective bronchodilation but also reflects the changes that may have occurred in dynamic hyperinflation.

Because P_D decays exponentially to P_S, the exact value assigned to P_S may depend on the duration of flow interruption. The point at which inspiratory flow first ceases (zero flow, ZF) invariably occurs before the plateau is fully achieved, so that the P_D minus P_S difference often exceeds

the P_D minus P_{ZF} difference by 10 to 20%. Values for end-inspiratory resistance computed using P_D minus P_{ZF} (Rmin) are therefore smaller than those computed using the full P_D minus P_S value, which includes pressure components related to volume redistribution and stress relaxation. The $V_t/(P_{ZF} - P_{ex})$ quotient yields an estimate of (inspiratory) dynamic compliance (C_{DYN}), a value invariably less than that commonly computed from the $V_t/(P_S - P_{ex})$ ratio (C_{STAT}). In normal subjects, R_{DYN}, which is a value influenced by tissue resistance as well as airway resistance, tends to remain stable or fall as flow rate increases, provided that airway opening pressure is measured beyond the tip of the endotracheal tube (Bates et al, 1985). In patients with airflow obstruction, however, both R_{DYN} and R_{STAT} demonstrate the expected rise with flow increases (Gottfried et al, 1985).

Expiratory Resistance

In obstructive disease, expiratory resistance (R_{ex}) exceeds inspiratory resistance (R_{in}), varies to a greater extent than does R_{in} during the course of the tidal cycle, and bears more direct relevance to air trapping (Rossi et al, 1985a; Gay et al, 1989). Although seldom computed, R_{ex} may be determined during passive exhalation from simultaneous recordings of exhaled airflow and tidal volume (V_t). A representative volume (V) is selected (for example, $V = \frac{1}{2}V_t$) and the corresponding flow ($\dot{V}$) recorded. From the estimated upstream alveolar pressure at volume V [$P_{alv(V)} \sim P_S - (V/C_{RS})$], expiratory flow resistance, the quotient of alveolar minus airway opening pressure (P_{ao}) and flow, can be approximated at that point from the expression:

$$R_{ex} = \frac{P_{alv(V)} - P_{ao}}{\dot{V}}$$

or

$$R_{ex} = \frac{P_S - [(V/C_{RS}) + P_{ao}]}{\dot{V}}$$

In theory, this method should provide a representative estimate of R_{ex}. No study is currently available, however, to test its validity against an alternative (plethysmographic or flow interruptive) method.

Once the static (inflation hold) pressure (P_S) is known and the corresponding C_{RS} value has been computed, expiratory resistance can also be estimated from the observed "time constant" of passive deflation. Ideally, the passive respiratory system deflates as a single compartment, allowing alveolar pressure to decay in purely exponential fashion from its starting value (P_S). If alveolar pressure, $P(t)$, is known at any time t after deflation begins:

$$P(t) \sim (P_S - PEEP)\, e^{-kt} + PEEP$$

where e is the base of natural logarithms (2.718), and k is the reciprocal of the expiratory time constant (τ). Solving this equation for $k = 1/R_xC$ estimates the time constant. When one time constant ($\tau = R_{ex}C$ sec) has elapsed since the onset of deflation, $1/e = 1/2.718$ or 37% of the starting volume (above PEEP) remains to be expelled. After three time constants, only 5% of the tidal volume remains. If both C_{RS} and the time constant (measured from a volume-time plot) are available, an average expiratory resistance can be computed from their quotient ($R_{ex} = \tau/C$).

In theory, this method for computing R_{ex} provides information unavailable from the inspiratory pressure data routinely used. The assumptions on which such estimates are based are often questionable, however, especially in patients with severe airflow obstruction. The lungs and chest wall rarely deflate as an ideal one-compartment system, and the expiratory pathway includes the external apparatus extending from endotracheal tube past the exhalation valve to the expiratory port, as well as the patient's airway. For these and other reasons, expiratory resistance values calculated from the τ/C ratio must be considered crude estimates, at best.

Flow Interruption Technique

The technique of interrupting expiratory airflow repeatedly may be used to determine the mechan-

ics of the respiratory system in acutely ill patients receiving mechanical ventilation (Gottfried et al, 1985). Following end-inspiratory airway occlusion, a series of brief (~ 0.2 sec) interruptions of expiratory flow is performed during passive deflation. Multiple post-interruption plateaus of airway pressure are thereby generated, yielding estimates of alveolar pressure that can be used in conjunction with flow and volume to compute R_{ex} and C_{RS}. The interrupter method can be applied to paralyzed or anesthetized patients, either manually or by using a highly responsive solenoid valve system. Flow interruption is not practical to apply to patients with high minute ventilation requirements or to those who respond by muscular contraction.

Although a post-interruption plateau is achieved almost immediately in most normal subjects and in patients with restrictive disease, patients with severe airflow obstruction exhibit a substantial delay before complete equilibration is achieved. Interestingly, those with dynamic expiratory flow limitation demonstrate high flow transients immediately after occlusion release (Gay et al, 1989). Other signs of dynamic airway compression include a linear and/or biphasic flow profile, as well as failure of added resistance to influence flow rate (Marini and Truwit, 1991). Such observations may have clinical relevance, in that expiratory airflow limitation during passive tidal deflation generally indicates severe disease, correlating with dynamic hyperinflation (Kimball et al, 1982; Marini and Truwit, 1991). Such flow limitation portends both a beneficial response to added PEEP and continued ventilator dependence (Gay et al, 1987; Gay et al, 1989). Flow-limiting dynamic airway compression during tidal breathing may also contribute directly to dyspnea (O'Donnell et al, 1987).

ENDOTRACHEAL TUBE AND EXPIRATORY VALVE RESISTANCE

The endotracheal tube is often a major determinant of the total resistance to airflow (Bates et al, 1985; Gottfried et al, 1985; Marini and Truwit, 1991). Depending on tube type, length, diameter, patency, and angulation, computed values for inspiratory resistance may be dominated by the resistive properties of the artificial airway. Tube resistance *in vivo* may be considerably higher than that of the same tube before insertion (Wright et al, 1989), which is a fact of particular importance for patients with copious airway secretions. Retained secretions may give rise to irregularities of the flow tracing that resolve after they are cleared (Jubran and Tobin, 1994). Marked flow dependence of resistance may also be demonstrated in certain patients, which is a phenomenon usually ascribed to turbulence developing in a narrow or partially occluded tube (Gottfried et al, 1985). If endogenous (bronchial) resistance must be determined precisely, airway pressure should be sensed beyond the carinal tip of the endotracheal tube. This can be done with an intra- or extraluminal catheter or with a tube specially designed for measuring pressure at this site (e.g., during jet ventilation). With the latter approach, the measured pressure may be influenced by Bernoulli effects at the tube orifice. During inspiration, pressure support can be used to effectively offset endotracheal tube resistance. During expiration, however, tube resistance must be overcome by elastic recoil or muscular forces.

Calculated pressure at the carinal end of the endotracheal tube has been used to regulate pressure in the expiratory circuit during both phases of the respiratory cycle, so as to compensate for expiratory (as well as inspiratory) endotracheal tube resistance (Guttmann et al, 1993). Although still in its development stages, this "automatic tube compensation" holds clear promise to reduce dyspnea and dynamic hyperinflation in predisposed patients. Expiratory resistance is influenced not only by the endotracheal (ET) tube and the endogenous properties of the airway, but also by the flow impedance of the exhalation valve.

AUTO-PEEP (INTRINSIC PEEP) EFFECT

Dynamic hyperinflation and the auto-PEEP phenomenon occur when insufficient time elapses between successive tidal inflations to re-establish the equilibrium position of the respiratory system (Pepe and Marini, 1982; Rossi et al, 1985). When a mechanical ventilator powers inflation, alveolar pressure remains continuously positive through both phases of the ventilatory cycle. Airflow does not cease at end-exhalation but continues very slowly as alveolar pressure gradually decompresses through critically narrowed airways. During apnea, as long as 40 seconds can elapse before flow completely stops. Auto-PEEP can be defined as the positive, flow-driving difference between alveolar and airway opening pressures at end-expiration (Fig. 10–7).

An auto-PEEP effect may be seen in virtually any circumstance causing a high demand for ventilation, even in patients without severe airflow obstruction. In patients without severe intrinsic airflow obstruction, auto-PEEP is largely the result of the high ventilation requirement, a shortened expiratory time, and the resistance offered by the ET tube and exhalation valve. Active muscular

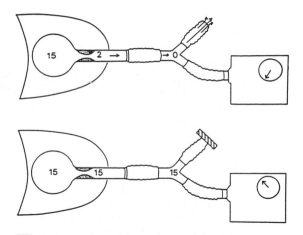

Figure 10–7
The auto-PEEP effect and its measurement by end-expiratory port occlusion. Auto-PEEP is defined as the positive-flow driving difference between alveolar pressure and applied pressure at end-exhalation. Auto-PEEP can be quantified by central airway pressure within 0.5 to 1.5 seconds of expiratory port occlusion at end-exhalation. (From Pepe PE, and Marini JJ: Occult positive end-expiratory pressure in mechanically ventilated patients with airflow obstruction. Am Rev Respir Dis 126:166–170, 1982. With permission.)

effort often contributes to the expiratory driving force and may cause alveolar pressure to remain positive at end-exhalation, even without notable hyperinflation (Fig. 10–8) (Ninane et al, 1993; Lessard et al, 1995). The auto-PEEP phenomenon has also been well described during high-frequency ventilation (Simon et al, 1984). High-frequency oscillation, which has an active expiratory phase, may be less predisposed to causing dynamic hyperinflation than is jet ventilation.

The auto-PEEP effect has numerous hemodynamic and mechanical consequences. Barotrauma is an obvious risk. Furthermore, the hemodynamic problems associated with the auto-PEEP effect under passive conditions may be more severe than those incurred with PEEP of a similar level because obstructive lung disease enhances (whereas restrictive disease impairs) transmission of alveolar pressure to the pleural space. Auto-PEEP also adds to the work of breathing, presenting an increased threshold load to spontaneous inspiration and depressing the effective triggering sensitivity of the ventilator (Fleury et al, 1985; Smith et al, 1987). The addition of counterbalancing positive end-expiratory pressure (PEEP or CPAP) to patients with quantifiable auto-PEEP and expiratory flow limitation may improve patient comfort, relieving dyspnea and the work of breathing with-

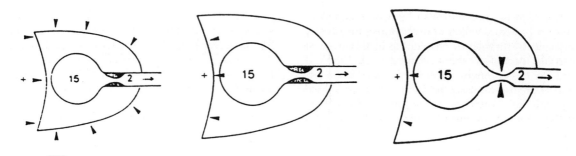

Figure 10–8
Three forms of auto-PEEP. Auto-PEEP can exist without dynamic hyperinflation (*left panel*) when vigorous expiratory muscle contraction persists to end-expiration. Under conditions of passive inflation, auto-PEEP implies dynamic hyperinflation either without (*middle*) or with (*right*) expiratory flow limitation. In the presence of dynamic airway collapse, the addition of a modest amount of PEEP may improve effective triggering sensitivity and work of breathing. (From Marini JJ: Lung mechanics in the adult respiratory distress syndrome. Recent conceptual advances and implications for management. Clin Chest Med 11(4):673–690, 1990. With permission.)

out markedly increasing lung volume or peak cycling pressure (Smith and Marini, 1988; Hoffman et al, 1989). If flow limitation is not present, however, adding PEEP simply presents a backpressure to expiratory gas flow and risks further hyperinflation without apparent benefit. Substituting PEEP for auto-PEEP may improve the distribution of ventilation in patients with markedly heterogeneous regional lung mechanics. As a general rule, PEEP more than sufficient to counterbalance auto-PEEP should not be added to patients with airflow obstruction. If peak static pressure rises significantly in response to PEEP, additional hyperinflation is implied, and adding PEEP may be ill advised.

Estimating Auto-PEEP

At the bedside, auto-PEEP can be estimated several ways (Table 10–1). Dynamic hyperinflation and auto-PEEP cause significant flow to persist to the very end of exhalation. Indeed, examination of the flow tracing gives a clear indication of the existence of auto-PEEP, but not its magnitude.

Table 10–1
Techniques for Estimating Auto-PEEP

- End-expiratory port occlusion
- Applied PEEP "counterbalancing"
- Post-maneuver change in P_s
- $P_s - [(V_T/C) + PEEP]$
- Proto-inspiratory "counterbalancing"
  Controlled (P_{aw})
  Spontaneous (P_{es})

Auto-PEEP (AP) is theoretically equivalent to the following expression:

$$AP = \frac{V_t}{[C(e^{t_e/RC} - 1)]}$$

where t_e is expiratory time and RC is the average exhalation time constant. If both end-expiratory resistance and flow are known, AP can be approximated as their quotient. Unfortunately, this is seldom the case. During passive ventilation, however, auto-PEEP can be measured by occluding the expiratory port of the ventilator at the end of the period allowed for exhalation between mechanical breaths (the end-expiratory port occlusion method) (Pepe and Marini, 1982). This value averages all end-expiratory alveolar pressures of open units, underestimating the highest and overestimating the lowest pressures that actually exist. Auto-PEEP estimated in this way does not reflect the actual degree of hyperinflation unless most airways are patent (*vide infra*). For accuracy, occlusion must occur at the appropriate time and persist for 0.5 seconds or longer—timing that is simplest to achieve during controlled ventilation. Delayed ventilator cycling can be achieved by markedly reducing frequency at the time of measurement. Several ventilators currently available facilitate prolongation of the exhalation phase by maintaining closure of the exhalation valve at the end of the set expiratory time, delaying the next breath and simplifying the measurement. A three-way valve can also be turned any time during expiration to close the inspiratory limb to the patient during inspiration while opening the ventilator to atmosphere. At the precise end of expiration, the ventilator's automated timed closure of the exhalation valve completes the occlusion for the duration of the inspiratory cycle (Gottfried et al, 1992). Total PEEP is then recorded as the occluded circuit pressure.

When a constant tidal volume is delivered to a passive subject, auto-PEEP must approximate the difference between end-inspiratory static pressure (plateau pressure) and the sum of (V_t/C and PEEP):

$$AP = P_S - \left(\frac{V_t}{C} + PEEP\right)$$

During passive constant flow conditions, C_{RS} can be estimated as the inverse of the average slope of the inspiratory airway pressure curve. P_{ZF} may be a more appropriate end-inspiratory value to use than P_S under dynamic conditions (without a pause applied). The validity of this assumption, however, has not been formally tested. When gas trapping is severe enough to cause complete airway closure at end-exhalation, estimating its severity and its response to intervention from the plateau pressure is more reliable than is expiratory port occlusion (Fig. 10–9) (Leatherman and Ravenscraft, 1996).

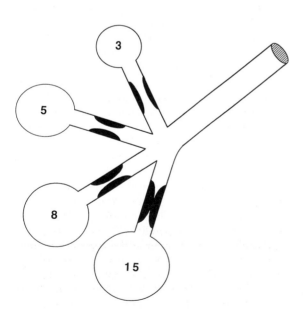

Figure 10–9
Regional variation in auto-PEEP. The greatest tendency for airway closure and gas trapping tends to occur in dependent regions. Although end-expiratory airway occlusion reflects the average auto-PEEP among open alveolar units, the highest levels of auto-PEEP are encountered by alveoli cut off from airway access. (From Marini JS and Wheeler AP: Critical Care Medicine, The Essentials, 2nd ed. Baltimore, Williams & Wilkins, 1997. With permission.)

Recording the change in peak static (plateau) pressure that occurs during passive ventilation, after exhalation time is dramatically prolonged, can be used to estimate auto-PEEP. Alternatively, because the pressure associated with dynamic hyperinflation is the quotient of trapped volume and compliance, recording the corresponding expelled volume change can provide similar information (Tuxen et al, 1992).

Alternative methods to quantify auto-PEEP directly require specialized sensing equipment and displays. During controlled inflation, auto-PEEP can theoretically be measured by noting the airway pressure at which inspiratory flow begins (Rossi et al, 1985a). During spontaneous efforts, the deflection of esophageal pressure needed to initiate inspiratory flow can be employed to quantify the pressure needed to counterbalance the expiratory action of elastic recoil. This counterbalancing pressure, however, tends to be lower than the auto-PEEP measured under passive conditions. The pressure required to initiate inspiratory flow is the pressure counterbalancing those units with the least AP.

Auto-PEEP can be estimated as the lowest PEEP level that causes a detectable increase in lung volume, measured by impedance plethysmography (Hoffman et al, 1989). For patients with dynamic airway compression, this suggestion may be approximately correct; for those without dynamic airway compression, it is unlikely to be correct (Ranieri et al, 1994). On average, lung volume begins to rise after PEEP has counterbalanced approximately 85% of the original auto-PEEP (Smith and Marini, 1988; Marini, 1989; Ranieri et al, 1994).

ESOPHAGEAL PRESSURE

With rare exception, fluctuations of global pleural pressure are sensed least invasively using a balloon catheter well positioned in the esophagus. Esophageal pressure (P_{es}) enables estimation of the force generated during spontaneous breathing and facilitates partitioning of transthoracic pressure into its lung and chest wall components during passive inflation. The esophagus is a convenient, but hardly ideal, site from which to measure pleural pressure. As can be surmised from its location beneath the heart, estimates of absolute pleural pressure and transpulmonary pressure obtained here, with the patient in the supine position, may not reflect those pertaining to other lung regions closest to the sternum. Indeed, the entire conformation of the lung, as well as the recorded P_{es}, changes with a shift in position to the upright, prone, or lateral decubitus.

Technique

P_{es} is measured with a latex balloon ($\sim$ 10 cm long) positioned in the lower or middle third of the esophagus (Macklem, 1974) and affixed to a multiperforated catheter stent. A spiral arrangement of the catheter holes is desirable. The 10-cm length samples an adequate portion of the esophagus while minimizing artifact. A shorter balloon can be influenced by regional pressure distortions arising near the heart and posterior mediastinum. A longer balloon may extend into the upper esophagus, which is a region that poorly reflects changes in global intrapleural pressure (Knowles et al, 1959; Macklem, 1974). A balloon volume of 0.2 to 0.5 cc transmits changes in intrathoracic pressure accurately during spontaneous cycles, whereas larger balloon volumes may stimulate esophageal contractions. To maintain catheter sensitivity during positive-pressure breathing cycles, however, a relatively large balloon volume (0.5–1.0 cc) is usually required. Larger volumes in this range prevent the balloon from collapsing against the catheter stent, damping the pressure signal.

In the upright position, P_{es} reflects the absolute value of global intrathoracic pressure with acceptable accuracy, but in the supine position P_{es} overestimates the average resting intrathoracic pressure. Because the esophagus is a posterior structure, the weight of the mediastinal contents on the sensing balloon produces this artifact, which may be reduced or eliminated by the patient's assuming the lateral decubitus position (Craven and Wood, 1981). Conversely, in the prone position, P_{es} underestimates average intrapleural pressure. Although P_{es} overestimates average pleural pressure in recumbency, *changes* in intrathoracic pressure are tracked well by a balloon catheter placed in appropriate position (Baydur et al, 1982). A coexisting nasogastric or feeding tube does not appear to influence the accuracy of P_{es} as a monitor of changes in pleural pressure. A multiperforated esophageal balloon catheter continues to reflect changes in intrathoracic pressure with accuracy acceptable for clinical purposes (Niknam et al, 1994).

To position the esophageal balloon during spontaneous breathing, the clinician must first pass it into the stomach, a site identified by positive deflections of pressure during forceful inspiratory efforts (sniff test). The balloon is then withdrawn gradually until negative pressure deflections first appear, signaling the entry of the uppermost hole of the balloon-enveloped portion of the catheter into the intrathoracic compartment. Multiperforated catheters tend to transmit the most negative pressure to which the balloon is exposed. The catheter is then withdrawn a distance equivalent to the balloon length ($\sim$ 10 cm) to ensure that the entire sensing area rests in the lower and mid-esophagus (Macklem 1974). Appropriate position can be confirmed by measuring airway and esophageal pressure deflections simultaneously during spontaneous efforts against an occluded airway (Baydur et al, 1982). When airway occlusion prevents gas from flowing into the lungs, no pressure can dissipate against resistance during breathing efforts and lung volume remains unchanged. It then follows that, on average, no pressure gradient develops between the occluded airway opening and the pleural space. Deflections of airway and esophageal pressure should therefore agree, to about 10% (Baydur et al, 1982). Precise balloon placement is difficult if spontaneous efforts are not present. Using approximate anatomic guidelines, the balloon tip is usually advanced about 35 to 40 cm from the nostril, depending on body habitus.

Combined nasogastric tube and esophageal balloon catheters that serve a dual clinical purpose have been commercially available for a number of years. These catheters appear to track changes in intrathoracic pressure quite well, while simultaneously providing a channel for aspirating stomach contents or administering liquid feedings (Gillespie, 1982).

Uses of Esophageal Pressure

Measurements of changes in esophageal pressure offer useful information when interpreting the end-expiratory wedge pressure under conditions of vigorous hyperpnea or elevated alveolar pressure (PEEP, auto-PEEP) (Marini, 1986). Moreover, the P_{es} tracing allows calculation of lung compliance, airway resistance, and auto-PEEP during spontaneous breathing and therefore helps partition the total impedance of the respiratory system into its lung and chest wall components. ΔP_{es} reflects the magnitude of patient effort during spontaneous or machine-aided breathing cycles. Although seldom employed clinically for this purpose, ΔP_{es} can be employed to compute the work of breathing across the lung and external circuit or the product of developed pressure and duration of inspiratory effort (the pressure-time product). Fluctuations in central venous pressure can be utilized for a similar purpose (Smiseth et al, 1984), but the vascular pressure tracing is variably damped and therefore yields a low-range estimate of effort.

TRANSDIAPHRAGMATIC PRESSURE

Transdiaphragmatic pressure (P_{di}), the difference between P_{es} and gastric pressure (P_{ga}), is generated

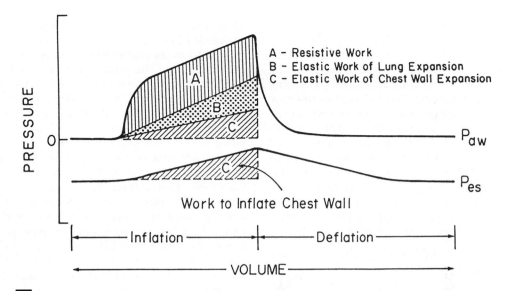

Figure 10–10
Work to inflate the lung and chest wall during a passive machine cycle delivered with constant flow. The pressure-volume area is composed of subcomponents related to various forms of frictional and elastic work. (From Marini JJ: Strategies to minimize breathing effort during mechanical ventilation. Crit Care Clin 6(3):635–661, 1990. With permission.)

by a single inspiratory muscle (the diaphragm) and is used primarily in the research setting to quantify effective diaphragmatic contractile force (Bellemare and Grassino, 1982). Although P_{di} is seldom utilized clinically, it is occasionally utilized in conjunction with phrenic nerve stimulation or voluntary effort (e.g., inspiration to total lung capacity, Müeller maneuver, forceful sniffing) to investigate the possibility of diaphragmatic paralysis.

INFLATION IMPEDANCE: VALUE OF CONTINUOUSLY MONITORING P_{aw}

In the intubated patient, a continuous tracing of airway pressure provides useful information commonly unobtained at the bedside. Many modern ventilators display airway pressure, flow, and volume—either as independent functions of time or plotted against one another in a "loop" format. When such monitoring options are not available, airway pressure can be measured with the transducer and display equipment normally used for ascertaining pressures in the pulmonary vasculature. An air-filled transducer dedicated to gas pressure measurement must be exclusively assigned to this purpose, however, to eliminate the risk of air embolism. Apart from enabling the estimation of R and C_{RS}, the wave form of inspiratory airway pressure traced during a controlled machine cycle provides a graphic representation of the inflation

work performed by the ventilator at that particular combination of tidal volume and flow settings (Fig. 10–10).

As noted, time and volume are linear analogues when inflation occurs passively under constant flow conditions. The slope of the airway pressure curve therefore reflects dynamic elastance the inverse of dynamic compliance), and the area under the pressure-time curve is proportional to the pressure-volume work performed per breath by the machine (Marini et al, 1986c). Under constant flow conditions, overdistention is detectable. The mean inflation pressure (P_i) is the work per liter of ventilation for the particular combination of tidal volume and flow settings. Provided that flow and tidal volume do not change, P_i indexes the average impedance to chest inflation. Under passive constant flow conditions, P_i can also be estimated from P_D and P_S without recording the pressure tracing by using the approximation:

$$\overline{P}_i = P_D - \frac{P_S - (PEEP + AP)]}{2}$$

Mean airway pressure (P_{aw}) for the *entire breathing cycle*, which is a value correlated with gas exchange efficiency, hemodynamic compromise, fluid retention, and incidence of barotrauma, can be estimated as the product of P_i and the inspiratory time fraction, adjusted for the effect of applied PEEP:

$$P_{\overline{aw}} = \overline{P}_i \left(\frac{t_i}{t_{tot}} \right) + PEEP \left(1 - \frac{t_i}{t_{tot}} \right)$$

As this equation implies, mean airway pressure can be altered in the clinical setting by changing the inspiratory time fraction (adjusting inspiratory flow if tidal volume and frequency are fixed), PEEP level, breathing impedance, or level of minute ventilation. Mean alveolar pressure (P_{alv}) deviates from mean airway pressure only when expiratory (R_x) and inspiratory (R_i) resistance differ significantly (Marini, 1990)(Fig. 10–11):

$$P_{\overline{alv}} = P_{\overline{aw}} + (R_x - R_i) \left(\frac{V_E}{60} \right)$$

As this equation implies, mean alveolar pressure may greatly exceed mean airway pressure under conditions of high minute ventilation and relatively high expiratory resistance.

MONITORING BREATHING EFFORT

Measures of Respiratory Muscle Activity

Oxygen Consumption of the Respiratory System (VO₂R)

Although the resting oxygen consumption rate of the ventilatory muscles during spontaneous breathing is usually less than 5% of the total body requirement, the energy cost of breathing during acute respiratory failure may raise that percentage tenfold (Field et al, 1982). Were it possible to do so, selectively measuring the oxygen consumption rate of the ventilatory pump (VO₂R) would estimate effort at the basic level of cellular metabolism. Although difficult to measure, VO₂R theoretically accounts for all factors that tax the respiratory muscles, integrating the stresses imposed by external workload (W_B) and those related to any lack of efficiency (E) of the conversion mechanism: $VO_2R = W_B/E$ (Roussos and Campbell, 1986). Two patients with different chest configurations, patterns of muscle activation, or degrees of coordination among the muscles of inspiration and expiration may perform identical external work but consume vastly different amounts of oxygen in the process. (See Chapter 6 for more details on respiratory muscles.)

Because VO₂R cannot be measured directly, total body oxygen consumption (VO₂) is tracked as ventilatory stresses (for example, resistance or CO_2 inhalation) are imposed or relieved. Without question, there is considerable "background-to-signal" and "noise-to-signal" variance in such computations, and consequently VO₂ does not lend itself to assessing breathing effort in the quasi-stable, critically ill patient. Providing high levels of inspired O_2 presents a major technical challenge. Unless extreme care is taken, these problems cannot be reliably overcome with present technology.

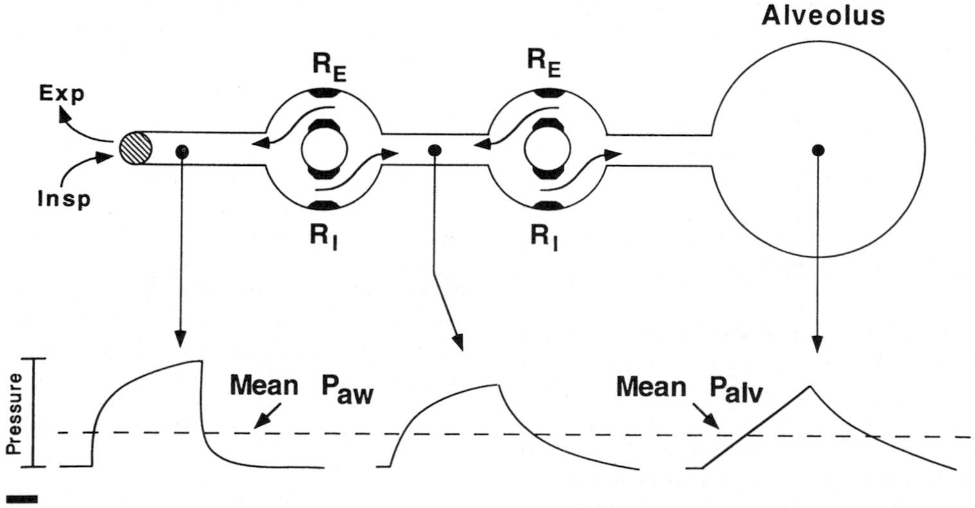

Figure 10–11
Relationship of mean airway pressure to mean alveolar pressure. In an airway in which inspiratory (Ri) and expiratory (Re) pressure losses are equivalent, the mean airway pressure averaged over the entire respiratory cycle should be equivalent at every point along the path, including the airway opening and alveolus. When Re is greater than Ri, mean alveolar pressure exceeds mean pressure at the airway opening. (From Marini JS and Wheeler AP: Critical Care Medicine, The Essentials, 2nd ed. Baltimore, Williams & Wilkins, 1977. With permission.)

Electromyography

In current intensive care unit practice, the combination of transcutaneous nerve stimulation and electromyography (EMG) recording is often chosen to monitor the depth of pharmacologic paralysis during mechanical ventilation. EMG can also be used to assess respiratory muscle activity. Although the amplitude of an integrated, rectified electromyographic signal has been reported to vary directly with the tension developed by the muscle it monitors (Bigland and Lippold, 1954), the force developed by a compound action potential of a given amplitude may change with the frequency of stimulation. In the laboratory setting, diaphragmatic EMG is best sensed by an electrode anchored at the gastroesophageal junction (Loring and Bruce, 1986). Unfortunately, such electrodes are difficult to position and cannot remain in place for long periods. Unless filtered out, the amplitude of the electrocardiographic (ECG) signal can complicate quantitative interpretation of the integrated value.

Surface EMG is more convenient, but specificity of the probe for the small area of underlying muscle limits its utility as a global measure of ventilatory effort. Furthermore, the integrated surface EMG fails to discriminate between activation of inspiratory and expiratory muscles, between tonic and phasic activity, or between respiratory and nonrespiratory muscle activity. Because the amplitude of the EMG varies widely with site preparation, electrode location, and patient anatomy, no absolute standards exist for comparing breathing effort among patients (Loring and Bruce, 1986). Like VO_2R, the EMG is limited to tracking *relative* changes in the activity of the ventilatory system. Despite these drawbacks, EMG of the sternocleidomastoid muscle, an accessory muscle of respiration activated only when the system is under significant stress, holds potential as a practical means of monitoring ventilatory effort (Moxham et al, 1980).

Direct Measures of External Mechanical Output

Work of Breathing

The mechanical work of breathing (defined by the laws of physics) and breathing effort are not synonymous terms. If the breathing pattern is inefficient, great effort can be expended without developing forceful pressures or accomplishing measurable external mechanical work. Nonetheless, certain pressures and volumes are precisely measurable, and for the same patient tend to fluctuate in the same direction as breathing effort.

QUANTIFYING TOTAL WORK OF CHEST INFLATION | The mechanical work of inspiration is performed when volume is moved by a pressure gradient applied across the lung. At any volume (V) above the equilibrium position, the total applied pressure difference (P_i) is distributed in accordance with the simplified "equation of motion" of the respiratory system (Otis et al, 1950):

$$P_i = R(\dot{V}) + \frac{V}{C}$$

The average pressure (P_i) developed during tidal inflation can be approximated:

$$P_i \sim R_i \left(\frac{V_t}{t_i} \right) + \frac{V_t}{2C} + P_{ex}$$

In this expression, P_{ex} is the end-expiratory alveolar pressure, and t_i and V_t are inspiratory time and tidal volume. P_i (the average trans-structural pressure) is numerically equivalent to the work per liter of ventilation (Marini 1987; 1990). Thus, if R_i, C, t_i, and V_t are known for the spontaneously breathing patient, the *external* work rate can be estimated. Work per tidal breath (W_B) can be quantified from the area enclosed within a plot of transmural inflation pressure (P_i) against inspired volume or from the integrated product of P_i and V:

$$W_B = \int_0^{t_i} P_i \dot{V} dt$$

Total inspiratory mechanical work per minute (power) is the product of P_i and V_E or of W_B and f, the breathing frequency. If inflation is achieved with constant flow, P_i is approximated by the inflation pressure at midcycle. With pressures and volumes expressed in their customary units, a convenient work unit is the joule or watt-second (1 joule $\sim$ 10 cm $H_2O \cdot$liter). One kilogram meter (KgM), another unit of work, equals about 10 joules.

To accurately estimate the work rate of spontaneous breathing, flow delivery during passive inflation must approximate the mean inspiratory flow rate and wave form of spontaneous breathing, and the delivered tidal volume must also be the same. Unfortunately, such preconditions are seldom accomplished without deep sedation or paralysis. A number of approximations appear to compensate satisfactorily for differences between machine-delivered and spontaneous cycles (Truwit et al, 1988).

Patient Work During Spontaneous and Machine-Aided Cycles

TRIGGERED VOLUME-LIMITED MACHINE CYCLES | During flow controlled, volume-cycled ventilation, patient effort has generally been assumed to be negligible whenever the machine aids the breathing cycle. This assumption is undoubtedly correct during controlled ventilation, but it is often invalid during patient-triggered, machine-assisted (assist-control) inflation (Marini et al 1985; 1986b). Relaxation does not occur abruptly once the machine cycle begins; rather, effort continues in proportion to respiratory drive and muscle strength (Marini et al, 1985; 1986b). The patient and machine work together to move the tidal volume at the specified rate. Assuming that similar external work is required to inflate the chest under passive and active conditions, the external work performed by the patient can be estimated from the difference in the machine's work component in these two circumstances (Fig. 10–12).

Similarity of the total mechanical workload can be assumed when impedance does not change and flow and tidal volume remain constant. When the ventilation requirement or sense of dyspnea is high, or when the ventilator is poorly adjusted, exertion levels during machine assistance may approach those of unsupported breathing. This fact is illustrated in a breath-by-breath comparison of the P_{es} during the spontaneous and machine-aided cycles of synchronized intermittent mandatory ventilation (SIMV). Interestingly, the impedance

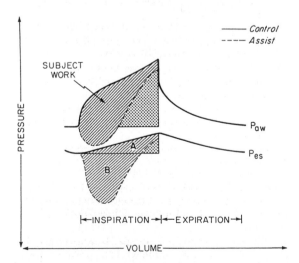

Figure 10–12
Two methods of computing subject work during machine-assisted cycles from active and passive plots of airway pressure (P_{aw}) and esophageal pressure (P_{es}). Area A represents subject work done across the chest wall, whereas area B represents subject work expended across the lung and external circuit. (Modified from Monitoring during mechanical ventilation. Clin Chest Med 9(1):73–100, 1988. With permission.)

characteristics of the chest (R and C) do not influence the patient's effort significantly during assist-control cycles, provided that the ventilator satisfies the patient's demand for inspiratory flow.

Any factor that amplifies respiratory drive adds to the patient's work of breathing during these triggered machine cycles. Trigger sensitivity, peak flow setting, tidal volume, and end-expiratory pressure are the key physician-controlled variables. Clues to patient exertion during triggered machine cycles are available from inspection of the deformed and variable airway pressure tracing. When an airway pressure tracing is not used, the only hint of vigorous inspiratory effort may be the stuttering rise of the ventilator's manometer needle toward its peak value, usually varying over time. P_D itself may not be far different from the expected value, as patient effort weakens while lung volume increases toward the end of the inflation cycle.

SPONTANEOUS BREATHING CYCLES | Although the work of breathing can be estimated utilizing the equation of motion, an esophageal balloon is required to directly measure mechanical work across the lung during spontaneous or pressure-supported breathing cycles. The fluctuation in the segment of pleural pressure tracing that spans inspiration tracks patient effort against the impedance of the lung and external circuit. Care must be taken to include any component attributable to auto-PEEP. When PEEP or CPAP is used, fluctuations of pressure should be referenced to the elevated baseline value of P_{es}. Inspiratory work can be quantified by electronically integrating the product of P_{es} and flow or by measuring the area enclosed within a plot of P_{es} against inspired volume. The work done in expanding the chest wall cannot be directly measured during active breathing and must be estimated from the published values of chest wall compliance or, preferably, from the inflation characteristic of the chest wall (P_{es} × V) traced during controlled (relaxed) inflation. Within physiologic limits, the pressure required to inflate the passive chest wall to a specified volume is largely independent of the flow profile.

PRESSURE-SUPPORTED CYCLES | During ventilation with pressure-support (PSV), the pressure contour theoretically remains unaltered from cycle to cycle, whereas the flow profile varies with changes in impedance and patient effort. Consequently, total work varies. Under these circumstances, airway pressure tracks only machine work and cannot be employed directly in assessing patient effort. The patient's component of the total inspiratory work of breathing can be gauged, nonetheless, by using plots of esophageal pressure and inspired volume during passive and pressure-supported inflations of similar depth and duration. The patient's work during the pressure supported breath can be roughly estimated as the difference between the total work required from the machine-patient system (gauged from the equation of motion) and the amount of work accomplished by the machine alone ($\sim P_S \times V_t$) (Jubran et al, 1995).

In patients with severe airflow obstruction, inspiratory flow may remain relatively constant throughout most of the inspiratory period, because pressure dissipates primarily against a relatively fixed resistance, and elastic recoil forces build only slowly. The patient may then be obligated to slow inspiration by expiratory muscular effort to meet the machine's flow offswitch criterion. This offswitch threshold is generally set at approximately 25% of the peak flow value, which would not be met passively until long after the patient's own inspiratory effort was terminated. Examination of the airway pressure tracing during pressure support ventilation can reveal the terminal elevation indicating expiratory effort (Fig. 10–13) (Jubran et al, 1995).

Pressure-Time Product (PTP) and Pressure-Time Index (PTI)

Isometric components of muscle tension, which consume oxygen without contributing to volume change, fail to register as externally measured work, accounting in large part for the lack of agreement between VO_2R and W_B (Roussos and Campbell, 1986). A pressure-time product (PTP $= P \times t_i$) parallels effort and VO_2R more closely than W_B because it includes the "isometric" component of muscle pressure and is less influenced by the impedance to contraction (McGregor and Becklake, 1961). Comparison of the mechanical work estimate with the pressure-time product during the intermittent unloading of SIMV brings these considerations into sharp relief (Marini et al, 1988). Here, calculation of workload would erroneously suggest effort to be greater during machine-aided cycles. In fact, for the dyspneic patient, the pressure time products are similar.

When P_i is referenced to the maximal isometric pressure that can be generated at FRC (P_{max}) by the fully cooperative patient and inspiratory time is expressed as a fraction of total cycle length (t_{tot}), a potentially helpful effort index is derived (Bellemare and Grassino, 1982; Roussos, 1985):

$$PTI = \overline{P_i}/P_{max} \times t_i/t_{tot}$$

PTI is also called tension time index and is utilized in assessing respiratory muscle function (see Chapter 6). Laboratory observations suggest that values of the PTI that exceed approximately 0.15 identify highly stressful breathing workloads that may induce fatigue. The PTI can therefore be regarded as an inverse indicator of endurance. Unfortunately, whereas P_i is relatively simple to estimate, P_{max} is very difficult to measure in critically ill patients. Techniques that enforce breathing effort, such as a one-way valve in conjunction with drive stimulation (e.g., by CO_2 inhalation) (Truwit and Marini, 1992), may eventually prove useful in this assessment.

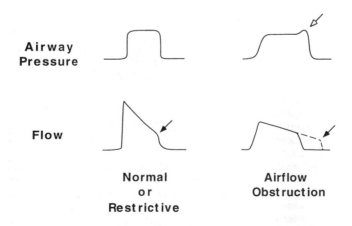

Airway Pressure

Flow

Normal or Restrictive

Airflow Obstruction

Figure 10–13

Airway pressure and flow profiles for patients with and without severe airflow obstruction receiving pressure support. Because inspiratory flow decelerates only slowly when the airway is obstructed, achieving the flow-based pressure cut-off criterion (*closed arrow*) may require expiratory effort, as reflected by the terminal rise in airway pressure (*open arrow*).

Influence of Auto-PEEP on W_B

Because pressure sufficient to counterbalance auto-PEEP must be applied before flow can be initiated, auto-PEEP (AP) imposes an inspiratory threshold load. Furthermore, a "block" of external work with the dimensions of AP and inspired volume (V_t) forms an important part of the total pressure-volume work described by the equation of motion:

$$W_B = \overline{P_i} \times V_t$$

$$W_B = R\left(\frac{V_t^2}{t_i}\right) + \left(\frac{V_t^2}{2C}\right) + (AP)(V_t)$$

During work calculations of triggered machine cycles, the additional work imposed by AP is accounted for in the proportional elevation of the baseline control curve. The threshold load imposed by AP effectively reduces the trigger sensitivity of the machine to a value equal to the sum of AP and the set value. In flow-limited patients, the judicious use of CPAP or PEEP can help restore trigger sensitivity and reduce work of breathing (Simkovitz et al, 1987; Smith et al, 1987; Smith and Marini, 1988; Marini, 1989).

SPIROMETRIC MEASUREMENTS

Vital Capacity

In *acute* disorders of neuromuscular function, vital capacity (VC) tends to be preserved relative to maximum inspiratory pressure (MIP) for two primary reasons. First, the pressure-volume relationship of the thorax is convex to the volume axis. Second, whereas many seriously ill patients can generate brief spikes of inspiratory pressure, few can or will sustain inspiratory effort long enough to achieve the plateau of their volume curve. Depending on the information desired from the VC, a "stacked" VC may be useful in this setting (Fig. 10–14) (Marini et al, 1986a).

The "stacking" technique measures volume on the inspiratory limb and employs a one-way valve to enable the patient to rest at an elevated volume between inspiratory efforts. The patient need not cooperate fully with testing—the naturally escalating inspiratory drive to breathe evokes forceful effort, especially when stimulated by inspired CO_2 or dead space rebreathing. For the same achieved volume, the peak esophageal pressures developed during breath stacking and standard inspiratory capacity (IC) maneuver are similar. Although a stacked VC may reflect the elastic properties of the lungs and chest wall more accurately than a conventional VC maneuver, it does not accurately reflect muscle strength. In fact, the breath-stacking technique may allow more effective incentive spirometry by extending the duration of therapeutic hyperinflation (Baker et al, 1990). A large discrepancy between the depth and duration of the conventional and breath-stacked VC may be seen in patients too weak, too uncooperative, or too air-hungry to sustain a single inspiratory effort.

As the supine position is assumed, VC falls by less than 20% in normal individuals and by only slightly more in patients with unilateral diaphragmatic paralysis. A positional change in VC greater than 30% suggests bilateral diaphragmatic dysfunction or paralysis, particularly if paradoxical abdominal motion and orthopnea are observed. Although fluoroscopy can help to detect *unilateral* diaphragmatic paralysis, there are many false-negative test results. Fluoroscopy is even more unreliable when both leaves of the diaphragm are dysfunctional. Diaphragmatic dysfunction can be confirmed utilizing esophageal and gastric pressure measurements to compute transdiaphragmatic pressure during deep breaths or forceful efforts (Table 10–2).

Other Spirometric Data

Few critically ill patients perform forced spirometry adequately. Nonetheless, measurements of

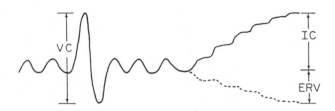

Figure 10–14
Vital capacity measured by conventional and "stacked" spirometry. Inspiratory capacity (IC) and expiratory reserve volume (ERV) can be measured using an appropriately directed one-way valve during spontaneous breathing. (From Marini JJ, Rodriguez RM, and Lamb VJ: Involuntary breath stacking. An alternative method for vital capacity estimation in poorly cooperative subjects. Am Rev Respir Dis 134:694–698, 1986. With permission.)

Table 10–2
Diaphragm Weakness

- Orthopnea
- Paradoxical abdominal motion
- ΔVC, sitting to supine >30%
- Transdiaphragmatic pressure
  - <25 cm H_2O at total lung capacity
  - <60 cm H_2O maximal

peak flow and FEV_1, which are useful in guiding management decisions, can generally be obtained in asthmatic patients and in those with exacerbated COPD. Furthermore, a great deal of helpful data is often available on the spirogram or flow tracing of tidal breathing. Persistent flow at end-expiration suggests auto-PEEP, and a linear or kinked flow profile suggests flow limitation during tidal exhalation (Truwit et al, 1988). A rippling flow contour suggests secretions retained in the central airway (Jubran and Tobin, 1994). During spontaneous ventilation, a ratio of frequency to tidal volume that exceeds 100 breaths/min per liter documents a pattern of rapid shallow breathing that is unlikely to be sustained and augurs poorly for weaning (Yang and Tobin, 1991). The ability of a patient to double resting minute ventilation indicates a considerable reserve of muscular power (Sahn et al, 1976). Delay of a ventilator-delivered breath during passive ventilation allows measurement of the volume of trapped gas (Tuxen and Lane, 1987).

MONITORING STRENGTH AND MUSCLE RESERVE

The output demanded of the ventilatory muscles is dictated by the product of V_E and the work or oxygen cost per liter of ventilation (discussed previously). The ability of the patient to sustain independent breathing, however, must not be judged on the basis of any absolute value for workload, but rather on workload interpreted against the background of muscular strength and endurance. Without full patient cooperation, it is questionable whether any measure of strength can reflect the full capability for pressure development. The two measures of respiratory muscle strength most commonly employed in the clinical setting are the VC and the MIP generated against an occluded airway (Godfrey and Campbell, 1968; Yang and Tobin, 1991; Truwit and Marini, 1992).

Maximal Inspiratory Pressure

Assuming full cooperation, a symmetrical reduction in inspiratory and expiratory maximal respi-

ratory pressures strongly suggests generalized muscle weakness. Although maximal expiratory pressures are seldom measured in critically ill patients, a good *qualitative* indication of expiratory muscle strength can sometimes be observed in the vigor of the coughing effort. When recording the MIP, lung volume should be trapped in the range between residual volume and FRC to optimize the mechanical advantage of the inspiratory muscles (Byrd and Hyatt, 1968; Black and Hyatt, 1969, 1971). In poorly cooperative patients, it is equally important to wait long enough to elicit a near-maximal increase in respiratory drive. When drive to breathe is strong, a one-way valve that blocks inspiration elicits a near-maximal effort (Marini et al, 1986; Truwit and Marini, 1992).

Approximately 20 seconds or 10 breathing efforts are required to elicit the maximal pressure response from a poorly cooperative patient (Marini et al, 1986d; Truwit and Marini, 1992). The patient must be neither overventilated nor overstressed before data recording, and occlusion of the airway must occur at FRC or lesser volume. Introducing a one-way valve that selectively permits expiration ensures that inspiratory efforts initiated late in the series occur at a volume between FRC and residual volume. With each breathing effort, additional air is pumped from the thorax, improving the mechanical advantage of the inspiratory muscles and amplifying respiratory drive (Godfrey and Campbell, 1968; Marini et al, 1986d). Measured in this way, the MIP of most patients on mechanical ventilation exceeds minus 40 mm Hg (-52 cm H_2O), even as they remain ventilator-dependent (Marini et al, 1986d; Truwit and Marini, 1992).

REFERENCES

Baker WL, Lamb VJ, and Marini JJ: Breath-stacking increases the depth and duration of chest expansion by incentive spirometry. Am Rev Respir Dis 141:343–346, 1990.

Bates JTM, Rossi A, and Milic-Emili J: Analysis of the behavior of the respiratory system with constant inspiratory flow. J Appl Physiol 58:1840–1848, 1985.

Baydur A, Behrakis K, Zin A, et al: A simple method for assessing the validity of esophageal balloon technique. Am Rev Respir Dis 126:788–791, 1982.

Bellemare F and Grassino A: Effect of pressure and timing of contraction on human diaphragm failure. J Appl Physiol 53:1190–1195, 1982.

Benito S and LeMaire F: Pulmonary pressure-volume relationship in acute respiratory distress syndrome in adults: Role of positive end-expiratory pressure. J Crit Care 5:27–34, 1990.

Bigland B and Lippold OCJ: The relation between force, velocity and integrated electrical activity in human muscles. J Physiol (London) 123:214–224, 1954.

Black LF and Hyatt RE: Maximal respiratory pressures. Normal values and relationship to age and sex. Am Rev Respir Dis 99:696–702, 1969.

Black LF and Hyatt RE: Maximal static respiratory pressure in generalized neuromuscular disease. Am Rev Respir Dis 103:641–650, 1971.

Blanch L, Fernandez R, Benito S, et al: Effect of PEEP on the arterial end-tidal carbon dioxide gradient. Chest 92:451–454, 1987.

Bone RC: Monitoring ventilatory mechanics in acute respiratory failure. Respir Care 28:597–603, 1983.

Byrd RB and Hyatt RE: Maximal static respiratory pressures in chronic obstructive lung disease. Am Rev Respir Dis 98:848–856, 1968.

Capps JS and Hicks GH: Monitoring non-gas respiratory variables during mechanical ventilation. Respir Care 32:558–571, 1987.

Chadha TS, Watson H, Birch S, et al: Validation of respiratory inductive plethysmography using different calibration procedures. Am Rev Respir Dis 125:644–649, 1982.

Chapin JC, Downs JB, Douglas ME, et al: Lung expansion, airway pressure transmission and positive end-expiratory pressure. Arch Surg 114:1193–1197, 1979.

Comroe JH: Physiology of respiration. Chicago, YearBook Medical Publishers, 1974, pp 104–105.

Craven KD and Wood LDH: Extrapericardial and esophageal pressures with positive end-expiratory pressure in dogs. J Appl Physiol 51:798–805, 1981.

Field S, Kelly SM, and Macklem PT: The oxygen cost of breathing in patients with cardiorespiratory disease. Am Rev Respir Dis 126:9–13, 1982.

Fleury BD, Murciano D, Talamo C, et al: Work of breathing in patients with chronic obstructive pulmonary disease in acute respiratory failure. Am Rev Respir Dis 131:822–827, 1985.

Gay PC, Rodarte JR, and Hubmyr RD: The effects of positive expiratory pressure on isovolumic flow and dynamic hyperinflation in patients receiving mechanical ventilation. Am Rev Respir Dis 139:621–626, 1989.

Gay PC, Rodarte JR, Tayyab M, et al: Evaluation of bronchodilator responsiveness in mechanically ventilated patients. Am Rev Respir Dis 136:880–885, 1987.

Gillespie DJ: Comparison of intraesophageal balloon pressure measurements with a nasogastric-esophageal balloon system in volunteers. Am Rev Respir Dis 126:583–585, 1982.

Godfrey S and Campbell EJM: The control of breath holding. Respir Physiol 4:385–400, 1968.

Gottfried SB, Reissman H, and Ranieri VM: A simple method for the measurement of intrinsic positive end-expiratory pressure during controlled and assisted modes of mechanical ventilation. Crit Care Med 20:621–629, 1992.

Gottfried SB, Rossi A, Higgs BD, et al: Noninvasive determination of respiratory system mechanics during mechanical ventilation for acute respiratory failure. Am Rev Respir Dis 131:672–677, 1985.

Guttmann J, Eberhard J, Gabry B, et al: Continuous calculation of intratracheal pressure in tracheally intubated patients. Anesthesiology 79(3):503–513, 1993.

Hoffman RA, Ershowsky P, and Krieger BP: Determination of auto-PEEP during spontaneous and controlled ventilation by monitoring dogs in end expiratory thoracic gas volume. Chest 96(3):613–616, 1989.

Jubran A and Tobin MJ: Use of flow-volume curves in detecting secretions in ventilator-dependent patients. Am J Respir Crit Care Med 150 (3):766–769, 1994.

Jubran A, Van de Graaff WB, and Tobin MJ. Variability of patient-ventilator obstructive pulmonary disease. Am J Respir Crit Care 152(1):129–136, 1995.

Katz JA, Zinn SE, Ozanne GM, et al: Pulmonary, chest wall, and lung-thorax elastances in acute respiratory failure. Chest 80:304–311, 1981.

Kimball WR, Leith DE, and Robins AG: Dynamic hyperinflation and ventilator dependence in chronic obstructive pulmonary disease. Am Rev Respir Dis 126:991–995, 1982.

Knowles JH, Henry SK, and Rahn H: Possible errors using esophageal balloon in determination of pressure-volume characteristics of the lung and thoracic cage. J Appl Physiol 14:525–530, 1959.

Lamy M, Fallat RJ, Koeniger E, et al: Pathologic features and mechanics of hypoxemia in adult respiratory distress syndrome. Am Rev Respir Dis 114:267–284, 1976.

Leatherman J and Ravenscraft S: Low measured auto-positive end-expiratory pressure during mechanical ventilation of patients with severe asthma: Hidden auto-positive end-expiratory pressure. Crit Care Med 24(3):541–546, 1996.

Lessard MR, Lofaso F, and Brochard L: Expiratory muscle activity increases intrinsic positive end expiratory pressure independently of dynamic hyperinflation in mechanically ventilated patients. Am J Respir Crit Care Med 151:562–569, 1995.

Loring SH and Bruce EW: Methods for study of the chest wall. In Fishman AP, Macklem PT, and Mead J (eds): Handbook of Physiology. Bethesda, American Physiological Society, 1986, pp 415–428.

McGregor M and Becklake M: The relationship of oxygen cost of breathing to respiratory mechanical work and respiratory force. J Clin Invest 40:971–980, 1961.

Macklem PT: Procedures for Standardized Measurements of Lung Mechanics. Bethesda, National Health Institute, Division of Lung Disease, 1974.

Marini JJ: Hemodynamic monitoring using the pulmonary artery catheter. Crit Care Clin 2(3):551–572, 1986.

Marini JJ: The role of the inspiratory circuit in the work of breathing during mechanical ventilation. Respir Care 32(6):419–430, 1987.

Marini JJ: Should PEEP be used in airflow obstruction? (editorial). Am Rev Respir Dis 140(1):1–3, 1989.

Marini JJ: Lung mechanics in the adult respiratory distress syndrome. Recent conceptual advances and implications for management. Clin Chest Med 11(4):673–690, 1990.

Marini JJ: Evolving concepts in the ventilatory management of ARDS. Clin Chest Med 17:269–292, 1996.

Marini JJ, Capps JS, and Culver BH: The inspiratory work of breathing during assisted mechanical ventilation. Chest 87(5):612–618, 1985.

Marini JJ, Rodriguez RM, and Lamb VJ: Involuntary breath stacking. An alternative method for vital capacity estimation in poorly cooperative subjects. Am Rev Respir Dis 134:694–698, 1986a.

Marini JJ, Rodriguez RM, and Lamb VJ: The inspiratory workload of patient-initiated mechanical ventilation. Am Rev Respir Dis 134:902–909, 1986b.

Marini JJ, Rodriguez RM, and Lamb VJ: Bedside estimation of the inspiratory work of breathing during mechanical ventilation. Chest 89(1):56–63, 1986c.

Marini JJ, Smith TC, and Lamb VJ: Estimation of inspiratory muscle strength in mechanically ventilated patients: The measurement of maximal inspiratory pressure. J Crit Care 1(1):32–38, 1986d.

Marini JJ, Smith TC, and Lamb VJ: External work output and force generation during synchronized intermittent mechanical ventilation. Effect of machine assistance on breathing effort. Am Rev Respir Dis 138:1169–1179, 1988.

Marini JJ and Truwit JD: Monitoring the respiratory system. In Schmidt GA (ed): Principles of Critical Care Medicine. New York, McGraw-Hill, 1991, pp 197–219.

Matamis D, LeMaire F, Harf A, et al: Total respiratory pressure volume curves in the adult respiratory distress syndrome. Chest 86:58–66, 1984.

Moxham J, Wiles CM, Newham D, et al: Sternomastoid muscle function and fatigue in man. Clin Sci Mol Med 59:463–468, 1980.

Niknam J, Chandra A, Adams AB, et al: Effect of nasogastric tube on esophageal pressure measurements in normal adults. Chest 6(1):137–141, 1994.

Ninane V, Yernault JC, and DeTroyer A: Intrinsic PEEP in patients with chronic obstructive pulmonary disease. Role of expiratory muscles. Am Rev Respir Dis 148:1037–1042, 1993.

O'Donnell DE, Sanii R, Anthonisen NR, and Younes M: Effect of dynamic airway compression on breathing pattern and respiratory sensation in severe chronic obstructive pulmonary disease. Am Rev Respir Dis 135:912–918, 1987.

O'Quin R, Marini JJ, Culver BH, and Butler J: Transmission of airway pressure to the pleural

space during lung edema and chest wall restriction. J Appl Physiol: Respirat Environ Exercise Physiol 59(4):1171–1177, 1985.

Otis AB, Fenn WO, and Rahn H: Mechanics of breathing in man. J Appl Physiol 2:592–607, 1950.

Pepe PE and Marini JJ: Occult positive end-expiratory pressure in mechanically ventilated patients with airflow obstruction. Am Rev Respir Dis 126:166–170, 1982.

Ranieri VM, Giulani R, Fiore T, et al: Volume-pressure curve of the respiratory system predicts effects of PEEP in ARDS: "Occlusion" versus "constant flow" technique. Am J Respir Crit Care Med 149:19–27, 1994.

Rossi A, Gottfried SB, Higgs BD, et al: Respiratory mechanics in mechanically ventilated patients with respiratory failure. J Appl Physiol 58:1849–1858, 1985a.

Rossi A, Gottfried SB, Zocchi L, et al: Measurement of static compliance of the total respiratory system in patients with acute respiratory failure during mechanical ventilation: The effect of intrinsic positive end-expiratory pressure. Am Rev Respir Dis 131:672–677, 1985b.

Roussos C: Energetics. In Roussos C, and Macklem PT (eds): The Thorax. New York: Marcel Dekker, 1985, pp 437–492.

Roussos C and Campbell EJM: Respiratory muscle energetics. In Fishman AP, Macklem PT, and Mead J (eds): Handbook of Physiology. Bethesda, American Physiological Society, 1986, pp 481–510.

Sahn SA, Lakshminarayan S, and Petty TL: Weaning from mechanical ventilation. JAMA 235:2208–2212, 1976.

Simkovitz P, Brown K, Goldberg P, et al: Interaction between intrinsic and externally applied PEEP during mechanical ventilation (abstract). Am Rev Respir Dis 135:A202, 1987.

Simon BA, Weinmann C, and Mitzner W: Mean airway pressure and alveolar pressure during high frequency ventilation. J Appl Physiol 57:1069–1078, 1984.

Smiseth OA, Refsum H, and Tyberg JV: Pericardial pressure assessed by right atrial pressure. A basis for calculation of left ventricular transmural pressure. Am Heart J 108:603–605, 1984.

Smith TC and Marini JJ: Impact of PEEP on lung mechanics and work of breathing in severe airflow obstruction. The effect of PEEP on Auto-PEEP. J Appl Physiol 65(4):1488–1499, 1988.

Smith TC, Marini JJ, and Lamb VJ: The inspiratory threshold load resulting from airtrapping during mechanical ventilation (abstract). Am Rev Respir Dis 135:A52, 1987.

Suter PM: Appropriate lung distention for gas exchange in ARDS. Chest 85:4–5, 1984.

Suter PM, Fairley HB, and Isenberg MD: Optimum end-expiratory pressure in patients with acute pulmonary failure. N Engl J Med 292:284–289, 1975.

Truwit JD and Marini JJ: Evaluation of thoracic

mechanics in the ventilated patient. Part 1: Primary measurements. J Crit Care 3(2):133–150, 1988.

Truwit JD and Marini JJ: Validation of a technique to assess maximal inspiratory pressure in poorly cooperative patients. Chest 102(4):1216–1219, 1992.

Truwit JD, Marini JJ, and Lamb VJ: The work of spontaneous breathing can be predicted noninvasively during mechanical ventilation (abstract). Am Rev Respir Dis 137:64, 1988.

Tuxen DV and Lane S: The effects of ventilatory pattern on hyperinflation, airway pressures, and circulation in mechanical ventilation of patients with severe airflow obstruction. Am Rev Respir Dis 136:872–879, 1987.

Tuxen DV, Williams TJ, Schienkestel CD, et al: Use of a measurement of pulmonary hyperinflation to control the level of mechanical ventilation in patients with acute severe asthma. Am Rev Respir Dis 146:1136–1142, 1992.

Wright PW, Marini JJ, and Bernard GR: In vitro versus in vivo comparison of endotracheal tube airflow resistance. Am Rev Respir Dis 140(1):10–16, 1989.

Yang KL and Tobin MJ: A prospective study of indexes predicting the outcome of trials of weaning from mechanical ventilation. N Engl J Med 324:1445–1450, 1991.

II

PRINCIPLES OF TREATMENT

CHAPTER

Principles of Mechanical Ventilation and Weaning

Stephen E. Lapinsky, M.B., B.Ch.

Arthur S. Slutsky, M.D.

GOALS OF MECHANICAL VENTILATION

PRIMUM NON NOCERE

Positive-pressure ventilation is a life-saving intervention necessary for the management of respiratory failure complicated by respiratory acidosis or severe hypoxemia. Although vital functions are supported during periods of respiratory failure, there are a number of potential adverse effects that may result in significant morbidity or even mortality. Complications may be associated with the insertion of an endotracheal tube; they may be related to the administration of positive pressure or to oxygen toxicity. Complications can also result from pharmacotherapy necessary to facilitate ventilation. These adverse effects are discussed in more detail below.

The presence of an endotracheal tube can result in local injury, but the major risk is that of nosocomial infection. Normal protective mechanisms are bypassed, causing colonization of the trachea, increasing the risk of pneumonia. High airway pressures as well as high inspired oxygen concentrations appear to cause alveolar damage. Although the precise mechanisms are not clear, ventilator-induced lung injury may be responsible for significant morbidity, prolonging the necessity for mechanical support. Positive pressure is also responsible for barotrauma (i.e., pneumothorax, pneumomediastinum, subcutaneous emphysema) and cardiovascular effects including hypotension and a reduction in cardiac output.

Given the significant hazards of endotracheal intubation and mechanical ventilation, an important management goal should be to minimize or prevent the adverse effects. One of the first issues to be addressed is whether ventilatory assistance is required and whether intubation is necessary. In many situations in which the patient has severe hypoxemia or cannot protect his airway, the decision may be relatively straightforward. However, in some instances the decision requires clinical judgment in which the risks of ventilation are weighed against the hazards of not ventilating the patient. The decision may be somewhat easier in those patients in whom noninvasive ventilation is an option. Patients with severe hypoxemia or severe shock or those who cannot protect their airway should be intubated. Greater clinical judgment is required in the patient with hypercapnia because isolated respiratory acidosis is usually not threatening in itself.

SUPPORT GAS EXCHANGE

A major application of ventilatory support is to optimize alveolar ventilation. In the patient with hypoventilation, mechanical ventilation takes over the function of respiratory muscles, correcting hypercapnia and respiratory acidosis. Although an acceptable goal is the normalization of $PaCO_2$ and pH, in some situations a higher-than-normal $PaCO_2$ may be accepted (permissive hypercapnia), particularly when alveolar ventilation is limited by high ventilation pressures. Ventilation is often necessary in the management of severe intractable hypoxemia, which may be improved by the delivery of inspired oxygen fractions greater than can be delivered by mask alone, as well as by the effect of positive pressure on lung volumes and alveolar recruitment. Adequate arterial oxygenation must be achieved using an inspired oxygen concentration that is not excessively high. Usually an oxygen saturation of greater than 90% is considered acceptable, and there is usually no advantage in aiming for higher levels of oxygenation.

The objective of ventilatory support should therefore be to improve respiratory acidosis and hypoxemia to an acceptable level, avoiding excessive inflation pressures and oxygen concentrations. Controlled hypoventilation with respiratory acidosis is generally well tolerated and avoids the necessity for high inflation pressures. Likewise, by monitoring parameters of oxygen delivery and tissue oxygenation, it may be possible to reduce the inspired oxygen tension to avoid toxicity.

OTHER OBJECTIVES

Mechanical ventilation has a number of beneficial physiologic effects on the respiratory system (Table 11–1). Positive pressure may be used to increase lung volumes, both at full inspiration and at end-expiration. Improved end-inspiratory lung volume may prevent or treat atelectasis and permits the recruitment of alveoli, with potential beneficial effects on oxygenation and lung compliance. Positive end-expiratory pressure increases functional residual capacity, correcting hypoxemia and maintaining alveolar recruitment. Ventilation acts also to unload ventilatory muscles, when the work of breathing is increased by high airway resistance or reduced lung compliance. Reduced respiratory muscle work results in a decreased cardiac output requirement for these muscles, which may account for up to 50% of oxygen consumption in acute respiratory failure. This is of particular benefit in the patient with myocardial ischemia or reduced oxygen delivery. Resting the respiratory muscles may also reverse the fatigue that may have been responsible for acute ventilatory failure (see Chapter 6).

Other clinical uses of mechanical ventilation are (1) to relieve the subjective sensation of respiratory distress; (2) to permit sedation or neuromuscular blockade in anesthesia; (3) to reduce intracranial pressure by controlled hyperventilation; and (4) to stabilize the chest wall in the presence of significant injury.

Table 11–1
Objectives of Mechanical Ventilation

Physiologic	Clinical
Avoid excessive lung stretch	Avoid iatrogenic lung injury
Modify gas exchange	
Arterial oxygenation	Reverse hypoxemia
Alveolar ventilation	Improve severe respiratory acidosis
	Permit anesthesia
	Reduce intracranial pressure
	Reduce respiratory distress
Increase lung volume	
End-expiratory volume (FRC)	Improve hypoxemia
End-inspiratory volume	Prevent/reverse atelectasis
	Stabilize chest wall
Reduce work of breathing	Reverse ventilatory muscle fatigue
	Decrease systemic/myocardial oxygen consumption

MECHANISMS OF MECHANICAL VENTILATION

PRESSURE AND VOLUME

Ventilation is achieved by the delivery of either predetermined volume or pressure to the lungs, on a regular or demand basis. Volume-controlled ventilation requires a preset tidal volume, traditionally one related to body weight (e.g., 10–15 ml/kg). However, in view of current concepts of pressure-related lung injury, lower volumes are now often used (Slutsky, 1993). This view is related also to the understanding that large regions of the lung may not be recruitable in patients with acute lung injury, and thus the use of large tidal volumes may result in overdistention and damage to the small volume of relatively normal lung. To minimize this risk, tidal volumes of 5 to 7 ml/kg are given to achieve an airway pressure no greater than 30 to 35 cm H_2O (Hickling et al, 1990). Pressure limits can be set on the ventilator at a level of about 40 cm H_2O. If airway pressure reaches this level, gas is released to prevent the airway pressure from exceeding that level, which is associated with sounding of a ventilator alarm.

Pressure-controlled ventilation differs from volume-controlled ventilation in that a level of airway pressure is set, with the delivered tidal volume being determined by pulmonary mechanics (Blanch et al, 1993). The duration of delivery of the pressure is preset as an inspiratory time (or as an inspiratory:expiratory [I:E] ratio and respiratory rate). The normal I:E ratio of about 1:2 may be adjusted based on oxygenation status and hemodynamics. Although the optimal pressure limit is not known, because of concerns of ventilator-induced lung injury, pressure is often set below 35 to 40 cm H_2O. The preset inspiratory pressure and inspiratory time and the patient's pulmonary resistance and compliance interact in a complex way to determine the tidal and minute volumes. The dynamics of pressure-controlled ventilation have been determined by mathematic modeling and validated experimentally (Burke et al, 1993). For a given preset pressure, tidal volume falls as ventilatory rate increases and minute ventilation increases to an upper limit, which is determined by lung mechanics. An optimal value for alveolar ventilation occurs at some level of ventilatory rate owing to the relative increase in dead space fraction as tidal volume decreases. Changes in total thoracic compliance affect tidal volume; a decrease in thoracic compliance results in a proportional decrease in tidal volume. Similarly, increased airway resistance decreases the delivered tidal volume, but this may be overcome by raising

the inspiratory time fraction to allow for pressure equilibration (see also Chapters 10 and 18).

TRIGGERING

The rate of ventilation may be a function of ventilator settings, spontaneous breathing, or a combination of both, depending on the mode. Synchronization of spontaneous breaths with delivered breaths is usually achieved by triggering the initiation of gas delivery by a small change in airway pressure (e.g., -0.5 to -2 cm H_2O). Insensitive triggering systems can impose substantial respiratory muscle loads, whereas an oversensitive system may produce spontaneous ventilator cycling. In patients with significant airflow obstruction, gas trapping can occur (often termed *dynamic hyperinflation,* or *intrinsic* or *auto-PEEP*), which may make the generation of even a small negative airway pressure difficult. The patient requires increased respiratory muscle work to overcome the positive alveolar pressure that exists at end-expiration, in order to create a negative triggering pressure. The clinician can help overcome this extra work of breathing by the administration of an equivalent external positive end-expiratory airway pressure (PEEP). Flow triggering, using small changes in airway flow, is available on some ventilators and may be more efficient than pressure triggering, but clinical benefits have not been demonstrated.

FLOW

The inspiratory flow rate and pattern of delivery must be set during volume-controlled ventilation, but they are determined by patient requirements with pressure-preset ventilatory modes. In the spontaneously breathing patient, the flow rate setting should match the patient's peak inspiratory demands, usually requiring from 40 to 100 l per minute. During controlled ventilation of a sedated or paralyzed patient, the flow rate can be used to establish the inspiratory time and manipulate the I:E ratio.

The inspiratory flow may be delivered in a variety of flow patterns, but no benefit in terms of oxygenation or work of breathing has been demonstrated between square-wave, sine-wave, or decelerating flow patterns. The flow profile influences the airway pressure wave form, a square-wave flow pattern producing a peaked pressure wave, with a high peak pressure and lower plateau or mean pressure. In contrast, a decelerating ramp inspiratory flow produces an almost square-wave pressure pattern, resembling that occurring in pressure-preset ventilation (Fig. 11–1). This pat-

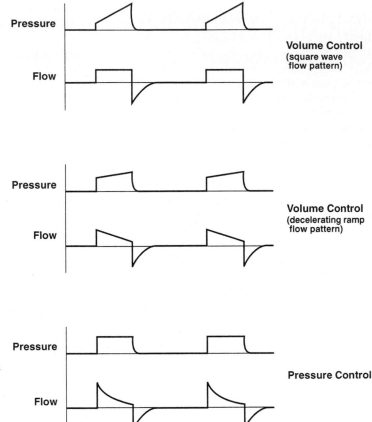

Figure 11–1
Schematic representation of airway pressure and flow during volume-controlled ventilation with a square-wave flow pattern, with a decelerating ramp flow pattern, and during pressure-controlled ventilation.

The square-wave volume-controlled tracings demonstrate a high peak airway pressure compared with that on the decelerating ramp tracing. During pressure-controlled ventilation the pressure remains constant, whereas flow decreases exponentially.

tern has the potential advantage of limiting peak pressure while optimizing mean airway pressure.

With pressure-targeted modes, the ventilator rapidly achieves and maintains the target pressure, producing an exponentially decelerating inspiratory flow pattern. Peak inspiratory flow rates are limited only by circuit resistance and the working pressure of the ventilator.

CYCLING

Gas flow at the end of inspiration can be terminated by reaching a preset volume, time, or flow rate. Volume cycling delivers a preset tidal volume, but additional patient effort is not rewarded with increased volume. Active expiratory effort by the patient during tidal volume delivery increases airway pressures. If the set pressure limit is reached, inspiratory flow is terminated.

Pressure-controlled ventilation uses time cycling, where the set airway pressure (and therefore gas delivery) is maintained for a preset inspiratory time. Additional patient effort during this time allows increased tidal volume, but the cycling time is not affected.

Pressure-support ventilation is a preset pressure mode that uses flow cycling. Airway pressure is maintained until inspiratory flow falls below a certain level (usually 25% of the peak inspiratory flow). This mode increases patient control over the delivered tidal volume and may improve patient-ventilator synchrony.

POSITIVE END-EXPIRATORY PRESSURE

Maintaining a positive pressure at end-expiration (PEEP) improves oxygenation by a number of mechanisms. Lung volume is recruited, mean airway pressure is elevated, and lung water is redistributed from interstitial space adjacent to the gas exchanging regions to the compliant perivascular interstitial space (Malo et al, 1984), all facilitating improvement in oxygenation. Pulmonary compliance may be improved, reducing airway pressures and decreasing work of breathing. The appropriate level of PEEP can be determined by optimizing the desired physiologic response, whether it is PaO_2, oxygen delivery, or lung compliance (Suter et al, 1975). In adult respiratory distress syndrome (ARDS) there is increasing evidence that PEEP should be set above the lower inflection point of the pressure-volume curve, usually a level of about 8 to 12 cm H_2O. The absence of PEEP may aggravate lung injury owing to the shear stresses associated with repeated opening and closing of alveoli (Muscedere et al, 1994). In patients with airflow limitation and auto-PEEP, increasing external PEEP facilitates triggering during spontaneous breathing and reduces work of breathing.

PEEP has a number of significant deleterious effects. Hemodynamic disturbances, characterized by decreased cardiac output and hypotension, occur as a result of reduced cardiac filling pressures, particularly in the volume-depleted patient. This disturbance may adversely affect oxygen delivery. The risk of barotrauma increases with rises in peak airway pressure, which may be affected by high levels of PEEP. The potential beneficial effects of higher levels of PEEP need to be weighed against these adverse effects.

INSPIRED OXYGEN CONCENTRATION

Because of the possibility of lung injury induced by a high inspired oxygen concentration (FIO_2), the lowest FIO_2 producing an acceptable PaO_2 should be selected. Exposure to an FIO_2 less than 0.5 is probably not of concern. Other determinants of PaO_2 that may be manipulated to reduce FIO_2 include mean airway pressure (by increasing PEEP, I:E ratio, or plateau pressure) and mixed venous oxygen saturation. The potential damaging effects of high airway pressure (or more correctly high lung stretch) must be balanced against those of a high FIO_2. Oxygenation may be improved by sedation with or without neuromuscular blockade, by facilitating ventilation, reducing airway pressures, and decreasing metabolic demands. Increasing cardiac output and therefore oxygen delivery augments tissue oxygenation and may increase PaO_2 by improving mixed venous oxygenation. It should be noted that currently the optimal balance between FIO_2, airway pressure, and ventilatory pattern for minimizing ventilatory-induced lung injury is not known.

NONINVASIVE VENTILATION

Ventilatory support is traditionally performed via an endotracheal tube, but there has been increasing interest in the noninvasive application of positive-pressure ventilation (Abou-Shala and Meduri, 1996). Endotracheal intubation carries the risk of significant complications, which can be avoided by a noninvasive approach. Complications include local damage to the pharynx, larynx, vocal cords, and trachea, and a predisposition to nosocomial pneumonia as a result of the loss of normal protective mechanisms. Intubation is uncomfortable and often requires deep sedation, with its own inherent complications. Noninvasive ventilation therefore has a number of advantages over conventional ventilatory methods (Table 11–2).

Noninvasive ventilation is achieved using a tight-fitting nasal or face mask attached to a positive-pressure source. Although the nasal mask is often well tolerated, the face mask is a more commonly used interface and is available in a variety of types and sizes. Some degree of leak commonly occurs, but this does not usually affect the efficacy of ventilation, particularly when pressure preset modes are used. These interfaces may be used with conventional ventilators, usually in a pressure-support mode although volume-controlled, pressure-controlled, and proportional-assist modes have been described. A number of simpler bilevel pressure-support devices are available, which provide adequate ventilation in a pressure-support mode with or without a backup rate. They have the advantage of simplicity and

---

Table 11–2
Advantages and Disadvantages of Noninvasive Ventilation

Advantages	Disadvantages
Avoid complications of intubations	Facial pressure necrosis
Local trauma	Mask interface leaks
Sedation	Aspiration risk
Nosocomial pneumonia	Inadequate tracheal toilet
Discomfort	Risk of disconnection hypoxemia
Vocal cord function intact	Increased monitoring may be required
Talk	Sometimes poorly tolerated
Cough	
Eat	
No extubation decisions	

low cost but do not have the monitoring capabilities of ventilators. The success of noninvasive ventilation often depends on the experience and perseverance of the medical personnel.

Noninvasive support can be considered in the patient who is protecting the airway and has adequate spontaneous respiratory effort, but is failing due to respiratory muscle fatigue or progressive hypoxemia. It is relatively contraindicated in the patient with a decreased level of consciousness, excessive secretions, or hemodynamic instability. Recent upper gastrointestinal anastomoses may be compromised if they are subjected to positive pressure. An adequate mask fit may not be possible in the edentulous patient or one with a facial injury or deformity. Noninvasive ventilation has a clear role to play in the management of patients with respiratory failure resulting from chronic obstructive airways disease, where a mortality benefit has been demonstrated (Bott et al, 1993; Brochard et al, 1995). Cardiogenic pulmonary edema can be treated by noninvasive continuous positive airway pressure (Bersten et al, 1991), and further benefit may be obtained using noninvasive ventilation. Other potential uses are for patients who refuse intubation and those who require short-term support.

Noninvasive ventilation is usually used for short-term ventilation, although support for several days to a week is feasible. The mask can be removed intermittently for feeding, communication, or patient comfort. Decisions regarding extubation are avoided by the ease of removal and reapplication of the mask interface. Although this mode of ventilatory support is promising, its exact role remains to be determined. Patients require close monitoring, and facilities for endotracheal intubation and conventional ventilation should be available.

PERMISSIVE HYPERCAPNIA

A major complication of the pressure-limited ventilatory strategy described earlier is alveolar hypoventilation and respiratory acidosis. The accumulating evidence of lung injury related to alveolar overdistension has generated a ventilatory strategy of controlled hypoventilation and permissive hypercapnia. This technique was first proposed in the management of acute severe asthma (Menitove and Goldring, 1983; Darioli and Perret, 1984) and has been applied to the management of patients with ARDS (Hickling et al, 1990).

Although many organ systems are affected by hypercapnia, results of animal studies and limited clinical literature suggest that the respiratory acidosis is usually well tolerated and may be an acceptable price to pay for the prevention of pulmonary overdistention. The major clinical effects are cardiopulmonary and neurologic. Hypercapnia and acidosis may decrease myocardial contractility, aggravate cardiac ischemia by a "steal" phenomenon due to vasodilation of normal vessels, and increase myocardial irritability and arrhythmias. Hypercapnia is also associated with sympathoadrenal stimulation, which is another potential danger in patients with coronary disease. Usually peripheral vasodilation with hypercapnia is associated with increased cardiac output. However, hypercapnia induces pulmonary arterial vasoconstriction. Vasoconstriction could decrease cardiac output in patients with impaired right ventricular systolic function.

The neurologic effects of hypercapnia are related to changes in pH, modification in cerebral blood flow, and elevation of the intracranial pressure. Carbon dioxide has direct neurologic depressant effects. Hypercapnia also affects blood flow and autoregulation within a number of other organs including the hepatic, renal, and intestinal circulation.

Human studies are reassuring in that they reveal hypercapnia to be generally well tolerated if adequate oxygenation is maintained. Studies of experimental exposure to hypercapnia demonstrate an increased respiratory drive and altered consciousness, but no adverse cardiovascular effects. Controlled hypoventilation with hypercapnia does not affect cardiac output, but pulmonary artery pressures may rise (Prys-Roberts et al, 1968; Viswanathan et al, 1970). A review of the experience of permissive hypercapnia in acute severe asthma demonstrates few adverse effects (Feihl and Perret, 1994). Levels of $PaCO_2$ up to 80 mm Hg (pH 7.15) are common, but in extreme cases, levels of $PaCO_2$ reach as high as 140 mm Hg with a pH as low as 7.0. Heavy sedation is usually mandatory to reduce the increased respiratory drive, preventing patient discomfort and ventilator dyssynchrony. Adequate inspired oxygen concentration must be ensured to avoid hypoxemia. Correction of acidosis is seldom required but may be considered at extremely low pH, although evidence of its utility is lacking. In accordance with the discussion earlier, hypercapnia is relatively contraindicated in patients with intracranial pathology, hypertensive disease, myocardial ischemia, hypovolemia, or pulmonary hypertension.

VENTILATORY MODES

With the introduction of numerous modes of ventilation over the years, there has been an increase in confusion as to the best strategy to use for ventilating patients. Frequently institutional culture and personal bias form the basis for choosing a particular ventilatory mode. However, based on sound physiologic principles, the pathophysiology of the particular disease process, and known risk factors, a rational choice of ventilatory mode can be made. Newer modes of ventilation require more sophistication on the part of the ventilator and a corresponding increase in cost. Studies, which include cost/benefit analysis, are clearly indicated to define the roles of newer and more sophisticated modes of ventilation, before they are widely instituted.

Assist-control Ventilation

Controlled ventilation is the simplest mode of ventilatory support, providing a predetermined tidal volume and rate regardless of patient effort or requirement (Fig. 11–2). However, this has the

disadvantage of asynchrony occurring between the patient's spontaneous efforts and the ventilated breaths. Neuromuscular blockade can overcome this problem but is associated with a number of potential problems, and suppression of spontaneous respiration may lead to atrophy of respiratory muscles. Assisted modes triggered by the patient's respiratory efforts are therefore more commonly used to synchronize patient and ventilator activity. In the assist-control mode, every breath is supported by the ventilator. A backup minimum rate is set, but each patient effort is rewarded by a ventilator breath. This mode may be used with volume-preset or pressure-preset ventilation. A potential disadvantage is that in patients with increased ventilatory drive (e.g., with pneumonia, sepsis, or ARDS), potentially high minute volumes can produce respiratory alkalosis and may worsen air trapping in patients with obstructive airways disease.

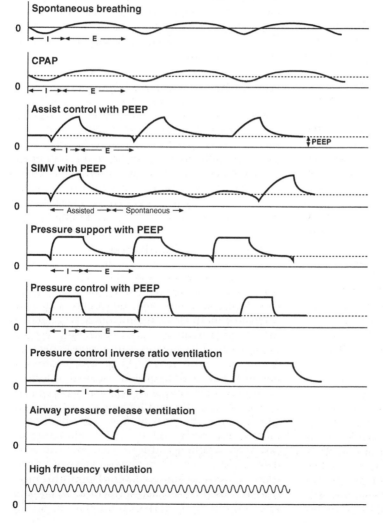

Figure 11–2
Airway pressure profiles during spontaneous breathing and various modes of mechanical ventilation. I indicates inspiratory phase and E expiratory phase. CPAP = continuous positive airway pressure; PEEP = positive end-expiratory pressure; SIMV = synchronized intermittent mandatory ventilation.

In the assist-control and pressure-control tracings, the first two breaths are triggered by patient effort, whereas the third breath is controlled because no spontaneous effort has occurred. During SIMV ventilation, spontaneous breathing occurs between ventilator breaths. The pressure support tracing demonstrates some variation in duration of the inspiratory phase due to flow cycling, as compared with the fixed inspiratory period of the time-cycled pressure-control mode. During pressure-controlled inverse ratio ventilation, the inspiratory period is prolonged and exceeds the expiratory period.

Synchronized Intermittent Mandatory Ventilation

This mode (SIMV) provides a preset number of ventilator breaths combined with the facility for spontaneous breathing not assisted by the ventilator (see Fig. 11–2). Ventilator breaths are patient-triggered and are therefore synchronized if spontaneous effort occurs, or are mandatory in the absence of such effort. Because of the advantage of allowing the patient to do a variable amount of respiratory work, and the security of backup ventilation, this mode of ventilation is often used in weaning. SIMV may be performed using volume- or pressure-preset ventilation. Spontaneous breaths may require significant work of breathing in the presence of high circuit or demand valve resistance. This extra work can be overcome to some degree by the use of pressure support (see later) during the spontaneous breaths.

Pressure-support Ventilation

Pressure-support ventilation is a pressure-preset, flow-cycled mode in which ventilatory support augments every spontaneous effort. The delivered pressure is triggered by patient effort and maintained until a specified decrease in inspiratory flow occurs. The patient therefore determines respiratory frequency and inspiratory time, with tidal volume being determined by the level of pressure set, patient effort, and pulmonary mechanics. This has the advantage of reducing dyssynchrony and optimizing patient control over ventilation. The ability to vary support from high pressure to near-spontaneous breathing make this a useful and effective weaning mode (Brochard et al, 1995). As described earlier, pressure support may be used to compensate for ventilator-induced work of breathing during spontaneous breathing in SIMV ventilation. These modes require spontaneous respiratory effort and do not guarantee a minimum tidal volume. An apnea backup facility is therefore advantageous. A mode similar to pressure-support ventilation is called volume-support ventilation, in which there is a preset minimum tidal volume.

Inverse Ratio Ventilation

Inverse ratio ventilation (IRV) involves prolongation of the inspiratory time until the I:E ratio is greater than 1. It has been used in an attempt to improve oxygenation. The rationale is that it is possible to increase mean airway pressure while minimizing end-inspiratory pressures. No controlled study has demonstrated an advantage and therefore no clear indications exist for the use of this mode of ventilation. IRV is most likely to be beneficial early in the disease process when there are still recruitable alveoli. Some patients do not respond to IRV. It has been suggested that nonresponse may occur when static thoracic compliance is less than 25 ml/cm H_2O (Gattinoni et al, 1984). It is not clear that IRV offers any distinct advantages over other approaches that increase mean airway pressure.

Proportional-assist Ventilation

This mode differs considerably from other ventilatory modes in that ventilator output is augmented in proportion to patient demand (Younes, 1992). The pressure delivered is increased in proportion to patient instantaneous effort throughout inspiration, giving the patient control of breathing pattern, tidal volume, inspiratory time, and flow pattern. The method has the advantage of increased comfort and preservation of respiratory control mechanisms. Spontaneous respiratory effort is necessary. This mode is being evaluated in intubated patients as well as being used as a mode for noninvasive ventilation.

Airway Pressure-release Ventilation

Pressure-release ventilation involves the administration of a continuous positive inflation pressure that is intermittently released (see Fig. 11–2). By periodically allowing airway and intrathoracic pressure to decrease, adverse cardiovascular effects are reduced. This mode is designed to assist the spontaneously breathing patient. No clear benefit has been demonstrated over conventional modes.

High-frequency Ventilation

The administration of small tidal volumes at high frequencies (100 to 3000/min) has the potential to reduce barotrauma and lung injury. Clinically applicable methods of high-frequency ventilation include high-frequency positive-pressure ventilation (60 to 120 breaths per minute), high-frequency jet ventilation (100 to 600 breaths per minute) and high-frequency oscillation (up to 3000 cycles per minute). The major physiologic difference is in the mechanism of gas transport, which occurs by coaxial flow, pendelluft, augmented dispersion, and molecular diffusion (Slutsky, 1988). Although there is no convincing data demonstrating a benefit of high-frequency jet ventilation over conventional ventilation, this mode has been used in the management of ARDS and tracheobronchial or tracheoesophageal fistula.

The effect of changes in ventilatory parameters on gas exchange may be different to conventional ventilation, and are influenced by the patient's respiratory mechanics. During high-frequency jet ventilation, alveolar ventilation is elevated by increasing driving pressure and by a reduction in frequency. In addition to changing inspired oxygen concentration, oxygenation may be improved by increasing the inspiratory time, which raises functional residual capacity. High-frequency ventilation carries risks related to the large flow rates and high driving pressures, which may cause air trapping and necrotizing tracheobronchitis. Because of gas trapping, high-frequency ventilation of any type should *not* be used in patients with obstructive airway disease.

SPECIFIC CONDITIONS

Adult Respiratory Distress Syndrome (ARDS)

Although there is no evidence that any ventilatory mode is superior to another in the management of patients with severe ARDS, recognition of the concept of iatrogenic lung injury has influenced ventilatory strategies (Kollef and Schuster, 1995). The outcome of ARDS has not changed dramatically over the past 20 years, although diagnostic criteria may be selecting more severely ill patients. The pathogenesis and outcome of ARDS is discussed in more detail in Chapter 18.

Current recommendations for ventilatory management in ARDS are to reduce plateau pressure even at the expense of an elevated $PaCO_2$, minimize FIO_2, and provide an adequate level of PEEP (Table 11–3). Lung injury in ARDS is not uniform, and the small fraction of compliant lung capable of gas exchange should be protected from excessive inflation pressure. If possible, plateau pressure should be limited to below 35 to 40 cm H_2O by reducing tidal volumes to 5 to 7 ml/kg. Because the pressure responsible for alveolar overdistention is the transpulmonary and not transrespiratory pressure, in the patient with a noncompliant chest wall (e.g., massive ascites), higher airway pressures may be accepted. Pressure limitation may be achieved in a number of ways, including conventional volume ventilation (often requiring sedation and paralysis), pressure-control ventilation with or without inverse ratio, or low-frequency positive-pressure ventilation with extracorporeal CO_2 removal. Low tidal volumes may result in alveolar hypoventilation and a rise in $PaCO_2$. The permissive hypercapnia is generally well tolerated, as described earlier.

Lung injury due to low airway pressure (inadequate PEEP) is becoming recognized as a potential cause of deterioration in ARDS. This observation is based largely on results of animal studies demonstrating significant lung injury during low-pressure ventilation without PEEP, which is likely to be due to the shear stresses associated with repeated opening and closing of alveoli (Muscedere et al, 1994). A level of PEEP should be chosen that is above the lower inflection point on the pressure-volume curve. An adequate level of PEEP is also essential to improve oxygenation and lung compliance. A randomized clinical trial using a strategy of PEEP greater than inflection point and limiting peak pressures has recently been shown to improve lung recovery and mortality in ARDS (Amato et al, 1995; 1996).

In addition to optimizing ventilatory settings, various other maneuvers have been used to improve oxygenation and alveolar ventilation. Use of the prone position may benefit oxygenation by a number of mechanisms, including increasing blood flow through well-aerated previously nonde-

---

Table 11–3
A Suggested Lung Protective Ventilatory Strategy

Tidal volume	5–7 ml/kg
PEEP	Usually 8–12 cm H_2O (keep above lower inflection point on static pressure-volume curve)
Recruitment maneuver	Inspiratory pause of 10–20 sec at 30–35 cm H_2O or periodic 12 ml/kg tidal volume breaths, to be used initially and after circuit disconnects
Airway pressure	Plateau pressure <35 cm H_2O unless high chest wall compliance (e.g., massive ascites)
Arterial PCO_2	Accept 50–80 mm Hg or higher if adequate oxygenation and pH>7.1

Data from Amato MBP, Barbas CSV, Medeiros DM, et al: Beneficial effects of the "open lung approach" with low distending pressures in acute respiratory distress syndrome. Am J Respir Crit Care Med 152:1835–1846, 1995; and Marini JJ: Pressure-targeted, lung-protective ventilatory support in acute lung injury. Chest 105[Suppl]:109S–114S, 1994.

pendent areas. Nitric oxide (NO) may have dramatic effects on oxygenation in a certain subset of patients. Although some of these patients have pulmonary hypertension, improvement in oxygenation with NO is not necessarily confined to these patients. Currently, tracheal insufflation of gas can be used to decrease dead space and reduce hypercapnia, or reduce the tidal volume required to achieve a given level of $PaCO_2$.

Obstructive Airway Disease

The predominant pathophysiologic abnormality in patients with obstructive airway disease is expiratory airflow limitation. This abnormality results in the development of hyperinflation and complications related to elevated intrathoracic pressure, such as barotrauma and hemodynamic collapse. Resistance to inspiration also occurs in asthmatics, resulting in markedly elevated peak airway pressures. The objective in mechanical ventilation should be to maximize expiratory time to reduce end-expiratory lung volume and auto-PEEP. This may be achieved by increasing inspiratory flow rates, although at the expense of increased peak airway pressures. It should be remembered that in patients with airways obstruction, there is a large inspiratory gradient between the proximal airway pressure measured in the ventilator circuit and pressure in peripheral airways likely to cause barotrauma. Thus, elevated peak inflation pressures measured in the ventilator circuit or even in the trachea are not necessarily transmitted to the alveolus; the risk of barotrauma is somewhat less than that for a similarly elevated plateau pressure. Hence, following plateau pressures is a better means for assessing the risk of barotrauma.

No evidence demonstrates an improved outcome with any particular ventilatory mode. Adequate peak flows should be set to meet patient demands and maximize expiratory time. Dynamic hyperinflation should be minimized; although increasing expiratory time is important, of most value is the reduction in minute volume to the lowest acceptable level. In severe airflow limitation this may require controlled hypoventilation with permissive hypercapnia. The development of hemodynamic compromise due to auto-PEEP should be managed by a reduction in minute volume and fluid therapy. Sedation and/or paralysis may be useful to reduce ventilation pressures and eliminate active expiration, which can cause airway collapse.

During weaning of the patient with obstructive airways disease, the presence of auto-PEEP may require increased work of breathing to trigger breaths. The increased work can be overcome by the application of extrinsic PEEP at a level lower than the measured auto-PEEP. PEEP above this level may aggravate the dynamic hyperinflation (Marini, 1989).

Bronchopleural Fistula

Although the majority of bronchopleural fistulae are physiologically insignificant, a large air leak can affect lung inflation and interfere with gas exchange. Treatment usually requires resolution of the underlying disease, although sometimes surgical repair may be possible. The objectives of ventilatory support are to ensure adequate ventilation but minimize inflation pressure to facilitate closure of the leak (Pierson, 1982).

No particular mode of ventilation has been shown to be more effective than another in the management of a bronchopleural fistula. Permissive hypercapnia may be necessary to minimize inspiratory pressures and reduce air leak. In the presence of a large air leak, high inspiratory flow rates with large tidal volumes may be necessary. Where difficulty is encountered in adequately achieving lung inflation, or when ventilation or oxygenation are inadequate, independent lung ventilation using two ventilators may be attempted. An alternative approach is the use of high-frequency jet ventilation.

TECHNICAL ASPECTS

Pneumatic Source

Delivery of gas by a ventilator requires a pressurized gas source, a means of blending an appropriate oxygen concentration, and a system for regulating pressure and flow. Air and oxygen are usually provided from a bulk gas delivery system, although some ventilators have internal compressors for air delivery. Air and oxygen are blended to achieve the desired concentration between 21 and 100% oxygen, using proportional valves or proportional solenoid valves. Some ventilators use an accumulator or mixing chamber before delivery of gas to the patient. This has potential disadvantages if used with a proximal NO delivery system, because the formation of toxic nitrogen dioxide is enhanced by prolonged contact between oxygen and NO.

Inspiratory flow and pressure may be regulated in a number of ways. Anesthesia machines commonly use a compressor-bellows system to deliver gas, and a piston is used in the proportional-assist ventilator. The newer microprocessor-controlled ventilators use various systems to control the flow of gas produced by the ventilator working pressure. A scissors valve controlled by a stepper motor can be used to regulate flow through a silicon tube, or proportional solenoids can control flow, functioning as either flow controllers or pressure controllers.

Monitoring

Modern microprocessor ventilators are capable of monitoring and generating an alarm on numerous patient and patient-ventilator variables. Multiple variables triggering false-positive alarms may produce many unnecessary alarms, ultimately resulting in medical personnel ignoring these warnings. Hierarchies of alarms, in terms of necessity for immediate response, have been developed. At the top of the hierarchy are loss of power, loss of gas source, apnea, and circuit-disconnect alarms. Pressure monitoring allows display of mean and peak pressures and facilitates circuit leak/disconnect and high-pressure alarms. Flow monitoring is achieved by a variety of methods and allows measurement of flow as well as volume, by integrating flow over time. This allows display of spontaneous and mechanical tidal and minute ventilation. Measurements based on pressure and flow recordings include graphs of pressure, flow, or volume versus time; pressure-volume and flow-volume loops; auto-PEEP measurements; and pulmonary system compliance estimation. Measurement of exhaled CO_2 may be used to estimate $PaCO_2$ and to calculate and monitor dead space.

Monitoring of a number of other nonventilator patient variables has become a standard of practice during mechanical ventilation (Marini, 1988). Pulse oximetry provides a continuous assessment of oxygenation and can be used to alert the medical staff to problems resulting in hypoxemia. Pulse oximetry reduces the need for evaluating arterial blood gases, but these are still required for assessment of acid-base status and $PaCO_2$. Transcutaneous measurement of CO_2 is available but not always accurate, particularly at higher levels. Invasive hemodynamic monitoring is sometimes used to optimize mechanical ventilation, particularly for assessing the effect of PEEP on cardiac output and oxygen delivery. Close clinical observation as well as standard intensive care monitoring such as by electrocardiogram (ECG) and blood pressure measurement remain an essential part of management (Table 11–4).

Humidification and Circuits

The ventilator circuit consists of components necessary for filtration and humidification of inspired gas, and tubing necessary for delivery of gas to the patient and for return of exhaled gas to the atmosphere. Endotracheal intubation bypasses the upper airways responsible for warming and humidifying inspired gas, and these functions must therefore occur in the ventilator circuit. Inadequate humidification may result in epithelial damage, loss of ciliary function, and mucosal ulceration. Several types of humidifiers may be used to condition inspired gas to a relative humidity of 95 to 100% at 32 to 34°C. Gas may simply be passed over a water surface (passover humidifier) or bubbled through water (cascade humidifier). The temperature of the water in all these systems can be servo-controlled, with a thermistor placed at the patient's proximal airway. Heated ventilator circuits can be used to more precisely control the temperature of the gas delivered to the patient and to prevent condensation occurring in the tubing. An important issue with regard to humidifiers is the resistance of the humidifier to gas

---

Table 11–4
Monitoring During Mechanical Ventilation

Ventilator Variables	Nonventilator Variables
Gas source, FIO_2	Gas exchange
Airway pressure	Arterial oxygen tension or saturation
Peak, plateau, mean	Arterial $PaCO_2$, pH
PEEP (external, auto)	Hemodynamic monitoring
Circuit disconnect/leak	Blood pressure
Pressure wave form	Cardiac output
Apnea	Oxygen delivery
Flow/volume	Urine output
Tidal volume	Chest radiograph
Minute volume	Endotracheal tube position
Respiratory frequency	Barotrauma, pneumonia
Flow wave form	ECG monitoring

flow, which may affect triggering and work of breathing. Artificial noses act as heat and moisture exchangers but have the disadvantage of increasing circuit resistance.

The ventilator circuit influences the efficacy of mechanical ventilation by contributing to airflow resistance, producing a compression volume, and contributing to the development of nosocomial pneumonia (see Chapter 21). Circuit resistance is important during spontaneous modes of ventilation, and endotracheal tube resistance plays a significant role (Bersten et al, 1989). Endotracheal tube resistance is especially important with smaller (≤8 mm internal diameter [ID]) endotracheal tubes and high flow rates associated with rapid breathing. The amount of effort required to activate gas delivery varies among the demand valves of different ventilators and may impose significant work of breathing. Some of the effects of circuit resistance may be overcome by low triggering sensitivity and rapid response times. Compression volume represents the volume of delivered tidal volume that is lost due to distention of the inspiratory circuit, and is affected by the volume of the circuit, the compliance of the tubing, and the pressure in the circuit. Compression volume may become clinically relevant at high inflation pressures with low tidal volumes. The displayed exhaled tidal volume overestimates the patient's tidal volume by an amount equal to the compression volume. Newer microprocessor ventilators can correct for this factor.

Mechanical ventilation in intubated patients is associated with a high risk of nosocomial infection, with significant morbidity and mortality. Traditionally ventilator circuits have been considered a potential cause, but contaminated condensate usually originates from the patient rather than the ventilator. Circuit changing protocols have evolved from daily to every 48 hours or even weekly. There is some evidence that circuit changes are unnecessary, unless the circuits are grossly contaminated (Dreyfuss et al, 1991).

COMPLICATIONS

INTUBATION

Endotracheal intubation may produce complications related to local trauma or tube misplacement. The disruption of normal protective mechanisms may predispose the patient to nosocomial infection. The nasal or oral route may be used for intubation, the nasal route improving comfort in some patients. However, there is an increased risk of bleeding on insertion of a nasal

tube, and sinusitis may occur as a result of ostial occlusion. Nasal tubes are usually narrower, increasing airway resistance. Glottic injury may occur during insertion of the endotracheal tube and as a result of prolonged intubation. High cuff inflation pressures (>25 cm H_2O) may cause ischemic ulceration, predisposing to glottic stenosis. Tracheostomy may provide some protection from glottic injury and is usually reserved for patients with an expected duration of ventilation greater than 2 to 3 weeks. This procedure has the benefits of enhancing patient comfort, improving secretion clearance, and allowing oral feeding. Potentially life-threatening complications of tracheostomy include extubation with loss of the airway in the early postoperative period and innominate artery hemorrhage as a later complication.

Malpositioning of the endotracheal tube, commonly into the right mainstem bronchus, produces overdistention of the ventilated lung and atelectasis on the nonintubated lung. This may result in hypoxemia, barotrauma, and hemodynamic compromise. Inadvertent extubation is a potentially dangerous complication, occurring commonly in the disoriented or uncooperative patient.

The presence of an artificial airway disrupts normal pulmonary protective mechanisms. Although gross aspiration is prevented by a cuffed endotracheal tube, pharyngeal secretions may nevertheless enter the trachea, resulting in colonization and increasing the risk for nosocomial pneumonia (Pingleton, 1988). The coughing mechanism and mucociliary escalator are impeded, encouraging the retention of secretions. Nosocomial pneumonia occurs in about 30% of patients being mechanically ventilated (the risk increasing with duration of ventilation), and is associated with an increased in mortality (Fagon et al, 1989).

POSITIVE PRESSURE

Barotrauma

High ventilating pressures and regional lung overdistention due to high tidal volumes can produce localized alveolar air leaks with the development of interstitial emphysema, leading to pneumothorax, pneumomediastinum, and subcutaneous emphysema. Lung cyst formation has been documented mainly in nondependent zones (Stewart et al, 1993). Susceptibility to barotrauma varies with lung compliance and the stage of disease, with an increased frequency after prolonged ventilation (Haake et al, 1987). Pre-existing acute and chronic lung disease predisposes to barotrauma.

Sudden respiratory distress associated with high ventilator pressures should alert the physician to the presence of a pneumothorax, particularly if it is associated with hemodynamic collapse. Chest radiograph diagnosis of a pneumothorax may occasionally be difficult because of the supine positioning of the patient. Management involves drainage of the pneumothorax via a percutaneous chest tube, but healing of injured lung may be delayed, resulting in a persistent bronchopleural fistula.

Ventilator-induced Lung Injury

A number of animal studies have demonstrated that large tidal volumes or high inflation pressures can produce or exacerbate lung injury (Dreyfuss et al, 1988; Parker et al, 1993). Pathologically, this is associated with granulocyte infiltration and changes of diffuse alveolar damage. It is becoming recognized that ARDS is not a diffuse disease, but it usually is a dependent airspace disease with nondependent areas of relatively normal lung (Gattinoni et al, 1988). The inflation capacity of the lung is markedly reduced, and overdistention of the aerated portion of the lung may produce alveolar damage. It is likely that overdistention rather than high pressure is responsible for the injurious effect. Ventilation with low tidal volumes (5 to 7 ml/kg), keeping peak airway pressure less than 35 cm H_2O, may be associated with less ventilator-induced injury and improved outcome (Hickling et al, 1990, 1994; Amato, 1995). The ventilatory strategies that have been used include permissive hypercapnia, inverse ratio ventilation, tracheal gas insufflation, extracorporeal CO_2 removal (ECCO$_2$R), and high-frequency ventilation. Adequate alveolar recruitment may necessitate initial or periodic inflations at maximal pressure (35 cm H_2O) with prolonged inspiratory pause and adequate PEEP to maintain recruited volume (Amato et al, 1995). PEEP may of itself be protective, reducing lung injury due to the shear stresses associated with repeated opening and closing of alveoli (Muscedere et al, 1994). A randomized controlled study of a pressure-limited ventilatory strategy has shown a clear benefit in terms of lung function, lung recovery, and outcome (Amato et al, 1995; 1996). Larger studies are currently in progress to confirm these findings.

Cardiovascular Effects

Chapter 4 reviews basic principles of heart-lung interactions relative to understanding changes in cardiac output during ventilation. Positive-pressure ventilation may impair cardiac output by reducing venous return and right ventricular preload (Pinsky, 1990). The degree to which alveolar pressure is transmitted to the pleural space is dependent on lung and chest wall compliance—hemodynamic effects are accentuated with compliant lungs and a stiff chest wall. Volume depletion and impaired cardiovascular reflexes aggravate the hemodynamic deterioration. The effects are noted most significantly in the patient with obstructive airway disease and auto-PEEP. Management involves a reduction in mean airway pressure and minute ventilation, concomitant with fluid resuscitation.

Sustained increases in intrathoracic pressure affect left ventricular function by reducing left ventricular afterload. In the presence of poor LV function, the cardiac output may increase in response to positive intrathoracic pressure, owing to the significant benefit of these afterloading decreasing effects. The increased cardiac output is most notable in patients with high filling pressures and is beneficial in the management of patients with heart failure (see Chapter 15).

Asynchrony

Increased work of breathing, hypoventilation, and barotrauma may result from poor interaction between the clinician-set ventilation pattern and the patient's natural breathing rhythm. Problems with patient-ventilator asynchrony, manifesting as the patient "fighting" the ventilator, occur more commonly with excessive circuit resistance, high triggering threshold, delayed ventilator response, and insufficient flow capacity to meet patient requirements. Demand valve function, response time, and triggering mechanisms vary between ventilators and may significantly influence efficacy. The mode of ventilation may also play a role, with synchronized modes (SIMV) having obvious advantages over controlled ventilation. The development of auto-PEEP increases the triggering threshold and contributes to increased work of breathing.

Slow inspiratory flow rates may be associated with increased work of breathing resulting from the patient's active inspiratory effort. Inadequate flow can be identified by examining the airway pressure versus time wave form (Tobin, 1994). A smooth convex appearance suggests adequate flow, whereas a scalloped tracing indicates inadequate flow (Fig. 11–3) relative to patient inspiratory effort. Ventilator-patient asynchrony may result when the patient begins expiration before the ventilator tidal volume has been delivered. Pressure-preset ventilatory modes allow flow rates to be determined by patient requirements, but these

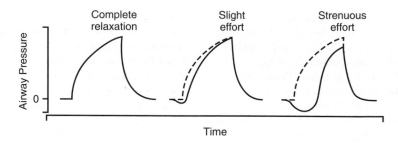

Figure 11–3

Airway pressure wave forms during assist-control ventilation. With no patient effort, a convex inspiratory pattern is present, but with increasing patient effort and inadequate inspiratory flow, a concave wave form is noted (From Tobin M: Mechanical ventilation. N Engl J Med 330:1058, copyright 1994; Massachusetts Medical Society.)

modes are also subject to problems and limitations. Rapid breathing rates can result in reduced tidal volumes, particularly with the development of auto-PEEP.

If maneuvers to correct patient-ventilator asynchrony fail, the final alternative is sedation and neuromuscular blockade. This eliminates the patient's contribution to ventilation and can reduce airway pressures, improve minute ventilation, and reduce oxygen consumption. These pharmacologic interventions nevertheless carry significant complications of their own (see later).

SEDATION AND PARALYSIS

Varying degrees of sedation are required during mechanical ventilation to allow patient comfort and reduce patient-ventilator asynchrony. Neuromuscular blockade immobilizes the patient and may be necessary to facilitate ventilatory strategies such as inverse ratio ventilation and permissive hypercapnia, or to reduce oxygen consumption. Sedative drugs often cause vasodilation and contribute to the hypotension and reduced cardiac output accompanying positive-pressure ventilation. Sedation and paralysis immobilize patients, subjecting them to the risks of pressure necrosis of the skin, deep venous thrombosis, retention of secretions, and atelectasis. Suppression of spontaneous respiratory efforts makes the patient totally dependent on the ventilator, and inadvertent disconnection from the ventilator can have disastrous consequences. Prompt attention must be given to ventilator alarms in this situation.

Immobilization can predispose to atrophy of muscles of respiration as well as peripheral musculature. A number of neuromuscular blocking agents have been associated with prolonged weakness persisting after withdrawal of treatment (Hansen-Flaschen et al, 1993). The mechanism is

unclear, but recommendations are to limit the depth of paralysis and allow frequent withdrawals from therapy. This phenomenon appears to be particularly common in asthmatics treated with muscle relaxants and corticosteroids (Douglass et al, 1992).

OTHER COMPLICATIONS

Various other complications may occur in patients on mechanical ventilation, which are related directly to this intervention, to the underlying illness, or to the ICU environment. Significant psychological stress and confusion may occur, which is related to sleep deprivation, pain, inability to communicate, and use of drugs. Renal dysfunction is believed to occur as a result of reduced intravascular volume, producing generalized fluid retention. The gastrointestinal effects of mechanical ventilation include bowel distention due to aerophagia, constipation due to drugs and immobility, and mucosal ulceration and bleeding. Increased intrathoracic pressure can elevate intracranial pressure and reduce cerebral perfusion. Venous thromboembolism and pressure necrosis of the skin may result from prolonged immobilization.

WEANING

Once the cause for acute respiratory failure has resolved, mechanical ventilation may be discontinued. In the patient with complete and rapid reversal of the predisposing cause, the ventilator may be disconnected after a trial of spontaneous breathing (e.g., T-piece trial). In those in whom recovery is incomplete, or after prolonged ventilation with loss of respiratory muscle strength and endurance, a period of gradual withdrawal or weaning is necessary.

Training periods of high-intensity work, followed by adequate periods of rest, may improve respiratory muscle function but can require several weeks. Fatigue must be avoided by close observation for signs of distress such as tachypnea, paradoxical abdominal motion, or respiratory alternans. Different techniques are available for the gradual withdrawal of ventilator support, each with potential advantages and disadvantages.

Appropriate timing of removal of the endotracheal tube is important in that early extubation may result in respiratory failure and necessitate reintubation, whereas unnecessarily prolonging intubation increases costs and the risk of complications. The ease of discontinuation and reapplication of ventilation with noninvasive ventilation or tracheostomy have significant benefits in this regard.

PREREQUISITES FOR WEANING

Respiratory Factors

The respiratory factors that determine the ability to discontinue mechanical ventilation are the capacity of the respiratory neuromuscular system to cope with the respiratory load and adequacy of oxygenation. Respiratory center and phrenic nerve dysfunction are uncommon problems, and the major site of failure is at the level of the respiratory muscles. Respiratory load is determined by respiratory resistance and compliance and the presence of auto-PEEP. Measurement of respiratory work and assessment of respiratory muscle fatigue are complex and are not of great clinical value. Clinically relevant measures that are used to assess the likelihood of weaning include tidal volume, respiratory rate, spontaneous minute ventilation, vital capacity, and maximal inspiratory force. In general, these factors are nonspecific and insensitive in predicting weaning success. Nevertheless, a low respiratory work load can be inferred by the presence of adequate gas exchange at a minute ventilation of less than 10 l/min and a respiratory rate of less than 25/min. The vital capacity and maximal inspiratory force may act as indices of muscle strength and the ability to cough and clear secretions. Various indices (Table 11–5) have been developed with varying predictive ability, such as the frequency/tidal volume ratio and an integrated index using compliance, rate, oxygenation, and pressure (Yang and Tobin, 1991).

By the time discontinuation of ventilation is considered, oxygenation problems have usually resolved. Although indices such as the PaO_2/FIO_2 ratio may be used, adequate oxygenation at an inspired oxygen concentration of less than 50% usually suffices.

Reversal or improvement in the respiratory problem necessitating ventilation is an obvious prerequisite for discontinuation of ventilation. It is equally important that secondary complications such as nosocomial pneumonia and heart failure have resolved before initiating weaning.

Airway Factors

Endotracheal intubation may have been performed to enable ventilation for respiratory failure, or to provide an adequate airway where airway patency was compromised or for tracheobronchial toilet. Before removal of the endotracheal tube, the upper airway and the patient's

---

Table 11–5
Parameters Used to Predict Weaning Success

Test	Value Predictive of Weaning Success	Positive Predictive Value	Negative Predictive Value
Minute ventilation	≤15 L/min	0.55	0.38
Respiratory frequency	≤38/min	0.65	0.77
Tidal volume	≥325 ml	0.73	0.94
Maximal inspiratory pressure	≤ −15 cm H_2O	0.59	1.0
PaO_2/PAO_2 ratio	≥0.35	0.59	0.53
Frequency/tidal volume	≤105 breath/min per liter	0.78	0.95
CROP score*	≥13 ml/breath per minute	0.71	0.70
Weaning index†	<4/min	0.96	0.95

Data from Jabour ER, Rabil DM, Truwit JD, et al: Evaluation of a new weaning index based on ventilatory endurance and the efficiency of gas exchange. Am Rev Respir Dis 144:531, 1991; and Yang KL, and Tobin MJ: A prospective study of indexes predicting the outcome of trials of weaning from mechanical ventilation. N Engl J Med 324:1445, 1991.

*CROP determined by dynamic compliance, maximum inspiratory pressure, rate, and oxygenation.

†Weaning index calculated from a modified pressure-time index and the minute ventilation required to attain a $PaCO_2$ of 40 mm Hg.

ability to clear secretions must be evaluated. This includes an assessment of the level of consciousness, upper airway edema, ability to cough, and quantity of secretions. Pre-existing airway problems must be alleviated before extubation.

Other Factors

Nonrespiratory factors may play an important role in failure to wean or to tolerate discontinuation of ventilation. Cardiovascular disease may have an impact on respiratory function, with impaired cardiovascular performance affecting oxygen supply to respiratory muscles. The development of pulmonary edema due to loss of positive intrathoracic pressure or to myocardial ischemia may be responsible for failure to wean.

Other factors to consider before discontinuing ventilation are the patient's level of consciousness and cooperation, and presence of unresolved nonrespiratory conditions, electrolyte disturbances, and nutritional status. Although much emphasis is given to respiratory variables, it is often these other issues that are responsible for unsuccessful weaning.

TECHNIQUES

Oxygenation support is often weaned before consideration is given to weaning ventilatory support. This involves a reduction of inspired oxygen concentration to a level that can easily be delivered by face mask (e.g., 50%) and reducing PEEP levels. PEEP is usually reduced slowly (e.g., in increments of 2–3 cm H_2O) to a level of about 5 cm H_2O while monitoring oxygen saturation. Ventilatory support is then gradually reduced by one of the methods described later, monitoring for signs of ventilatory distress or fatigue, such as tachypnea, agitation, diaphoresis, or respiratory acidosis.

Until recently few data were available comparing the various weaning modes. However, two randomized studies have addressed this issue. Weaning failure occurred less commonly and weaning duration was shorter using pressure-support weaning, compared with SIMV or T-piece weaning, in a study of 109 patients (Brochard et al, 1994). In contrast, in another study of 130 patients, a daily 2-hour T-piece trial was demonstrated to have a lower failure rate and duration of ventilation than other weaning modes (Esteban et al, 1995). The different outcomes of these studies most likely is related to differences in protocols for weaning and the objective criteria for extubation and weaning failure. Thus, further studies are needed to draw firm conclusions concerning the best mode of weaning under different circumstances.

T-piece Weaning

Weaning using a T-piece involves discontinuation of ventilation with the patient being allowed to breathe spontaneously through the endotracheal tube by means of a T-piece. The duration of the intermittent T-piece trials is gradually increased (e.g., 30 minutes, 60 minutes), ensuring that the patient does not develop fatigue. Adequate rest periods must be allowed between trials. The aim is to increase respiratory muscle strength and endurance until the patient can tolerate unassisted spontaneous breathing. The T-piece provides no support to overcome ventilator circuit resistance. Alternatively, a daily 2-hour T-piece trial can be used to assess the patient's ability to sustain spontaneous breathing and to decide whether to extubate or continue ventilation for a further 24 hours (Esteban et al, 1995).

SIMV Weaning

An alternative approach involves using SIMV and gradually reducing the ventilator rate, with the patient gradually increasing the amount of respiratory work performed. The rate of decrease in the SIMV is determined by clinical assessment and arterial blood gas levels. Although the ventilator provides support during this gradual weaning, breathing through the demand valve of the IMV circuit can produce a significant increase in work of breathing. Prolonged periods of breathing at low ventilator rates can result in muscle fatigue, which must be avoided.

Pressure-support Weaning

Pressure-support weaning involves gradually reducing the level of pressure delivered, allowing the patient to take over an increasing amount of respiratory work. Pressure may be reduced by 2 cm H_2O several times daily, while staff assess the patient for signs of fatigue. The pressure support is reduced to a level that is believed to overcome ventilator-induced work of breathing (circuit and valve resistance), at which point extubation is considered. This level of pressure support varies between about 5 and 12 cm H_2O, depending on the ventilator and endotracheal tube size. In practice, weaning protocols combining SIMV and pressure support are commonly used.

REFERENCES

Abou-Shala N and Meduri U: Noninvasive mechanical ventilation in patients with acute respiratory failure. Crit Care Med 24:705–715, 1996.

Amato MBP, Barbas CSV, Medeiros DM, et al: Beneficial effects of the "open lung approach" with low distending pressures in acute respiratory distress syndrome. Am J Respir Crit Care Med 152:1835–1846, 1995.

Amato MBP, Barbas CSV, Medeiros DM, et al: Improved survival in ARDS: Beneficial effects of a lung protective strategy. Am J Respir Crit Care Med 153:A531, 1996.

Bersten AD, Rutten AJ, Vedig AE, and Skowronski GA: Additional work of breathing imposed by endotracheal tubes, breathing circuits, and intensive care ventilators. Crit Care Med 17:671–677, 1989.

Bersten AD, Holt AW, Vedig AE, et al: Treatment of severe cardiogenic pulmonary edema with continuous positive airway pressure delivered by face mask. N Engl J Med 325:1825–1830, 1991.

Blanch PB, Jones M, Layon AJ, and Camner N: Pressure-preset ventilation. Part 1: Physiologic and mechanical considerations. Chest 104:590–599, 1993.

Bott J, Carroll MP, Conway JH, et al: Randomised controlled trial of nasal ventilation in acute ventilatory failure due to chronic obstructive airways disease. Lancet 341:1555–1557, 1993.

Brochard L, Rauss A, Benito S, et al: Comparison of three methods of gradual withdrawal from ventilatory support during weaning from mechanical ventilation. Am J Respir Crit Care Med 150:896–903, 1994.

Brochard L, Mancebo J, Wysocki M, et al: Noninvasive ventilation for acute exacerbations of chronic obstructive pulmonary disease. N Engl J Med 333:817–822, 1995.

Burke WC, Crooke PS, Marcy TW, et al: Comparison of mathematical and mechanical models of pressure-controlled ventilation. J Appl Physiol 74:922–933, 1993.

Darioli R and Perret C: Mechanical controlled hypoventilation in status asthmaticus. Am Rev Respir Dis 129:385–387, 1984.

Douglass JA, Tuxen DV, Horne M, et al: Myopathy in severe asthma. Am Rev Respir Dis 146:517–519, 1992.

Dreyfuss D, Soler P, Basset G, et al: High inflation pressure pulmonary edema. Respective effects of high airway pressure, high tidal volume, and positive end-expiratory pressure. Am Rev Respir Dis 137:1159–1164, 1988.

Dreyfuss D, Djedaini K, Weber P, et al: Prospective study of nosocomial pneumonia and of patient and circuit colonization during mechanical ventilation with circuit changes every 48 hours versus no change. Am Rev Respir Dis 143:738–743, 1991.

Esteban A, Frutos F, Tobin MJ, et al: A comparison of four methods of weaning patients from mechanical ventilation. N Engl J Med 332:345–350, 1995.

Fagon JY, Chastre J, Domart Y, et al: Nosocomial pneumonia in patients receiving continuous mechanical ventilation: Prospective analysis of 52 episodes with use of a protected specimen brush and quantitative culture techniques. Am Rev Respir Dis 139:877–884, 1989.

Feihl F and Perret C: Permissive hypercapnia: How permissive should we be? Am J Respir Crit Care Med 150:1722–1737, 1994.

Gattinoni L, Pesenti A, Caspani ML, et al: The role of static lung compliance in the management of severe ARDS unresponsive to conventional treatment. Intensive Care Med 10:121–126, 1984.

Gattinoni L, Pesenti A, Bombino M, et al: Relationships between lung computed tomographic density, gas exchange, and PEEP in acute respiratory failure. Anesthesiology 69:824–832, 1988.

Haake R, Schlichtig R, Ulstad DR, et al: Barotrauma. Pathophysiology, risk factors, and prevention. Chest 91:608–613, 1987.

Hansen-Flaschen J, Cowen J, and Raps EC: Neuromuscular blockade in the intensive care unit. More than we bargained for. Am Rev Respir Dis 147:234–236, 1993.

Hickling KG, Henderson SJ, and Jackson R: Low mortality associated with low volume pressure limited ventilation with permissive hypercapnia in severe adult respiratory distress syndrome. Intensive Care Med 16:372–377, 1990.

Hickling KG, Walsh J, Henderson S, and Jackson R: Low mortality rate in adult respiratory distress syndrome using low-volume, pressure limited ventilation with permissive hypercapnia: A prospective study. Crit Care Med 22:1568–1578, 1994.

Jabour ER, Rabil DM, Truwit JD, et al: Evaluation of a new weaning index based on ventilatory endurance and the efficiency of gas exchange. Am Rev Respir Dis 144:531, 1991.

Kollef MH and Schuster DP: The acute respiratory distress syndrome. N Engl J Med 332:27–37, 1995.

Malo J, Ali J, and Wood LD: How does positive end-expiratory pressure reduce intrapulmonary shunt in canine pulmonary edema? J Appl Physiol 57:1002–1010, 1984.

Marini JJ: Monitoring during mechanical ventilation. Clin Chest Med 9:73–100, 1988.

Marini JJ: Should PEEP be used in airflow obstruction? Am Rev Respir Dis 140:1–3, 1989.

Marini JJ: Pressure-targeted, lung-protective ventilatory support in acute lung injury. Chest 105[Suppl]:109S–114S, 1994.

Marini JJ, Crooke PS, and Truwit JD: Determinants and limits of pressure-preset ventilation: A mathematical model of pressure control. J Appl Physiol 67:1081–1092, 1989.

Menitove SM and Goldring RM: Combined ventilator and bicarbonate strategy in the management of status asthmaticus. Am J Med 74:898–901, 1983.

Muscedere JG, Mullen JBM, Gan K, and Slutsky AS: Tidal ventilation at low airway pressures can augment lung injury. Am J Respir Crit Care Med 149:1327–1334, 1994.

Parker JC, Hernandez LA, and Peevy KJ: Mechanisms of ventilator induced lung injury. Crit Care Med 21:131–143, 1993.

Pierson DJ: Persistent bronchopleural air leak during mechanical ventilation. Respir Care 27:408, 1982.

Pingleton SK: Complications of acute respiratory failure. Am Rev Respir Dis 137:1463–1493, 1988.

Pinsky MR: The effects of mechanical ventilation on the cardiovascular system. Crit Care Clin 6:663–678, 1990.

Prys-Roberts C, Kelman GR, Greenbaum R, et al: Hemodynamics and alveolar-arterial PO_2 differences at varying $PaCO_2$ in anesthetized man. J Appl Physiol 25:80–87, 1968.

Slutsky AS: Nonconventional methods of ventilation. Am Rev Respir Dis 138:175–183, 1988.

Slutsky AS: Mechanical ventilation. Chest 104:1833–1859, 1993.

Stewart TE, Toth JL, Higgins RJ, et al: Barotrauma in severe ARDS is greatest in non dependent lung regions: Evaluation by computed tomography. Crit Care Med 21:S284, 1993.

Suter PM, Fairley HB, and Isenberg MD: Optimum end-expiratory airway pressure in patients with acute pulmonary failure. N Engl J Med 292:284–289, 1975.

Tobin M: Mechanical ventilation. N Engl J Med 330:1058, 1994.

Viswanathan R, Lodi ST, Subramian S, et al: Pulmonary vascular response to ventilation hypercapnia in man: Contribution of hypercapnia and hypoxia to vascular response to ischemia. Clin Sci 39:203–222, 1970.

Yang KL and Tobin MJ: A prospective study of indexes predicting the outcome of trials of weaning from mechanical ventilation. N Engl J Med 324:1445, 1991.

Younes M: Proportional assist ventilation, a new approach to ventilatory support. Am Rev Respir Dis 145:114–120, 1992.

CHAPTER 12

Ventilatory Control in the Critical Care Setting

Peggy McGinnis Simon, M.D.

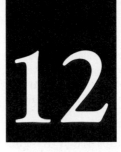

The rate and intensity of patients' inspiratory efforts vary not only over time but also from breath to breath. The respiratory controller's responses to mechanical ventilation depend on both the mode and settings of ventilation. During controlled mechanical ventilation (CMV), the machine breaths are ventilator-initiated, whereas during assisted ventilation, the machine breaths are triggered by the patient's inspiratory efforts.

In the clinical setting, mechanical ventilation in the assist-control mode becomes CMV when patients are paralyzed or hyperventilated (particularly during non-rapid eye movement [NREM] sleep). In general, CMV is not a clinically useful mode in an unsedated patient for the obvious reasons: lack of patient comfort, frequent poor patient-ventilator synchrony, and increased work of breathing. Another drawback is minute ventilation that remains constant despite changing patient needs. However, CMV (by disabling sensitivity/trigger mechanisms) has been useful in studying respiratory controller responses of humans to periodic imposed lung inflations that are externally controlled. Control is achieved by setting constant machine tidal volume, inspiratory flow, and machine rate, therefore eliminating feedback-response interactions.

Patients are usually placed on an assist mode with a mandatory backup rate. Depending on the backup rate, patients alternate between assisted breaths (i.e., patient-triggered breaths) and controlled breaths. To date, information is lacking on the effect of alternating between patient-initiated and machine-initiated breaths on respiratory controller output and, ultimately, on ventilation.

Assist modes of ventilation have also been useful in the laboratory setting to examine the response of the respiratory controller when it is under the influence of feedback. Feedback as related to both active movement of the lung by contraction of inspiratory muscles and passive movement of air into the lungs by pressure generated from the ventilator are examined. To the extent that the output of the ventilator can influence the output of the respiratory pump and the output of the pump on that of the ventilator, there is considerable interaction between patient and ventilator. Studies of mechanically ventilated humans show that we have begun to gain additional insight into the interaction between the mechanical ventilator and the respiratory controller.

This chapter reviews that which is known about human respiratory control system responses to mechanical ventilation. The following sections provide the background for the major thrust of this review, which is to examine feedback response interactions (i.e., the interactive effects between the output of the ventilator and the output of the respiratory pump).

REVIEW OF NEURAL CONTROL OF BREATHING

Much of the available information on neural control of breathing has been derived from anesthetized animals. Our knowledge of respiratory control in normal humans is limited, but even scantier is the available information on respiratory control in patients with lung disease undergoing ventilatory support. The following is a brief review of the aspects of neural control of breathing relevant to patient-ventilator interactions.

RESPIRATORY RHYTHM AND PATTERN FORMATION

Populations of neurons that play a role in the generation of respiratory rhythm and in the formation of respiratory pattern have been identified in specific areas of the brainstem, but the mechanisms by which respiratory rhythm is generated are not entirely understood. Rhythm generation is the initial step in producing a patterned respiratory motor output. Models of respiratory rhythm generation range from "pacemaker"-driven to "neuronal networks" to hybrids of each model (Feldman and Smith, 1995; Feldman et al, 1990).

A network of medullary premotor neurons, the so-called central pattern generator for respiration, drives and coordinates the activity of respiratory motor neurons. Its output is modified by chemoreceptive and mechanoreceptive feedback. Whereas chemosensory input is important in regulating alveolar ventilation appropriate for acid-base homeostasis, mechanosensory signals are critical in adjusting, adapting, and integrating breathing with other brain and body activity.

Two separate control systems with different feedback are thought to exist: one system is charged with the initiation of the rhythm of respiration (timing) and the other is responsible for shaping the burst of activity (respiratory drive) as

it is developing (Feldman et al, 1990). The concept that neurons mediating changes in timing or rhythm are separate and anatomically distinct from those involved in modulating amplitude of motor activity or respiratory drive is still a presumption.

RESPIRATORY MOTONEURONS

Respiratory muscles are controlled by various motoneuron groups distributed in the brainstem and spinal cord. The respiratory motoneuron groups include spinal motoneurons that innervate pumping muscles (e.g., the diaphragm, intercostal, and abdominal muscles) and the cranial motoneurons that innervate muscles responsible for modulating airway resistance (e.g., laryngeal, pharyngeal, and bronchial muscles). The distribution of various types of input from brainstem central pattern generators may be relatively uniform or they may be selective for a specific respiratory motoneuron group or pool. Although monosynaptic input from the medullary respiratory group provides the major source of respiratory drive, polysynaptic input from sources such as propriospinal interneurons and nonrespiratory input from the cortex have also been identified (see the section on wakefulness vs. sleep effects).

DEFINING RESPIRATORY MOTOR OUTPUT AND DRIVE

To a neurobiologist, the amplitude or rate of rise in inspiratory neural activity and the timing of the respiratory phases are separate functions of the respiratory pattern generator, which are controlled by distinct systems. Phase switching or timing of the respiratory cycle is mediated by premotor neurons whose activity is shaped by mechanosensory feedback, whereas the rate of rise in motor activity is controlled by premotor neurons whose activity is shaped by chemosensory feedback. The use of terms such as *respiratory motor output* frequently ignores the distinction between these neuronal types. Throughout this chapter, the term *respiratory drive* is used to describe the rate of increase in inspiratory neural activity. The term *respiratory motor output* is synonymous with integrated neural output to the respiratory pump.

CHEMICAL FEEDBACK

Chemoreceptor feedback is essential to the regulation of breathing. Humans have two types of chemoreceptors that maintain chemical homeostasis. The carotid bodies are peripherally located and sense changes in oxygen (PaO_2), carbon dioxide ($PaCO_2$), and acid-base (pH) status of the arterial blood. They are particularly important in stimulating ventilation when PaO_2 is reduced. The second type of chemoreceptor is believed to be located on the ventrolateral surface of the medulla and is especially sensitive to changes in interstitial brain fluid pH from fluctuations in $PaCO_2$.

Ventilation rises in response to an increase in chemoreceptor activity, usually through a combination of increases in rate and tidal volume. In general, increasing the ventilation of normal, spontaneously breathing humans from resting levels up to moderate levels of stimulation elicits primarily a tidal volume response. With higher levels of respiratory stimulation, changes in respiratory rate (i.e., a frequency response) predominates. Both the mechanical properties of the respiratory system and gain of the vagal reflex influence the breathing pattern response to chemical stimuli. The extent to which these factors influence breathing responses in patients on ventilatory support needs further study.

Whether the patient's response to chemical stimuli is predominantly a frequency or tidal volume response is of particular importance to the way in which the patient interacts with the mechanical ventilator. Less is known about how mechanically ventilated patients respond to chemical stimuli (hypoxia, hypercapnia, and acidemia—i.e., frequency vs. tidal volume response). However, it is reasonable to infer that ventilatory support modes that allow tidal volume to rise in response to increases in inspiratory effort permit greater patient control over the $PaCO_2$. This topic is discussed in more detail under the section on effect of ventilator settings on ventilatory control.

MECHANOSENSORY FEEDBACK

Respiratory controller responses (such as respiratory rate and magnitude of respiratory muscle activation) are influenced by a wide array of reflexes originating from mechanoreceptors present in the airways, lung parenchyma, and chest wall. "Irritant" receptors in the airway stimulated by inhaled chemicals, particulates, or changes in bronchial smooth muscle can produce cough and may augment inspiration ("sighs") to maintain patent airways. Unmyelinated so-called C-fiber endings in the lung parenchyma cause tachypnea when they are stimulated by interstitial fluid.

Vagal Reflexes

Slowly adapting pulmonary stretch receptors (PSR) in the lung and airway sense the magnitude and rate of lung stretch via changes in transpulmonary pressure. PSR have been shown to have substantial effects on the rate and depth of breathing in animals (Petrillo et al, 1983; Vibert et al, 1981). Changes in tidal volume have reciprocal effects on inspiratory activity (i.e., as tidal volume decreases, inspiratory duration increases and when tidal volume increases, inspiratory duration decreases).

Although the relative importance of vagal influences on breathing in humans remains a topic of debate, the classic responses referred to as Breuer-Hering (BH) reflexes have been well described in humans. BH reflexes can be abolished by vagal blockade (Guz et al, 1964) and are absent in patients with lungs vagally denervated from transplantation (Iber et al, 1995).

Because BH reflexes in humans operate during single lung inflations, vagal afferent nerves are likely to mediate breathing responses during repeated lung inflations delivered by a mechanical ventilator. There is circumstantial evidence that vagal feedback may shape patient-ventilator interactions inasmuch as respiratory rhythms of anesthetized and sleeping humans can be entrained to a ventilator (Graves et al, 1986; Zurob et al, 1996), whereas entrainment mechanisms are severely impaired in patients following lung transplantation (Habel et al, 1996). This topic is discussed further in the section on principles of entrainment.

Whether reaching or exceeding a volume threshold during single lung inflations is required for BH mechanisms to be operative is still debated. Most studies on humans report a volume threshold of 1.0 to 1.5 liter (Polacheck et al, 1980; Iber et al, 1995) before a single inflation produces prolongation of expiratory time. On the other hand, the volume threshold may substantially underestimate the sensitivity to dynamic lung inflation, as suggested by the significant inspiratory prolongation achieved with obstructed normal tidal breaths in anesthetized (Guz et al, 1964) or sleeping humans (Iatridis and Iber, 1993). Regardless, it is unclear whether a threshold that holds for a single lung inflation is pertinent for volume-related modulation of respiratory rate during mechanical ventilation.

Effects of tidal volume on respiratory rate (vagal volume-related feedback) during mechanical ventilation cannot be extrapolated from breath timing responses to single lung inflations without considering the phase relationships between inspiratory neural activity and the machine inflation cycle. Machine inflations that last longer than the inspiratory neural activity (neural T_I, duration of inspiration) and the machine inflation cycle (machine T_I—i.e., machine T_I>neural T_I) delay the onset of the next inspiratory effort (T_E is prolonged); hence, these machine inflations have a tendency to slow the rate of breathing. Machine inflations that precede neural T_I and coincide with the end of inspiratory activity tend to shorten neural T_I; hence, these machine inflations have a tendency to increase the rate of breathing.

When operative in a patient on pressure-assist ventilation, vagal feedback may not only modulate respiratory rate but may also mitigate changes in tidal volume with changes in level of support. For example, an increase in the level of support for a patient on pressure-assist ventilation tends to reduce both inspiratory time and peak inspiratory activity (i.e., an increase in tidal volume reduces inspiratory activity). Because peak inspiratory effort affects tidal volume in pressure-assist modes, it follows that tidal volume does not increase as much as it might otherwise from an increase in the level of support. Likewise, a reduction in the level of pressure support tends to increase both inspiratory time and peak inspiratory activity. As a result of an increase in peak inspiratory effort, tidal volume may not decrease as much as it might otherwise from a reduction in the level of support.

Continuous elevation of lung volume (e.g., by dynamic hyperinflation, addition of positive end-expiratory pressure [PEEP], or with a deliberate large lung inflation) results in prolongation of expiratory time or a slowing of rate. The presence of this vagal reflex during the application of PEEP during mechanical ventilation tends to modulate the elevation of lung volume by promoting more complete emptying via prolongation of expiratory time and recruitment of expiratory muscles. This vagal reflex may also explain the slowing effect of high tidal volumes (large lung inflations) on rate in patients ventilated in a volume-preset mode (see the section on effect of volume and pressure).

Chest Wall Reflexes

Chest wall mechanoreceptors (joint, tendon, and spindle receptors) provide input to the respiratory neurons concerning the forces exerted by the respiratory muscles and the movements of the chest wall. Electrical stimulation of intercostal nerves during inspiration shortens inspiratory time and increases frequency (Remmers, 1970). There is substantial evidence that the tachypnea associated with an elastic load is mediated by a reflex originating in the chest wall (Axen et al, 1983; Puddy and Younes, 1981). Studies in animals with vagotomies suggest that the gain in the response is dependent on the level of consciousness (i.e., the gain of the response is most pronounced during wakefulness) (Clark and von Euler, 1972; Grunstein et al, 1973).

When operative, vagal and chest wall reflexes can have opposing influences on frequency in response to a load or reduction in tidal volume. Vagal feedback promotes a slowing of rate while chest wall feedback promotes a higher rate. For example, patients with restrictive respiratory disorders have a faster respiratory rate than normal humans (Rebuck and Slutsky, 1986). If vagal volume feedback is operative, smaller tidal volumes result in slower rates. The net effect of sensory input from the vagus versus intercostal on respiratory rate may differ depending on the underlying disease. Furthermore, alterations in the mechanical properties produced by disease may change the gain of these reflexes during ventilatory support (Stroetz et al, 1996). Although the balance of these reflexes in ventilated patients is not known, it can be expected that they may differ depending on the underlying disease and clinical setting. The mechanisms of load-related tachypnea are relevant to mechanical ventilation and the concept of "unloading" (i.e., the removal of a mechanical load from the respiratory muscles).

Wakefulness Versus Sleep Effects

The effect of mechanical ventilation on respiratory motor output can be quite different in wakefulness versus sleep. Significant effects of sleep on the ventilatory response to selected sensory inputs have been shown by the hypocapnia-induced apneic threshold (Dempsey and Skatrud, 1986) and the loss of immediate compensation to imposed mechanical loads (Henke et al, 1992). Results of several studies have shown significant differences between wakefulness and NREM sleep in the way the output of the ventilator influences the output of the respiratory pump (Ingrassia et al, 1991; Simon et al, 1993; Tobert et al, 1997; Wies et al, 1994; Zurob et al, 1996). Changes in volume, airway pressure, and flow are readily perceived in awake humans. These sensory perceptions can evoke behavioral respiratory responses, the intent of which is to enhance comfort. It is important to recognize the potential influences of behavioral responses when interpreting changes in breathing patterns of patients receiving ventilatory support.

The removal of the wakefulness drive during NREM sleep causes a significant reduction in inspiratory drive and leads to ventilatory instability. When the $PaCO_2$ of a sleeping volunteer is lowered by mechanically augmenting tidal volume, inspiratory motor output declines. Apnea can occur during or after cessation of mechanical hyperventilation (Henke et al, 1988; Leevers et al, 1994). A reduction in the intensity of inspiratory efforts during volume-assist ventilation may cause uncoupling of machine breaths and inspiratory efforts (Tobert et al, 1997). Similar degrees of erratic, periodic breathing have been observed in sleeping subjects during pressure-support ventilation (Rajagopalan et al, 1996). In summary, during wakefulness, behavioral/learning influences can dominate, whereas during sleep, inhibitory feedback effects (particularly those that are chemically mediated) are unmasked. Differences in ventilatory control between wakefulness and sleep and their relevancy to patient-ventilator interactions are discussed throughout the chapter.

BREATHING RESPONSES TO CONTROLLED MECHANICAL VENTILATION

PRINCIPLES OF ENTRAINMENT

Entrainment of inspiratory muscle activity to an extrinsic periodic stimulus, such as intermittent machine breaths, is one example of the interactions between a mechanical ventilator and the respiratory control system. Entrainment of spontaneous breathing to periodic machine breaths implies a fixed temporal relationship between the machine breath and the inspiratory effort (Fig. 12–1). Entrainment patterns of the respiratory pump to a mechanical ventilator have been examined in anesthetized animals (Muzzin et al, 1992; Petrillo and Glass, 1983, 1984). In those studies, the duration and magnitude of the mechanical stimulus and the phase of the respiratory cycle to which it was delivered appeared to be important determinants in altering inherent rhythm.

Coupling of the patient's inherent respiratory pattern to the machine cycle is an indicator of entrainment or synchronization with the ventilator. Although entrainment has been less extensively studied in humans, the ability of the respiratory controller to reset its rhythm in response to machine-imposed lung inflations has been examined at different ventilator settings during anesthesia (Graves et al, 1986), wakefulness (Wies et al, 1994), and NREM sleep (Zurob et al, 1996). In general, the results of studies from anesthetized normal volunteers are similar to those of anesthetized animal preparations. One-to-one entrainment (each machine breath is coupled with one spontaneous respiratory effort with a fixed phase between the two rhythms) (see Fig. 12–1) was observed at ventilator rates in a range of ±40% of spontaneous breathing frequencies. During wakefulness, the range of machine rates over which 1:1 entrainment occurred in normal volunteers during mechanical ventilation was greater than during NREM sleep (Wies et al, 1994; Zurob et al, 1996). Cortical influences appear to facilitate resetting of the respiratory rhythm to maintain a 1:1 entrainment pattern, perhaps as an adaptive strategy to avoid discomfort associated with patient-ventilator dyssynchrony.

The magnitude of the stimulus (i.e., the depth of the lung inflation [tidal volume]) influences the ease with which the respiratory controller can reset its inherent rhythm in response to changes in machine rate. This is illustrated in Fig. 12–2, which shows that the range of machine rates in which 1:1 entrainment was observed in normal subjects during mechanical ventilation was greater at the higher tidal volume settings (Graves et al, 1986; Wies et al, 1994).

Although one may predict that an increase in respiratory drive would reduce the capacity of the respiratory controller to entrain its rhythm to machine breaths, CO_2 tension has not been shown to affect entrainment patterns in normal

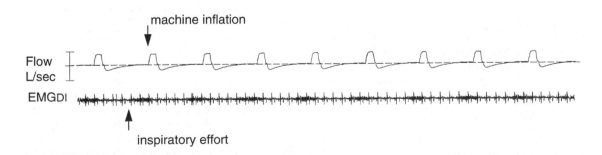

Figure 12–1
Stable temporal relationship between inspiratory efforts and machine inflations. The diaphragm contractions (EMG_{DI}) occur at a consistent time relative to the ventilator cycle. This example shows a 1:1 entrainment pattern (i.e., one effort for each machine cycle).

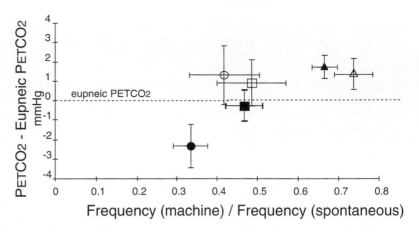

Figure 12–2
The effect of tidal volume on the lower range of machine rates (normalized to the spontaneous rate) that results in loss of 1:1 entrainment in five awake, normal subjects with *(open symbols)* and without *(closed symbols)* CO_2 supplementation. $\triangle$ = spontaneous tidal volume; $\square$ = 1.3 × spontaneous tidal volume; $\circ$ = 1.5 × spontaneous tidal volume.

sleeping subjects during mechanical ventilation. Figure 12–3 illustrates the effect of CO_2 supplementation on the entrainment pattern of one normal subject during NREM sleep, when machine frequency was varied during volume-preset mechanical ventilation with disabled trigger mechanisms (controlled mechanical ventilation). Each data point represents an inspiratory effort defined by its phase relationship to the machine breath (phase angle) at each machine frequency. To define the phase relationship between ventilator-delivered breaths and spontaneous inspiratory efforts, each ventilator cycle spanned 360° with phase angles between −180° and +180°; onset of machine inflation was assigned a value of 0° (Fig. 12–4). The subject's spontaneous rate (f_s), which had been measured in the assist-control mode, is shown at two different CO_2 conditions (see Fig. 12–3). As the machine rate was decreased below f_s by 2 to 3 breaths per minute (bpm), the respiratory controller slowed its respiratory rate to maintain 1:1 entrainment, denoted by the narrow distribution of phase angles. The response was similar under both isocapnic and

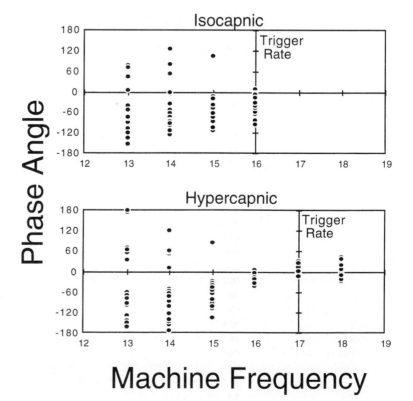

Figure 12–3
The rate at which 1:1 entrainment was lost is shown for an individual sleeping subject during isocapnic and hypercapnic conditions. The loss of 1:1 entrainment occurred at two to three breaths below trigger rate during controlled volume-cycled ventilation; there was no difference between the CO_2 conditions. Each data point represents an inspiratory effort defined by its relationship to the machine breath (phase angle) at each machine frequency.

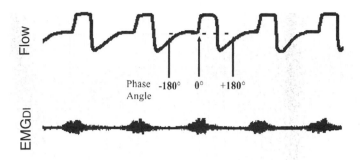

Figure 12–4
Onset of machine inflation was assigned a value of 0° with a ventilator cycle spanning 360° from −180° to +180°. Any inspiratory effort associated with a particular inflation would therefore have a phase angle between −180° and +180°. A phase angle of 0° indicates that both inflation and EMG onset occurred at the same time. When EMG onset occurs before machine inflation, the frequency is between −180° and 0°; when EMG onset occurs after machine inflation, the frequency is between 0° and +180°.

hypercapnic conditions (PetCO$_2$ 3 mm Hg above eupnea). It is possible that resetting mechanisms are not affected by changes in respiratory drive until higher levels are reached. This observation is similar to normal spontaneously breathing humans, in whom moderate levels of stimulation elicit primarily a tidal volume response, and only at higher levels do changes in respiratory rate predominate.

Entrainment is thought to be mediated via vagal afferent nerves (Petrillo, 1983; 1984). In animals, entrainment to a ventilator is lost following bilateral vagotomy (Vibert et al, 1981). A study of lung transplant recipients with bilateral vagal denervation who were mechanically ventilated during NREM sleep showed either no unitary phase relationship between spontaneous efforts and machine breaths or a 1:1 entrainment pattern at a restricted range of machine rates above their spontaneous breathing frequencies (Habel et al, 1996). In intact humans, neural T$_I$ is shorter when the inspiratory effort coincides with the onset of the machine inflation (Fig. 12–5). In contrast, neural T$_I$ is longer when the inspiratory effort begins during the expiratory phase of the machine cycle (not shown in figure). The neural T$_I$ of vagally denervated patients was not altered by its relationship to the machine cycle (see Fig. 12–5). These observations in animals and humans suggest that vagal afferent nerves are important in mediating entrainment of the respiratory rhythm to a mechanical ventilator.

These studies have significant implications in our understanding of asynchrony between patient efforts and machine breaths during mechanical ventilation.

Lack of synchrony, or uncoupling, between patient efforts and machine breaths is a common problem in the management of mechanically ventilated patients with respiratory failure (see the section on clinical relevance of adverse patient-ventilator interactions). This uncoupling can be viewed as an impasse in the interaction between two competing oscillators: the ventilator and the patient's respiratory rhythm and pattern generator. Unavoidable limitations in sensing algorithms and response times prevent the machine from adjusting its output to patient demand. However, equally important is the failure of the respiratory control system to adjust its output, which may reflect constraints in the resetting of respiratory rhythms in response to the mechanical ventilator.

For example, Figure 12–6 shows a recording from a sleeping, mechanically ventilated patient with severe chronic obstructive pulmonary disease (COPD). Individual tracings include those of the rib cage and abdomen displacements (with Respitrace), nasal mask pressure, oxygen saturation, estimated flow from a BiPAP device, and one representative electroencephalogram (EEG) lead. Note that the nasal ventilator failed to recognize patient efforts on multiple occasions (wasted efforts) and that the phase relationships between ventilator and thoracic excursions are variable. In contrast is the example shown in Figure 12–7, which demonstrates the ease with which the ventilatory pump of a patient with amyotrophic lateral sclerosis can be captured and ventilation augmented with nasal positive-pressure ventilation.

The observation that patients with COPD have more asynchronous events is one explanation for the variable success of noninvasive nocturnal mechanical ventilation (NNMV) in preventing daytime hypoventilation and CO$_2$ retention. On the contrary, patients with chronic

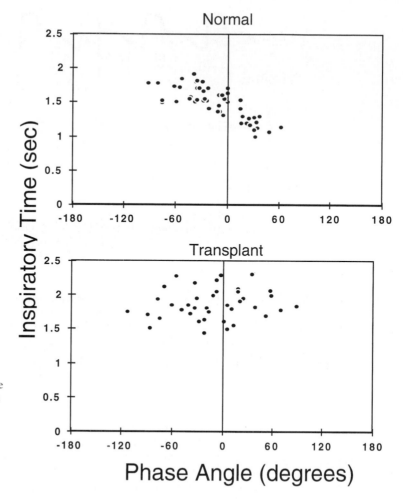

Figure 12–5
In normal subjects, muscle inspiratory time is shorter for those inspiratory efforts that extend into the machine inflation cycle. In lung transplant recipients, muscle inspiratory time is not affected by the relationship of inspiratory efforts to the machine inflation cycle.

respiratory failure from neuromuscular disease have shown improvement in daytime CO_2 retention and a reduction in symptoms following the institution of NNMV.

INHIBITION OF INSPIRATORY MUSCLE ACTIVITY

Profound reduction or even abolishment of phasic inspiratory muscle activity during mechanical ventilation is another respiratory controller response to mechanical ventilation (Altose et al, 1986; Manchanda et al, 1996; Prechter et al, 1990; Simon et al, 1991, 1993). Inhibition of respiratory motor output during prolonged mechanical ventilation in wakefulness and NREM sleep has been shown to be highly sensitive to changes in ventilator tidal volume, frequency, and a combination of both (Altose et al, 1986; Simon et al, 1991; Manchanda et al, 1996). The absence of inspiratory effort in these studies was based on the loss of (EMG_{DI}) and the stable configuration

of mouth pressure and expiratory wave form (Fig. 12–8). Inhibition of inspiratory effort in intubated patients in the intensive care unit (ICU), awake and sleep, during controlled mechanical ventilation using similar settings has also been shown (Ingrassia et al, 1991; Prechter et al, 1990).

There is conflicting evidence (Fink, 1961; Patrick et al, 1995) concerning the capacity for achieving purely passive conditions during mechanical ventilation in wakefulness, and, once achieved, the prevalence of post-hyperventilation apnea. Unlike NREM sleep, during wakefulness, the reduction in inspiratory drive is not a simple consequence of hypocapnia, but is intimately linked to neuromechanical as well as behavioral feedback (Banzett et al, 1996). Under these conditions, CO_2 supplementation has very little effect on inspiratory motor output unless end-tidal CO_2 tension reaches normocapnic or mildly hypercapnic levels. In wakefulness, at least part of the effects of prolonged mechanical ventilation may be attributed simply to the promotion of subject

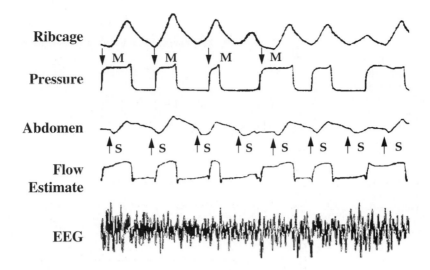

Figure 12–6
Rib cage and abdominal displacements were measured with respiratory inductive plethysmography; the flow estimate is the leak-adjusted flow estimate of the BiPAP device. Downward arrows (M) indicate timed or nontriggered machine breaths (i.e., breaths that are machine-initiated, not those initiated in response to patient effort). Upward arrows (S) identify the patient's own spontaneous inspiratory efforts. There is a variable phase relationship between ventilator breaths and thoracic excursions, and the ventilator failed to recognize patient efforts on multiple occasions.

habituation to the ventilator and, therefore, relaxation. The effect of duration of mechanical ventilation on the control of breathing has not been studied systematically to date, but it may play a major role in accounting for some of the differences reported among studies in terms of the inhibitory effects of mechanical ventilation during wakefulness and sleep.

CO_2 supplementation during mechanical ventilation has been used in patients with respiratory failure during passive mechanical hyperventilation to measure CO_2 recruitment threshold or

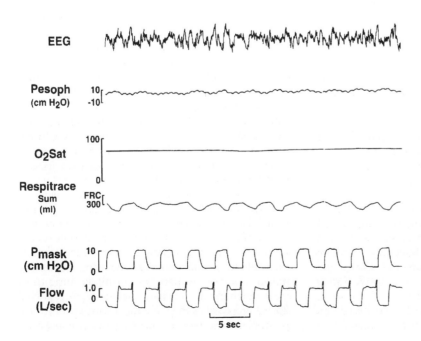

Figure 12–7
This is a recording of values for a patient with amyotrophic lateral sclerosis with individual tracings including EEG, esophageal pressure, oxygen saturation, approximate tidal volume from Respitrace, pressure at mask, and flow. Note the ease at which the respiratory oscillator can be captured.

Figure 12–8
Representative tracing from a normal subject showing the effect of increasing frequency (tidal volume held constant at 1.0 l) on inspiratory muscle activity during controlled mechanical ventilation, as evidenced by the changes in diaphragm EMG (EMG_{DI}), mouth pressure (P_M), and expiratory flow. Isocapnic conditions are maintained. (*Left*) period of spontaneous breathing; (*middle*) period of persistent inspiratory effort at a frequency (f) of 8, 10, 12 breaths per minute (bpm); (*right*) cessation of inspiratory muscle activity after f increased to 13 bpm (inhibition frequency).

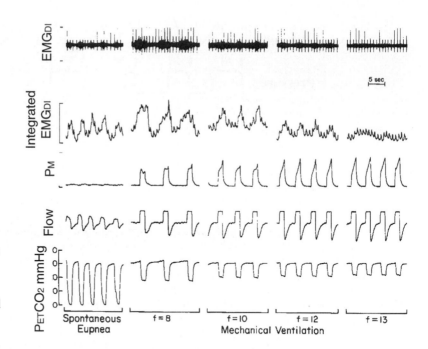

apparent CO_2 setpoint of the unloaded respiratory pump (Dunn et al, 1991; Prechter et al, 1990). Results of these studies, which examine the level of CO_2 required to reactivate inspiratory muscle activity, suggest that the CO_2 sensitivity varies considerably among patients and indicate that at conventional ventilator settings many patients are being overventilated (Dunn et al, 1991). This interpretation is consistent with observations on breathing pattern responses to pressure-support ventilation in contrast to proportional-assist ventilation (Marantz et al, 1996).

Mechanical ventilation has been proposed as a way to decrease the mechanical load on the respiratory muscles and therefore "rest" the muscles. In humans, unloading has been assessed by measuring the effects of pressure-assist or volume-assist ventilation on respiratory muscle electromyogram (EMG) or pleural pressure. A reduction in phasic inspiratory muscle activity provides evidence for unloading of the inspiratory muscles. Analysis of pressure and flow wave forms and direct measurement of electrical activity from an inspiratory muscle (e.g., the diaphragm, EMG_{DI}) to assess persistence of inspiratory muscle contraction or inspiratory effort and inherent timing with the machine breaths are important tools to evaluate patient-ventilator interactions and, therefore, the work of breathing (Brochard et al, 1987, 1989; Flick et al, 1989; Marini et al, 1985, 1986a, 1986b, 1988; Ward et al, 1988).

Although an earlier study by Rochester and coworkers (1977) demonstrated that assisted ventilation in patients with chronic respiratory failure markedly diminished diaphragmatic and accessory inspiratory muscle activity, several authors (Flick et al, 1989; Marini et al, 1985, 1986b; Pearle and Simmons, 1982; Tan and Simmons, 1979; Ward et al, 1988) have cited variations in airway pressure and measurements of the mechanical work of breathing as evidence of continued inspiratory muscle contraction throughout a machine-delivered breath. These studies have largely examined the mechanical work of breathing during mechanical ventilation in the acutely ill ventilator-dependent patient. Marini and coworkers showed significant activity of the respiratory muscles that persisted throughout both patient-initiated ventilator cycles (Marini et al, 1985, 1986a) and synchronized intermittent mechanical ventilation (Marini et al, 1988) at levels that can tax ventilatory reserve. These studies have demonstrated the importance of examining patient-ventilator interactions during the selection and reassessment of ventilation mode and machine settings in the ventilator-dependent patient.

Several studies by Brochard and coworkers (1987, 1989, 1990) have demonstrated reduction in diaphragm and sternocleidomastoid muscle activity during inspiratory pressure support via a face mask in COPD patients with acute respiratory failure. Similar observations using inspiratory pressure support in patients during weaning trials from mechanical ventilation have been reported (Brochard et al, 1989). Patients with chronic respiratory failure have achieved partial suppression of EMG activity of the diaphragm (Belman et al, 1990; Carrey et al, 1990; Celli et al, 1989; Goldstein et al, 1987, 1991; Shapiro et al, 1992) and sternocleidomastoid (Carrey et al, 1990) when undergoing nocturnal noninvasive ventilation, both intermittent negative- and positive-pressure mechanical ventilation. The type of ventilator and the settings used to match or augment minute ventilation varied widely among those studies (Belman et al, 1990; Carrey et al, 1990; Celli et al, 1989; Goldstein et al, 1987, 1991; Shapiro et al, 1992). Few studies used reduction of diaphragm EMG as an endpoint to setting the ventilator.

The benefit of suppressing or silencing respiratory muscles with mechanical ventilation to treat acute or chronic respiratory failure has not been proved, although it is a plausible hypothesis that "resting" fatigued muscles is a desirable goal (Braun et al, 1983; Cropp and Dimarco, 1987; Gutierrez et al, 1988; Rochester et al, 1977). There is alternative data to suggest that respiratory muscles require conditioning (Braun and Marino, 1984; Luce et al, 1981; MacIntyre and Leatherman, 1989; Weisman et al, 1983).

The goals of treatment with mechanical ventilation depend on the individual's cause of respiratory failure and the clinical setting (i.e., acute, recovering, or chronic). For example, a patient recovering from acute respiratory failure may need ventilator support that allows for respiratory muscle conditioning or gradual increases in the work of breathing. Therefore, silencing respiratory muscles may not be beneficial for that patient during that particular phase of ventilator dependency. Proportional-assist ventilation may be a useful alternate mode of ventilation in this group of patients.

MEMORY CHARACTERISTICS OF THE RESPIRATORY CONTROLLER

What happens when mechanical inhibitory input (i.e., mechanical ventilation) is removed in humans? Apnea has been observed after the cessation of passive hyperventilation during anesthesia (Fink, 1961; Hanks et al, 1961) and NREM sleep (Datta et al, 1991; Henke et al, 1988; Skatrud and Dempsey, 1983). However, the phenomenon of apnea occurring after passive hyperventilation in awake humans is less clear. The generation of apnea after discontinuation of passive hyperventilation was inconsistently observed in normal subjects during wakefulness (Datta et al, 1991; Fink, 1961; Skatrud and Dempsey, 1983) or not at all (Puddy et al, 1996). From these observations, Puddy and coworkers (1996) argued that

apnea during controlled mechanical ventilation in awake subjects is due to both the tidal volume and rate settings being higher than the subject's tidal volume and frequency demands, rather than the existence of built-in neuromechanical feedback that suppresses respiratory drive. Results from these studies suggest that a reduction or absence of ventilatory output during and after removal of a mechanical stimulus is critically dependent on hypocapnia and the removal of the wakefulness stimulus.

In contrast, Leevers and coworkers (1993, 1994) have shown that apneic periods can occur after cessation of normocapnic or slightly hypercapnic controlled mechanical ventilation after a period of loss of inspiratory activity during both wakefulness and sleep in normal subjects (Fig. 12–9). These observations suggest that neither the sleep state nor hypocapnia is required to observe apnea after discontinuation of mechanical inhibitory feedback. Persistence of apnea after normocapnic mechanical ventilation was similarly found in vagally denervated lung transplant patients, suggesting that vagal feedback is not required (Leevers et al, 1993). Differences between studies on the occurrence of apnea during the state of wakefulness may be explained at least in part by subject habituation to the ventilator and, therefore, relaxation. Furthermore, these studies differed concerning the duration of mechanical ventilation. The fundamental effects of the duration of repeated sensory input may also be important.

The mechanisms responsible for continued apnea after cessation of mechanical ventilation are not entirely clear. Terms such as *hysteresis*, *memory*, or *inertia* have been used interchangeably in the literature to describe a lag in the excitation and relaxation of the neural control system. The continued apnea that persists after the inhibitory stimulus is removed may represent an inherent inertia characteristic of the control system operating at the level of pattern generation of respiratory motor output. Once the neural output to the respiratory muscles is profoundly reduced by sensory inhibition, it becomes more difficult to restore phasic respiration. Alternatively, this apnea-initiating mechanism may be a memory phenomenon, reflecting the persistence of mechanical inhibition related to volume and frequency involved in the initiation of inhibition during mechanical ventilation.

Inertia or memory in the respiratory controller has both excitatory (Eldridge, 1973, 1976) and inhibitory (Karczewski et al, 1975; Lawson, 1981) effects on ventilatory output after stimulus offset. An example is the ventilatory response in humans

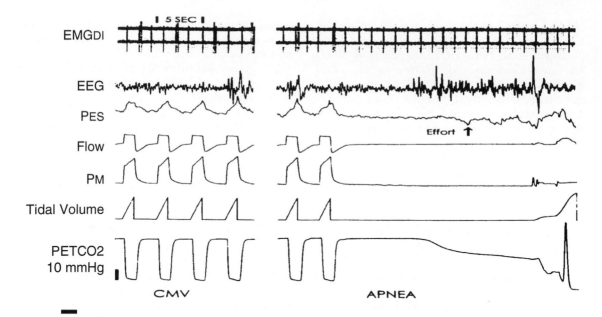

Figure 12–9

Representative tracing from a normal subject in NREM sleep showing EEG, diaphragm EMG (EMG_{DI}), volume, mouth pressure (P_M), flow, and $PetCO_2$ during spontaneous eupnea, isocapnic mechanical ventilation, and the period after the mechanical ventilator is disconnected. The ventilator was first put in the assist-control mode with the subject setting the machine rate, then changed to controlled mechanical ventilation (CMV) before disconnecting the ventilator. Note the period of inspiratory muscle inhibition before cessation of mechanical ventilation and the substantial expiratory time prolongation when mechanical ventilation was removed. (From Leevers AM, Simon PM, and Dempsey JA: Apnea after normocapnic mechanical ventilation during NREM sleep. J Appl Physiol 77:2079–2085, 1994. With permission from the American Physiological Society.)

during both wakefulness and NREM sleep to increasing and decreasing levels of $PetCO_2$ during mechanical ventilation (Simon et al, 1992). The $PetCO_2$ required to recruit inactive inspiratory muscles was greater than eupneic $PetCO_2$ and greater than the $PetCO_2$ required to inhibit inspiratory muscle activity once it was restored during mechanical ventilation (Simon et al, 1992).

Many important questions need to be addressed that are related to these features of the respiratory controller. Is there a "resetting" of the respiratory rhythm after a prolonged period of mechanical ventilation? Is the tachypnea that is frequently observed after patients are removed from the ventilator the result not only of changes in load but also of a resetting of the respiratory pattern generator initiated during mechanical ventilation? Despite the use of prolonged mechanical ventilation in the treatment of respiratory failure, little is known about the effect of repetitive periodic mechanical input on ventilatory control.

EFFECT OF VENTILATOR SETTINGS ON VENTILATORY CONTROL

EFFECT OF VOLUME AND PRESSURE

Mechanical ventilation in a volume preset mode eliminates a person's ability to regulate CO_2 stores by adjusting tidal volume. Consequently, if the machine-delivered tidal volume exceeds that demanded, the arterial CO_2 tension ($PaCO_2$) falls unless the respiratory rate declines as well.

Several observations suggest that changes in ventilator tidal volume affect respiratory rate. Tidal volume effects have been observed in awake and sleeping normal volunteers during volume-preset ventilation (Puddy and Younes, 1992; Puddy et al, 1996; Tobert et al, 1997). Figure 12–10 illustrates the average relationships between tidal volume settings, respiratory rate, and end-tidal CO_2 tension in eight *awake*, mechanically ventilated volunteers (Tobert et al, 1997). In this experiment, inspiratory flow had been set

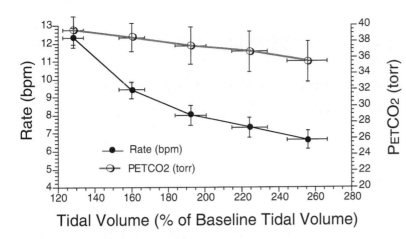

Figure 12–10
Effect of tidal volume on respiratory rate and $PetCO_2$ at a constant inspiratory flow is shown. Mean respiratory rates ($\pm$SEM) of all eight awake subjects (*closed circles*) and the mean $PetCO_2$ ($\pm$SEM) (*open circles*) are plotted for each tidal volume setting. Although respiratory rate falls from 12.3 to 6.7 bpm as tidal volume increases, this fall is insufficient to prevent hypocapnia.

to 40 l/min and kept constant at all tidal volume settings. Baseline tidal volume ranged from 0.6 to 0.8 liters. Two findings are of note: (1) increasing tidal volume above baseline slowed the rate of breathing; and (2) the fall in rate was insufficient to prevent hypocapnia.

CO_2 maintenance has no effect on the tidal volume/rate relationship in awake humans (Puddy et al, 1996; Tobert et al, 1997). This observation is shown in Figure 12–11, in which the tidal volume/rate response curve of Figure 12–10 can be compared with an average response curve that had been measured under isocapnic conditions. There is no difference between the curves. A number of investigators have shown that awake volunteers do not maintain normal CO_2 homeostasis during either volume- or pressure-preset ventilation (Lofaso et al, 1992; Morrell et al, 1993; Puddy and Younes, 1992; Puddy et al, 1996; Scheid et al, 1994). This observation is consistent with the data of Figure 12–10, implying that "unphysiologically" high tidal volume or pressure support settings may place tachypneic patients at risk for ventilator-induced respiratory alkalosis.

In contrast to wakefulness, during sleep hypocapnia has profound consequences on inspiratory drive (Rajagopalan et al, 1996; Tobert et al, 1997). Minute volume normally falls during the transition from wakefulness to sleep, resulting in an increase in $PaCO_2$ between 3 and 8 mm Hg (Phillipson and Bowes, 1986). The fall in ventilation during sleep reflects the removal of the wakefulness stimulus combined with an increase in upper airway resistance and lack of immediate load compensation. Therefore, when the $PaCO_2$ of a sleeping volunteer is lowered by mechanically augmenting tidal volume, inspiratory motor output declines and breathing becomes irregular (Tobert et al, 1997).

The author and coworkers recently reported

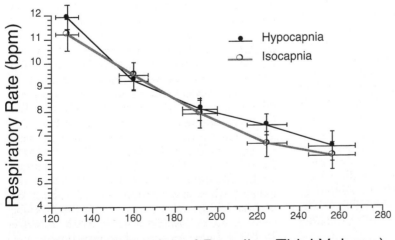

Figure 12–11
Effect of tidal volume on respiratory rate at a constant inspiratory flow during wakefulness when inspired CO_2 is added to maintain eupneic $PetCO_2$ (isocapnia) and when inspired CO_2 equals 0 (hypocapnia). Mean respiratory rates ($\pm$SEM) of all eight awake subjects are plotted for each tidal volume setting under both hypocapnic (*closed circles*) and isocapnic (*open circles*) conditions. Note that the effect of tidal volume on respiratory rate is similar among the different CO_2 conditions.

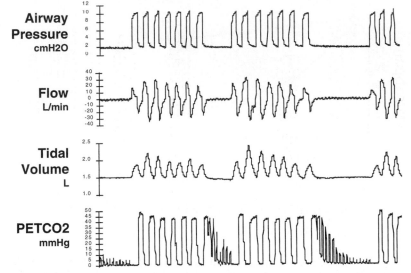

Figure 12–12
Example of ventilator-induced periodic breathing in a sleeping normal volunteer. Mechanical ventilation was provided through a nasal mask using a bilevel pressure device (BiPAP, Respironics) set to deliver an inspiratory pressure of 10 cm H_2O. The panel labeled PetCO$_2$ shows the CO_2 tension in one of the nares.

reductions in respiratory rate in sleeping volunteers during ventilation with as little as 5 cm H_2O positive inspiratory pressure (Rajagopalan et al, 1996). Uncoupling between neural and machine T_1 is uncommon at inspiratory pressures below 10 cm H_2O (Rajagopalan et al, 1996). Application of an inspiratory positive airway pressure (IPAP) of 10 cm H_2O can cause periodic breathing (Rajagopalan et al, 1996). An example of ventilator-induced breathing instability in a sleeping volunteer is shown in Figure 12–12. CO_2 supplementation to the inspired gas prevents ventilator-induced disordered breathing during sleep (Tobert et al, 1997), suggesting that the responsible mechanism is at least in part a hypocapnia-mediated reduction in inspiratory drive.

Tidal volume effects on rate can be readily documented in intubated patients with lung disease (Stroetz et al, 1996), as well as in vagally denervated lung transplant recipients both during wakefulness and sleep under isocapnic conditions.* These observations suggest that nonvagal pathways may also play a role in determining respiratory rate during mechanical ventilation. Lung stretch receptors are not the only receptors capable of sensing changes in tidal volume settings. Volume-related feedback from either the rib cage or diaphragm has also been shown to modulate breathing in animals (Bolser et al, 1987). Furthermore, ventilation through a nasal mask can stimulate pressure-, flow-, and temperature- (humidity-) sensitive receptors of skin, nasophar-

ynx and oropharynx, larynx, and proximal airways. Although these receptors have been shown to affect breathing under specific experimental conditions (Easton et al, 1985; Mathew et al, 1982; Speck, 1987), their activation does not produce BH responses in sleeping humans in the absence of vagal afferent discharge from the lung (Iber et al, 1995). Nor does bypassing upper airway receptors with an endotracheal tube seem to affect the tidal volume/rate response (Stroetz et al, 1996).

EFFECT OF FLOW

Not all studies have demonstrated as substantial tidal volume effects on respiratory rate as those shown in Figures 12–10 and 12–11 (Puddy et al, 1996; Scheid et al, 1994). Confounding factors, such as the choice of flow rates, flow profiles, machine T_1 settings, posture, and patient-ventilator interface, may be responsible for this discrepancy in results. The ventilator flow setting is an important determinant of inspiratory drive and timing. Clinicians have known for some time that increasing inspiratory flow reduces patient effort when the ventilator flow setting fails to meet the patient's demand (Marini et al, 1985). More recently, it has been shown that the amplitude of the inspiratory effort and the respiratory rate increase when flow settings exceed subject demand (Georgopoulos et al, 1996a, 1996b; Habel et al, 1995; Puddy and Younes, 1992; Tobert et al, 1997). Increasing flow at a given tidal volume shortens T_1, and peak lung volume is reached

---

*P.M. Simon, unpublished observations

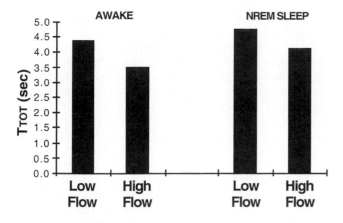

Figure 12–13

Effect of low (25 l/min) versus high (64 l/min) inspiratory flow rate on breath duration (T_{TOT}) in three bilateral vagally denervated patients following lung transplant during both wakefulness and NREM sleep. Note that T_{TOT} decreases (respiratory rate increases) at the higher flow rate ($p < 0.04$). The flow effect appears attenuated but is present during NREM sleep.

earlier. Inhibitory vagal feedback and its decay relative to breath onset occur before the flow (and T_I) changes. Therefore, any increase in expiratory time is not sufficient to compensate for the reduction in T_I; hence, respiratory rate increases. These observations are consistent with results from experiments on anesthetized dogs demonstrating changes in phrenic nerve discharge rates that correspond to changes in inspiratory flow (Pack et al, 1981).

The mechanisms mediating the effect of inspiratory flow rate on respiratory rate remains obscure. Puddy and Younes (1992) studied the response to changes in inspiratory flow rate in humans and demonstrated that in awake normal subjects mechanically ventilated on a volume-preset mode, increases in flow rate had an excitatory effect on respiratory frequency. They showed that the response was largely complete within one breath, suggesting a neural origin for the effect. This response is not affected by breathing route, temperature of inspired gas, or tidal volume at which the response is studied (Georgopoulos et al, 1996a). The rate response to changes in flow rate has been shown to be present during NREM sleep; whether the effect is attenuated during NREM sleep depends on the study (Georgopoulos et al, 1996b; Tobert et al, 1997). The flow effect on rate has also been observed in lung transplant recipients with bilateral vagal denervation during both wakefulness (Mitrouska et al, 1996; P.M. Simon, unpublished observations) and NREM sleep* (Fig. 12–13). Furthermore, the excitatory effects of inspiratory flow rate on respiratory motor output have been shown in awake quadriplegics with intercostal denervation (Mitrouska et al, 1996). These studies suggest that the excitatory effects of inspiratory flow on respiratory output are not mediated through intercostal and pulmonary vagal afferent nerves.

EFFECT OF DIFFERENT MODES ON VENTILATORY CONTROL AND THE MANAGEMENT OF RESPIRATORY FAILURE

An exciting development in the management of patients with chronic respiratory failure has been the use of noninvasive positive-pressure ventilation (NPPV) at night (Meyer and Hill, 1994). Improvements in daytime CO_2 retention and symptoms of hypoventilation have been achieved with the use of NPPV in patients with neuromuscular diseases, chest wall abnormalities, obstructive sleep apnea, and primary alveolar hypoventilation (Meyer and Hill, 1994). Studies are less convincing for efficacy of NPPV in patients with COPD (Meyer and Hill, 1994). Mechanisms proposed to explain the beneficial effects of nocturnal NPPV include alleviated respiratory muscle fatigue, reset respiratory center sensitivity to CO_2, improved lung compliance because of decreased atelectasis, increased upper airway dimensions, or some combination of them (Martin and Sanders, 1995; Meyer and Hill, 1994). Regardless of which mechanisms are responsible for improvement with NPPV, it is likely that augmentation of ventilation is required.

Questions remain about when and how to optimally implement NPPV. These questions cannot be answered from prior studies in patients receiving NPPV because of vast differences in study design including underlying disease, equipment, modes of ventilation, and ventilator settings. In my experience, patients are usually reluctant to start NPPV unless they are symptomatic. Most often they become symptomatic only when

---

*P.M. Simon, unpublished observations

there is significant impairment in daytime gas exchange.

How should the ventilator be set to augment minute ventilation? Pressure- or volume-preset breaths can be delivered via a full face mask, nasal mask, or mouthpiece. During nasal positive-pressure ventilation, the pressure applied to the respiratory system equals the sum of the machine-delivered pressure and the inspiratory muscle-derived pressure; when patient-triggered, the relative contribution changes with the timing of the machine breath. Because the impedance of the respiratory system is determined by its resistive and elastic properties, higher pressures are required to overcome the impedance of the respiratory system in patients with high upper airway resistance, noncompliant lungs or a stiff chest wall, obstructive airways and hyperinflation, or when machine breaths are delivered during the exhalation phase.

Upper airway resistance increases when state changes from wakefulness to NREM sleep (Henke et al, 1992). This is not a major problem in a mechanically ventilated patient whose upper airway is bypassed with an endotracheal tube or a tracheostomy. Furthermore, during wakefulness, cortical influences can adjust breathing pattern to avoid discomfort (e.g., increase inspiratory activity or alter timing to facilitate a machine breath). However, in sleeping patients receiving NPPV, there is a limit to the amount of pressure or volume delivered that, when exceeded, can lead to a leak around the mask and/or a startle response with arousal. If the ventilator is set and patient-ventilator interactions are observed during wakefulness, the changes in respiratory impedance related to state differences are not appreciated. These problems may go unrecognized. When setting the ventilator, differences in the response of the ventilatory control system to nasal positive-pressure breathing related to state of consciousness cannot be ignored.

The effect on ventilation of machine breaths delivered in the absence of an inspiratory effort in both awake and sleeping normal volunteers during controlled volume- and pressure-cycled mechanical ventilation via a nasal mask has been previously examined. Rodenstein's group noted progressive narrowing of the glottic aperture in normal subjects with increasing levels of passive hyperventilation with volume- and pressure-preset NPPV, which resulted in progressive reductions in delivered ventilation (Jounieaux et al, 1995a, 1995b; Parreira et al, 1996). The narrowing of the upper airway to timed volume- or pressure-cycled breaths was worse during NREM sleep than during wakefulness. Increased upper airway resistance from narrowing of the glottic aperture can

produce mask leaks that lead to desaturation and sleep disruption.

It is not clear whether minute ventilation can be effectively augmented during sleep when the ventilator is set so that the patient has to trigger each breath (i.e., without a timed backup rate). When the $PaCO_2$ of a sleeping volunteer is lowered by mechanically augmenting tidal volume, inspiratory motor output declines (Dempsey and Skatrud, 1986; Henke et al, 1988; Skatrud and Dempsey, 1983). A reduction in the intensity of inspiratory efforts during volume-assist ventilation can cause uncoupling of machine breaths and inspiratory efforts (Tobert et al, 1997). Similar degrees of erratic, periodic breathing have been observed in sleeping subjects during pressure-support ventilation (Younes, 1993). Whether the concept that maintenance of CO_2 homeostasis during NREM sleep prevents augmentation of minute ventilation is applicable to patients with chronic respiratory failure is not known. Marantz and coworkers (1996) showed that ventilator-dependent patients on proportional-assist ventilation did not change their minute ventilation as the level of support was altered between near-maximal and lowest tolerable.

CLINICAL RELEVANCE OF ADVERSE PATIENT-VENTILATOR INTERACTIONS

Virtually all modern mechanical ventilators possess sensing mechanisms so that their output can be coordinated with the patient's inspiratory effort. Sensing algorithms respond either to the airway pressure or the flow signal and, depending on ventilator mode, regulate machine on-switch and off-switch mechanisms. Failure to detect or respond to an inspiratory effort may cause uncoupling of patient and machine output (i.e., patient-ventilator asynchrony).

Patient-ventilator asynchrony is common in intubated patients and is almost always present in patients during NPPV (see Fig. 12–6). Although patient-ventilator asynchrony seems undesirable, it has yet to be shown that it is an impairment to recovery from respiratory failure. To address the implications of patient-ventilator asynchrony, it is necessary to consider whether (a) it is caused by inadequacies of available ventilator technology; (b) it is a result of respiratory system disease; or (c) it is a reflection of normal physiologic mechanisms.

Figure 12–6 illustrates patient-ventilator asynchrony during NPPV with a bilevel pressure device (BiPAP, Respironics, Inc.) in a sleeping patient with COPD. Several observations should be noted: (1) there is no consistent relationship between machine and spontaneous breaths; (2) chest wall displacement (and presumably ventilation) is largest when machine and spontaneous breaths are initiated in close temporal proximity; and (3) a machine breath that is initiated during spontaneous expiration is ineffective in raising lung volume.

Because patients with COPD are prone to dynamic hyperinflation, they are particularly susceptible to patient-ventilator asynchrony. In the presence of dynamic hyperinflation, the alveolar pressure at end-expiration (i.e., the recoil pressure of the respiratory system) is greater than atmospheric pressure, thereby adding an elastic load to the inspiratory muscles (Gay et al, 1989; Milic-Emili et al, 1987; Pepe and Marini, 1982). The inspiratory muscles must generate a pressure that counterbalances the increased elastic recoil before they can begin to inflate the lungs. In addition, these muscles require a greater neural drive to generate pressure because at high lung volumes neuromechanical coupling is impaired (Hubmayr et al, 1989; Smith and Bellemare, 1987). This impairment is due to a reduction in inspiratory muscle length during hyperinflation, reducing the muscles' ability to generate force. The primary muscle of inspiration, the diaphragm, flattens, resulting in a reduction in its mechanical efficiency as a pressure generator (Roussos and Macklem, 1977).

A number of inferences concerning the implications of patient-ventilator asynchrony can be made. Augmentation of minute ventilation above spontaneous breathing requires synchronization between patient effort and machine output. During sleep, hypocapnia limits the amount by which minute ventilation can be augmented when the ventilator is set in the spontaneous (patient-triggered) mode (Dempsey and Skatrud, 1986; Henke et al, 1988; Rajagopalan et al, 1996). During wakefulness, it is easy to overventilate a patient because inspiratory drive is much less dependent on CO_2 than it is during sleep (Lofaso et al, 1992; Morrell et al, 1993; Puddy et al, 1996; Scheid et al, 1994; Tobert et al, 1997). The implications of patient-ventilator asynchrony differ, depending on the level of inspiratory drive. In the presence of a low drive state, patient-ventilator asynchrony is a manifestation of relative hypocapnia and inspiratory unloading; therefore, changes in ventilator settings may not be required. In the presence of a high drive state, patient-ventilator asynchrony reflects either machine sensing failure or abnormal lung mechanics, or both. In contrast,

sedation or changes in ventilator settings may be required in this case.

REFERENCES

Altose MD, Castele RJ, Connors AF Jr, et al: Effects of volume and frequency of mechanical ventilation on respiratory activity in humans. Respir Physiol 66:171–180, 1986.

Axen KS, Sperber-Haas S, Hass F, et al: Ventilatory adjustments during sustained mechanical loading in conscious humans. J Appl Physiol 55:1211–1218, 1983.

Banzett RB, Lansing RW, Evans KC, et al: Stimulus-response characteristics of CO_2-induced air hunger in normal subjects. Respir Physiol 103:19–31, 1996.

Belman MJ, Soo Hoo GW, Kuei JH, et al: Efficacy of positive vs negative pressure ventilation in unloading the respiratory muscles. Chest 98:850–856, 1990.

Bolser DC, Lindsey BG, and Shannon R: Medullary inspiratory activity: Influence of intercostal tendon organs and muscle spindle endings. J Appl Physiol 62:1046–1056, 1987.

Braun NMT, Faulkner J, Hughes RL, et al: When should respiratory muscle be exercised? Chest 84:76–84, 1983.

Braun NMT and Marino WD: Effect of daily intermittent rest of respiratory muscles in patients with severe chronic airflow limitation (CAL). Chest 85:59S–60S, 1984.

Brochard L, Harf A, Lorino H, et al: Inspiratory pressure support prevents diaphragmatic fatigue during weaning from mechanical ventilation. Am Rev Respir Dis 139:513–521, 1989.

Brochard L, Isabey D, Piquet J, et al: Reversal of acute exacerbations of chronic obstructive lung disease by inspiratory assistance with a face mask. N Engl J Med 323:1523–1530, 1990.

Brochard L, Pluskwa F, and Lemaire F: Improved efficacy of spontaneous breathing with inspiratory pressure support. Am Rev Respir Dis 136:411–415, 1987.

Carrey Z, Gottfried SB, and Levy RD: Ventilatory muscle support in respiratory failure with nasal positive pressure ventilation. Chest 97:150–158, 1990.

Celli B, Lee H, Criner G, et al: Controlled trial of external negative pressure ventilation in patients with severe chronic airflow obstruction. Am Rev Respir Dis 140:1251–1256, 1989.

Clark FJ and von Euler C: On the regulation of depth and rate of breathing. J Physiol 222:267–295, 1972.

Cropp A and Dimarco AF: Effects of intermittent negative pressure ventilation on respiratory muscle function in patients with severe chronic obstructive pulmonary disease. Am Rev Respir Dis 135:1056–1061, 1987.

Datta AK, Shea SA, Horner RL, et al: The influence

of induced hypocapnia and sleep on the endogenous respiratory rhythm in humans. J Physiol 440:17–33, 1991.

Dempsey JA and Skatrud JB: A sleep-induced apneic threshold and its consequences. Am Rev Respir Dis 133:1163–1170, 1986.

Dunn WF, Nelson SB, and Hubmayr RD: The control of breathing during weaning from mechanical ventilation. Chest 100:754–761, 1991.

Easton PA, Jadue C, Arnup ME, et al: Effects of upper or lower airway anesthesia on hypercapnic ventilation in humans. J Appl Physiol 59:1090–1097, 1985.

Eldridge FL: Posthyperventilation breathing: Different effects of active and passive hyperventilation. J Appl Physiol 34:422–430, 1973.

Eldridge FL: Central neural stimulation of respiration in unanesthetized decerebrate cats. J Appl Physiol 40:23–28, 1976.

Feldman JL and Smith JC: Neural control of respiratory pattern in mammals: An overview. In Dempsey JA and Pack AI (eds): Regulation of Breathing. Lung Biology in Health and Disease 79:39–64, 1995.

Feldman JL, Smith JC, Ellenberger HH, et al: Neurogenesis of respiratory rhythm and pattern: Emerging concepts. Am J Physiol 28:R879–R886, 1990.

Fink BR: Influence of cerebral activity in wakefulness on regulation of breathing. J Appl Physiol 16:15–20, 1961.

Flick GR, Bellamy PE, and Simmons DH: Diaphragmatic contraction during assisted mechanical ventilation. Chest 96:130–135, 1989.

Gay PC, Rodarte JR, and Hubmayr RD: The effects of positive expiratory pressure on isovolume flow and dynamic hyperinflation in patients receiving mechanical ventilation. Am Rev Respir Dis 139:621–626, 1989.

Georgopoulos D, Mitrouska I, Bshouty Z, et al: Effects of breathing route, temperature and volume of inspired gas, and airway anesthesia on the response of respiratory output to varying inspiratory flow. Am J Respir Crit Care Med 153:168–175, 1996a.

Georgopoulos D, Mitrouska I, Bshouty Z, et al: Effect of non-REM sleep on the response of respiratory output to varying inspiratory flow. Am J Respir Crit Care Med 153:1624–1630, 1996b.

Goldstein RS, De Rosie J, Avendano MA, et al: Influence of noninvasive positive pressure ventilation on inspiratory muscles. Chest 99:408–415, 1991.

Goldstein RS, Molotiu N, Skrastins R, et al: Reversal of sleep-induced hypoventilation and chronic respiratory failure by nocturnal negative pressure ventilation in patients with restrictive ventilatory impairment. Am Rev Respir Dis 135:1049–1055, 1987.

Graves C, Glass L, Laporta D, et al: Respiratory phase locking during mechanical ventilation in anesthetized human subjects. Am J Physiol 250:R902–R909, 1986.

Grunstein MM, Younes M, and Milic-Emili J: Control of tidal volume and respiratory frequency in anesthetized cats. J Appl Physiol 35:463–476, 1973.

Gutierrez M, Beroiza T, Contreras G, et al: Weekly cuirass ventilation improves blood gases and inspiratory muscle strength in patients with chronic air-flow limitation and hypercarbia. Am Rev Respir Dis 138:617–623, 1988.

Guz A, Noble MIM, Trenchard D, et al: Studies on the vagus nerves in man: Their role in respiratory and circulatory control. Clin Sci 27:293–304, 1964.

Habel AM, Hubmayr RD, and Simon PM: Role of vagal feedback in the entrainment of the respiratory rhythm in sleeping humans to a mechanical ventilator. Am J Respir Crit Care Med 153:A775, 1996.

Habel AM, Simon PM, Stroetz RW, et al: Effects of inspiratory flow on respiratory rate in sleeping normals during mechanical ventilation. Chest 108:99S, 1995.

Hanks EC, Ngai SH, and Fink BR: The respiratory threshold for carbon dioxide in anesthetized man: Determination of carbon dioxide threshold during halothane anesthesia. Anesthesiology 22:393–397, 1961.

Henke KG, Arias A, Skatrud JB, et al: Inhibition of inspiratory muscle activity during sleep. Chemical and nonchemical influences. Am Rev Respir Dis 138:8–15, 1988.

Henke KG, Badr MS, Skatrud JB, et al: Load compensation and respiratory muscle function during sleep. J Appl Physiol 72:1221–1234, 1992.

Hubmayr RD, Litchy WJ, Gay PC, et al: Transdiaphragmatic twitch pressure: Effects of lung volume and chest wall shape. Am Rev Respir Dis 139:647–652, 1989.

Iatridis A and Iber C: The effect of lung denervation on the reflex response to inspiratory resistive loads during sleep. Am Rev Respir Dis 147:A954, 1993.

Iber C, Simon P, Skatrud JB, et al: The Breuer-Hering reflex in humans: Effects of pulmonary denervation and hypocapnia. J Appl Physiol 152:217–224, 1995.

Ingrassia TS III, Nelson SB, Harris CD, et al: Influence of sleep state on CO_2 responsiveness: A study of the unloaded respiratory pump in humans. Am Rev Respir Dis 144:1125–1129, 1991.

Jounieaux V, Aubert G, Dury M, et al: Effects of nasal positive-pressure hyperventilation on the glottis in normal awake subjects. J Appl Physiol 79:176–185, 1995a.

Jounieaux V, Aubert G, Dury M, et al: Effects of nasal positive-pressure hyperventilation on the glottis in normal sleeping subjects. J Appl Physiol 79:186–193, 1995b.

Karczewski WA, Budzinska K, Gromysz H, et al: Some responses of the respiratory complex to stimulation of its vagal and mesencephalic inputs.

Respiratory Center and Afferent Systems INSERM 59:107–115, 1975.

Lawson EE: Prolonged central respiratory inhibition following reflex-induced apnea. J Appl Physiol 50:874–879, 1981.

Leevers AM, Simon PM, and Dempsey JA: Apnea after normocapnic mechanical ventilation during NREM sleep. J Appl Physiol 77:2079–2085, 1994.

Leevers AM, Simon PM, Xi L, et al: Apnoea following normocapnic mechanical ventilation in awake mammals: A demonstration of control system inertia. J Physiol 472:749–768, 1993.

Lofaso F, Isabey D, Lorino H, et al: Respiratory response to positive and negative inspiratory pressure in humans. Respir Physiol 89:75–88, 1992.

Luce JM, Pierson DJ, and Hudson LD: Intermittent mandatory ventilation. Chest 79:678–685, 1981.

MacIntyre NR and Leatherman NE: Mechanical loads on the ventilatory muscles: A theoretical analysis. Am Rev Respir Dis 139:968–973, 1989.

Manchanda S, Leevers AM, Wilson CR, et al: Frequency and volume thresholds for inhibition of inspiratory motor output during mechanical ventilation. Respir Physiol 105:1–16, 1996.

Marantz S, Patrick W, Webster K, et al: Response of ventilator-dependent patients to different levels of proportional assist. J Appl Physiol 80:397–403, 1996.

Marini JJ, Capps JS, and Culver BH: The inspiratory work of breathing during assisted mechanical ventilation. Chest 87:612–618, 1985.

Marini JJ, Rodriguez RM, and Lamb V: Bedside estimation of the inspiratory work of breathing during mechanical ventilation. Chest 89:56–63, 1986a.

Marini JJ, Rodriguez RM, and Lamb V. The inspiratory workload of patient-initiated mechanical ventilation. Am Rev Respir Dis 134:902–909, 1986b.

Marini JJ, Smith TC, and Lamb VJ: External work output and force generation during synchronized intermittent mechanical ventilation: Effect of machine assistance on breathing effort. Am Rev Respir Dis 138:1169–1179, 1988.

Martin TJ and Sanders MH: Chronic alveolar hypoventilation: A review for the clinician. Sleep 18:617–634, 1995.

Mathew OP, Abu-Osba YK, and Thach BT: Influence of upper airway pressure changes on respiratory frequency. Respir Physiol 49:223–233, 1982.

Meyer TJ and Hill NJ: Noninvasive positive pressure ventilation to treat respiratory failure. Ann Intern Med 120:760–770, 1994.

Milic-Emili J, Gottfried SB, and Rossi A: Dynamic hyperinflation: Intrinsic PEEP and its ramifications in patients with respiratory failure. In Vincent JL (ed): Update in Intensive Care and Emergency Medicine: Update 1987. New York, Springer-Verlag, 1987, pp 192–198.

Mitrouska I, Georgopoulos D, Younes M, et al: Effects of pulmonary and intercostal denervation on the response of respiratory output to varying inspiratory flow. Am J Respir Crit Care Med 153:A775, 1996.

Morrell MJ, Shea SA, Adams L, et al: Effect of inspiratory support upon breathing in humans during wakefulness and sleep. Respir Physiol 93:57–70, 1993.

Muzzin S, Baconnier P, and Benchetrit G: Entrainment of respiratory rhythm by periodic lung inflation: Effect of airflow rate and duration. Am J Physiol 263:R292–R300, 1992.

Pack AI, Delaney RG, and Fishman AP: Augmentation of phrenic neural activity by increased rates of lung inflation. J Appl Physiol 50:149–161, 1981.

Parreira VF, Jounieaux V, Aubert G, et al: Nasal two-level positive-pressure ventilation in normal subjects: Effects on the glottis and ventilation. Am J Respir Crit Care Med 153:1616–1623, 1996.

Patrick W, Webster K, Puddy A, et al: Respiratory response to CO_2 in the hypocapnic range in awake humans. J Appl Physiol 79:2058–2068, 1995;

Pearle JL and Simmons DH: Ventilatory and neuromuscular responses to inspiratory positive pressure during CO_2 breathing. Respiration 43:277–284, 1982.

Pepe PE and Marini JJ. Occult positive end-expiratory pressure in mechanically ventilated patients with airflow obstruction: The auto-PEEP effect. Am Rev Respir Dis 126:166–170, 1982.

Petrillo GA and Glass L: A theory for phase locking of respiration in cats to a mechanical ventilator. Am J Physiol 246:R311–R320, 1984.

Petrillo GA, Glass L, and Trippenbach T: Phase locking of the respiratory rhythm in cats to a mechanical ventilator. Can J Physiol Pharmacol 61:599–607, 1983.

Phillipson EA and Bowes G: Control of breathing during sleep. In Handbook of Physiology, Section 3, Vol 2: The respiratory system. Part 2: Control of breathing. Bethesda, MD, American Physiological Society, 1986, pp 649–690.

Polacheck J, Strong R, Arens J, et al: Phasic vagal influence on inspiratory motor output in anesthetized human subjects. J Appl Physiol 49:609–619, 1980.

Prechter GC, Nelson SB, and Hubmayr RD: The ventilatory recruitment threshold for carbon dioxide. Am Rev Respir Dis 141:758–764, 1990.

Puddy A, Patrick W, Webster K, et al: Respiratory control during volume-cycled ventilation in normal humans. J Appl Physiol 80:1749–1758, 1996.

Puddy A and Younes M: Effect of slowly increasing elastic load on breathing in conscious humans. J Appl Physiol 70:1277–1283, 1981.

Puddy A and Younes M: Effect of inspiratory flow rate on respiratory output in normal subjects. Am Rev Respir Dis 146:787–789, 1992.

Rajagopalan N, Simon PM, Gay PC, et al: Effects of nasal BiPAP on breathing in normal sleeping humans. Am J Respir Crit Care Med 153:A371, 1996.

Rebuck AS and Slutsky AS: Control of breathing in disease of the respiratory tract and lungs. In Handbook of Physiology; Section 3. The Respiratory System. Control of Breathing, Vol 2. Bethesda, MD, American Physiological Society, 1986, pp 771–791.

Remmers JE: Inhibition of inspiratory activity by intercostal muscle afferents. Respir Physiol 10:358–383, 1970.

Rochester DF, Braun NMT, and Laine S: Diaphragmatic energy expenditure in chronic respiratory failure: The effect of assisted ventilation with body respirators. Am J Med 63:223–232, 1977.

Roussos C and Macklem P: Diaphragmatic fatigue in man. J Appl Physiol 43:189–197, 1977.

Scheid P, Lofaso F, Isabey D, et al: Respiratory response to inhaled CO_2 during positive inspiratory pressure in humans. J Appl Physiol 77:876–882, 1994.

Shapiro SH, Ernst P, Gray-Donald K, et al: Effect of negative pressure ventilation in severe pulmonary disease. Lancet 340:1425–1429, 1992.

Simon PM, Dempsey JA, Griffin D, et al: Effect of sleep on respiratory muscle activity during mechanical ventilation. Am Rev Respir Dis 147:32–37, 1993.

Simon PM, Skatrud JB, Badr MF, et al: Role of airway mechanoreceptors in the inhibition of inspiration during mechanical ventilation in humans. Am Rev Respir Dis 144:1033–1041, 1991.

Simon PM, Skatrud JB, Landry DM, et al: Level of chemical stimuli at initiation and termination of apnea in humans. Am Rev Respir Dis 145:A406, 1992.

Skatrud JB, and Dempsey JA: Interaction of sleep state and chemical stimuli in sustaining rhythmic ventilation. J Appl Physiol 55:813–822, 1983.

Smith J, and Bellemare F: Effect of lung volume on in vivo contraction characteristics of human diaphragm. J Appl Physiol 62:1893–1900, 1987.

Speck DF: Supraspinal involvement in the phrenic-to-phrenic inhibitory reflex. Brain Res 414:169–172, 1987.

Stroetz RW, Simon PM, and Hubmayr RD: Effect of lung disease on the relationship between ventilator tidal volume and respiratory timing. Am J Respir Crit Care Med 153:A379, 1996.

Tan CSH, and Simmons DH: Effect of assisted mechanical ventilation on arterial carbon dioxide tension of normal anesthetized dogs. Lung 156:255–264, 1979.

Tobert DG, Simon PM, Stroetz RW, et al: The determinants of respiratory rate during mechanical ventilation. Am J Respir Crit Care Med, 155:485–492, 1997.

Vibert J-F, Caille D, and Segundo JP: Respiratory oscillator entrainment by periodic vagal afferents. Biol Cybern 41:119–130, 1981.

Ward ME, Corbeil C, Gibbons W, et al: Optimization of respiratory muscle relaxation during mechanical ventilation. Anesthesiology 69:29–35, 1988.

Weisman IM, Rinaldo JE, Roges RM, et al: Intermittent mandatory ventilation. Am Rev Respir Dis 127:641–647, 1983.

Wies WM, Simon PM, Tobert DG, et al: Entrainment pattern of inspiratory activity in awake human subjects during controlled mechanical ventilation. Chest 106:69S, 1994.

Younes M: Patient-ventilator interactions with pressure-assisted modalities of ventilatory support. Semin Respir Med 14:299–321, 1993.

Zurob A, Simon P, Wies W, et al: Effect of CO_2 on entrainment of the respiratory rhythm to a mechanical ventilator in sleeping humans. FASEB J 10:A641, 1996.

C H A P T E R

Critical Care Radiology

Peter G. Herman, M.D.

Arfa Khan, M.D.

In the United States most acute care hospitals have a specialized intensive care unit (ICU). In larger institutions the critical care areas also are subspecialized according to the clinical services responsible for patients' care. It is the usual practice in most ICUs to obtain a routine, daily, bedside chest radiograph. Very often the routine radiographs are obtained early in the morning and, therefore, are available for review at the time of the morning rounds. The justification of this practice is based on several considerations: it is difficult and sometimes impossible to clinically evaluate and communicate with an ICU patient, and malposition of the support and monitoring devices is frequent (Goodman and Putnam, 1992; Herman, 1983; Wechsler et al, 1988). In the assessment of the patient's cardiopulmonary status, the chest radiograph can be essential. The necessity of this practice, however, has been frequently questioned based on economic considerations and the concern of exposing the patient and the environment to unnecessary radiation. Numerous studies investigated the utility of the bedside chest radiograph based on the impact on patient management (Bekemeyer et al, 1985; Greenbaum and Marschall, 1982; Henschke et al, 1983). The consensus from these studies indicates that approximately 30% of the routine radiographs do, indeed, have an impact on the patients' management and thereby justify this practice (Bekemeyer et al, 1985; Greenbaum and Marschall, 1982; Henschke et al, 1983; Hall et al, 1991).

Imaging of the critically ill, however, is not limited to the confines of an ICU. Patients frequently require computed tomography (CT) (Gross and Spizarny, 1994), occasionally magnetic resonance imaging (MRI), and nuclear medicine studies for various vascular and nonvascular interventional procedures.

BEDSIDE RADIOGRAPHIC TECHNOLOGY

ICU bedside radiography was once similar to the radiographic technique used for other purposes. A standard radiographic film is exposed in a cassette, and the films are processed in the routine manner.

Digital (Fraser et al, 1989) or computed radiography (CR) has been increasingly introduced in ICUs (Blume and Jost, 1992; Marglin et al, 1990; Saito et al, 1988). The CR technology employs an imaging plate that is coated with a photo-stimuable phosphor. Following exposure to x-rays, this imaging plate develops a latent image. Subsequently, the latent image is scanned by laser reader; the emitted light from the image is converted into an electrical signal. This electrical signal is eventually converted into digital information. Depending on the characteristics of the system, digital images of various resolutions can be obtained.

Compared to standard technologies, CR results in images with a much wider dynamic range and with automatic density control. CR technology has the capability of further digital image processing, which can modify and often improve the final image. Using this technique, under- and overexposure are less likely. Magnified images and black and white reversal images can also be obtained (Fig. 13–1). Image contrast can be changed. On the negative side, CR images are lower in spatial resolution. Most observer performance studies, however, have shown no difference in the ability to detect normal structures and common abnormalities (Jennings et al, 1992; Maguire et al, 1994; Niklason et al, 1993; Thompson et al, 1989). The CR image can be immediately viewed on dedicated work stations, which very often are located within the ICU areas (Humphrey et al, 1993). In addition to the work stations, laser printed copies of the CRs can be viewed and filed in a manner similar to that for standard radiographs.

Digital images can be stored on magnetic or optical disks and eventually entered into a central picture archiving and communication system (Ravin, 1990). A single bedside chest radiograph contains approximately five megabytes of information, which, however, can be subsequently further compressed.

The added benefit of digital imaging is the ability to distribute the images through a local area network, or possibly through telephone lines to patient care areas and physicians' offices (Bellon et al, 1994). Because CR eliminates the need

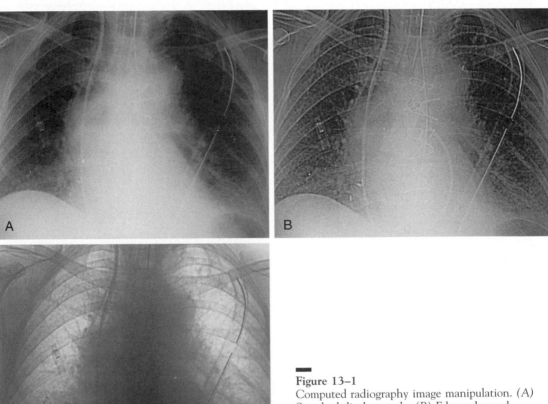

Figure 13–1
Computed radiography image manipulation. (A) Standard display mode. (B) Edge-enhanced display. The tubes and lines are better visualized. (C) Black and white reversal mode. The visibility of the bones, mediastinal structures, and some of the tubes and lines is improved.

for development and processing of x-ray films, the images are available for clinical assessment far sooner than those with the standard technology (Bellon et al, 1994).

One disadvantage of the digital system is that only the current and most recent previous images are usually available on the work stations. This is due to limits on the amount of memory available for data storage.

In radiology departments where CR is currently not available it is very useful to place a motorized viewer in close proximity to the ICU, where all the current images on the ICU patients can be centrally displayed.

ORGANIZATION OF THE ICU RADIOLOGY SERVICE

Because of the special needs of the critical care units, it is important that a separate radiology supervisory structure be established. The radiology supervisor has to ensure the proper maintenance of the equipment, training of the staff, and quality of the images obtained. The imaging service has to have a very close working relationship with the patient care providers within the units.

It is desirable that the radiologist who reviews the ICU studies be familiar with the patients and have regular interaction with the clinical care team. It is very important to have immediate transmission of all significant observations obtained on the radiograph to the patient care team.

Working in the critical care areas is often stressful for radiologic technologists. Critically ill patients are unable to cooperate, and various support systems also interfere with the movement and positioning of the patients. It is desirable to identify a group of technologists who are personally interested and devoted to the critical care setting and can establish good working relationships with the nurses.

EQUIPMENT CONSIDERATIONS

The most commonly used portable radiographic units are usually constant-potential battery operated or capacitor discharge systems. Their maximal output is usually 110 kV and 400 MA. It is desirable to have a long x-ray tube stand that permits the maintenance of a 48-inch distance between the film cassette and x-ray tube.

RADIOGRAPHIC TECHNIQUE

An important technical consideration is to maintain the consistency of the bedside radiographs. Because daily changes have to be assessed, it is important that positioning of the patients be maintained. The exposure factors should not be changed. The optical density of the images has to be comparable. It is recommended that a technique book be maintained by the technologists recording the position, distance, and exposure factors used. Additional information regarding the patients' ventilatory status can also be included, such as the amount of positive end-expiratory pressure (PEEP) (Goodman and Putnam, 1992; Zimmerman et al, 1979). Recording PEEP may aid later correlation between changes in clinical and ventilatory status and radiographic findings. It is important that the portable units be frequently checked to ensure that they have well-functioning collimators.

PATIENT POSITIONING

In ICUs, most of the routine bedside radiographs are obtained with the patient in the supine, anteroposterior (AP) position at 48-inch target-to-film distance. For patients who are able to sit up, a posteroanterior (PA) radiograph is obtained while the patient is sitting on the edge of the bed hugging the cassette. Lateral decubitus views are obtained for evaluation of pleural effusion and occasionally for pneumothorax. The lateral decubitus view can be helpful to assess the appearance of the lungs on the nondependent side.

Occasionally, in less severely ill patients, a 6-foot erect PA radiograph can also be obtained. For routine daily studies we prefer a properly positioned and exposed supine radiograph over a semierect and/or erect radiograph, which may be compromised by motion or obliquity. Lateral chest films could be particularly useful to clarify the position of various tubes and lines (Brandstetter et al, 1994), such as the endotracheal (ET) tube or central venous pressure (CVP) line.

In addition to the patient's name, date, unit number, and time of examination, the inclinometer reading indicating the patient's position is desirable. If the patient is on a ventilator with PEEP, the amount of PEEP should be noted. In patients with Swan-Ganz catheters, the pulmonary wedge pressure obtained at the time of the radiograph can be helpful in correlating the physiologic and radiographic information. We recommend that radiographs be obtained with the patient in deep inspiration because the maximal amount of air provides a good contrast for assessment of the lung. In the critical care area such inspiration, however, is often not always feasible. Furthermore, it should be remembered that most often films are taken at functional residual capacity (end-expiration) in patients on ventilators, which is considerably smaller than total lung capacity (greatest lung volume) used in most films. At a distance of 48 inches on an AP film, there is an approximately 10 to 15% magnification in the width of the mediastinal structures. However, even when allowing for magnification, the assessment of the cardiac size is not to be considered reliable for the AP projection.

Limiting the radiation exposure for both the patient and the personnel is an important consideration. Proper collimation and careful technique significantly limit the radiation outside of the field. The technologists should be at least six feet from the mobile radiographic unit. With the appropriate safeguards the occupational exposure of the staff is minimal and is within the established safety standards.

RADIOLOGY OF SUPPORT AND MONITORING DEVICES

In routine daily ICU chest radiographs, approximately 20% of the tubes and lines are found to be malpositioned (Hunter, 1995). ET tubes, CVP lines, and Swan-Ganz lines are most often displaced. Recognizing the inappropriate position of these lines on the routine radiograph prevents serious complications, which can follow improper placement (Hall et al, 1991; Henschke et al, 1983; Pasternack and O'Cain, 1983).

ENDOTRACHEAL TUBE

The adult trachea is approximately 12 cm in length, and the optimal position of the tip of the endotracheal tube should be in the midtrachea, approximately 5 to 7 cm from the carina while the patient's neck is in the neutral position. During flexion and extension of the neck, however, there is considerable excursion of the tip, which can move caudally during flexion and cephalad during extension by several centimeters (Conrady et al, 1976). Although the carina is not always easily visible, the oblique direction of the left mainstem bronchus can often be recognized and its junction with the trachea used as the marker of the carina. The carina is commonly at the level of the T5/T6 thoracic vertebrae. A common problem with the placement of the ET is a downward displacement of the tube into the right mainstem bronchus. Intubation of the right mainstem bronchus can eventually lead to atelectasis of the nonventilated left lung (Fig. 13–2). Upward misplacement of the endotracheal tube eventually may result in extubation and can cause damage to the larynx. A rare event is inadvertent

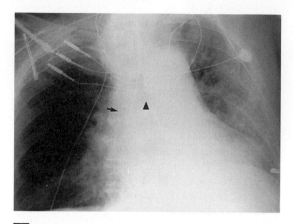

Figure 13–2
Malposition of an endotracheal tube (ETT). The arrow points to the tip of the tube, which is within the right mainstem bronchus. The arrowhead indicates the position of the carina. Note the retrocardiac opacity, which is indicative of impending left lung atelectasis.

insertion of the ET into the pharynx or the esophagus. If there is any question about the endotracheal placement, a lateral radiograph should be immediately obtained.

Perforation of the trachea is uncommon and usually involves the posterior membranous wall. Perforation can result in pneumomediastinum, pneumothorax, and subcutaneous emphysema. The presence of these signs should raise suspicion of misplacement of the ET tube. In cases of tracheal perforation, particularly when it is limited to the adjacent mediastinum, malposition may be more difficult to detect. The slightly oblique direction of the ET tube can be a suggestive sign. Thoracic CT can be very helpful to make the definitive diagnosis.

Prolonged endotracheal intubation may result in pressure necrosis of the tracheal wall. Since the introduction of the high-volume, low-pressure cuffs this complication is less frequent. Bulging of the ET cuff, projecting of the cuff outside of the tracheal outline, and cuff-to-tracheal ratio over 1.5 are useful radiologic signs of potential pressure necrosis of the trachea (Khan et al, 1976) (Fig. 13–3). In patients who require long-term ventilation, tracheostomy is often performed. The stoma is usually located at the level of the second and third tracheal cartilage. Immediately following tracheostomy, the tracheostomy tube should be parallel with the axis of the trachea. The position of the trachea and the tracheostomy tube is not dependent on the position of the patient's neck. Similar to ETs, the cuff of the tracheostomy tube should not distend the tracheal wall.

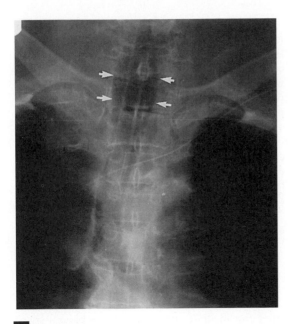

Figure 13–3
ETT cuff overdistention. Arrows indicate the air within the overdistended cuff of the ETT. The increased width of the cuff is indicative of potential damage to the tracheal wall.

Both ETs and tracheostomy tubes may cause tracheostenosis or tracheomalacia. In current practice, if these are suspected the radiologic examination of choice is CT. Spiral or helical CT is particularly useful and provides an exquisite image of the trachea. Following the removal of the tracheostomy tube, tracheostenosis may occur at the level of the stoma as a consequence of granulation tissue. If the stenosis is below the stoma and extends over several tracheal cartilages it is usually related to overdistention of the cuff. Tracheomalacia is a result of the destruction of the tracheal wall when associated with secondary ulcerations and infection.

CHEST TUBE

Thoracotomy tubes, or pleural drainage tubes, are introduced for the relief of pneumothorax or pleural effusion, and possibly empyema. The optimal position of the thoracotomy tube to drain pleural effusions should be in the lower posterior pleural space. To treat pneumothorax, the thoracotomy tube is best positioned in the anterior-superior pleural space. Occasionally the thoracotomy tube is buried within the fissures, which may interfere with its proper function. If there is a question about the proper positioning of the thoracotomy, an additional lateral view should be obtained.

Following removal of chest tubes, a linear opacity on the chest radiograph usually represents residual pleural reaction and is usually of no significance.

NASOGASTRIC TUBES

In ICUs, nasogastric tubes are commonly employed. One purpose is to suction gastric contents, and some modified nasogastric tubes are used for feeding. It is important that the tip of the nasogastric tube pass into the stomach. Most of the nasogastric tubes have side holes at the distal 2 to 10 cm. When the nasogastric tube is properly positioned, all the side holes should be within the stomach. If they are inadvertently in the esophagus they may cause aspiration. Feeding tubes also have fenestrations. Often the tip of the feeding tube is densely radiopaque, thus aiding assessment of position.

There are complications associated with the insertion of a feeding tube. Often the feeding tubes are passed using a stiffening wire, aiding the placement of the tube. If the wire exits through a side hole it may perforate the esophagus or the stomach. Because patients in the ICU frequently cannot swallow, these tubes may be mistakenly inserted through the glottis into the trachea. The inadvertent insertion of the feeding or nasogastric tube into the tracheobronchial tree can result in life-threatening aspiration (Stark, 1982; Woodall et al, 1987) (Figs. 13–4, 13–5). If it is clearly established that the feeding tube is not in the

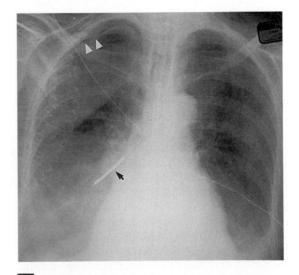

Figure 13–4
Malposition of a feeding tube. The arrow indicates the radiopaque tip of the feeding tube, which was placed inadvertently in the right lower lobe bronchus. There is associated pneumothorax (*arrowheads*).

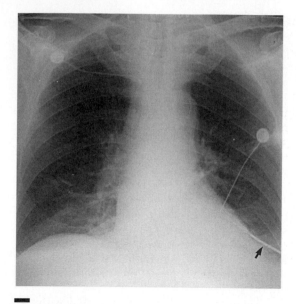

Figure 13–5
Malposition of a feeding tube. The arrow indicates the radiopaque tip of a feeding tube, which was placed inadvertently in the left lower lobe bronchus.

tracheobronchial tree, injection of a small amount of diluted barium can verify its exact position. Because low-pressure endotracheal cuffs are commonly used, there is little resistance to a nasogastric tube that is inadvertently passed into the trachea. If esophageal perforation is suspected, the examination of choice is thoracic CT. During the routine review of the chest radiographs it is important to note deviations of the nasogastric tubes because they can indicate displacement resulting from a mediastinal mass or hemorrhage.

CARDIOVASCULAR DEVICES

Central lines are one of the most commonly employed devices in the ICU (Handel and Ravin, 1983). Central lines, in addition to monitoring cardiovascular performance, can be used for intravenous administration of fluids. Most of the lines are radiopaque; some, however, tend to be faint on film and it is difficult to establish their exact position. The central catheters are usually inserted through the subclavian or internal jugular vein. The desired location of the tip of the central line is in the superior vena cava; however, location at the junction of the brachiocephalic veins and the superior vena cava may be acceptable. The right brachiocephalic vein is vertical in its orientation; the left is horizontal, crossing the mediastinum from left to right. The brachiocephalic veins and the superior vena cava contain no valves. The

junction between the superior vena cava and the left brachiocephalic vein is usually at the level of the first intercostal space. If, on a lateral view, the central line is positioned posteriorly, it may be within the azygos arch. Left-sided superior vena cava is present in somewhat less than 1% of the population, but more than half of these individuals have double superior vena cava and both eventually drain into the right atrium (Fig. 13–6). A common malposition of the central line is upward displacement into the jugular vein (Fig. 13–7). If the line enters the right atrium, eventually it may be positioned within the coronary sinus.

Intracardiac placement of the central line is undesirable. It may result in cardiac perforation. Eventually it may enter the pericardial space and result in cardiac tamponade, although this complication is rare. Passage of the central line through the tricuspid valve can cause cardiac arrhythmias. If the central line perforates, it can enter the mediastinum or even the pleural space (Mitchell and Clark, 1979) (Fig. 13–8). Fluoroscopy and injection of a small amount of contrast material may be very helpful to verify the position of the central line. During the insertion of the central line, pneumothorax may occur as often as 12% of the time. The pneumothorax may be delayed in appearance. Central lines that are in place for long periods may cause thrombosis in the surrounding vessel. All lines remaining in place for a long duration may cause infectious complications.

SWAN-GANZ CATHETER

The Swan-Ganz catheter is a balloon-tipped, flow-directed catheter that is usually positioned within the left or right main pulmonary artery while the balloon is deflated (McCloud and Putnam, 1975). Following inflation of the balloon, the pulmonary arterial occlusion (wedge) pressure can be obtained by establishing a continuous column of blood between the catheter tip and the left atrium through the pulmonary microcirculation. In supine patients the ideal position of the inflated balloon tip should be in the lower zone of the lungs. If the tip of the catheter is too distal, thrombosis and infarction of the involved segment may result (Fig. 13–9). These complications are usually recognized as a patchy opacity in the areas supplied by the pulmonary artery in the region of the tip of the Swan-Ganz catheter. Withdrawal of the catheter to a proximal position usually is sufficient to treat this event. Rarely, other complications may occur, which may be infection, septic emboli, and cardiac arrhythmias.

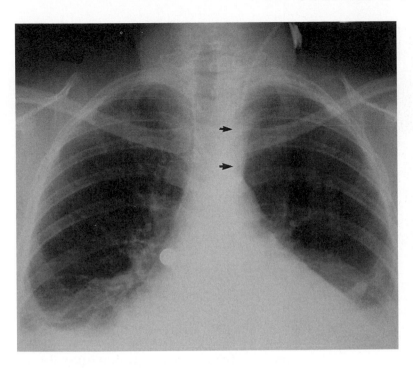

Figure 13–6
Malposition of a venous
catheter. Arrows outline a
central venous catheter
introduced from the left side
descending along the left side
of the mediastinum. It is
located within a persistent left
superior vena cava.

INTRA-AORTIC COUNTER PULSATION BALLOON (IACB)

The IACB is a large-bore catheter usually introduced from through the femoral artery. It is advanced through the upper descending thoracic aorta. A 20-cm-long inflatable balloon surrounds the distal end of the catheter. The balloon is inflated during diastole and deflated during systole by electrocardiographic gating. The desired posi-

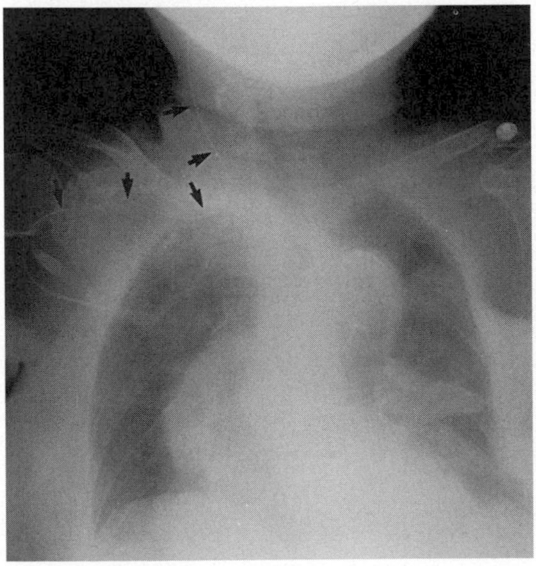

Figure 13–7
Malposition of a venous catheter. Arrows outline the course of a right subclavian catheter. Note that instead of entering the superior vena cava, the catheter has turned cephalad into the jugular vein.

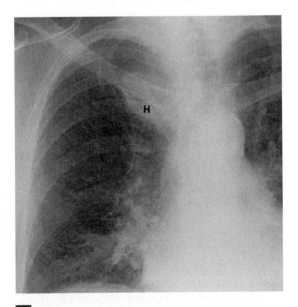

Figure 13–8
Mediastinal hematoma following insertion of central line. A poorly defined opacity is adjacent to the right upper mediastinal border, causing deviation to the trachea to left. It appeared suddenly following an attempt of central venous catheter placement. The opacity represents a hematoma (H).

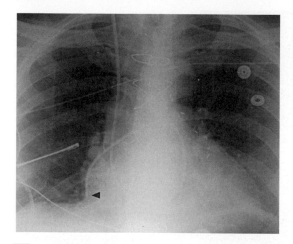

Figure 13–9
Malposition of a Swan-Ganz catheter. The arrowhead indicates the distal end of the Swan-Ganz catheter, which is located too far distally within a subsegmental pulmonary artery. Subsequently, the patient developed a pulmonary infarction adjacent to the tip of the Swan-Ganz catheter.

tion of the IACB is in the aorta distal to the left subclavian artery. If the catheter is too proximal it may enter the left subclavian artery or even reach within the aortic arch, which can create cerebral embolism (Fig. 13–10).

TRANSVENOUS PACEMAKERS

The electrode is advanced through the jugular or subclavian vein intracardially and should be near the apex of the right ventricle. There are common malpositions of electrodes; they may terminate in the coronary sinus or in the right atrium. To recognize malposition within the coronary sinus, a lateral chest radiograph is required, which verifies that instead of the anterior curvature toward the apex of the right ventricle the electrode is pointing posteriorly (Herman, 1983).

Myocardial perforation may be associated with placement of pacemakers. The tip of the electrode can project outside of the confines of the heart. CT can be helpful to verify the exact position of the tip of the electrode (Fig. 13–11).

CARDIOPULMONARY DISEASE

The radiographic evaluation of cardiopulmonary problems in critically ill patients is often difficult for a number of reasons. Portable radiographs do not provide the resolution and reproducibility achieved by stationary equipment. The lung and cardiac abnormalities visualized are frequently the

result of more than one disease process. The acute disease may be superimposed on a chronic lung disease. In addition, the radiographic appearance of cardiopulmonary disease may be altered by various support and monitoring devices as well as therapeutic maneuvers. Serial radiographs must be viewed not only for day-to-day change, but also for more general trends. It is common to see no radiographic change from one day to the next, whereas very definite trends may be apparent when films are viewed serially over several days. Additional views like lateral, oblique, or lateral decubitus films, and even CT scans, may be needed to clarify the disease process.

ATELECTASIS

The most common radiographic abnormality in the ICU is atelectasis. It is especially common in the postoperative period. Various factors, sometimes multiple, contribute to atelectasis in ICU patients. These include hypoventilation due to central ventilatory depression, surgery, or trauma, and retained bronchial secretions resulting from

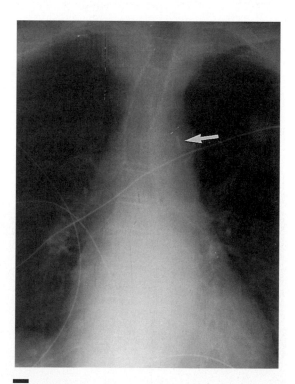

Figure 13–10
Intra-aortic counter-pulsation balloon (IACB) malposition. The arrow points to the distal end of the IACB. Because of the high position of the tip, the balloon may obstruct the left subclavian artery.

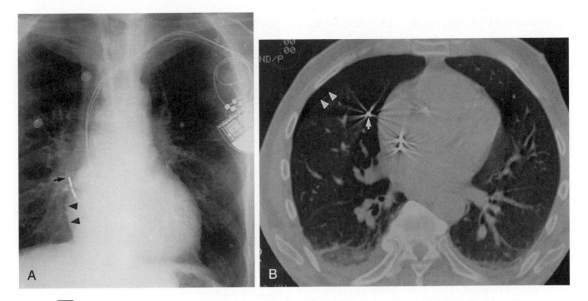

Figure 13–11
Myocardial perforation by pacemaker wire. (A) The arrow points to the tip of the atrial pacing electrode, which is projecting beyond the right atrial wall (*arrowheads*). (B) CT scan shows the catheter tip in the pleural space (*arrow*) and the presence of pneumothorax (*arrowheads*).

decreased ability to cough and diminished mucociliary clearance, especially in intubated patients. The radiographic evidence of atelectasis varies from a slight decrease in lung volume without visible infiltrate to complete opacification and collapse of the segment, lobe, or lung (Fig. 13–12). Subsegmental or plate-like atelectasis appears as linear densities parallel or oblique to the diaphragm. Segmental or lobar atelectasis may be patchy and ill-defined and difficult to differentiate from pneumonia. The direct signs of atelectasis

are lack of aeration with shift of interlobar fissure and blurring of bronchovascular markings as a consequence of volume loss. Indirect signs include shift of the mediastinum (including nasogastric tube, if present), displacement of the hilum, and elevation of the diaphragm. Atelectasis is most common and most severe in the left lower lobe, which may be related to extrinsic pressure on the left lower lobe bronchus by the heart in supine, bed-ridden patients (Shevland et al, 1983).

Left lower lobe atelectasis typically presents

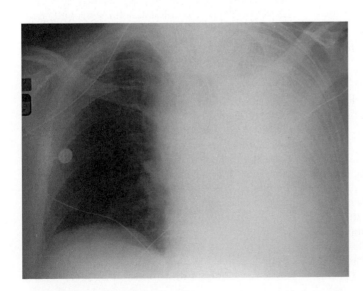

Figure 13–12
Total opacification of the left lung resulting from atelectasis. The mediastinum is shifted to the left. A mucous plug in the left mainstem bronchus was responsible for the atelectasis.

as a retrocardiac density with obliteration of the medial part of the left hemidiaphragm and descending aorta, elevation of the diaphragm, depression of the left hilum, shift of the mediastinum, and hyperaeration of the left upper lobe. However, the diagnosis of left lower lobe atelectasis may be difficult from a supine portable radiograph. Its presence may be overlooked on an underpenetrated image. Obliteration of the medial part of the left diaphragm is not always a reliable sign of left lower lobe atelectasis, because the atelectasis may also be silhouetted by the heart itself on supine or semierect radiographs. An x-ray beam not perfectly perpendicular to the dome of the diaphragm also causes indistinct left hemidiaphragm, which is a finding known as *pseudoconsolidation* (Zylak et al, 1988). The presence or absence of air bronchograms in an area of atelectases is a helpful indicator of the cause of atelectasis and represents approximate site of obstruction. The presence of an air bronchogram in an area of atelectasis rules out endobronchial obstruction, such as mucous plug, clot, or tumor and, conversely, absence of air bronchograms usually suggests endobronchial obstruction. This has important consequences. For example, patients with endobronchial obstruction and persistent atelectasis often benefit from bronchoscopy (Marini et al, 1979).

PNEUMONIA

Lung infection occurs in 10 to 20% of ICU patients. The majority of lung infections in ICU patients are hospital-acquired or nosocomial infection and they differ significantly from community-acquired infections. The majority of community-acquired infections are due to viruses, mycoplasmic organisms, or gram-positive cocci, whereas the majority of nosocomial infections are due to gram-negative aerobes, such as *Klebsiella*, *Escherichia coli* and *Pseudomonas* species or to anaerobic organisms associated with aspiration.

Pseudomonas aeruginosa is a particularly virulent nosocomial organism causing pneumonia. *P. aeruginosa* pneumonia usually appears as a diffuse nodular bilateral lower lobe infiltrates that rapidly progress to involve most of the lung. A bilaterally symmetrical pattern simulating pulmonary edema is not uncommon. The nodules rapidly coalesce into large confluent areas, and at this stage abscess formation may be seen (Fig. 13–13). Unilateral infiltrates, interstitial infiltrates, or pleural effusions are uncommon findings. Pneumonia due to *P. aeruginosa* septicemia also initially appears with discrete nodules, but rapidly progresses to present

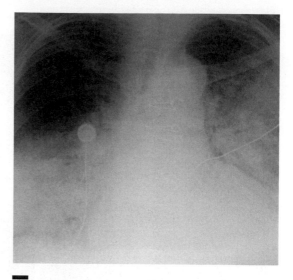

Figure 13–13
Bilateral *Pseudomonas* pneumonia due to aspirated infected secretions. Bilateral diffuse airspace infiltrates mimic the appearance of pulmonary edema and adult respiratory distress syndrome (ARDS).

a picture similar to that of the primary pneumonic form.

The portable chest radiograph appears to be of limited value for the diagnosis of pneumonia in the mechanically ventilated patient, with a diagnostic accuracy of about 50% because radiologic patterns suggestive of pneumonia are often associated with other conditions. New or persistent focal opacities are suggestive of pneumonia, but often noninfectious disorders such as atelectasis, bland aspiration, pulmonary hemorrhage, infarction, atypical cardiogenic pulmonary edema, asymmetrical adult respiratory distress syndrome (ARDS), loculated pleural effusion, and neoplasms all may have a radiographic appearance similar to that of pneumonia. Alternatively, a focal opacity due to pneumonia may be incorrectly interpreted to represent a noninfectious disorder. Moreover, mechanically ventilated patients may suffer simultaneously from more than one pulmonary abnormality (e.g., pneumonia and atelectasis). Infection may involve previously collapsed lung and, conversely, pneumonia predisposes the patient to develop atelectasis by mucous plugging of both small and large airways with abundant viscous secretions. Similarly, presence of atelectasis adjacent to a pleural effusion may be mistaken for pneumonia or obscure or underlying pneumonia (Goodman and Putnam, 1992).

A negative reading of a radiograph does not totally exclude significant infection. CT has been particularly helpful in demonstrating focal consolidation not visible on portable radiographs and in differentiating pneumonia from other noninfectious opacities (e.g., atelectasis, tumor, loculated fluid) (Fig. 13–14).

Complications of nosocomial infections are common and may present as abscess, empyema, and bronchopleural fistula. Differentiation between lung abscess and air-containing loculated empyema is usually not possible on AP radiograph only, and a lateral radiograph is also required. In general, pleural air collections occur along the posterior chest wall. On AP projection they have a long air-fluid level that is not dense, whereas on lateral projection the air-fluid level is relatively short and dense. The air-fluid level in empyema usually touches the chest wall (Fig. 13–15). An air-fluid level crossing the fissure also indicates a pleural collection. Conversely, the air-fluid level in a lung abscess is of the same length on an AP and lateral radiograph; it does not reach the chest wall and it does not cross the fissure. Abscess is usually spherical, whereas empyemas are long and oval (Goodman and Putnam, 1992). When diag-

nosis is obscure on conventional radiographs, CT scan often helps in the differentiation. On CT scan (Waite et al, 1990), empyema tends to be oval and forms obtuse angles with the chest wall. Empyemas act like a space-occupying lesion and cause displacement of the adjacent lung. Lung abscesses, on the other hand, are spherical and form an acute angle with the chest wall. They do not act as space-occupying lesions, and the bronchovascular markings usually continue into the abscess. The walls of empyema are smooth and may enhance with administration of intravenous contrast material. The walls of an abscess tend to be ragged. Loculated pleural collections usually need drainage. Drainage under imaging guidance is usually more successful and less traumatic than conventional thoracostomy placement (Westcott, 1985).

ASPIRATION SYNDROMES

Aspiration pneumonitis is another frequent cause of pulmonary infiltrates in the ICU patient. Pre-

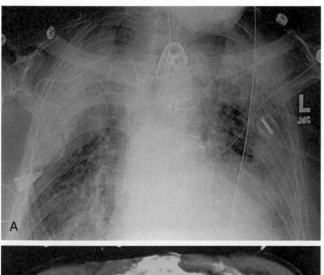

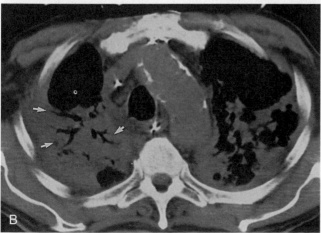

Figure 13–14
Consolidation versus empyema. (A) Chest radiograph shows a right upper lobe opacity believed to be loculated fluid. (B) CT scan shows presence of consolidation with air bronchograms (arrows) without loculated fluid.

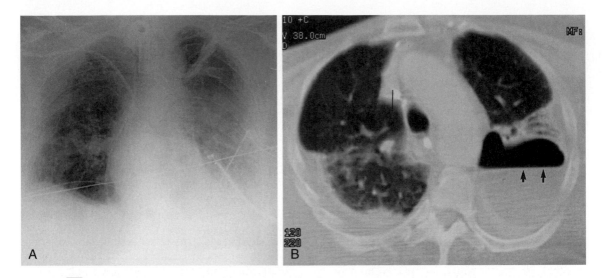

Figure 13–15
Empyema on chest radiograph versus computed tomography (CT) scan. (A) Portable chest radiograph shows left pleural effusion. (B) CT scan at the level of aortic arch shows a large empyema adjacent to posterior chest wall with air-fluid level (*arrows*). Because of the patient's supine position, this air-fluid level is not visible on the chest radiograph.

disposing factors include general anesthesia, decreased consciousness, neuromuscular disorder, esophageal disease, and the presence of nasogastric or endotracheal tubes. Pulmonary disease may be produced by the aspiration of toxic fluids, bland fluids, or particles or secretions contaminated with heavy inocula of organisms from the upper airway. The clinical and radiographic course depends on the nature of the material aspirated. The only common denominator is the breakdown of normal protective mechanisms of the pharynx and larynx.

ASPIRATION OF TOXIC FLUIDS

Aspiration of low pH gastric fluid is the most common cause of chemical pneumonitis (Mendelson's syndrome) in ICU patients and may occur as a massive single event or as multiple small aspirations. Within 1 to 2 hours after aspiration of low pH gastric juice, the patient exhibits fever, tachycardia, rales, and hypoxia. The initial radiographic appearance of chemical pneumonitis is variable, but the radiograph usually demonstrates rapidly progressive alveolar infiltrates that are most often bilateral or predominantly right-sided. The volume of aspirate may have a bearing on the extent of pulmonary infiltrates that develop. After the first 24 to 36 hours, radiographic and clinical improvement should be evident. Complete clearing may require 1 to 2 weeks.

Bilateral aspiration pneumonia may be diffi-cult to differentiate radiographically from cardiogenic pulmonary edema. A normal-sized heart and lack of upper lobe vascular distention favor the diagnosis of aspiration pneumonia. Aspiration must be distinguished from congestive heart failure. Chemical pneumonitis may be complicated by bacterial infection and abscess or empyema formation in about 25% of patients. Clinically, infection is suspected if the patient's condition suddenly worsens. The lung infiltrates either stabilize or worsen, with evidence of abscess formation of pleural effusion. Repeated small aspirations of gastric contents usually occur at night and are difficult to diagnose. In older or debilitated patients, recurrent bouts of lower lobe atelectasis, pneumonitis, or cavitation without apparent cause should lead one to consider this diagnosis.

ASPIRATION OF BLAND FLUID

Aspiration of fluids such as blood, water, barium, and neutralized gastric contents does not cause chemical pneumonitis. The radiograph is normal unless large volumes of fluid are aspirated. The infiltrate, if present, corresponds to the physical presence of the aspirated material and rapidly disappears following coughing or suctioning.

ASPIRATION OF INFECTED SECRETIONS

The upper airways of hospitalized patients are frequently colonized by various saprophytic and pathogenic organisms. Aspiration of infected secretions may lead to an indolent or recurrent pneumonia. The radiographic appearance of infiltrates is nonspecific. The infiltrates are located in gravity-dependent segments, such as the posterior segment of upper lobes and superior and posterior basal segment of lower lobes. Cavitation and empyema are frequent, and healing is often slow.

PULMONARY EDEMA

Chest radiography is the most commonly used noninvasive technique for assessing the presence or absence of pulmonary edema in critically ill patients. Physiologically there are two main types of pulmonary edema: (1) hydrostatic edema, which includes edema due to heart failure, and that due to fluid overload; (2) increased permeability of the pulmonary alveolar-capillary membrane, as occurs in acute lung injury (Aberle et al., 1988) (see Chapters 1, 3, 18, 19). To optimally treat acutely ill patients with pulmonary edema, it is important to differentiate hydrostatic or cardiogenic edema from the increased permeability or noncardiogenic edema. Although chest radiography is important in the management of pulmonary edema, it cannot be relied upon exclusively, and its findings should be interpreted in

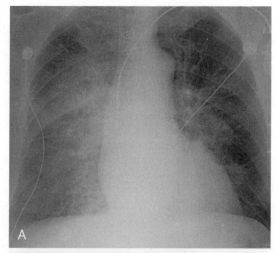

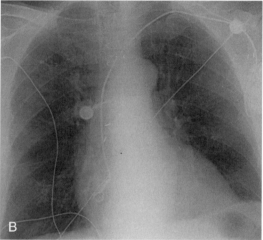

Figure 13–17
Asymmetric interstitial pulmonary edema. (A) Note the increased vascularity and the perivascular and perihilar haze, which is more pronounced on the right side. (B) Rapid clearing of pulmonary edema 10 hours later.

light of all other available clinical information (Milne and Pistolesi, 1990; Staub, 1980).

In hydrostatic pulmonary edema, the edema fluid is a transudate that is low in protein. The first site of accumulation of fluid is in the interstitial space (Figs. 13–16, 13–17) surrounding the blood vessels and bronchi. Interstitial pulmonary edema is visible on chest radiographs even before it can be detected clinically, because at this stage there is little or no fluid within the alveoli, and, therefore, the clinician does not hear any rales. Interstitial pulmonary edema is characterized by perihilar haze, peribronchial cuffing, increase in size and blurring of vascular markings, increased artery-bronchus ratio, septal lines (Kerley B line),

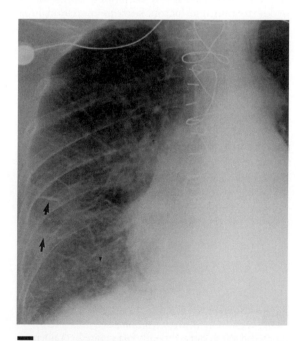

Figure 13–16
Interstitial pulmonary edema. Arrows point to the thickened interlobular septae (Kerley B lines).

and fluid in the fissure. As fluid progressively accumulates and saturates the interstitial space, alveolar edema develops. The edema is usually central in distribution. In increased permeability edema, the fluid is high in protein and may not flow from the extravasated site into the interstitial space, but may flood the alveolar space. This may explain the relative absence of peribronchial cuffing and septal lines and the infrequent occurrence of pleural effusion in patients with permeability edema. The distribution of increased permeability edema is patchy and peripheral and heart size is usually normal. The radiographic distinction between cardiogenic and noncardiogenic edema can be difficult.

Atypical pulmonary edema may have asymmetric or unilateral distribution (see Fig. 13–17). This arrangement is usually the result of preexisting underlying lung disease such as emphysema, pulmonary embolism, interstitial fibrosis, and prior radiation. Atypical pulmonary edema frequently simulates other acute pulmonary disorders such as pneumonia. Interval change of serial radiographs and clinical information helps in differential diagnosis.

ADULT RESPIRATORY DISTRESS SYNDROME

ARDS is a syndrome recognized by a clinical, functional, and radiographic tetrad: (1) acute, severe and progressive respiratory distress; (2) hypoxemia; (3) increased stiffness of the lung leading to acute respiratory failure; and (4) diffuse radiographic lung opacification. Lung injury leading to ARDS may affect capillary endothelial or alveolar epithelial lining cells. Common causes of acute lung injury include sepsis, aspiration of gastric contents, pneumonia, hypovolemic shock, drug toxicity, multiple system trauma, severe burns, and disorders necessitating multiple blood transfusions. Mortality rates are high and frequently reflect the associated development of extrathoracic organ system failure. There is variable involvement of the cardiovascular, renal, hepatic, hematologic, and central nervous systems.

There are three morphologic stages of acute alveolar damage that produce characteristic clinical, functional, and radiographic findings.

Stage 1 occurs in the first 12 to 24 hours. During the earliest and most transient stage of ARDS, there is capillary congestion, endothelial swelling, and extensive microatelectasis. A radiograph at this stage most often shows shallow inspiration with elevated diaphragms and clear lungs. When the inciting condition is associated with an underlying pulmonary process such as aspiration, lung opacification may be present at the outset. In the early phase of ARDS, the cause of respiratory distress may be unclear and may require differentiation from other conditions associated with acute respiratory distress and clear lungs such as central or musculoskeletal hypoventilation, acute airway obstruction, and massive pulmonary embolism.

Stage 2 occurs at (1 to 5 days). This stage is characterized by fluid leakage, fibrin deposition, and hyaline membrane lining the alveoli. The chest radiograph typically shows bilateral, diffuse, poorly marginated confluent opacities with or without air bronchograms, which is consistent with increased permeability edema (Fig. 13–18). The size of the heart and the caliber of the pulmonary vessels are normal. Consolidation, which may be more patchy at the outset of stage 2, usually becomes grossly uniform and indistinguishable from that of cardiogenic pulmonary edema. Detailed hemodynamic study and response to therapeutic trials of diuresis may be necessary to differentiate ARDS from hydrostatic edema. CT shows that consolidation in ARDS is often patchy, regional, or gravitationally distributed even when it appears uniform on the radiograph (Tagliabue et al, 1994).

Stage 3 occurs after 5 days. Alveolar flooding is replaced by hyperplasia of type II pneumocytes and collagen deposition. Functional impairment is due to multiple factors such as increased lung stiffness, ventilation-perfusion imbalance, diffu-

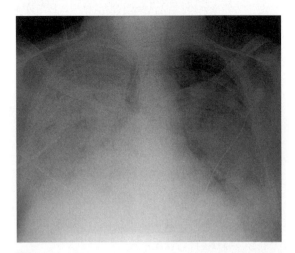

Figure 13–18
Acute respiratory distress syndrome secondary to sepsis. Bilateral, diffuse, poorly marginated confluent opacities, which are indistinguishable from the appearance of cardiogenic pulmonary edema or bilateral pneumonia.

sion impairment, and capillary bed destruction. Radiographic consolidation becomes less dense and the appearance more of "ground glass" as the edema fluid is replaced by collagen deposition by alveolar cell hyperplasia (Green, 1987).

The prognosis of ARDS is greatly affected by the development of major complications such as lung barotrauma, nosocomial infection, sepsis, hemorrhage, and multisystem failure. One of the feared complications of mechanical ventilation in ARDS is barotrauma (see Chapter 18). Portable radiographs should be scrutinized for evidence of interstitial emphysema, subpleural air cysts, pneumomediastinum, subcutaneous emphysema, and pneumothorax.

Nosocomial infection as a complication of ARDS may be overlooked on chest radiographs. Suggestive signs include accentuated regions of consolidation and discrete macrocystic lung abscesses. Most survivors appear to have a good chance for full recovery of respiratory function within 4 to 12 months. The chest radiograph may appear normal or show residual opacities (11%) or hyperinflation (8%).

ABNORMAL THORACIC AIR IN THE CRITICALLY ILL PATIENT

Extra alveolar air collections are a frequent and potentially lethal problem in the ICU. Positive-pressure therapy, closed-chest massage, and subclavian vein catheterization are the three most frequently implicated procedures. The incidence of barotrauma in patients receiving mechanical ventilation has been reported to be between 4 and 15%, and the rate increases as mean airway pressure increases (Zwilick et al, 1974).

Identification and localization of abnormal intrathoracic air collection may be difficult or even impossible in the supine patient. Additional evaluation by radiographs made with the patient in the erect or decubitus position may be helpful but difficult to obtain at the bedside. CT is rarely necessary but is by far the most accurate method of identifying and localizing abnormal air collections.

PNEUMOTHORAX

Pneumothorax is a common emergency in patients supported by mechanical ventilation, with an incidence rate of up to 25% (Greene et al, 1977; Khan et al, 1990). Air may reach the pleural surface following pneumomediastinum or may enter directly into the pleural space from rupture of alveoli or air cysts. Pneumothorax can also be a complication of invasive procedures, such as central venous catheterization, endotracheal intubation, and feeding tube placement (Silvani et al, 1993).

The radiographic appearance of pneumothorax varies with changes in patient positioning, size of the pneumothorax, and presence of intrapleural adhesions. The typical finding on an upright chest radiograph is a superolateral lucency outlined medially by a thin white visceral pleural line that parallels the chest wall (Fig. 13–19). In the supine position, the intrapleural air collects in the anteromedial and subpulmonic regions, because in this position the regions are the most nondependent portions of the pleural space (Tocino et al, 1985). Pleural air in the anterior costophrenic sulcus may produce hyperlucency over the upper abdomen or an unusually deep and sharp lateral costophrenic sulcus—the so-called deep sulcus sign, which may be the only sign of pneumothorax in the supine critically ill patient in the ICU (Gordon, 1980) (Fig. 13–20). The presence of visceral-to-parietal pleural adhesions or decreased lung compliance (e.g., in ARDS) may produce an unusual appearance such as subpulmonic or intrafissural air collection. When in doubt, a lateral decubitus film

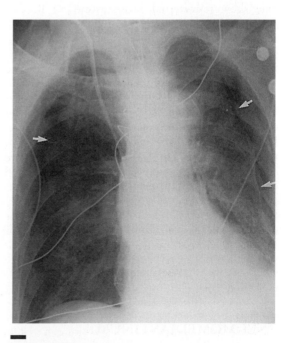

Figure 13–19
Bilateral pneumothorax. The arrows point to the fine visceral pleural line between the pleural air and the lung bilaterally, which is indicative of pneumothoraces.

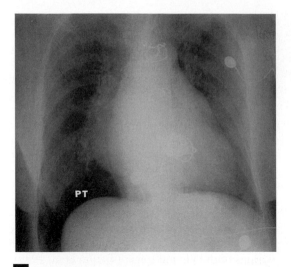

Figure 13–20
Pneumothorax in the supine position. A supine bedside chest radiograph shows a hyperlucent area above the right hemidiaphragm with deep and sharp lateral costophrenic sulcus—the *deep sulcus sign* of pneumothorax (PT) on a supine film. The pneumothorax followed an attempted subclavian catheter insertion on the right.

with the side in question elevated may show air between lung and ribs. If the patient cannot be moved, horizontal crosstable lateral radiographs may show retrosternal lucency and air in the sternodiaphragmatic angle. CT, however, is more sensitive than plain radiographs in detecting pneumothoraces, particularly in the supine patient (Tocino and Miller, 1987).

Tension pneumothorax is a clinical diagnosis, and treatment should not await radiographic confirmation. The radiograph usually shows the presence of pneumothorax with total collapse of the lung and a shift of the heart and mediastinum to the opposite side (Fig. 13–21). Because of pleural adhesions and gas trapping in ARDS, total lung collapse and mediastinal shift may be absent in the presence of tension pneumothorax. Additional findings of flat or inverted hemidiaphragm, displacement of the anterior junction line and azygoesophageal recess to the contralateral side, and flattening of the heart border and other vascular structures confirm the diagnosis (Gobien et al, 1982).

PNEUMOMEDIASTINUM

In critically ill patients, pneumomediastinum results from positive-pressure ventilation with secondary overdistention and rupture of intraparen-

chymal alveoli, with subsequent dissection of air along the peribronchovascular interstitium into the mediastinum (the Macklin effect). Other causes of mediastinal air include disruption of the esophagus, trachea, or central bronchi; blunt chest trauma; coughing; or vomiting. Pneumomediastinum may also occur as a consequence of dissection of air along the facial planes from the peritoneal cavity, retroperitoneum, or neck (Cylark et al, 1984). Radiographic signs of pneumomediastinum are (1) a lucent band around the heart and mediastinum, delineated by a thin white line laterally, comprised of visceral and parietal pleura (Fig. 13–22). A similar appearance may be produced by the so-called kinetic halo—a radiolucency seen around the heart border resulting either from the milking action of the structures in motion against the lung or an optical illusion, which is called the Mach effect (Lane et al, 1976). This halo can be differentiated from pneumomediastinum by the absence of the white line produced by displaced pleura. (2) Continuous diaphragm sign is air extending beneath the pericardium and above the central portion of the diaphragm allowing visualization of the entire length of the diaphragm, producing the sign (Levin, 1973). (3) On the lateral radiograph, vertically oriented lucencies, which are sharply radiolucent, outline the ascending aorta, great vessels, thymus, or prevertebral soft tissues. (4) Air in soft tissues of the neck or retroperitoneum offers indirect confirmation of a pneumomediastinum.

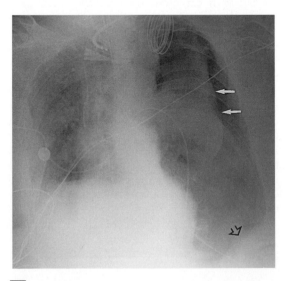

Figure 13–21
Tension pneumothorax. Arrows point to the collapsed left lung. The open arrow indicates the depression of the left hemidiaphragm. Note that the mediastinum is shifted to the contralateral (right) side.

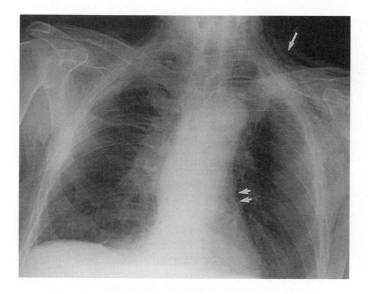

Figure 13–22
Pneumomediastinum. Arrows point to a lucent band adjacent to the heart and left side of mediastinum, which is delineated by a thin white line. Note the associated subcutaneous emphysema (*single arrow*).

PNEUMOPERICARDIUM

Pneumopericardium, which is most often seen in the premature newborn receiving mechanical ventilation for respiratory distress syndrome, is an uncommon finding in the adult. In the adult ICU patient, air in the pericardium is frequently found after coronary bypass surgery.

The radiographic features of pneumopericardium are classic, with a band of radiolucency surrounding the lateral and diaphragmatic portions of the heart (Fig. 13–23). The presence of air beneath the heart and above the diaphragm produces a continuous diaphragm sign similar to

that seen in pneumomediastinum. In distinction to pneumomediastinum, the collection of air in the pneumopericardium surrounds the heart and does not extend above the superior pericardial recess, which reflects the root of the aorta and pulmonary artery. Pneumopericardium does not usually cause ill effects, but if the pericardial air is under tension, cardiac tamponade may occur.

PULMONARY INTERSTITIAL EMPHYSEMA

Sudden and increased intra-alveolar pressure leads to sustained rupture of the alveolar wall. The air dissects along the peribronchovascular sheaths and interlobular septa, leading to pulmonary interstitial emphysema. The early radiographic sign of pulmonary interstitial emphysema (PIE) is the sudden development of irregular radiolucent mottling and linear shadows radiating from the hila to the periphery of the lung, which is likened to a so-called disorganized air bronchogram (Fig. 13–24). These lucencies do not taper or branch as they progress peripherally, differentiating them from air bronchogram. A pathognomonic but rare sign of PIE is the visualization of a radiolucent halo of air around a pulmonary vessel (Westcott and Cole, 1974). The interstitial air may accumulate in the loose connective tissue under the pleural surfaces and can be recognized on radiographs as round or oval subpleural air cysts, measuring up to 5 mm in size. Although any radiographic manifestation of PIE should be considered a precursor of pneumothorax, subpleural air cysts represent the finding most likely to forecast the pneumothorax. As a general rule, PIE changes rapidly.

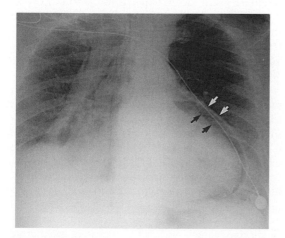

Figure 13–23
Pneumopericardium. The heart is outlined by the air separated from the lung by the parietal pericardium (*arrows*).

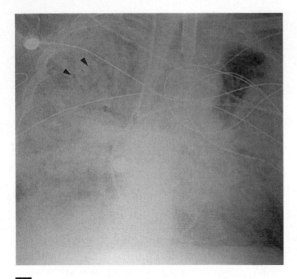

Figure 13–24
Pulmonary interstitial emphysema. A patient with ARDS who has been on positive end-expiratory pressure (PEEP) breathing for several days. The arrowheads point to small interstitial air collections, which are likened to a "disorganized" air bronchogram and indicative of interstitial pulmonary emphysema.

Frequently it appears and disappears within several hours. When it persists for several days, it often proves to be irreversible. At times PIE may be difficult to differentiate from lung consolidation with underlying emphysema. However, most cases of PIE are seen in younger age groups, and it is more extensive in the central and lower portion of the lungs, unlike emphysema which is more severe in the upper lobes. Early recognition of PIE is fundamental to ventilatory management, and its progression should be monitored with daily chest radiographs correlated with clinical information.

SUBCUTANEOUS EMPHYSEMA

Air from the mediastinum can extend along facial planes into subcutaneous tissue of the neck and chest wall, as well as the abdominal wall. Subcutaneous air in the neck and shoulder may also be due to local trauma (tracheostomy). Subcutaneous emphysema in patients receiving mechanical ventilation is often the first radiographic sign of barotrauma, because the underlying pneumomediastinum and pneumothorax may not be visible on a supine radiograph. Subcutaneous emphysema is a usually benign event that resolves as pneumomediastinum and pneumothorax resolve. Progressive or persistent subcutaneous emphysema appears as sharply etched linear radiolucencies that parallel the tissue planes or multiple lucent bubbles in the soft tissues. Individual muscle masses or muscle slips are often visible. Extensive subcutaneous emphysema of the chest wall may mimic alveolar disease or conversely may obscure true parenchymal disease. The lucent lines may mimic pneumothorax. In such cases, CT of the chest can be of great help to evaluate the presence of parenchymal disease or pneumothorax.

PULMONARY THROMBOEMBOLISM

Pulmonary thromboembolism (PE) is estimated as the third most common cause of death in the United States. It is important in the ICUs because many patients have multiple risk factors predisposing them to thromboembolism.

Perfusion ventilation lung scans identify the probability of PE based on the size and number of the perfusion defects and whether or not they coincide with matching ventilation defects (Kelley et al, 1991). A normal ventilation perfusion scan effectively rules out a pulmonary embolism and a low probability scan with low clinical suspicion makes pulmonary embolism unlikely (less than 4%). A positive-perfusion ventilation scan with high clinical suspicion makes pulmonary embolism very highly probable (96%). The reliability of ventilation perfusion scan was recently investigated in the Prospective Investigation of Pulmonary Embolism Diagnosis (PIOPED) study (PIOPED, 1990). The PIOPED gold standard for diagnosing pulmonary embolism is selective pulmonary angiography. Most pulmonary emboli originate from deep venous thrombosis (DVT) primarily in the lower extremity. DVT can be investigated with impedance plethysmography, ultrasound and, eventually, with lower extremity venography.

The advent of spiral (helical) CT and electron-beam CT made it more practical to perform pulmonary CT angiography to detect clots within the pulmonary arteries. Spiral CT technology permits continuous travel of the patient through the CT gantry, significantly reducing the time of the examination (Fig. 13–25). It eliminates respiratory misregistration and provides continuous visualization of the entire thorax using CT angiography. Remy-Jardin and coworkers (1992) reported 100% sensitivity, 96% specificity, 95% positive predictive value, and 100% negative predictive value. There was essentially complete agreement between angiography and CT findings to the level of the segmental pulmonary arteries. Goodman and coworkers (1995) however, found that if the

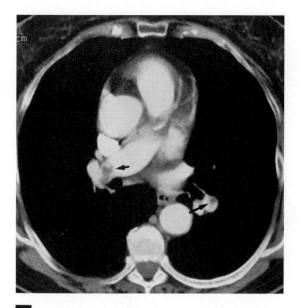

Figure 13–25
CT pulmonary angiogram (CTPA). Arrows point to filling defects in the right main pulmonary artery and left lower lobe segmental artery. These filling defects, resulting from pulmonary thromboembolism, resolved on follow-up CTPA after appropriate anticoagulant therapy.

subsegmental smaller pulmonary vessels are also included in the evaluation, the sensitivity of CT angiography decreases to 63%. Rossum and co-workers (1994), however, again found high sensitivity and specificity for CT angiography.

CT angiography can have a significant role in detection of intraluminal clots, which can be particularly important in patients in the intensive care setting. Because CT offers the benefit of evaluating the entire thorax, CT angiography requires a relatively speedy injection (2–5 ml/sec) of low-iodine-concentration contrast material (approximately 30%). Interpretation of CT angiography requires some experience. Pitfalls in the interpretation include beam-hardening artifacts from the densely opacified superior vena cava. Lymph nodes adjacent to the pulmonary arteries may mimic a filling defect (Remy-Jardin et al, 1994).

MRI is another potentially noninvasive method of identifying pulmonary artery clots (Gefter et al, 1995). MRI is usually unsuitable, however, for patients in the ICU, where monitoring devices and support systems very often make MRI impractical.

A diagnostic algorithm in the ICU setting should include perfusion ventilation scanning; however, because of coexisting pulmonary and other thoracic abnormalities, this technique may have limited value. Evaluation for DVT with compression ultrasound may preclude the necessity for direct studies of the pulmonary arteries. It is likely that CT angiography will play an increasing role and will subsequently reduce the number of patients requiring standard contrast pulmonary angiography.

POSTOPERATIVE CHEST

Following lung surgery, any unexpected radiographic appearance may indicate complications.

Following pneumonectomy the remaining lung expands, and in the immediate postoperative period the pneumonectomy space is vacant. In the ensuing days the mediastinum gradually shifts toward the operated side. The speed of fluid accumulation varies during the first week, and the lower half of the hemithorax usually fills with fluid. It may take several weeks before the entire pneumonectomy space is filled with fluid. Following lobectomy there is usually only minimal mediastinal shift and elevation of the diaphragm on the operated side. Air leaks are not uncommon but they usually subside within days.

Postoperative morbidity following lung surgery includes atelectasis, pneumonia, acute respiratory failure, or cardiac decompensation. Empyema is relatively rare. The infectious complications occur usually within days of surgery. Bronchopleural fistula is a serious complication that manifests itself with progressive pneumothorax. Postoperative bleeding complications may become manifest, with rapid expansion of the mediastinum or opacification of the hemithorax (Fig. 13–26). Herniation of the heart through a pericardial defect is a serious complication that may occur following radical pneumonectomy. Postoperative air may be still present within the pericardial sac. Lobar torsion is rare but may occur following right upper lobe lobectomy. The upward-displaced right middle lobe may rotate around its bronchovascular pedicle, resulting in severe engorgement of the veins, which often leads to pulmonary gangrene.

AORTIC DISSECTION

Acute aortic dissection is a life-threatening emergency requiring prompt diagnosis and often surgical treatment. The clinical presentation is usually suggestive of the diagnosis. More than 95% of patients have chest pain, which can be anterior or posterior. Hypertension, the most common predisposing condition, is present in 90% of patients. Other predisposing factors include cystic medial

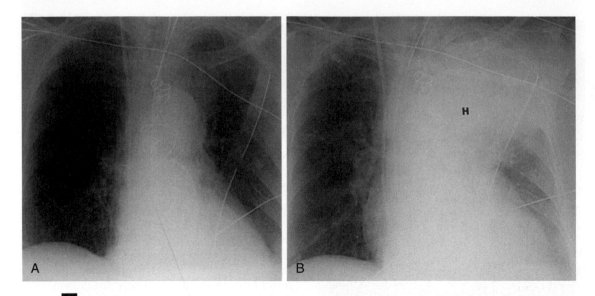

Figure 13–26
Postoperative hematoma. (A) Normal post-CABG radiograph. (B) Twenty-four hours following CABG, a rapidly expanding opacity in the left upper hemithorax is the result of a mediastinal hematoma (H).

necrosis, coarctation, congenital aortic stenosis, bicuspid aortic valve, and pregnancy (Slater and Desanctis, 1976).

The Stanford classification system (Daily et al, 1970) divides aortic dissections anatomically into two types on the basis of location. A dissection in which there is involvement of ascending aorta, regardless of site of entry, is defined as type A, which includes DeBakey types I and II (DeBakey et al, 1962). All aortic dissections that do not involve ascending aorta are defined as type B, including DeBakey type III dissection.

Type A dissections are considered surgical emergencies because they may dissect proximally to cause pericardial effusion and tamponade, acute aortic insufficiency, or acute myocardial infarction. Type B dissections can be treated successfully with medical therapy alone. The diagnostic information sought in patients with aortic dissection includes confirming the presence of dissection, involvement of ascending aorta, extent of dissection, sites of entry and re-entry, thrombosis in the false lumen, branch vessel involvement, aortic insufficiency, pericardial effusion, and coronary artery involvement (Cigarroa et al, 1993). Optimal care of patients with aortic dissection requires a prompt diagnosis. There are many diagnostic technologies, each with associated availability, accuracy, cost, and limitations.

CHEST RADIOGRAPHY

Chest radiograph is fundamental, not for the specific diagnosis, but to evaluate possible congestive heart failure, mediastinal widening, displacement of calcification in the aortic wall, or other unsuspected abnormalities.

COMPUTED TOMOGRAPHY

CT is a rapid, relatively noninvasive, and readily available method for evaluation of aortic dissection, with a sensitivity of 93.8% and specificity of 87.1% (Nienabacher et al, 1993). The diagnosis of aortic dissection is based on visualizing an intimal flap, with identification of true and false lumen (Figs. 13–27 and 13–28). Secondary findings include increased attenuation of the acutely thrombosed false lumen on noncontrast CT, internal displacement of intimal calcification, mediastinal or pericardial hematoma, and delayed enhancement of false lumen. Ischemia or infarction of organs supplied by branch vessels from the false lumen is an important secondary finding.

Strict adherence to technically well-performed studies is important. A routine "chest CT with contrast" may not be sufficient for this specific purpose. Helical CT has a higher sensitivity and specificity than conventional CT for diagnosis of aortic dissection, which is reported up to 100% in one series. With helical (spiral) CT, the scans are achieved at a much higher level of circulating contrast material because of the rapidity of scanning. In addition, two-dimensional and three-dimensional reconstructions can be performed to better define the relevant anatomy (Zeman et al, 1995). Helical CT is superior to other

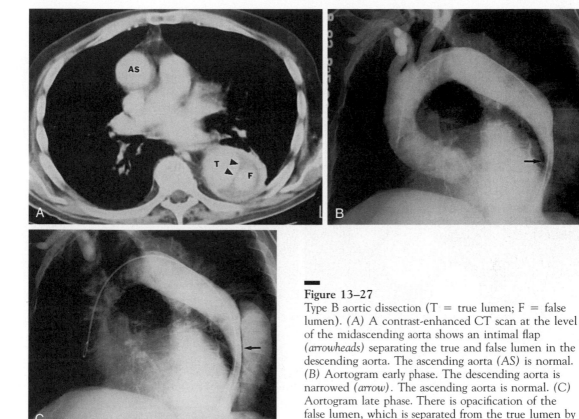

Figure 13–27
Type B aortic dissection (T = true lumen; F = false lumen). (A) A contrast-enhanced CT scan at the level of the midascending aorta shows an intimal flap (*arrowheads*) separating the true and false lumen in the descending aorta. The ascending aorta (AS) is normal. (B) Aortogram early phase. The descending aorta is narrowed (*arrow*). The ascending aorta is normal. (C) Aortogram late phase. There is opacification of the false lumen, which is separated from the true lumen by the intima (*arrow*).

imaging modalities like MRI and transesophageal echocardiography for assessment of the supraaortic branches (Sommer et al, 1995). With helical CT, a scan is obtained from above the aortic arch (to include the origin of the great vessels) to below the aortic valve. The table travel is about 20 cm in 30 sec, obtaining a volume that offers a true reconstructive slice thickness of less than 10 mm with no interslice gaps. The contrast is injected at 3 to 5 ml/min through an 18 to 20-gauge intracath in an antecubital vein. In addition to axial images, multiplanar reformations are obtained in coronal, sagittal, and sagittal oblique orientations, simulating a thoracic aortogram and aiding the diagnosis as well as pictorially communicating the information to clinicians and surgeons. The drawback of CT is that it does not evaluate for associated complications such as aortic regurgitation or coronary artery occlusion.

MAGNETIC RESONANCE IMAGING

MRI has been used in the diagnosis of aortic dissection since 1983 (Herfkens et al, 1983). MRI is 95 to 100% sensitive and 90 to 100% specific for the detection of aortic dissection (Laissy et al, 1995). Aortic dissection is diagnosed with the use of MRI by visualization of the intimal flap separating the true and false channels of the aorta. The flowing blood in the true lumen generally produces little or no signal at MRI, whereas the false lumen is variable in signal intensity, depending on the velocity of blood flow and the presence or absence of intraluminal thrombus. Multiplanar views can be obtained, simulating aortograms. Intimal calcification is usually not visible on MRI. MRI does not reliably provide information about the involvement of coronary arteries. Although MRI may provide some information about the arch vessel involvement, the imaging of these vessels is poorer in quality than that obtained with aortography.

With the use of flow-sensitive sequences, physiologic information can be obtained. Cine MRI methods allow evaluation of the aortic valve with a sensitivity of 83% (Nienabacher et al, 1993). This technique rapidly supplies images that are referenced to a simultaneously recorded electrocardiogram and then used to simulate real-time cardiac imaging. As with CT, MRI findings support the diagnosis of aortic dissection, including pericardial or pleural effusion, mediastinal

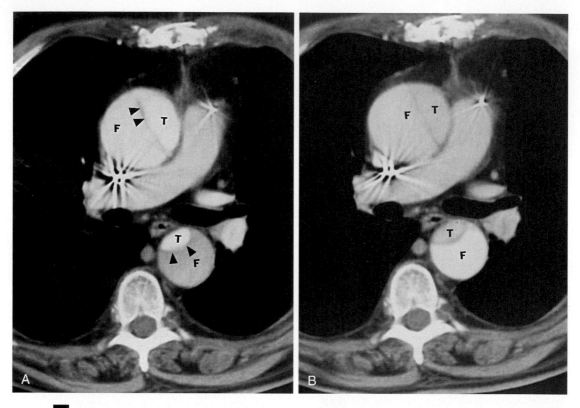

Figure 13–28
Type A aortic dissection. A single-level dynamic CT scan at the level of the midascending aorta. (T = true lumen; F = false lumen). (A) Early phase. (B) Late phase. Opacification of the true and false lumen separated by intimal flap (*arrowheads*) involving both the ascending and descending aorta. The true lumen opacifies earlier than the false lumen.

hemorrhage, and aortic wall thickening (Wolff et al, 1991).

The advantages of MRI include lack of ionizing radiation, lack of requirement for contrast media, and capability of direct multiplanar imaging. However, in the patient with suspected aortic dissection, MRI is often not obtained because of limited scanner availability, long scanning time, and paramagnetic life support equipment (e.g., pacemakers). Currently MRI is most often considered for the elective evaluation of less acutely ill patients or for postoperative follow-up.

TRANSESOPHAGEAL ECHOCARDIOGRAPHY AND TRANSTHORACIC ULTRASONOGRAPHY

Transesophageal echocardiography (TEE) and transthoracic ultrasonography (TT-US) are noninvasive modalities that provide both physiologic information and anatomic detail. TEE is superior to TT-US, although it is not as readily available; TEE is more costly and requires patient sedation and esophageal intubation. The sensitivity and

specificity of TEE for detection of aortic dissection is reported to be 85 to 95% and 59 to 85%, respectively. The echocardiographic criterion of aortic dissection is presence of an undulating intimal flap in the aorta. TEE can image the entire thoracic aorta except for the distal transverse arch, which may be partially obscured by the trachea. TEE can also depict the entry sites into false lumen, thrombi, pericardial effusion, aortic valve, and the entire heart. Visualization of heart is important in evaluating potential cardiac complications of dissection, such as aortic regurgitation, pericardial effusion, and myocardial ischemia (Fisher et al, 1994). TEE can be performed at the bedside in locations such as the emergency room or the ICU, precluding movement of critically ill patients. TEE is contraindicated in patients with known esophageal disease, and it may not be tolerated in 3% of patients (Cigarroa et al, 1993).

AORTOGRAPHY

Thoracic aortography has been considered as the gold standard for diagnosis of aortic dissection for many years. With respect to identification of aortic dissection, aortography has a sensitivity of 86 to 88% and a specificity of 75 to 94% (Amour et al, 1988). As with other techniques, the classic feature of aortic dissection at aortography is an intimal flap (see Fig. 13–27). False-negative aortograms may occur in cases of thrombosis of the false lumen and faint opacification of the false lumen. False-negative readings may also occur when the intimal flap is not perpendicular to the x-ray beam and therefore is not visualized. Aortography is an invasive procedure requiring femoral puncture and use of contrast media. At present, angiography is reserved for cases of indeterminate findings on other imaging modalities.

Selecting a method of imaging in suspected aortic dissection depends on the clinical condition of the patient; diagnostic information needed; accuracy of diagnostic information obtained; and availability, length of time involved, safety, and cost of the study. In some institutions, TEE is the preferred method of choice because of its accuracy, safety, speed, and convenience. Although MRI may be less practical than TEE for evaluation of patients with suspected aortic dissection, it is nonetheless very well suited for patients with stable or long-term dissection. In many hospitals, CT is the diagnostic method of choice in the evaluation of patients with suspected aortic dissection, with a sensitivity and specificity comparable to those of TEE and MRI. Aortography, which is an accurate technique for evaluating patients with aortic dissection, should be reserved for patients who have indeterminate results on noninvasive imaging techniques. In the final analysis, each institution determines its own best method of approaching the diagnosis of aortic dissection on the basis of available human and material resources.

REFERENCES

Aberle DR, Wiener-kronish JP, Webb WR, et al: Hydrostatic versus increased permeability edema: Diagnosis based on radiographic criteria in critically ill patients. Radiology 168:73, 1988.

Amour T, Gutierrez F, Levitt R, and McKnight R: CT diagnosis of type A aortic dissections not demonstrated by aortography. J Comp Assist Tomog 12:963, 1988.

Bekemeyer WB, Crapo RO, Calhoon S, et al: Efficacy of chest radiography in a respiratory intensive care unit—a prospective study. Chest 88:691, 1985.

Bellon E, Feron M, Marchal G, et al: Design for user efficiency in a dedicated ICU viewing station. Med Inf (Lond) 19(2):161, 1994.

Bellon E, Houtput W, Bijnens B, et al: Combining fast response and low cost in an intensive care unit viewing station. J Digit Imaging 7(2):91–94, 1994.

Blume H and Jost RG: Chest imaging within the radiology department by means of photostimulable phosphor computed radiography: A review. J Digit Imaging 5(2):67, 1992.

Brandstetter RD, Garcia JC, Majumder M, and Chisolm A: The benefit of lateral radiographs in an intensive care unit. Chest 105(2):560, 1994.

Cigarroa JE, Isselbacher EM, DeSantis RW, and Eagle K: Diagnostic imaging in the evaluation of suspected aortic dissection. N Engl J Med 328:35, 1993.

Conrady PA, Goodman LR, Lainge F, and Singer M: Alteration of endotracheal tube position. Flexion and extension of neck. Crit Care Med 4:8, 1976.

Cylark D, Milne EWC, and Imray TJ: Pneumomediastinum: A diagnostic problem. Crit Rev Diagn Imaging 23:75, 1984.

Daily PO, Trueblood HW, Stinson EB, and Wuerflein RD: Management of acute aortic dissections. Am J Thorac Surg 10:234, 1970.

DeBakey ME, Henly WS, Cooley DA, et al: Surgical management of dissecting aneurysm of the aorta. J Thorac Cardiovasc Surg 49:130, 1962.

Fisher ER, Stern EJ, Godwin JD II, et al: Acute aortic dissection: Typical and atypical imaging features. Radiographics 14:1263, 1994.

Fraser RG, Sanders C, Barnes GT, et al: Digital imaging of the chest. Radiology 171:297, 1989.

Gefter WB, Hatabu H, Holland GA, et al: Pulmonary thromboembolism: Recent developments in diagnosis with CT and MR imaging. Radiology 197:561, 1995.

Gobien RP, Reines HD, and Schabel SJ: Localized tension pneumothorax: Unrecognized form of barotrauma in adult respiratory distress syndrome. Radiology 142:15, 1982.

Goodman LR, Curtin JJ, Mewissen MW, et al: Detection of pulmonary embolism in patients with unresolved clinical and scintigraphic diagnosis: Helical CT versus angiography. AJR Am J Roentgenol 164:1369, 1995.

Goodman LR and Putnam CE: Critical Care Radiology, 3rd ed. Philadelphia, WB Saunders, 1992.

Gordon R: The deep sulcus sign. Radiology 136:25, 1980.

Green R: Adult respiratory distress syndrome. Acute alveolar damage. Radiology 163:57, 1987.

Greenbaum DM and Marschall KE: The value of routine daily chest X-rays in intubated patients in the medical intensive care unit. Crit Care Med 10:29, 1982.

Greene R, McLoud TC, and Stark P: Pneumothorax. Semin Roentgenol 12:315, 1977.

Gross BH and Spizarny DL: Computed tomography of the chest in the intensive care unit. Crit Care Clin 10(2):267, 1994.

Hall JB, White SR, and Karrison T: Efficacy of daily routine chest radiographs in intubated, mechanically ventilated patients. Crit Care Med 19(5):689, 1991.

Handel DB and Ravin CE: The ICU chest film. Cardiopulmonary monitoring and assist devices. Cardiol Clin 1(4):711, 1983.

Henschke CL, Pasternack GS, Schroeder S, et al: Bedside chest radiography: Diagnostic efficacy. Radiology 149:23, 1983.

Herfkens RJ, Higgins CB, Hricak H, et al: Nuclear magnetic resonance imaging of the cardiovascular system, normal and pathologic findings. Radiology 147:749, 1983.

Herman PG (ed): Iatrogenic Thoracic Complications. New York, Springer-Verlag, 1983.

Humphrey LM, Fitzpatrick K, Attalah N, and Ravin CE: Time comparison of intensive care units with and without digital viewing systems. J Digit Imaging 6(1):37, 1993.

Hunter TB: Tubes, lines, catheters, and other interesting devices. Curr Probl Diagn Radiol 24(2):53, 1995.

Jennings P, Padley SP, and Hansell DM: Portable chest radiography in intensive care: a comparison of computed and conventional radiography. Br J Radiol 65(778):852, 1992.

Kelley MA, Carson JL, Palevsky HI, and Schwartz JS: Diagnosing pulmonary embolism: New facts and strategies. Ann Intern Med 114:300, 1991.

Khan A, Noma S, and Herman PG: Iatrogenic diseases of the lung. Postgrad Radiol 10:219, 1990.

Khan F, Reddy N, and Khan A: Cuff-trachea ratio as an indicator of tracheal damage (abstract). Chest 70:431, 1976.

Laissy J-P, Blanc F, Soyer P, et al: Thoracic aortic dissection: Diagnosis with transesophageal echocardiography versus MR imaging. Radiology 194:331, 1995.

Lane EF, Proto AV, and Philips TW: Mach bands and density perception. Radiology 121:9, 1976.

Levin B: The continuous diaphragm sign. Clin Radiol 24:337, 1973.

McCloud TC and Putnam CE: Radiology of the Swan-Ganz catheter and associated pulmonary complications. Radiology 116:19, 1975.

Maguire WM, Herman PG, Khan A, et al: Interobserver agreement using computed radiography in the adult intensive care unit. Acad Radiol 1:10, 1994.

Marglin SI, Rowberg AH, and Godwin JD: Preliminary experience with portable digital imaging for intensive care radiography. J Thorac Imaging 5(1):49, 1990.

Marini JJ, Pierson DJ, and Hudson LD: Acute lobar atelectasis: A prospective comparison of fiberoptic bronchoscopy and respiratory therapy. Am Rev Respir Dis 149:971, 1979.

Milne EN and Pistolesi M: Pulmonary edema—cardiac and noncardiac. In Putman CT (ed): Diagnostic Imaging of the Lung. New York, Marcel Dekker, 1990.

Mitchell SE and Clark RA: Complications of central venous catheterization. AJR Am J Roentgenol 133:467, 1979.

Nienabacher CA, von Kodolitsch Y, Nicolas V, et al: The diagnosis of thoracic aortic dissection by non-invasive procedures. N Engl J Med 328:1, 1993.

Niklason LT, Chan HP, Cascade PN, et al: Portable chest imaging: Comparison of storage phosphor digital, asymmetric screen-film, and conventional screen-film systems. Radiology 186(2):387, 1993.

Pasternack G and O'Cain CF. Thoracic complications of respiratory intensive care. In Herman PG (ed): Iatrogenic Thoracic Complications. New York, Springer-Verlag, 1983.

PIOPED investigators: Value of the ventilation/perfusion scan in acute pulmonary embolism: Results of the prospective investigation of pulmonary embolism diagnosis (PIOPED). JAMA 263:2753, 1990.

Ravin CE: Initial experience with automatic image transmission to an intensive care unit using picture archiving and communications system technology. J Digit Imaging 3(3):195, 1990.

Remy-Jardin M, Duyck P, Remy J, et al: Anatomy of hilar lymph nodes as shown on spiral CT angiograms (abstract). Radiology 193:338, 1994.

Remy-Jardin M, Remy J, Wattinner L, and Gibraud F: Central pulmonary thromboembolism: Diagnosis with spiral volumetric CT with the single-breath-hold technique—comparison with pulmonary angiography. Radiology 185:381, 1992.

Rossum AV, Keift G, Trevrniet F, et al: Spiral volumetric CT in patients with clinical suspicion of pulmonary embolism (abstract). Radiology 193:262, 1994.

Saito H, Kurashina T, Ishibashi T, et al: Digital radiography in an intensive care unit. Clin Radiol 39(2):127, 1988.

Shevland J, Hirelman MT, Huang KA, and Kealey GP: Lobar collapse in surgical intensive care unit. Br J Radiol 56:531, 1983.

Silvani P, Colombo S, Cabrini L, et al: Conventional radiology and computerized axial tomography in the diagnosis of pneumothorax in intensive therapy. Retrospective study of 2 years of activity. Minerva Anestesiol 59(9):427, 1993.

Slater EE and Desanctis RW: The clinical recognition of dissecting aneurysm. Am J Med 60:623, 1976.

Sommer T, Fehske W, von Smekal A, et al: Spiral computerized tomography, multiplane transesophageal echocardiography and magnetic resonance imaging in the diagnosis of thoracic aortic dissection. Rofo Fortschr Geb Rontgenstr Neuen Bildgeb Verfahr 162(2):104, 1995.

Stark P: Inadvertent nasogastric tube insertion into tracheobronchial tree. Radiology 142:239, 1982.

Staub NC: The pathogenesis of pulmonary edema. Prog Cardiovasc Dis 23:53, 1980.

Tagliabue M, Casella TC, Zincone GE, et al: CT and chest radiography in the evaluation of adult respiratory distress syndrome. Acta Radiol 35(3):230, 1994.

Thompson MJ, Kubicka RA, and Smith C: Evaluation

of cardiopulmonary devices on chest radiographs: Digital vs analog radiographs. AJR Am J Roentgenol 153(6):1165, 1989.

Tocino I and Miller MH: Computed tomography in blunt chest trauma. J Thorac Imaging 2:18, 1987.

Tocino IM, Miller MH, and Fairfax WR: Distribution of pneumothorax in supine and semi-recumbant critically ill adults. AJR Am J Roentgenol 144:901, 1985.

Waite RJ, Carbonneau RJ, Balikian J, et al: Parietal pleural changes in empyema: Appearances at CT. Radiology 175:145, 1990.

Wechsler RJ, Steiner RM, and Kinori I: Monitoring the monitors: The radiology of thoracic catheters, wires and tubes. Semin Roentgenol 23:61, 1988.

Westcott JL: Percutaneous catheter drainage of pleural effusion and empyema. AJR Am J Roentgenol 144:1189, 1985.

Westcott JL and Cole SR: Interstitial pulmonary emphysema in children and adults: roentgenographic features. Radiology 111:367–378, 1974.

Wolff KA, Herold CT, Parravano JC, and Zerhouni EA: Aortic dissection: Atypical patterns seen on MR imaging. Radiology 181:489, 1991.

Woodall BH, Winfield DF, and Bisset GS III: Inadvertent tracheobronchial placement of feeding tubes. Radiology 165:727, 1987.

Zeman RK, Berman PM, Silverman PM, et al: Diagnosis of aortic dissection: Value of helical CT with multiplanar reformation and three-dimensional rendering. AJR Am J Roentgenol 164(6):1375, 1995.

Zimmerman JE, Groodman LR, and Shahvari MBG: Effect of mechanical ventilation and positive end-expiratory pressure (PEEP) on chest radiograph. AJR Am J Roentgenol 133:811, 1979.

Zwilick CW, Pierson DJ, Creagh CE, et al: Complications of assisted ventilation. A prospective study of 354 consecutive episodes. Am J Med 57:161, 1974.

Zylak CJ, Littleton JT, and Durizch ML: Illusory consolidation of the left lower lobe: A pitfall of portable radiography. Radiology 167:653, 1988.

Cardiopulmonary Resuscitation

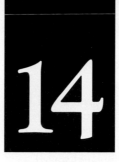

Warren R. Summer, M.D.

Peter M.C. DeBlieux, M.D.

The standards and guidelines for cardiopulmonary resuscitation (CPR) and emergency cardiac care (ECC) were last revised in 1992, representing an update of the recommendations published in 1974 and revised in 1980, and again in 1986 (Kerber et al, 1992). Guideline updates are an attempt to improve knowledge and performance levels of all rescuers, and to make it easier for rescuers working together to coordinate their efforts and provide a framework for continued research.

Although the CPR standardized procedures continue to be modified, there are many areas of insufficient data, which are preventing the determination of the best way to accomplish a particular objective. Exciting investigations in CPR are taking place at numerous institutions, and it must be remembered that standardization is not the equivalent of optimization. The Advanced Cardiac Life Support (ACLS) treatment algorithms present summaries of recommendations and cannot convey all clinical decision points (Einagle et al, 1988). Algorithms and guidelines are always a compromise between complex clinical realities and user-friendly clinical overviews. Deviations from guidelines may be warranted when a trained medical provider proficient in CPR and ECC recognizes that some modification is in the best interest of the patient.

In addition to refinement of CPR techniques, emphasis has been placed on cost-effectiveness, medicolegal obligations, and moral issues related to resuscitation efforts. In this chapter, we review the ethical considerations, current guidelines for treatment of cardiac arrest and CPR, mechanisms that are believed to control cardiac output during the cardiac arrest, airways management, determinants of vital organ blood flow during CPR, controversies, and future directions for improving CPR.

HISTORIC BACKGROUND

Resuscitation and the restorative properties of air blown into the lungs have existed from the earliest times (Hermreck, 1988) and may well be the basis for the biblical quotation (II Kings 4:34–55) when Elisha resuscitated the child of a Shunammite woman:

> "And he went up, and lay upon the child and put his mouth upon his mouth, and his eyes upon his eyes, and his hands upon his hands, and he stretched himself upon the child, and the flesh of the child waxed warm. Then he returned, and walked in the house to and fro, and went up and stretched himself upon him, and the child sneezed seven times, and the child opened his eyes."

In 1740, the Academy of Science in Paris promulgated the first standardized recommendations for techniques of CPR when it certified the method of mouth-to-mouth breathing as the treatment of choice for victims of drowning (Debard, 1980). The use of the mouth-to-mouth ventilation as a means of resuscitation fell into disfavor in the next century for two primary reasons. One concern was that expired gas concentrations were inadequate for oxygenation, a belief that is now known to be invalid, and the other centered on the undesirable aesthetics of intimate contact with a stranger and the fear of contagion. The latter concern has persisted and actually has grown stronger in the twentieth century with the appreciation of acquired immunodeficiency syndrome (AIDS) and the concern of exposure to others' bodily fluids. During the nineteenth century and early twentieth century, several manual techniques were developed using direct thoracic compression either anteriorly or posteriorly in an attempt to ventilate the lungs of drowning victims. These techniques used chest compression for active expiration and allowed passive recoil of the chest wall to produce inspiration, aided by elevation and extension of the arms while placing the patient in the lateral decubitus position. In the late 1950s, it was clearly established by Safar and colleagues with clinical arterial blood gas measurements that chest compression arm-lift techniques were ineffective in producing alveolar ventilation, whereas mouth-to-mouth ventilation was highly effective (Beyar R, et al).

The impetus of our current techniques for CPR arrived from an effort to treat electrical workers who sustained accidental electrocution, leading to ventricular fibrillation (Kouwenhaven et al, 1973). Animal studies demonstrated that ventricular fibrillation could be reversed by a second shock, or "countershock." Initially, these studies were not undertaken by physicians, but rather by Kouwehaven, an electrical engineer, who developed a defibrillator to reverse electrically induced ventricular fibrillation (Hooker et al, 1933). In the 1950s, it was appreciated that

cardiac arrest after acute myocardial infarction commonly was associated with ventricular fibrillation, and Zoll and associates developed and implemented the external cardiac defibrillator (Zoll et al, 1956).

A fortuitous event occurred in Kouwehaven's laboratory when his assistant, Knickerbocker, noted that every time he applied the defibrillator paddles with great force to the chest of the dog, there was a rise in the animal's arterial blood pressure. After this observation, Kouwehaven, in association with Jude, a surgical resident, and Knickerbocker developed the *first* acceptable technique of closed-chest compressions, allowing successful resuscitation in animal models and in patients with ventricular fibrillation. It is ironic that the very same technique, chest compressions, which had been ineffective in sustaining ventilation during cardiopulmonary arrest, was effective in sustaining circulation, and that these discoveries were made by two teams of researchers in the same city, working in independent hospitals, nearly simultaneously.

ETHICAL CONSIDERATIONS

The most profound challenge to health care professionals' participation in resuscitation in the mid and late 1990s will be the process of addressing issues of futility. The 1992 guidelines acknowledge the general ineffectiveness and, in some cases, the inappropriateness of resuscitation efforts, recognizing that cessation of a heartbeat often represents the terminal event of a terminal state. Health care providers must develop guidelines and protocols by which terminally ill patients can receive care and support, but be allowed to experience a natural death devoid of inappropriate resuscitative efforts.

The AMA has formed a group called the Task Force on Quality Care at the End of Life whose mission is to define futile treatment and identify how patients and physicians can mutually agree upon a treatment plan. The task force identifies that physicians have an obligation to relieve pain and suffering and to promote the dignity and autonomy of dying patients in their care. This obligation includes providing effective palliative treatment, even though it may hasten death. Managed care may offer and stress opportunities for hospice and home health care in their health care plans to improve autonomy for dying patients and their families.

To meet these ends, a number of medical and lay groups are working toward a common goal, matching patient preferences with realistic medical options. The Study to Understand Prognoses and Preferences for Outcomes and Risks of Treatments (SUPPORT) documented care offered to critically ill patients and the interactions of these patients' physicians. The researchers discovered that doctors were unaware of their patients' desire to withhold CPR 47% of the time. The SUPPORT group (1995) reported that 46% of do-not-resuscitate (DNR) orders were not written until a day or two before the patient's death, which intimates poor advance planning in end-of-life decision. Other issues include the documentation of DNR orders, role of procedure-specific DNR orders, and cost of enforcing DNR orders on all appropriate patients. The cost of DNR orders has not been fully evaluated, but admission to a hospital with a established nonresuscitation order appears to be cost-effective (Maksoud et al, 1993). Cost efficiency is less clear for DNR orders instituted during the management process.

Miranda (1994) investigated quality-of-life issues after resuscitation. An impairment in the ability to resume work and a delayed effect on mental functioning was not noted when compared with age- and comorbid-matched controls.

The Patient Self Determination Act of 1991 has addressed the issues of advanced directives, organ and tissue donation, and withdrawal of life support, but tougher issues of medical futility, allocating resources, and termination of resuscitation efforts have yet to be addressed and incorporated into standard practice guidelines. Cugliari and associates (1995) have investigated the timeliness of obtaining advanced directives. They argue strongly for distributing information on the advance directives to patients before their admission to the hospital. Forty percent of those patients receiving advance directives by mail before admission completed their proxies, as compared with 3% of those receiving the information for the first time upon admission.

Outcome from CPR is closely dependent on the prior health of the patient and the clinical status at the time of arrest (Table 14–1). Many medical patients, especially those in the intensive care setting, have little chance of recovery after cardiac arrest. It has been suggested that most patients receiving active resuscitation with ventilation and pharmacologic agents are inappropriate candidates for CPR (Table 14–2).

CURRENT STANDARDS FOR CARDIOPULMONARY RESUSCITATION

To standardize various techniques, the National Conference on Cardiopulmonary Resuscitation (CPR) and Emergency Cardiac Care (ECC) have published their recommendations with periodic updates in 1974, 1980, 1986, and again in 1992. Advanced cardiac life support (ACLS) includes

Table 14–1
Factors Influencing Outcome in CPR

Factor	Favorable Outcome	Unfavorable Outcome
Rhythm	Ventricular tachycardia/fibrillation	Asystole
		Bradycardia
		Pulseless electrical activity
Site of arrest	Non-ICU telemetry	ICU medical med/surg floor
Witnessed arrest	Yes	No
Prior fitness (not age per se)	Active	Skilled nursing facility
Co-morbidity*	None	Pneumonia, cancer
		Hypotension, AIDS
CPR duration	<15 min	>15 min
CPR delay in onset	<2.5 min	>2.5 min
Pre-arrest		
Glasgow coma scale	>10	<8
Hemoglobin	Normal	Low
Temperature	Normal	High
Blood glucose	Normal	High
Lactic acidosis	Absent	Present
During arrest		
pH	Normal	>7.6
ET_{CO_2} (mm Hg)	>15	<8

*Critically ill patients, especially septic patients, rarely survive to leave the hospital following CPR.

Table 14–2
Criteria for Terminating Resuscitation

Failure to achieve any return of spontaneous circulation within 25 minutes of ACLS institution has been proposed as a criterion for terminating resuscitation in the prehospital setting. Proposed guidelines for terminating an inpatient resuscitation suggest that all of the following four criteria must be met:

1. Prolonged attempt of 20 to 30 minutes without resumption of spontaneous circulation
2. Adequate ACLS (IV, airway, drugs, electricity) during the resuscitation period
3. Terminal rhythms: Pulseless electrical activity (PEA) and asystole
4. Normothermia

---

basic life support (BLS) techniques plus the use of adjuvant equipment to support ventilation, intravenous fluid infusion, drug administration, diagnosis of cardiac rhythm, defibrillation, control of subsequent arrhythmias, and post-CPR care. These procedures are guided by a physician, or by previously defined hospital policies.

Consensus panels have modified the approach to the management of cardiac arrest for advanced life support in the critical care setting. There has been a formulation of a classification of therapeutic interventions in CPR and ECC based on the strength of the supporting scientific evidence as evaluated by the 1992 National Conference on CPR and ECC.

Class I. A therapeutic option that is usually indicated, always acceptable, and considered useful and effective

Class II. A therapeutic option that is acceptable, is of uncertain efficacy, and may be controversial

Class IIa. A therapeutic option for which the weight of evidence is in favor of its usefulness and efficacy

Class IIb. A therapeutic option that is not well established by evidence, but may be helpful and probably is not harmful

Class III. A therapeutic option that is inappropriate, is without scientific supporting data, and may be harmful

Important changes in ACLS recommended by the 1992 National Conference on CPR and ECC include:

1. Change of intravenous fluids from 5% dextrose in water (D_5W) to normal saline (NS) for resuscitation

2. Total dose of atropine has been increased to 3 mg

3. Adenosine has been approved for therapy in paroxysmal supraventricular tachycardia

4. Epinephrine 5 mg or 0.1 mg/kg if the initial 1-mg dosage has failed as a IIb recommendation (this is discussed later under Vasoactive Therapy)

5. Pulseless electrical activity (PEA) has supplanted the electromechanical dissociation algorithm

6. Magnesium is of probable benefit as treatment for torsades de pointes, refractory ventricular fibrillation, and ventricular dysrhythmia associated with hypomagnesemia.

Final decision by the Conference on Standards and Guidelines took into account not only those techniques that were considered most correct, but also those that would be best used safely and effectively in an integrated approach that could be taught to most individuals needing to learn the procedures. These guidelines should be considered reasonable for the management of cardiac arrest, with the realization that definitive data are lacking in many areas and that new information is reported regularly. The greatest problems in the management of cardiac arrest in the critical care unit are often the result of inadequate organization and delineation of responsibilities during the resuscitation effort. Written policy designating lines of responsibility during cardiac arrest can partially alleviate these problems. Unfortunately, frequent practice is the surest method for developing and maintaining competence.

MECHANISM OF CARDIOPULMONARY RESUSCITATION

At the time that CPR by closed-chest cardiac massage was first developed, it was assumed that blood flow was generated by the direct compression of the heart between the sternum and the vertebral bodies. It was presumed that the ventricles were compressed to a greater extent than the atria, and therefore there was closure of the atrioventricular valves, leading to forward systemic pulmonary arterial blood flow. When the compression was released, the right and left sides of the heart were filled by passive venous return from the compliant regions of the peripheral circulation and the pulmonary circulation. Some early investigators, notably Weale and Rothwell-Jackson (1962), questioned this mechanism because right atrial pressure and arterial pressure rose the same amount during chest compression. The elevation of arterial pressure was only a transmission of elevated intrathoracic pressure to the peripheral vessels without a gradient for peripheral blood flow. Not long after that, however, it was demonstrated with indicator-dilution that there was blood flow during CPR that amounted to 0.3 to 1.7 l/min in humans (Cugliari et al, 1995).

Criley and associates found that blood flow could be maintained in asystolic humans by rhythmic coughing (Criley et al, 1986; Niemann et al, 1980). The explanation for these findings was not clear until the seminal work of Rudikoff and associates (1980) noted that carotid blood flow was difficult to generate with chest compression in patients with flail chests but was easier to generate in patients with hyperinflated chests. Rudikoff and colleagues (1980) extended these observations in a series of experiments that led them to conclude that blood flow during CPR must be accomplished by a generalized increase in intrathoracic pressure, causing blood to move from vascular structures of the thorax to the peripheral circulation. When the compression was released, blood flowed from the peripheral structures and returned back into the thorax. The flow of blood was thought to be maintained in an antegrade direction by valves in the veins or heart, preventing regurgitant flow (Feneley et al, 1988).

The *thoracic pump theory* has received widespread support from a number of experimental findings (Paraskos, 1986a). The pressure rise in all of the intrathoracic blood-containing structures is approximately equal to the pressure within the chest cavity. Techniques that augment pleural pressure have included simultaneous ventilation and compression, binding of the abdomen to prevent onward displacement of the diaphragm, and clamping of the airway during compression (Capparelli et al, 1989; Chandra et al, 1980, 1981b, 1981c; Harris et al, 1967; Koehler et al, 1983; Niemann et al, 1994; Redding et al, 1971).

Techniques utilizing pneumatic binders that cause a generalized increase in thorax surface pressure have been successful for closed-chest cardiac resuscitation in animals (Halperin et al, 1993; Luce et al, 1983; Ralston et al, 1982; Schleien et al, 1989). Possibly the best supporting evidence for the thoracic pump theory is the demonstration that mechanical ventilation alone without chest compression raises intrathoracic pressure and produces effective forward blood flow (Passerini et al, 1988). The advent of an active compression-decompression device for resuscitation also argues well for the thoracic pump theory.

Results of radionuclide, echocardiographic, and angiographic studies have all indicated that during compression of the chest, blood moves from the pulmonary capillary bed through the left ventricle to the peripheral circulation, whereas during release of the compression, blood moves from the peripheral circulation into the pulmonary circulation (Cohen et al, 1982; Neimann et al, 1994; Rich et al, 1981; Werner et al, 1981). During compression, there is no closure of the atrioventricular valves at a time when blood is flowing antegrade out of the left ventricle. Niemann and colleagues (1994) showed with cineangiography that during compression of the chest, the heart shifted away from the area of compression and that forward blood flow occurred without appreciable distortion or change in the size of the left ventricular cavity. During compression, blood moves from the pulmonary circuit forward into the left atrium. During relaxation, blood flowed from the vena cava through the chambers in the right side of the heart antegrade.

Werner and colleagues (1981) demonstrated with two-dimensional echocardiography that there was no closure of the mitral valve during compression. The aortic valve opened during compression, whereas the pulmonic valve tended to close. They found little change in left ventricular cross-sectional area during compression. Rich and colleagues (1981) and Werner and colleagues (1981) also used two-dimensional echocardiography to visualize the heart during CPR in human subjects. These investigators found that the left ventricular cross-sectional area changed little during compression and that compression was accompanied by opening of both the aortic and mitral valves, suggesting that the left ventricle acted as a simple conduit for blood flowing from the pulmonary vessels.

Weisfeldt's group documented that during compression of the chest in experimentally fibrillated dogs, radiolabeled albumin moved from the right side of the heart to the pulmonary circulation during the relaxation phase, whereas blood moved from the left pulmonary venous circuit into the left side of the heart during the compression phase (Cohen et al, 1992). These studies have all been consistent with the belief that the heart is not directly compressed during closed-chest CPR. They indicate that during compression of the chest, the major blood flow is achieved through translocation of blood from the pulmonary vasculature into the peripheral vasculature, with the left side of the heart acting as a passive conduit (Paraskos 1986b; Schleien et al, 1989). This theory is directly challenged by Boczar and associates, who detail the benefits of open cardiac massage in refractory human arrest (Boczar et al, 1995). Thirty percent of the patients manifested a return of spontaneous circulation.

A markedly significant difference in coronary perfusion pressures can be measured during open chest massage. Clinical trials comparing efficacy of standard CPR with open cardiac massage have not been performed to date, but current animal and human studies are intriguing.

Forceful rhythmic coughing can generate systolic pressure comparable with that of normal cardiac activity and sustained cardiac output during asystole (Criley et al, 1986; Niemann et al, 1980). The temporary effectiveness of this maneuver has been demonstrated by maintenance of consciousness and presumable cerebral circulation in the presence of asystole and by recording of peripheral pulsed Doppler flow in the systemic vessels during coughs interposed between cardiac systoles in subjects with sinus bradycardia (Cary et al, 1978).

The evidence may seem convincing that blood flow during CPR can result from the generalized increase in pleural pressure rather than from direct cardiac compression, but all investigators do not find similar results, nor do they all reach similar conclusions. Under certain circumstances there is good evidence for direct compression of the heart. This is demonstrable by increasing the extent of compression and may be influenced by the size and the configuration of the thorax (Halperin et al, 1986; Neimann et al, 1994). Using a canine model of high-impulse sternal compression, Maier and associates (1986) reported peak cardiac and vascular pressures two to four times greater than corresponding intrathoracic pressure. The finding in chronically instrumented dogs that compression of the thorax caused distortion of the heart in the axis of compression suggests that forces are exerted unevenly on the surface of the heart. O'Quinn and colleagues (1984) confirmed that the pressures during manual CPR are not uniform on the surface of the heart, with greater pressures in axis of compression. In contrast, simultaneous compression of the chest with a pneumatic vest and airway occlusion led to almost uniform pressure changes on the surface of the heart and pleural space (Newton et al, 1988).

Whether CPR blood flow is the result of direct cardiac compression or a generalized increase in pleural pressure is no longer a compelling controversy. The bulk of evidence is that both mechanisms may occur, and both mechanisms may effectively generate blood flow, depending on the technique used, duration of the resuscitation, and anatomy and pathology of the patient (Ducas et al, 1983; Safar et al, 1988; Stacpoole, 1986; Sylvester et al, 1983). In some patients a continuum may exist, with the cardiac compression mechanism early on, followed by the thoracic pump mechanism (Raessler et al, 1988).

THORACOABDOMINAL MECHANICS AND CARDIOPULMONARY RESUSCITATION

Localized compression of the rib cage deforms the thorax and leads to a reduction in lung volume below its resting level. The airway and abdominal diaphragmatic compartments provide two degrees of freedom for the thorax. If the airway is open and the diaphragm is allowed to descend freely, the only mechanism for generating an increase in pleural pressure is the resistance of the lung to deformation.

A goal of CPR by the thoracic pump mechanism is to develop large elevations of pleural pressure around all of the structures in the thorax and to distribute this elevation of pleural pressure more uniformly. Theoretically, the greater the elevation of pleural pressure, the greater the blood flow. A more even application of pressure leads to less deformation of the thorax, lungs, and abdominal viscera. A more even application should minimize local trauma. Several strategies have been applied to achieve these goals. By maintaining a constant lung volume during chest compression, alveolar pressure increases the same amount as pleural pressure, assuming constant elastic properties of the lung (constant transpulmonary pressure at a particular lung volume) (Ben-Haim et al, 1988).

Another approach to increasing pleural pressure relative to body surface pressure is not compression of the rib cage, but rather compression of the abdomen. If the lung is held at constant resting volume, the diaphragm has little or no tension. Without active or passive tension of the diaphragm, no transdiaphragmatic pressure can be generated. Any increase in abdominal pressure may thus be transmitted in full to the pleural space. This technique mimics "cough-CPR," in which the closure of the glottis is accompanied by an increase in both abdominal and pleural pressure (Neimann et al, 1980).

AIRWAY MANAGEMENT IN CARDIOPULMONARY RESUSCITATION

The time-honored dictum of the ABCs of cardiopulmonary resuscitation has been challenged by

Fukui and associates and may soon be coined the "CABs" (circulation, airway, and breathing) of CPR (Noc et al, 1995). By questioning the need for positive-pressure ventilation during cardiopulmonary resuscitation, a series of porcine resuscitation experiments have identified the absence of a marked treatment benefit by alternating compressions with ventilation, versus chest compressions alone. Chest compressions and spontaneous gaspings produce minute ventilations up to 5 liters during resuscitative efforts. Bystander resuscitation is difficult to master and far more challenging to teach, and the possibility of simplifying technique is attractive.

Airway maintenance in cardiopulmonary resuscitation is ideally achieved by endotracheal intubation by direct laryngoscopy, but this is a technique that requires a certain expertise that many have not mastered. A number of alternative options for securing airway maintenance have emerged and include endotracheal intubation with lighted stylet, transtracheal ventilation, laryngeal mask airway, and esophageal tracheal Combitube.

The esophageal tracheal Combitube (ETC) is a double-lumen tube approved by the Food and Drug Administration in 1988. The first lumen of the ETC is open at the proximal end and closed at the distal end, with a number of perforations approximately halfway along its length. The second lumen is open at both ends. The large pharyngeal inflatable balloon is affixed to the proximal end, and a smaller inflatable balloon is attached to the distal end. The ETC is gently, blindly inserted into the patient's mouth. The larger, proximal, pharyngeal 100-ml balloon is inflated; then the smaller, distal 15-ml balloon is inflated. This technique results in correct esophageal placement in 96 to 98% of cases (Reed, 1995). Following placement, ventilations are performed through the blind-ended lumen, and confirmation of pulmonary ventilation is made. If this technique is unsuccessful, ventilation through the second lumen is attempted, with subsequent placement confirmed by the presence of bilateral breath sounds. Failing this second attempt, the tube is removed and placement is attempted again.

The laryngeal mask airway (LMA) is a device popularized in Europe as an adequate airway for general anesthesia, but data on this equipment during resuscitation are limited. This airway tool fits over the larynx similar to the way an oxygen face mask fits on the face. The LMA is oval-shaped with an inflatable balloon surrounding the periphery and a tube attached, leading to a gas source. Inserted uninflated, the LMA rests in the oropharynx with the convex surface abutting the hard palate. Next, the LMA is advanced until the distal tip abuts the upper esophageal sphincter. The cuff is then inflated. Hence, the cuff rests above the larynx, sealing the airway, and the upper portion of the mask is located posterior to the base of the tongue. The mask and cuff are too large to advance into the airway, and the device is fitted with "ribs," which prevent the epiglottis from falling into and occluding the airway. Millions of general anesthesia cases have been conducted worldwide using this device, and success rates are marked after even brief training episodes in nurses, paramedics, medical students, and paramedical students.

STRATEGIES TO IMPROVE CARDIOPULMONARY RESUSCITATION

THEORETICAL MODEL OF CARDIOPULMONARY RESUSCITATION BLOOD FLOW

In understanding the blood flow mechanisms of CPR, a hydraulic model is beneficial to determine the parameters that optimize blood flow. Figure 14–1 delineates a model of the circulation as two compliant regions, one containing all the thoracic structures and the other containing all of the peripheral vascular structures (see Chapters 4 and 5 for similar circulatory models). There are two lumped parameter compliances connected by two lumped parameter conduits with characteristics of resistance and collapsibility that are contained partly within the thorax and partly outside the thorax. These two conduits are connected by one-way valves that prevent retrograde flow, much like those in the heart and venous system. At the moment when active circulation stops, the pressure within the two compliant regions equilibrate at the mean systemic pressure, or at the static pressure of the circulation. When the pressure is raised around the thoracic compartment, blood moves from the thorax into the peripheral compartment. During relaxation, or lowering of pleural pressure, blood returns from the peripheral compartment back to the thoracic vessels.

VOLUME

When pleural pressure has been raised sufficiently to cause flow limitation during compression and lowered sufficiently to cause flow limitation during filling, there is an advantage to further increase pleural pressure swings. The drainage volume,

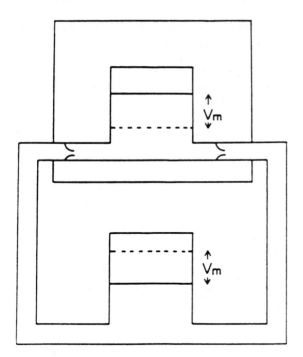

Figure 14–1

The upper reservoir represents the thoracic blood volume surrounded by a pressurized chamber. The lower reservoir represents the peripheral vascular compliance. Each of the conduits is a collapsible tube with resistance partitioned between segments inside and outside the thorax. One-way valves represent the cardiac and venous valves and ensure unidirectional flow. Vm is the total volume that would leave one reservoir and enter the other reservoir when the pressure is changed from conditions of filling to conditions of emptying, and the system is allowed to equilibrate.

however, can be increased by adding blood volume, stiffening the complaint vascular structures, or preventing the collapsibility of the conduits (Yin et al, 1982). Whether increasing blood volume improves CPR blood flow depends on whether flow limitation is present and may account for conflicting findings on this point. Although total blood flow is likely to increase by raising the volume in the central circulation (pulmonary vessels and heart), large increments of fluid may reduce vital organ perfusion by raising the back pressure to forward flow, or causing tissue congestion and elevated resistance to microvascular perfusion, or oxygen (O_2) diffusion.

PRESSURE AND VOLUME

Central blood volume can also be improved, theoretically, by abdominal compression when in cycle. Such "countermassage" or interposed ab-

dominal compression combined with chest compression (IAC-CPR) has been shown to increase mean diastolic aortic pressure, cerebral and coronary flow, peripheral O_2 delivery and cardiac output, and short-term survival in animal models (Ohomoto et al, 1976; McDonald, 1985; Voorhees et al, 1983, 1984; Ward et al, 1989). This technique probably has an additional mechanism for increasing mean and diastolic aortic pressure other than the possibility of volume-priming the intrathoracic pump. Compression of the abdominal aorta during chest recoil may propel blood retrograde toward the heart and brain, similar to the action of an intra-aortic balloon pump. A theoretical analysis of IAC-CPR based on fundamental properties of the cardiovascular system provides a rational basis for flow augmentation during CPR (Babbs et al, 1984a).

In contrast, Einagle and associates (1988) found no difference between early and late modes of interposed abdominal compression and concluded that increased carotid blood flow in a dog model was caused by increased pressure in a common thoracoabdominal unit. All peak intravascular pressures occurred during abdominal compression, producing a more effective "systole." The peak pressures of the right atria and thoracic aorta approximated each other, however, and the average coronary perfusion pressure remained only 20 mm Hg.

Initially, IAC-CPR results were conflicting; IAC-CPR did not improve cardiac and central nervous system (CNS) function or long-term survival compared with standard CPR in animal models and failed to show a difference in outcome compared with standard CPR in a prehospital study (Mateer et al, 1985). Howard and associates (1987) found that IAC-CPR offered some advantage in improving diastolic and mean arterial venous pressure difference across the coronary circulation in patients; the small differences were thought to be unlikely to improve survival rates appreciably (Howard et al, 1987). Data from our group has demonstrated that IAC-CPR improves end-tidal PECO$_2$ compared with standard CPR, and is associated with an increased return of spontaneous circulation in 33 patients arriving with nontraumatic cardiac arrest in the emergency department (Ward et al, 1989). Most current data suggest that IAC may improve meaningful survival following in hospital cardiac arrest (Sack et al, 1992).

VASCULAR RESISTANCE

An approach to increasing CPR blood flow is to reduce the time constants of drainage by decreasing the vascular resistance or compliance. Methods of doing this can rely on pharmacologic agents, such as sympathomimetics, that reduce vascular capacitance and resistance (Brown et al, 1987; Holmes et al, 1980; Michael et al, 1984; Redding et al, 1963; Schleien et al, 1989). Maneuvers, such as administering adrenergic drugs or occluding the descending aorta, which direct flow away from the compliant splanchnic circulation, have a similar effect (Permutt et al, 1975; Sylvester et al, 1983). Increasing the compliance of either the thoracic or peripheral compartments raises the mobile volume, but also has the effect of lengthening the time constants of drainage. Lengthening time constants of drainage is not a very effective strategy to improve CPR blood flow.

DUTY CYCLE AND HEART RATE

Data from Taylor and associates (1977) and from Fitzgerald and associates (Feneley et al, 1988) support the importance of optimizing the duty cycle of CPR, but with little effect of increasing the frequency of compression beyond a threshold value. Maier and colleagues (1984) have found that increasing the frequency of compression optimizes blood flow when the compression time is brief and held constant, which is a strategy similar to lengthening the duty cycle (the time compression is taking place during each cycle of compression/decompression). In a variety of models, we have found little effect of increasing the frequency of compression beyond a rate of 20 cycles/min, but we have observed an optimal duty cycle at approximately 0.6 (Wise et al, 1982; 1983). Based on these observations, CPR training should emphasize less the proper timing of compression, and emphasize more the proper duty cycle of compression (Weisfeldt et al, 1986). Unfortunately, it is also clear that one best duty cycle cannot be designated for all subjects. Rather, the duty cycle depends on the characteristics of the peripheral and thoracic circulations at the time of the cardiac arrest.

A third strategy to increase CPR blood flow is to increase the heart rate. This is the major strategy to increase blood flow by the cardiac compression model. Although sufficient data are not yet available on the more rapid resuscitative compression rates, neurologic outcome, long-term survival, and higher cardiac outputs have been reported at increased compression rates in humans (Maier et al, 1986). Compression rates of 2 Hz have been reported to increase cardiac output and coronary blood flow in a vest CPR canine model and with manual compression (Ben-Haim et al, 1989; Fenely et al, 1988).

The National Conference of Standards and Guidelines for Cardiopulmonary Resuscitation and Emergency Cardiac Care have recommended a compression rate of 90 to 100 beats/min with a 50% relative compression duration. The decision to use the high rates seems to be related to perceived ease of performing manual compression at 90 to 100 beats/min, and is based on preliminary data in patients (Swenson et al, 1988). In addition, a study comparing mean end-tidal carbon dioxide levels at compression rates of 80 and 120 beats/min revealed a slight but significant improvement of end-tidal carbon dioxide evident at the higher compression rate. In a CPR mannequin, it was found that greater compression force is necessary to sustain similar sternal displacements when the rate is increased due to a rate-limited fall in compression duration, suggesting that the controversy on recommended rate is not settled.

BLOOD FLOW TO VITAL ORGANS

Although maintenance of total cardiac output is a major goal in CPR, the criterion for success is the salvage of the patient for eventual discharge from medical care. With in-hospital cardiopulmonary arrest, approximately 55% of patients are successfully resuscitated, 15 to 25% are discharged alive, and 4 to 20% have long-term survival (Burns et al, 1989; George et al, 1989; Tresch et al, 1989). The extent of prearrest morbidity has a major role in survival after cardiopulmonary arrest, and age does not (Kerber et al, 1983; Standards and Guidelines, 1986).

Factors that adversely effect outcome in CPR are listed in Table 14–1. Because the salvage rate from CPR is critically dependent on the total time of cardiac arrest before the institution of spontaneous cardiac activity, immediate measures that restore spontaneous cardiac activity should take precedence over cardiac massage (Howard et al, 1987; Schleien et al, 1986). These measures include correction of ventricular arrhythmias with electrical, pharmacologic, or mechanical cardioversion; treatment of complete heart block with drugs or electrical pacing; treatment of severe metabolic or electrolyte imbalance, such as acidemia, hyperkalemia, hypoglycemia; and relief of asphyxia due to airway obstruction or muscular paralysis. At present, CPR is only a temporizing measure until definitive treatment can be undertaken. It is less important to maintain perfusion to all vascular beds than to prevent irreversible damage to the brain and heart by directing adequate blood flow to these organs. With the current techniques of CPR, as many as one of five survivors of cardiac arrest has serious permanent brain damage (Lumpkin et al, 1982). We shall therefore consider the special characteristics of blood flow to the brain and heart during CPR.

Cerebral Blood Flow

Although the traditional teaching is that irreversible brain damage occurs within 4 to 6 minutes of anoxia, isolated neurons on the periphery of ischemic areas are more tolerant of anoxia than was previously suspected, showing complete recovery after as long as 20 to 60 minutes of anoxia (White et al, 1984; Kelly et al, 1993). Postischemic damage to the brain may involve spasm of the cerebral vessels, leading to postischemic hypoperfusion, release of O_2 free radicals from injured tissue, neuronal intracellular calcium overload, or release of an excitatory neurotoxic neurotransmitter (Kelly et al, 1993; Schleien et al, 1989; White et al, 1984;). Little is known about the efficacy of different modes of CPR on salvage of cerebral function, but various pharmacologic techniques have been suggested to reduce cerebral O_2 consumption and preserve cerebral function during cardiac arrest (Rolfsen et al, 1989). These techniques include calcium channel antagonists, O_2 free radical scavengers, transient postresuscitation hypertension, retrograde arterial perfusion with low-viscosity solutions, anticoagulation, hypothermia, barbiturate coma, neutrophil adherence receptor blockers, hyperosmotic solutions, antiplatelet aggregating factors, anti-leukocyte adhesion antibodies, ganglioside therapy, and N-methyl-D-aspartate (NMDA) receptor antagonists (Safar et al, 1988; Kelly et al, 1983). These techniques are still in the experimental stage and, although controversial, some show considerable promise.

Much of the experimental work that has been conducted with CPR has used common carotid blood flow as an index of cerebral perfusion. The determinants of cerebral blood flow can differ from those of carotid blood flow, however (Rogers, 1981; Schleien et al, 1989). The perfusion of the brain is determined by the gradient between arterial pressure and either intracranial or jugular venous pressure (whichever is higher). The intracranial pressure surrounding the vessels acts analogously to alveolar pressure in the lung, causing vascular closure whenever surrounding pressure exceeds intravascular pressure.

Chest compression causes elevation of intracranial pressure owing to the translocation of blood from the thorax into the rigid cranium. Koehler and colleagues (1983) and Luce and colleague (1983) have shown that simultaneous compression and ventilation with abdominal binding causes an improvement in cerebral perfusion pressure and blood flow compared with conventional techniques of CPR. Cerebral perfusion could be kept at approximately one third of the control value. In contrast, Michael and associates (1984) showed that abdominal binding, although it increased common carotid blood flow and arterial pressure, had a deleterious effect on cerebral blood flow due to the increase in intracranial and jugular venous pressures. Ditchey (1982) found that excessive volume loading may be detrimental to cerebral blood flow, presumably due to the development of cerebral edema or shunting of blood through extracerebral vessels. The most successful techniques to maintain cerebral blood flow include high-pressure vest inflation, piston compression, or large doses of epinephrine. These procedures produced cerebral blood flow approaching the normal level and excellent survival in dogs and piglets (Halperin et al, 1986; Schleien et al, 1986). This level of perfusion is adequate to maintain viability of brain tissue (Steen et al, 1979).

Coronary Blood Flow

Although cardiac work is negligible during cardiac arrest, basal myocardial O_2 consumption remains at about 30 to 40% of control during ventricular fibrillation (Livesay et al, 1978). If coronary blood flow is insufficient to meet this demand, the likelihood of successful defibrillation is diminished. Studies in animals have shown widely varying estimates for coronary blood flow during CPR, ranging from less than 1% (Ditchey et al, 1982) to 100% (Halperin et al, 1986) of the control value. There is also a sharp reduction in coronary blood flow over time during a cardiac arrest, falling from 31% of normal to 5% of normal within the first 20 minutes. This time-dependent decline in coronary blood flow can be mitigated with the use of epinephrine (Michael et al, 1984).

The most effective techniques for eliciting coronary blood flow have used direct heart compression, or deformation of the thorax, and employ a force of more than 250 lbs, which requires a mechanical assist device or a very large rescuer (McDonald, 1982). During CPR, as during normal circulation, coronary blood flow occurs mainly during diastole. The upstream driving pressure for coronary blood flow is the aortic diastolic pressure during the relaxation, or the decompression, phase. It is less clear what constitutes the effective back pressure to coronary blood flow during CPR. In isolated perfused hearts with fibrillation, the effective coronary back pressure is higher than venous pressure due to myocardial tissue pressure, but in animal studies of CPR without external perfusion, the right atrial pressure appears to be the effective coronary back pressure (Ditchey et al, 1982).

The upstream driving pressure for coronary blood flow is generated by the elastic recoil pressure of the aorta, which is stored from the previous compression. The techniques of CPR that cause the greatest volume of blood to remain in the thoracic aorta during the relaxation phase of CPR are the techniques that provide the greatest diastolic aortic pressure and, therefore, the greatest coronary blood flow. Under conditions of CPR, in which blood flow is caused by a generalized increase in pleural pressure, the factors that raise stroke volume lead to a reduction in the volume of blood left in all of the thoracic vessels, including the aorta. Thus, the maneuvers that increase peripheral blood flow have a deleterious effect on coronary blood flow. In contrast, during direct cardiac compression, when the pressure around the heart increases more than the pressure around the aorta, maneuvers that raise stroke volume lead to more aortic diastolic blood volume and improved coronary blood flow (Swenson et al, 1988). This effect may account for the finding by Luce and associates (1983) that CPR performed with a piston compression device over the sternum (which may, in part, compress the heart) improved coronary blood flow compared with that performed with an inflatable vest, although cerebral blood flows were similar. Improved coronary blood flow is likely to be the major advantage of direct open chest cardiac compression over closed chest CPR.

The efficacy of epinephrine in improving CPR coronary blood flow is probably related to the increase in aortic diastolic pressure caused by the decrease in diastolic peripheral run-off (Schleien et al, 1989). Binding of the abdomen has a deleterious effect on coronary blood flow owing to the elevation of right arterial pressure (Michael et al, 1984; Niemann et al, 1994; Sanders et al, 1982). Babbs has suggested, however, that the diastolic thoracic aorta can be maintained with a higher volume by compression of the abdomen during diastole, augmenting coronary blood flow (Babbs et al, 1984b; Babbs et al, 1986). Several studies have shown a salutary effect of diastolic abdomen compression on CPR blood flow, coronary perfusion pressure, and cardiac output (Babbs et al, 1984b; Bircher et al, 1984; Coletti et al, 1983; Ohomoto et al, 1976; Ralston et al, 1982; Steen et al, 1979). Data demonstrate that active compression-decompression (ACD) improves cardiac output and coro-

nary perfusion pressure during human resuscitation (Shultz et al, 1994).

ADJUVANT METHODS TO AID BLOOD FLOW

Volume infusion has been found to increase CPR blood flow in some but not all studies (Ditchey et al, 1984; Harris et al, 1967; Passerini et al, 1988). One model of CPR predicts that an increase in volume will improve blood flow by raising the critical transmural pressure at which collapse occurs. Peripheral vascular resistance, or compliance, may change with volume infusion, however, obviating the model's predictions (Ditchey et al, 1984). Furthermore, volume-related increases in total flow may not reflect vital organ perfusion because volume loading may raise right atrial pressure to the same extent as aortic pressure, limiting perfusion gradients for coronary or cerebral blood flow.

Volume loading has been reported to cause hemodynamic deterioration after major pulmonary embolism because of ventricular interaction mediated by a left-side septal shift, increased pericardial pressure, and reduced left ventricular transmural pressure (preload) (Belenkie et al, 1989). Ventricular interdependence produced through volume overload may have a role during CPR. Clinically, pulmonary artery mean pressure and pulmonary capillary wedge pressure have been found to rise considerably during CPR in humans, and clinical evidence of pulmonary edema has been found in 30% of short-term survivors of CPR (Ornato JP, et al, 1985). In light of clinical experimental data, it appears that overly liberal infusion of fluid during CPR is not beneficial to patients who are already euvolemic. Fluid overload may result in reduced specific organ blood flow and pulmonary edema.

In the clinical context of CPR and ACLS, glucose-containing fluids are no longer given routinely for drug administration. At present, with the clinical risk and unfavorable outcome data of hypoglycemia clear, the recommendation is for normal saline as the resuscitation fluid of choice (Kelly et al, 1993). Glucose supplementation is reserved for those patients with documented hypoglycemia.

VASOACTIVE THERAPY

Epinephrine is considered to be the vasopressor agent of choice in the treatment of cardiac arrest. Redding and associates (1963), using a dog model of CPR, showed that epinephrine improved the success rate of resuscitation. This improvement correlated with an increase in aortic diastolic pressure (Lindner et al, 1989). The restoration of spontaneous heartbeat has been shown to result from alpha-adrenergic receptor stimulation (Lindner et al, 1989). Michael and associates (1984) showed that the effects of epinephrine appear to be caused by peripheral noncerebral and nonmyocardial vasoconstriction with development of higher perfusion pressure to the heart and brain. In contrast, blood flow to the gut and kidney is decreased despite higher aortic pressure.

Epinephrine also has beta-adrenergic effects on the heart that may increase contractibility and wall tension with a resultant rise in myocardial O_2 consumption (Ditchey et al, 1988). Intramyocardial wall pressure is high during fibrillation, thus reducing myocardial perfusion. If epinephrine increases wall tension further during fibrillation, myocardial O_2 supply may be impaired along with the heightened demand. Successful resuscitation has been performed with pure alpha-adrenergic agents with equivalent success rates to those of epinephrine in some reports, but not in all (Schleien et al, 1989). Norepinephrine with marked alpha and beta$_1$ activity, but with weak beta$_2$ activity, has been reported in a porcine model of CPR to be superior in equal doses to epinephrine in the treatment of ventricular fibrillation (Lindner et al, 1989; Robinson et al, 1989).

The optimal dose and method of administration of vasoactive drugs during CPR still has to be determined. Increasing doses of epinephrine from 20 to 2,000 μg/kg has produced inconsistent results. Several studies do suggest that dosages of epinephrine, higher than those usually recommended, may improve blood flow to vital organ (Brown et al, 1986). Anecdotal success as well as significant dose-dependent vasopressor and $PetCO_2$ responses during CPR in humans have been reported (Koscove et al, 1988; Gonzalez et al, 1989). Myocardial O_2 demand, however, has been noted to increase significantly with higher doses of epinephrine, so that the balance between the supply and demand with higher dosing is unclear.

Clear regimens for dosing epinephrine have been suggested. Epinephrine 1 mg by intravenous (IV) push remains the recommendation of choice, with subsequent 1-mg dosages given at 3- to 5-minute intervals (Textbook of Advanced Cardiac Life Support, 1994; Wise et al, 1987). The use of higher dosages of epinephrine is considered acceptable and possibly helpful, according to the 1992 guidelines. Two large adult clinical trials published in 1992 failed to demonstrate any difference in the rate of return of spontaneous circulation, survival to hospital admission, survival to hospital discharge, or neurologic outcome be-

tween patients treated with a standard dose of epinephrine and those treated with a high dose (Brown et al, 1992; Rivers et al, 1994; Stiell et al, 1992). Rivers and associates (1994) have outlined the post-resuscitative detrimental effects of epinephrine administration in out-of-hospital arrests. Reductions in O_2 delivery and consumption are correlated with the total cumulative dose given. These results have not been consistent in the pediatric resuscitation literature, in which high-dose epinephrine has provided a higher return of spontaneous circulation rate and a better long-term outcome in cardiac arrest (Goetting et al, 1991). Current high-dose regimens should be reserved for second-line therapy only and include

High: Epinephrine 0.1 mg/kg, IV push every 3 to 5 minutes

Escalating: Epinephrine 1 mg–3 mg–5 mg, IV push, 3 minutes apart.

SODIUM BICARBONATE

Sodium bicarbonate ($NaHCO_3$) is no longer a mainstay of drug therapy during CPR. This subject has been debated vigorously (Narins et al, 1986; Stacpoole, 1986). Guerci and associates (1986) did not find a beneficial effect in $NaHCO_3$ resuscitation of a dog model compared with saline resuscitation. Currently, $NaHCO_3$ is no longer recommended for routine administration by the American Heart Association (Textbook of Advanced Cardiac Life Support, 1994; Wise et al, 1987).

During CPR, most patients have near-normal arterial pH with a frequent respiratory acidosis, or mixed acidosis on the venous side of the circulation. The pH appears to be significantly lower, and the $PaCO_2$ appears to be significantly higher in the myocardial venous blood compared with pooled mixed venous blood (Capparelli et al, 1989). More myocardial lactate is produced than systemic lactate during CPR, contributing to the metabolic acidosis observed in the myocardial venous outflow. A select few instances are well documented citing the benefits of $NaHCO_3$ therapy during resuscitation; these include known hyperkalemia, metabolic acidosis responsive to bicarbonate therapy, tricyclic antidepressant overdose, and cocaine overdose in patients presenting with wide complex tachydysrhythmia.

MONITORING EFFECTIVENESS OF CARDIOPULMONARY RESUSCITATION

A number of investigators have correlated the outcome of CPR with mean aortic and aortic diastolic aortic pressure. Higher diastolic aortic pressure correlates with better coronary perfusion pressure and coronary blood flow, as long as right atrial pressure does not rise as much or more than aortic pressure (Ditchey et al, 1982; Coletti et al, 1983, Neimann et al, 1994; Redding, 1971; Swenson et al, 1988).

Arterial pH and $PaCO_2$ generally do not correlate with clinical outcome except in extreme situations. High arterial pH (above 7.6) is associated with failure to defibrillate and a clinically poor outcome. Large amounts of lactic acidosis predict unsuccessful results of CPR and probably reflect premorbid conditions or a prolonged delay in beginning resuscitation. Mixed venous pH and $PaCO_2$ often demonstrate significantly different values from arterial measurements (Weil et al, 1986), but have not been shown to correlate with initial success or failure of CPR. Mixed venous lactate levels are similar to arterial measurements.

Failure to eliminate CO_2 produced from both residual aerobic metabolism and buffering of anaerobically produced lactic acid has been correlated with inadequate pulmonary blood flow and cardiac output. This failure results in a high mixed venous CO_2 and a low end-tidal CO_2 tension ($PetCO_2$) (Gudipati et al, 1988). In animal models, the onset of ventricular fibrillation is associated with a rapid decrease in $PetCO_2$ which is significantly increased during precordial comparison. The change in $PetCO_2$ correlates with measured systemic blood flow and coronary artery perfusion pressure during CPR and has been reported to serve as a noninvasive measure of pulmonary blood flow and therefore effective CPR (Gudipati et al, 1988; Sanders, 1989; Trevins et al, 1985). This measurement has also been shown to predict successful outcome during CPR and immediately identifies the restoration of spontaneous circulation (Gudipati et al, 1988; Ward et al, 1989).

Gazmuri and associates (1989), in a porcine model of cardiac arrest, have shown a close correlation among $PetCO_2$, cardiac output, coronary perfusion pressures, and $PaCO_2$ being depressed during poor forward blood flow. After successful resuscitation, there is a marked increase in $PaCO_2$ corresponding with an increase in $PetCO_2$. Both $PaCO_2$ and $PetCO_2$ may serve as indicators of effective CPR and are prognostic for cardiac resuscitation under conditions of adequate constant ventilation and airway distribution. A very low initial $PetCO_2$ or $PaCO_2$ may indicate either poor blood flow or lack of CO_2 production (death).

CONCLUSIONS

The understanding of the mechanics, pharmacology, epidemiology, and physiology of CPR has increased tremendously. The optimal techniques for support of the circulation during cardiac arrest are not well established and require individualization for different clinical circumstances. Although standardization of techniques for CPR is a useful device for training large numbers of the general population to provide bystanders with assistance, little rational basis exists for the unquestioning application of these "standard" techniques. In contrast, the application of new methods of CPR in humans requires not only a strong basis in animal experimentation, but also careful consideration of the ethics of informed consent in the setting of cardiac arrest. We believe that the understanding of basic principles and usual outcomes enables the physician to individualize the treatment of cardiac arrest and maximize results.

REFERENCES

Babbs CF, Ralston SH, and Geddes LA: Theoretical advantages of abdominal counter pulsation in CPR as demonstrated in a simple electrical model of the circulation. Ann Emerg Med 13:660–667, 1984a.

Babbs CF and Tacker WA: Cardiopulmonary resuscitation with interposed abdominal compression. Circulation 74[Suppl IV]:37–41, 1986.

Babbs CF, Tacker WA, Paris RL, et al: CPR with simultaneous compression and ventilation at high airway pressure in 4 animal models. Crit Care Med 10:501–504, 1982.

Babbs CF, Weaver JC, Ralston S, et al: Cardiac, thoracic, and abdominal pump mechanisms in cardiopulmonary resuscitation. Am J Emerg Med 2:299–308, 1984b.

Belenkie I, Dani R, Smith ER, and Tyberg JV: Effects of volume loading during experimental acute pulmonary embolism. Circulation 80:178–188, 1989.

Ben-Haim SA, Shofti R, Ostrow B, and Dinner V: Effect of vest cardiopulmonary resuscitation rate of cardia output and coronary blood flow. Crit Care Med 17:768–772, 1989.

Ben-Haim SA, Shofti R, and Saidel GM: Effects of airway occlusion during cardiopulmonary resuscitation. J Crit Care 3:240–248, 1988.

Beyar R, Kishon Y, Dinnar U, et al: Cardiopulmonary resuscitation by intrathoracic pressure variation—in vivo studies and computer simulation. Angiology 35:71–77, 1984.

Bircher NG and Abramson NS: Interposed abdominal compression CPR (IAC-CPR): A glimmer of hope. Am J Emerg Med 2:177–178, 1984.

Boczar ME, Howard MA, Rivers EP, et al: A technique revisited: Hemodynamic comparison of closed chest and open chest cardiac massage during human CPR. Crit Care Med 23:498–503, 1995.

Brown CG, Martin DR, Pepe PE, et al: A comparison of standard-dose and high-dose epinephrine in cardiac arrest outside the hospital. N Engl J Med 327:1051–1055, 1992.

Brown CG, Werman HA, Davis EA, et al: Comparative effects of graded doses of epinephrine on regional brain blood flow during CPR in a swine model. Ann Emerg Med 15:1138, 1986.

Brown CG, Werman HA, Davis EA, et al: The effects of graded doses of epinephrine on regional myocardial blood flow by cardiopulmonary resuscitation in swine. Circulation 71:491–497, 1987.

Burns R, Graney MJ, and Nichols LO: Prediction of in-hospital cardiopulmonary arrest outcome. Arch Intern Med 149:1318–1321, 1989.

Capparelli EV, Chow MSS, Kluger J, et al: Differences in systemic and myocardial blood acid base status during cardiopulmonary resuscitation. Crit Care Med 17:442–446, 1989.

Cary J, Ross BK, Krugmire R, et al: Coughing causes systemic blood flow. Chest 74[Suppl]:332–333, 1978.

Chandra N, Cohen JM, and Tsitlik J: Negative airway pressure between compressions augments carotid flow during CPR. Circulation 60(II):46, 1979.

Chandra N, Guerci A, Weisfeldt ML, et al: Contrasts between intrathoracic pressures during external chest compression and cardiac massage. Crit Care Med 9:789–792, 1981a.

Chandra N, Rudikoff J, and Weisfeldt ML: Simultaneous chest compression and ventilation at high airway pressure during cardiopulmonary resuscitation. Lancet 1:175–178, 1980.

Chandra N, Snyder LD, and Weisfeldt ML: Abdominal binding during cardiopulmonary resuscitation in man. JAMA 246:351–353, 1981b.

Chandra N, Weisfeldt ML, Tsitlik J, et al: Augmentation of carotid flow during cardiopulmonary resuscitation by ventilation at high airway pressure simultaneous with chest compression. Am J Cardiol 48:1053–1063, 1981c.

Cohen JM, Chandra N, Alderson PO, et al: Timing of pulmonary and systemic blood flow during intermittent high intrathoracic pressure cardiopulmonary resuscitation in the dog. Am J Cardiol 49:1883–1889, 1982.

Cohen TJ, Kelly MD, Tucker KJ, et al: Active compression-decompression resuscitation: A novel method of cardiopulmonary resuscitation. Am Heart J 124:1145–1150, 1992.

Coletti RH, Kashel PS, and Bragman D: Abdominal counterpulsation: Effects on canine coronary and carotid blood flow. Circulation 68:226–231, 1983.

Criley JM, Blaufuss AH, and Kissel GL: Cough-induced cardiac compression. JAMA 236:1246–1250, 1976.

Criley JM, Niemann JT, Rosborough LP, and Hausknecht M: Modification of cardiopulmonary resuscitation based on cough. Circulation 74[Suppl IV]:42–58, 1986.

Cugliari A, Miller T, and Sobal J: Factors promoting completion of advanced directives in the hospitals. Arch Intern Med 155:1893–1898, 1995.

Debard ML: The history of cardiopulmonary resuscitation. Ann Emerg Med 9:273–275, 1980.

Ditchey RV and Lindenfeld J: Potential adverse effects of volume loading on perfusion of vital organs during closed chest resuscitation. Circulation 69:181–189, 1984.

Ditchey RV and Lindenfeld J: Failure of epinephrine to improve the balance between myocardial oxygen supply and demand during closed chest resuscitation in dogs. Circulation 78:381–389, 1988.

Ditchey RV, Windler JV, and Rhodes CA: Relative lack of coronary blood flow during closed chest compressions in dogs. Circulation 66:297–302, 1982.

Ditchey RV, Windler JV, and Rhodes CA: Relative lack of coronary blood flow during closed chest resuscitation in dogs. Circulation 69:181–189, 1984.

Ducas J, Oussos CH, Karsardis C, et al: Thoracoabdominal mechanics during resuscitation maneuvers. Chest 84:446–451, 1983.

Einagle V, Bertrand F, Wise RA, et al: Interposed abdominal compression and carotid blood flow during cardiopulmonary resuscitation. Chest 93:1206–1212, 1988.

Feneley MP, Maier GW, Gaynor MW, et al: Sequence of mitral valve motion and transmitral blood flow during manual cardiopulmonary resuscitation in dogs. Circulation 76:363–375, 1987.

Feneley MP, Maier GW, Kern KB, et al: Influence on compression rate on initial success of resuscitation and 24 hour survival after prolonged cardiopulmonary resuscitation in dogs. Circulation 77:240–250, 1988.

Gazmuri RJ, Von Planta M, Weil MH, et al: Arterial P_{CO_2} as an indicator of systemic perfusion during cardiopulmonary resuscitation. Crit Care Med 17:237–248, 1989.

George AL, Folk BP III, Crecelius PL, et al: Pre-arrest morbidity and other correlates of survival after in-hospital cardiopulmonary arrest. Am J Med 87:28–33, 1989.

Goetting MG and Paradis NA: High-dose epinephrine improves outcome from pediatric cardiac arrest. Ann Emerg Med 20:22–26, 1991.

Gonzalez ER, Ornato JP, Richmond V, et al: Dose-dependent vasopressor response to epinephrine during CPR in human beings. Ann Emerg Med 18:920–926, 1989.

Gudipati CV, Weil MH, Bisera J, et al: Expired carbon dioxide: A noninvasive monitor of cardiopulmonary resuscitation. Circulation 77:234–239, 1988.

Guerci AD, Chandra N, Johnson E, et al: Failure of sodium bicarbonate to improve resuscitation from ventricular fibrillation in dog. Circulation 74[Suppl IV]:75–79, 1986.

Halperin HR, Guerci AD, Chandra N, et al: Vest inflation without simultaneous ventilation during cardiac arrest in dogs. Circulation 74:1407–1415, 1986.

Halperin HR, Tsitlik JE, Gelfand M, et al: A preliminary study of cardiopulmonary resuscitation by circumferential compression of the chest with use of a pneumatic vest. N Engl J Med 329:762–768, 1993.

Halperin HR, Weiss JL, Guerci AD, et al: Cyclic elevation of intrathoracic pressure can close the mitral valve during cardiac arrest in dogs. Circulation 78:754–760, 1988.

Harris LC, Kirmili B, and Safar P: Augmentation of artificial circulation during cardiopulmonary resuscitation. Anesthesiology 28:730–734, 1967.

Hermreck AS: The history of cardiopulmonary resuscitation. Am J Surg 156:430–436, 1988.

Holmes FR, Babbs CR, Voorhees WD, et al: Influence of adrenergic drugs upon vital organ perfusion during CPR. Crit Care Med 8:137–140, 1980.

Hooker DR, Kouwenhaven WB, and Longworthy OR: The effect of alternating currents on the heart. Am J Physiol 103:444–454, 1933.

Howard M, Carrubba C, Foss F, et al: Interposed abdominal compression CPR: Its effects on parameters of coronary perfusion in human subjects. Ann Emerg Med 16:253–259, 1987.

Kerber RE, Jensen SR, Gascho JA, et al: Determinants of defibrillation: Prospective analysis of 183 patients. Am J Cardiol 52:739–745, 1983.

Kelly BJ and Luce JM: Current concepts in cerebral protection. Chest 103:1246–1254, 1993.

Kerber RE, Ornato JP, Brown DD, et al: Guidelines for cardiopulmonary resuscitation and emergency cardiac care. JAMA 268:2172–2183, 1992.

Koehler RC, Chandra N, Guerci A, et al: Augmentation of cerebral perfusion by simultaneous chest compression and lung inflation with abdominal binding after cardiac arrest in dogs. Circulation 67:266–274, 1983.

Koscove EM, Norman MD, Norman A, and Paradis MD: Successful resuscitation from cardiac arrest using high-dose epinephrine therapy: Report of two cases. JAMA 259:3031–3034, 1988.

Kouwenhaven WB, Jude JR, and Knickerbocker GG: Closed chest cardiac massage. JAMA 173:1064–1067, 1960.

Kouwenhaven WB, Longworthy OR: Cardiopulmonary resuscitation: An account of forty-five years of research. Johns Hopkins Med J 132:186–193, 1973.

Lindner KH and Ahnefeld FW: Comparison of epinephrine and norepinephrine in the treatment of asphyxial or fibrillatory cardiac arrest in a porcine model. Crit Care Med 17:437–441, 1989.

Livesay JJ, Follette D, Fey KH, et al: Optimizing myocardial supply/demand balance with alpha-adrenergic drugs during cardiopulmonary resuscitation. J Thorac Cardiovasc Surg 76:244–251, 1978.

Luce JM, Ross BK, O'Quinn RJ, et al: Regional blood flow during cardiopulmonary resuscitation in dogs using simultaneous and non-simultaneous compression and ventilation. Circulation 67:258–264, 1983.

Lumpkin JR and Safar P: Brain resuscitation after cardiac arrest. In Harwood AL (ed): Cardiopulmonary Resuscitation. Baltimore, Williams & Wilkins, 1982, pp 55–68.

McDonald JL: Systolic and mean arterial pressures during manual and mechanical CPR in humans. Am Emerg Med 11:292–295, 1982.

McDonald JL: Effect of interposed abdominal compression during CPR on central arterial and venous pressure. Am J Emerg Med 3:156–159, 1985.

Maier GW, Newton JR, Wolfeda S, and Tyson GS: The influence of manual chest compression rate on hemodynamic support during cardiac arrest: High-impulse cardiopulmonary resuscitation. Circulation 74[Suppl IV]:51–59, 1986.

Maier GW, Tyson GS, Olsen CO, et al: The physiology of external cardiac massage: High impulse cardiopulmonary resuscitation. Circulation 70:86–101, 1984.

Maksoud A, Jahnigen DW, Skibinski CI: Do not resuscitate orders and the cost of death. Arch Intern Med 153:1249–1253, 1993.

Mateer JR, Steven HA, Thompson BM, et al: Pre-hospital IAC-CPR versus standard CPR. Am J Emerg Med 3:143–147, 1985.

Michael J, Guerci A, Hoehler R, et al: Mechanisms by which epinephrine augments cerebral and myocardial perfusion during cardiopulmonary resuscitation. Circulation 69:822–835, 1984.

Miranda DR: Quality of life after cardiopulmonary resuscitation. Chest 106:524–530, 1994.

Narins GG and Cohen JJ: Bicarbonate therapy for organic acidosis: The case for continued use. Ann Intern Med 150:615–618, 1986.

Newton JR, Glower DD, Wolfe JA, et al: A physiologic comparison of external cardiac massage techniques. J Thorac Cardiovasc Surg 95:892–901, 1988.

Niemann JT, Rosborough J, Hausknect M, et al: Cough-CPR. Documentation of systemic perfusion in man and in an experimental model: A "window" to the mechanism of blood flow in external CPR. Crit Care Med 8:141–146, 1980.

Niemann JT, Rosborough J, Ung S, and Criley JM: Hemodynamic effects of continuous abdominal binding during cardiac arrest and resuscitation. Am J Cardiol 53:269–274, 1994.

Noc M, Weil MH, Tang W, et al: Mechanical ventilation may not be essential for initial cardiopulmonary resuscitation. Chest 108:821–827, 1995.

O'Quinn R, Culver B, and Butler J: Juxtacardiac, ventricular and airway pressures during CPR (abstract). Am Rev Respir Dis 129[Suppl]:A335, 1984.

Ohomoto T, Miura I, and Konno S: A new method of external cardiac massage to improve diastolic augmentation and prolong survival time. Ann Thorac Surg 21:284–290, 1976.

Ornato JP, Ryschon TW, Gonzalez ER, and Bredthaver

JL: Rapid changes in pulmonary vascular hemodynamics with pulmonary edema during cardiopulmonary resuscitation. Am J Emerg Med 3:237–242, 1985.

Paraskos JA: Cardiovascular pharmacology. III: Atropine, calcium; calcium blockers, and β-blockers. Circulation 74[Suppl IV]:86–89, 1986a.

Paraskos JA: External compression without adjuncts. Circulation 74[Suppl IV]:33–36, 1986b.

Passerini L, Wise RA, Roussas C, and Magder S: Maintenance of circulation without chest compression during CPR. J Crit Care 3:96–102, 1988.

Permutt S and Caldini P: Regulation of cardiac output by the circuit: Venous return. In Raines J, Noordergraaf A, Baan J (eds): Cardiovascular System Dynamics. Cambridge, MA, MIT Press, 1975.

Raessler KL, Kern KB, Sanders AB, et al: Aortic and right atrial systolic pressures during cardiopulmonary resuscitation: A potential indicator of the mechanism of blood flow. Am Heart J 115:1021–1029, 1988.

Ralston SH, Babbs CF, and Niebauer MJ: Cardiopulmonary resuscitation with interposed abdominal compression in dogs. Anesth Analg 61:645–651, 1982.

Redding JS: Abdominal compression in cardiopulmonary resuscitation. Anesth Analg 50:668–675, 1971.

Redding JS and Pearson JW: Evolution of drugs for cardiac resuscitation. Anesth Analg 24:203–208, 1963.

Reed AP: Current concepts in airway management for cardiopulmonary resuscitation. Mayo Clin Proc 70:1172–1184, 1995.

Rich S, Wix HL, and Shapiro EP: Clinical assessment of heart chamber size and valve motion during cardiopulmonary resuscitation by two-dimensional echocardiography. Am Heart J 102:368–373, 1981.

Rivers EP, Wortsman J, Rady MY, et al: The effect of the total cumulative epinephrine dose administered during human CPR on hemodynamic, oxygen transport, and utilization variables in the postresuscitation period. Chest 106:1499–1507, 1994.

Robinson LA, Brown CG, Jenkins J, et al: The effects of norepinephrine versus epinephrine on myocardial hemodynamics during CPR. Ann Emerg Med 18:336–340, 1989.

Rogers MC: Cerebral blood flow during cardiopulmonary resuscitation. Anesth Analg 60:73–75, 1981.

Rolfsen ML and Davis WR: Cerebral function and preservation during cardiac arrest. Crit Care Med 17:283–291, 1989.

Rudikoff MT, Maughan WL, Effron M, et al: Mechanisms of blood flow during cardiopulmonary resuscitation. Circulation 61:345–352, 1980.

Sack JB, Kesselbrenner MB, and Bregman D: Survival from in-hospital cardiac arrest with interposed abdominal counterpulsation during cardiopulmonary resuscitation. JAMA 267:379–385, 1992.

Safar P: On the history of modern resuscitation. Crit Care Med 24:S3–S11, 1996.

Safar P and Bircher NG: Cardiopulmonary Cerebral Resuscitation, 3rd ed. Philadelphia, WB Saunders, 1988, pp 229–276.

Safar P, Escarraga LA, and Elain JO: A comparison of mouth-to-mouth and mouth-to-airway methods of artificial respiration with the crest-pressure arm-lift methods. N Engl J Med 258:671–677, 1958.

Sanders AB: End-tidal carbon dioxide monitoring during cardiopulmonary resuscitation: A prognostic indicator for survival. JAMA 262:1347–1351, 1989.

Sanders AB, Erby GA, Alferness C, et al: Failure of one method of simultaneous chest compression, ventilation and abdominal binding during CPR. Crit Care Med 10:509–513, 1982.

Schleien CL, Berkowitz ID, Traystman R, and Rogers MC: Controversial issues in cardiopulmonary resuscitation. Circulation 78:809–817, 1986.

Schleien CL, Dean JM, Hochler RC, et al: Effect of epinephrine on cerebral and myocardial perfusion in an infant animal preparation of cardiopulmonary resuscitation. Anesthesiology 71:133–149, 1989.

Shultz JJ, Coffeen P, Sweeney M, et al: Evaluation of standard and active compression-decompression CPR in an acute human model of ventricular fibrillation. Circulation 89:684–693, 1994.

Stacpoole PW: Lactic acidosis: The case against bicarbonate therapy. Ann Intern Med 104:276–279, 1986.

Standards and guidelines for cardiopulmonary resuscitation and emergency cardiac arrest. JAMA 225:2905–2932, 1986.

Steen PA, Milde JM, and Michenfelder JD: Incomplete versus complete cerebral ischemia: Improved outcome with minimal blood flow. Ann Neurol 6:389, 1979.

Stiell IG, Hebert PC, Weitzmann BN, et al: High-dose epinephrine in adult cardiac arrest. N Engl J Med 327(15):1045–1050, 1992.

Support Principal Investigators: A Controlled Trial to Improve Care for Seriously Ill Hospitalized Patients. JAMA 274:1591–1598, 1995.

Swenson RD, Weaver D, Niskanen RA, et al: Hemodynamics in humans during conventional and experimental methods of cardiopulmonary resuscitation. Circulation 78:630–639, 1988.

Sylvester JT, Goldberg HS, and Permutt S: The role of the vasculature in the regulation of cardiac output. Clin Chest Med 4:111–125, 1983.

Taylor GJ, Theber WM, Greene HL, et al: Importance of prolonged compression during cardiopulmonary resuscitation in man. N Engl J Med 296:1515–1517, 1977.

Textbook of Advanced Cardiac Life Support. American Heart Association, 1994.

Tresch DD, Thakur RK, Hoffruan RG, et al: Should

the elderly be resuscitated following out-of-hospital arrest? Am J Med 86:145–149, 1989.

Trevins RP, Bisera J, Weil MH, et al: End-tidal CO$_2$ as a guide to successful cardiopulmonary resuscitation: A preliminary report. Crit Care Med 13:910–911, 1985.

Voorhees WD, Niebauer MJ, and Babbs CF: Improved oxygen delivery during cardiopulmonary resuscitation with interposed abdominal compression. Ann Emerg Med 12:128–135, 1983.

Voorhees WD, Ralston SH, and Babbs CF: Regional blood flow during cardiopulmonary resuscitation with abdominal counterpulsation in dog. Am J Emerg Med 2:123–127, 1984.

Ward KR, Sullivan RJ, Zelenak RR, and Summer WR: A comparison of interposed abdominal compression CPR and standard CPR by monitoring end-tidal pCO$_2$. Ann Emerg Med 18:831–837, 1989.

Weale FE and Rothwell-Jackson RL: The efficiency of cardiac massage. Lancet 1:990–992, 1962.

Weil MH, Rackow EC, Trevino R, et al: Difference in acid-base state between venous and arterial blood during CPR. N Engl J Med 315:153–156, 1986.

Weisfeldt ML and Halperin HR: Cardiopulmonary resuscitation: Beyond cardiac massage. Circulation 74:443–448, 1986.

Werner JA, Greene L, Janko C, et al: Visualization of cardiac valve motion in man during external chest compression using two dimension echocardiography. Circulation 63:1417–1421, 1981.

White BC, Widgenstein JC, Winegar CD: Brain ischemia anoxia: Mechanism of injury. JAMA 251:1586–1589, 1984.

Wise RA and Summer WR: Pulmonary mechanics and artificial support of the arrested circulation. Clin Chest Med 4:189–198, 1983.

Wise RA and Summer WR: Cardiopulmonary resuscitation. Cardiopulmonary Crit Care 335–337, 1987.

Wise RA, Taylor WR, Pinsky MR, et al: Effect of duty cycle and frequency on blood flow in a model of cardiopulmonary resuscitation (CPR). Fed Proc 41:1608, 1982.

Yin FCP, Cohen JM, Tsitlik J, et al: Role of carotid artery resistance to collapse during high intrathoracic pressure CPR. Am J Physiol 243:H259–H267, 1982.

Zoll PM, Linethal AJ, and Gibson W: Termination of ventricular fibrillation in man by externally placed electric countershock. N Engl J Med 254:727–732, 1956.

C H A P T E R

Pharmacologic and Ventilatory Support of the Circulation in Critically Ill Patients

15

Alan Multz, M.D.

Steven M. Scharf, M.D., Ph.D.

Shock is a clinical syndrome characterized by hypoperfusion. When shock occurs, a very complex and complicated series of events ensues that creates the pathophysiology as we see it clinically.

One classification of shock is based on the underlying pathophysiology (Weil and Shubin, 1972). Shock may be classified as being the result of inadequate venous return (hypovolemic), poor cardiac function (cardiogenic), and arterial vasodilation. The first two categories correspond to the venous return and cardiac function curves in the classic venous return/cardiac output (CO) scheme (see Chapters 4 and 5). Vasodilatory shock, of which sepsis is the most common cause, is due to extreme arterial vasodilation in the presence of adequate or even supranormal cardiac output (CO). Because there is evidence of end-organ dysfunction with sepsis, it is often considered that blood flow is distributed such that end-organ capillary blood flow is reduced even though overall CO is increased. Hence, the term *maldistributive* is often applied to this type of shock. Cardiogenic shock may be due to a number of causes that can depress the Starling function curve. These include myocardial depression, valvular dysfunction, and massive acute obstruction of the pulmonary artery due to pulmonary embolus. The latter has been called *obstructive shock* and is considered separately.

All forms of shock are clinically manifested by hypotension, evidence of tissue hypoperfusion, and cellular hypoxia. Tissue hypoperfusion is characterized by abnormal end-organ function. Clinical manifestations of shock include oliguria and renal insufficiency, hepatic dysfunction, change in mental status, gastrointestinal dysfunction, and increased serum lactate. Lactic acidosis is due to anaerobic metabolism on a cellular level from tissue and cellular hypoxia.

In this chapter, we consider several controversies pertaining to the management of shock in the critical care setting. These include the role of crystalloid versus colloid fluid therapy in shock, vasoactive substances for support of the blood pressure in cardiogenic and septic shock, antimediator therapy in septic shock, pharmacologic support in massive pulmonary embolus, and ventilatory maneuvers to increase CO with myocardial failure. It is not our purpose to give an exhaustive review of these controversies—such a review is beyond the scope of our chapter. We do attempt, however, to pinpoint where some of the controversies lie. A number of modern controversies concerning support of the failing circulation are actually re-examinations of older therapies, some of which had been discarded and some of which have been accepted with little critical evaluation. At any rate, it is clear that there will be changes in the routine clinical management of the failing circulation in the near future.

CRYSTALLOID VERSUS COLLOID FLUID THERAPY IN HYPOVOLEMIC AND SEPTIC SHOCK

Hypovolemic shock is very common and occurs in patients who have sustained trauma, those who have had massive hemorrhage, or those who are severely dehydrated. It can also be seen in disease with large extravascular fluid losses such as pancreatitis, severe burns, and small or large bowel obstruction, or intra-abdominal catastrophe associated with the development of peritonitis. Hypotension is associated with decreased blood volume. The latter decreases mean circulatory pressure and, hence, decreases the gradient for venous return from the periphery to the right heart (see Chapters 4 and 5). There is a significant reduction in total oxygen transport ($TO_2 = CO \times$ arterial O_2 content) in the setting of relatively normal oxygen demand. In severe hemorrhage, a reduction in hemoglobin also contributes to the reduction in TO_2. Along with decreased CO, there is a decrease in capillary blood volume.

Figure 15–1 demonstrates the effect of hemorrhage on CO and arterial blood pressure. Because of baroreceptor reflexes, the effects of decreasing CO are buffered. Thus, decreases in blood pressure underestimate the severity of the drop in peripheral O_2 delivery. With worsening shock, as blood pressure begins to drop below the autoregulatory range (60–80 mm Hg), coronary blood flow may become compromised. This cardiogenic component puts the heart at risk for ischemic injury and can serve to decrease CO even further. With progression of shock, cardiac function deteriorates over hours. Eventually the heart becomes the determining factor as to whether or not shock is reversible.

Besides baroreceptor-mediated sympathoadrenal responses and decreased coronary blood flow (in severe shock), other factors are important in determining the outcome of the shock state. With

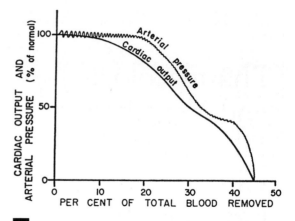

Figure 15–1
The effect of acute hemorrhage on cardiac output and arterial pressure. Note that about 10% of the blood volume may be lost without a significant hemodynamic effect. Note also that arterial pressure is maintained longer than cardiac output in a person with an acute hemorrhage. (From Guyton AC: Textbook of Medical Physiology. Philadelphia, WB Saunders, 1976, p 358. With permission.)

decreasing cerebral perfusion there is a brainstem-mediated sympathoadrenal response called the *ischemic* response, which is activated at very low blood pressures, usually less than 50 mm Hg. Mediators from the kidney, most significantly related to the renin-angiotensin axis leading to angiotensin release, buffer the effects of shock. Angiotensin is itself a potent vasoconstrictor, and renin release leads to conservation of salt and water in an attempt to increase blood volume.

Controversy exists as to what is the most appropriate way to replace volume in nonhemorrhagic hypovolemic shock (Davies, 1989; Ross and Angaran, 1984; Vincent, 1991; Wagner and D'Amelio, 1993). The crystalloid-colloid controversy centers on three major issues. First, when crystalloids alone are used, very large volumes are often required because most of the infused solutions leak into the extravascular space. Indeed, crystalloids can be considered to be an infusion into the entire extracellular—including intravascular and extravascular—fluid space rather than only the intravascular fluid space. This is a potential advantage when extracellular fluid depletion is part of the shock syndrome, such as with hypovolemic shock. Second, there is a biologic cost to the patient from the sequestration of extravascular fluid as edema when there is no component of extravascular extracellular fluid depletion. Hence, the risk of pulmonary edema is generally considered greater with crystalloid than with colloid infusions. Third, there is the issue of cost-effectiveness, because colloid solutions are more expensive than crystalloid solutions.

The crystalloids in current use are generally normal saline and Ringer's lactate solution. The colloids include albumin, hetastarch, pentastarch, and dextrans. Many studies have compared the efficacy of hetastarch, albumin, and crystalloid in the treatment of shock. The current literature is often difficult to evaluate because of problems like small sample sizes, inhomogeneous patient cohorts, and differences in clinical end points. In one meta-analysis, Velanovich (1989) examined the results of eight trials comparing clinical efficacy of crystalloids and colloids in both trauma and nontrauma patients. It was concluded that in trauma patients the mortality rate for crystalloid resuscitation was 12.3% less than that for colloid resuscitation. In nontrauma patients, the opposite trend was found—the mortality rate for colloid resuscitation was 7.8% less than that for crystalloid resuscitation. Neither of these differences was statistically significant, and the studies cannot be regarded as conclusive.

Many other clinical investigations have examined the use of different fluids in various types of shock. Puri and coworkers (1981) found that hetastarch increased the pulmonary capillary wedge pressure (P_w), cardiac index, and mean arterial pressure without respiratory complications in patients with hypovolemic, septic, or cardiogenic shock. Using a cohort of 26 patients, Haupt and Rackow (1982) compared hetastarch, albumin, and normal saline. The patients had either hypovolemic, septic, or cardiogenic shock, and all solutions were given to maintain P_w between 10 and 15 mm Hg for 24 hours. An increase in colloid oncotic pressure was noted after administration of 1 liter of both hetastarch and albumin, but to a 25% greater extent with the hetastarch. In contrast, 1 liter of saline decreased colloid oncotic pressure by 12%. Almost three to four times the amount of saline was required to keep P_w at the desired level than was necessary with either albumin or hetastarch ($p<.05$ for all comparisons).

Puri and coworkers (1983) directly compared hetastarch and albumin in patients with hypovolemia due to multiple etiologies including sepsis, trauma, and surgery. With similar volumes infused, all hemodynamic variables were comparable except for left ventricular stroke work index, which increased to twice the baseline value with infusion of hetastarch as compared with albumin. Rackow and coworkers (1983) performed a similar trial in 26 consecutive patients with hypovolemic shock of various etiologies, comparing hetastarch, albumin, and normal saline. Two to four times

the amount of crystalloid as colloid were required to achieve equivalent hemodynamic responses. A significantly higher incidence of pulmonary edema (88% versus 22%) was seen in those resuscitated with crystalloid. There were no significant differences in the response to the two types of colloid (albumin and hetastarch).

To summarize, there are few convincing data to indicate an advantage of crystalloid or colloid resuscitation for hypovolemic shock. The major limitation of many trials is heterogeneity of the patient population and small sample sizes. For the treatment of hypovolemic shock, both types of solutions are associated with certain real and theoretical advantages and disadvantages. Thus, in the light of the current state of the art, therapy must be individualized. Regarding cost, crystalloid is the least expensive, 5% albumin is the most expensive, and hetastarch is somewhere between.

In septic shock, although CO may be elevated, there is maldistribution of blood flow with relative underperfusion of critical vascular beds in end organs. Hence, this type of shock has been called *distributive*. Furthermore, increased capillary permeability can lead to substantial volume loss from intravascular to extravascular compartments.

Extravascular volume may be considered to be "unstressed" and does not contribute to venous return or CO. Thus, from one point of view, septic shock can be considered a type of hypovolemic shock. Furthermore, changes in venous capacitance with pooling of blood in unstressed compartments and excess insensible losses of fluids contribute to redistribution of blood volume from stressed to unstressed compartments (see Chapter 19). Early septic shock is characterized by a drop in mean circulatory pressure, decreased CO, and hypotension (Blain et al, 1970; Rackow et al, 1987). The characteristic hyperdynamic state of sepsis is usually seen only after fluid resuscitation.

During the hypodynamic phase of septic shock, therapy using fluids is commonly the treatment of choice. As in the case of hypovolemic shock, controversy exists as to the relative efficacy of crystalloids versus colloids (Hauser et al, 1980; Rackow et al, 1983; Ross and Angaran 1984; Shoemaker 1987; Virgilio et al, 1979). Figure 15–2 illustrates data from one such study (Rackow et al, 1983) comparing 6% hetastarch, 0.9% normal saline, and 5% albumin. There were no significant differences in hemodynamic responses in patients given the three types of fluids. As in the case of hypovolemic shock, there are few differences related to the type of fluid given. Differences do exist in the volume required to achieve equivalent hemodynamic results. Fluid requirements described by Rackow and coworkers

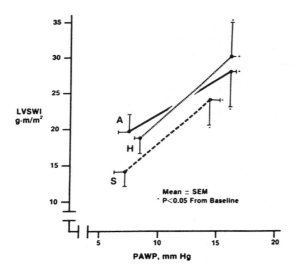

Figure 15-2
Hemodynamic effects of fluid challenge with 6% hydroxyethyl starch (H), 5% albumin (A), and 0.9% normal saline (S). The pulmonary arterial wedge pressure (PAWP) and left ventricular stroke work index (LVSWI) both significantly improved. (From Rackow EC, Falk JL, Fein IA, et al: Fluid resuscitation in circulatory shock: A comparison of the cardiorespiratory effects of albumin, hetastarch, and saline solution in patients with hypovolemia and septic shock. Crit Care Med 11:839–850, 1983. With permission.)

were 1 to 2 liters for colloid resuscitation and up to as much as 8 liters in crystalloid resuscitation. These large fluid requirements may persist for days after the onset of septic shock.

The specific goals of fluid resuscitation in septic shock remain controversial. On a cellular level, the treatment endpoint is to reverse tissue hypoxia, diminish anaerobic metabolism, and improve tissue perfusion. Early work by Duff and coworkers (1969) and Siegel and coworkers (1967) suggested an imbalance between O_2 transport and O_2 consumption in septic shock. Other studies demonstrated transport-dependent O_2 uptake in septic shock. This concept was termed the *pathologic supply-dependency relationship* (Astiz et al, 1987; Gilbert et al, 1986; Haupt et al, 1985). According to this notion, in sepsis, peripheral utilization of O_2 is dependent on transport of O_2 over a range in which O_2 utilization is transport-independent in normals (Dantzker and Gutierrez, 1989). This concept has been the basis for a treatment strategy geared to maximizing O_2 transport, by maximizing CO and mixed venous O_2 saturation (Shoemaker et al, 1986–1989). For example, Packman and Rackow (1983) have recommended infusion of fluid until "maximum" CO

and TO_2 have been achieved. This was defined as having occurred when P_w was 12 to 15 mm Hg. Figure 15–3 is from this work and demonstrates increased left ventricular stroke work index with P_w brought up to this range. In fact, Shoemaker and coworkers demonstrated that in postoperative patients, increasing CO and TO_2 to supranormal levels improved mortality rate.

The concept of "pushing" TO_2 to supranormal levels has been tested in randomized trials in other clinical settings. Hayes and coworkers (1994) performed a randomized trial evaluating the effects of increasing O_2 transport in critically ill patients with inotropic therapy. The in-hospital mortality of the treatment group was actually greater than of the control group (54 versus 34%). Gattinoni and coworkers (1995) performed a large randomized controlled trial comparing results in two treatment groups. In one group, O_2 transport was maintained at a high level, defined as cardiac index greater than 4.5 l/min/m² with mixed venous O_2 saturation 70% or higher or arterial-mixed venous A-V O_2 difference less than 20%. In the other group (control), cardiac index was maintained in the normal range, defined as 2.5 to 3.5 l/min/m². This study showed no differences in mortality or morbidity between the treatment groups, suggesting no beneficial effect in critically ill patients by increasing O_2 transport to greater than normal levels. Hence, there are few data from randomized controlled trials supporting the concept that increasing TO_2 (usually by increasing CO) to greater than normal levels has a beneficial effect on the outcome of septic shock.

VASOPRESSOR SUPPORT IN CARDIOGENIC SHOCK

Cardiogenic shock occurs most frequently in the setting of acute myocardial infarction (see Chapter 16) and complicates 5 to 10% of all cases of patients with myocardial infarctions admitted to hospitals. There is a clear correlation between the amount of damaged myocardium and the chance of developing cardiogenic shock. Chances of developing cardiogenic shock are high when greater than 40% of the left ventricular myocardium is damaged (Alonso et al, 1973; Page et al, 1971). Forrester and coworkers (1976) described hemodynamic subsets of acute myocardial infarction based on measurements of cardiac index and P_w. For a low cardiac index (≤2.2 l/min/m²), the mortality rate was 74%. Despite the newest technologies in cardiology and cardiac surgery, the mortality rate from cardiogenic shock remains quite high. Arterial hypotension in cardiogenic shock is usually due to a reduction in CO. As in

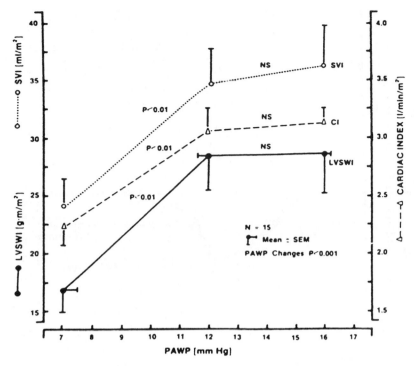

Figure 15–3
Changes in stroke volume index (SVI), left ventricular stroke work index (LVSWI), and cardiac index (CI), as fluid resuscitation is performed and pulmonary arterial wedge pressure (PAWP) increases. Elevation of the PAWP to 16 ± 0.9 mm Hg was not associated with increases in CI, SVI, LVSWI, and mean arterial pressure (MAP). (From Packman MI and Rackow EC: Optimum left heart filling pressure during fluid resuscitation of patients with hypovolemic and septic shock. Crit Care Med 11:165–169, 1983. With permission.)

hemodynamic shock and acute cor pulmonale, the relationship between peripheral O_2 consumption and TO_2 in cardiogenic shock is characterized by a reduction in TO_2 in the setting of a relatively normal O_2 consumption.

With cardiogenic shock, the Starling function curve shifts downward to the right (Figure 15–4). Compensatory sympathetic reflexes buffer these changes somewhat. Sympathoadrenal reflexes act to maintain blood pressure by leading to vasoconstriction and improving myocardial contractility. In contrast, sustained sympathetic stimulation may have adverse effects on myocardial function. Sustained vasoconstriction, although necessary for maintaining blood pressure, increases left ventricular afterload by increasing the resistive component of left ventricular impedance. This change can lead to increased myocardial O_2 demand. Sustained β-1 stimulation can lead to increased myocardial O_2 demand in contracting tissue as well. In the presence of limited coronary flow reserve, as in the "border zone" of the infarction, myocardial O_2 supply/demand ratios can change unfavorably, and infarction size can even be increased (Daly and Sole, 1990; Swedberg et al, 1990).

A very complicated series of physiologic derangements accounts for the clinical manifestations of cardiogenic shock. In addition to depressed contractility (see Chapter 7) ischemia is associated with a decrease in left ventricular com-

pliance (Bertrand et al, 1979; Bigger et al, 1984; Glantz and Parmley, 1978). Acute mitral valve dysfunction, interventricular septal defect, brady- and tachyarrhythmias, and rupture of the free wall of the left ventricle are secondary complications of myocardial infarction that can decrease cardiac pumping ability without a reduction in myocardial contractility *per se*. Metabolic acidosis, hypoxemia, and concomitant use of medications with a negative inotropic effect may all contribute to the clinical deterioration of the patient in cardiogenic shock (Braunwald et al, 1984; Smith et al, 1988).

Vasopressor catecholamines work via stimulation of adenyl cyclase to increase production of cyclic adenosine monophosphate (cAMP). These medications are often used in the initial treatment of cardiogenic shock in an attempt to raise blood pressure and CO as well as to lower pulmonary microvascular pressures to reduce pulmonary congestion. Effects of the vasoactive catecholamines are often dose-dependent. For example, at doses between 5 and 10 μg/kg/min, dopamine is a mild β_1 agonist and increases stroke volume, heart rate, and CO. Little vasodilation is produced by this drug due to low β_2 activity. At doses between 10 and 20 μg/kg/min, α_1 receptors are stimulated, which results in peripheral vasoconstriction contributing to an increase in blood pressure (Goldberg et al, 1977; Marcus et al, 1991).

Ichard and coworkers (1983) demonstrated

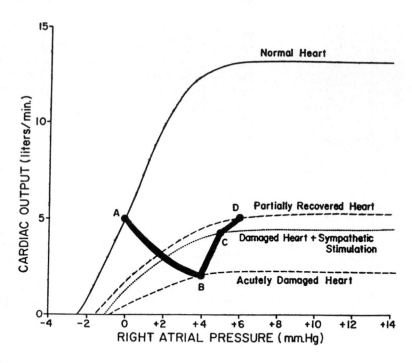

Figure 15–4
Changes in cardiac output and right atrial pressure following an acute myocardial infarction. Point A is the normal state. Point B occurs within seconds of acute myocardial disease. Point C represents the compensatory effect of the sympathetic nervous system, and point D represents the status of the partially recovered heart after an acute myocardial infarction. (From Guyton AC: Textbook of Medical Physiology. Philadelphia, WB Saunders, 1976, p 333. With permission.)

that dopamine is useful in patients with decreased left ventricular function as demonstrated by high left ventricular end diastolic volumes, pulmonary congestion, and clinical shock state. Holzer and coworkers (1973) demonstrated both improved overall hemodynamics and renal function in cardiogenic shock patients. This finding was attributed to both its positive inotropic effects and local vasodilating effects in the splanchnic and renal vessels. Arnold and coworkers (1985) addressed the question of extension of infarction size with dopamine. These investigators found no adverse effects on infarction size or overall cardiac function.

Norepinephrine is the other catecholamine vasopressor agent used in circulatory support. It has both α and β agonist properties, with minimal β_2 agonist effects. Its primary effect is to increase blood pressure due to arterial vasoconstriction. In cardiogenic shock, arterial vasoconstriction can lead to a decrease in CO. Hence, when used in cardiogenic shock, it is frequently combined with dobutamine or another inotropic agent (Abrams et al, 1973). Muller and coworkers (1970) studied norepinephrine in cardiogenic shock. It was used in their study to augment diastolic blood pressure and hence aid in coronary perfusion. Contractility also increased. Neither positive nor adverse effects on the clinical outcome, however, were observed.

Dobutamine is a relatively selective agonist for β_1 receptors, which results in an increase in CO combined with a decrease in systemic vascular resistance and, hence, left ventricular afterload.

This effect leads to decreased left ventricular end diastolic pressure and increased stroke work. Other effects include an increase in heart rate. Because systemic vasodilation is combined with increased CO, the effect on blood pressure is variable (Sonnenblick et al, 1979). As a result of increases in heart rate and stroke work, myocardial O_2 consumption and coronary blood flow demand rise with dobutamine (Bendersky et al, 1981). Although this effect may be considered to be dangerous in the setting of acute myocardial infarction, Maekawa and coworkers (1983) demonstrated improved left ventricular performance without increasing the enzymatically assessed infarction area.

Caution is urged when dobutamine is administered to patients with severe coronary artery disease. For example, Goldstein (1985) showed that although dobutamine raises blood flow in patients with coronary artery disease, these increases are inhomogeneous (Goldstein, 1985). Presumably, myocardial blood flow did not increase in areas served by critically stenotic vessels. In addition, Gillespie and coworkers (1977) showed that 22% of patients receiving doses of dobutamine (up to 15 μg/kg/min) with coronary artery disease demonstrated myocardial lactate production, suggesting myocardial ischemia. Two separate groups have compiled data to suggest that the ischemic potential of dobutamine may be related to increasing the heart rate and, hence, myocardial O_2 demand (Vatner and Baig, 1979; Willerson et al, 1976).

Amrinone is an inotropic agent that works by inhibiting the enzyme phosphodiesterase III, the result of which is to increase cAMP levels. This medication also causes arterial and venous vasodilation and, hence, reduces both preload and afterload. This drug has a substantial positive effect on CO in the absence of changes in heart rate and blood pressure (Klein et al, 1981; LeJemtel et al, 1979) and is associated with decreased pulmonary arterial pressures and P_w (Benotti et al, 1978; Mancini et al, 1985). In contrast to catecholamine inotropic agents, decreases in myocardial O_2 consumption of the magnitude of 20 to 30% have been measured with amrinone (Baim et al, 1985; Benotti et al, 1980). In the setting of acute myocardial infarction complicated by cardiogenic shock, amrinone increased CO and decreased P_w and systemic vascular resistance (SVR) (Taylor et al, 1985; Verma et al, 1985). Because there appears to be little if any tachyphylaxis to amrinone, the beneficial hemodynamic effects may persist longer than those of the catecholamine pressors (Klein et al, 1981).

The use of dobutamine and amrinone together has been studied as well, but not in the setting of cardiogenic shock. The concomitant administration of these agents makes sense because cAMP levels are increased both by enhancing synthesis (catecholamines) and inhibiting breakdown (phosphodiesterase inhibitors). Indeed, a synergistic effect on CO and dP/dt and a decrease in P_w have been noted (Gage et al, 1986; Uretsky et al, 1987). Table 15–1 summarizes the characteristics of the commonly used vasopressors in shock.

The last class of drugs in the treatment of cardiogenic shock are the vasodilators, of which intravenous nitroglycerin and sodium nitroprusside are the most commonly used preparations. Nitroglycerin decreases venous return and pulmonary arterial occlusion pressure (P_w) as well as blood pressure. Sodium nitroprusside acts as a nitric oxide (NO) donor and leads to arterial vasodilation. This effect in turn decreases the impedance to left ventricular (LV) ejection and hence LV afterload. In the setting of LV failure both with and without acute myocardial infarction, this action of sodium nitroprusside increases both CO and stroke volume and leads to decreased P_w. Generally a vasodilator is contraindicated in the shock state because further drops in blood pressure may worsen peripheral organ function and may decrease coronary arterial perfusion. Nitroprusside has been used in severe cardiogenic shock, however, in combination with an intra-aortic balloon pump to maintain coronary blood flow (Chaterjee et al, 1976; Franciosa et al, 1972; Plamer and Lasseter, 1975). Ischemia-induced reductions in left ventricular diastolic compliance may improve with both nitroprusside and nitroglycerin, hence improving diastolic filling.

The future holds other possible treatments for some of the other known substances and mediators released in cardiogenic shock. These include atrial natriuretic peptide and antidiuretic hormone, both of which are elevated in cardiogenic shock. Other treatments aimed at the compensatory mechanisms mediated via the sympathetic nervous system or the renin-angiotensin-aldosterone system may also soon be on the forefront of therapy for cardiogenic shock.

SUPPORT OF THE CIRCULATION IN SEPTIC SHOCK—VASOPRESSORS AND ANTIMEDIATOR THERAPY

Septic shock generally occurs over hours to days and is due to effects of bacteria, fungi, viruses, or protozoa, and the various toxins these microorganisms produce. Septic shock also results from various inflammatory mediators released by host cells in response to infection, such as tumor necrosis factor (TNF), interleukin-1 (IL-1), or eicosanoids to name a few (see Chapter 1). The reduction in blood pressure in septic shock is primarily due to a reduction in arterial vascular resistance.

Table 15–1
Characteristics of Vasopressors for Shock

Pressor	Dose	Beta$_1$ Effect	Alpha Effect	Dopamine Effect	Beta$_2$ Effect
Dopamine	1–3 µg/kg/min	None	None	Yes + + +	Yes + +
Dopamine	5–10 µg/kg/min	Yes + +	Yes +	None	Yes + +
Dopamine	10–20 µg/kg/min	Yes + +/+ + +	Yes + + +	None	None
Norepinephrine	2–8 µg/kg/min	Yes + +/+ + +	Yes + + + +	None	None
Phenylephrine	20–200 µg/min	None	Yes + + + +	None	None
Epinephrine	1–8 µg/min	Yes + + + +	Yes + + + +	None	Yes + +

Thus, hypotension is accompanied by low cardiac filling pressures, high CO (see earlier and Chapter 19), and decreased systemic vascular resistance. Myocardial function is often depressed in septic shock, which is an occurrence that complicates the hemodynamic findings. Although left ventricular dilation is often observed with septic shock, in a small number of septic patients the left ventricle fails to dilate. In these patients, the Starling mechanism is unavailable to compensate for depressed myocardial function, and severe reductions in CO can occur (Parker et al, 1984, 1989).

Numerous pharmacologic approaches to septic shock exist, with each interaction aimed at a different pathophysiologic event and each with a different goal for treatment. Furthermore, therapy must be directed against the underlying pathologic process (i.e., the infection) (Kreger et al, 1980). For example, in a canine model of septic shock, dogs receiving both antibiotics and vasopressor agents had a much higher survival rate (43%) than those receiving either therapy alone (13%) or no therapy at all (0%) (Natanson et al, 1988).

Fluid resuscitation for septic shock is addressed earlier. Dopamine is often given as the initial vasopressor of choice in septic shock unresponsive to fluid challenge. The vasoconstrictive properties of dopamine may decrease perfusion and lead to ischemia of end organs in septic shock, however, as has been demonstrated for hemorrhagic shock (Segfal et al, 1992). Ruokonen and coworkers (1993) suggested that patients with septic shock receiving dopamine may have an increased splanchnic O_2 requirement. This, coupled with increased arteriovenous shunting, which may reduce capillary blood flow, may account for hastening of gut ischemia with dopamine.

Norepinephrine has been re-evaluated as initial therapy in septic shock.

Earlier, it was feared that norepinephrine would induce vasoconstriction and alter end organ, especially renal blood flow. In septic patients who had not responded to volume resuscitation, antibiotics and dopamine, however, Desjars and coworkers (1987) demonstrated increased blood pressure and systemic vascular resistance and maintenance of urine flow with norepinephrine. The favorable effect of norepinephrine on renal function was demonstrated again in later studies (Desjars, 1989; Martin et al, 1990). Hence, norepinephrine did not worsen renal ischemia in patients with septic shock and may even be beneficial. In another study (Meadows et al, 1988), patients with septic shock were fluid resuscitated and then given dopamine or dobutamine or a combination of those two agents. If hypotension

remained unresponsive, the addition of norepinephrine led to increases in mean arterial pressure and systemic vascular resistance.

In a prospective and randomized trial, Martin and coworkers (1993) compared dopamine and norepinephrine for the treatment of septic shock. Only 31% of the patients in the dopamine treatment group compared with 93% of the norepinephrine group reached the defined hemodynamic endpoints. In addition, 10 of 11 patients who did not reach the end points with dopamine did achieve treatment goals when norepinephrine was added to the treatment regimen. Marik and Mohedin (1994) compared the effects of dopamine and norepinephrine on systemic and splanchnic O_2 utilization in patients with septic shock. Gastric tonometry was used to assess endorgan (splanchnic) function. Although hemodynamic responses were similar in the two groups, only the norepinephrine-treated group demonstrated increased gastric intramucosal pH compared with the dopamine group, implying that norepinephrine may improve splanchnic tissue oxygenation in septic shock or that dopamine may worsen that process. Thus, the weight of available evidence suggests that norepinephrine has to be given at least equal consideration as the primary pressor of choice for the treatment of hypotension and hypoperfusion in septic shock. Other vasopressors including phenylephrine and epinephrine are also being re-examined for use in the treatment of septic shock, reflecting the ongoing controversy that continues to exist in this area.

Most of the work in the pharmacologic approach to treating septic shock involves antimediator therapy. Table 15–2 summarizes some examples of antimediator therapy in septic shock. The spectrum of agents has been wide and quite varied. Initial studies were performed to evaluate the therapeutic efficacy of antibodies to endotoxin. In one study, a polyclonal antibody against *Escherichia coli* J5 was studied in gram-negative septic shock. Mortality rates were identical in the control and treatment groups (50% and 49%, respectively) (Calandra et al, 1988).

Assuming that a highly specific antibody would be more effective, the therapeutic efficacy of monoclonal preparations was evaluated. These monoclonal antibodies were directed against the lipid A portion of endotoxin. The first such monoclonal antibody was E5. The first clinical trial in patients with gram-negative sepsis showed that only patients who did not have shock demonstrated improved mortality and resolution of organ dysfunction (Greenman et al, 1991). A second E5 trial was subsequently performed in

Table 15–2
Some Examples of Mediator Therapy for Shock

Antiendotoxin Therapy	Anticytokine Therapy	Nitric Oxide	Antilipid Therapy	Antiadhesion Molecule Therapy
MAb HA-1A	MAbs to TNF	Nitric oxide synthase inhibitors L-NMMA	PAF antagonists BN 502021	MAb (1B4) to CD18
MAb to E5	IL-1 receptor antagonists		Leukotriene antagonists	MAb to IL-8
MAb to CD14	MAb to IL-6		Cyclooxygenase inhibitors	MAb to ELAM
LPS antagonists (Lipid 406, Lipid X)	MAb to IFN-gamma Corticosteroids		Lipoxygenase inhibitors Thromboxane A_2 inhibitors	MAb to P/E selectin
	Soluble TNF receptors		Thromboxane synthetase inhibitors —ketoconazole	

patients who did not have refractory shock. No improvement in mortality over 30 days was seen in the treatment group when compared with results in the control group. The lack of benefit on survival was independent of the presence of organ failure in addition to the gram-negative sepsis (Bone et al, 1995).

The second monoclonal antibody to endotoxin to be evaluated was HA-1A. In patients with gram-negative septic shock, no difference in mortality was found (33% treatment versus 32% control). In fact, those patients with gram-positive sepsis had a higher mortality rate, and this drug was withdrawn from the market (McCloskey et al, 1994).

A considerable amount of work has been done investigating anticytokine therapy in the treatment of septic shock. Strategies aimed at interleukin-1 receptors and TNF have been the most extensively studied. One promising agent, currently in phase-3 clinical trials, is monoclonal murine IgG anti-TNF antibody. In one randomized, double-blind, multicenter trial of anti-TNF antibodies, there was no overall mortality benefit. Although there was a trend toward improved survival in the patients with severe septic shock 3 days following onset of therapy, the difference was not maintained at 28 days (Abraham et al, 1995; Exley et al, 1990; Fisher et al, 1993b). Interleukin-1 is another cytokine known to be involved in the pathophysiology of septic shock. Early phase-3 trial data suggest a dose-related reduction in both morbidity and mortality in patients treated with human recombinant interleukin-1 receptor antagonists with sepsis (Fisher et al, 1993a, 1994).

Nitric oxide (NO) plays a central role in the endothelial regulation of vascular tone as well as several other physiological processes. Additionally, NO is thought to be a major cause of hypotension in septic shock (Moncada and Higgs, 1993). Normally, NO is formed in endothelial cells from L-arginine by a calcium-dependent constitutive NO synthase (cNOS). From there it diffuses to nearby smooth muscle cells and stimulates the formation of cyclic guanosine monophosphate, which then leads to smooth muscle relaxation. Following the introduction of endotoxin and certain cytokines, a calcium-independent isoform of NO synthase (iNOS) is induced in endothelium and smooth muscle cells, which accelerates the process of vascular dilation that is resistant to vasoconstrictor therapy. In septic shock, the increase in NO synthesis is related to the degree of hypotension, suggesting a causal relationship. In addition, excess NO synthesis appears to lead to decreased myocardial contractility (Stamler et al, 1993), which is another complication of septic shock. Thus, it appears logical to treat the hypotension of septic shock with NOS inhibitors.

In animal models of sepsis (Cobb et al, 1992; Kilbourn et al, 1990, 1995; Klabude and Ritger, 1991; Lorente et al, 1993) and in human septic shock (Lin et al, 1994; Petros et al, 1991, 1995), administration of NOS inhibitors leads to an increase in arterial blood pressure. This is usually associated with a decrease in CO and often evidence of myocardial dysfunction (Lorente et al, 1993). Increased mortality in animal models is reported as well (Cobb et al, 1992). Hypotension in association with decreased CO following the initial vasoconstrictive effect of NOS is reported by some investigators in animal models (Nava et al, 1991; Wright et al, 1992).

One putative mechanism for decreased CO and worsening myocardial contractility is coronary vasoconstriction caused by NOS. Cohen and coworkers (1996) compared the effects of the NOS inhibitor N^G-nitro-L-arginine (L-NAME) with fluid resuscitation in a canine model of endotoxin infusion. They specifically evaluated the myocardial effects of these two modes of therapy. They found that arterial pressure could be raised by the same extent with L-NAME as with fluid therapy. With fluids, CO, coronary blood flow, and myocardial O_2 consumption were increased. With L-NAME, CO was unchanged or decreased relative to control. There was no evidence of myocardial ischemia or of any adverse effects on myocardial function with L-NAME. Although NOS inhibition did not cause coronary vasoconstriction in this animal model, much work remains to be done to evaluate the effects of NOS inhibition on peripheral organ function before the place of this form of therapy in septic shock can be defined. One variant to this approach is the use of specific inhibitors of iNOS, which is induced with sepsis. The use of this specific inhibitor may act to preserve "background" NO production by allowing continuing action of cNOS, but may block excessive vasodilation with sepsis owing to enhanced iNOS activity.

Therapy directed against other mediators of the sepsis syndrome have been and are being evaluated (Lee et al, 1989). To date, results of therapy directed against specific inflammatory mediators of the sepsis syndrome have been disappointing. Such therapy has not substantially improved mortality in septic patients. It may be that the demonstration of dramatic effects may await the results of newer, more specific agents; larger trials; or the definition of the subgroups of patients that can expect benefit. As reviewed in Chapter 1, the complexity of the inflammatory pathway may preclude significant benefit from therapy directed at only one of many components.

SUPPORT OF THE FAILING CIRCULATION WITH ACUTE COR PULMONALE

McGinn and White (1935) used the term *acute cor pulmonale* to describe right heart strain resulting from acute pulmonary hypertension. Although massive pulmonary embolism is the best-known cause of acute cor pulmonale, the same syndrome can be the result of any clinical entity acutely and severely increasing pulmonary vascular resistance. This includes sepsis and ventilation with high airway pressures in the presence of adult respiratory distress syndrome.

The right ventricle is often said to be a "volume pump," whereas the left ventricle is said to be a "pressure pump." This implies something different about the properties of the two ventricles. Right and left ventricular contraction are remarkably similar. When normalized for peak pressure, the time course of right and left ventricular isovolumic pressure development are virtually superimposable. Indeed, the determinants of right ventricular function are the same as those of left ventricular function, namely, preload, afterload, and contractility (see Chapter 7). The stress over the right ventricle during contraction represents the afterload.

Just as for the left, right ventricular contraction can be viewed as a series of time-varying elastances, a concept that had been developed for the left ventricle. For the right, as for the left ventricle, the instantaneous pressure-volume relationship may be expressed as

$$P_t = E_t (V_t - V_0)$$

where P_t is the pressure at any given time in the cardiac cycle, E_t is the slope of the pressure-volume curve at time t, V_t is ventricular volume at time t, and V_0 is the volume intercept of the regression line. E_t, the maximal systolic elastance, is a measure of ventricular contractility, which is relatively independent of pre or afterload.

These concepts, developed and validated for the left ventricle both in isolated load clamped heart preparations and in *in situ* preparations, generally also apply to the right ventricle with some slight modifications. First, pulmonary arterial pressure only represents part of the hydraulic load placed on the right ventricle (afterload) during contraction. A substantial part of the total hydraulic load is represented by the elastance of the pulmonary arterial circulation. The total hydraulic load placed on the right ventricle is more properly represented by the input impedance of the pulmonary circulation (Murgo et al, 1984). Second, end-systole is more difficult to define for the right than for the left ventricle because the left ventricle end-ejection and end-contraction correspond fairly well. For the right ventricle, there is a bit of slip in that the ventricle continues to eject for a short time after end-contraction. Furthermore, there are slight differences in end-systolic volume, depending on whether contraction is isovolumic or isotonic (Maughan, 1989). Practically speaking, however, these quantitative differences do not negate the concept of the end-systolic pressure-volume curve being an important measure of ventricular contractile function.

RIGHT VENTRICULAR RESPONSE TO ACUTELY INCREASED AFTERLOAD—THE PHYSIOLOGY OF ACUTE COR PULMONALE

Investigators have assessed the ability of the right ventricle to tolerate increased afterload by graded occlusions of the pulmonary artery or injection of glass beads or other small particles into the distal pulmonary bed (reviewed in Scharf et al, 1986). These two models are not strictly comparable because the hydraulic load produced by main pulmonary arterial constriction is greater than that produced by microvascular embolization (Calvin et al, 1985). The principles governing load tolerance are the same. Numerous studies have confirmed that a previously normal right ventricle (RV) can tolerate an acute rise in systolic pressure produced by a rise in afterload of up to approximately 55 to 60 mm Hg (mean pressure 40 mm Hg) without producing circulatory failure (reviewed in Scharf et al, 1986). Small increases in pulmonary arterial pressure beyond this point lead to circulatory collapse even if there is no further change in pulmonary arterial diameter (Ghignone et al, 1984). Conversely, if systemic arterial pressure is increased by occlusion of the descending aorta or infusion of pressors, the degree to which right ventricular systolic pressure can be increased without producing circulatory collapse is greater (Cooper et al, 1975; Ghignone et al, 1984; Scharf et al, 1986). This finding illustrates the interaction between systemic and pulmonary factors in determining the response of the RV to increased afterload.

The mechanisms of right ventricular failure with acute increases in afterload remain controversial (Weidman et al, 1989). The right coronary artery, which supplies the right ventricular free wall, originates in the aorta. Because the perfusion pressure gradient for right coronary arterial flow is the difference between aortic and right ventricular diastolic pressure, decreased aortic pressure reduces the gradient for right ventricular coronary flow. Brooks and coworkers (1971) first demonstrated that right coronary occlusion reduced right ventricular load tolerance. Other studies have addressed the issue of right coronary flow during progressive pulmonary hypertension. Manohar and coworkers (1981) demonstrated increased right coronary blood flow during progressive pulmonary arterial occlusion in spite of the fact that there was a decrease in the driving pressure for

flow (i.e., there was right coronary autoregulation). Of course, increasing right ventricular end-diastolic pressure with greater afterload further reduces the gradient for coronary perfusion. A number of investigators (Gold and Bache, 1982; Manohar et al, 1981; Reller et al, 1992) have demonstrated that with infusion of a vasodilator there is an increase in right coronary flow during progressive pulmonary arterial occlusion. This revealed that coronary flow was not at the limits of its vasodilator reserve when right ventricular failure occurred. In contrast, coronary flow failed to increase proportionally to right ventricular myocardial O_2 demand as measured by tension-time index (Scharf et al, 1986) or rate-pressure product (Reller et al, 1992), suggesting that coronary flow inadequately compensates for increased O_2 demand. Some studies have demonstrated the appearance of biochemical markers of ischemia with pulmonary arterial occlusion (Gold and Bache, 1982; Vlahakes et al, 1981).

Scharf and coworkers (1986) failed to find a decrease in intramyocardial pH with pulmonary arterial occlusion leading to circulatory collapse, suggesting that ischemia is not a necessary condition for right ventricular failure with increased afterload.

Whatever the mechanism for deterioration of right ventricular function with progressive occlusion of the pulmonary artery, as aortic pressure falls with decreased CO, a point is reached where arterial pressure falls. This arterial pressure drop reduces the perfusion gradient for right coronary flow, which in turn may lead to a decrease in CO, further reducing arterial pressure and closing the vicious circle of right ventricular failure.

Diagnosis and specific therapy of acute right ventricular failure should be instituted as rapidly as feasible while supportive measures are being instituted (ACCP Consensus Statement on Pulmonary Embolism, 1996). This approach includes the use of thrombolytic therapy (Urokinase Pulmonary Embolism Trial, 1973; Urokinase-Streptokinase Pulmonary Embolism Trial, 1974). Percutaneous transvenous embolectomy may be a consideration in the subgroup of patients who have a contraindication to thrombolysis (Greenfield and Langham, 1984; Timsit et al, 1991). The issues discussed earlier have direct clinical relevance in the assessment and treatment of acute right ventricular failure. First, the presence of sustained right ventricular systolic pressures greater than 55 to 60 mm Hg means that pulmonary hypertension cannot have been acute because the normal RV cannot sustain systolic pressures greater than this level. Second, whether ischemia is involved or not, one should view right ventricular failure in the light of the balance between myocardial O_2 supply and demand. At the point of the highest tolerable right ventricular afterload, the administration of agents that increase cardiac contractility may be ineffective or even dangerous because they increase myocardial O_2 demand (Molloy et al, 1984).

We favor volume infusion in patients who are dehydrated and/or in whom central venous pressure is reduced. Massive volume infusion when right ventricular afterload is severely elevated may actually worsen failure and produce circulatory decompensation (Ghignone et al, 1984).

Support measures should be directed toward maintaining aortic pressure and hence coronary flow. Vasoconstrictor agents, such as Neo-Synephrine or norepinephrine, are probably preferable to agents that increase myocardial contractility and heart rate while producing arterial vasodilation, such as isoproterenol or dobutamine (Ghignone et al, 1984; Molloy et al, 1984; Prewitt and Ghignone, 1983). Although there are few clinical data in humans evaluating specific pressors in the treatment of massive pulmonary embolism, there is at least one report (Bourlain et al, 1993) of epinephrine being useful in patients with shock complicating a massive pulmonary embolism that was resistant to treatment with volume, dobutamine, norepinephrine, and thrombolysis. The investigators suggested that epinephrine is a more effective β_1 agonist than dobutamine with much less β_2 activity and comparable α-vasoconstrictive effects to norepinephrine.

The mechanism by which increasing aortic pressure leads to improved right ventricular function is not clear. Although it may be thought that increased perfusion pressure could lead to increased right coronary flow, this has not been shown to be the case (Scharf et al, 1986). In fact, the important principle for preserving CO seems to be increased aortic pressure *per se*, whether by pharmacologic (Ghignone et al, 1984; Molloy et al, 1984) or physical means (Scharf et al, 1986; Spotnitz et al, 1971). Although it is possible that increased aortic pressure allows for improved perfusion of the endocardial layers of the myocardium, the absence of an increase in coronary flow with increased aortic pressure may mean that another mechanism must be sought.

The ventricles exhibit two major types of mechanical interaction, which are sometimes called serial and parallel. Serial interactions are those that are related to the effects of right-on-left ventricular output. If right ventricular output drops, left ventricular output must of necessity drop as well. Parallel interactions refer to those interactions arising from the fact that the two ventricles are actually part of one structure; they contain common muscle bands, are located within the same pericardial sac, and, most important, share a common septum. Parallel diastolic interactions have been discussed in Chapter 4. Briefly, increased end-diastolic volume in one ventricle leads to a decrease in the filling of the other. During systole, the contraction of one ventricle actually aids the contraction of the other. These systolic interactions are extremely important for the right ventricle. It has been demonstrated (Farrar et al, 1993; Little et al, 1984; Maughan and Oikawa, 1987; Yamaguchi et al, 1993) that up to one third of the developed right ventricular systolic pressure actually results from left ventricular contraction. Scharf (1994) analyzed the relative gain in systolic right ventricular pressure produced from increasing aortic pressure during progressive occlusion of the pulmonary artery. He concluded that the known systolic interactions between left and right ventricles could have accounted for the earlier findings that raising aortic pressure increases right ventricular load tolerance. Thus, the reported beneficial effect of increasing aortic pressure on right ventricular function with severely elevated afterload may have been due to systolic mechanical interactions between the ventricles and may have been unrelated to changes in coronary flow.

RESPIRATORY SUPPORT OF THE FAILING HEART

In Chapter 5, the effects of changes in intrathoracic pressure on cardiac function are reviewed. In particular, the increase in impedance to LV ejection observed with decreased intrathoracic pressure was emphasized. Of course, the converse is true, namely that increasing intrathoracic pressure may aid the function of the failing LV. This observation may work in two ways. First, changes in intrathoracic pressure may be transmitted to the thoracic aorta (McIntyre and Scharf, 1989; Scharf et al, 1980). Increasing intrathoracic pressure raises intra-aortic pressure relative the rest of the arterial system, which in turn leads to the efflux of blood from the thorax. Such a response is especially important in young individuals in whom the aorta is relatively compliant (Lichtenstein et al, 1985). Of course, this efflux occurs in the great veins of the chest and the right atrium as well as in the arterial system, a change that hinders venous return into the chest. If intrathoracic pressure falls periodically, blood moves back into the chest via the veins but, because of the presence of the aortic valve, hardly at all via the arteries. Thus, with periodic increases in intrathoracic pressure, there is net movement of blood from the venous to the arterial system. This notion has been called the *thoracic pump* and is one of the mechanisms by which "cardiac" massage aids in supporting the circulation (Hausknecht et al, 1984; Rudikoff et al, 1980).

A good illustration of the role of the thoracic pump is the finding that repetitive cough can sustain the circulation in patients who have undergone sudden ventricular fibrillation, obviating the need for cardiac massage until definitive therapy (cardioversion) can be instituted (Criley et al, 1976). If increases in intrathoracic pressure were timed by gating to ventricular diastole, theoretically blood flows from the aorta into the extrathoracic arterial system during this phase of the cardiac cycle. At the next ventricular systole, the LV therefore ejects into a relatively empty aorta, and ejection is augmented. This may be the mechanism by which increases in intrathoracic pressure timed to diastole lead to increased stroke volume in the failing heart (Fessler et al, 1988; Lichtenstein et al, 1985; Pinsky et al, 1986). In contrast, with aortic emptying, aortic input impedance increases. This change increases LV afterload and may limit the rise in stroke volume observed with diastolic phasic elevations in intrathoracic pressure. Current work emphasizing the role of *systolic* phased increases in intrathoracic pressure is considered later.

EFFECTS OF INCREASED CARDIAC SURFACE PRESSURE ON CORONARY BLOOD FLOW

When cardiac surface pressure increases relative to aortic pressure, the effect is to decrease the gradient for perfusion of these vessels. This occurs if increased cardiac surface pressure raises the critical closing pressure of the surface vessels or if transmitted changes in right atrial pressure raise the back pressure to coronary perfusion. Indeed, Fessler and coworkers (1990) demonstrated decreased coronary perfusion in an isolated heart preparation in which cardiac surface pressure was increased relative to aortic pressure. They could demonstrate the onset of ischemia and worsening of cardiac function when the perfusion pressure gradient became low enough. However, these adverse effects were seen only when cardiac surface pressure increased to 60 mm Hg or more. At lower levels of cardiac surface pressure, improved left ventricular function consistent with the afterload-reducing effects of increased intrathoracic pressure were observed.

A number of workers have studied the effects of mechanical ventilation and increased positive end-expiratory pressure (PEEP) on coronary blood flow and left ventricular function in animals and in patients with heart disease. At least two animal studies (Tucker and Murray, 1973; Venus and Jacobs, 1984) demonstrated that with positive end-expiratory pressure (PEEP) coronary blood flow falls out of proportion to decreases in cardiac work. These studies suggest caution regarding the use of increased cardiac surface pressure to support the circulation in patients with active ischemic heart disease.

In humans following coronary bypass graft, Tittley and coworkers (1985) demonstrated decreased lactate utilization in 17 of 33 patients at 15 cm H_2O PEEP. They concluded that "ischemic metabolism" was observed in many patients on PEEP with limited coronary flow reserve. On the other hand, in animal studies, when cardiac surface pressure was increased only during cardiac systole, coronary flow changes were proportional to decreased cardiac work (Hassapoyannes et al, 1991). This observation may indicate that gating-increased intrathoracic pressure to systole minimizes the ischemia-producing potential. However, the authors caution that because aortic diastolic pressure decreased, a limit may exist to the benefit of this procedure.

We have reviewed coronary flow effects at this point because the variable effects of increasing intrathoracic pressure reported in the literature may be because these effects often are not accounted for in the interpretation of the data. Other reasons for varying interpretations of the data are that experimental conditions vary widely from deeply anesthetized animals to unanesthetized sedated or unsedated humans in clinical situations. The effects of anesthetics on sympathoadrenal and other reflex homeostatic mechanisms need to be remembered when trying to generalize between studies. Furthermore, the presence or absence of paralysis means that the effects of a given maneuver on intrathoracic pressure are far from constant.

EFFECTS OF CONTINUOUS POSITIVE AIRWAY PRESSURE (CPAP) IN CONGESTIVE HEART FAILURE

CPAP ventilatory support refers to the application of pressure to the airway of the spontaneously breathing patient throughout all phases of respiration. This mode of support is old and has been used since at least the beginning of the century (Bunnel, 1912). Poulton and Oxon (1936) reported a CPAP device made from spare vacuum cleaner parts to treat various forms of respiratory distress including congestive heart failure. Subsequently, CPAP has become an acceptable mode of treatment of cardiogenic and noncardiogenic pulmonary edema (Duncan et al, 1986; Gregory et al, 1971; Perel et al, 1983; Pery et al, 1991; Räsänen et al, 1985a; Venus et al, 1979). It is well documented that in these conditions, CPAP leads to increased arterial PO_2, decreased work of breathing (Naughton et al, 1995c; Pery et al, 1991; Räsänen et al, 1985b), and small increases in arterial PCO_2 (Perel et al, 1983). The concept that CPAP can actually improve the function of the failing heart beyond improving gas exchange and ventilatory mechanics is far more controversial.

CPAP can raise intrathoracic pressure because of increased lung volumes. The amount by which intrathoracic pressure increases depends on pulmonary and chest wall compliance, which are in turn influenced by the clinical disease and activation of the muscles of expiration. As thoroughly reviewed in Chapters 4 and 5, this increase in intrathoracic pressure should act to decrease venous return. Thus, any effects of CPAP on cardiac function should be understood in the context of the tendency for venous return to decrease.

CPAP is the most common treatment for the obstructive sleep apnea syndrome. Clinical observations in patients on CPAP for sleep apnea who also have congestive heart failure have suggested improved left ventricular function (Malone et al, 1991). Patients with stable congestive heart failure and nocturnal Cheyne-Stokes respiration who receive nocturnal CPAP have been shown to demonstrate improvement in New York State Heart cardiac functional class and increased left ventricular ejection fraction compared with controls (Naughton et al, 1995b). These studies suggest long-term improvement with nocturnal CPAP in daytime cardiac function comparable to that reported in many vasodilator trials. In a follow-up study, Naughton and coworkers (1995a) demonstrated that long-term CPAP therapy in patients with congestive heart failure was associated with decreased baseline sympathetic nerve activity. This outcome may reflect improved CO, decreased sleep fragmentation, or improved nocturnal oxygenation. Sympathoadrenal withdrawal may, by lessening the vasoconstriction associated with heart failure, lead to unloading of the left ventricle, thereby improving functional and clinical status. In contrast, two uncontrolled, small, patient trials failed to demonstrate significant daytime improvement in indices of left ventricular function with nocturnal CPAP (Buckle et al, 1992; Davies et al, 1993). The Davies study actually demonstrated deterioration in three patients.

Although the reason for the difference in conclusions is not clear, differences in baseline cardiac function and autonomic function may be responsible. This uncertainty argues for large-scale standardized trials of nocturnal CPAP in the treatment of congestive heart failure.

The question of the acute effects of CPAP on cardiac, specifically left ventricular, function has been investigated as well. In 22 stable patients with dilated cardiomyopathy, Bradley and coworkers (1992) reported increased CO following the application of 5 cm H_2O CPAP. Improvement was observed only when the baseline pulmonary occlusion ("wedge") pressure was 12 mm Hg or higher. In patients in whom the baseline pulmonary occlusion pressure was less than 12 mm Hg, CO decreased. Others (Baratz et al, 1992; Pery et al, 1991; Räsänen et al, 1985a) have also demonstrated improved CO in at least some patients with acute congestive heart failure. Although not systematically studied, the impression seems to be that patients with the poorest baseline left ventricular function improve the most. Nevertheless, a large-scale systematic trial of CPAP for treating congestive heart failure in critical care situations is clearly needed.

One of the problems with studying the effects of CPAP in clinical situations is the difficulty in controlling for potentially confounding variables such as medication use, other clinical conditions, and other therapy. Animal studies have been performed to try to elucidate the conditions under which CO improves with CPAP, as well as the mechanisms that account for this improvement demonstrated in CO with CPAP. Genovese and coworkers (1994) studied the effects of CPAP up to 20 cm H_2O on sedated pigs that had been previously instrumented for measurements of aortic flow, left ventricular pressure, and left ventricular volume. Under normal conditions, increasing CPAP was associated with decreased CO, decreased left ventricular preload, and no change in contractility or ejection fraction. When the animals were made hypervolemic by massive transfusion of hetastarch, baseline left ventricular end-diastolic pressure was increased to 0.25 mm Hg and CO increased at CPAP 5 cm H_2O compared with baseline. It then decreased to a value not different than baseline by CPAP 20 cm H_2O. The increase in CO observed at the lowest level of CPAP was associated with greater left ventricular ejection fraction and decreased left ventricular end-systolic volume with no change in end-diastolic volume. No changes in contractility or heart rate were noted. The differences between normo- and hypervolemic animals were understood in terms of the different effects on venous return and cardiac function. In normovolemic animals, effects on cardiac function are less important than effects on venous return. In hypervolemic animals in which venous return reserve is high, positive effects of CPAP on cardiac function lead to increased CO, especially at the lowest levels of CPAP when venous return effects are minimal.

The same group studied the effects of CPAP in pigs in which congestive heart failure had been induced by 7 to 10 days of rapid LV pacing (Genovese et al, 1995). A similar increase in CO was seen at the lowest level of CPAP, although to a greater degree than had been observed in the normal hearts. Although CO decreased by CPAP of 15 cm H_2O, it remained above baseline. The most intriguing aspect of the study was that following removal of CPAP, there was a secondary rise in CO that lasted for 20 to 60 minutes. These points are summarized in Figure 15–5, which illustrates the effects of CPAP in pigs with normal

hearts and in pigs with congestive heart failure. Note that even when baseline CO was elevated (hypervolemia) there was a further increase in CO with low-level CPAP. The secondary increase in CO following removal of CPAP in congestive heart failure is illustrated as well.

These observations suggest that CPAP-induced increases in CO do not depend on baseline CO or left ventricular function, but rather on left ventricular dilation. They also suggest that although there may be a common mechanism at work, probably additional mechanisms are at work for congestive heart failure. This observation is also illustrated by the finding that in congestive heart failure there is an increase in left ventricular dP/dt, suggesting greater contractility (Genovese et al, 1995).

Congestive heart failure is known to be associated with an increase in sympathoadrenal tone and alterations in autonomic function (Bristow et al, 1982; Cohn et al, 1984; Daly and Sole, 1990; Swedberg et al, 1990). Thus, CPAP can be associated with altered sympathoadrenal reflexes, which would contribute to increases in CO. Either increased myocardial inotropy or decreased arterial sympathetic tone and vasodilation as postulated by Naughton and coworkers (1995c) may therefore be responsible. These changes could persist beyond the removal of CPAP, which leads to the secondary persistent increase in CPAP observed. That stimulation of the myocardium plays a role in the CPAP and post-CPAP increases in CO in congestive heart failure is suggested by the observations that left ventricular dP/dt rises when measured with CPAP use and in the post-CPAP period, after the pressure has been removed (Genovese et al, 1995). The heart rate rises post-CPAP as well. These reflexes probably play a contributory but not a primary role, because CO increases in the hypervolemic animals.

To assess the role of sympathoadrenal stimulation in the CPAP-induced increases in CO, our group measured plasma norepinephrine levels in the experiments shown in Figure 15–5. Plasma norepinephrine was used as an index of overall sympathetic nerve activity (Cohn et al, 1984) and does not reflect regional changes. Figure 15–6 shows the results of these studies (Scharf et al, 1996). Note that baseline plasma norepinephrine levels were increased in the hypervolemic normals and the congestive heart failure animals. In spite of similar increases in CO with low-level CPAP (see Fig. 15–5), plasma norepinephrine changed in opposite directions with hypervolemia and congestive heart failure. Thus, these data suggest that the role of overall sympathoadrenal stimulation in CPAP-associated increases in CO is at best

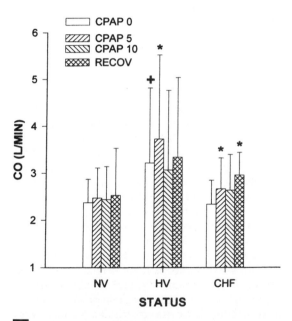

Figure 15–5
Effects of CPAP to 10 cm H_2O on cardiac output (CO) in normal pigs under normovolemic (pulmonary occlusion pressure ≈8 mm Hg) and hypervolemic (pulmonary occlusion pressure ≈18 mm Hg), and in pigs in which cardiomyopathy had been induced by 7 days of rapid ventricular pacing. NV = normovolemia, HV = hypervolemia, CHF = congestive heart failure. For difference from baseline* = $p < 0.05$ (oneway ANOVA). (From Scharf SM, Chen L, Slamowitz D, Rao PS: Effects of continuous positive airway pressure on cardiac output and plasma norepinephrine in sedated pigs. J Crit Care 11:57–64, 1996. With permission.)

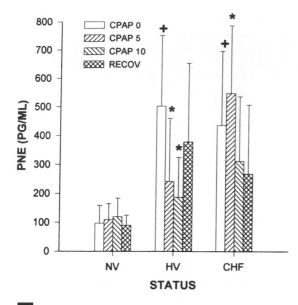

Figure 15–6
Effect of CPAP on plasma norepinephrine levels (PNE) in the studies illustrated in Figure 15–1. Note the different responses to CPAP in the hypervolemic normals and the congestive heart failure animals. (See the legend in Figure 15–1.) (From Scharf SM, Chen L, Slamowitz D, Rao PS: Effects of continuous positive airway pressure on cardiac output and plasma norepinephrine in sedated pigs. J Crit Care 11:57–64, 1996. With permission.)

secondary. Furthermore, there was no suggestion that the post-CPAP increase in CO in congestive heart failure was due to greater overall sympathetic nerve tone. Either there were changes in regional sympathetic tone to the heart (Daly and Sole, 1990) or the fact that there had been some improvement in cardiac function associated with decreased left ventricular volumes (Genovese et al, 1995) led to persistent increases in CO once the inhibiting effects of CPAP on venous return were removed. Thus, CPAP administration in congestive heart failure may be somewhat analogous to intermittent therapy with inotropic infusions, which lead to persistently improved cardiac function when therapy is withdrawn (Gibelin et al, 1990).

Because changes in sympathoadrenal tone do not appear to explain the increase in CO seen with CPAP in normal hypervolemic and myopathic animals, explanations based on mechanics have been proposed. One explanation is based on the principle that increasing intrathoracic pressure can act to unload the left ventricle (see Chapter 5 for a complete review of the effects of intrathoracic pressure on LV function). If cardiac

surface pressure increased relative to left ventricular end-systolic pressure, end-systolic transmural pressure, which is a measure of systolic wall stress, would decrease and CO could increase.

Huberfeld and coworkers (1995) measured left ventricular surface pressure and esophageal pressure and calculated left ventricular transmural pressures in normal and hypervolemic pigs. They found that, as expected, in normovolemic animals left ventricular surface pressure increased and left ventricular end-systolic transmural pressure tended to decrease at the higher levels of CPAP. In hypervolemic animals, although esophageal pressure increased, left ventricular surface pressure actually *decreased* with increasing CPAP, and there were no changes in end-systolic transmural pressure. Although it may seem surprising that increasing intrathoracic (esophageal) pressure may occur at the same time that cardiac surface pressure decreases, a similar effect on cardiac surface pressure has been observed when PEEP is applied during cardiac congestion (Cabrera et al, 1989). This finding was explained by assuming that left ventricular surface pressure was equal to the arithmetic sum of pericardial fossa (= intrathoracic) pressure and pericardial elastic recoil pressure:

$$P_{LVS} = P_{PR} + P_{PF}$$

where P_{LVS} is LV surface pressure, P_{PR} is pericardial elastic recoil pressure, and P_{PF} is pericardial fossa pressure. Furthermore, it was assumed that CPAP had some other salutary effect on left ventricular function leading to a decrease in end-diastolic and end-systolic volumes (see later). Under normovolemic conditions, when heart volume is relatively low, the pericardium is relatively relaxed. Reduction in cardiac volume causes relatively little decrease in pericardial elastic recoil pressure, which is more than offset by increased pericardial fossa pressure. Under hypervolemic conditions, pericardial constraint is increased. Because of increased heart volume, the pericardium is on the relatively stiff portion of its pressure-volume curve. Thus, decreases in cardiac volume with CPAP cause large decreases in pericardial elastic recoil pressure, which more than offsets the CPAP-associated increase in pericardial fossa pressure. Under these circumstances, LV surface pressure decreases.

Why does cardiac volume decrease with CPAP in hypervolemia and congestive heart failure? It cannot be due to a decrease in venous return *per se* because venous return (equal to CO in the steady state) increases at low level CPAP. One possible explanation is in general that when CO increases with CPAP there is associated vasodilation and systemic vascular resistance decreases

(Fig. 15–7). Possibly CPAP is associated with reflex vasodilation, either through withdrawal of sympathetic tone to resistance vessels (in spite of inconstant changes in overall sympathetic nerve activity) or activation of parasympathetic vasodilator mechanisms. In contrast, vasodilation may be secondary to increased CO possibly mediated via the baroreceptors. An alternative mechanism is that with increased intrathoracic pressure there is shift of volume out of intrathoracic reservoirs including the LV. The volume transferred from intra- to extrathoracic compartments is equal to

$$(\Delta P_{ITP})(C_{ET})$$

where ΔP_{ITP} is the change in intrathoracic pressure with CPAP and C_{ET} is the lumped compliance of the extrathoracic reservoirs (see Chapter 5). This change would lead to equal decreases in left ventricular end-diastolic and end-systolic transmural pressures. Under normovolemic conditions, when end-diastolic compliance is greater than end-systolic compliance, left ventricular end-diastolic volume decreases more than end-systolic volume and stroke volume decreases.

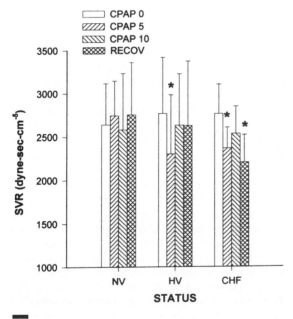

Figure 15–7
Effect of CPAP under the various conditions shown in Figures 15–1 and 15–2 on systemic vascular resistance (SVR). Note that under the conditions when cardiac output increases with CPAP (Figure 15–5), SVR decreases. (From Scharf SM, Chen L, Slamowitz D, Rao PS: Effects of continuous positive airway pressure on cardiac output and plasma norepinephrine in sedated pigs. J Crit Care 11:57–64, 1996. With permission.)

When the left ventricle is at the limits of its diastolic distension (hypervolemia, congestive heart failure), end-diastolic compliance is actually less than end-systolic compliance (Permutt and Wise, 1987). Under these circumstances, for equal reductions in transmural pressure, end-systolic volume decreases less than end-diastolic volume, and stroke volume increases. Thus, the application of CPAP may be analogous to the application of tourniquets or phlebotomy, in which stroke volume decreases in normals but may increase in patients with severe congestive heart failure (Howarth et al, 1946; McMichael and Sharpey-Schaefer, 1944).

To summarize, low-level CPAP can lead to clinical improvement in patients with congestive heart failure. This improvement may last beyond the time over which CPAP is actually applied. Although part of this effect is related to better respiratory function (greater gas exchange, decreased work of breathing), there are definitely patients in whom CO and left ventricular function are improved. This subset of patients is likely to be that group with the most compromised baseline cardiac function, probably those in whom the heart is close to the limits of diastolic distension. The mechanisms leading to improved CO are not unequivocally known, but left ventricular unloading by vasodilation, transfer of volume out of the thorax, and possibly sympathetic stimulation may be involved. Further investigation will improve patient selection and provide clearer clinical guidelines for the application of this form of therapy.

IMPROVING CO EJECTION BY USING THE MECHANICAL VENTILATOR

As noted earlier and reviewed thoroughly in Chapter 5, when intrathoracic pressure is increased relative to left ventricular end-systolic pressure, end-systolic transmural pressure decreases. This decreases effective afterload. Although normal hearts are relatively afterload-insensitive, in the case of failing hearts, a decrease in afterload can substantially aid ejection. Indeed, the mechanical ventilator, which increases intrathoracic pressure, can be utilized as a cardiac assist device.

In 1982, Grace and Greenbaum reported on the effects of mechanical ventilation with PEEP in patients with cardiac failure. They found that 3 to 5 cm H_2O PEEP raised CO by a mean of 500 ml/min in those patients with a pulmonary occlusion pressure 19 mm Hg or greater and either had no effect or decreased CO in those in whom the occlusion pressure was lower. Mathru and coworkers (1982) studied patients after cardiopulmonary bypass and compared controlled ventilation with intermittent mandatory ventilation (IMV) and IMV + 5 cm H_2O PEEP. In patients with severe congestive heart failure (LV end-diastolic pressure >16 mm Hg), institution of IMV led to decreased CO and increased pulmonary occlusion pressure. Adding PEEP to IMV reversed the trend and led to increased CO and decreased pulmonary occlusion pressure. These studies illustrate the principle that performing maneuvers that increase mean intrathoracic pressure can improve CO in patients with cardiac failure.

Pinsky and coworkers (1983) produced experimental cardiac failure in dogs by administering large doses of propranolol. They used large tidal volumes (30 ml/kg) and chest and abdominal binding to exaggerate inspiratory swings in intrathoracic pressure. They were able to demonstrate an upward shift in the Frank-Starling function curve compared with the baseline state. Pinsky and Summer (1983) reported using a similar system in mechanically ventilated patients with cardiogenic shock. They applied binders to the chest and abdomen sufficiently to increase esophageal pressure by 5 mm Hg during inspiration but not to change end-expiratory esophageal pressure. In five of seven patients CO increased. There was no correlation between baseline pulmonary occlusion pressure and the response to increased intrathoracic pressure. In an accompanying editorial Robotham (1983) coined the term *ventilatory assisted myocardial performance* or VAMP to describe the use of positive pressure ventilators to support the failing heart.

CARDIAC CYCLE–SPECIFIC INCREASES IN INTRATHORACIC PRESSURE

One problem with high tidal volume ventilation with chest wall binding is the effect of these maneuvers on venous return. If circulating blood volume is low (i.e., the patient is hypovolemic), as discussed earlier, the effects on venous return may outweigh those on cardiac function, and CO may fall. Furthermore, the effects on CO are always tempered by those on venous return when intrathoracic pressure is increased throughout all phases of the cardiac cycle.

Large tidal volume ventilation may also be problematic in the critical care unit for the point of view of gas exchange. Large tidal volumes may entail overventilation and severe respiratory alkalosis. The larger the tidal volume the greater the risk of barotrauma. To address the problem of the balance between the beneficial effects of increased intrathoracic pressure on cardiac function and its detrimental effects on venous return, the use of cardiac cycle–specific increases in intrathoracic pressure was instituted by Pinsky and colleagues. This approach attempts to limit the increases in intrathoracic pressure to that phase of the cardiac cycle when it would do the most good (i.e., during systole).

In an early study, Pinsky and coworkers studied (1985) phasic increases in intrathoracic pressure in anesthetized dogs with propranolol induced heart failure. Pressure pulses were produced by a jet ventilator and exaggerated by respiratory binding. They altered respiratory timing and duty cycle while maintaining constant mean intrathoracic pressure. With normal cardiac function, stroke volume decreased (venous return effects). However, when cardiac function was compromised (left ventricular filling pressure >17 mm Hg), stroke volume increased with the institution of the pressure pulses. Furthermore, the changes in intrathoracic pressure can account for all observable changes in steady-state hemodynamics, independent of the respiratory timing.

In a later study (Pinsky et al, 1986) the jet ventilator pulses were synchronized to early and late systole and diastole. The pulses timed to systole had the greatest positive effect on stroke volume in heart failure. In cardiac transplant candidates, Pinsky and coworkers (1987) showed that jet ventilation timed to occur with upstroke of arterial pressure produced significant increases in CO compared with baseline, whereas there were no changes when the jet was not synchronized to the cardiac cycle. These results suggest that data from the animal studies could be extrapolated to human diseases and that the key is timing of the jet pulse to occur in synchrony with left ventricular ejection.

Using a mathematical analysis, Beyer and coworkers (1989) predicted that maximal flow augmentation occurred when the onset of the increase in intrathoracic pressure is simultaneous with the onset of LV isovolumic contraction and has a duration of 400 msec. The magnitude of flow augmentation is a function of the amplitude of the rise in intrathoracic pressure. These predictions were borne out by experiments in anesthetized dogs in which pressure was increased by a rapidly inflating/deflating vest. They found that there was a little further flow augmentation when the rise in intrathoracic pressure was more than 30 to 40 mm Hg. Because this method can be applied easily and noninvasively, it has great potential for cardiac assist.

Stein and coworkers (1990) found that both systolic and diastolic timed jet pulses can lead to increased LV stroke volume, but that systolic increases were greater than diastolic. Thus, even if LV contractility is normal when mitral regurgitation impedes forward LV flow, increased intrathoracic pressure raises LV ejection.

Peters and Ihle (1992) evaluated the effects of single and repetitive increases in intrathoracic pressure produced by external vest inflation in anesthetized dogs under a variety of conditions. Although single inflations coupled to late systole led stroke volume augmentation, repetitive inflations coupled to all cardiac phases led to nonspecific flow augmentation. This effect was not seen following adrenergic blockade. Thus, the effects of cyclic increases in intrathoracic pressure were related to changes in sympathoadrenal tone rather than increases in intrathoracic pressure *per se*. As with CPAP, the role of sympathoadrenal tone in this form of cardiac assist required further elucidation. These workers suggested that previous results with jet ventilation were due to increases in lung volume and direct mechanical heart-lung interactions rather than increases in intrathoracic pressure *per se*. That is, direct compression of the heart with the jet ventilator gave the cardiac assist. One can only agree with these investigators who concluded that "there remain several unsolved issues with respect to assisting a failing heart by pleural pressure increments."

VENTILATORY ASSIST OF THE FAILING HEART—CONCLUSIONS

Numerous factors govern the cardiac and peripheral circulatory response to ventilatory maneuvers in patients with normal and failing hearts. Therefore, it should not be surprising that without carefully specifying conditions, different studies may appear to lead to different conclusions. Although the balance between venous return and improved cardiac function has been viewed as a key factor determining the effects of increased intrathoracic pressure on CO, other factors such as arterial compliance, autonomic tone, coronary blood flow, and coupling of central and peripheral circulatory components may play an important role. At least some patients with failing hearts respond to ventilatory maneuvers such as CPAP, PEEP, and cyclic increases in intrathoracic pressure. Because effective nonpharmacologic therapy for poor cardiac function offers many advantages, it is advantageous for further careful evaluation of role of ventilatory support in caring for the acutely ill patient.

REFERENCES

Abraham E, Wunderink R, Silverman H, et al: Efficacy and safety of monoclonal antibody to human tumor necrosis factor alpha in patients with sepsis syndrome: A randomized, controlled, double-blind, multicenter clinical trial. JAMA 273:934–941, 1995.

Abrams E, Forrester JS, Chaterjee K, et al: Variability in response to norepinephrine in acute myocardial infarction. Am J Cardiol 32:919–923, 1973.

ACCP Consensus Committee on Pulmonary Embolism: Opinions regarding the diagnosis and management of venous thromboembolic disease. Chest 109:233–237, 1996.

Alonso DR, Scheidt S, Post M, et al: Pathophysiology of cardiogenic shock: Quantification of myocardial necrosis, clinical, pathologic and electrocardiographic correlations. Circulation 45:588–593, 1973.

Arnold JMO, Braunwald E, Sandor T, and Kloner RA: Inotropic stimulation of reperfused myocardium with dopamine. Effects on infarct size and myocardial function. J Am Coll Cardiol 6:1026, 1985.

Astiz ME, Rackow EC, Falk JL, et al: Oxygen delivery and consumption in patients with hyperdynamic septic shock. Crit Care Med 15:26–28, 1987.

Baim DS: Effects of amrinone on myocardial energetics in severe congestive heart failure. Am J Cardiol 96:16–18, 1985.

Baratz DM, Westbrook PR, Shah PK, and Mohsenifar Z: Effect of nasal continuous positive airway pressure on cardiac output and oxygen delivery in patients with congestive heart failure. Chest 102:1397–1401, 1992.

Bendersky R, Chaterjee K, Parmley WW, et al: Dobutamine in chronic ischemic heart failure: Alterations in left ventricular function and coronary hemodynamics. Am J Cardiol 48:554–558, 1981.

Benotti JR, Grossman W, Braunwald E, et al: Hemodynamic assessment of amrinone: A new inotropic agent. N Engl J Med 299:1373–1377, 1978.

Benotti JR, Grossman W, Braunwald E, et al: Effects of amrinone on myocardial energy metabolism and hemodynamics in patients with severe congestive heart failure due to coronary artery disease. Circulation 62:28–34, 1980.

Bertrand M, Rousseau MF, LaBlanche JM, et al: Cineangiographic assessment of left ventricular function in the acute phase of transmural myocardial infarction. Am J Cardiol 43:472–480, 1979.

Beyer R, Halperin HR, Tsitlik J, et al: Circulatory assistance by intrathoracic pressure variations: Optimization and mechanisms studied by a mathematical model in relation to experimental data. Circ Res 64:703–720, 1989.

Bigger JT, Fleiss JL, Kleiger R, et al: The relationship among ventricular arrhythmias, left ventricular dysfunction and mortality in the two years after myocardial infarction. Circulation 69:250–258, 1984.

Blain C, Anderson T, Pietras R, et al: Immediate

hemodynamic effects of gram-negative vs. gram-positive bacteremia in man. Arch Intern Med 126:260–265, 1970.

Bone RC, Balk RA, Fein AM, et al: A second large controlled clinical study of E5, a monoclonal antibody to endotoxin: Results of a prospective, multicenter, randomized, controlled trial. Crit Care Med 23:994–1006, 1995.

Bourlain T, Lanotte R, Legras A, and Perrotin D: Efficacy of epinephrine therapy in shock complicating pulmonary embolism. Chest 104:300–302, 1993.

Bradley TD, Holloway RM, McLaughlin PR, et al: Cardiac output response to continuous positive airway pressure in congestive heart failure. Am Rev Respir Dis 145:377–382, 1992.

Braunwald E, Sonnenblick EH, and Ross JR: Contraction of the normal heart. In Braunwald E (ed): Heart Disease: A Textbook of Cardiovascular Medicine, 2nd ed. Philadelphia, WB Saunders, 1984, pp 409–446.

Bristow MR, Ginsburg P, Minobe W, et al: Decreased catecholamine sensitivity and β-adrenergic receptor density in failing human hearts. N Engl J Med 307:205–211, 1982.

Brooks H, Kirk ES, Vokanas PS, et al: Performance of the right ventricle under stress: Relation to right coronary flow. J Clin Invest 50:2176–2183, 1971.

Buckle P, Millar R, and Kryger M: The effect of short-term CPAP on Cheyne-Stokes respiration on congestive heart failure. Chest 103:3–7, 1992.

Bunnel S: The use of nitrous oxide and oxygen to maintain anesthesia and positive pressure for thoracic surgery. JAMA 58:835–840, 1912.

Cabrera MR, Nakamura GE, Mantague DA, and Cole RP: Effect of airway pressure on pericardial pressure. Am Rev Respir Dis 140:659–667, 1989.

Calandra T, Glauser MP, Schellenkens J, et al: Treatment of gram-negative septic shock with human IgG antibody to Escherichia coli J5: A prospective double-blind, randomized study. J Infect Dis 158:312–319, 1988.

Calvin JE, Baer RW, and Glantz SA: Pulmonary artery constriction produces a greater load than lung microvascular injury in the open chest dog. Circ Res 56:40–48, 1985.

Chaterjee K, Swan HJC, Kaushik VS, et al: Effects of vasodilator therapy for severe pump failure in acute myocardial infarction on short-term and late prognosis. Circulation 53:797–802, 1976.

Cobb P, Natanson C, Hoffman W, et al: N^G-amino-L-arginine, an inhibitor of nitric oxide synthase, raises vascular resistance by increases mortality rates in awake canines challenged with endotoxin. J Exp Med 176:1175–1182, 1992.

Cohen RI, Huberfeld S, Genovese J, et al: A comparison between the acute effects of nitric oxide synthase inhibition and fluid resuscitation on myocardial function and metabolism in endotoxemic dogs. J Crit Care 11:27–36, 1996.

Cohn JN, Levine TB, Oliveri MT, et al: Plasma norepinephrine as a guide to prognosis in patients with chronic congestive heart failure. N Engl J Med 311:819–823, 1984.

Cooper N, Brazier J, and Buckley G: Effects of systemic-pulmonary shunts on regional blood flow in experimental pulmonary stenosis. J Thorac Cardiovasc Surg 70:166–172, 1975.

Criley JM, Blaufuss AH, and Kissel GL: Cough-induced cardiac compression. JAMA 236:1246–1250, 1976.

Daly PA and Sole MJ: Myocardial catecholamines and the pathophysiology of heart failure. Circulation 82(Suppl 1):I35–I43, 1990.

Dantzker DR and Gutierrez G: Effects of circulatory failure on pulmonary and tissue gas exchange. In Scharf SM and Cassidy SS (eds): Heart-Lung Interactions in Health and Disease. New York, Marcel Dekker, 1989, pp 983–1019.

Davies MJ: Crystalloid or colloid: Does it matter. J Clin Anesth 1:467–471, 1989.

Davies RJO, Harrington KJ, Ormerod OJM, and Stradling JR: Nasal continuous positive airway pressure in chronic heart failure with sleep-disordered breathing. Am Rev Respir Dis 147:630–634, 1993.

Desjars P, Pinaud M, Bugnon D, and Tasseau F: Norepinephrine therapy has no deleterious renal effects in human septic shock. Crit Care Med 17:426–429, 1989.

Desjars P, Pinaud M, Potel G, et al: A reappraisal of norepinephrine therapy in human septic shock. Crit Care Med 15:134–137, 1987.

Duff JH, Groves AC, McLean APH, et al: Defective oxygen consumption in septic shock. Surg Gynecol Obstet 128:1051–1066, 1969.

Duncan AW, Oh TE, Hillman DR: PEEP and CPAP. Anaesth Intensive Care 14:236–250, 1986.

Exley AR, Cohen J, Buurman W, et al: Monoclonal antibody to TNF in severe septic shock. Lancet 1:1275–1277, 1990.

Farrar DJ, Woodard JC, and Chow E. Pacing-induced dilated cardiomyopathy increases left-to-right ventricular systolic interaction. Circulation 88:720–725, 1993.

Fessler HE, Brower RG, Wise R, et al: Positive pleural pressure decreases coronary perfusion. Am J Physiol 258:H814–H820, 1990.

Fessler HE, Brower RG, Wise RA, and Permutt S: Mechanism of reduced LV afterload by systolic and diastolic positive pleural pressure. J Appl Physiol 65:1244–1250, 1988.

Fisher CJ, Dhainaut J-F, Pribble JP, et al: A phase III multicenter trial of human recombinant interleukin-1 receptor antagonist (IL-1ra) in the treatment of patients with sepsis syndrome [abstract]. Lymphokine Cytokine Res 12:390A, 1993a.

Fisher CJ, Opal SM, Dhainaut J-F, et al: Influence of anti-TNF monoclonal antibody on cytokine levels in patients with sepsis. Crit Care Med 21:318–327, 1993b.

Fisher CJ, Slotman GJ, Opal SM, et al: Initial evaluation of human recombinant interleukin-1 receptor antagonist in the treatment of sepsis syndrome: A randomized, open-label, placebo-controlled, multicenter trial. The IL-1ra sepsis syndrome study group. Crit Care Med 22:12–21, 1994.

Forrester JS, Diamond G, Chaterjee K, et al: Medical therapy of acute myocardial infarction by application of hemodynamic subsets. N Engl J Med 295:1404–1413, 1976.

Franciosa JB, Buiha NM, Limas CJ, et al: Improved left ventricular function during nitroprusside infusion in acute myocardial infarction. Lancet 1:650–654, 1972.

Gage J, Rutman J, Lucido D, et al: Additive effects of dobutamine and amrinone on myocardial contractility and ventricular performance in patients with severe heart failure. Circulation 74:367–373, 1986.

Gattinoni L, Brazzi L, Pelosi P, et al: A trial of goal-oriented hemodynamic therapy in critically ill patients. N Engl J Med 333:1025–1032, 1995.

Genovese J, Huberfeld S, Tarasiuk A, et al: Effects of CPAP on cardiac output in pigs with pacing-induced congestive heart failure. Am J Respir Crit Care Med 152:1847–1853, 1995.

Genovese J, Moskowitz M, Tarasiuk A, et al: Effects of CPAP on cardiac output in normal and hypervolemic unanesthetized pigs. Am J Respir Crit Care Med 150:752–758, 1994.

Ghignone M, Girling L, and Prewitt RM: Volume expansion vs noradrenaline in treatment of a low cardiac output complicating an acute increase in right ventricular afterload in dogs. Anesthesiology 60:48–55, 1984.

Gibelin P, Sbirrazzuoli V, Drici M, et al: Effects of short-term administration of dobutamine on left ventricular performance, exercise capacity, norepinephrine levels and lymphocyte adrenergic receptor density in congestive heart failure. Cardiovasc Drugs Ther 4:1105–1111, 1990.

Gilbert EM, Haupt MT, Mandanas RY, et al: The effect of fluid loading, blood transfusion and catecholamine infusion on oxygen delivery and consumption in patients with sepsis. Am Rev Respir Dis 134:873–878, 1986.

Gillespie TA, Ambos HD, Sobel BE, et al: Effects of dobutamine in patients with acute myocardial infarction. Am J Cardiol 39:588–594, 1977.

Glantz SA and Parmley WW: Factors which affect the diastolic pressure-volume curve. Circ Res 42:171–180, 1978.

Gold FL and Bache RJ: Transmural right ventricular blood flow during acute pulmonary artery hypertension in the sedated dog. Circ Res 51:196–204, 1982.

Goldberg LI, Hsleh YY, and Resnekov L: Newer catecholamines for treatment of heart failure and shock: An update on dopamine and a first look at dobutamine. Prog Cardiovasc Dis 19:327–340, 1977.

Goldstein RA: Clinical effects of intravenous amrinone in patients with congestive heart failure. Am J Cardiol 56:B16–B18, 1985.

Grace MD and Greenbaum DM: Cardiac performance in response to PEEP in patients with cardiac dysfunction. Crit Care Med 10:358–360, 1982.

Greenfield LJ and Langham MR: Surgical approaches to thromboembolism. Br J Surg 71:968–970, 1984.

Greenman RL, Schein RMH, Martin MA, et al: A controlled clinical trial of E5[7] murine monoclonal IgM antibody to endotoxin in the treatment of gram-negative sepsis. JAMA 266:1097–1102, 1991.

Gregory GA, Kitterman JA, Phibbs RH, et al: Treatment of idiopathic respiratory distress syndrome with continuous positive airway pressure. N Engl J Med 284:1333–1337, 1971.

Guyton AC: Textbook of Medical Physiology. Philadelphia, WB Saunders, 1976, pp 333 and 358.

Hassapoyannes C, Harper JF, Stuck LM, et al: Effects of systole-specific pericardial pressure increases on coronary flow. J Appl Physiol 71:104–111, 1991.

Haupt MT, Gilbert EM, and Carlson RW: Fluid loading increases oxygen consumption in septic patients with lactic acidosis. Am Rev Respir Dis 131:912–916, 1985.

Haupt MT and Rackow EC: Colloid osmotic pressure and fluid resuscitation with hetastarch, albumin and saline solutions. Crit Care Med 10:159–162, 1982.

Hauser CJ, Shoemaker WC, Turpin I, et al: Oxygen transport response to colloids and crystalloids in critically ill surgical patients. Surg Gynecol Obstet 150:811–816, 1980.

Hausknecht M, Brower R, Wise R, and Permutt S: The contribution of left ventricular stroke volume to CPR blood flow depends upon the duty cycle. Am J Emerg Med 2:350–351, 1984.

Hayes MA, Timmins AC, Yau EHS, et al: Elevation of systemic oxygen delivery in the treatment of critically ill patients. N Engl J Med 330:1717–1722, 1994.

Holzer J, Karliner JS, O'Rourke RA, et al: Effectiveness of dopamine in patients with cardiogenic shock. Am J Cardiol 32:79, 1973.

Howarth S, McMichael J, and Sharpey-Schaefer EP: Effects of venesection in low output heart failure. Clin Sci 6:41–50, 1946.

Huberfeld S, Genovese A, Tarasiuk A, and Scharf SM: Effects of CPAP on pericardial pressure, transmural left ventricular pressure and respiratory mechanics in hypervolemic unanesthetized pigs. Am J Respir Crit Care Med 152:142–147, 1995.

Ichard C, Ricome JL, Rimailho A, et al: Combined hemodynamic effects of dopamine and dobutamine in cardiogenic shock. Circulation 67:620–625, 1983.

Kilbourn RG, Fonseca GA, Griffith OW, et al: N[G]-methyl-L-arginine, an inhibitor of nitric oxide synthase, reverses interleukin-2 induced hypotension. Crit Care Med 23:1018–1024, 1995.

Kilbourn RG, Jobran A, Cross S, et al: Reversal of endotoxin mediated shock by N[G]-methyl-L-arginine, an inhibitor of nitric oxide synthesis.

Biochem Biophys Res Comm 127:1132–1138, 1990.

Klabude R and Ritger R: N^G-monomethyl-L-arginine restores arterial blood pressure by reducing cardiac output in a canine model of endotoxic shock. Biochem Biophys Res Comm 128:1135–1140, 1991.

Klein NA, Siskind SJ, Frishman WH, et al: Hemodynamic comparison of intravenous amrinone and dobutamine in patients with chronic congestive heart failure. Am J Cardiol 48:170–175, 1981.

Kreger BE, Craven DE, and McCabe WR: Gram-negative bacteremia. IV. Re-evaluation of clinical features and treatment in 612 patients. Am J Med 68:344–355, 1980.

Lee R, Lotze M, Skibber J, et al: Cardiorespiratory effects of immunotherapy with interleukin-2. J Clin Oncol 7:7–20, 1989.

LeJemtel TH, Keung E, Sonnenblick EH, et al: Amrinone: A new non-glycoside, non-adrenergic cardiotonic agent effective in the treatment of intractable myocardial failure in man. Circulation 59:1098–1104, 1979.

Lichtenstein SV, Slutsky A, and Salerno TA: Noninvasive right and left ventricular assist. Surg Forum 36:306–310, 1985.

Lin PJ, Chang C-H, and Chang J-P: Reversal of refractory hypotension in septic shock by inhibitor of nitric oxide synthase. Chest 106:626–629, 1994.

Little WC, Badke FR, and O'Rourke RA: Effect of right ventricular pressure-volume relationship before and after chronic right ventricular pressure overload in dogs without pericardia. Circ Res 54:719–730, 1984.

Lorente J, Landin L, Renes E, et al: Role of nitric oxide in the hemodynamic changes of sepsis. Crit Care Med 21:759–767, 1993.

McCloskey RV, Straube RC, Sanders C, et al: Treatment of septic shock with human monoclonal HA-1A. Ann Intern Med 121:1–5, 1994.

McGinn S and White PD: Acute cor pulmonale resulting from pulmonary embolism. JAMA 104:1473–1478, 1935.

McIntyre K and Scharf SM: The use of Valsalva's and Mueller's maneuvers as diagnostic tests for coronary artery disease. In Scharf SM and Cassidy SS (eds): Heart-Lung Interactions in Health and Disease. New York, Marcel Dekker, 1989, pp 1021–1046.

McMichael J and Sharpey-Schaefer EP: The action of intravenous digoxin in man. Q J Med 13:123, 1944.

Maekawa K, Liang C-S, and Hood WB Jr: Comparison of dobutamine and dopamine in acute myocardial infarction. Effects of systemic hemodynamics, plasma catecholamines, blood flow and infarct size. Circulation 67:750–754, 1983.

Malone S, Liu PP, Holloway R, et al: Obstructive sleep apnoea in patients with dilated cardiomyopathy: Effect of continuous positive airway pressure. Lancet 338:1480–1484, 1991.

Mancini D, LeJemtel TH, and Sonnenblick EH: Intravenous use of amrinone for treatment of the failing heart. Am J Cardiol 56:8B, 1985.

Manohar M, Tranquili WJ, Parks C, et al: Regional myocardial blood flow and coronary vasodilator reserve during acute right ventricular failure due to pressure overload in swine. J Surg Res 31:382–391, 1981.

Marcus FI, Opie LH, and Sonnenblick EH: Digitalis, sympathomimetics and inotropic dilators. In Opie LH (ed): Drugs for the Heart, 3rd ed. Philadelphia, WB Saunders, pp 91–110, 1991.

Marik PE and Mohedin M: The contrasting effects of dopamine and norepinephrine on systemic and splanchnic oxygen utilization in hyperdynamic sepsis. JAMA 272:1354–1375, 1994.

Martin C, Eon B, Saux P, et al: Renal effects of norepinephrine used to treat septic shock patients. Crit Care Med 18:282–285, 1990.

Martin C, Panazian L, Perrine G, et al: Norepinephrine or dopamine for treatment of hyperdynamic septic shock. Chest 103:1826–1831, 1993.

Mathru M, Rao TLK, El-Etr AA, and Pifarre R: Hemodynamic response to changes in ventilatory patterns in patients with normal and poor left ventricular reserve. Crit Care Med 10:423–426, 1982.

Maughan WL and Oikawa RY: Right ventricular function. In Scharf SM and Cassidy SF (eds): Heart-Lung Interactions in Health and Disease. New York, Marcel Dekker, 1989, pp 179–220.

Meadows D, Edwards D, Wilkens RG, and Nightingale P: Reversal of intractable septic shock with norepinephrine therapy. Crit Care Med 16:663–666, 1988.

Molloy WD, Girley L, Prewitt RM, et al: Treatment of shock in a canine model of pulmonary embolus. Am Rev Respir Dis 130:870–874, 1984.

Moncada S and Higgs SA: The L-arginine nitric oxide pathway. N Engl J Med 329:2002–2012, 1993.

Muller H, Ayres SM, Gregory JJ, et al: Hemodynamics, coronary blood flow and myocardial metabolism in coronary shock response to L-norepinephrine and isoproterenol. J Clin Invest 49:1885, 1970.

Murgo JP and Westerhof N: Input impedance of the pulmonary arterial system in normal man. Circ Res 54:666–672, 1984.

Natanson C, Danner RL, Alein GL, et al: Antibiotics, fluids and dopamine in a lethal canine model of septic shock: effects on survival [abstract]. Clin Res 36:372A, 1988.

Naughton ML, Benard DC, Liu PP, et al: Effects of nasal CPAP on sympathetic activity in patients with heart failure and central sleep apnea. Am J Respir Crit Care Med 152:473–479, 1995a.

Naughton ML, Liu PP, Benard DC, et al: Treatment of congestive heart failure and Cheyne-Stokes respiration during sleep by continuous positive airway pressure. Am J Respir Crit Care Med 151:92–97, 1995b.

Naughton ML, Rahman MA, Hara K, et al: Effects of continuous positive airway pressure on intrathoracic and left ventricular transmural pressure in congestive heart failure. Circulation 91:1725–1731, 1995c.

Nava E, Palmer R, and Moncada S: Inhibition of nitric oxide synthesis in septic shock: How much is beneficial? Lancet 338:1555–1558, 1991.

Packman MI and Rackow EC: Optimum left heart filling pressure during fluid resuscitation of patients with hypovolemic and septic shock. Crit Care Med 11:165–169, 1983.

Page D, Caulfield JB, Kastor JA, et al: Myocardial changes associated with cardiogenic shock. N Engl J Med 285:133, 1971.

Parker MM, Shelhamer JH, Bacharach SL, et al: Profound but reversible myocardial depression in patients with septic shock. Ann Intern Med 100:483–90, 1984.

Parker MM, Sulfrendini AF, Natanson C, et al: Responses of left ventricular function in survivors and nonsurvivors of septic shock. J Crit Care 4:19–25, 1989.

Perel A, Williamson DC, and Modell JH: Effectiveness of CPAP by mask for pulmonary edema associated with hypercarbia. Intensive Care Med 9:17–19, 1983.

Permutt S and Wise RA: The control of cardiac output through coupling of heart and blood vessels. In Yin FCP (ed): Ventricular/Vascular Coupling. New York, Springer-Verlag, 1987, pp 159–179.

Pery N, Payen D, and Pinsky MR: Monitoring the effect of CPAP on left ventricular function using continuous mixed-blood saturation. Chest 99:512–513, 1991.

Peters J and Ihle P: ECG synchronized thoracic vest inflation during autonomic blockade, myocardial ischemia or cardiac arrest. J Appl Physiol 73:2263–2273, 1992.

Petros A, Bennett D, and Vallance P: Effect of nitric oxide synthase inhibitors on hypotension in patients with septic shock. Lancet 338:8782–8783, 1991.

Petros A, Lamb G, Leone A, et al: Effects of nitric oxide synthase inhibitor in humans with septic shock. Cardiovasc Res 28:34–39, 1994.

Pinsky MR, Marquez J, Martin D, and Klain M: Ventricular assist by cardiac cycle-specific increases in intrathoracic pressure. Chest 91:709–715, 1987.

Pinsky MR, Matuschuk GM, Bernardi L, and Klain M: Hemodynamic specific increases in intrathoracic pressure. J Appl Physiol 60:604–612, 1986.

Pinsky MR, Mataschuk GM, and Klain M: Determinants of cardiac augmentation by elevations in intrathoracic pressure. J Appl Physiol 58:1189–1198, 1985.

Pinsky MR and Summer WR: Cardiac augmentation by phasic high intrathoracic pressure support. Chest 84:370–375, 1983.

Pinsky MR, Summer WR, Wise RA, et al: Augmentation of cardiac function by elevation of intrathoracic pressure. J Appl Physiol 54:950–955, 1983.

Plamer RP and Lasseter KC: Sodium nitroprusside. N Engl J Med 292:294–297, 1975.

Poulton EP and Oxon DM: Left-sided failure with pulmonary oedema. Lancet 2:981–983, 1936.

Prewitt RM and Ghignone RM: Treatment of right ventricular dysfunction in acute respiratory failure. Crit Care Med 11:346–352, 1983.

Puri VK, Howard M, Paidipaty BB, and Singh S: Resuscitation in hypovolemia and shock: A prospective study of hydroxyethyl starch and albumin. Crit Care Med 11:518–23, 1983.

Puri VK, Paidipaty B, and White L: Hydroxyethyl starch for resuscitation of patients with hypovolemia and shock. Crit Care Med 9:833–837, 1981.

Rackow EC, Falk JL, Fein IA, et al: Fluid resuscitation in circulatory shock: A comparison of the cardiorespiratory effects of albumin, hetastarch, and saline solutions in patients with hypovolemic and septic shock. Crit Care Med 11:839–850, 1983.

Rackow EC, Kaufman B, Falk J, et al: Hemodynamic response to fluid repletion in patients with septic shock. Circ Shock 22:11–22, 1987.

Räsänen J, Heikkilä J, Downs J, et al: Continuous positive airway pressure by face mask in acute cardiogenic pulmonary edema. Am J Cardiol 55:296–300, 1985a.

Räsänen J, Vaisanen IT, Heikkilä J, et al: Acute myocardial infarction complicated by left ventricular dysfunction and respiratory failure: The effects of continuous positive airway pressure. Chest 87:158–162, 1985b.

Reller MD, Morton MJ, Giraud GD, et al: Severe right ventricular pressure loading in fetal sheep augments global myocardial blood flow to submaximal levels. Circulation 86:581–588, 1992.

Robotham JL: Ventilatory-assisted myocardial performance (VAMP). Chest 84:366, 1983.

Ross AD and Angaran DM: Colloids vs. crystalloids in a continuing controversy. Drug Intell Clin Pharm 18:202–212, 1984.

Rudikoff MT, Maughan WL, Effron M, et al: Mechanisms of blood flow during cardiopulmonary resuscitation. Circulation 61:345–352, 1980.

Ruokonen E, Takala J, Kari A, et al: Regional blood flow and oxygen transport in septic shock. Crit Care Med 21:1296–1303, 1993.

Scharf SM: Right ventricular load tolerance: Role of left ventricular function. Perspectives en réanimation, Les Interactions cardio-pulmonaires. Société de réanimation de langue français, Arnette, Paris, 1994, pp 17–28.

Scharf SM, Brown R, Saunders NA, and Green LH: Hemodynamic effects of positive pressure inflation. J Appl Physiol 49:124–131, 1980.

Scharf SM, Chen L, Slamowitz D, and Rao PS: Effects of continuous positive airway pressure on cardiac output and plasma norepinephrine in sedated pigs. J Crit Care 11:57–64, 1996.

Scharf SM, Warner KG, Josa M, et al: Load tolerance of the right ventricle: Effect of increased aortic pressure. J Crit Care 1:163–173, 1986.

Segfal JM, Phang PT, and Walley KP: Low-dose dopamine hastens the onset of gut ischemia in a porcine model of hemorrhagic shock. J Appl Physiol 73:1159–1164, 1992.

Shoemaker WC: Relation of oxygen transport patterns to the pathophysiology and therapy of shock states. Intensive Care Med 13:230–243, 1987.

Shoemaker WC, Appel PL, and Kram HB: Hemodynamic and oxygen transport effects of dobutamine in critically ill general surgical patients. Crit Care Med 14:1032–1037, 1986.

Shoemaker WC, Appel PL, Kram HB, et al: Prospective trial of supranormal values of survivors as therapeutic goals in high-risk surgical patients. Chest 94:1176–1186, 1988.

Shoemaker WC, Appel PL, Kram HB, et al: Comparison of hemodynamics and oxygen transport effects of dopamine and dobutamine in critically ill patients. Chest 96:120–126, 1989.

Siegel JH, Greenspan M, and Del Guercio LRM: Abnormal vascular tone, defective oxygen transport and myocardial failure in human septic shock. Ann Surg 165:505–517, 1967.

Smith TW, Braunwald E, and Kelly RA: The management of heart failure. In Braunwald E (ed): Heart Disease: A Textbook of Cardiovascular Medicine, 3rd ed. Philadelphia, WB Saunders, pp 485–543, 1988.

Sonnenblick EH, Frishman WH, and LeJemtel TH: Dobutamine. A new synthetic cardioactive sympathetic amine. N Engl J Med 300:17–22, 1979.

Spotnitz HM, Berman MA, and Epstein SE: Pathophysiology and experimental treatment of acute pulmonary embolism. Am Heart J 82:511–520, 1971.

Stamler J, Loh E, Roddy M-A, et al: Nitric oxide regulates basal systemic and pulmonary vascular resistance in healthy humans. Circulation 89:2035–2040, 1993.

Stein KL, Kramer DJ, Killian A, and Pinsky MR: Hemodynamic effects of synchronous high-frequency jet ventilation in mitral regurgitation. J Appl Physiol 69:2120–2125, 1990.

Swedberg KP, Enroth J, Kjekshus J, and Wilhelmsen L: Hormones regulating cardiovascular function in patients with severe CHF and their relation to mortality. Circulation 82:1730–1736. 1990.

Taylor SH, Verma SP, Hussain M, et al: Intravenous amrinone in left ventricular failure complicated by acute myocardial infarction. Am J Cardiol 56:29B, 1985.

Timsit J, Reynaud P, Meyer G, et al: Pulmonary embolectomy by catheter device in massive pulmonary embolism. Chest 100:655–658, 1991.

Tittley JG, Fremes SE, Weisel RD, et al: Hemodynamic and myocardial metabolic consequences of PEEP. Chest 88:496–502, 1985.

Tucker HJ and Murray JF: Effects of end-expiratory pressure on organ blood flow in normal and diseased dogs. J Appl Physiol 34:573–577, 1973.

Uretsky BF, Lawless CE, Verbalis JG, et al: Combined therapy with dobutamine and amrinone in severe heart failure: Improved hemodynamics and increased activation of the renin-angiotensin system with combined intravenous therapy. Chest 92:657, 1987.

Urokinase Pulmonary Embolism Trial: A cooperative study. Circulation 47[Suppl II]:1–103, 1973.

Urokinase-Streptokinase Pulmonary Embolism Trial, Phase 2 results: A cooperative study. JAMA 229:1606–1613, 1974.

Vatner SF and Baig H: Importance of heart rate in determining the effects of sympathomimetic amines on regional myocardial infarction and blood flow in conscious dogs with acute myocardial ischemia. Circ Res 45:793–803, 1979.

Velanovich V: Crystalloid versus colloid fluid resuscitation: A meta analysis of mortality. Surgery 105:65–71, 1989.

Venus B and Jacobs HK: Alterations in regional myocardial blood flows during different levels of positive end-expiratory pressure. Crit Care Med 12:96–102, 1984.

Venus B, Jacobs HK, and Lim L: Treatment of the adult respiratory distress syndrome with continuous positive airway pressure. Chest 76:257–264, 1979.

Verma SP, Silke B, and Taylor SH: Hemodynamic dose-response effects of amrinone in left ventricular failure complicating myocardial infarction. Br J Clin Pharmacol 19:540P, 1985.

Vincent JL: Fluids for resuscitation. Br J Anaesth 67:185–193, 1991.

Virgilio RW, Rice CL, Smith DE, et al: Crystalloid vs. colloid resuscitation: Is one better? Surgery 85:129–139, 1979.

Vlahakes GJ, Turley K, and Hoffman JIE: The pathophysiology of failure in acute right ventricular hypertension: Hemodynamics and biochemical correlations. Circulation 63:87–95, 1981.

Wagner BKJ and D'Amelio LF: Pharmacologic and clinical considerations in selecting crystalloid, colloidal and oxygen-carrying resuscitation fluids, part 2. Clin Pharmacol 12:415–428, 1993.

Weidman HP and Matthay RA: The management of cor pulmonale. In Scharf SM and Cassidy SS (eds): Heart-Lung Interactions in Health and Disease. New York, Marcel Dekker, 1989, pp 915–981.

Weil M and Shubin H: Proposed reclassification of shock states with special reference to distributive defects. In Hinshaw L and Cox B (eds): The Fundamental Mechanisms of Shock. New York, Plenum Press, 1972, pp 13–23.

Willerson JT, Hutton I, Watson JT, et al: Influence of

dobutamine on regional myocardial blood flow and ventricle performance during acute and chronic myocardial ischemia in dogs. Circulation 53:828–833, 1976.

Wright C, Rees D, and Moncada S: Protective and pathological roles of nitric oxide in endotoxic shock. Cardiovasc Res 26:48–57, 1992.

Yamaguchi S, Li KS, Harasawa H, et al: The left ventricle affects the duration of right ventricular ejection. Cardiovasc Res 27:211–215, 1993.

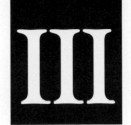

SPECIFIC
DISORDERS

C H A P T E R

Acute Myocardial Infarction

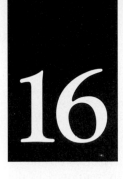

Ira L. Weg, M.D.

Monty M. Bodenheimer, M.D.

As the end of the twentieth century approaches, progress is being made against the mortality and disability engendered by coronary artery disease. Whether changes in cardiology practice attributable to new understandings of ischemic heart disease are responsible for the decline in mortality is debatable. It is clear that the cardiovascular death rate from 1982 to 1992 has declined by over 24%, faster than the corresponding overall death rate (Heart and Stroke Facts, 1995).

This decade saw the increasing use of megatrials as a useful research tool to test hypotheses based on newer concepts of the pathophysiology of myocardial infarction. As a result, we have a huge body of data not only on studied subjects but on those registered and not given the targeted course of therapy. One may consider, for example, that the patients who present with acute myocardial infarction late in the course of the attack and receive neither thrombolysis nor primary angioplasty are, in many ways, modeled by the placebo groups of the early thrombolysis megatrials. The achievements of the megatrials drew hitherto unappreciated attention to weaknesses in the basic understanding of the myocardial infarction process.

Management of the patient with an acute myocardial infarction through the 1950s and into the 1960s was essentially that of control of ischemic pain, coupled with long periods of bed rest to allow healing of the infarct. Recognition of the critical importance of early ventricular arrhythmias as a cause of death in the 1960s led to the development of intensive monitoring and both pharmacologic and electrical cardioversion—the key resuscitative step—which resulted in the saving of many lives that otherwise would have been lost to ventricular fibrillation. Preservation of myocardium was in its infancy. The focus of experimental and clinical studies was to devise ways to reduce oxygen demand and thereby limit infarction size. This focus is illustrated by one of the earliest megatrials, the First International Study of Infarct Survival (ISIS Collaborative Group, 1986), which examined the roles of early beta blockade and decreased oxygen demand to improve survival.

Of central importance to the fundamental

change in approach was the recognition that thrombus formation at the site of a ruptured plaque is the crucial event in the genesis of myocardial infarction. As an outgrowth of studies to determine the effectiveness of emergent aortocoronary bypass surgery in myocardial infarction, DeWood and coworkers (1980) reported on the results of coronary arteriography performed in the early hours of myocardial infarction. They demonstrated that 87% of the infarction-related coronary arteries studied within 4 hours were completely occluded. However, when patients were studied later, between 12 and 24 hours after the onset of symptoms, only 65% of the infarction-related coronaries were occluded. The knowledge that the infarction-related coronary arteries recanalized over the early hours of myocardial infarction completely altered the approach to treatment, placing it squarely in a new era when thrombolysis and angioplasty assume critical therapeutic roles.

As a result, today's clinician must approach the patient with acute myocardial infarction with an orderly, systematic algorithm of care. In addition, the clinician must ensure that the delivery of care in his or her practice environment is adequate to allow these modern algorithms to be put into place quickly and smoothly. The immediate requirements for the clinician are to make the diagnosis of myocardial infarction and, simultaneously, decide whether and what mode of reperfusion will be pursued over the next hour. As soon as the diagnosis of a putative myocardial infarction is made, and while any reperfusion therapy is in preparation, the clinician must ensure that certain adjunctive therapies are initiated without delay.

THE INITIAL FEW MINUTES

The first few "platinum minutes" of the first "golden hour" are key to the success of the present approach to rapid identification, diagnosis, and treatment of myocardial infarction. Unfortunately, the system of care is crippled by the patient's delay in seeking care, the so-called symptoms-to-door interval. The National Registry of Myocardial Infarction (Rogers et al, 1994) reported a median time of 130 minutes from chest pain onset to arrival at the emergency department in the years 1990 to 1993. Patients treated with thrombolytic drugs arrived at a median of 95 minutes, and those not treated arrived at 180 minutes. The median delay increased in older patients, with patients older than 75 years presenting at a median delay of 2.5 hours. Only 26%

presented within 1 hour of symptoms (Maynard et al, 1995). Recognizing that the symptoms-to-door time is the greatest drag on the delivery of acute cardiac care, public education and awareness programs are essential to improving outcome.

Once the patient has entered the system, hospitals can and must implement changes to identify the systems-related slowdowns in the "door-to-drug" intervals that result in late delivery of reperfusion therapy. A suspicion supported by the history and electrocardiographic confirmation remains the basis for the diagnosis of myocardial infarction. As is discussed later, the electrocardiographic changes are the most important feature in the early diagnosis of myocardial infarction because they, as well as the patient's overall state, determine the course of therapy. The patient often first describes the event to the emergency services dispatcher, paramedic, family member, or triage nurse. At any of these levels, the mere suspicion of myocardial infarction should activate mechanisms designed to confirm its presence.

ELECTROCARDIOGRAPHY

An electrocardiogram (ECG) should be performed immediately in any patient presenting with symptoms suggesting myocardial infarction, which, for the purposes of discussion, is henceforth called *chest pain*. Triage personnel should be instructed to routinely order this safe and inexpensive test without a requirement for consultation with a physician. The importance of the ECG in making the diagnosis of myocardial infarction depends not only on the test's result but also on its timing. Kline found that door-to-data time was 11 minutes, identifying the ECG as an important limiting factor in the delivery of reperfusion therapy (Kline et al, 1992).

Where it has been available, transmission of an ECG tracing by cellular telephone allows the emergency department staff to corral the resources that will be called upon over the next few minutes. Nonetheless, this intervention is beyond the reach of many localities. Even in the absence of telephone transmission, patients receive faster treatment if paramedics in the field are directed to identify the clinical and ECG findings that make reperfusion therapy appropriate (Weaver et al, 1993).

Although it is an extremely valuable test, the ECG lacks sensitivity. The Gruppo Italiano per lo Studio della Streptochinasi nell' Infarto Miocardico (GISSI-1) criteria have been widely accepted as reasonable electrocardiographic support for the rapid diagnosis of acute myocardial infarction in anticipation of reperfusion therapy. These include

(1) 1 mm or greater ST segment elevation in any limb lead or (2) 2 mm or greater ST segment elevation in any precordial lead (Gruppo Italiano per lo Studio della Streptochinasi nell' Infarto Miocardico, 1986). Mair and coworkers found that the electrocardiographic pattern of "probable myocardial infarction" was a more informative test than any of the cardiac enzymes during the first 3 hours after onset of chest pain. The ECG criteria used by Mair were essentially the GISSI-1 criteria, with the addition of a tall R anteriorly with S-T depression compatible with posterior myocardial infarction and hyperacute T waves (Mair et al, 1995b).

Adding a requirement that more than one lead be positive may restrict the use of therapy to a smaller population, as may adding more S-T elevation to the criteria. No data at present support the use of thrombolysis in patients who do not have S-T elevation or, where clinically appropriate, left bundle branch block. Indeed, data from GISSI-1 demonstrated that there was no benefit of thrombolysis with S-T depression.

HISTORY AND PHYSICAL EXAMINATION

Chest pain, or perhaps *discomfort* as a more exact descriptive term, is present in 85% of patients with myocardial infarction. The classic description of the discomfort is as a crushing pain, tightness, or pressure in the mid or left chest. The pain is described as burning or knifelike in a significant number of patients. Lee and coworkers (1985) found that 59% of patients with proven myocardial infarction complained of pressure in the chest, but 17% complained of burning or stabbing pain. Reproduction of pain by palpation does not exclude the presence of myocardial infarction, and in Lee's study 8% of patients with fully or partially reproducible pain had evidence of myocardial infarction. Particularly in the elderly, shortness of breath is a more likely complaint (Bayer and Chadha, 1986). It has been suggested that women, more frequently than men, present with symptoms other than chest pain (Fiebach et al, 1990).

Radiation of chest pain to the arms, shoulders, back, neck, jaw, or epigastrium is common and increases the diagnostic value of the symptom complex. Radiation pattern is most valuable in the patient with retrosternal chest pain and/or ECG changes. In their absence, or in association with less typical types of chest pain, the sensitivity of radiation is diminished. Aortic dissection, for example, may occur with "tearing" chest pain radiating to the back.

Associated symptoms—nausea, vomiting, dia-phoresis, dyspnea, dizziness or lightheadedness, and palpitations—are frequently reported early in myocardial infarction. Any one of these should serve as a flag, particularly in the elderly patient, as a stand-alone symptom of myocardial infarction.

PHYSICAL EXAMINATION

Although there is no single physical finding characteristic of myocardial infarction, the common picture is of a patient in significant discomfort and appearing acutely ill. The vital signs are helpful for the most part in assessing the patient's immediate stability and in dictating the therapeutic plan, rather than serving as a diagnostic tool.

Attention should be paid to the presence of congestive heart failure and overall hemodynamic stability, particularly in the early moments of the attack. These criteria have been used to prognosticate as well as assist in selection of patients for thrombolysis. In GISSI-1, only those patients falling within Killip class I and II benefited from thrombolytic therapy (Gruppo Italiano per lo Studio della Streptochinasi nell' Infarto Miocardico, 1986). Patients with more severe hemodynamic compromise may have greater benefit from primary angioplasty and intra-aortic balloon counterpulsation than from thrombolysis.

Presence of a systolic heart murmur, in contrast, points the physician in another direction altogether. Evaluation for acute mitral regurgitation or ventricular septal rupture should be pursued with strong consideration for emergent surgical treatment.

CARDIAC ENZYMES

The so-called cardiac enzymes serve as biochemical markers for myocardial injury. The chemical tests rely on the release of a marker substance that must rise over a critical threshold before the assay has any value. They are readily and rapidly available and easy for clinicians to use, and these points have been their attraction. Their value is sometimes overrated, because they lack specificity and/or sensitivity, and results are generally available too late to contribute to the decision for reperfusion therapy. Newer tests as well as combinations of various assays may offer improved accuracy and perhaps earlier confirmation of the presence of infarction. Nonetheless, because the infarction process occurs gradually over time, indices of cell destruction probably will never be as useful as indices of cell-level ischemia.

Creatine Kinase and CK-MB

Three isoenzymes of creatine kinase (CK) are known, but the major clinically utilized fractions are MM and MB. The MB isoenzyme has been the standard for the diagnosis of myocardial infarction over the last several years. Although the characteristic pattern of rise and fall of CK and its CK isoenzyme CK-MB levels confirm the diagnosis of myocardial infarction, the level of the first enzyme drawn on arrival in the emergency department is usually not elevated. The characteristic enzyme pattern demonstrates a rise in CK level within 4 to 8 hours after admission (recognizing that this represents a varying interval from actual onset of the infarction), reaching a peak in most patients by about 12 to 20 hours, but earlier with large infarctions or with reperfusion. Indeed, one should never wait for the return of the cardiac enzymes as currently obtained to initiate thrombolysis, because this jeopardizes the survival of salvageable myocardium. The classic sampling times at 0, 8, and 16 hours have been questioned, and regimens involving more frequent sampling over a shorter time period are being investigated.

A problem with the CK-MB assay is that the enzyme is released from sources other than the heart, when these organs (such as the prostate) are subjected to trauma or surgery; it is also released in normal marathon runners and in patients with muscular dystrophy (Lee and Goldman, 1986). In addition, very high levels of CK release, such as in rhabdomyolysis, or impaired excretion or metabolism, such as in renal failure, may result in confusing levels of CK-MB as well. In the trauma patient with myocardial damage, a large release of CK may mimic myocardial infarction. The clinician must be able to ascertain with some certainty, based on the clinical context, whether an elevation in CK-MB truly reflects myocardial infarction or whether it is a value representing another muscle process.

Creatine Kinase Isoforms

The two clinically useful CK isoenzymes each have subforms that are effectual in the diagnosis of myocardial infarction. These subforms are essentially the same in enzymatic activity, but their electrophoretic migration patterns are changed by modification of a terminal lysine molecule at the carboxy terminal of the M and B chains. Puleo and coworkers (1994) found that measurement of CK-MB isoforms had a twofold increase in specificity at 6 hours compared with CK-MB alone in patients admitted for myocardial infarction.

MYOGLOBIN

Myoglobin is a small molecule that is ubiquitous in muscle tissue. When investigators evaluate patients with known myocardial infarction using myoglobin as a marker, it has a fairly high sensitivity (de Winter et al, 1995). Because it may be released from skeletal muscle, or because it may not be cleared if renal function is abnormal, it is not very specific for the diagnosis of myocardial infarction in indeterminate populations. Serum carbonic anhydrase III concentration may be used to localize the myoglobin rise to myocardium or skeletal muscle, because this cytoplasmic protein fails to increase with myocardial injury but increases along with myoglobin when skeletal muscle is damaged. Where it is being used to confirm a clinically suspected diagnosis, the rapid rise of myoglobin in serum, reaching a peak in 1.5 to 2 hours, makes it a valuable adjunct in the diagnostic process. It probably should not be used as a single determination, because the level may rise and fall over the first hours of a myocardial infarction with staccato episodes of ischemia; thus, a single negative value may not exclude infarction.

De Winter and coworkers evaluated the negative predictive values of CK-MB, troponin T, and myoglobin in patients admitted to an emergency department to rule out myocardial infarction, using the CK-MB as the standard (de Winter et al, 1995). In this study, myoglobin was a better early marker for myocardial infarction than CK-MB (utilizing an immunochemical assay measuring CK mass) or troponin T (Fig. 16–1). Its negative predictive value (NPV) declined after 6 hours, essentially indicating a decrease in the trustworthiness of the assay after this time, whereas the NPV of the other tests continued to increase, reaching the 90 to 99% range, depending on assay. This finding has an important implication: considering the delay found in patient arrival at the emergency department, myoglobin may be a good assay that is impractical for many patients, particularly the elderly, who arrive too late to take advantage of the test's value in eliminating the diagnosis of myocardial infarction.

TROPONINS

The troponin complex is composed of three proteins, troponin T, troponin I, and troponin C. Cardiac troponin T and troponin I are contractile apparatus proteins that have amino acid sequences unique to cardiac muscle, and thus assays using monoclonal antibodies can readily target these proteins. Rapid assays for cardiac troponin T and I have been made commercially available.

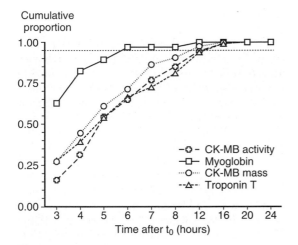

Figure 16–1
Plot of the proportion of patients with acute myocardial infarction who have a sample of CK-MB activity, CK-MB mass, myoglobin, and troponin T that is above the upper reference limit of normal. Of the four markers studied, myoglobin was the earliest to significantly rise beyond this point. (From de Winter RJ, Koster RW, Sturk A, Sanders GT: Value of myoglobin, troponin T, and CK-MB mass in ruling out an acute myocardial infarction in the Emergency Room. Circulation 92:3401–3407, 1995. Reproduced with permission. Copyright 1995 American Heart Association.)

Troponin T level rises somewhat earlier than CK-MB level, being found in serum as early as 3.5 hours after infarction, but later than myoglobin. As noted earlier, de Winter and coworkers found that troponin T had a good NPV, with a positive predictive value that was not appreciably better than that of CK-MB (de Winter et al, 1995). Troponin T is capable of documenting myocardial infarction in patients in whom the event may have occurred some days before admission, because it remains elevated for several days. It is not as helpful in making the rapid diagnosis of myocardial infarction because of the time required to perform the analysis, and thus values cannot guide reperfusion decisions. The performance of troponin I immunoassay is more rapid, and it is therefore more suitable for the triage of chest pain patients (Keffer, 1996). Its cost is higher than that of CK-MB, however.

There are no head-to-head trials of both troponins in myocardial infarction. Mair and coworkers reported equivalent sensitivities for both markers (Mair et al, 1995a). Despite de Winter's study demonstrating a rising NPV for several biomarkers, other studies have found the specificity of troponin T to be 60 to 70%, with elevation in unstable angina as well as in myocardial infarction (Katus et al, 1991; Bakker et al, 1994). Data do indicate that in unstable angina defined as a normal CK-MB, elevated troponin T is a marker for increased risk of cardiac death or myocardial infarction (Lindahl et al, 1996). This marker may have a high sensitivity for small infarctions that do not cause elevation of CK-MB level. Elevation of troponin T level with normal troponin I was reported in patients with renal disease, however, suggesting a lower specificity for the T form when used in unselected populations (Bhayana et al, 1995).

THERAPY IN MYOCARDIAL INFARCTION

REPERFUSION

In 1912, Herrick described coronary thrombosis as a cause of myocardial infarction. The determination based on postmortem examinations that the atheroma had something to do with the overall course of coronary disease, as well as the debut of angiography, which allowed cardiologists to assess the degree of atheroma in coronary vessels *in vivo*, changed the course of thinking about coronary disease in the middle part of this century. Although a dynamic component superimposed on the static atheroma was postulated as a proximate cause of an acute myocardial infarction, the mechanism of this conversion was widely disputed. Although others had emphasized the role of coronary thrombosis, an evaluation of patients after infarction by DeWood and coworkers was fortuitous in noticing that coronary obstructions decreased over the first 24 hours following infarction, suggesting that the dynamic component was acute thrombus formation superimposed on the fixed component (DeWood et al, 1980). This study was instrumental in focusing efforts on eliminating the thrombus that actually seemed to trigger the acute infarction, and the modern age of reperfusion therapy was born.

Thrombolytic agents had already been used for various purposes, but Rentrop and coworkers first used intracoronary streptokinase in an attempt to lyse coronary thrombus (Rentrop et al, 1981). The Western Washington Intracoronary Streptokinase Trial demonstrated a significant difference for 30-day mortality in patients who were reperfused at an average of 31 minutes from the start of therapy as compared with patients who were not successfully reperfused (3.7% vs. 11.2%, p=0.02) (Kennedy et al, 1983, 1985; Kennedy, 1995). No corresponding improvement in global left ventricular function was found. After 1 year, the difference in mortality for the streptokinase and control groups was not significant (8.2% vs. 14.7%, p = .10). When perfusion status was analyzed for the streptokinase group alone, the percentage with survival was 98% at 1 year for patients with complete reperfusion, as compared with 85% for treated patients with no reperfusion. Perplexingly, at the time, patients with partial reperfusion had an even lower 1-year survival (77%). It is now accepted that immediate, aggressive invasive therapy that is inadequate to restore full patency to an occluded coronary artery may cause or may be associated with a variety of complications as well as possible further damage to the ventricle (Kennedy, 1995).

INTRAVENOUS CORONARY THROMBOLYSIS

Intracoronary thrombolysis indeed proved successful at opening closed coronary arteries, but with the disadvantage of an early invasive procedure. Difficult logistics made intracoronary thrombolysis the property of centers that had aggressive catheterization facilities and delayed the time to initiation of the therapy. As a result, the role of intravenous thrombolytics, which had been largely abandoned, was re-evaluated. Interestingly, similar issues of relative efficacy and logistics cloud the role of catheter-based revascularization versus intravenous thrombolytics to this day (see later).

Efficacy of Intravenous Thrombolysis

The GISSI-1 investigators were the first to conclusively demonstrate that intravenous (IV) administration of streptokinase was accompanied by improved survival of patients with acute myocardial infarction (Gruppo Italiano per lo Studio della Streptochinasi nell' Infarto Miocardico [GISSI], 1986). The GISSI-1 investigators studied 11,806 patients admitted within 12 hours after onset of symptoms and reported an 18% overall decrease in mortality at 21 days in the streptokinase-treated group. The improvement was time-related, with the greatest improvement (a 23% decline) in the subgroup treated within 3 hours. There was a less significant improvement, 17%, in the group treated within 3 to 6 hours after the onset of symptoms (Fig. 16–2). An analysis of patients treated within 1 hour found a reduction of in-hospital mortality of 47%. Of note, Killip class 1 and 2 patients, patients with anterior myocardial infarction, and patients younger than 65 were identified as the major subgroups achieving improvements in rates of mortality. Most patients were not treated with heparin or antiplatelet agents in the GISSI-1 trial. Considering that streptokinase was the agent used, this omission was probably of minor significance, as is discussed in the section on antithrombotic adjunctive therapy.

All of the major trials since GISSI-1 have shown improved survival after IV administration of thrombolytic drugs. The Fibrinolytic Therapy

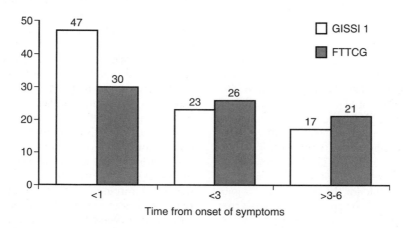

Figure 16–2
Effect of fibrinolytic therapy on decrease in mortality in patients treated with fibrinolytic drug versus placebo; comparison of GISSI-1 and Fibrinolytic Therapy Trialists Collaborative Group (FTTCG) data. GISSI-1 was one of the trials reviewed by the FTTCG investigators. Note that despite the difference in size between these two studies (11,806 patients in GISSI-1 versus 58,600 patients analyzed by FTTCG), the overall mortality at each time from onset of symptoms is similar.

Trialists Group reviewed nine trials of thrombolytic therapy in a meta-analysis format (including the aforementioned GISSI-1 and ISIS-3, to be discussed later). The agents in the studies differed, of course, and the study design varied as well. The conclusion was that fibrinolytic therapy reduced overall mortality by 18% at 35 days, a highly significant impact (Fibrinolytic Therapy Trialists Group, 1994). This benefit was seen despite a highly significant excess of deaths on the day of randomization, which are the so-called early hazards attributed to cardiac rupture, electromechanical dissociation, and congestive heart failure, and a small but significant excess of strokes on days 0 to 1, generally due to cerebral hemorrhage. There was benefit in patients with both anterior and inferior infarctions with S-T elevation at all ages and in either gender. The earlier the patient was treated, the greater the benefit—in the same order of magnitude as in GISSI-1 (Fig. 16–3).

Choice of Thrombolytic Agent

Which agent improved the mortality statistics most favorably? Several comparative trials have examined the relative efficacies of streptokinase versus recombinant tissue plasminogen activator, tPA. In the GISSI-2 trial (Gruppo Italiano per lo Studio della Sopravvivenza nell' Infarto Miocardico, 1990) as well as the Third International Study of Infarct Survival (ISIS-3 [Third Interna-

tional Study of Infarct Survival] Collaborative Group, 1992), there was no difference between streptokinase or tPA for in-hospital or late mortality. In both of these studies, the mortality rates were of the same order of magnitude and rose slightly over the few months after discharge, which is similar to the prethrombolytic era asymptotic curve for Q-wave infarctions. In both trials, tPA caused a significant excess of strokes in the range of 4 per 1000 patients, as well as an excess of cerebral hemorrhage, although cerebral hemorrhage achieved statistical significance only in ISIS-3.

Among the criticisms of GISSI-2 and ISIS-3 was the use of subcutaneous heparin even in the tPA group, which was considered suboptimal to prevent early reocclusion. The Global Utilization of Streptokinase and Tissue Plasminogen Activator for Occluded Coronary Arteries (GUSTO) Investigators (1993) randomized 41,021 patients to four treatment arms within 6 hours of symptoms. The two "conventional" study arms included an accelerated tPA dosage regimen with immediate IV heparin and a streptokinase regimen, also with immediate IV heparin. The other two arms included a combined streptokinase and tPA regimen with immediate IV heparin and a conventional streptokinase regimen but with delayed subcutaneous heparin.

As far as the thrombolytic regimen was concerned, the group with accelerated tPA/IV heparin had the lowest mortality of the four regimens, 6.3%, albeit with a significant excess of stroke and cerebral hemorrhage, which were almost twofold those of the streptokinase/subcutaneous heparin group (0.94% vs. 0.49%). As is discussed later regarding anticoagulation and antithrombins, there was a disadvantage to subcutaneous heparin in the streptokinase dosing arm, with more hemorrhage noted.

Analysis of some prespecified subgroups indicated that patients younger than 75 years old, presenting within 4 hours and with anterior wall myocardial infarction, achieved maximal benefit from therapy with accelerated tPA/IV heparin, as compared with streptokinase/subcutaneous heparin treatment. There was an increase in hemorrhagic stroke in the population older than 75 years, and this increase narrowed the absolute difference between the two agents. Although there were differences between the drugs related to time to treatment, the differences narrowed as the time grew later, and the mortality benefit with tPA compared with streptokinase (SK) essentially disappeared at more than 6 hours after symptom onset.

The GUSTO-1 angiographic substudy (The

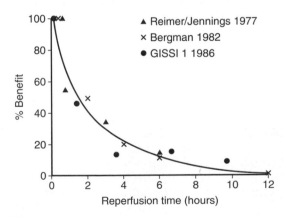

Figure 16–3
Plot of the benefit anticipated by the interval between coronary occlusion and reperfusion in GISSI-1 and two animal studies, demonstrating the similarity between anticipated and clinical results. (From Tiefenbrunn AJ, Sobel BE: Timing of coronary recanalization: paradigms, paradoxes, and pertinence. Circulation 85:2314, 1992. Reproduced with permission. Copyright 1992 American Heart Association.)

GUSTO-1 Angiographic Investigators, 1993; Simes et al, 1995) provided at least a partial explanation of the improved survival with tPA given early. Achievement of TIMI grade 3 flow (Table 16–1) at 90 minutes regardless of treatment regimen was associated with a 30-day mortality rate of 4.0% as compared with 8.4% for TIMI grade 0 flow at 90 minutes. Importantly, at 90 minutes, coronary patency at the level of TIMI grade 3 flow was higher in the tPA/IV heparin group compared with the SK/subcutaneous heparin group (54% vs. 29%); at 180 minutes, SK showed nearly equivalent patency to tPA. Furthermore, by 90 minutes, only 19% of the accelerated tPA group had level 0 or 1 flow. This data suggests that early restoration of complete flow was associated with a better survival and that this degree of reperfusion was more likely to be attained with tPA.

Consistent with early reports from the Western Washington Study, partial restoration of flow was far less successful. Even TIMI grade 2 flow was associated with a 30-day survival that was not significantly different from that of patients with TIMI grade 0 flow.

As a reminder of the tremendous potential of rapid reperfusion of the infarction-related coronary artery, a comparison of the data gathered by the GISSI investigators in 1986 with the GUSTO-1 angiographic substudy data is illuminating (Fig. 16–4). In GISSI-1, the mortality was in the range of 9% when SK was delivered less than 3 hours from onset of symptoms and nearly 12% when delivered from 3 to 6 hours from onset. In comparison, GUSTO found a 30-day mortality of as little as 4.0% in patients who had TIMI grade 3 flow at 90 minutes.

Time of Latest Treatment

How late can one treat with thrombolytic drugs and still obtain benefit from thrombolysis? The Late Assessment of Thrombolytic Efficacy (LATE) Study randomized 5711 patients to tPA

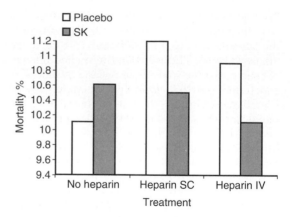

Figure 16–4
A small improvement in mortality was seen in patients treated with intravenous heparin in GISSI-1 as compared with response to subcutaneous heparin or no heparin at all. (From Gruppo Italiano per lo Studio della Streptochinasi nell' Infarto Miocardico: Effectiveness of intravenous thrombolytic treatment in acute myocardial infarction. Lancet 2:397–401, 1986. With permission. Copyright by The Lancet Ltd, 1986.)

treatment (not given in the accelerated dosage, but rather in the conventional 3-hour infusion) at 6 to 24 hours after symptoms (LATE Study Group, 1993). There was a 14.1% relative reduction in mortality with tPA at 35 days, but the absolute mortality was fairly low in both groups, 10.3% with placebo and 8.9% with tPA. The 35-day mortality for tPA was essentially unchanged for those treated earlier than 12 hours (8.9%), as compared with mortality in patients treated later than 12 hours (8.7%); however, the placebo-treated patients demonstrated a higher 35-day mortality rate (12.0%) for the earlier treatment as compared with 9.2% in the later treatment group.

The significant benefit for tPA comes in the context of an inflated mortality rate for the early-treated placebo group. The relative risk reduction for the patients treated with tPA from 12 to 24 hours after symptom onset was fairly low (5.4%), suggesting very little difference between treatment regimens when treatment is delayed and raising the issue of cost-effectiveness. Moreover, survival was similar for tPA given from 6 to 24 hours after onset and placebo administered after 12 hours, suggesting that there was no real effect seen with treatment after 6 hours. This finding is consistent with the GUSTO angiographic substudy. Benefit requires early and complete restoration of flow. Time is (indeed) muscle.

A vast literature has developed in the aftermath of the publication of the ISIS-3, GISSI-2,

Table 16–1
TIMI Perfusion Grades

0	Absent antegrade flow
1	Incomplete filling of the distal vessel
2	Complete opacification, delayed washout
3	Normal vessel flow

From The TIMI Study Group: The Thrombolysis in Myocardial Infarction (TIMI) trial. N Engl J Med 312:932–936, 1985. Copyright 1985. Massachusetts Medical Society. All rights reserved.

and GUSTO studies, deconstructing them based on the dissimilarities of the study designs, heparin regimen, and subgroup analysis (Ridker et al, 1993; Lee et al, 1994; Ridker et al, 1994). All are united in certain key conclusions. The *sine qua non* of reduction of mortality is in the wider utilization of thrombolytic drugs, regardless of which specific agent is chosen (Hennekens et al, 1995). It is incumbent upon the physician caring for patients with myocardial infarction to ensure that, early in the course of management, the role of thrombolysis is actively considered. It is equally incumbent upon the health care organization to ensure that this therapy can be delivered promptly and safely in an appropriately monitored environment. It is incumbent upon the early responders to the scene of a patient with myocardial infarction to ensure prompt transport of that patient to the most appropriate environment for delivery of reperfusion therapy.

Cost Analysis

In the current health care environment, cost is a major issue in the clinical decision for use of any therapy, and in the case of thrombolysis, the wide disparity between the costs of the two major drugs (approximately $2500 for tPA versus $400 for SK) makes the situation more complicated. A cost analysis from GUSTO data (Mark et al, 1995) used a social perspective (i.e., the benefit to society as a whole) to identify relevant costs and expressed the cost per year of life saved. The investigators found that tPA was cost-effective, but less so in patients younger than 40 years of age and the subgroup of patients with inferior wall myocardial infarction less than 60 years of age. The American College of Chest Physicians (ACCP) Consensus Conference notes that although individual decisions about the use of tPA versus SK should consider the cost-effectiveness of the drug chosen based on the varying benefit to the specific group being considered, tPA appeared to be reasonably cost-effective in patients younger than 75 years of age with large infarctions when administered within 6 hours of onset of myocardial infarction (Cairns et al, 1995b).

In summary, coronary thrombolysis is an effective therapy when it is administered within 6 hours or less from the onset of symptoms of myocardial infarction. Its value is diminished and its risks are similar to those of early administration when it is given from 6 to 12 hours after onset of symptoms, but it may be useful in some patients who are continuing to have active ischemia or for those with a stuttering presentation. Although thrombolysis has benefit for infarctions with S-T

elevation in the anterior and inferior electrocardiographic areas, it has little value for infarctions characterized with S-T depression alone. There is no contraindication to its use in patients who are older than 75 years of age. To be maximally effective, thrombolytics must be administered with as little delay as possible after the patient's arrival in the emergency department.

PRIMARY ANGIOPLASTY IN MYOCARDIAL INFARCTION

Considering the pathogenesis of myocardial infarction as a plaque that fissures and develops an overlying thrombus, it is not surprising that a combined attack on the thrombus, with thrombolytic drugs, and on the plaque, with angioplasty, was an attractive concept. Bringing the concept to actualization has been more difficult, for, as in the Western Washington intracoronary trials, the logistics involved in performing this procedure promptly are daunting. The three variants of the technique are administration of a thrombolytic followed by immediate angioplasty, which is seldom performed at present; "rescue angioplasty"; and primary angioplasty without thrombolytics, which is the most commonly performed of the acute invasive procedures.

Immediate Angioplasty

What was initially called *immediate angioplasty*, but perhaps is better termed *adjunctive angioplasty*, refers to the routine performance of angioplasty after the administration of a thrombolytic agent. The Thrombolysis and Angioplasty in Myocardial Infarction (TAMI) and the Thrombolysis in Myocardial Infarction Phase II (TIMI II) megatrials found this approach to be associated with a worse outcome (Topol et al, 1987; The TIMI Study Group, 1989).

TAMI examined the outcomes of patients who had been treated with 150 mg of tPA within 4 hours (mean, 2.95 hours) of onset of myocardial infarction. For those in whom catheterization demonstrated TIMI grade 2 or 3 flow but with residual stenosis in the infarction-related coronary artery, randomization to immediate or elective (7–10 days) angioplasty was performed. The results showed that, despite successful dilation in 86% of patients, the mortality in the immediate-treatment group was 4.0%, whereas that in the elective-treatment group was 1.0%. In addition, immediate angioplasty did not improve global or regional left ventricular function or decrease recurrent ischemic events. Moreover, this lack of benefit was seen despite only 35% of the patients in the elective group actually undergoing angioplasty at days 7 to 10, although there was a 16% crossover rate to emergency angioplasty in the elective-treatment group because of recurrent ischemia, mostly within 24 hours of presentation.

In TIMI II, patients treated with tPA had angiography at 18 to 48 hours ("immediate") after onset of myocardial infarction or conservative therapy with crossover to angiography if there was ischemia during the hospitalization. Because of this design, the immediate-treatment group received catheterization at a mean of 32.5 hours after the infarction, or nearly 1½ days (vs. about 90 minutes in TAMI-1). Of this group, nearly 54% underwent attempted angioplasty. In contrast, the conservatively treated group ultimately underwent angiography within 14 days, and 13% required angioplasty. The invasive strategy resulted in a statistically insignificant increase in death and reinfarction. In addition, there was no benefit in left ventricular function. Of note, subgroup analysis failed to identify who may benefit from immediate angioplasty.

Rescue Angioplasty

From 20 to 30% of patients who receive IV thrombolytics fail to achieve reperfusion. GUSTO-1 showed that, using the most successful regimen, which was accelerated tPA, only 54% had TIMI grade 3 flow at 90 minutes, leaving 46% with less than optimal results. The TAMI-5 study included a group of patients who had cardiac catheterization after failed thrombolysis (residual TIMI grade 0–1 flow) compared with a group undergoing delayed elective predischarge catheterization. There was a trend toward higher TIMI grade 2 and 3 patency at the time of leaving the catheterization laboratory (greater than 94%) and predischarge (94%) in the aggressive strategy group and significant improvement in wall motion and clinical outcome parameters (Califf et al, 1991). However, even the delayed catheterization strategy resulted in 90% predischarge patency.

To date, only one randomized comparison of rescue angioplasty with conservative therapy (Ellis et al, 1994) has been performed. Patients with anterior wall myocardial infarction were randomized an average of 4.5 hours after onset of pain to emergency percutaneous transluminal coronary angioplasty (PTCA) if TIMI 0 or 1 flow was seen in the left anterior descending coronary artery after treatment with thrombolytic agents. Angioplasty restored coronary patency, which persisted to the time of discharge, in 92% compared with 42% for the conservatively treated group. There was no statistical difference at 30 days in ejection fraction, mortality, congestive heart failure (CHF), or ventricular tachycardia. A clinical difference in the event rates (5.1% vs. 9.6% for death and 1.3% vs. 7.0% for CHF) in the angioplasty versus conservative treatment group was seen. Thus, the ultimate role of rescue angioplasty remains unclear. Because only coronary arteriography can accurately identify failure of thrombolysis, logistical considerations severely limit widespread application of rescue angioplasty.

Primary Angioplasty

A more central role is evolving for primary or direct angioplasty, defined as angioplasty performed immediately after myocardial infarction as a primary means of achieving reperfusion. Although adjunctive therapy with heparin and aspirin is used, no thrombolytics are administered. Results for this technique are improving because of technical advances such as stents, which, contrary to early fears of exacerbating thrombus formation, seem to decrease the incidence of problematic results after the performance of PTCA. In comparison, as in the studies of intracoronary thrombolysis, the often overwhelming logistics may be the rate-limiting step. Indeed, this approach assumes rapid and appropriate selection of patients combined with immediate availability of interventional cardiologists at all times of the day and night. In the absence of massive infusions of resources, this approach will remain limited in application (Lange and Hillis, 1993).

To date, the largest randomized investigation of the efficacy of primary angioplasty is the Primary Angioplasty in Myocardial Infarction (PAMI) Trial (Grines et al, 1993). In this trial, 395 patients were randomized to treatment with tPA or to angiography and planned angioplasty. Reperfusion was achieved in 99% of the angioplasty group. There were no strokes in the PTCA treatment group, compared with a 2.0% incidence of hemorrhagic stroke in the patients receiving thrombolysis (a surprisingly high number), all of whom died. There was an overall trend toward lower mortality (2.6% vs. 6.5%) and reinfarction rates (2.6% vs. 6.5%) with primary angioplasty, but the mortality was significantly lower only in the PTCA subgroup classified as "not low risk," 2.0% versus 10.4% in the tPA treatment group. Recurrent ischemia, in which the investigators included reinfarction, showed a significant difference in favor of PTCA (10.3% vs. 28.0%). Half of the PTCA-treated patients underwent repeat catheterization, but 84% of the tPA-treated patients ultimately underwent catheterization because of recurrent ischemia. Rescue angioplasty was required in 7% of tPA-treated patients. Importantly, from a logistical point of view, the time from randomization to start of treatment was longer in the PTCA-treated group, 60 minutes versus 32 minutes for tPA; however, time from symptom onset to resolution of pain was shorter for PTCA than for tPA treatment by more than 1 hour (290 vs. 354 minutes), demonstrating that the entire PTCA procedure is more expeditious, obtaining reperfusion faster than tPA. The hospital stay was shorter in the PTCA group than in the tPA treatment group (7.5 vs. 8.4 days).

A much smaller study from the Mayo Clinic (Gibbons et al, 1993) examined myocardial salvage as assessed by sestamibi radionuclide injection before initiating reperfusion therapy in 108 patients randomized to treatment with immediate PTCA or tPA (in the double-stranded form, duteplase). There was no difference in mortality. More myocardium appeared to be salvaged in the PTCA treatment group, but the difference was insignificant between the two groups. When the data were adjusted to account for the greater number of anterior wall myocardial infarctions in the thrombolysis group, there was no difference between the groups. Recurrent ischemia requiring revascularization (coronary artery bypass graft [CABG] surgery or PTCA) developed in 36% of thrombolysis-assigned patients.

The Zwolle study (Zijlstra et al, 1993) randomized 142 patients with acute myocardial infarction to receive SK or immediate PTCA. With a time to balloon inflation similar to that in PAMI, the incidence of recurrent ischemia was significantly lower in patients with PTCA, with fewer complications or required procedures.

A number of nonrandomized trials have compared primary PTCA with thrombolysis. A meta-analysis was performed in an attempt to assess the results of these studies, and the results showed lower mortality and reinfarction rates for PTCA (Michels and Yusuf, 1995). The investigators cautioned that only two of the trials reviewed found a benefit for PTCA in left ventricular function and that the highly specialized milieu of the participating centers made the extrapolation of the overall results to general cardiac practice difficult.

The relative cost has been evaluated by the Mayo study investigators (Reeder et al, 1994). Indirect costs were not measured in dollars; there was a significant increase for the thrombolysis group for the number of "late" procedures in which crossover reperfusion therapy was initiated after 24 hours, usually angiography/PTCA in the tPA-treated patients. Despite this increase, the dollar amount of the direct costs of the hospitalization, approximated from hospital and professional fee charges, did not differ between the two groups. Substitution of SK for tPA further reduced the mean cost for the thrombolysis group. This is not surprising, but the model used was different from the analysis used by GUSTO, as noted previously (Mark et al, 1995).

The AHA/ACC Task Force (AHA/ACC Taskforce Report, 1993) has recommended primary angioplasty for patients who are

Less than 6 hours after onset of myocardial infarction
Within 6–12 hours but have continued ischemic symptoms
In cardiogenic shock within 12 hours of onset

Where possible, primary angioplasty is an important modality and may be superior to thrombolysis. The bottom line is the provision of some form of effective reperfusion therapy as soon and as safely as possible. If primary angioplasty will result in delay, it is unlikely that the patient will benefit and, in fact, is likely to suffer greater myocardial loss by being denied immediate thrombolysis. The enemy of good is better if better requires time-wasting logistics.

ACE INHIBITORS IN MYOCARDIAL INFARCTION

Angiotensin-converting enzyme (ACE) inhibitors have assumed a central role in the management of patients with myocardial infarction for immediate as well as long-term therapy. Although the understanding of the mechanism of their benefit is undergoing radical change, that they have benefit is well accepted.

Left ventricular dilation is a major pathophysiologic component of systolic left ventricular dysfunction, and ventricular size and function are important predictors of survival after myocardial infarction (White et al, 1987; Multicenter Diltiazem Postinfarction Trial Research Group, 1988). Infarct expansion, which is the process of stretching and thinning of necrotic infarcted myocardium, is an early process that is found in humans and in animal research preparations as early as 3 days after myocardial infarction. Left ventricular dilation begins in the peri-infarction period and continues for months (Pfeffer et al, 1988). This process, called remodeling, involves myocyte "slippage" (rearrangement of the myocyte bundles) and myocyte lengthening and thinning. Hypertrophy occurs during this period, mediated in part by angiotensin II, and serves as a compensatory reaction to the increased wall stress (Lonn et al, 1994).

Gaudron and coworkers found that myocardial infarction patients with limited left ventricular dilation had increasing ventricular volumes up to 4 weeks after myocardial infarction, and then stabilized. Presumably, the ventricular enlargement was a compensatory mechanism. A second group with large myocardial infarctions continued to have an increase in left ventricular volume progressively over a 3-year period and a decreased ejection fraction and cardiac index concurrently with rising pulmonary wedge pressure (Gaudron et al, 1993).

Several large trials have shown the efficacy of ACE inhibition in patients with varying degrees of left ventricular dysfunction. The Survival and Ventricular Enlargement (SAVE) Trial looked at the efficacy of captopril in 2231 patients with anterior myocardial infarction and an ejection fraction less than 40%. Treatment began, on average, 11 days after the myocardial infarction. A 19% reduction in mortality was found (Pfeffer et al, 1992). Interestingly, a post hoc analysis noted a decrease in the number of recurrent myocardial infarctions in the captopril group as compared with the placebo treatment group, suggesting that captopril's benefit derives from its less well-known anti-ischemic effects as well as its well-known use as a vasodilator (Rutherford et al, 1994). The Acute Infarction Ramipril Efficacy Study (AIRE) showed that ACE inhibitors other than captopril demonstrated efficacy as well, even when administration was delayed to the second to ninth day after infarction in patients with CHF, which is a high-risk population (The Acute Infarction Ramipril Efficacy Study Investigators, 1993).

The optimal time to begin therapy with ACE inhibitors has been controversial. When administered intravenously, ACE inhibition did not fare well. The Second Cooperative New Scandinavian Enalapril Survival Study (CONSENSUS II) ad-ministered enalaprilat IV within 24 hours of onset of myocardial infarction in a relatively low-risk group. The study was terminated early by the study's safety committee after preliminary analysis suggested that there seemed to be no difference between the drug and placebo and that there may be a harmful effect, particularly in elderly patients with early hypotensive responses (Swedberg et al, 1992).

In the Survival of Myocardial Infarction Long Term Evaluation (SMILE), oral zofenopril was started at a mean of 15 hours after symptoms in patients with anterior wall myocardial infarction who did not receive thrombolysis, which is a rather high-risk group in the present era. Interestingly, despite discontinuing therapy at 6 weeks, a 25% reduction in mortality risk was sustained to 1 year (Ambrosioni et al, 1995).

Less—but real—risk reduction was found in two megatrials of oral ACE inhibitors in all patients with suspected myocardial infarction. These lower risk patients started treatment within 1 day after myocardial infarction. GISSI-3 (Gruppo Italiano per lo Studio della Sopravvivenza nell' Infarto Miocardico, 1994) and ISIS-4 (ISIS-4 Collaborative Group, 1995) both found benefit for ACE inhibitor–treated patients, with GISSI-3 demonstrating 11% and ISIS-4 showing 7% risk reduction. The benefit in these low-risk groups was substantially lower than in the higher risk SMILE group.

A consensus committee of investigators (Latini et al, 1995) from the major trials has suggested a set of principles useful in ACE inhibitor therapy after myocardial infarction (Table 16–2).

BETA BLOCKERS

Since their introduction in the 1960s, beta adrenergic blocking agents have been applied to cardiac

---

Table 16–2
Guidelines for Use of ACE Inhibitors After Myocardial Infarction

Patients with signs and symptoms of LV dysfunction should be treated, perhaps lifelong

Early (first 24 hours) treatment is appropriate for patients with acute MI in the absence of contraindications and with favorable hemodynamic status. However, subgroups with greater efficacy have not been identified

ACE inhibitor treatment may be discontinued after 4 to 6 weeks if LV dysfunction is not apparent, even if the patient is asymptomatic

Doses of medication are individualized, but study doses should be targeted. The patient's LV function should be re-evaluated after 4 to 6 months

There has been no additional risk demonstrated for the elderly or for women

Adapted from Latini R, Maggioni AP, Flather M, et al: ACE inhibitor use in patients with myocardial infarction: Summary of evidence from clinical trials. Circulation 92:3132–3137, 1995. Reproduced with permission. Copyright 1995 American Heart Association.

disease in a variety of clinical circumstances. It was hoped in the 1960s and 1970s that potent block of sympathetic outflow would decrease infarction size and thus mortality in the acute period after myocardial infarction. The design of the trials of the 1960s used different doses, times from symptom onset to dosing, and duration of therapy. Although the larger trials of these agents completed in the 1970s show a consistent pattern of survival benefit, controversy still surrounds their early IV use and their incremental value in patients treated with reperfusion techniques.

Intravenous Beta-Blocker Therapy

A meta-analysis of 27 randomized studies performed in the pre-thrombolytic era compared results in 27,500 patients who were given beta-blockers or placebo (Yusuf et al, 1988b). The analysis showed a 13% reduction in mortality in the first week of treatment, with the reduction most marked in the first 2 days (25%). The reduction in mortality was attributed to prevention of cardiac rupture and ventricular fibrillation. This analysis added support to the practice of starting beta-blockers early in the peri-infarction period, at least for patients not being treated with thrombolytics.

The largest of the trials included in the meta-analysis, the ISIS-1 trial (ISIS Collaborative Group, 1986), prospectively tested the addition of beta-blockers to the acute treatment regimen of patients not treated with thrombolytics. The investigators randomized 16,027 patients into active or control treatment groups. The control group was not given placebo. The active treatment group was given 5 mg of atenolol IV followed by a second dose 10 minutes later. Oral atenolol was then given until discharge. There was a 15% mortality difference between the atenolol group and the control group (2p<.04), with the benefit observed over the first day. The decrease in mortality with atenolol was most marked in females and in patients over 65 years old. The reduction in mortality in ISIS-1 was partially attributed to a decrease in the incidence of myocardial rupture (ISIS-1 Collaborative Group, 1988). Death from ventricular fibrillation was also less common in the atenolol group (5 vs. 13 patients), but bradycardia/asystole was more common (10 vs. 3 patients).

Can beta-blockers serve as anti-arrhythmics in the post-myocardial infarction period—at the price of the bradycardia commensurate with effective beta blockade? The question of the anti-arrhythmicity of beta blockade had been studied before ISIS. The early Goteburg trial (Ryden et al,

1983) randomized 1395 patients with suspected myocardial infarction to receive metoprolol or placebo at a mean of 11 hours after onset of symptoms. There were nearly three times as many cases of ventricular fibrillation over the entire hospital period in the placebo group than in the metoprolol group (17 vs. 6 patients, p<.05).

With the advent of thrombolytic therapy, the value of beta blockade has again been questioned. Does beta blockade have a role in the patient treated with thrombolysis? Unfortunately, only the Thrombolysis in Myocardial Infarction Phase II Trial (TIMI-2) has addressed this question, and even then in a limited fashion (The TIMI Study Group, 1989; Roberts et al, 1991).

The primary goal of the TIMI-2 trial was to compare results of early catheterization and PTCA to symptom-driven PTCA in patients treated with thrombolytic agents. Specifically, the trial assessed the possible reduction in reocclusion, rethrombosis, and reinfarction by routine coronary arteriography and PTCA performed 18 to 48 hours after the initiation of thrombolytic therapy. The TIMI 2B substudy enrolled 1434 eligible patients into an immediate metoprolol treatment group or a deferred beta-blocker therapy group, with oral metoprolol administered on day 6 and thereafter to all patients. The groups were randomized to receive invasive and conservative strategies, as well. There was no difference in the primary end point, which was global left ventricular ejection fraction at discharge, or in the secondary end points, death or reinfarction at any time of follow-up, in either the IV or deferred beta-blocker therapy groups. A highly statistically significant benefit was seen for immediate metoprolol in recurrent ischemia (p=.005) and a smaller benefit was seen for nonfatal reinfarction (p=.02). This benefit was lost, however, by 6 weeks (TIMI, 1989). When reperfusion with tPA was performed within the first 2 hours after onset of symptoms, benefit was observed for immediate beta-blockers solely in the combined secondary end points of reinfarction or death at 6 weeks (but not at 6 days or at 1 year) compared with results in the patients for whom metoprolol treatment was deferred (5.4% vs. 13.7%, p<.007).

Overall, results of the study suggested that beta-blocker therapy can be safely administered in patients with acute myocardial infarction who were being treated with reperfusion to obtain the short-term benefits of decreased myocardial ischemia and reinfarction, but not to decrease the incidence of death. Administration of beta-blockers did not seem to convey any meaningful benefit over prompt reperfusion therapy itself. Some data in this study raised warning flags. Decreased blood pressure or clinical signs of decreased perfusion were experienced in the IV beta-blocker group somewhat more frequently than in the deferred group (33.2% vs. 28.4%, p = 0.05).

Based on these data, guidelines published by the American College of Cardiology (ACC) and the American Heart Association (AHA) in 1990 (Gunnar et al, 1990) recommend IV beta-blockers in patients with acute myocardial infarction who present with reflex tachycardia or systolic hypertension, continuing or recurrent ischemic pain, or atrial fibrillation, and in those with no contraindication to taking this class of drug. It was recommended that other patients with myocardial infarction with no contraindications be given a class IIA recommendation (i.e., acceptable but of uncertain efficacy, with the weight of evidence in favor of usefulness) for routine early IV beta blockade. These guidelines are in process of revision at present and are due to be reissued in 1996.

Long-term Beta Blockade for Secondary Prevention

In addition to the meta-analysis mentioned earlier, several placebo-controlled trials support beta blockade begun in the early phase of myocardial infarction and continued for periods of months to years. These studies, which were mostly performed in the prethrombolytic era, found improvement in survival and a decrease in reinfarction for at least several months after the myocardial infarction (Yusuf et al, 1988b). The Beta-Blocker Heart Attack Trial Research Group (BHAT), using fixed doses of propranolol, 180 or 240 mg/day, demonstrated a 28% decrease in mortality over 2 years as compared with a placebo group (9.8% vs. 7.2%). There was no risk reduction in patients with "nontransmural" myocardial infarction (Beta-Blocker Heart Attack Trial Research Group, 1982).

The combined ACC and AHA class I recommendations for long-term beta blockade include all but low-risk patients, with therapy continuing for at least 2 years. The low-risk patients are included as a class IIA (see earlier) recommendation if there is no contraindication and with consideration for potential side effects.

Usage Patterns

Do cardiologists use beta-blockers in acute myocardial infarction? Data from the National Registry of Myocardial Infarction (NRMI) as well as studies from other countries suggest that they do not, at least as much as they should or could.

NRMI found that, in patients who had received thrombolytics, 17% received IV and 36% oral beta-blockers. For the group who had not received thrombolytic therapy, 30 and 42% received IV or oral beta-blocker therapy (Rogers et al, 1994). In GUSTO, however, nearly half of the patients received IV beta-blockers and 71% received oral beta-blockers (Pilote et al, 1995). The GUSTO investigators found a marked regional difference in myocardial infarction management with a range of 55 to 81% utilization of beta-blockers across the United States. Brand and coworkers reported fewer than 50% of eligible patients received beta-blockers in a study of insurance claims from 17 network–model health plans in 10 states (Brand et al, 1995).

Our recommendations are long-term (at least 2 years) oral beta blockade in nearly all patients, particularly those deemed to be at high risk, and IV beta blockade only in selected moderate-risk patients treated with thrombolytics with no contraindications to beta blockade, who are not undergoing revascularization.

ADJUNCTIVE THERAPY

A coronary thrombus forms when a coronary atheromatous plaque ruptures. When a plaque ruptures, subendothelial collagen is exposed and tissue factor is released, causing the aggregation of platelets, the generation of thrombin, arachidonic acid, and thromboxane A_2, and ultimately the formation of a "red" thrombus. Plaque rupture is a complex process. The fibrous cap of the soft atheroma is stressed at its weakest point—the area of attachment to the normal intimal wall. The cap is thinnest at this point and most heavily infiltrated with foam cells that weaken the local tissue. This site is an easy target for various metalloproteinases and other proteolytic enzymes secreted by local macrophages. Plaques that rupture are indeed not the heavily calcified, thick atheromas but those that are relatively small, often causing less than 50% luminal stenosis on angiography (Little et al, 1988).

A focus of therapy has been the more efficacious use of available agents and development of new agents that will limit this process, preventing ongoing thrombus formation.

Thrombin and Antithrombin Agents

Thrombin is a critical nexus in the pathogenesis of the acute coronary syndrome and is the central actor in the "thrombin hypothesis." It plays several roles in the thrombotic process. It is the most potent platelet activating stimulus and is not inhibited by aspirin's effect on platelets. Thrombin may cause platelet aggregation despite aspirin. Thrombin has a direct chemotactic effect on monocytes, converts fibrinogen to fibrin, and activates factor XIII— the factor that enhances the crosslinking of the fibrin clot, thus stabilizing it and solidifying it. A paradox in the use of thrombolytic agents is that it may lead to increased amounts of thrombin in the peri-infarction period, thereby serving as procoagulants.

Heparin

Heparin is currently the most readily available antithrombin agent. Heparin has a high affinity for binding to antithrombin III, inducing a conformational change in the antithrombin III molecule, accelerating its binding to thrombin, factor Xa, and factor IXa. Heparin serves as a template to bring antithrombin III in proximity to thrombin, thus forming a ternary complex. It also binds to antithrombin III without forming a ternary complex to inhibit factor Xa. When thrombin is bound in clots, its heparin binding site is not accessible, and heparin is prevented from "passivating" (the opposite of activate, implying a process of inactivation and inhibition) the active thrombotic lesion by inhibiting thrombin's effects. This, as well as its molecular heterogeneity causing biologic variability, limits heparin's abilities as the ultimate anti-thrombin agent.

Heparin in adjunctive treatment of patients who have received tPA is essentially noncontroversial at this time. Several angiographic studies have shown improved patency with IV heparin and tPA, although these results are usually seen in the presence of aspirin. GUSTO-1 compared treatment with tPA and full-dose IV heparin to treatment with SK and either IV or subcutaneous heparin, finding that tPA with heparin resulted in better 90-minute patency and improved survival in this group (The GUSTO Investigators, 1993).

There is still considerable controversy over the use of heparin with SK. In both GISSI-1 and ISIS-2, anticoagulant treatment was not specifically part of the study design. Indeed, in GISSI-1 there was no difference in the group treated with anticoagulation as compared with the group treated without it. The ISIS-2 data demonstrate a slightly lower mortality in the IV heparin group than in the subcutaneous heparin group and the no-heparin treatment group, for patients treated with SK alone. Of note, the mortality rate of the placebo–no heparin group was lower than that for placebo with heparin and was equivalent to that with SK–IV heparin treatment.

In both GISSI-2 and ISIS-3, all patients were randomized to treatment with fibrinolysis and received subcutaneous heparin no earlier than 4 to 24 hours after symptom onset. Heparin had no effect on survival, reinfarction, or stroke incidence, but the incidence of bleeding was increased.

The timing and administration of heparin has been much criticized in the United States, where early IV heparin is favored. As a result, GUSTO-1 compared results of treatment SK and delayed subcutaneous heparin to treatment with SK and immediate IV heparin, finding no difference between mortality or hemorrhagic stroke rates. The ACCP Consensus Panel concluded that patients treated with SK should receive IV heparin only in situations of high risk for systemic or venous thromboembolism. Patients receiving tPA should be administered IV heparin to maintain the activated partial thromboplastin time (aPTT) at 1.5 to 2 times control for about 48 hours. After 48 hours, aspirin alone suffices to inhibit reocclusion.

Because of the risk of systemic and pulmonary embolism, anticoagulation with at least low-dose heparin (7500 U subcutaneous every 12 hours) has been recommended by the ACCP Consensus Panel (Cairns et al, 1995b). In particular, the panel recommended that patients deemed to be at high risk for systemic or pulmonary embolism, including patients with anterior Q-wave infarctions, congestive heart failure, or severe left ventricular dysfunction; evidence on echocardiography of a mural thrombus; atrial fibrillation; or a previous embolic event should receive IV heparin, followed by warfarin for up to 3 months.

Other Antithrombin Agents

The direct thrombin inhibitors bind to thrombin without the intervention of antithrombin III. Hirudin is a naturally occurring 65 amino acid polypeptide originally derived from the leech but now manufactured, using recombinant deoxyribonucleic acid (DNA) technology, in the desulfatoform, resulting in less affinity for thrombin than in the native form. Hirulog (Biogen, Cambridge, MA) is a smaller synthetic polypeptide. These compounds bind both to the substrate recognition center and to the active catalytic site on the thrombin molecule. The effects of Hirulog are more transient than those of hirudin with a shorter half life; nonetheless, both have a more consistent effect on the aPTT than does heparin.

Two other new antithrombin agents, PPACK (D-phenylalanyl-L-propyl-L-arginyl chloromethylketone) and argatroban, work by binding to the active catalytic site of thrombin. They have less specificity for thrombin than do hirudin and Hirulog.

Preliminary data on the direct thrombin inhibitors suggest that these are potentially beneficial adjuncts to thrombolytic drugs. Hirudin was efficacious in restoring TIMI grade 3 flow in the TIMI-5, TIMI-6, and HIT-1 trials. The toxic-to-therapeutic ratio is quite small. In the TIMI-9A, GUSTO-IIA, and HIT-3 trials, hirudin was associated with an increase in intracranial hemorrhage, requiring a change in the dosing schedule for the TIMI-9B and GUSTO-IIB configurations (Antman, 1994; Neuhaus et al, 1994; The Global Use of Strategies to Open Occluded Coronary Arteries [GUSTO] IIA Investigators, 1994). Preliminary results of the GUSTO IIB study showed a reduction in deaths and myocardial infarctions over the first 24 hours after administration, but at 30 days, there was no significant benefit compared with heparin-treated patients.

Hirulog has been studied in conjunction with SK, comparing it with heparin. The results appear promising, but more work must be done to clarify the clinically effective dose.

Warfarin

Even before the use of thrombolytic drugs in myocardial infarction, numerous studies examined the use of anticoagulants in the peri-infarction period. However, only three studies were large enough to affect clinical practice, and in each of these, the study design included oral anticoagulation. The Bronx Municipal Hospital Center Trial (Drapkin and Merskey, 1972) was the only trial to find a statistically significant decline in all-cause mortality in 1136 patients who received heparin 5000 U IV followed by subcutaneous heparin for the next 2 days. Only 61% of these patients were proved to have a myocardial infarction. There was no effect on reinfarction, pulmonary embolus, or stroke. The influence of the short-term oral anticoagulation in this study is debatable.

The Anticoagulation in the Secondary Prevention of Events in Coronary Thrombosis (ASPECT) Research Group is a contemporary long-term study of anticoagulation after myocardial infarction. Although the patients were treated with nicoumalone or phenprocoumon rather than warfarin, the study found higher event-free survival (83% vs. 76%; p<.001) and a significant risk reduction (59%) for reinfarction in the anticoagulated group (Anticoagulation in the Secondary Prevention of Events in Coronary Thrombosis [ASPECT] Research Group, 1994).

Although warfarin does appear beneficial after myocardial infarction, we recommend aspirin as the agent of choice until such time as randomized trials show the superiority of warfarin. Indeed, preliminary data from the Coumadin Aspirin Reinfarction Study showed no benefit of low-dose warfarin combined with aspirin compared with aspirin alone in preventing death, nonfatal myocardial infarction, or stroke. Clearly, more data are required to better answer this question.

ANTIPLATELET DRUGS IN MYOCARDIAL INFARCTION

Aspirin is an irreversible inhibitor of platelet cyclo-oxygenase, an enzyme critical in the process leading to the formation of the potent platelet aggregating agent and vasoconstrictor, thromboxane A_2. Aspirin is not effective against other strong agonists of platelet aggregation, including thrombin, collagen, and platelet-activating factor. When platelet activation is established by these agonists, glycoprotein (GP) IIb/IIIa receptors appear on the platelet surface and are bound to fibrinogen or von Willebrand factor, crosslinking the platelets to one another. Novel agents are now available to block the GP IIa/IIIb receptors, offering the possibility of more completely inhibiting this final common pathway step in platelet aggregation.

Aspirin

ISIS-2 was designed to answer the question of the value of aspirin therapy (162.5 mg/day, enteric coated) in comparison with SK in 17,187 patients with myocardial infarction. It demonstrated a 21% risk reduction for 5-week mortality with aspirin alone and a 40% risk reduction with aspirin added to SK. The risks of nonfatal infarction and stroke were reduced by nearly 50%, although minor bleeding increased slightly as well. Importantly, the time of administration of aspirin did not interfere with its benefits: if given within 24 hours from onset of symptoms its effect was equivalent. Whether this was a primary effect of aspirin or a secondary prevention effect is not clear.

The exact dose required was not clear from ISIS-2. The inhibitory effect on cyclooxygenase is obtained with small doses, on the order of 20 to 40 mg. It appears reasonable to treat with a minimum of 162 mg when the patient arrives in the Emergency Department but not to exceed 325 mg, because of increasing risk of gastric toxicity. Certainly, when used in conjunction with SK, there is no special benefit from administering both drugs together. Rather, the aspirin may be given later if not administered on arrival, as long as there is a check in the system to ensure that aspirin is not inadvertently omitted.

Integrins

An inhibitor of the GP IIb/IIIa receptor, abciximab (ReoPro, Lilly), was approved for use in angioplasty based on data demonstrating a 35% reduction in ischemic complications in high-risk cases (The EPIC Investigators, 1994). This drug, the Fab fragment of the monoclonal antibody 7E3, binds to the GP IIb/IIIa receptors and blocks them, preventing the crosslinking of fibrinogen and von Willebrand factor between platelets. Studies in acute myocardial infarction are progressing with abciximab, as well as with other GP IIb/IIIa receptor blocking agents such as the hexapeptide Integrelin.

OTHER ADJUNCTIVE AGENTS

Magnesium

On the basis of several small studies suggesting that magnesium may have efficacy in myocardial infarction, two large trials were performed but came to opposite conclusions. The LIMIT-2 trial randomized over 2300 patients to receive either magnesium sulfate or placebo for 24 hours after myocardial infarction. The result in the magnesium group was better than in the placebo group, with a relative reduction in mortality of 25%, from 7.8 to 10.3% (Woods et al, 1992). In contrast, the ISIS-4 trial (ISIS Collaborative Group, 1995) found no difference between the magnesium treatment group and the placebo treatment group for 35-day mortality.

The discrepancy between the positive results for LIMIT-2 as compared with those of ISIS-4 has been extensively argued (Antman, 1995). In ISIS-4, magnesium was administered later in the course, after the administration of thrombolytic agents but perhaps after reperfusion injury had already occurred. A large subset of patients in ISIS-4 had the magnesium administered at about the time of reperfusion, and they would have been expected therefore to have derived benefit, if some were to be had.

Nitrates

Intravenous Nitroglycerin

Nitroglycerin has been a mainstay of antianginal therapy for over 100 years, although its IV use for acute myocardial infarction was not advised until 1981 when the United States Food and Drug Administration approved it. On a mechanistic basis, there seems to be a rationale for nitroglycerin. At infusion rates averaging 37 μg/min, Flaherty found that nitroglycerin reduces left ventricular cnd-diastolic pressure (preload), which decreases left ventricular wall stress and thus oxygen demand (Flaherty et al, 1975). At slightly higher doses (averaging 57 μg/min), it lowered afterload by causing arterial vasodilatation, again reducing oxygen demand (Flaherty et al, 1976). It may improve myocardial oxygen supply by augmenting coronary collateral blood flow, reversing coronary vasoconstriction or vasospasm, improving endothelial function, and enlarging the lumen at the site of coronary stenoses.

Manipulation of afterload and preload are integral to the treatment of acute myocardial infarction, but this manipulation can lead to the major complications of nitroglycerin therapy, which are hypotension and tachycardia. Lowering coronary perfusion pressure with any vasodilator may provoke ischemia (Bodenheimer et al, 1981), and right ventricular infarction is associated with a hemodynamic picture in which preload is critically reduced. The concomitant administration of ACE inhibitors and the tachycardia-blunting effects of beta-blockers may help to confuse the clinical picture further, as may the tachycardia related to fever, anxiety, CHF, or pericarditis. The drug must be given in a monitored environment and patients' hemodynamic status should be carefully observed to ensure that problems with preload and afterload are not magnified. "Low-dose" infusions are given, beginning at 5 μg/min and increasing every 2–5 minutes, or more carefully if required, until mean arterial pressure is decreased by 10% or symptoms (particularly chest pain) abate. The usual maximal dose with this regimen is 200 μg/min (Jugdutt, 1992).

Intravenous nitroglycerin was not considered as an adjunctive therapy for myocardial infarction until several studies in the late 1970s and early 1980s suggested that it had some benefit in decreasing infarction size. These studies used indirect measurements of left ventricular damage, such as CK release and S-T elevation to make this determination (Flaherty et al, 1976). Most short-term studies of mortality showed no advantage for IV nitroglycerin, but data pooled by Yusuf and coworkers demonstrated a 35% reduction in mortality with this therapy (Yusuf et al, 1988a). Thus, indications for IV nitroglycerin include control of chest pain due to ongoing or recurrent ischemia, congestive heart failure, and lowering of mean arterial pressure in the hypertensive infarction patient.

Oral Nitrates

Two megatrials examined the role of oral nitrates in acute myocardial infarction. Both ISIS-4 (ISIS-4 Collaborative Group, 1995) and GISSI-3 (Gruppo Italiano per lo Studio della Sopravvivenza nell' Infarto Miocardico, 1994) assessed the efficacy of ACE inhibitors as well as nitrates (isosorbide mononitrate in ISIS-4 and IV nitroglycerin followed by transdermal nitroglycerin in GISSI-3) on mortality, with GISSI-3 also evaluating echocardiographic measures of left ventricular function. There was no effect of either preparation on the end points. This result has been explained by noting that the patients randomized in these trials were a relatively low-risk group, with mortality rates in the range of 7%. In addition, it is argued, the doses in the studies were low, and the effects of the ACE inhibitors may have masked any positive benefits from the oral nitrates. Nonetheless, it is clear that for most patients with myocardial infarction, there is no role for the routine use of oral nitrates in the routine care of a patient. Patients with recurrent ischemia or hypertension may be managed with other, more beneficial medications—ACE inhibitors are a strong first choice—without incurring the expense and potential risk of the nitrates.

HEMODYNAMIC AND MECHANICAL PROBLEMS IN MYOCARDIAL INFARCTION

The injury to the myocardium during acute infarction results in a region that is threatened not only by the dysfunction of damaged contractile elements resulting in systolic and diastolic dysfunction but by the disruption of tissue, particularly collagen, that permits an element of weakness in the affected wall (Whittaker et al, 1991). Thus, the major mechanical complications of myocardial infarction include cardiogenic shock and rupture of various myocardial sites. The contributions of thrombolytic therapy and the possible improvement with drug therapy, specifically beta blockade, are discussed in the appropriate sections.

CARDIOGENIC SHOCK

The diagnosis of cardiogenic shock is often not subtle. The patient appears to be hypoperfused, with decreased urine output (usually less than 20 ml/hr), vasoconstriction, tachycardia (heart rate greater than 100), and hypotension (systolic pressure less than 90 mm Hg). The lungs may be congested, as detected either on auscultation or on chest radiograms, or they may be normal. This distinction has led to the hemodynamic subset approach developed in the 1970s and found useful up to the present time. In this scheme, four hemodynamic subsets are defined (Table 16–3). The patient in shock, or at least hypotensive after acute myocardial infarction, usually belongs to subset III or IV (i.e., low cardiac output with either no pulmonary congestion or in congestive heart failure). A more difficult and significantly more subtle presenting picture is the patient whose mental status has become somewhat clouded or agitated, which is often at first thought to be caused by lidocaine or by a psychological reaction to the stress of the critical care unit or the illness. It is important to exclude other reasons for this presentation such as volume depletion, sepsis, or bleeding (the latter being a problem that is especially confusing in patients who have undergone invasive testing). It is of utmost importance to determine if a new systolic cardiac murmur is present, because, as is discussed later, this suggests a potentially correctable complication in which a different clinical algorithm may be applied.

Although some patients with cardiogenic shock and no clinical evidence of myocardial rupture do not require invasive hemodynamic monitoring, many are more carefully and exactly managed with this technique. In some patients, the examination itself brings a degree of risk (e.g., patients with left bundle branch block in whom passage of a pulmonary artery catheter may cause complete heart block, or patients with emphysema in whom even a small pneumothorax may cause abrupt respiratory failure). The clinician must judge whether the benefit of invasive monitoring outweighs the risk. The pulmonary artery catheter provides the managing physician with data that assist in the overall assessment of the patient's hemodynamic picture, including cardiac output, systemic vascular resistance, and pulmonary wedge pressure tracing. The wedge pressure is a "proxy" for direct left atrial pressure, and the

Table 16–3
Hemodynamic Subsets

Subset	Cardiac Index (l/min/m²)	PWP (mm Hg)
I	>2.2	<18
II	>2.2	>18
III	<2.2	<18
IV	<2.2	>18

PWP = pulmonary wedge pressure

wave form transmitted from this chamber may demonstrate the pattern of mitral insufficiency or of cardiac tamponade from unsuspected chamber rupture.

The patient in whom the cardiac output measurement demonstrates a low cardiac output should undergo treatment with inotropic agents as well as vasoconstrictors, as required. Unfortunately, these drugs, although effective in some patients in a circumscribed way, are limited by the ischemic and infarcted state of the myocardium itself.

Dobutamine, an intravenously administered inotropic agent, works by direct stimulation of adrenergic receptors. It may cause vasodilation, resulting in a fall in blood pressure; however, an improvement in stroke volume and cardiac output may be associated with no change or even an increase in blood pressure in some patients. Its advantage in patients with myocardial infarction is that it can be titrated fairly easily and that it does not cause much tachycardia.

Milrinone is an inotropic agent that requires less titration than dobutamine but may cause a more significant hypotensive response. Its advantage is that it does not increase myocardial oxygen demand to the same degree as dobutamine and dopamine (Grose et al, 1986). This advantage may be helpful in the myocardial infarction patient who frequently has other coronary occlusions and thus in whom an increase in oxygen demand may worsen ischemia and further depress myocardial function in other cardiac regions.

Dopamine has a well-known variable effect on cardiac adrenergic receptors. It also may cause significant tachycardia. When given in the norepinephrine range (greater than 10 µg/kg per minute), it is probably worthwhile to substitute norepinephrine.

Despite the best use of inotropic agents combined with invasive monitoring, the prognosis of cardiogenic shock remains abysmal. The GUSTO investigators found that the in-hospital and 30-day mortality for patients who developed cardiogenic shock was about 56%, as compared with 3% for those who did not develop this complication (Holmes et al, 1995). As a result, emergent PTCA has been suggested to improve the outcome in these patients, although the risk is high in the event of failure to reperfuse (Lee et al, 1991; Klein, 1992; Seydoux et al, 1992). Treatment with thrombolytic agents decreased the frequency of development of this complication, but did not affect the mortality in GUSTO-I. In those patients who had angioplasty—only 19% of the entire group—the mortality rate was decreased, 31% versus 61% in those patients who had shock but did not undergo angioplasty (Holmes et al, 1995).

Intra-aortic balloon pumping (IABP) is a seemingly attractive alternative for adjunctive treatment of patients in cardiogenic shock. It provides a method of reducing afterload as well as maintaining a diastolic blood pressure adequate to perfuse the coronary vessels, without lowering systolic blood pressure, as do the vasodilating drugs. This therapy, although successful in improving the patient's hemodynamic picture, does not improve survival (Gacioch et al, 1992). In contrast, in patients with a mechanical lesion or in whom life-threatening lesions have been identified and reperfusion therapy, particularly coronary artery bypass surgery, is being planned, IABP has been shown to be helpful. IABP relies on an intact aorta and aortic valve and is contraindicated in aortic regurgitation, in pre-existing vasodilated states such as sepsis, and in aortic dissection. Severe occlusive peripheral vascular disease is not a contraindication but constrains the availability of vascular access.

RIGHT VENTRICULAR INFARCTION

Rarely occurring alone, right ventricular myocardial infarction is a result of a proximal occlusion of the right coronary artery. Some degree of right ventricular myocardial infarction may be detected in up to 50% of inferior wall myocardial infarctions. The diagnosis is usually made in the context of an inferior wall myocardial infarction, often accompanied by S-T elevations in the right ventricular precordial leads, V_3R and V_4R. The elevation of the S-T segment in V_4R is the most predictive finding for right ventricular infarction (Kinch and Ryan, 1994). Clinically, patients may present with signs of right-sided pressure elevation with dilated jugular veins, as well as hypotension and clear lung fields. The hemodynamic tracings classically demonstrate that the right atrial pressure is often more elevated than the pulmonary wedge pressure. The right ventricular pressure tracing may demonstrate the "dip and plateau" characteristic of restrictive cardiomyopathy and constrictive pericarditis, but usually the clinical setting makes the diagnosis of right ventricular myocardial infarction clear. The wave form may be broad, bifid, and slow in its upstroke. An echocardiogram may demonstrate a dilated, poorly functioning right ventricle.

Because of diminished right ventricular pump function, the patient's diminished left ventricular preload may be optimized by volume infusions guided by pulmonary artery catheterization. Inotropic support with dobutamine may be required to maintain cardiac output and control hypotension. In many patients, their use may be discontinued when the volume load is adequate. Preload-reducing drugs such as nitrates and morphine may complicate the hemodynamic picture, although these preparations may be required for control of pain or relief of heart failure.

As is true for left ventricular infarction, the prognosis for right ventricular infarction is dependent on the extent of pump dysfunction, particularly over the long term. In-hospital mortality has been reported as high as 31% (Zehender et al, 1993). Eventually, most patients with right ventricular myocardial infarction have recovery of right ventricular function.

MECHANICAL LESIONS AND RUPTURE

Disruption of a necrotic scar, sometimes stressed further by hemorrhage resulting from reperfusion, is seen by critical care clinicians, usually in a patient previously recovering uneventfully from myocardial infarction who suddenly develops acute pulmonary edema and cardiac arrest. The three lesions most characteristic of this presentation are acute mitral regurgitation, acute ventricular septal rupture, and perforation of the left ventricular free wall.

Acute mitral regurgitation and ventricular septal rupture share a common clinical finding in the patient with acute or subacute hemodynamic deterioration: the new systolic murmur. Indeed, simple auscultation of the heart in patients with myocardial infarction may detect the new murmur while its hemodynamic burden is not yet overpowering, prompting an emergency echocardiographic study. Although echocardiography may be overused in many clinical settings, obtaining this examination for the diagnosis of the new systolic murmur in acute myocardial infarction is desirable. Acute mitral regurgitation is usually caused by partial or total papillary muscle rupture with the hemodynamic burden dependent on the level of the rupture. Complete transection is usually overwhelming to the patient, whereas rupture of the tip or head of the muscle is more hemodynamically tolerable. Acute mitral regurgitation accounts for about 5% of all infarction deaths and occurs more frequently with inferior rather than anterior myocardial infarction (Wei et al, 1979). Unlike the anterolateral papillary muscle, which has a dual circulation from left anterior descending and left circumflex arteries, the posteromedial papillary muscle has a blood supply derived from the posterior descending coronary artery alone. This makes it much more susceptible to single-vessel coronary obstruction. The time of occurrence was often between 2 and 7 days in the prethrombolytic era (Wei et al, 1979), but studies of patients receiving thrombolytics suggest that this therapy may accelerate the occurrence of the rupture (Becker et al, 1995). Treatment of this lesion includes prompt hemodynamic stabilization, intra-aortic balloon pumping, and rapid surgical therapy.

Although the diagnosis and treatment of ventricular septal rupture is similar to that of acute papillary muscle rupture, the clinical features of the former are somewhat different. Acute rupture of the septum occurs perhaps more frequently than does papillary muscle rupture, although this may be because it is more hemodynamically tolerable. Acute septal rupture occurs in both anterior and inferior wall myocardial infarction with similar frequency. Although the murmur is similar, presenting in both cases as a holosystolic murmur, the murmur in ventricular septal rupture may demonstrate a thrill over the precordium more frequently than in acute mitral regurgitation. The location of the murmur is usually not helpful. The characteristic finding of an oxygen saturation step-up of 1.0 vol% from right atrium to pulmonary artery on pulmonary artery catheterization confirms the diagnosis that has often already been made using the echocardiogram. Sampling should be done in all three right heart chambers and an arterial sample or a reliable pulse oximetry reading should be obtained.

The most sudden manifestation of myocardial disruption is that of free wall rupture, which accounts for about 10% of deaths from acute myocardial infarction. It is classically said to occur more frequently in women than in men, although in the thrombolytic era this may not be the case (Oliva et al, 1993; Becker et al, 1995). There may be a role for hypertension as the trigger for the tear (Oliva et al, 1993). Free wall rupture occurs less commonly in hypertrophied ventricles than in those with normal wall thickness, probably because of the greater collagen content in the hypertrophied walls as well as the bulk of myocardium. The diagnosis of free wall rupture is usually made with the patient *in extremis*, if an echocardiogram can be performed or if empiric thoracotomy is performed. Despite this approach, the condition has an exceedingly high mortality.

Pseudoaneurysm is a special case of free wall rupture. This is an incomplete rupture that has become sealed off by thrombus, hematoma, and pericardium. There is a persisting communication with the ventricular cavity, and the neck of the communication can often be detected with echocardiography. In this condition, prompt surgical repair with or without coronary bypass grafting may be lifesaving, because complete rupture generally ensues.

CONCLUSIONS AND PERSPECTIVE

With the explosion in the knowledge base on the pathogenesis, diagnosis, and treatment of myocardial infarction, fundamental changes have been introduced into clinical practice. The emphasis today is on rapid identification and referral of patients to appropriate facilities with adequate resources to promptly evaluate and intervene on behalf of the patient. The resources required are intensive and expensive, both in human and financial terms.

Nonetheless, it is clear that certain principles in the initial assessment apply. The physician must be prepared to address chest pain promptly and aggressively and to consider ischemic heart disease when "anginal equivalents" such as dyspnea or arrhythmia are the presenting symptoms. Facilities must ensure that triage and assessment procedures allow prompt patient attention and rapid access to confirmatory diagnostic means. In addition, the facility and physicians must jointly ensure that their response to the patient with suspected myocardial infarction is appropriate and decisive. Although many cases occur in which a specific form of therapy is preferred, either thrombolysis or acute angioplasty, often no absolute indications exist for one or the other approach. The consideration must be to do that which is available, whether on-site or in another accessible facility, with the greatest alacrity.

The physician must also be prepared for the subacute and chronic management of myocardial infarction. Adjunctive therapies must be considered early in the course of the myocardial infarction and initiated when appropriate, so that (1) the patient's length of stay in the hospital is minimized and (2) proper risk stratification is applied in a timely fashion. The physician should also bear in mind the potentially negative effects of the therapies that are applied, whether they are the risk of rupture related to thrombolytics or the exacerbation of heart failure with beta-blockers. Although rare, as described earlier, these complications are iatrogenic; their prompt recognition is critical.

What of the future? Clearly, there is a burgeoning interest in newer means of dissolving or removing clot that seem to offer greater safety with increased success. Technical advances, such as stents, show promise to permit better long-term success for aggressive interventions. Length of stay in the hospital is decreasing. Ultimately, however, there is a great deal of prevention that must still be initiated by the physician and patient. It is too early to say whether the new medical environment that is emerging will enhance the interaction that is required for this crucial component to be realized.

REFERENCES

AHA/ACC Taskforce Report: Guidelines for percutaneous transluminal coronary angioplasty: A report of the American College of Cardiology/American Heart Association Task Force on assessment of diagnostic and therapeutic procedures. JACC 22:2033–2054, 1993.

Ambrosioni E, Borghi C, Magnani B for the Survival of Myocardial Infarction Long Term Evaluation (SMILE) Investigators: The effect of the angiotensin-converting enzyme inhibitor zofenopril on mortality and morbidity after anterior myocardial infarction. N Engl J Med 332:80–85, 1995.

Anticoagulation in the Secondary Prevention of Events in Coronary Thrombosis (ASPECT) Research Group: Effect of long-term anticoagulant treatment on mortality and cardiovascular morbidity after myocardial infarction. Lancet 343:499–503, 1994.

Antman EM: Magnesium in acute MI: Timing is critical. Circulation 92:2367–2372, 1995.

Antman EM for the TIMI 9A Investigators: Hirudin in acute myocardial infarction: Safety report from the Thrombolysis and Thrombin Inhibition in Myocardial Infarction (TIMI) 9A trial. Circulation 90:1624–1630, 1994.

Bakker AJ, Koelemay MJW, Gorgels JPMC, et al: Troponin T and myoglobin at admission: Value of early diagnosis of acute myocardial infarction. Eur Heart J 15:45–53, 1994.

Bayer AJ and Chadha JS: Changing presentation of MI with increasing old age. J Am Geriatr Soc 34:263–266, 1986.

Becker RC, Charlesworth A, Wilcox RG, et al: Cardiac rupture associated with thrombolytic therapy: Impact of time to treatment in the late assessment of thrombolytic efficacy (LATE) study. J Am Coll Cardiol 25:1063–1068, 1995.

Bergmann SR, Lerch RA, Fox KAA, et al: Temporal dependence of beneficial effects of coronary thrombolysis characterized by positron tomography. Am J Med 73:573–581, 1982.

Beta-Blocker Heart Attack Trial Research Group: A randomized trial of propranolol in patients with acute myocardial infarction: I. Mortality Results. JAMA 247:1707–1714, 1982.

Bhayana V, Gougoulias T, Cohoe S, and Henderson AR: Discordance between results for troponin T and troponin I in renal disease. Clin Chem 41:312–317, 1995.

Bodenheimer MM, Ramanthan K, Banka VS, et al: Effect of progressive pressure reduction with nitroprusside on acute myocardial infarction in humans: Determination of optimal afterload. Ann Intern Med 94:435–439, 1981.

Brand DA, Newcomer LN, Freiburger A, and Tian H: Cardiologists' practice compared with practice guidelines: Use of beta-blockade after acute myocardial infarction. JACC 26:1432–1436, 1995.

Cairns JA, Fuster V, Gore J, et al: Coronary thrombolysis. Chest 108[Suppl]:401S–423S, 1995a.

Cairns JA, Lewis HD, Meade TW, et al: Antithrombotic agents in coronary artery disease. Chest 108[Suppl]:380S–400S, 1995b.

Califf RM, Topol EJ, Stack RS, Ellis SG, et al for the TAMI Study Group: Evaluation of combination thrombolytic therapy and timing of cardiac catheterization in acute myocardial infarction: Results of Thrombolysis and Angioplasty in Myocardial Infarction—Phase 5 randomized trial. Circulation 83:1543–1556, 1991.

De Winter RJ, Koster RW, Sturk A, and Sanders GT: Value of myoglobin, troponin T and CK-MB mass in ruling out an acute myocardial infarction in the Emergency Room. Circulation 92:3401–3407, 1995.

DeWood MA, Spores J, Notske R, et al: Prevalence of total coronary occlusion during the early hours of transmural myocardial infarction. N Engl J Med 303:897–902, 1980.

Drapkin A and Merskey C: Anticoagulant therapy after myocardial infarction: Relation of therapeutic benefit to patients' age, sex and severity of infarction. JAMA 222:541–548, 1972.

Ellis SG, da Silva ER, Heyndrickx G, Talley JD, et al for the RESCUE investigators: Randomized comparison of rescue angioplasty with conservative management of patients with early failure of thrombolysis for acute anterior myocardial infarction. Circulation 90:2280–2284, 1994.

Fibrinolytic Therapy Trialists Group: Indications for fibrinolytic therapy in suspected acute myocardial infarction: Collaborative overview of early mortality and major morbidity results from all randomised trials of more than 1000 patients. Lancet 343:311–322, 1994.

Fiebach NH, Viscoli CM, and Horwitz RI: Differences between women and men in survival after myocardial infarction: Biology or methodology? JAMA 263:1092–1096, 1990.

Flaherty JT, Come PC, Baird MG, et al: Effects of intravenous nitroglycerin on left ventricular function and ST segment changes in acute myocardial infarction. Br Heart J 38:612–621, 1976.

Flaherty JT, Reid PR, Kelly DT, et al: Intravenous nitroglycerin in acute myocardial infarction. Circulation 51:132, 1975.

Gacioch GM, Ellis SG, Lee L, et al: Cardiogenic shock complicating acute myocardial infarction: The use of coronary angioplasty and the integration of the new support devices into

patient management. J Am Coll Cardiol 19:647–653, 1992.

Gaudron P, Eilles C, Kugler I, and Ertl G: Progressive left ventricular dysfunction and remodeling after myocardial infarction. Circulation 87:755–763, 1993.

Gibbons RJ, Holmes DR, Reeder GS, et al: Immediate angioplasty compared with the administration of a thrombolytic agent followed by conservative treatment for myocardial infarction. N Engl J Med 328:685–691, 1993.

Grines CL, Browne KF, Marco J, et al: A comparison of immediate angioplasty with thrombolytic therapy for acute myocardial infarction. N Engl J Med 328:673–679, 1993.

Grose R, Strain J, Greenberg M, and LeJemtel TH: Systemic and coronary effects of milrinone and dobutamine in congestive heart failure. J Am Coll Cardiol 7:1107–1113, 1986.

Gruppo Italiano per lo Studio della Sopravvivenza nell' Infarto Miocardico: GISSI-2: A factorial randomised trial of alteplase versus streptokinase and heparin versus no heparin among 12 490 patients with acute myocardial infarction. Lancet 336:65–71, 1990.

Gruppo Italiano per lo Studio della Sopravvivenza nell' Infarto Miocardico: GISSI-3: Effects of lisinopril and transdermal glyceryl trinitrate singly and together on 6-week mortality and ventricular function after acute myocardial infarction. Lancet 343:1115–1122, 1994.

Gruppo Italiano per lo Studio della Streptochinasi nell' Infarto Miocardico: Effectiveness of intravenous thrombolytic treatment in acute myocardial infarction. Lancet 2:397–401, 1986.

Gunnar RM, Bourdillon PDV, Dixon DW, et al: Guidelines for the early management of patients with acute myocardial infarction. JACC 16:249–292, 1990; Circulation 82:664–707, 1990.

Heart and Stroke Facts: 1995 Statistical Supplement, American Heart Association, 1995.

Hennekens CH, O'Donnell CJ, Ridker PM, and Marder VJ: Current issues concerning thrombolytic therapy for acute myocardial infarction. JACC 25[Suppl]:18S–22S, 1995.

Herrick JB: Clinical features of sudden obstruction of the coronary arteries. JAMA 59:2015–2020, 1912.

Holmes DR, Bates ER, Kleiman NS, et al: Contemporary reperfusion therapy for cardiogenic shock: The GUSTO-I trial experience. J Am Coll Cardiol 26:668–674, 1995.

ISIS Collaborative Group: Randomised trial of intravenous atenolol among 16,027 cases of suspected acute myocardial infarction: ISIS-1. Lancet 2:57–66, 1986.

ISIS Collaborative Group: ISIS-4: A randomized factorial trial assessing early oral captopril, oral mononitrate and intravenous magnesium sulphate in 58,050 patients with suspected myocardial infarction. Lancet 345:669–685, 1995.

ISIS-1 Collaborative Group: Mechanisms for the early mortality reduction produced by beta blockade started early in acute myocardial infarction: ISIS-1. Lancet 1:921–923, 1988.

ISIS-3 (Third International Study of Infarct Survival) Collaborative Group: ISIS-3: A randomised comparison of streptokinase vs tissue plasminogen activator vs anistreplase and of aspirin plus heparin vs aspirin alone among 41,299 cases of suspected myocardial infarction. Lancet 339:753–770, 1992.

ISIS-4 Collaborative Group: ISIS-4: A randomised factorial trial assessing early captopril, oral mononitrate and intravenous magnesium sulphate in 58,050 patients with suspected myocardial infarction. Lancet 345:669–685, 1995.

Jugdutt BI: Role of nitrates after acute myocardial infarction. Am J Cardiol 70:82B–87B, 1992.

Katus HA, Remppis A, Neumann FJ, et al: Diagnostic efficiency of troponin T measurements in acute myocardial infarction. Circulation 83:902–912, 1991.

Keffer JH: Myocardial markers of injury; evolution and insights. Am J Clin Pathol 105:305–320, 1996.

Kennedy JW: Optimal management of acute myocardial infarction requires early and complete reperfusion. Circulation 91:1905–1907, 1995.

Kennedy JW, Ritchie JL, Davis KB, et al: The Western Washington randomized trial of intracoronary streptokinase in acute myocardial infarction. N Engl J Med 312:1073–1078, 1985.

Kennedy JW, Ritchie JL, Davis KB, and Fritz JK: Western Washington randomized trial of intracoronary streptokinase in acute myocardial infarction. N Engl J Med 309:1477–1482, 1983.

Kinch JW and Ryan TJ: Right ventricular infarction. N Engl J Med 330:1211–1217, 1994.

Klein LW: Optimal therapy for cardiogenic shock; the emerging role of coronary angioplasty. J Am Coll Cardiol 19:654–656, 1992.

Kline EM, Smith DD, Martin JS, et al: In-hospital treatment delays in patients treated with thrombolytic therapy; a report of the GUSTO time to treatment substudy. Circulation 86(4[Suppl 1]):I–702, 1992.

Lange RA and Hillis LD: Immediate angioplasty for acute myocardial infarction. N Engl J Med 328:726–728, 1993.

LATE Study Group: Late assessment of thrombolytic efficacy (LATE) study with alteplase 6–24 hours after onset of acute myocardial infarction. Lancet 342:759–766, 1993.

Latini R, Maggioni AP, Flather M, et al: ACE inhibitor use in patients with myocardial infarction: Summary of evidence from clinical trials. Circulation 92:3132–3137, 1995.

Lee KL, Califf RM, Simes J, et al: Holding GUSTO up to the light. Ann Intern Med 120:876–881, 1994.

Lee L, Erbel R, Brown TM, et al: Multicenter registry of angioplasty therapy of cardiogenic shock: Initial and long-term survival. J Am Coll Cardiol 17:599–603, 1991.

Lee TH, Cook EF, Weisberg M, et al: Acute chest pain in the emergency room; identification and examination of low-risk patients. Arch Intern Med 145:65–69, 1985.

Lee TH and Goldman L: Serum enzyme assays in the diagnosis of acute myocardial infarction: Recommendations based on a quantitative analysis. Ann Intern Med 105:221–233, 1986.

Lindahl B, Venge P, Wallentin L for the FRISC Study Group: Relation between troponin T and the risk of subsequent cardiac events in unstable coronary artery disease. Circulation 93:1651–1657, 1996.

Little WC, Constantinescu M, Applegate RJ, et al: Can coronary angiography predict the site of a subsequent myocardial infarction in patients with mild-to-moderate coronary artery disease? Circulation 78:1157–1166, 1988.

Lonn EM, Yusuf S, Jha P, et al: Emerging role of angiotensin-converting enzyme inhibitors in cardiac and vascular protection. Circulation 90:2056–2069, 1994.

Mair J, Morandell D, Genser N, et al: Equivalent early sensitivities of myoglobin, creatine kinase MB mass, creatine kinase isoform ratios and cardiac troponins I and T for acute myocardial infarction. Clin Chem 41:1266–1272, 1995a.

Mair J, Smidt J, Lechleitner P, et al: A decision tree for the early diagnosis of acute myocardial infarction in nontraumatic chest pain patients at hospital admission. Chest 108:1502–1509, 1995b.

Mark DB, Hlatky MA, Califf RM, et al: Cost effectiveness of thrombolytic therapy with tissue plasminogen activator as compared with streptokinase for acute myocardial infarction. N Engl J Med 332:1418–1424, 1995.

Maynard C, Weaver WD, Lambrew C, et al: Factors influencing the time to administration of thrombolytic therapy with recombinant tissue plasminogen activator (data from the National Registry of Myocardial Infarction). Am J Cardiol 76:548–552, 1995.

Michels KB and Yusuf S: Does PTCA in acute myocardial infarction affect mortality and reinfarction rates? A quantitative overview (meta-analysis) of the randomized clinical trials. Circulation 91:476–485, 1995.

Multicenter Diltiazem Postinfarction Trial Research Group: The effect of diltiazem on mortality and reinfarction after myocardial infarction. N Engl J Med 319:385–392, 1988.

Neuhaus KL, Essen RV, Tebbe U, et al: Safety observations from the pilot phase of the randomized r-hirudin for improvement of thrombolysis (HIT-III) study. Circulation 90:1638–1642, 1994.

Oliva PB, Hammill SC, and Edwards WD: Cardiac rupture, a clinically predictable complication of acute myocardial infarction: Report of 70 cases with clinicopathologic correlations. J Am Coll Cardiol 22:720–726, 1993.

Pfeffer MA, Braunwald E, Moyé LA, et al on behalf of the SAVE Investigators: Effect of captopril on mortality and morbidity in patients with left ventricular dysfunction after myocardial infarction. Results of the Survival and

Ventricular Enlargement Trial. N Engl J Med 327:669–677, 1992.

Pfeffer MA, Lamas GA, Vaughan DE, et al: Effect of captopril on progressive ventricular dilation after anterior myocardial infarction. N Engl J Med 319:80–86, 1988.

Pilote L, Califf RM, Sapp S, et al: Regional variation across the United States in the management of acute myocardial infarction. N Engl J Med 333:565–572, 1995.

Puleo P, Meyer D, Wathen C, et al: Use of a rapid assay of subforms of creatine kinase MB to diagnose or rule out acute myocardial infarction. N Engl J Med 331:561–566, 1994.

Reeder GS, Bailey KR, Gersh BJ, and Holmes DR: Cost comparison of immediate angioplasty versus thrombolysis followed by conservative therapy for acute myocardial infarction: A prospective randomized trial. Mayo Clin Proc 69:5–12, 1994.

Reimer KA, Lowe JE, Rasmussen MM, and Jennings RB: The wave front phenomenon of ischemic cell death: I. Myocardial infarct size vs. duration of coronary occlusion in dogs. Circulation 56:786–794, 1977.

Rentrop P, Blancke H, Karsch KR, et al: Selective intracoronary thrombolysis in acute myocardial infarction and unstable angina pectoris. Circulation 63:307–317, 1981.

Ridker PM, O'Donnell C, Marder VJ, and Hennekens CH: Large-scale trials of thrombolytic therapy for acute myocardial infarction. Ann Intern Med 119:530–532, 1993.

Ridker PM, O'Donnell CJ, Marder VJ, and Hennekens CH: A response to "holding GUSTO up to the light." Ann Intern Med 120:882–885, 1994.

Roberts R, Rogers WJ, Mueller HS, et al: Immediate versus deferred β-blockade following thrombolytic therapy in patients with acute myocardial infarction: Results of the thrombolysis in myocardial infarction (TIMI) II-B Study. Circulation 83:422–437, 1991.

Rogers WJ, Bowlby LJ, Chandra NC, et al: Treatment of myocardial infarction in the United States (1990 to 1993): Observations from the National Registry of Myocardial Infarction. Circulation 90:2103–2114, 1994.

Rutherford JD, Pfeffer MA, Moyé LA, et al on behalf of the SAVE Investigators: Effects of captopril on ischemic events after myocardial infarction. Results of the Survival and Ventricular Enlargement Trial. Circulation 990:1731–1738, 1994.

Ryden L, Ariniego R, Arnman K, et al: A double blind trial of metoprolol in acute myocardial infarction. N Engl J Med 308:614–618, 1983.

Seydoux C, Goy J-J, Beuret P, et al: Effectiveness of percutaneous transluminal angioplasty in cardiogenic shock during acute myocardial infarction. Am J Cardiol 69:968–969, 1992.

Simes RJ, Topol EJ, Holmes DR, et al: Link between the angiographic substudy and mortality outcomes in a large randomized trial of myocardial reperfusion: Importance of early and complete infarct artery reperfusion. Circulation 91:1923–1928, 1995.

Swedberg K, Held P, Kjekshus J, et al on behalf of the CONSENSUS II study group: Effects of the early administration of enalapril on mortality in patients with acute myocardial infarction. N Engl J Med 327:678–684, 1992.

The Acute Infarction Ramipril Efficacy Study Investigators: Effect of ramipril on mortality and morbidity of survivors of acute myocardial infarction with clinical evidence of heart failure. Lancet 342:821–828, 1993.

The EPIC Investigators: Use of a monoclonal antibody directed against the platelet glycoprotein IIb/IIIa receptor in high-risk coronary angioplasty. N Engl J Med 330:956–961, 1994.

The Global Use of Strategies to Open Occluded Coronary Arteries (GUSTO) IIA Investigators: Randomized trial of intravenous heparin versus recombinant hirudin for acute coronary syndromes. Circulation 90:1631–1637, 1994.

The GUSTO Investigators: An international randomized trial comparing four thrombolytic strategies for acute myocardial infarction. N Engl J Med 329:673–682, 1993.

The GUSTO-1 Angiographic Investigators: The effects of tissue plasminogen activator, streptokinase, or both on coronary artery patency, ventricular function, and survival after myocardial infarction. N Engl J Med 329:1615–1622, 1993.

The TIMI Study Group: The Thrombolysis in Myocardial Infarction (TIMI) trial. N Engl J Med 312:932–936, 1985.

The TIMI Study Group: Comparison of invasive and conservative strategies after treatment with intravenous tissue plasminogen activator in acute myocardial infarction: Results of the Thrombolysis in Myocardial Infarction (TIMI) Phase II trial. N Engl J Med 320:618–627, 1989.

Tiefenbrunn AJ and Sobel BE: Timing of coronary recanalization: paradigms, paradoxes, and pertinence. Circulation 85:2311–2315, 1992.

Topol EJ, Califf RM, George BS, et al: A randomized trial of immediate versus delayed elective angioplasty after intravenous tissue plasminogen activator in acute myocardial infarction. N Engl J Med 317:581–588, 1987.

Weaver WD, Cerqueira M, Hallstrom AP, et al: Prehospital-initiated vs. hospital-initiated thrombolytic therapy. The Myocardial Infarction Triage and Intervention Trial. JAMA 270:1211–1216, 1993.

Wei JY, Hutchins GM, and Bulkley BH: Papillary muscle rupture in fatal acute myocardial infarction: A potentially treatable form of cardiogenic shock. Ann Intern Med 90:149–153, 1979.

White HD, Norris RM, Brown MA, et al: Left ventricular end-systolic volume as the major determinant of survival after recovery from myocardial infarction. Circulation 76:44–51, 1987.

Whittaker P, Boughner DR, and Kloner RA: Role of collagen in acute myocardial infarct expansion. Circulation 84:2123–2134, 1991.

Woods KL, Fletcher S, Roffe C, et al: Intravenous magnesium sulphate in suspected acute myocardial infarction: Results of the Second Leicester Intravenous Magnesium Intervention Trial (LIMIT-2). Lancet 339:1553–1558, 1992.

Yusuf S, Collins R, MacMahon S, et al: Effect of intravenous nitrates on mortality in acute myocardial infarction: An overview of the randomized trials. Lancet 1:1088–1092, 1988a.

Yusuf S, Wittes J, and Friedman L: Overview of results of randomized clinical trials in heart disease. JAMA 260:2088–2093, 1988b.

Zehender M, Kasper W, and Kauder E: Right ventricular infarction as an independent predictor of prognosis after acute inferior myocardial infarction. N Engl J Med 328:981–988, 1993.

Zijlstra F, de Boer MJ, Hoorntje JCA, et al: A comparison of immediate coronary angioplasty with intravenous streptokinase in acute myocardial infarction. N Engl J Med 328:680–684, 1993.

Cardiac Rhythm Disorders in the Critical Care Setting: Pathophysiology, Diagnosis, and Management

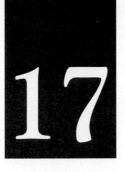

Noel G. Boyle, M.D., Ph.D.

Steven J. Evans, M.D.

This chapter is a review of the arrhythmias commonly seen in patients monitored in the ICU setting. The aim is to discuss the approach to diagnosis and management of the most common arrhythmias rather than provide a comprehensive review of all possible arrhythmias. Arrhythmias resulting from underlying cardiac disease may be exacerbated or new arrhythmias may develop in the intensive care unit (ICU) setting because patients often develop renal insufficiency, hepatic insufficiency, respiratory compromise, or gastrointestinal dysfunction, which can lead to metabolic abnormalities and toxic drug levels.

APPROACH TO ARRHYTHMIAS IN THE ICU

The initial approach to any arrhythmia in the ICU is to determine whether the patient's hemodynamic status is stable or unstable. If the patient's condition is hemodynamically unstable, immediate synchronized cardioversion or defibrillation is appropriate for tachyarrhythmias. In the case of bradyarrhythmias associated with hypotension that do not respond to atropine, temporary transcutaneous or transvenous pacing is indicated. Two commonly encountered arrhythmias that require specific therapy are torsades de pointes (a form of ventricular tachycardia), which should be treated with IV magnesium, isoproterenol, and/or temporary pacing, and tachycardias in the setting of digoxin toxicity, which respond to digoxin antibody (Fab) fragments (see later).

In the patient whose condition is stable, a focused history and physical examination together with a review of laboratory and other data should be performed. Underlying ischemic or valvular cardiac disease may predispose the patient to ventricular or atrial arrhythmias, whereas conduction abnormalities may indicate fibrosis around the atrioventricular (AV) node or valvular calcification. Noncardiac conditions such as pulmonary and thyroid disease may precipitate atrial arrhythmias. Drug history and a review of the medication sheets are critical. Drugs that are normally well tolerated may rapidly accumulate to toxic levels in patients with hepatic or renal insufficiency or in elderly patients; digoxin and theophylline are among the most common examples. The proarrhythmic effect of commonly used antiarrhythmic drugs is also frequently seen in the ICU setting in the patient with hepatic or renal impairment and other metabolic disturbances. Class IA (e.g., quinidine and procainamide) and class III (particularly sotalol) drugs are associated with QT prolongation and a form of ventricular tachycardia known as torsades de pointes (Table 17–1).

Physical examination should be focused particularly on the patient's hemodynamic, cardiac, and respiratory status but should briefly include evaluation of all organ systems. A parkinsonian tremor may explain the flutter-like activity on a telemetry tracing or an electrocardiogram (ECG). It is important in the patient whose condition is stable to obtain a 12-lead ECG during the arrhythmia and to save all rhythm strips, particularly those showing initiation and termination of the arrhythmia for later review. A baseline ECG either before or following the arrhythmia may provide valuable information by indicating underlying cardiac disease, QT prolongation, or electrolyte abnormality.

Laboratory evaluation should provide electrolyte and drug levels, a complete blood count, and a blood gas evaluation. Hypokalemia, hyperkalemia, hypocalcemia, and hypercalcemia and other metabolic abnormalities have all been implicated in arrhythmogenesis. Many ICU patients have a pulmonary artery catheter in place, and the available data on cardiac output, pulmonary artery wedge pressure, and systemic vascular resistance should be reviewed. The chest radiograph is sometimes overlooked, yet it often provides invaluable information concerning the underlying pulmonary status. Echocardiography can be performed in the ICU setting and provides information on underlying structural heart disease, ventricular function, wall motion abnormalities, chamber sizes, valvular abnormalities, and pressure gradients.

When an ICU patient develops an unexplained arrhythmia, rapid evaluation of the patient together with a review of medications and electrolytes often provides the means to a simple solution such as discontinuation of a medication or correction of metabolic abnormalities.

TACHYARRHYTHMIAS

Three distinct mechanisms have been shown to underlie tachyarrhythmias: reentry, triggered activity, and abnormal automaticity (Janse, 1993). Knowledge of the mechanism underlying an arrhythmia can help in the choice of drug or other therapy.

Reentry is the most common mechanism underlying supraventricular and ventricular arrhythmias. In this situation, two distinct pathways with different conduction properties must be present, which are connected proximally and distally. In the case of atrioventricular nodal reentrant tachycardia (AVNRT), in which the tachycardia circuit is believed to be confined within the AV node,

Table 17–1
Vaughan Williams Classification, Kinetics, and ECG Effects of Common Antiarrhythmic Drugs

Class	Agent	Half Life (Hours)	Therapeutic Range (μg/ml)	Route of Elimination	ECG Effects
IA	Quinidine	5–7	3–6	Hepatic	Prolongs QRS, QTc
	Procainamide	3–5	3–10	Renal	Prolongs QRS, QTc
	Disopyramide	8–9	2–5	Hep./Renal	Prolongs QRS, QTc
IB	Lidocaine	1–2	2–4	Hepatic	Prolongs QRS
	Mexiletine	10–12	0.5–2.0	Hepatic	Prolongs QRS
	Tocainide	15	3–5	Hepatic	Prolongs QRS
IC	Flecainide	20	0.4–1.0	Hepatic	Prolongs QRS
	Encainide	3–4	0.5–1.0	Hepatic	Prolongs QRS
	Propafenone	2–10	0.6–1.0	Hepatic	Prolongs QRS
II	Propranolol	4–6		Hepatic	Prolongs PR
	Esmolol	9 min		Hepatic	Prolongs PR
	Lopressor	3–7		Hepatic	Prolongs PR
III	Sotalol	12		Renal	Prolongs QTc
	Amiodarone	26–107 days	1.0–2.5	Hepatic	Prolongs QTc
IV	Diltiazem	3.5–5		Hepatic	Prolongs PR
	Verapamil	3–8		Hepatic	Prolongs PR

the two limbs of the circuit are known as the "fast" and "slow" AV nodal pathways. Tachycardia is initiated when there is antegrade (forward) block in the fast pathway, antegrade conduction over the slow pathway, followed by retrograde (reverse) conduction over the fast pathway. Tachycardia is then maintained by antegrade conduction (Fig. 17–1).

Other examples of tachycardias due to reentry are atrioventricular reentrant tachycardia (AVRT) seen in the Wolff-Parkinson-White (WPW) syndrome, atrial flutter, and ventricular tachycardias in the setting of coronary artery disease (Fig. 17–2). Arrhythmias with this mechanism respond to class IA, IC, and III antiarrhythmic drugs. Those that involve the AV node as part of the circuit can be treated with AV nodal blocking agents such as beta-blockers or calcium channel blockers. In addition, radiofrequency catheter ablation can provide a cure for reentrant arrhythmias by permanently interrupting the reentrant circuit.

Triggered activity is defined as pacemaker activity that requires at least one preceding impulse or action potential. The arrhythmia is generated by oscillations in the cardiac cell membrane po-

tential known as *afterdepolarizations*. When these occur in the repolarization phase they are designated as *early afterdepolarizations* and when they occur after repolarization is completed they are known as *late afterdepolarizations*. Examples are torsades de pointes resulting from early afterdepolarizations and some types of idiopathic ventricular tachycardia (VT), such as exercise-induced right ventricular outflow tract VT from late afterdepolarizations. Beta-blockers and calcium channel blockers are the most effective agents for triggered arrhythmias; however, if VT is suspected, calcium channel blockers should not in general be used (see later); rather, lidocaine is the drug of first choice.

Abnormal automaticity is defined by spontaneous depolarization occurring in cells that do not normally exhibit spontaneous diastolic depolarization, such as working atrial and ventricular muscle. When the resting membrane potential is reduced by some pathologic process such as ischemia, diastolic depolarization may occur. Examples include ectopic atrial tachycardias, ventricular arrhythmias during the first few days after myocardial infarction, and fascicular tachycardia in the setting of digoxin toxicity (Table 17–2). Lido-

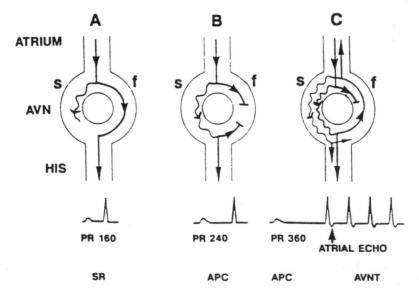

Figure 17–1
Mechanism of reentry within the atrioventricular (AV) node. The AV node is functionally divided into two pathways, slow (s) and fast (f). (A) During sinus rhythm the impulse preferentially conducts over the fast pathway. (B) A premature impulse finds the fast pathway refractory and conducts over the slow pathway, resulting in a longer PR interval. (C) Reentry is established when the fast pathway conducts retrograde, producing an atrial "echo" beat. When this pattern continues, a reentrant tachycardia is generated. (From Wellens, HJJ: Supraventricular tachycardias. In Willerson JT, and Cohn JN (eds): Cardiovascular Medicine. New York, Churchill Livingstone, 1995, p 1338. With permission.)

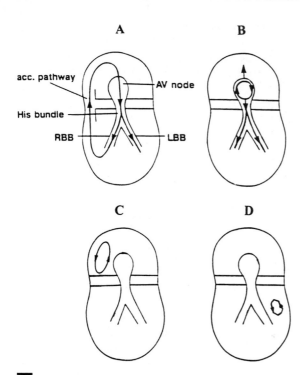

Figure 17–2
Schematics of reentrant tachycardias. *(A)* Atrioventricular reentrant tachycardia (AVRT). In the reentrant circuit shown, there is antegrade conduction over the normal conduction system with retrograde conduction over a right-sided bypass tract. *(B)* AV nodal reentrant tachycardia (AVNRT), wherein the reentrant circuit is located within the AV node. *(C)* Atrial flutter with the reentrant circuit located within the right atrium. *(D)* Ventricular tachycardia, wherein the reentrant circuit is associated with scar tissue in the left ventricle. (Adapted from Wellens HJJ: Supraventricular tachycardias. In Willerson JT, and Cohn JN (eds): Cardiovascular Medicine. New York, Churchill Livingstone, 1995, p 1337. With permission.)

caine, beta-blockers, and calcium channel blockers are useful in this setting.

SUPRAVENTRICULAR ARRHYTHMIAS

SINUS TACHYCARDIA

Sinus tachycardia is recognized on telemetry as P wave, QRS, and T wave complexes identical to those in sinus rhythm, with a rate conventionally defined as greater than 100 beats per minute (bpm). Almost invariably, sinus tachycardia in the ICU setting is a consequence of the underlying disease process. Treatment therefore should be directed to the underlying disease process and not at the sinus tachycardia, which is a secondary process. Although beta-blockers may be appropriate in a patient with acute myocardial infarction displaying sinus tachycardia because of the proven survival benefit they confer, they should be avoided in the patient with sinus tachycardia in the setting of congestive heart failure and low ejection fraction. The syndrome of inappropriate sinus tachycardia is typically seen in healthy young women and is not an appropriate diagnosis in the ICU setting (Lee et al, 1994).

ATRIAL FIBRILLATION

Atrial fibrillation is one of the most common cardiac arrhythmias both inside and outside the ICU setting. Current management strategies are evolving rapidly; however, little consensus yet exists on the use of individual drugs or other methods of treatment (Falk et al, 1992). Atrial fibrillation results from reentry of multiple wavelets within the atrium, causing a very rapid and disorganized atrial rhythm. These impulses bombard the AV node and are randomly conducted to the ventricle with rates that may approach 200 bpm. The arrhythmia is usually diagnosed by irregular R-R intervals and absence of discernible P waves.

Multiple underlying conditions may predispose a patient to atrial fibrillation in the ICU setting. Underlying cardiac causes such as ischemic heart disease, congestive heart failure, hypertensive heart disease, valvular heart disease, pericarditis, and postcardiac surgery are common. Noncardiac-associated conditions frequently include pulmonary disease, thyrotoxicosis, and alcohol intoxication. Baseline evaluation of the patient should include a 12-lead ECG, thyroid function tests, electrolyte and drug levels, chest radiograph, and echocardiogram.

The approach to the treatment of atrial fibrillation can be divided into three parts: (1)

Table 17–2
Arrhythmias Associated With Digoxin Toxicity

Sinoatrial exit block or arrest
First, second, or third degree AV block
Atrial tachycardia with 2:1 AV block
Atrial fibrillation with a slow, regularized ventricular rate
Nonparoxysmal junctional rhythm
Frequent ventricular premature complexes
Ventricular bigeminy and trigeminy
Fascicular tachycardia/bidirectional tachycardia
Ventricular tachycardia

achievement of rate control with an AV nodal blocking drug tailored to the individual patient; (2) consideration of cardioversion, either chemical or electrical; and (3) review of the need for anticoagulation versus contraindications in the individual patient.

Multiple AV nodal blocking agents can be used to achieve rate control, including digoxin, beta-blockers, and calcium channel blockers. A ventricular rate less than 100 per minute is generally described as "controlled" (Fig. 17–3). Digoxin has long been the first choice of many physicians for treating atrial fibrillation. Although it is an effective drug at slowing the ventricular rate through its effect on increasing vagal tone, it is of no proven value in achieving chemical cardioversion (Falk et al, 1987). The narrow therapeutic range for digoxin (1–2 ng/ml), makes it a less favorable choice for most patients in the ICU setting, particularly in the elderly and in those with renal insufficiency. The positive inotropic effect may benefit patients with heart failure. The commonly used approach of giving a total of 1 mg intravenously (IV) in 0.25 mg increments followed by additional IV doses of 0.125 to 0.25 mg IV may often result in toxic levels before rate control is achieved. Indeed, many elderly patients admitted to the ICU may be hospitalized as a result of digoxin toxicity, which is a condition presenting an interesting and challenging array of arrhythmias (to be discussed in detail later).

Beta-blockers provide a selection of effective drugs for rate control that can be tailored to individual ICU patients with differing conditions. Propranolol, metoprolol, and atenolol can all be given intravenously for initial rate control and later be given orally. Intravenous esmolol, with its very short half life, can be used if there is a concern regarding side effects such as in patients with congestive heart failure. Beta-blockers are generally contraindicated in patients with a history of asthma, diabetes mellitus, and peripheral vascular disease.

Calcium channel blockers are also very effective drugs for rate control in patients with atrial fibrillation. Both verapamil and diltiazem are effective and can be given intravenously or orally; diltiazem can also be given as an infusion and titrated to achieve the desired rate control effect. Both agents can precipitate congestive heart failure in patients with left ventricular dysfunction.

Depending on the patient's clinical condition and the chronicity of the atrial fibrillation, electrical or chemical cardioversion may be utilized to achieve sinus rhythm. Patients with new-onset atrial fibrillation (less than 48–72 hours) who are hemodynamically unstable should be treated with prompt chemical or direct current (DC) cardioversion. DC cardioversion of atrial fibrillation is unlikely to be successful with less than 200 J as the initial synchronized shock. The shock can be delivered via electrode pads in the anterior-apical or apical-posterior position. These can also be used to provide backup transcutaneous bradycardia pacing.

When digoxin is given as the agent for achieving rate control it is important to exclude digoxin toxicity before attempting DC cardioversion, because affected patients may develop profound bradycardia following cardioversion. In general, DC cardioversion should not be performed in patients with high (>2.5 ng/ml) digoxin levels unless the hemodynamic situation is unstable (Ditchey and Karliner, 1981). External bradycardia pacing should be available; consideration should also be given to inserting a temporary transvenous pacing wire. If DC cardioversion is initially unsuccessful, it can be tried again following loading with an antiarrhythmic drug (Lundstrom and Ryden, 1988). In the emergent situation, a short-acting benzodiazepine such as midazolam in increments of 0.5 mg can be used for sedation; in the less emergent situation sedation by the anesthesia service, using either propofol or etomidate (less cardiodepressant) is effective.

The multiplicity of antiarrhythmic drugs used in chemical cardioversion of atrial fibrillation reflects the overall lack of efficacy of these drugs both in acutely converting atrial fibrillation to sinus rhythm and in maintaining sinus rhythm (Fuchs and Podrid, 1992). Quinidine sulfate has been used for over 40 years as the antiarrhythmic drug of first choice in treating atrial fibrillation. The usual approach has been to administer 200 mg at 4- to 6-hour intervals for 24 hours followed with a sustained-release formulation such as quinidine gluconate (Quinaglute) at 8-hour intervals. Quinaglute contains 202 mg of quinidine base in each 324 mg tablet, whereas each 300-mg tablet of quinidine sulfate (Quinidex) contains 249 mg of quinidine alkaloid. Intravenous quinidine is available, but is rarely used because of its hypotensive side effects. The most common side effects with quinidine are nausea and diarrhea; they may sometimes be avoided by changing from one preparation to another. Proarrhythmias such as VT and torsades de pointes, which is discussed later, represent more serious side effects.

Procainamide is particularly useful in the ICU setting for the acute conversion of atrial fibrillation to sinus rhythm. The loading dose is 10 to 15 mg/kg given IV; the infusion rate should be as rapid as possible to avoid hypotension, but not greater than 50 mg/min. Hypotension oc-

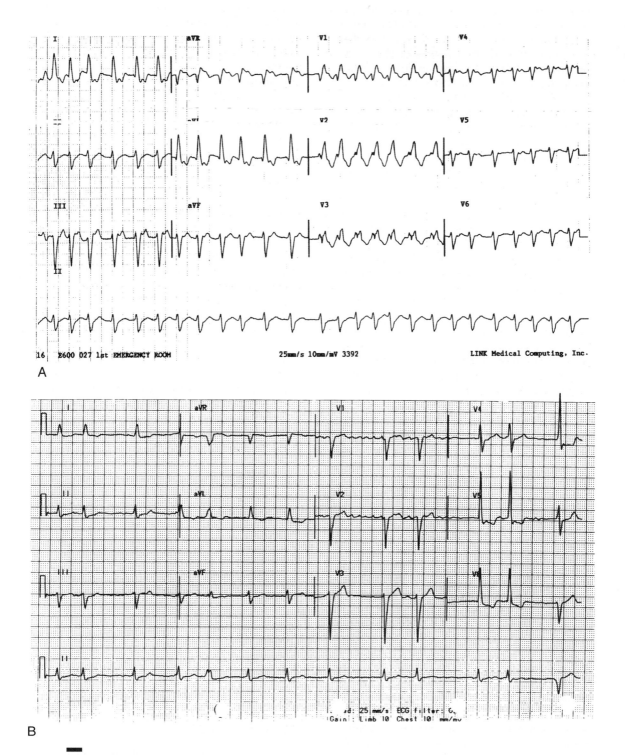

A

B

Figure 17–3
(A) Atrial fibrillation with rapid ventricular rate, averaging 150/min; the QRS shows a right bundle branch block, left anterior hemiblock pattern. (B) Atrial fibrillation with a controlled ventricular rate averaging 75/min; voltage criteria for left ventricular hypertrophy are present.

curring during infusion can be managed by slowing the infusion rate and administering intravenous fluids. The infusion should also be slowed or terminated if significant QRS or QT prolongation occurs, if second or third degree AV block develops, or if new ventricular arrhythmias occur. The usual maintenance dose is 1 to 4 mg/min; however, if the patient's arrhythmia does not convert during or shortly after the infusion, chemical cardioversion with procainamide alone is unlikely to be effective. Blood levels of procainamide needed for acute chemical cardioversion are on the order of 8 μg/ml. The usual total daily dose of oral procainamide is 2000 to 4000 mg. If long-term therapy is undertaken, it must be remembered that procainamide is hepatically metabolized by acetylation and slow acetylators (approximately 20% of population) are more likely to develop antinuclear antibodies and lupus.

Amiodarone is increasingly being administered in the pharmacologic treatment of atrial fibrillation. The drug can be loaded orally or via nasogastric (NG) tube and is highly effective in chemical cardioversion and in maintaining sinus rhythm in patients with atrial fibrillation. Our current practice is to use a loading dose of 5 g (given as 800 mg TID for 2 days), which in general is well tolerated, followed by a maintenance dose of 200 mg/day (Evans et al, 1992). Dosing may need to be adjusted in the setting of bradycardia, and the common side effect of nausea can be diminished if the drug is given with food. Thyroid function tests, liver function tests, chest radiographs, and pulmonary function tests should be obtained before commencing amiodarone therapy; however, the well-known thyroid, hepatic, and pulmonary side effects of amiodarone are rarely seen with a maintenance dose of 200 mg/day.

Several other antiarrhythmic drugs can be given in the treatment of atrial fibrillation (Fuchs and Podrid, 1992). The class IC agents flecainide and propafenone are effective in maintaining sinus rhythm but may cause bradycardia, decreased cardiac output, and proarrhythmia. Sotalol is a class III agent which is more effective than the class I agents in maintaining sinus rhythm but is associated with a dose-related incidence of torsades de pointes.

Anticoagulation with heparin should be started in all patients developing atrial fibrillation unless there is a contraindication. Current practice is to proceed to chemical or electrical cardioversion in patients in whom the duration of atrial fibrillation is less than 72 hours; if the duration of atrial fibrillation is unknown or is greater than 72 hours, transesophageal echocardiography

(TEE) should be performed to exclude atrial thrombi before cardioversion. This approach has been shown to be safe and to yield a low incidence of stroke, similar to that seen with the alternative approach of deferring cardioversion until after a 3-week period of anticoagulation with coumadin (Manning et al, 1995). In addition, cardioversion of atrial fibrillation to sinus rhythm early in the hospital course may result in significant hemodynamic improvement in many ICU patients. When there is no contraindication, and when the duration of atrial fibrillation is unknown, anticoagulation is usually maintained for 8 to 12 weeks after cardioversion to allow for the return of atrial mechanical function (Manning et al, 1994).

Atrial fibrillation in the patient with WPW syndrome can present an emergency situation. If atrial fibrillation develops in a patient in whom the bypass tract has a short refractory period, it is possible for the atrial activity to conduct rapidly to the ventricles and provoke ventricular fibrillation (Klein et al, 1979). This usually presents as a wide complex tachycardia with varying RR intervals and with QRS complexes of varying morphologies. The treatment of choice in this situation is DC cardioversion, even in a patient who appears to be tolerating the arrhythmia, because rapid hemodynamic collapse may develop. Sedation should be given before cardioversion, as needed. Cardiac electrophysiologic consultation should be obtained because radiofrequency catheter ablation of the bypass tract is a curative procedure for these patients.

Our current approach to new onset atrial fibrillation in the ICU is as follows: laboratory and imaging studies are obtained as detailed earlier, a beta-blocker or calcium channel blocker is used to achieve rate control, and anticoagulation with heparin is initiated. If the patient is hemodynamically stable, chemical cardioversion is attempted with intravenous procainamide; if this is unsuccessful, we proceed immediately to loading with amiodarone, 5 g over 48 hours, and then to DC cardioversion within 72 hours if necessary. The choice and duration of maintenance therapy depend on the individual patient, clinical setting, and underlying condition.

ATRIAL FLUTTER

Atrial flutter is recognized by the characteristic flutter waves at a rate of 250 to 350 per minute and a ventricular rate dependent on the degree of atrioventricular conduction, which is often half the atrial rate, typically 125 to 175 per minute (Fig. 17–4). Electrophysiologic mapping studies

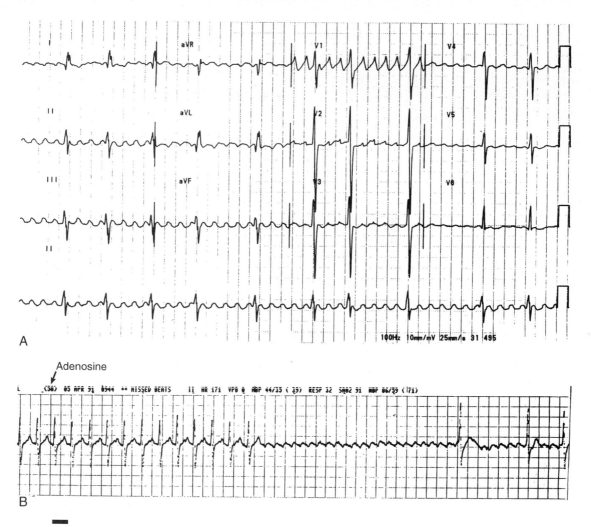

Figure 17–4
(A) Atrial flutter with variable atrioventricular (AV) block. (B) A supraventricular tachycardia, with a rate approximately 160/min, is shown at the left of the tracing. Following administration of intravenous adenosine, there is AV nodal block revealing the underlying atrial flutter.

have shown that atrial flutter is a macroreentrant arrhythmia with the circuit typically located in the right atrium (Waldo, 1990). Frequently, atrial fibrillation and flutter coexist in the same patient. Atrial flutter can be subdivided into typical (type I) with atrial rates of 250 to 350 per minute, and atypical (type II) with atrial rates greater than 350 per minute. This distinction is important clinically because type I atrial flutter can often be converted to sinus rhythm with atrial overdrive pacing, whereas type II cannot. The treatment of choice for atrial flutter is DC cardioversion. Although atrial flutter does not have the same thrombogenic potential as atrial fibrillation, it is common practice to obtain a TEE before cardioversion if the duration of atrial flutter is greater than 72 hours. Alternatively a 3-week period of

anticoagulation with coumadin may be undertaken before cardioversion. The same antiarrhythmic drugs used to maintain sinus rhythm in atrial fibrillation may also be used in atrial flutter. Radiofrequency catheter ablation is now an option for curative treatment of typical atrial flutter (Feld et al, 1992).

PAROXYSMAL SUPRAVENTRICULAR TACHYCARDIA

Paroxysmal supraventricular tachycardia defines a group of reentrant tachycardias, which includes atrioventricular nodal reentrant tachycardia (AVNRT), atrioventricular reentrant tachycardia (AVRT) in the presence of a concealed bypass tract (i.e., conducting only in the retrograde direction), and atrioventricular reentrant tachycardia in the presence of a manifest bypass tract (WPW syndrome) (Prystowsky and Klein, 1994) (see Fig. 17–2). The electocardiographic hallmark of these tachycardias is the narrow complex tachycardia (QRS duration <120 ms) with rates of 150 to 280 per minute. P waves may occur before, within, or after the QRS complex.

In atrioventricular nodal reentrant tachycardia, reentry occurs within the AV node, usually with antegrade conduction over a slow and retrograde conduction over a fast AV nodal pathway (Figs. 17–1 and 17–5). In atrioventricular reentrant tachycardia, antegrade conduction is usually via the AV node and retrograde conduction via the bypass tract (Figs. 17–2A and 17–6). The differential diagnosis includes atrial tachycardia (Fig. 17–7) and atrial flutter with 2:1 block (see Fig. 17–4B). These arrhythmias may become manifest for the first time (i.e., the patient has not previously had arrhythmias, or the arrhythmias were not previously documented) or may occur more frequently in the acutely ill ICU patient.

Because of its unique pharmacokinetics, intravenous adenosine is the treatment of choice to terminate these arrhythmias in the ICU setting (DiMarco, 1983). The method of administration is important because the drug has a half life of approximately 10 seconds; a bolus of 6 mg is administered over 1 to 2 seconds followed by a rapid saline flush. If the tachycardia does not terminate, this drug can be repeated with a 12-mg bolus after 5 minutes. The mechanism of action is to block conduction in the AV node; rarely, some atrial and ventricular tachycardias also terminate with adenosine. Adenosine should be administered cautiously in asthmatic patients because it may exacerbate bronchospasm; however, adverse effects are very short-lived and usually are not serious. In some cases, adenosine may also provide diagnostic information regarding the mechanism of the tachycardia. For example, if AV block occurs before termination of the tachycardia and P waves or flutter waves can be seen, AVRT and AVNRT are excluded (see Fig. 17–4B).

Alternative treatment options include verapamil given in incremental 2.5- to 5-mg IV doses, which also acts by slowing conduction in the AV node; however, it must be given with caution in patients with left ventricular dysfunction. Diltiazem is an alternative, but with the same precautions as for verapamil. Procainamide (50 mg/min IV to a total dose of 1000 mg) may also be used in the acute setting and causes tachycardia termination by conduction block in the bypass tract in patients with atrioventricular reentrant tachycardia (AVRT). Ultimately, the treatment of choice for these patients is now electrophysiologic study and radiofrequency catheter ablation.

ECTOPIC ATRIAL TACHYCARDIA

Ectopic atrial tachycardia is characterized by P waves of a single morphology, but with a different axis to that in sinus rhythm, indicating that the focus is not the sinus node. Atrial tachycardia may be paroxysmal or incessant, and the mechanism is usually an automatic focus within the atria. After the onset, the tachycardia may display a characteristic shortening of the P-P intervals known as a "warm-up" phase. Most adults with this arrhythmia do not have underlying heart disease; however, in some patients the tachycardia may provoke cardiomyopathy. When treatment of an underlying condition or discontinuation of provocative agents such as beta-agonists does not resolve the tachycardia, beta-blockers or calcium channel blockers may help to control the ventricular rate, but they rarely suppress the tachycardia. Class I antiarrhythmic drugs and amiodarone have been given with limited success in some patients, but the treatment of choice in resistant cases is now radiofrequency catheter ablation (Lesh et al, 1994). As discussed later, atrial tachycardia in the setting of digoxin toxicity should be treated with digoxin-specific antibody fragments.

MULTIFOCAL ATRIAL TACHYCARDIA

Multifocal atrial tachycardia is characterized by an atrial rate between 100 and 160 per minute and the presence of P waves with at least three distinct morphologies (Kastor, 1994). Notably, it is rarely encountered outside the acute medical care or postoperative situation. It is important to distinguish this rhythm from atrial fibrillation, because therapy should be directed at the underlying cause and agents such as digoxin frequently produce only drug toxicity.

Common causes include exacerbation of chronic obstructive pulmonary disease; pneumonia; metabolic disorders such as acidosis, hypokalemia, or hypomagnesemia; and theophylline toxicity. With amelioration of these factors, the rate is frequently controlled and the arrhythmia may resolve. This treatment method parallels the approach to sinus tachycardia, which is often seen in similar situations. If ventricular rate control is required, for example in a patient with unstable angina, beta-blockers or calcium channel blockers can be administered for rate control until the underlying condition is improved.

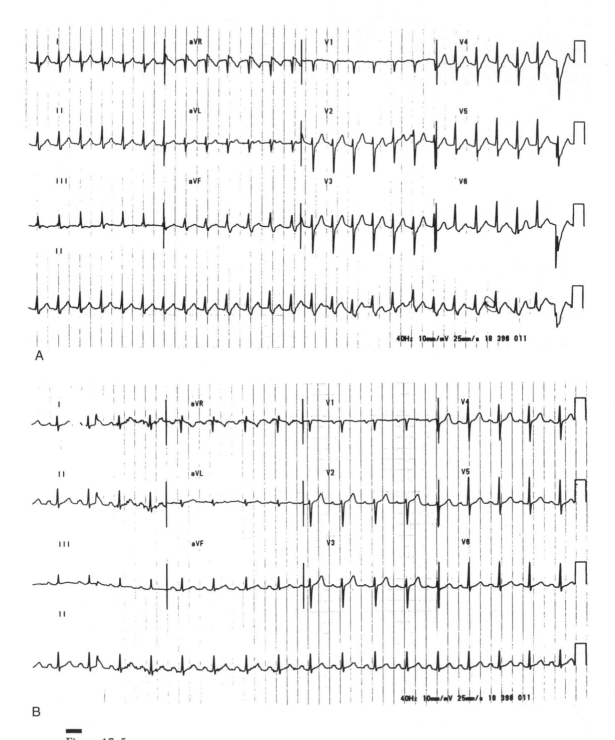

Figure 17–5
(A) Supraventricular tachycardia with a rate of approximately 160/min. Note the pseudo S waves in lead II and the pseudo R′ wave in lead V1, which represent retrograde P waves and suggest AV nodal reentrant tachycardia (AVNRT) as the mechanism. (B) Tracing from the same patient following conversion to sinus rhythm.

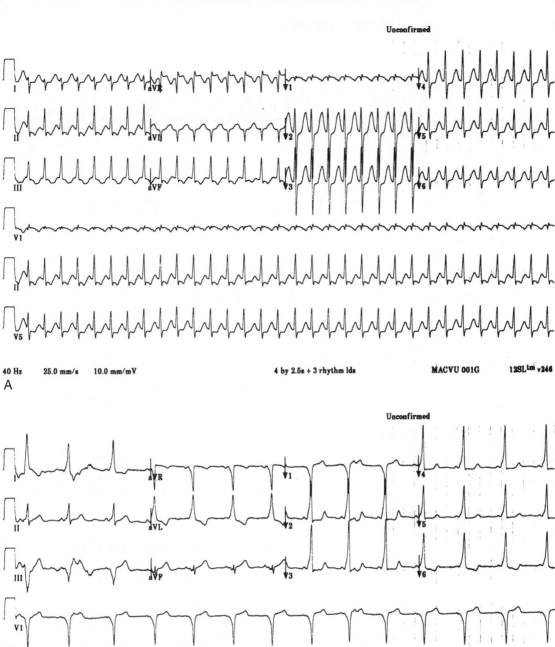

40 Hz   25.0 mm/s   10.0 mm/mV   4 by 2.5s + 3 rhythm lds   MACVU 001G   12SL^{tm} v246

A

40 Hz   25.0 mm/s   10.0 mm/mV   4 by 2.5s + 3 rhythm lds   MACVU 001G   12SL^{tm} v246

B

Figure 17–6
(A) Orthodromic (i.e., antegrade conduction over the normal conduction system and retrograde conduction over the bypass tract) atrioventricular reentrant tachycardia (AVRT). The tachycardia was terminated with verapamil. (B) 12-lead ECG in the same patient following conversion to sinus rhythm showing the classic Wolff-Parkinson-White pattern of short PR interval, widened QRS and delta wave. Note the presence of pseudo Q waves, seen here in the inferior leads, which means that prior myocardial infarction cannot generally be diagnosed in the presence of WPW.

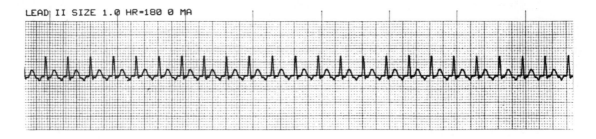

Figure 17–7
Supraventricular tachycardia rhythm strip. Discrete P waves are present, which is consistent with an atrial tachycardia whereas negative P waves in lead II suggest a low atrial focus.

DIGOXIN TOXICITY

Digoxin toxicity remains a common cause of arrhythmia requiring admission of patients to the ICU, and it still occurs in the ICU setting despite monitoring (Fisch and Knobel, 1985). It has been reported in up to 20% of hospitalized patients taking the drug. Digoxin levels commonly increase in the ICU patient with renal failure or as a result of drug interactions. Classic symptoms such as nausea, visual disturbances, and neurologic symptoms may be difficult to detect or may be absent in the ICU patient. The first sign may be the development of a new arrhythmia.

The mechanism of digoxin-induced arrhythmias may be either delayed or blocked impulse conduction, enhanced impulse formation, or both. Thus, a wide range of arrhythmias can be seen in the patient with digoxin toxicity (Fig. 17–8A–E). Ectopic impulse formation can occur in the atrium, AV node, or ventricle and block may occur in the sinoatrial (SA) or AV nodes. Paroxysmal atrial tachycardia with atrial rates from 140 to 250 per minute with 2:1 AV nodal conduction (so-called PAT with block) represents the classic arrhythmia of digoxin toxicity (Fig. 17–8A). Usually the P waves are of a different morphology than those of sinus rhythm, indicating that the ectopic rhythm is originating from a source other than the sinus node. Nonparoxysmal (i.e., gradual speed-up and slow-down) junctional tachycardia usually has a ventricular rate of 70 to 140 per minute with ventriculoatrial dissociation (Fig. 17–8D). Fascicular tachycardia usually has a right bundle branch block pattern and may also have a bidirectional pattern (alternating right and left axis deviation); the rate is typically 90 to 100 per minute (Fig. 17–8C). The tachycardia results from triggered activity due to delayed afterdepolarizations in the Purkinje tissues.

Digoxin toxicity may also occur in a patient with a "therapeutic" digoxin level. In the case of minor toxicity, which may be an asymptomatic patient with a slow ventricular response or occasional ectopy, discontinuation of digoxin may be adequate treatment. For serious bradyarrhythmias or tachyarrhythmias, or in digoxin overdoses with very elevated levels, digoxin antibodies should be used (Hickey et al, 1991). Digoxin antibodies are administered intravenously over a 15- to 30-minute period and are rapidly effective. The dose administered is calculated according to a formula taking into account both the serum digoxin level and the patient's weight. Note that because serum digoxin levels measure both free and bound digoxin, there is no value in measuring the serum digoxin level once digoxin antibodies have been given because the level remains elevated. Hemodialysis and peritoneal dialysis are both ineffective in removing digoxin.

VENTRICULAR ARRHYTHMIAS

VENTRICULAR PREMATURE BEATS

Ventricular premature beats (VPBs) are common and may be found in 40 to 75% of normal individuals (Bigger, 1994). They increase in frequency with age and with the presence and degree of heart disease. In the asymptomatic individual with no cardiac abnormality, ventricular ectopy is not associated with an additional risk of increased cardiac death. In individuals with underlying heart disease, frequent ventricular ectopy correlates with an increased risk of sudden death and is additive to the risks associated with left ventricular dysfunction. With the exception of symptom relief in some patients, there is no proven benefit to treating VPBs with antiarrhythmic drugs. In fact, some patients may even have a worse outcome because of the proarrhythmic effects of these drugs. Attention should be directed to the underlying condition, and in particular metabolic abnormalities should be corrected and potentially proarrhythmic drugs discontinued.

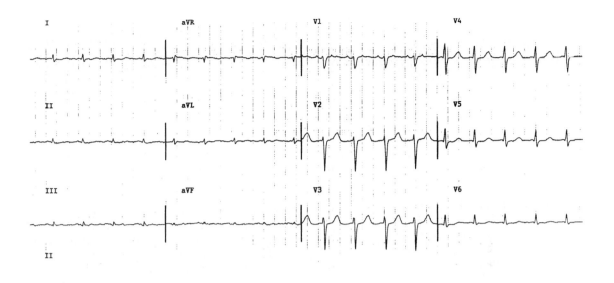

16   E600 027 1st EMERGENCY ROOM   25mm/s 10mm/mV 1386

A

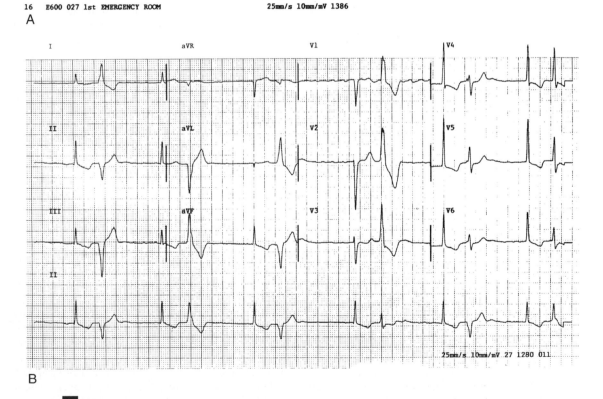

B

Figure 17–8
Selection of arrhythmias seen in digoxin toxicity (levels varied from 1.5 to 3.2).
(A) Paroxysmal atrial tachycardia with 2:1 block (best seen in lead V1). (B) Ventricular
bigeminy with underlying atrial fibrillation.

Illustration continued on following page

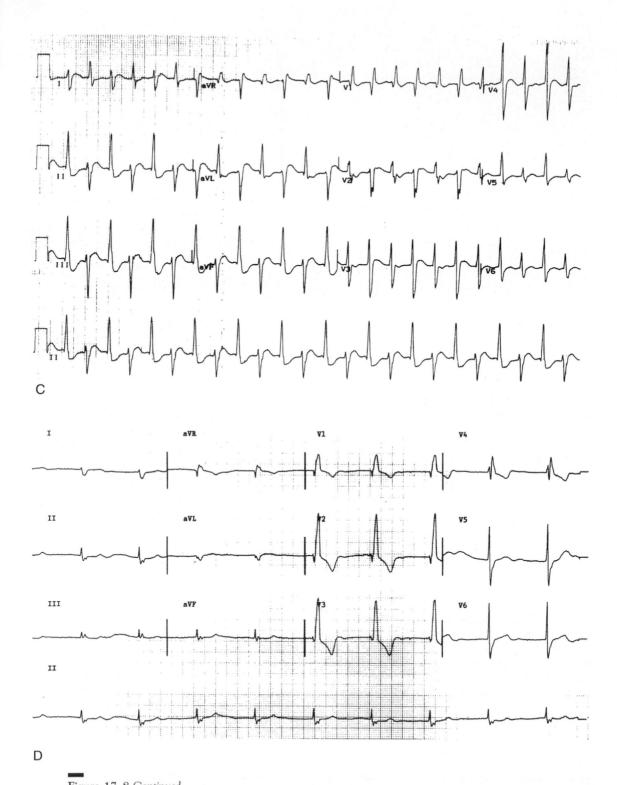

Figure 17–8 *Continued*
(C) 'Bidirectional tachycardia' with alternating left anterior and left posterior hemiblock. (D) Junctional rhythm.

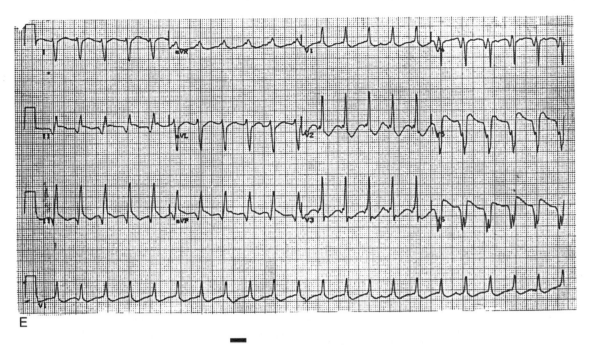

Figure 17–8 *Continued*
(E) Fascicular tachycardia.

NONSUSTAINED VENTRICULAR TACHYCARDIA

Nonsustained VT is defined as three or more ventricular beats with a rate greater than 100 per minute and a duration less than 30 seconds, not requiring intervention (Hsia and Buxton, 1993). In most cases, nonsustained VT is relatively brief in duration and often lasts less than ten beats, frequently with rates less than 160 per minute. Episodes may be highly variable in terms of rate and duration, and the morphology may be monomorphic or polymorphic (Fig. 17–9). Such episodes are common in patients with underlying structural heart disease, but rarely occur in patients with normal hearts. Most patients are asymptomatic, and the arrhythmia is noted incidentally during telemetry monitoring. Symptoms may include palpitations and presyncope. In general, unless the patient is symptomatic, no specific treatment is indicated; however, electrolyte levels should be checked and medications reviewed for possible proarrhythmic effects.

Lidocaine is commonly given in the ICU to treat nonsustained VT, but the benefits remain uncertain. It may increase the risk of asystole in patients with recent infarction. In the early phase of myocardial infarction (less than 72 hours) the occurrence of nonsustained VT is of no long-term prognostic significance. The significance of late phase (after 72 hours) nonsustained VT depends strongly on the underlying pathology and ejection fraction. Patients with a normal ejection fraction and nonsustained VT have been found to have a lower risk of sudden cardiac death than those with ejection fraction of less than 40%. Beta-blockers are indicated in patients after myocardial infarction when tolerated and have been shown to increase long-term survival. The role of antiarrhythmic drugs and/or implantable cardiac defibrillators (ICD) in these patients remains controversial and is the subject of several ongoing clinical trials (Moss, 1993).

MONOMORPHIC VENTRICULAR TACHYCARDIA

Monomorphic VT occurring in the ICU is most frequently the result of a reentrant arrhythmia in patients with prior myocardial infarction (Josephson, 1993). Triggered activity or abnormal automaticity may be the mechanism in patients with active ischemia, idiopathic cardiomyopathy, and digoxin toxicity. In the acute situation with hemodynamic compromise, immediate DC cardioversion is indicated. If the patient is hemodynamically stable, a 12-lead ECG and laboratory evaluation should be obtained. For patients with sustained monomorphic VT and a history of coronary artery disease, the initial drug of choice is intravenous lidocaine. A bolus of 1.0 to 1.5 mg/kg should be administered and an IV infusion at

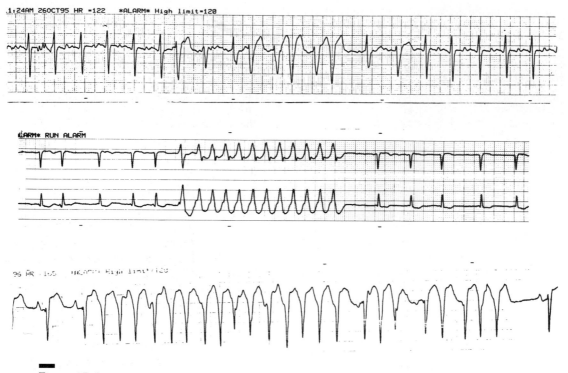

Figure 17–9
Examples of nonsustained ventricular tachycardia recorded on telemetry strips in three different patients. Note that the duration and rate of the tachycardia can vary widely.

1 to 4 mg/min started; this can be followed in 5 to 10 minutes by a second bolus of 0.5 mg/kg, while continuing the infusion. The therapeutic plasma level for lidocaine is 2 to 4 μg/ml. Toxic effects, especially those of the central nervous system, become evident at levels above 4 μg/ml, and are more likely in elderly patients and those with heart failure and hepatic insufficiency. Careful clinical monitoring of the patient is important, and the drug should be discontinued immediately if there is evidence of toxicity such as drowsiness, agitation, slurred speech, confusion, and, in more severe cases, seizures or coma.

If lidocaine is ineffective, procainamide can be tried. The loading dose of procainamide is 15 mg/kg given at a rate of up to 50 mg/min. Blood pressure should be monitored every 1 to 2 minutes during loading because hypotension is a common side effect; hypotension usually responds to decreasing the infusion rate and the administration of IV fluids.

The usual maintenance dose of procainamide is 1 to 4 mg/min. The therapeutic range for procainamide is 3 to 10 μg/ml, and toxicity is likely if this exceeds 15 μg/ml. The active metabolite N-acetyl procainamide (NAPA) can have potential proarrhythmic effects and negative inotropic

effects if the level exceeds 30 μg/ml, and its level should also be monitored. Because procainamide and NAPA are renally cleared, these effects are most likely in patients with renal insufficiency. The patient should be monitored carefully for clinical or ECG evidence of toxicity, including symptomatic sinus bradycardia, second degree heart block, increase in QRS duration of more than 25%, QTc of greater than 500 ms, or development of torsades de pointes. The development of hemodynamically unstable VT or torsades de pointes during or subsequent to procainamide loading should always be anticipated, and prompt cardioversion with at least a 200 J synchronized shock should be performed. If the rhythm degenerates to ventricular fibrillation, an immediate 360 J asynchronized shock should be delivered. Bretylium, given in boluses of 5–10 mg/kg IV at 20-minute intervals, may also be used for refractory episodes of VT. Hypotension, most often orthostatic, is the most common side effect.

Intravenous amiodarone has been approved by the Food and Drug Administration for treating ventricular tachyarrhythmias (Naccarelli et al, 1995). The currently recommended dosing schedule is an infusion of 150 mg over the first 10 minutes (15 mg/min) followed by an infusion of

1 mg/min for the next 6 hours; the maintenance infusion is 0.5 mg/min. Hypotension and bradycardia are the most significant side effects during infusion and usually respond to decreasing the infusion rate and volume repletion. Proarrhythmia is rare. Although there are isolated case reports of adult respiratory distress syndrome and hepatocellular necrosis in patients receiving intravenous amiodarone, the well-known pulmonary, hepatic, and thyroid side effects of long-term oral amiodarone therapy are usually not of concern in the ICU setting.

Amiodarone is eliminated primarily by hepatic metabolism with biliary excretion. Although no adjustment in the intravenous dosage has been defined for patients with hepatic or cardiac abnormalities, long-term amiodarone therapy is best avoided in patients with chronic hepatic and pulmonary diseases, if possible. Amiodarone has clinically important drug interactions including increased digoxin levels and inhibition of warfarin metabolism, leading to increased prothrombin

time. In addition, monomorphic VT can often be terminated by overdrive pacing, as shown in Figure 17–10. When the acute episode is controlled, a cardiology or an electrophysiology consultation should be obtained. Definitive treatment may include drug therapy guided by electrophysiologic testing, radiofrequency catheter ablation, or defibrillator implantation (Josephson, 1993).

POLYMORPHIC VENTRICULAR TACHYCARDIA

Polymorphic VT is usually observed in the setting of ongoing myocardial ischemia or infarction, but it may also be observed in cardiomyopathy and as a proarrhythmic effect in patients taking class I and III antiarrhythmic drugs (Horowitz, 1994). Lidocaine is the antiarrhythmic agent of choice because of its demonstrated efficacy in treating ischemia-related ventricular arrhythmias. Alternative antiarrhythmic agents are intravenous procainamide and amiodarone, as discussed earlier. In

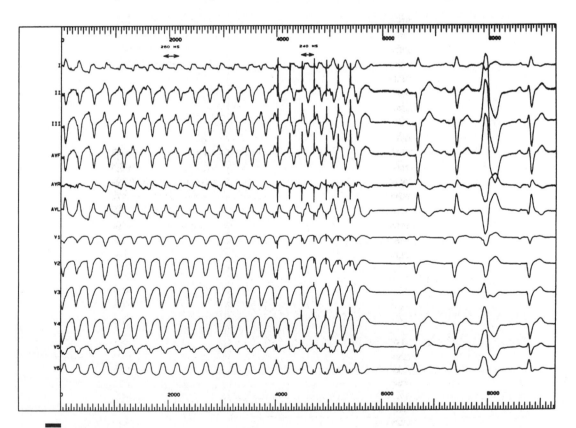

Figure 17–10
Termination of monomorphic ventricular tachycardia with overdrive pacing. The ventricular tachycardia rate is 230 bpm (cycle length = 260 ms). Overdrive ventricular pacing was attempted as the tachycardia was hemodynamically tolerated; pacing at the faster rate of 250 bpm (cycle length = 240 ms) captures the ventricle after the third paced beat and terminates the tachycardia. (Numbers on the x-axis are in milliseconds.)

most cases, defibrillation is required to terminate sustained polymorphic VT, because this condition is usually hemodynamically unstable (Fig. 17–11). Treatment should be directed to any underlying ischemia, including the use of nitrates, aspirin, beta-blockers, calcium channel blockers, and thrombolytics or angioplasty in the case of acute infarction.

TORSADES DE POINTES

Torsades de pointes is a form of polymorphic VT that is seen in the setting of either acquired or genetic QT prolongation (Horowitz, 1994). The term, which translates from the French as "twisting of points," was used by Dessertenne in his original report in 1966 to describe the rotating axis of the QRS complex (Dessertenne, 1966). The acquired form is by far the most likely encountered in the ICU setting.

The mechanism of the arrhythmia in the case of acquired long QT syndrome is postulated to be triggered activity due to early afterdepolarizations (Jackman et al, 1988). The most common etiolo-

gies of QT prolongation in the ICU setting are class IA and class III antiarrhythmic drugs and metabolic abnormalities such as hypokalemia. Episodes of torsades de pointes may be asymptomatic and nonsustained or may lead to cardiac arrest. In the acquired form of long QT syndrome, a pause is frequently noted on the ECG recording before the onset of torsades de pointes (Fig. 17–12).

As defined, torsades de pointes requires the presence of QT prolongation, although this prolongation may be minimal. An ECG during the baseline rhythm should therefore be inspected for the QT duration. The importance of making the correct diagnosis with torsades de pointes must be emphasized. Although antiarrhythmic drugs may be appropriate in episodes of polymorphic VT with a normal QT at baseline, they will most likely make the situation worse for patients with torsades de pointes. In the acute care situation, magnesium sulfate IV, 2 g of 50% solution, should be given (regardless of serum magnesium level), and can be repeated at 10- to 15-minute intervals, as required (Tzivoni et al, 1988), in addition to intravenous lidocaine. In the acquired (pause-

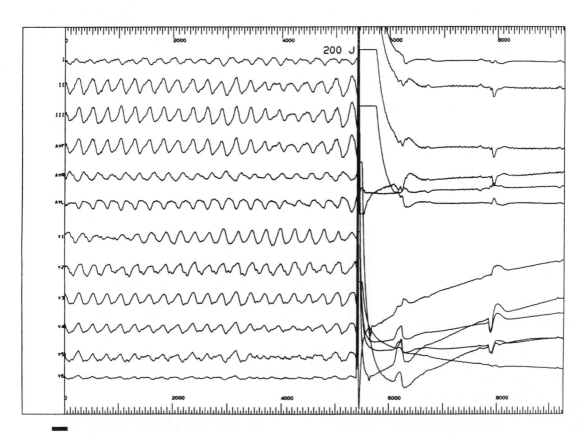

Figure 17–11

Termination of polymorphic ventricular tachycardia with a 200 J shock. Overdrive pacing was not attempted because of hemodynamic collapse. (Numbers on the x-axis are in milliseconds.)

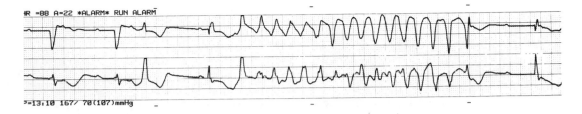

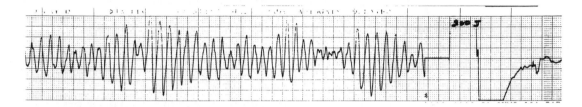

Figure 17–12
Torsades de pointes. *(Upper tracing)* Classic long-short cycle onset, with a nonsustained episode of torsades de pointes. *(Lower tracing)* Example of sustained torsades de pointes requiring cardioversion.

dependent) form of torsades de pointes, temporary transvenous pacing or isoproterenol should be administered to increase the heart rate to 90 to 100 bpm, which results in a rate-related shortening of the QT interval and diminishes the potential for further episodes. Prevention, however, is the key to treatment.

Metabolic abnormalities should be corrected, and drugs that prolong the QT interval should be discontinued. In addition to class I and III antiarrhythmic agents, other drugs that can prolong QT interval should be discontinued in this setting and include erythromycin, ketoconazole, tricyclic antidepressants (Fig. 17–13), phenothiazines, and certain antihistamines. In the case of genetic long QT syndrome, a different therapeutic approach is required, which often includes a combination of beta-blockers, permanent pacemaker, sympathetic ganglionectomy, or implantable defibrillator.

VENTRICULAR FIBRILLATION

Ventricular fibrillation occurs most commonly as a terminal event in the setting of coronary artery disease. It may also occur in many other cardiac diseases such as cardiomyopathy, valvular heart disease, congenital heart disease, and the WPW syndrome. In patients resuscitated from cardiac arrest, approximately 75% have had ventricular fibrillation, with bradycardia and asystole occurring in the remainder. VT often precedes the

onset of ventricular fibrillation. The ECG is characterized by irregular undulations of varying amplitude without discernible QRS complexes. Hemodynamic collapse always results, and the arrhythmia is uniformly fatal in 3 to 5 minutes unless promptly treated. Immediate nonsynchronized DC electrical shock with at least 200 J is mandatory. Cardiopulmonary resuscitation should be initiated.

The importance of rapid defibrillation must be emphasized, because the longer ventricular fibrillation is present the greater the energy required for successful defibrillation. Current American Heart Association advanced cardiac life support protocols advise repeating defibrillation a total of at least three times with energies up to 360 J. It is then appropriate to try epinephrine, 0.5 to 1.0 mg (5–10 ml of 1:10,000 solution), because this drug may allow a subsequent defibrillation attempt to be successful. Epinephrine can be repeated at 5-minute intervals and lidocaine, bretylium, and amiodarone can also be given. Patients who survive a cardiac arrest should be referred for cardiac electrophysiology consultation. The majority of these patients are now treated with an implantable cardioverter-defibrillator.

PROARRHYTHMIC EFFECTS OF ANTIARRHYTHMIC DRUGS

Proarrhythmia is defined as a new arrhythmia or significant worsening of an existing arrhythmia in

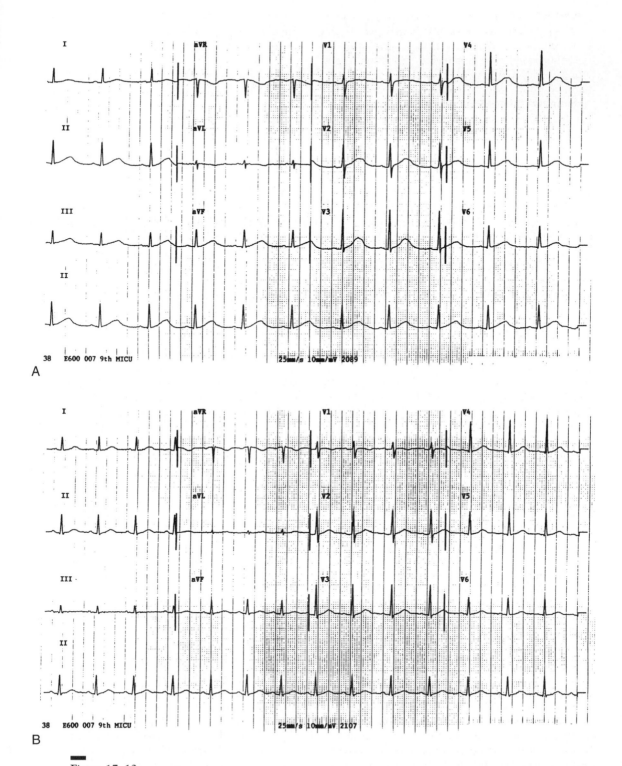

Figure 17–13
(A) QT prolongation (~600 ms) in a patient with tricyclic antidepressant overdose; (B) Baseline ECG in the same patient.

a patient receiving antiarrhythmic drugs. Antiarrhythmic drugs may be double-edged swords and can occasionally cause new arrhythmias more serious than those being treated (Goodman and Peter, 1995). In addition new bradycardias or conduction disease may develop. Sinus node dysfunction may occur as a result of administration of beta-blockers, calcium channel blockers, flecainide, sotalol, or amiodarone. Combinations of AV nodal blocking agents such as digoxin and beta-blockers are most likely to cause AV block. Adenosine is highly effective in terminating reentrant supraventricular tachycardias. It may also induce atrial fibrillation, although this is usually nonsustained. Occasionally drugs used to treat atrial flutter, such as quinidine, flecainide, and propafenone, may slow the flutter rate, but if concurrent AV nodal suppression is not administered, they may cause conversion of 2:1 AV conduction to 1:1 AV conduction, leading to a faster ventricular rate.

Ventricular proarrhythmia is the most serious side effect of antiarrhythmic drug therapy. It is most common in patients with underlying heart disease, and often (but not always) occurs in the initial period of antiarrhythmic drug therapy. This problem was highlighted by the results of the Cardiac Arrhythmia Suppression Trial (CAST) (Echt et al, 1991), which demonstrated a higher incidence of arrhythmic death in patients treated with flecainide and encainide than in controls; other studies have reported an incidence of proarrhythmia as high as 30% with these agents. Ventricular proarrhythmic effects may range from worsening of a previous ventricular arrhythmia to new-onset sustained VT, torsades de pointes, or ventricular fibrillation. In general, the class IC agents encainide and flecainide demonstrate the highest incidence of ventricular proarrhythmia, followed by the class IA agents quinidine, procainamide, and disopyramide and the class III agents sotalol and amiodarone. Notably, proarrhythmia is rare with the class IB agents lidocaine and mexiletine.

If a patient being treated with antiarrhythmic drugs experiences a worsening of the baseline arrhythmia, it is important to exclude metabolic imbalance and active ischemia. Drug levels should also be measured when possible. If the levels are in a therapeutic range or higher, the drug should be discontinued. Proarrhythmic effects, however, may not be dose-related, as in the case of quinidine-induced torsades de pointes. Frequent episodes of VT may require treatment with intravenous agents such as lidocaine or cardioversion, and pressor support may be needed in the case of hemodynamic compromise. Once the patient's condition has stabilized, alternative pharmacologic or nonpharmacologic therapy can be considered.

VENTRICULAR VERSUS SUPRAVENTRICULAR ARRHYTHMIAS

APPROACH TO DIAGNOSIS OF WIDE COMPLEX TACHYCARDIA IN THE ICU

One of the most common diagnostic dilemmas in the ICU setting is the treatment of a wide complex (QRS >0.12s) tachycardia. The differential diagnosis can be simplified to supraventricular tachycardia (SVT) with a functional or preexisting bundle branch block, supraventricular tachycardia with antegrade conduction over an accessory pathway (antidromic tachycardia), and VT. When the tachycardia is associated with hemodynamic compromise, cardioversion is appropriate as the first line of therapy. Knowledge of the mechanism of the tachycardia is not required. If the patient is hemodynamically stable, a 12-lead ECG should be obtained, if possible. ICU patients may also present with a wide complex tachycardia that is hemodynamically stable. A 12-lead ECG should always be obtained in any patient whose condition is stable before any treatment is given. In general, all wide complex tachycardia should initially be regarded as VT until proved otherwise. In particular, calcium channel blockers such as verapamil should not be given unless VT has been definitely excluded. Verapamil-mediated peripheral vasodilation and reflex sympathetic discharge–mediated tachycardia acceleration may lead to hemodynamic collapse in patients with VT. Lidocaine or procainamide can be administered initially in patients whose condition is stable, as previously discussed; if drug therapy is ineffective or if there is hemodynamic instability, prompt cardioversion is indicated.

The clinical history is a highly useful criterion in the diagnosis of wide complex tachycardia. Akhtar has pointed out that in patients presenting with a wide complex tachycardia, 98% of those with a history of prior myocardial infarction have VT (Akhtar et al, 1988). Patients with VT tend to be older than those with SVT, but there is a significant degree of overlap. In the younger patient with wide complex tachycardia, particularly those younger than 20 years without a history of congenital or other structural heart disease, the more likely diagnosis is SVT, especially that associated with a bypass tract.

The physical examination is also important

and may provide diagnostic information. Of note, heart rate and blood pressure can vary widely in both SVT and VT and hence cannot be used in the differentiation. When present in a wide complex tachycardia, AV dissociation, as indicated by the presence of cannon 'a' waves in the jugular venous pulse, a variable first heart sound, or P waves dissociated from the QRS on the ECG, is diagnostic for VT. AV dissociation is present in approximately 70% of cases of VT but very rarely in SVT. Note, however, that the absence of AV dissociation is not helpful in excluding VT as the mechanism.

Carotid sinus massage results in increased vagal tone and may either terminate a reentrant supraventricular tachycardia involving the atrioventricular node (such as AVNRT or AVRT) or may cause transient AV block, revealing an underlying atrial tachycardia or atrial flutter. In rare cases, carotid sinus massage terminates VT. The response to antiarrhythmic agents is helpful, but not diagnostic. A response to adenosine suggests SVT, whereas a response to lidocaine favors VT. Some forms of VT are sensitive to adenosine (e.g., exercise-induced VT originating from the right ventricular outflow tract).

As previously mentioned, it is valuable to obtain a 12-lead ECG in the hemodynamically stable patient before starting therapy. The 12-lead ECG findings that favor VT include a QRS duration greater than 140 ms, extreme left axis deviation, and AV dissociation (Table 17–3). Comparison with a prior ECG obtained during sinus rhythm can be very helpful. A marked change in morphology or a significant shift in axis also suggests VT. Fusion beats (morphology intermediate between sinus beat and ventricular complex) and capture beats (complex similar to sinus beats) can be seen with VTs at slower rates and are features of AV dissociation. Specific morphologic criteria favoring VT have also been developed for both right bundle branch block (lead V_1 predominantly positive) and left bundle branch block (lead V_1 predominantly negative) wide complex tachycardias (see Table 17–3).

The classic criteria, however, have limitations. For example, AV dissociation is clearly seen in approximately 20% of ventricular tachycardias. The stepwise algorithm of Brugada is designed so that a positive answer at any step is diagnostic of VT with a specificity of greater than 98% (Brugada et al, 1991). Further steps can then be omitted when a previous one is answered positively. In the first step, all the precordial leads are inspected for the presence or absence of an RS complex; if an RS complex cannot be identified in any precordial lead, the diagnosis of VT can be made with 100% specificity. If an RS is present in any of the precordial leads, one proceeds to step 2. If the RS interval (measured from the onset of the R wave to the deepest part of the S wave) is greater than 100 ms, the diagnosis of VT can be made with 98% specificity; otherwise, proceed to step 3. If AV dissociation is clearly present, this finding is 100% specific for VT. If none of the criteria in steps 1 to 3 is met, we proceed to step 4, which is to apply the morphology criteria for V_1-positive (RBBB) and V_1-nega-

---

Table 17–3
Criteria for Ventricular Tachycardia

Classic Criteria

1. QRS duration >0.14 sec
2. Superior QRS axis
3. AV dissociation, fusion, and capture beats
4. Morphologic criteria in precordial leads (see later)

Brugada's Criteria

1. Absence of an RS complex in leads V_1 to V_6
2. Onset of R wave to nadir of S wave greater than 100 ms in any precordial lead
3. AV dissociation, fusion, and capture beats
4. Morphology criteria in precordial leads (see later)

Morphology Criteria (in Precordial Leads)

RBBB pattern		LBBB pattern	
V_1	Monophasic or biphasic R	V_2	R >30 ms notch on S downstroke onset R to nadir S >70 ms
V_6	R/S <1	V_6	any Q wave

tive (LBBB) wide complex QRS tachycardias. For diagnosing VT, both the lead V_1 (V_2) and the lead V_6 criteria must be fulfilled, otherwise an SVT is assumed. These workers have reported an overall specificity of 96.5% and a sensitivity of 98.6% for all four steps of this algorithm. Examples of VTs with RBBB and LBBB morphologies are shown in Figure 17–14.

EFFECTS OF ELECTROLYTE DISORDERS

Electrolyte disorders are common in the ICU setting. The presence of ECG changes may often be the first indication of a particular metabolic abnormality, hence the importance in recognizing these changes (Rardon and Fisch, 1994).

Hypokalemia is characterized by flattening of the T wave and presence of a U wave, particularly when the amplitude of the U wave exceeds the amplitude of the T wave. With more severe hypokalemia, the ST segment may become depressed, the QRS widens slightly, and the P wave or PR interval prolongs. This pattern is nonspecific and may also be seen with antiarrhythmic drugs, digoxin, and in left ventricular hypertrophy. Hypokalemia may also promote supraventricular or ventricular ectopy.

The earliest electrocardiographic manifestations of hyperkalemia are symmetrically peaked or tented T waves, which occur as the potassium level approaches 6.0 mEq/l. When the level exceeds 7.0 mEq/l, the P wave flattens, the PR interval prolongs, the QRS widens, and the T waves become very prominent (Fig. 17–15). At levels above 10 mEq/l, the QRS and T wave blend together to produce a pattern simulating a sine wave. Both acidosis and hyponatremia augment the electrocardiographic changes of hyperkalemia. The differential for tall peaked T waves includes subendocardial ischemia and cerebrovascular accidents. In general, these T waves are broad-based and the QT is prolonged, whereas in hyperkalemia the T waves are narrow-based and the QT is normal. When coexistent hypocalcemia or hypomagnesemia is present, the QT interval prolongs as well. Hyperkalemia may also produce various bradyarrhythmias or levels of AV block, sinus arrest, or asystole. In other cases, tachyarrhythmias, from extrasystoles to VT and ventricular fibrillation, may occur. The rate of potassium elevation appears to influence the type of arrhythmia produced, with slower increases in potassium more likely to produce block and rapid elevations in potassium more likely to produce ventricular ectopic rhythms.

Hypercalcemia is characterized by a decrease in duration of the ST segment, and the T wave may actually begin at the end of the QRS complex. This change also produces a decrease in the QT interval. The QT has not been found to correlate with the serum calcium. Cardiac arrhythmias resulting from hypercalcemia are unusual. Hypocalcemia prolongs the ST segment with a resultant increase in the QT interval. Hypocalcemia is frequently seen combined with hyperkalemia in the patient with chronic renal failure, producing a combination of prolongation of the ST segment with a tented T wave.

BRADYARRHYTHMIAS

Bradyarrhythmias arise owing to either failure of impulse formation (as in sinus node dysfunction) or failure of conduction (as in AV nodal or His-Purkinje system disease) (Prystowsky et al, 1994). The cause may be solely from cardiac factors, but in many ICU patients other factors such as drugs, metabolic disorders, hypothyroidism, or hypothermia contribute. Many patients are asymptomatic, but when symptoms due to hypoperfusion occur, treatment is indicated. The first step in management is to increase the heart rate, which may be achieved with either a parasympatholytic drug such as atropine or a sympathomimetic drug such as isoproterenol. Doses of atropine less than 0.3 mg may cause a centrally mediated bradycardia and should be avoided, whereas sympathomimetics should be used cautiously in patients with suspected cardiac ischemia. Temporary pacing and circulatory support may be needed when there is no response to atropine, as in complete heart block. External temporary pacing is helpful for short periods until a transvenous temporary pacer can be inserted. Often, stopping an offending drug such as an AV nodal blocking agent causes resolution of the bradycardia or heart block. When bradycardia persists, cardiology consultation should be obtained to evaluate the need for permanent pacing.

Sinus bradycardia may be physiologic (e.g., in athletic individuals) or pathologic. Although sinus bradycardia is defined as less than 60 bpm, it is rarely considered pathologic unless the rate is persistently under 50 bpm. Sinus bradycardia is commonly associated with some degree of sinus arrhythmia. Sinoatrial block refers to abnormal conduction of an impulse from the sinus node to the atrium. A sudden sinus pause in which the length of the pause is an exact multiple of the PP interval suggests Mobitz type 2 sinus node exit block. A progressive shortening of the PP and RR intervals before the loss of the P wave and QRS

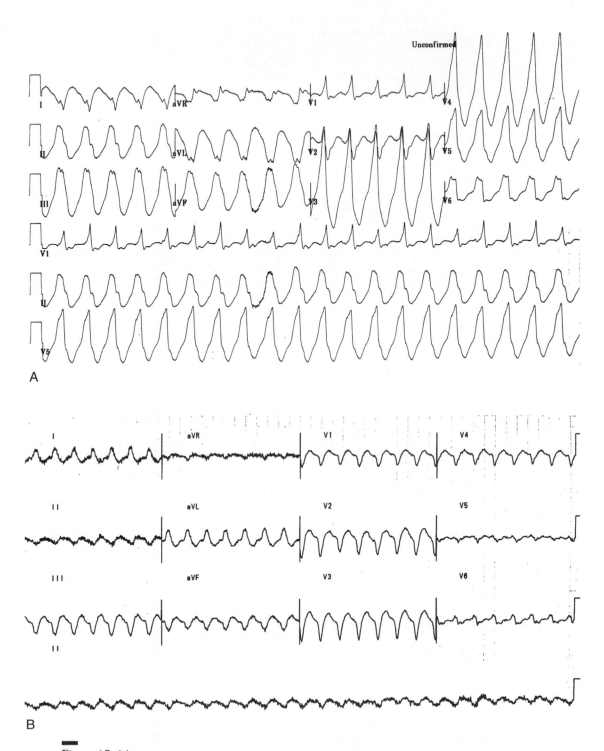

Figure 17–14
Wide complex tachycardias: *(A)* Ventricular tachycardia with a right bundle branch block pattern. VA dissociation is best seen in lead V1. *(B)* Ventricular tachycardia with a left bundle branch block pattern. Note the notch on the downstroke of the QS wave in lead V2; VA dissociation is also seen in multiple leads.

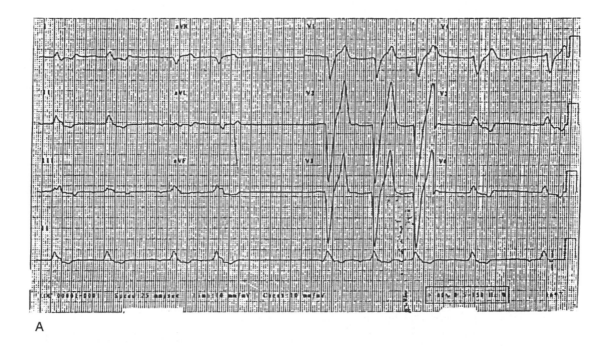

A

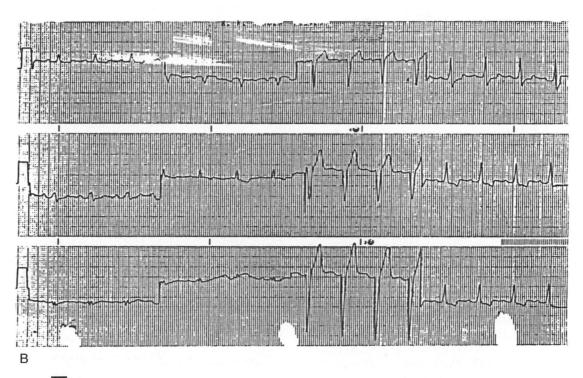

B

Figure 17–15
Hyperkalemia. (A) 12-lead ECG in a patient presenting with acute renal failure and a potassium
level of 9.0. Note the prominent T waves and widened QRS. The underlying rhythm is
wandering atrial pacemaker with AV block and junctional beats. (B) 12-lead ECG in the same
patient after dialysis; potassium level is 5.0. Note the decrease in T wave amplitude and QRS
duration; the rhythm is now sinus rhythm.

complex suggests Mobitz type I sinus node exit block.

Sinus arrest refers to an asystolic pause arbitrarily defined as greater than 2 seconds. It may be terminated by a sinus beat or by a lower escape beat. The distinction between sinus arrest and sinus exit block frequently cannot be made and, practically, is not important. Sick sinus syndrome, also known as *tachy-brady syndrome*, is characterized by sinus node dysfunction, episodes of supraventricular tachycardia, and abnormalities of intra-atrial and AV nodal conduction (Fig. 17–16). The atrial tachyarrhythmias may be atrial fibrillation, atrial flutter, or atrial tachycardia. Often an episode of atrial tachyarrhythmia terminates abruptly and is followed by a pause, presumably due to overdrive suppression of the sinus node. Tachy-brady syndrome in ICU patients may often be transient, resulting from a combination of hypoxia, metabolic abnormalities, and drug effects. If the syndrome persists once these abnormalities are corrected, a combination of antiarrhythmic drugs and permanent pacemaker is usually required.

AV nodal block is defined by delayed or absent conduction from the atria to the ventricles. The approach to treating a patient with AV nodal conduction disease should be based on three factors: the symptoms, the degree of conduction block, and the site of conduction block. The degree of AV conduction block has been traditionally classified as first, second, or third degree (Fig. 17–17). All forms of AV conduction disturbance cannot be defined in this classification, and two further categories may be added. The current electrocardiographic classification of AV block is as follows:

1. First degree AV block is defined as a prolongation of the PR interval beyond 0.2 seconds. The term is a misnomer because no P waves are actually blocked but rather there is a conduction delay from the atria to the ventricles.

2. Second degree AV block is defined as intermittent failure to conduct a single P wave. In type I second degree AV block (Wenckebach), there is progressive prolongation of the PR interval before the blocked P wave, whereas in type II second degree AV block the PR intervals are constant before the blocked P wave.

3. AV block with a 2:1 conduction ratio where the Mobitz classification system cannot be applied.

4. Advanced or high-grade AV block, where multiple P waves are blocked, but complete AV block is not present.

5. Third degree AV block (complete AV

block) is a failure of all P waves to conduct to the ventricle, resulting in complete dissociation between the P waves and the QRS complexes.

For any degree of AV conduction block, the site of the block may occur in the AV node or His-Purkinje system. Mobitz type I with a narrow QRS and a prolonged PR interval on the conducted beats suggests that the site of block is most likely in the AV node. A Mobitz type II pattern in association with a bundle branch block or an intraventricular conduction delay and a relatively normal PR during the conducted beats usually places the level of block in His-Purkinje system. For third degree heart block, a narrow QRS complex with an escape rate of 40 per minute or greater favors a diagnosis of block within the AV node; block within the His bundle or Purkinje system is characterized by a wide QRS complex with an escape rate less than 40 per minute. Noninvasive maneuvers also help differentiate the site of block. Exercise, isoproterenol, or atropine tend to improve AV nodal conduction, but have no effect or may worsen the conduction ratio in His-Purkinje (infranodal) conduction disease (Table 17–4). Vagal maneuvers or beta-blockers tend to worsen AV nodal block but do not affect or may improve conduction in infranodal disease. Slowing conduction through the AV node may allow the His-Purkinje tissue to recover from refractoriness and so improve the overall conduction ratio. There are patients, however, in whom the site of block cannot be determined without an electrophysiologic study.

As previously mentioned, the treatment of heart block in the ICU patient depends on the symptoms, the degree of block, and the site of block. Drugs that depress the AV node such as calcium channel blockers, beta-blockers, and digoxin are a common cause of heart block, and these agents should be discontinued whenever possible. Mobitz type I block is also commonly

---

Table 17–4
Noninvasive Differentiation of AV Nodal Versus Infranodal Block

Agent	AV nodal	Infranodal
Exercise/ isoproterenol	Improves	No change/ worsens
Atropine	Improves	No change/ worsens
Vagal maneuvers	Worsens	No change/ improves
Beta-blockers	Worsens	No change/ improves

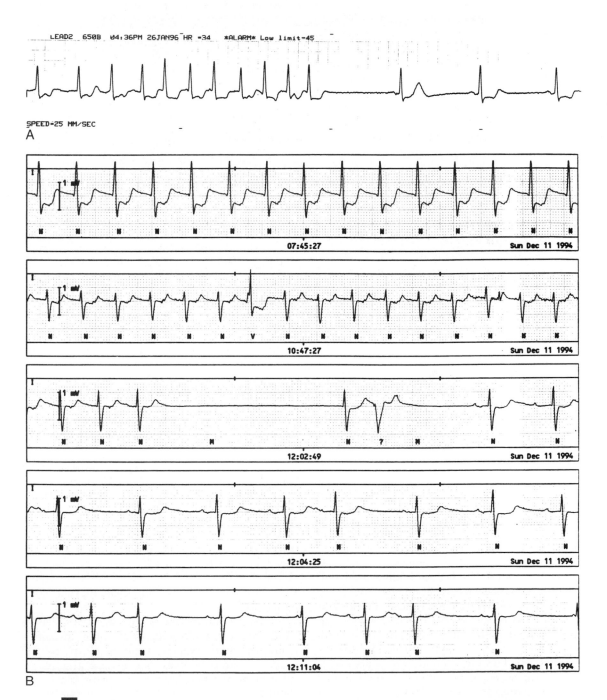

Figure 17–16
Tachy-brady syndrome. *(A)* Episode of atrial fibrillation terminating with sinus bradycardia at rate
of 35/min. *(B)* Serial rhythm strips from the same patient showing *(from top)*: junctional
tachycardia; atrial fibrillation; sinus pause; sinus bradycardia with first degree AV block.

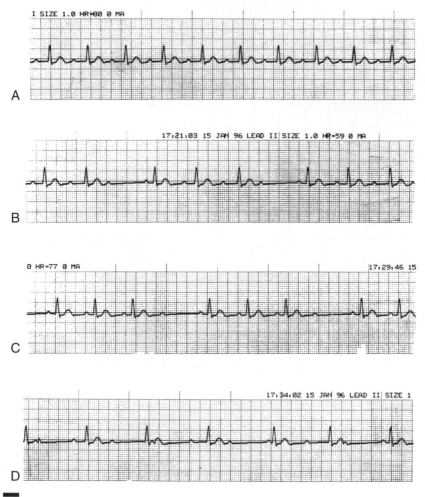

Figure 17–17
Heart block. (A) First-degree. (B) Second-degree (Mobitz type I). (C) Second-degree (Mobitz II). (D) Third-degree.

seen in the presence of an acute inferior myocardial infarction; here, as in general for first degree and Mobitz type I block, temporary pacing is not required unless the patient is unresponsive to atropine, is hypotensive, or is symptomatic.

Patients with first degree heart block with associated left bundle branch block or bifascicular block (right bundle branch block with left anterior or left posterior hemiblock) usually have a damaged His-Purkinje conduction system. Although temporary pacing is generally not required in this situation, it is important to be aware that agents that further slow conduction in the His-Purkinje system such as procainamide may cause progression to complete heart block. Mobitz type II second degree block almost always occurs in the His-Purkinje system, and the QRS morphology frequently displays a bundle branch pattern. When this type of block occurs in a critically ill

patient, a temporary pacemaker is required because of the likelihood of progressing to complete heart block without an adequate escape rhythm. If the block persists once possible causative agents have been discontinued, a permanent pacemaker is required.

Hypervagotonic states are sometimes seen in ICU patients undergoing suctioning and may cause transient complete heart block in the AV node. If atropine does not reverse the block, placement of a temporary pacing wire may be required.

Temporary cardiac pacing is usually indicated in patients with symptomatic bradycardia or heart block unresponsive to medical therapy (Wood, 1995). External units with transcutaneous pacing can be utilized to support a patient pending placement of a temporary transvenous pacemaker.

Table 17–5 summarizes the indications for

Table 17–5
Indications for Temporary Transvenous Pacing

General
  Symptomatic bradycardia or heart block
    refractory to medical therapy
  Third degree AV block with wide QRS
    escape rhythm or ventricular rate <50/min
Prophylactic
  New AV block or new bundle branch block
    in the setting of endocarditis, particularly
    of the aortic valve
  Cardioversion in the setting of sick sinus
    syndrome (transcutaneous also acceptable)
  Risk of temporary bradycardia due to drugs
  Postoperative—cardiac surgery
In patients with acute myocardial infarction
  Asystole
  Complete heart block (third degree)
  Mobitz type II second degree AV block
  New left bundle branch block
  New bifascicular block (either alternating
    RBBB and LBBB or RBBB with left
    anterior or left posterior hemiblock)
  Marked sinus bradycardia or sinus pauses
    despite atropine
  Mobitz type I second degree AV block with
    bradycardia and hypotension unresponsive
    to atropine

placement of temporary pacing in the ICU setting. In addition to Mobitz type 2 second degree block or complete heart block, new LBBB or bifascicular block developing in the setting of acute myocardial infarction usually indicates a large anteroseptal infarction, and temporary pacing is indicated. Permanent pacing is usually indicated with persistent Mobitz type 2 or complete heart block. Occasionally, prophylactic temporary pacing is necessary to allow treatment with pharmacologic agents, which may exacerbate bradycardia, such as beta-blockers in acute myocardial infarction or antiarrhythmics drugs in ventricular ectopy. Temporary pacing may also be used in the treatment of tachycardias as in the suppression of torsades de pointes or in the pace termination of typical atrial flutter or VT. Note that temporary pacing is contraindicated in the setting of bradycardia associated with hypothermia because it may precipitate refractory ventricular fibrillation.

CONCLUSIONS

1. Do not panic when presented with management of a wide complex tachycardia! The initial approach to any arrhythmia is to evaluate the patient's hemodynamic status. VT may present as a hemodynamically stable wide complex tachycardia, but may rapidly become unstable. If the patient becomes hemodynamically unstable, immediate synchronized cardioversion, for VT, or defibrillation, for ventricular fibrillation, is necessary, and knowledge of the mechanism of the arrhythmia is not needed.

2. The clinical history is as useful in diagnosing VT as a detailed analysis of the 12-lead ECG. A history of prior myocardial infarction makes the diagnosis of VT virtually certain. In one study of patients presenting with a wide complex tachycardia, 98% with a history of prior myocardial infarction had VT, whereas only 2% had supraventricular tachycardia (Akhtar et al, 1988).

3. Administration of calcium channel blockers in common (coronary artery disease–associated) VT may cause hemodynamic deterioration, acceleration of the tachycardia, or degeneration to ventricular fibrillation. Always treat a wide complex tachycardia as VT until the condition is proved otherwise. Use lidocaine or procainamide; do not use calcium channel blockers.

4. Before starting drug therapy for VT, have a defibrillator ready for operation and make sure a crash cart and intubation equipment are in the room. Remember that procainamide may cause hypotension, and if hypotension does not rapidly respond to decreasing infusion rate and IV fluid bolus, proceed to cardioversion without delay.

5. In patients receiving antiarrhythmic drugs who develop worsening of their arrhythmia or new arrhythmias, think of proarrhythmic effects of the drug—and stop it. Recall also that lidocaine toxicity causes mental status changes, and the dosage should be decreased or the drug discontinued in these so affected patients.

6. Digoxin is no better than placebo in converting atrial fibrillation to sinus rhythm. Patients with renal insufficiency and the elderly are more prone to develop digoxin toxicity. When new conduction abnormalities or tachyarrhythmias develop in a patient on digoxin, suspect digoxin toxicity.

7. Amiodarone's interaction with digoxin and coumadin may cause elevated digoxin levels and prolonged prothrombin time (PT). It is our practice to decrease the dose of digoxin by half and follow the PT carefully when using these drugs concomitantly.

8. Always save rhythm strips, particularly those showing the initiation and termination of tachycardia, and the response to any maneuvers or drugs. A 12-lead ECG should always be obtained if possible for stable tachyarrhythmias.

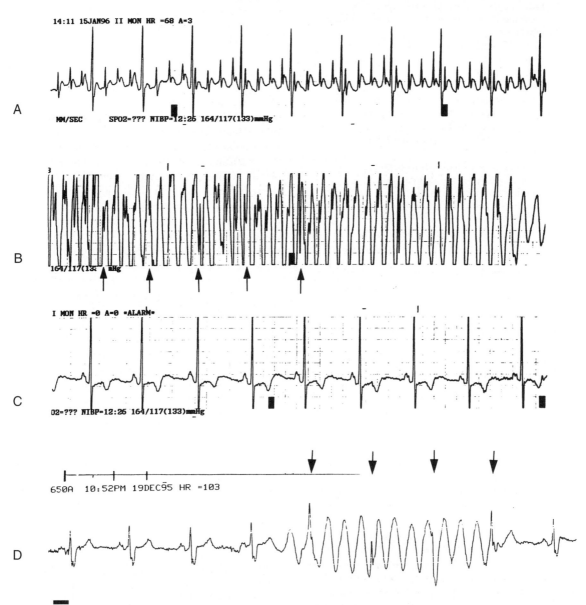

Figure 17–18
Artifact tracings in an elderly patient with Parkinson's disease. (A) Artifact mimicking atrial
flutter. (B) Artifact mimicking polymorphic ventricular tachycardia/ventricular fibrillation, with
the underlying QRS complexes arrowed. (C) The patient's underlying sinus rhythm. (D) Artifact
tracing from a different patient mimicking nonsustained ventricular tachycardia.

Table 17–6
Acute Management of Common Arrhythmias

Arrhythmia	Approach to Management

Bradycardia	Without hemodynamic compromise
	   Observe for first degree and Mobitz type I block
	   Transcutaneous or transvenous pacemaker for Mobitz 2 or third degree AV block
	With hemodynamic compromise
	   Atropine 0.5 mg IV
	   Transcutaneous pacemaker until transvenous possible
	   Consider dopamine or isoproterenol infusions

Narrow complex Tachycardia (QRS <120 ms)	Atrial flutter or fibrillation
	   Rate control—beta or Ca channel blocker, digoxin
	   Cardioversion—procainamide 20–30 mg/min to maximal dose of 15 mg/kg; quinidine; electrical (if duration <48 hours)
	   Anticoagulation
	For hemodynamic instability, cardiovert with 100 J or 200 J
	SVT (AVNRT, AVRT, Atrial tachycardia)
	   Adenosine 6 mg IV; may repeat with 12 mg and 18 mg
	   Verapamil 2.5–5 mg IV
	For hemodynamic instability, cardiovert with 50 J or 100 J

Wide complex Tachycardia (QRS >120 ms)	Treat as ventricular tachycardia unless certain of other etiology
	   Lidocaine 1–1.5 mg/kg IV;
	   Procainamide 20–30 mg/min IV to max dose of 15 mg/kg;
	   Bretylium 5–10 mg/kg IV;
	   Consider amiodarone IV (loading dose 15 mg/min for the first ten minutes, then 1 mg/min over next 6 hours)
	For hemodynamic instability, cardiovert with 200 J, 300 J, 360 J

Ventricular fibrillation/ pulseless ventricular tachycardia	CPR, O_2, intubate, IV Defibrillate 200 J, 300 J, 360 J Epinephrine 1 mg IV; repeat q 3–5 min Continue management per ACLS protocols
Asystole/ electromechanical dissociation (EMD)	CPR, O_2, intubate, IV Consider transcutaneous pacer immediately in asystole if available Epinephrine 1 mg IV; repeat at 3- to 5-min intervals Atropine 1 mg IV; repeat at 3- to 5-min intervals Establish and treat cause if possible (e.g. hypoxemia, pulmonary embolus, cardiac tamponade, acute MI, hypovolemia, hypothermia, drug overdose) Consider sodium bicarbonate 1 mEq/kg in acidosis

The above table is not designed to serve as a guide to Advanced Cardiac Life Support (ACLS). Readers should refer to the Guidelines for Cardiopulmonary Resuscitation and Emergency Cardiac Care of the American Heart Association published in the Journal of the American Medical Association 268: 2171–2303, 1992.

9. Artifact may sometimes simulate arrhythmias in the ICU patient. A Parkinsonian tremor may mimic atrial flutter, whereas movement artifact may mimic VT. In the latter case, the native QRS complex can be traced through the artifact (Fig. 17–18).

Table 17–6 provides an overview of the management of common acute arrhythmias.

REFERENCES

Akhtar M, Shenasa M, Jazayeri M, et al: Wide complex QRS tachycardia: Re-appraisal of a common clinical problem. Ann Intern Med 109:905, 1988.

Bigger JT: Ventricular premature complexes. In Kastor JA (ed): Arrhythmias. Philadelphia, WB Saunders, 1994, p 310.

Brugada P, Brugada J, Mont L, et al: A new approach to the differential of a regular tachycardia with a wide QRS complex. Circulation 62:1303, 1991.

Dessertenne F: La tachycardie ventriculaire a deux foyers opposes variables. Arch Mal Coeur 59:263, 1966.

DiMarco JP: Adenosine; electrophysiologic effects and therapeutic use for terminating paroxysmal supraventricular tachycardia. Circulation 68:1254, 1983.

Ditchey RV and Karliner JS: Safety of electrical

cardioversion in patients with digitalis toxicity. Ann Intern Med 95:676, 1981.

Echt DS, Leibson PR, Mitchell LB, et al: Mortality and morbidity in patients receiving encainide, flecainide or placebo: The Cardiac Arrhythmia Suppression Trial. N Engl J Med 324:781, 1991.

Evans SJL, Myers M, Zaher C, et al: High dose oral amiodarone loading: Electrophysiologic effects and clinical tolerance. J Am Coll Cardiol 19:169, 1992.

Falk RH, Knowlton AA, Bernard SA, et al: Digoxin for converting recent onset atrial fibrillation to sinus rhythm: A randomized, double blind trial. Ann Intern Med 106:503, 1987.

Falk RH and Podrid P (eds): Atrial Fibrillation Mechanisms and Management. New York, Raven Press, 1992.

Feld G, Fleck P, Chen PS, et al: Radiofrequency catheter ablation for the treatment of human type I atrial flutter. Circulation 86:1223, 1992.

Fisch C and Knobel SB: Digitalis cardiotoxicity. J Am Coll Cardiol 5:91A, 1985.

Fuchs T and Podrid PJ: Pharmacologic therapy for reversion of atrial fibrillation and maintenance of sinus rhythm. In Falk RH, and Podrid P (eds): Atrial Fibrillation Mechanisms and Management. Raven Press, New York, 1992, p 233.

Goodman JS and Peter CT: Proarrhythmia: Primum non nocere. In Mandel WJ (ed): Cardiac Arrhythmias, 3rd ed. Philadelphia, JB Lippincott, 1995, p 173.

Hickey AR, Wegner TL, Carpenter VP, et al: Digoxin immune Fab therapy in the management of digitalis intoxication. J Am Coll Cardiol 17:590, 1991.

Horowitz LN: Polymorphic ventricular tachycardia including torsade de pointes. In Kastor JA (ed): Arrhythmias. Philadelphia, WB Saunders, 1994, p 376.

Hsia HH and Buxton AE: Work-up and management of patients with sustained and nonsustained ventricular tachycardias. Cardiol Clin 11(1):21, 1993.

Jackman WM, Friday KJ, Anderson JL, et al: The long QT syndromes: A critical review, new clinical observations and a unifying hypothesis. Prog Cardiovasc Dis 31:115, 1988.

Janse MM: Mechanisms of Arrhythmias. Mount Kisco, NY, Futura Publishing, 1993.

Josephson ME: Clinical Cardiac Electrophysiology: Techniques and Interpretations, 2nd ed. Philadelphia, Lee & Febiger, 1993.

Kastor JA: Arrhythmias. Philadelphia, WB Saunders, 1994, p 133.

Klein GJ, Bashore T, Sellers TD, et al: Ventricular fibrillation in the Wolff-Parkinson-White syndrome. N Engl J Med 301:1080, 1979.

Lee JR, Grogin HR, Fitzpatrick AP, et al: Sinus node modification for inappropriate sinus tachycardia. J Am Coll Cardiol 82:155A, 1994.

Lesh MD, Van Hare GF, Epstein LE, et al: Radiofrequency catheter ablation of atrial arrhythmias: Results and mechanisms. Circulation 89:1974, 1994.

Lundstrom T and Ryden L: Chronic atrial fibrillation: Long term results of direct current cardioversion. Acta Med Scand 223:53, 1988.

Manning WJ, Silverman DI, Katz SE, et al: Impaired left atrial mechanical function after cardioversion: Relation to the duration of atrial fibrillation. J Am Coll Cardiol 23:1535, 1994.

Manning WJ, Silverman DI, Keighley CS, et al: Transesophageal echocardiography facilitated early cardioversion from atrial fibrillation using short-term anticoagulation: Final results of a prospective 4.5 year study. J Am Coll Cardiol 25:1354, 1995.

Moss AJ: Influence of the implantable cardioverter defibrillator on survival: Retrospective studies and prospective trials. Prog Cardiovasc Dis 36:85, 1993.

Naccarelli GV and Jalal S: Intravenous amiodarone: Another option in the acute management of sustained ventricular tachyarrhythmias. Circulation 92:3154, 1995.

Prystowsky EN and Klein GJ: Cardiac Arrhythmias: An Integrated Approach for the Clinician. New York, McGraw-Hill, 1994, pp 99 and 211.

Rardon DP and Fisch C: Electrolytes and the heart. In Schlant RC, and Alexander RW (eds): Hurst's The Heart, 8th ed. New York, McGraw-Hill, 1994.

Tzivoni D, Keren A, Cohen AM: Treatment of torsade de pointes with magnesium sulfate. Circulation 77:392, 1988.

Waldo AL: Atrial flutter: New directions in management and mechanism. Circulation 81:1142, 1990.

Wood MA: Temporary cardiac pacing. In Ellenborgen KA, Kay GN, and Wilkoff BL (eds): Clinical Cardiac Pacing. Philadelphia, WB Saunders, 1995, p 759.

Acute Respiratory Distress Syndrome

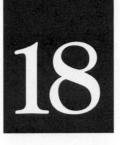

Daniel P. Schuster, M.D.

Marin H. Kollef, M.D.

DEFINITION

The American Thoracic Society and the European Society of Intensive Care Medicine (ATS-ESICM) have recommended that so-called acute lung injury (ALI) be defined as "a syndrome of inflammation and increasing permeability that is associated with a constellation of clinical, radiologic, and physiologic abnormalities that cannot be explained by, but may coexist with, left atrial or pulmonary capillary hypertension" (Bernard et al, 1994). The acute respiratory distress syndrome (ARDS), then, is simply defined as a particularly severe form of ALI (see Chapter 1), based principally on how severely oxygenation is affected (Table 18–1).

Although this definition lends itself to operational criteria that are easily implemented, it has also been challenged as nonspecific (the causes of abnormal oxygenation are multifactorial and are not limited to those due to lung injury alone) and insensitive (patients with lung injury *and* pulmonary capillary hypertension for any reason are automatically excluded). Accordingly, an alternative view has been presented (Schuster, 1995): ARDS is viewed as a *specific type* of lung injury (albeit a severe one with diverse causes), characterized by pathologic structural changes (in this case, known as *diffuse alveolar damage* [DAD]) (see Pathology, later), which is associated with a breakdown in the barrier and gas exchange functions of the lung. The result is proteinaceous alveolar edema and severe hypoxemia—both clinical hallmarks of ARDS (see Table 18–1). Although this definition may be more rigorous, its criteria are not as easily implemented as that for the criteria of the ATS-ESICM conference.

DIAGNOSIS

Patients with ARDS have severe respiratory distress (dyspnea, tachypnea) associated with the acute onset of diffuse infiltrates on chest radiographs, and hypoxemia. So do patients with many other pulmonary syndromes. To diagnose ARDS definitively, these signs and symptoms must be linked with the presence of DAD and increased

Table 18–1
Definitions and Diagnostic Criteria

	Lung Injury		ARDS	
	ATS-ESICM recommendation	Our recommendation	ATS-ESICM recommendation	Our recommendation
Definitions	"Syndrome of inflammation and increased permeability . . . [not due to] pulmonary capillary hypertension"	Significant deterioration in lung function associated with characteristic pathology	Severe ALI	Specific type of ALI
Criteria	Acute onset bilateral radiographic infiltrates PaO_2/FIO_2 <300 No evidence for CHF	Depends on condition	ALI criteria, but PaO_2/FIO_2 <200	Bilateral radiographic infiltrates, increased pulmonary vascular permeability, diffuse alveolar damage
Quantitation	LIS; general scoring systems	Depends on condition	LIS, general scoring systems	Measure of vascular permeability; general scoring systems

ATS = American Thoracic Society; ESICM = European Society of Intensive Care Medicine; ALI = acute lung injury; ARDS = acute respiratory distress syndrome; CHF = congestive heart failure; LIS = lung injury score

vascular permeability (see Table 18–1). Because therapy does not yet depend on knowing whether permeability is abnormal or DAD is present (which requires expensive and invasive testing), the diagnosis of ARDS is still usually made by inference, employing operational criteria similar to those suggested by the ATS-ESICM consensus conference (see Table 18–1).

Even so, the diagnosis of ARDS can be difficult; any process that can cause alveolar filling can mimic ARDS: any alveolar hemorrhage syndrome, other acute inflammatory processes such as pneumonia, and other causes of pulmonary edema. Without pathology laboratory demonstration of DAD (Meyrick, 1986; Tomashefski, 1990) and without direct evidence of increased pulmonary vascular permeability (Kaplan, 1991), the diagnosis of ARDS can be made with certainty only if these other processes can be excluded, or if in retrospect the pulmonary infiltrates failed to clear despite treatment for these other conditions.

QUANTIFYING SEVERITY

Currently, the most popular method of quantifying "injury" in ARDS is to generate a score based on the degree of hypoxemia, the extent of pulmonary infiltrates on a chest radiograph, and the respiratory system compliance measurement (Murray et al, 1988) (Table 18–2). Although easy to obtain, virtually no objective data support such widespread use of this scoring system as a measure

of severity. Because the pathophysiology of the three main components of this score is linked, it would be surprising if they had individual discriminatory value. A direct measure of pulmonary vascular permeability is probably a better index of alveolar damage (Schuster, 1995), whereas generalized intensive care unit (ICU) scoring systems may be better predictors of overall outcome (Schuster, 1992).

EPIDEMIOLOGY

There is no evidence that ARDS is more common among patients of a certain age, gender, or race. Its exact incidence is controversial, perhaps because of the problems just cited with definition and diagnosis. A figure of 75 affected persons in 100,000 population per year is often cited, but other estimates are only one-tenth to one-twentieth as large (Lewandowski et al, 1995). In any individual ICU, the incidence of ARDS probably

Table 18–2
Components of Lung Injury Score (LIS)

- Extent of involvement on chest radiograph
- PaO_2/FIO_2 value
- Amount of PEEP
- Respiratory system compliance

Range of values for each component: 0–4
Arbitrarily, ARDS = LIS >2.5

reflects the relative frequency of various "risk factors" often associated with the syndrome (see the section on pathogenesis).

PRESENTATION

ARDS is not difficult to recognize when a patient, without pre-existing or coexisting conditions that mimic or obscure otherwise typical signs and symptoms, develops acute respiratory distress and bilateral alveolar infiltrates on a chest radiograph following an appropriate clinical event. The inhalation of a toxic gas (see Chapter 25) or the ingestion of certain drugs in toxic doses, severe viral pneumonia, and aspiration of gastric contents during resuscitation from cardiac arrest are all examples of well-defined events that can cause ARDS in otherwise healthy individuals.

Interestingly, the onset of respiratory distress is often delayed by several hours (and sometimes by as many as 1–3 days) from the actual inciting event. No explanation for this delay, or for why it varies among individuals, has ever been developed with supporting evidence, although it is widely suspected that time is needed for upregulation of inflammatory mediators. Even so, 80% of patients who develop ARDS do so within the first 24 hours after the onset of the inciting event (Fowler et al, 1985).

Another interesting and still inadequately explained aspect is that respiratory symptoms often precede the full development of infiltrates on the chest radiograph. Alveolar infiltrates invariably develop within several hours of the onset of symptoms.

Respiratory symptoms other than dyspnea and tachypnea are uncommon. Obviously, significant fever, cough, and purulent sputum suggest primary pneumonia instead of ARDS. With audible wheezing and pleuritic pain, one should consider alternative diagnoses. Of course, symptoms of congestive heart failure also suggest a different etiology for pulmonary edema.

The most dramatic and consistent aspects of the physical examination include tachypnea, tachycardia, signs of increased work of breathing (intercostal muscle retraction and use of other accessory muscles of respiration during inspiratory effort), and occasionally cyanosis. With such signs, the patient may be extremely agitated, even in the absence of a primary neurologic condition. Hypotension and signs of shock are present only if they are due to an associated condition such as sepsis or massive trauma. Likewise, fever may not be prominent unless the associated condition is related to infection. On pulmonary examination, "dry" crackles (rales) may be heard throughout the lung fields, although the chest examination may be surprisingly normal despite severe alveolar infiltrates on the chest radiograph. End-expiratory wheezes can often be heard, but frank airway obstruction with a prolonged expiratory time is not. Pleural friction rubs are also rare. At the time of presentation, the rest of the physical examination is usually normal unless other organ systems are involved by pre-existing or coexisting disease.

CHEST RADIOGRAPHY AND OTHER TESTS

The initial abnormal radiograph may show only a bilateral perihilar haze with linear opacities extending from the hilum, which is consistent with interstitial edema. As alveolar flooding develops in some areas, the linear opacities coalesce into areas consistent with alveolar filling. If alveolar filling progresses, more of the lung parenchyma becomes involved radiographically, occasionally progressing to near-total "white-out" of both lung fields (Fig. 18–1). Although always bilateral, the actual extent of lung involvement in many cases, of course, is much less dramatic.

The appearance of radiographic shadows within the lung parenchyma can be identical to that in congestive heart failure, although at least one group has concluded that the densities tend to be more peripheral and less gravitationally oriented (from apex to base in the semirecumbent or supine position) than those in typical heart

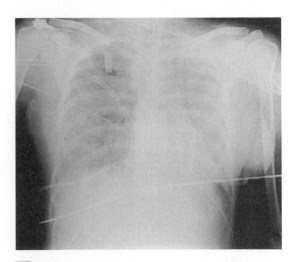

Figure 18–1
Portable chest radiograph showing classic diffuse bilateral interstitial and alveolar infiltrates of a patient with early adult respiratory distress syndrome (ARDS), creating a picture of near-total "white-out."

failure (Milne et al, 1985). More important, when pre-existing or coexisting heart disease or intravascular fluid overload is absent, other radiographic signs of congestive failure, such as cardiomegaly, perfusion redistribution, peribronchial cuffing, peripheral septal lines (Kerley B lines), and pleural effusions, are absent. Although these distinctions are conceptually useful, overlap is common and distinctions between cardiogenic and noncardiogenic causes can be difficult in individual cases.

Computed tomography (CT) has been utilized to evaluate the ventral-dorsal distribution of pulmonary infiltrates in supine or prone patients with ARDS (Bone, 1993; Gattinoni et al, 1986). Surprisingly, although the infiltrates are always bilateral and diffuse, parenchymal densities are usually greater in dorsal than ventral lung regions in supine patients (Fig. 18–2). Because some of these infiltrates resolve when patients are repositioned into the prone position, atelectasis is thought to be an important cause for such regional inhomogeneity. Although ventral-dorsal gradients in lung density may be detected with CT, the increases in vascular permeability are more evenly distributed (Sandiford et al, 1995). CT often reveals evidence for barotrauma that was otherwise unsuspected from conventional portable radiography.

Measurements of gas exchange, although absolutely vital to management, are rarely of help diagnostically. Not uncommonly, the initial arterial blood studies show respiratory alkalosis and varying degrees of hypoxemia. Finger pulse oximetry shows arterial desaturation in proportion to the extent of arterial hypoxemia. The hypoxemia is often relatively resistant to supplemental oxygen (i.e., little improvement occurs when O_2 is administered by nasal prongs or face mask). Indeed, such "refractory" hypoxemia is a classic sign of ARDS, indicating that intrapulmonary shunting is an important, and often the principal, cause for the hypoxemia (Fig. 18–3) (see Chapter 2). As alveolar edema accumulates, hypoxemia continues to worsen and mechanical ventilatory support becomes necessary. Other routine laboratory tests are not expected to be abnormal, unless they reflect abnormalities resulting from associated conditions.

Bronchoalveolar lavage (BAL), protected

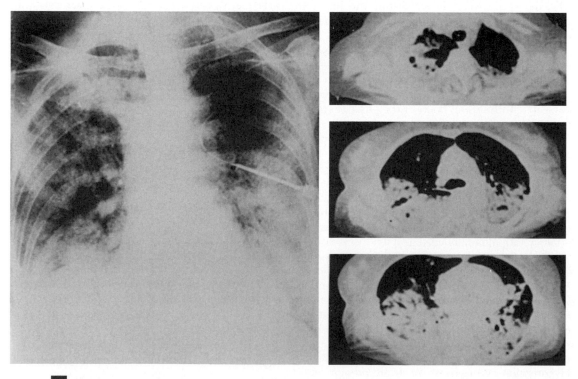

Figure 18–2
Portable chest radiograph and accompanying computed tomography scans emphasizing the nonhomogeneous and dorsally dependent infiltrates present in some patients with ARDS. (From Bombino M, Gattinoni L, Torresin A, et al: The value of portable chest roentgenography in adult respiratory distress syndrome. Chest 100:762–769, 1991. With permission.)

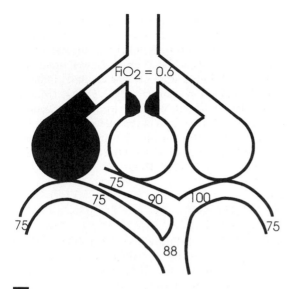

Figure 18–3
Schematic representation of intrapulmonary shunt. Normally, ventilation and perfusion are well matched. However, with the development of ARDS, blood flowing past lung units that are not ventilated (*left unit*) because of alveolar edema or atelectasis remains deoxygenated ("shunt"), regardless of FiO_2. Other units, those with low ventilation relative to perfusion (*middle unit*), allow some improvement in postcapillary oxygenation, especially with enriched oxygen in the inspired gas. Numbers represent the oxygen saturation of blood perfusing the depicted lung units.

specimen brushing of the airways, and transbronchial biopsy are often performed in patients with ARDS to evaluate whether nosocomial bacterial superinfection may be the cause of new radiographic infiltrates or persistent fever, or to rule out opportunistic infection (Leeper, 1993). In the absence of infection, the most prominent finding from lavage specimens is an increased number of polymorphonuclear leukocytes, composing as much as 80% of the total cell population (normal is <5%) (Fig. 18–4). Occasionally, eosinophilia can also be prominent, with important implications for therapy (see the section on steroid therapy). Although various investigations indicate that these studies can be performed safely, the proper role for them in diagnostic algorithms has not been clearly elucidated.

Hemodynamic monitoring via pulmonary artery catheterization is common in ARDS and is often initiated within hours of presentation. Although pulmonary edema, high cardiac output, and low ventricular filling pressures are *characteristic* of ARDS, partially treated intravascular volume overload and so-called flash pulmonary

edema (in which filling pressures are elevated only during a period of coronary ischemia and then resolve before pulmonary artery catheterization is performed) are examples of clinical problems that can cause confusion with the expected hemodynamics of ARDS. Likewise, although pulmonary edema classically develops in ARDS with normal pulmonary hydrostatic pressures, intracardiac filling pressures can nevertheless be elevated artifactually (for instance, by increased intrathoracic pressures) or as a result of therapy (for instance, by volume administration for hypotension). In turn, cardiac function can be depressed (for example, by acidosis, hypoxia, or depressant factors associated with sepsis). In our opinion, although hemodynamic monitoring can be quite valuable for *therapeutic* decision-making (and even this point is controversial), its *diagnostic* value in ARDS is greatly overemphasized.

Changes in respiratory mechanics (i.e., measurements of respiratory system compliance [C_{rs}] or work of breathing) can readily be evaluated in ARDS patients (Marini, 1990). To fully characterize C_{rs}, quasistatic pressure-volume curves can be determined (Matamis et al, 1984), although for accuracy the data must be obtained with nearly perfect patient-ventilator interaction. In ARDS, this interaction may require heavy seda-

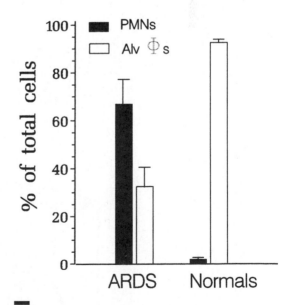

Figure 18–4
Change in the composition of bronchoalveolar lavage fluid in patients with ARDS compared with that in normal volunteers. PMNs = polymorphonuclear white blood cells. Alv øs = alveolar macrophages. (Data from Marinelli WA and Ingbar DH: Diagnosis and management of acute lung injury. Clin Chest Med 15(3):517–546, 1994.)

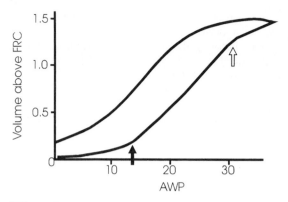

Figure 18–5
Schematic representation of airway pressure (AWP)–volume inflation (*lower*) and –deflation (*upper*) curves in early ARDS. Lung volume above functional residual capacity (FRC) is displayed on the ordinate. Curves such as these can be obtained by injecting 100-ml aliquots of air into a patient's lungs from a "super syringe" (Matamis et al, 1984), beginning at functional residual capacity, and measuring the airway pressure (AWP) at each step until either 1600 ml of air (or so) or a plateau airway pressure of 30 to 35 cm H_2O is reached. In early ARDS, lung volume changes little as airway pressure increases above FRC until a lower inflection point is reached (indicating recruitable lung and improved "compliance," *closed arrow*). At high lung volumes, the lung is maximally recruited and additional injected gas raises pressure disproportionately (upper inflection point, *open arrow*). In late ARDS, no lower inflection point may be detectable.

tion or muscle relaxation with paralytic agents. Nevertheless, the data may be especially valuable in planning ventilator support (see the section on lung protective strategies under mechanical ventilatory support, later).

When performed properly, the curves that result from these maneuvers often show lower and upper inflection points on the inflation limb of the curve, representing, initially, significant recruitment of new lung units (lower inflection point), and then a state of near-maximal inflation (upper inflection point) (Fig. 18–5) (Marini, 1990; 1993). Even without formally measuring C_{rs}, useful information can be inferred from simple inspection of the airway pressure curve during mechanical ventilation (see the section on lung mechanics, later) (Fig. 18–6).

PATHOLOGY

The pathology of diffuse alveolar damage (DAD) changes dynamically as ARDS evolves and resolves (Meyrick, 1986; Tomashefski, 1990). The changes that develop are conveniently divided into phases: exudative (days 1–3), proliferative (days 3–7), and fibrotic (after 1 week). These times, of course, are approximate, and characteristic features in each phase often overlap. The initial pathologic abnormalities are interstitial swelling, proteinaceous alveolar edema, hemorrhage, and fibrin deposition. Basement membrane disruption and denudation, especially of alveolar epithelial cells, can be seen with electron microscopy. After 1 to 2 days, hyaline membranes (sloughed alveolar cellular debris mixed with fibrin) are commonly observed by light microscopy (Fig. 18–7). Cellular infiltrate may be minimal or may be dominated by neutrophils. Fibrin thrombi can be seen in some of the alveolar capillaries and small pulmonary arteries.

Even though the type-I alveolar epithelial cell covers 95% of the alveolar surface, it is still a terminally differentiated cell that cannot regenerate. Instead, several days after the onset of ARDS, it is the type-II cell (the cell responsible

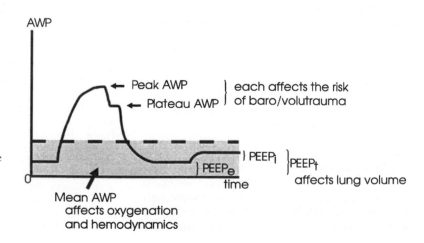

Figure 18–6
Schematic representation of the airway pressure (AWP)–time curve. $PEEP_e$, $PEEP_i$, and $PEEP_t$ = extrinsic, intrinsic, and total positive end-expiratory pressure, respectively.

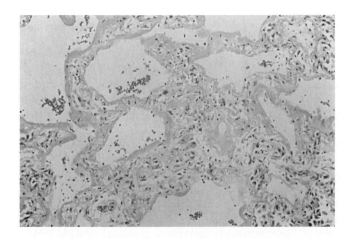

Figure 18–7
Low-power micrograph of diffuse alveolar damage, showing inflammatory cell infiltrate and hyaline membranes.

for surfactant production) that proliferates and then differentiates into new type-I cells to reline the alveolar walls. An area of active research has addressed the question of how proliferating type-II cells eventually reduce their number via apoptosis ("programmed" cell death) to re-establish a normal cell–surface area relationship (Puybasset et al, 1995).

Usually, after approximately 1 week, most of the alveolar edema has resolved, hyaline membranes are much less prominent, mononuclear cells have replaced the neutrophilic infiltrate, and fibroblasts are proliferating within the interstitium, depositing new collagen. Eventually, this healing of injured tissue may result in lung fibrosis, but the extent to which scarring develops is enormously variable. When parenchymal fibrosis does develop, intimal fibrosis and medial hypertrophy of pulmonary arterioles, along with complete obliteration of portions of the vascular bed, are also common.

Lung fibrosis in ARDS is often referred to as "interstitial" because structures between airspaces appear to be markedly widened by fibrotic material. Newer immunohistochemical techniques have revealed, however, that this fibrosis is often the result of either alveolar collapse or *intra*-alveolar fibrosis, in which the proteinaceous edema and cellular debris of the exudative stage have been incorporated into the alveolar wall. Actual deposition of new collagen within the interstitial space *per se* appears to be relatively uncommon (Crouch, 1990; McDonald, 1991).

PATHOGENESIS

A long list of agents, mediators, and conditions is associated with ARDS, undoubtedly reflecting the fact that the lung can be injured by toxic agents

after exposure from either the airways or bloodstream. Although many isolated cases of so-called ARDS are certainly examples of noncardiogenic pulmonary edema, actual DAD has not always been documented.

The causes of ARDS are often categorized as direct or indirect (i.e., whether the initiating mediator is known or whether a host response seems to be required for injury to develop) (Table 18–3). Direct causes of lung injury (e.g., pulmonary aspiration) are more likely to result in ARDS than indirect ones. In contrast, indirect mechanisms (e.g., from sepsis) are more common overall as causes of ARDS (Fowler et al, 1983; Hudson et al, 1995; Pepe et al, 1982; Sloane et al, 1992).

The risk of developing ARDS increases as the number of potential causes (sometimes alternatively called *risk factors*) increase (Hudson et al, 1995; Milberg et al, 1995; Sloane et al, 1992). Indeed, because sepsis (now generally referred to as systemic inflammatory response syndrome, or SIRS) is so often suspected as an underlying contributor, many physicians begin to treat ARDS with antibiotics as soon as infection is considered a likely diagnostic possibility. When sepsis pre-

Table 18–3
Common Conditions Associated With ARDS

Direct	Indirect
Aspiration	Sepsis
Toxic gas inhalation	SIRS
Lung contusion	Nonthoracic trauma
Lung infection	Massive transfusion
	Burns
	Pancreatitis
	Drug overdose

SIRS = systemic inflammatory response syndrome

cedes ARDS in hospitalized patients, the abdomen is often the source of infection; when sepsis develops in a patient with established ARDS, the source is usually nosocomial pulmonary infection (Bell et al, 1983; Montgomery et al, 1985; Seidenfeld et al, 1986).

When ARDS develops outside the hospital in an otherwise healthy patient (absent obvious massive trauma or burns), the most likely causes are viral infection, illicit drug ingestion, toxic gas inhalation, and gastric aspiration after some other event that caused a change in the level of consciousness (e.g., a seizure or a cardiac arrest). In contrast, when ARDS develops in a hospitalized patient, the most likely cause is either the systemic inflammatory response syndrome (including sepsis) or gastric aspiration.

EXUDATIVE PHASE

The exact mechanism of damage to the pulmonary endothelium and epithelium, even when initiated by so-called direct means, is still unknown. The most likely agents of damage are various reactive oxygen species and proteases (Deby-Dupont et al, 1991), and the neutrophil is the most likely source for their production. Also to be considered are whether and to what extent normal body defenses (oxygen radical scavengers, antiproteases) are depleted, inactivated, or overwhelmed.

The mechanisms by which neutrophils attach to endothelial cells via adhesion molecules have been the focus of enormous interest: If adhesion can be prevented, injury may be reduced or eliminated (Bevilacqua and Nelson, 1993). Neutrophils (and other cells) can also release a variety of arachidonic acid metabolites. Although these eicosanoids, as chemoattractants, can markedly affect the development and course of lung injury by their vasoactive or proinflammatory effects, they themselves are probably not responsible for increased permeability or cell damage.

ARDS can develop in patients with severe neutropenia (Matthay and Wiener-Kronish, 1990). It is possible, if not likely, that other cells residing within the lungs (e.g., tissue macrophages) can produce toxic molecules. Alternatively, some molecules, such as endotoxin, tumor necrosis factor, interleukins, or platelet activating factor, may be able to initiate membrane damage directly, by as yet uncertain mechanisms.

FIBROPROLIFERATIVE PHASE

After neutrophils are activated, they not only release potentially toxic products along endothe-lial surfaces, but they also migrate into the lung interstitium, where they can damage resident cells and release mediators, such as leukotriene B_4, which act as chemoattractants for other inflammatory cells. These cells, along with alveolar macrophages, are in part responsible for the orderly removal of cellular debris and for the orderly repair of damaged alveolar epithelium. In some patients, however, the repair process is *disordered*, and the result is an exuberant fibrosis that eventually makes gas exchange ineffective and inefficient.

Why one patient experiences complete resolution of lung injury and another develops extensive fibrosis is unknown (Marinelli et al, 1990). The basement membrane acts as a scaffold upon which replicating type-II pneumocytes can migrate and differentiate into new type-I cells to reestablish a normal alveolar lining (Crouch, 1990). Hence, an intact basement membrane is probably essential to normal repair. If the initial injury causes significant basement membrane disruption, normal cells cannot be expected to breach the large gaps that develop, and the spaces are filled by scar tissue instead (Crouch, 1990).

Endothelial injury causes the platelets to be sequestered, the coagulation cascade to be initiated, and microthrombi to develop (Jones et al, 1992). Severe fibrosis is associated with concomitant progressive occlusion and obliteration of the pulmonary vascular bed. Pulmonary arterial filling defects have been found in ARDS, but how these resolve and/or affect the resolution of the injured lung parenchyma is unknown (Jones et al, 1992). The balance (or imbalance) between procoagulant and fibrinolytic systems within the alveolar space may be an important factor affecting fibroproliferative repair.

PATHOPHYSIOLOGY

DEVELOPMENT AND RESOLUTION OF PULMONARY EDEMA

The normal extravascular water content of the lung is less than 500 ml (Sivak and Wiedemann, 1986). Modest additional amounts of extravascular water can usually be accommodated within the interstitium without significant physiologic disturbance. Because interstitial widening does not seriously compromise the thin portion of the alveolocapillary interface, interstitial edema alone generally has little effect on gas exchange. The interstitial compartment cannot expand indefinitely, however. When the extravascular lung water content approximately doubles, alveolar edema usually develops, and gas exchange is compromised (Bongard et al, 1984). The principal mechanism responsible for the development of pulmonary edema in ARDS is increased vascular permeability, although the sequence of events seems to be different for the development of interstitial versus alveolar edema (Staub, 1974, 1978).

Much less is known about how pulmonary edema resolves than about how it is generated (Matthay, 1985). The resolution of pulmonary edema is not simply a reversal of how it developed. Pulmonary edema can and probably does resolve via several pathways: lymphatics, pulmonary circulation, bronchial circulation, airways, and pleural space. The quantitative importance of each probably depends on several factors, including the rapidity with which edema develops, nature of the edema fluid, and amount of fluid that accumulates. Other factors that may affect the resolution of pulmonary edema include whether vascular permeability is normal and which therapeutic measures are employed (e.g., mechanical ventilation with PEEP) that may interfere with resolution by certain routes (e.g., the lymphatics).

The clearance of proteinaceous alveolar edema (as in ARDS) is especially interesting. Matthay and coworkers have shown that as the edema leaves the alveolar compartment, the protein concentration increases; further clearance is slower but is not halted (Matthay et al, 1985; Matthay and Wiener-Kronish, 1990). The fact that clearance continues despite the unfavorable oncotic pressure gradient suggests that clearance to some degree is dependent on an active transport process (Berthiaume et al, 1988). Indeed, Matthay and coworkers have reported that patients with ARDS who increase the protein concentration in alveolar lavage fluid (implying intact epithelial transport) have a better prognosis than those patients who do not (Matthay and Wiener-Kronish, 1990). It remains to be determined whether these observations can be confirmed and generalized, but they do hold promise that therapeutic interventions to improve edema resolution are plausible.

Even less understood is how the protein in the alveolar space is cleared. Although potential mechanisms include diffusion, mucociliary clearance, and transcellular transport, it seems likely that much of the protein is incorporated as hyaline membranes into the rest of the inflammatory exudate that accompanies the increased permeability edema of ARDS. Accordingly, clearance by alveolar macrophages seems to be the most likely, albeit still unproven, route.

GAS EXCHANGE

An important cause of the hypoxemia is extensive right-to-left intrapulmonary shunting of blood flow (see Fig. 18–3), which in ARDS may approach 25 to 50% of the cardiac output (Dantzker et al, 1979). For any given amount of alveolar involvement, the amount of shunt is greater if vessels supplying these regions are vasodilated (e.g., by prostaglandins) instead of vasoconstricted (e.g., by hypoxia).

LUNG MECHANICS

In ARDS, the change in lung volume for a given change in transpulmonary pressure is markedly reduced (from >80 ml/cm H_2O to sometimes <20 ml/cm H_2O). This change in respiratory system "compliance," reflected as higher inflation pressures, can be attributed to the reduction in aeratable lung in the early stages of ARDS and not to any change in the intrinsic elastic properties of lung tissue (Marini, 1990).

Because airway resistance is usually only modestly elevated in ARDS, *peak* airway pressures at maximal inflation should be only a few cm H_2O above the *plateau* pressure (see Fig. 18–6). In the early stages of ARDS, peak and plateau airway pressures greater than 40 to 45 cm H_2O (above the upper inflection point on the lung pressure-volume curve, see Fig. 18–5) often indicate the possibility of alveolar overdistention, with an attendant increased risk of barotrauma. Because alveolar overdistention (and not pressure-induced disruption *per se*) is now thought by many to be primarily responsible for airway pressure–associated injury in ARDS, the term *volutrauma* (instead of barotrauma) is preferred by some.

Equal in importance to avoiding alveolar overdistention may be the importance of avoiding cyclic opening and closing of atelectatic and injured lung units when ventilating below the lower inflection point on the lung pressure-volume curve (see Fig. 18–5) (Marini, 1995). This goal, if important, can usually be accomplished with PEEP levels of 10 to 15 cm H_2O, but occasionally higher levels may be necessary.

PULMONARY HEMODYNAMICS

Pulmonary hypertension is common in ARDS, but pulmonary blood pressure is usually only mildly to moderately elevated. Some patients do eventually develop right ventricular failure, and the prognosis in patients with significant elevations in pulmonary vascular resistance is worse than in those with lesser degrees of pulmonary hypertension. This observation has led some to attempt therapeutic reductions in pulmonary vascular resistance (see the section on pharmacologic therapies, later).

The causes of pulmonary hypertension in ARDS are multifactorial (Jones et al, 1992). Vasoconstriction due to alveolar hypoxia or other vasoactive mediators like thromboxane and endothelin, and intravascular obstruction from platelet thrombi or perivascular edema, probably dominate at first. Later, sustained or worsening pulmonary hypertension probably reflects the degree to which fibrosis is responsible for the obliteration of the vascular bed. Thus, the poor prognosis associated with late pulmonary hypertension in ARDS may simply reflect the severity of fibrosis.

THERAPY

GENERAL MEASURES

Because there are no specific measures to correct either the permeability abnormality or the injurious inflammatory reaction in ARDS, clinical management primarily involves supportive measures aimed at maintaining cellular and physiologic functions (e.g., gas exchange, organ perfusion, aerobic metabolism) while the acute lung injury resolves. These measures should include mechanical ventilatory support with oxygen, antibiotics for infection, nutritional support, and hemodynamic monitoring when necessary to guide fluid management and cardiovascular support (Table 18–4). Although few supportive therapies have been evaluated in a rigorous scientific fashion, an evidence-based approach can still be used to develop a reasonably rational therapeutic plan. A comprehensive review of current therapy employing this approach has been done (Kollef and Schuster, 1995).

NONPHARMACOLOGIC THERAPIES

Mechanical Ventilation

Patient-specific, physiologically targeted goals should be used to guide ventilator settings instead of routine ordering strategies (MacIntyre, 1993; Marini and Kelsen, 1992; Schuster, 1990; Slutsky, 1993). Our own priorities are to first preserve arterial oxygen saturation (i.e., SaO_2 ≥0.9), and then to prevent complications from elevated airway pressures (AWPs) (i.e., peak AWP >40–45 cm H_2O or transalveolar pressures >35 cm H_2O), from high inspired oxygen concentrations (i.e., $FIO2$ >0.6), or unnecessary atelectasis (PEEP <10 cm H_2O in most cases). Some refer to this as a lung-protective strategy (Slutsky, 1993). Our overall approach is similar to that recommended by Marinelli and Ingbar (1994) (Fig. 18–8).

Table 18–4
Summary Recommendations for Supportive Therapies in ARDS

Routine therapies
  Mechanical ventilation
  • Least FIO_2 (goal: <0.6)
  • TV to keep P_{plat} <35 cm H_2O (usually 6–10 ml/kg)
  • PEEP above lower inflection point (usually 8–15 cm H_2O)
Fluid restriction/diuresis when possible
  • Least wedge consistent with adequate cardiac output
Cardiovascular support
  • Hgb >9–10 g/100 ml
  • Inotropic support when necessary
  • Hemodynamic monitoring commonly
Nutritional support early in course
Antibiotics for proven or highly likely infection
"Rescue" therapies (for inadequate PaO_2 or excessive AWP) (in approximate order of preference)
  Neuromuscular blockade
  Permissive hypercapnea
  IRV
  Inhaled NO
  Prone position
  TGI
  ECMO/ECCO$_2$R

TV = tidal volume; P_{plat} = plateau pressure; Hgb = hemoglobin; IRV = inverse ratio ventilation; NO = nitric oxide; TGI = tracheal gas insufflation; ECMO = extracorporeal membrane oxygenation; ECCO$_2$R = extracorporeal CO_2 removal

The key elements of this strategy are to (1) recruit as many functional lung units as possible, (2) maintain their patency throughout the respiratory cycle, and (3) avoid alveolar overdistention (Marini, 1993; Tsuno et al, 1991). Accordingly, given the shape of the pressure-volume curve in early ARDS (with lower and upper inflection points), some experts believe that the ventilator should be adjusted to keep airway pressure between these two points (see Fig. 18–5). Early, but still limited, clinical data seem to show that outcomes may be favorably affected by adopting this approach (Amato et al, 1995).

We agree with the trend toward smaller tidal volumes (6–10 ml/kg) rather than the traditional larger volumes of 12 to 15 ml/kg. More specifically, we recommend that the initial tidal volume be 10 ml/kg, and that it be reduced if the transalveolar pressure (i.e., static inflation or plateau pressure) is greater than 35 cm H_2O (usually corresponding to a peak AWP >40–45 cm H_2O). Higher static inflation pressures are allowed if lung fibrosis is present, and higher peak pressures

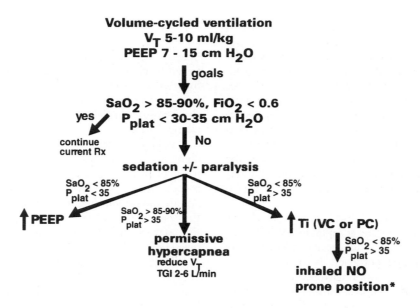

Figure 18–8
Suggested algorithm for providing mechanical ventilatory support to ARDS patients, based on a "lung protective" strategy (Marini JJ: New options for the ventilatory management of acute lung injury. New Horiz 1:489–503, 1993). FiO_2 = forced inspiratory oxygen, SaO_2 = oxygen saturation in arterial blood, V_T = tidal volume, PEEP = positive end-expiratory pressure, P_{plat} = plateau airway pressure, Rx = therapy, Ti = inspiratory time, VC = volume controlled, PC = pressure controlled, NO = nitric oxide, TGI = tracheal gas insufflation. * = some would use the prone position at an earlier stage. (Modified from Marinelli WA, and Ingbar DH: Diagnosis and management of acute lung injury. Clin Chest Med 15(3):517–546, 1994. With permission.)

are tolerated if airways resistance (e.g., bronchospasm) is present (Albert, 1995). Alternatively, the quasistatic pressure-volume curve itself may be determined (Matamis et al, 1984) to optimize tidal volume selection. If very small tidal volumes (i.e., <6–8 ml/kg) are administered, it may be advantageous (although still not proved) to give periodic breaths of larger size (i.e., ≥10 ml/kg) two to three times per minute to prevent the development of atelectasis. Although differing in some specifics, the reported approach by Amato and coworkers is similar (Amato et al, 1995).

Although this strategy seeks to minimize secondary lung injury caused by atelectasis or alveolar overdistention, it should not become an excuse to use an FIO_2 that is unnecessarily high. Although the upper limit for an FIO_2 that can be administered safely in already injured lung is unknown, the lung-protective strategy outlined earlier can be implemented with an FIO_2 at or below the conventional "upper limit" of 0.6 in the majority of cases (Amato et al, 1995). The key to achieving this dual set of goals (limited alveolar plateau pressure and limited $FIO2$) is recognizing that improved oxygenation is principally dependent on the *mean* airway pressure (see Fig. 18–6).

Positive PEEP is just one of several methods

to increase mean airway pressure with the twin goals of recruiting previously nonventilated lung and maintaining patency of these same units once recruited. Unfortunately, despite utilization of PEEP for more than two decades, the optimal end points for deciding how much PEEP (or other methods of increasing mean airway pressure, for that matter) are not established. Two approaches are made most commonly, and in our view, given the dearth of scientific data, either is acceptable. One of these strategies is empiric. PEEP is applied in increments of 3 to 5 cm H_2O until the desired physiologic goal is reached. These include acceptable arterial oxygenation (i.e., SaO_2 ≥0.9), relatively nontoxic levels of FIO_2 (i.e., FIO_2 ≤0.6) acceptable airway pressures, and improvement (or at least no reduction) in systemic oxygen delivery (from PEEP-associated decreases in cardiac output) (Marini, 1993). In general, we do not recommend exceeding 15 cm H_2O. Others, of course, believe that higher PEEP levels can be justified, especially if they are needed to exceed the pressure inflection point on the pulmonary pressure-volume curve.

The alternative approach to titrating PEEP seeks to keep the end-expiratory lung volume above the lower inflection point of the static pressure-volume curve (see Fig. 18–5). In most patients, this goal is achieved with PEEP levels between 8 and 15 cm H_2O, although levels above this may be necessary in some patients. Technically, the measured PEEP level should include both intrinsic and extrinsic PEEP, but in most cases, especially with the advent of permissive hypercapnea (see the section on mechanical ventilation, later), intrinsic PEEP is usually not very important in ARDS. In later stages of ARDS, the lower inflection point is often absent, and targeting the level of PEEP to ablate an inflection point is not possible.

When this level of PEEP does not achieve adequate oxygenation at acceptable levels of FIO_2 and airway pressure, additional measures are necessary. Our first approach is to try so-called controlled hypoventilation with permissive hypercapnia (Marini, 1993). With this approach, hypoventilation and hypercapnia are allowed because gradual increases in $PaCO_2$ (even as high as 100 mm Hg) are usually well tolerated, especially if significant acidosis (i.e., pH <7.20–7.25) does not occur. Buffer administration can be used if more severe acidosis develops, or, in centers with the appropriate experience, extracorporeal CO_2 removal can be used. By itself, the reduction in ventilatory rate allows more time for exhalation, thereby reducing the level of auto-PEEP and mean AWP. Therefore, permissive hypercapnea makes it easier to initiate ventilatory modes like inverse ratio ventilation (see the next section).

Even if oxygenation and FIO_2 goals are being met, excessively high AWP may still be present, requiring ventilator adjustments that result in hypercapnia. For instance, many patients with ARDS develop plateau pressures exceeding pressures at the upper inflection point, even with tidal volumes of 10 ml/kg or less (Roupie et al, 1995). Reducing the tidal volume by 20 to 30% lowers the plateau pressure below the upper inflection point, but also is accompanied by a significant rise in the $PaCO_2$ (Roupie et al, 1995). Uncontrolled studies that employ a similar strategy appear to show reduced patient mortality compared with predicted mortality rates (Hickling et al, 1990, 1994). Validation of these results in prospective, controlled studies is needed.

Inverse ratio ventilation (IRV) is one method of increasing mean airway pressure without further increasing peak alveolar pressures (Marcy and Marini, 1991). IRV can be used in both pressure-controlled and volume-controlled modes (Tharratt et al, 1988).

The fundamental distinction between pressure-controlled IRV and volume-controlled IRV is that in the former, airway pressure is controlled whereas airflow and tidal volume are allowed to change; in the latter, airflow and thus tidal volume are controlled whereas airway pressure is allowed to change. Under circumstances of changing resistance and compliance properties of the lung (e.g., bronchospasm, pulmonary edema), the pressure-controlled mode of IRV produces changes in airflow and tidal volume. In contrast, the volume-controlled mode of IRV results in changing airway pressures. A volume-controlled mode of IRV is preferred if the therapeutic goal is to maintain a preset level of minute ventilation despite changes in lung impedance. Alternatively, the pressure-controlled mode of administering IRV is preferred if the intent is to limit airway pressure and prevent alveolar overdistention.

Theoretically, pressure-controlled IRV should be safer because excessive alveolar pressures, by definition, can be avoided (Tharratt et al, 1988). Little evidence exists yet that ARDS patients as a whole benefit from IRV (Mercat et al, 1993). Therefore, we do not recommend that IRV be used for routine management of ARDS. Instead, when acceptable arterial oxygenation cannot be achieved with PEEP 15 cm H_2O or less or when the use of PEEP is associated with excessive airway pressures despite attempts at permissive hypercapnea, we use IRV in an attempt to salvage oxygenation without excessive airway pressure (see Fig. 18–8). Pressure-controlled IRV or volume-controlled IRV with a decelerating inspiratory flow produces approximately similar flow patterns. The principal advantage of pressure-controlled IRV in this setting is simply greater control of alveolar plateau pressures. With either form of IRV, increasing the inspiratory time over which intrathoracic pressure is raised can have a substantial detrimental effect on venous return and cardiac output.

Airway pressure release ventilation (APRV) and high frequency ventilation (HFV) are additional methods of mechanical ventilatory support with the goal of recruiting and stabilizing collapsed lung units (Villar et al, 1990). Studies with APRV are still too limited to allow a specific evidence-based recommendation, and studies of HFV in patients with ARDS have not shown significant advantage over conventional forms of mechanical ventilation (Holzapfel et al, 1987). In fact, in patients with concomitant airway disease, HFV may lead to severe hyperinflation and may be dangerous. Therefore, we cannot recommend use of either of these modes routinely in ARDS until more favorable data become available.

Tracheal gas insufflation (TGI) is a supplementary technique, especially if low ventilatory rates are being utilized, to improve the ventilatory efficiency of small tidal volumes delivered by conventional techniques (by washing out the "dead space") (Ravenscraft et al, 1993). During TGI, a flow of fresh gas (2–14 l/min) is applied through a small-lumen catheter at the level of the carina, bypassing the anatomic dead space. This technique is best employed in a research setting at present.

Yet another strategy, which is currently under active investigation, is perfluorocarbon-associated gas exchange (i.e., partial liquid ventilation [PLV]), in which the gaseous residual capacity of the lung is replaced with perfluorocarbon liquid, and tidal breaths are delivered by a conventional ventilator (Gauger et al, 1996; Hirschl et al, 1996; Leach et al, 1993). The higher density of the perfluorocarbon liquid (about twice that of water) may aid in opening up dependent atelectatic areas and in literally removing proinflammatory debris from the alveolar space while maintaining satisfactory oxygenation. This exciting technique will certainly be aggressively evaluated over the next few years.

Extracorporeal Respiratory Support (ERS)

Two forms of ERS have been evaluated in ARDS patients: extracorporeal membrane oxygenation (ECMO) and extracorporeal CO_2 removal (EC-CO_2R). A prospective trial of ECMO failed to show any survival benefit compared with conventional mechanical ventilation (Zapol et al, 1979), although it is still used in some centers for support of the most severely affected ARDS patients.

ECCO$_2$R is still frequently utilized in Europe. In the United States, no survival advantage was found in a study of ECCO$_2$R-treated ARDS patients (Morris et al, 1994).

The intravenous gas exchange catheter (IVOX) is a potentially less invasive option for augmenting gas exchange (Conrad et al, 1993). To date, the reported experience with IVOX has been limited to case series of patients with severe ARDS and has not been rigorously evaluated.

Patient Positioning

Because lung infiltrates in ARDS can be distributed nonuniformly (see Fig. 18–2), positional changes can at times improve oxygenation by changing the distribution of perfusion. Indeed, the prone position significantly improves oxygenation in up to 50% of patients with ARDS. The best mechanism to explain the improvement in gas exchange with prone positioning is improved ventilation to dorsal lung units while maintaining ventilation in ventral lung units and perfusion to

all lung regions (Lamm et al, 1994). It may be difficult to routinely position patients in the prone position, although such problems can often be overcome with cooperation between medical, nursing, and other professional staff members. Accurate predictors of patient response to repositioning are currently unavailable. Hypotension, desaturation, and arrhythmias may occur transiently with prone positioning but are usually self-limiting. The optimal frequency of repositioning is also unknown but probably is best done at least once daily. Prone positioning technique should be limited to those willing to familiarize themselves with its use and potential problems.

Fluid Management

Even though pulmonary edema in ARDS is due to increased vascular permeability, intravascular hydrostatic forces are still a contributing factor. Several clinical studies indicate that pulmonary function and outcome are better in patients who lose weight or in whom the wedge pressure falls as a result of diuresis or fluid restriction. Investigators in one prospective trial arrived at a similar conclusion: A clinical strategy of fluid restriction and diuresis was associated with a reduced amount of pulmonary edema and time requiring mechanical ventilation, although patients with congestive heart failure and volume overload as well as ARDS were included in the study (Mitchell et al, 1992) (Figs. 18–9, 18–10). The strategy of early diuresis and fluid restriction tested in this study was not associated with a higher incidence of complications, such as renal failure and hemodynamic compromise (Mitchell et al, 1992). Thus, these data support the strategy of relative fluid restriction when possible, especially during the first few days after onset of ARDS, while carefully monitoring (and correcting if possible) compromise in end-organ function due to hemodynamic compromise. We usually attempt to achieve a net negative fluid balance of 500 to 1500 ml, as long as hemodynamics and indices of renal function are adequately preserved. The benefits of continuing fluid restriction or diuresis for more than 3 or 4 days are unclear. Central hemodynamic monitoring often is necessary to determine appropriate fluid management, given the hemodynamic variability among patients.

PHARMACOLOGIC THERAPIES

Many therapeutic agents have been tried as treatment for prevention of ARDS. Unfortunately, none has yet met with success, although a few are still promising. Particularly disappointing has

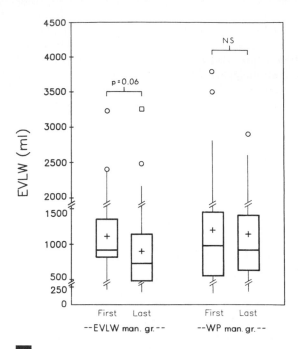

Figure 18–9

Box plots of first versus last extravascular lung water (EVLW) measurement from a study of fluid management in 101 patients with severe pulmonary edema (Mitchell et al, 1992). Patients' status was managed either with a protocol incorporating EVLW measurements (EVLW) that emphasized fluid restriction/diuresis or with wedge pressure measurements (WP). Boxes represent 25 to 75% quartiles. Middle line in each box represents the median value, and the + sign represents the mean value. "Whiskers" above and below each box represent values within 1.5 times the interquartile range. Circle = outlier with three times the interquartile range; square = outlier beyond this point (p = 0.06 by comparison of median values using the Wilcoxon test). NS = not significant. (From Mitchell JP, Calandrino FS, et al: Improved outcome based on fluid management in critically ill patients requiring pulmonary artery catheterization. Am Rev Respir Dis 145(5):990–998, 1992. With permission.)

been the lack of effect of prostaglandin E_1 (Bone et al, 1989b), exogenous surfactant (Anzueto et al, 1994), selective digestive decontamination, the antioxidant N-acetylcysteine, and various antiendotoxin and anticytokine drugs (Kollef and Schuster, 1995). Other drugs currently being evaluated, which may still prove to be of some value, include the vasoconstrictor almitrine, ketoconazole (as a thromboxane synthesis inhibitor), nonsteroidal anti-inflammatory agents like ibuprofen, and the phosphodiesterase inhibitor pentoxifylline. New delivery systems, like liposome encapsulation, may make it possible to give drugs, like

PGE_1, more effectively and efficiently intracellularly. When otherwise given intravenously, these have unacceptable vasoactive effects (Abraham et al, 1996).

Corticosteroids

Patients with ARDS, as a whole, clearly do not benefit from high-dose corticosteroids early in the disease process (Bernard et al, 1987; Bone et al, 1987). A few patients with ARDS have high numbers of eosinophils in their blood and lungs (as assayed by BAL); these patients can have a dramatic response to early steroid treatment (Allen et al, 1989). These patients may also have a form of eosinophilic pneumonia.

Anecdotal reports also suggest that corticosteroids may be helpful if administered during the fibroproliferative phase of ARDS (7–10 days after onset) (Meduri et al, 1994a). If a prolonged course of corticosteroids is to be administered for ARDS during the fibroproliferative phase, we recommend that systemic infection be excluded or adequately treated *first*. Thereafter, 2 to 5 mg/kg of methylprednisolone per day (in divided doses) can be tried, tapering the dose over the next 1 to 2 weeks based on the clinical response. If a beneficial response seems to occur (improved oxygenation, clearing of chest radiographic infiltrates), 0.5 to 1.0 mg/kg per day of steroid can be continued until extubation, with additional slow tapering thereafter. More definitive recommendations cannot be made until a steroid protocol has been studied in a prospective, placebo-controlled, randomized trial.

Nitric Oxide

Inhaled NO can act as a selective pulmonary vasodilator in both humans and animals when inhaled in concentrations of 5 to 80 ppm (Frostell et al, 1993; Rossaint et al, 1993). The rapid binding of NO to hemoglobin, for which it has a high affinity, prevents any significant systemic vasodilation. In ARDS, inhaled NO can reduce pulmonary artery pressures and intrapulmonary shunt, increase the PaO_2/FIO_2 ratio, and leave mean arterial pressure and cardiac output unchanged (Puybasset et al, 1995; Rossaint et al, 1993). These effects can be maintained even for many weeks. Lower concentrations seem overall to be as effective as higher ones. As with many other ARDS treatments, individual responses can sometimes be much more dramatic than group responses. It seems likely that inhaled NO will become part of the therapeutic armamentarium, especially for those patients with excessively increased pulmo-

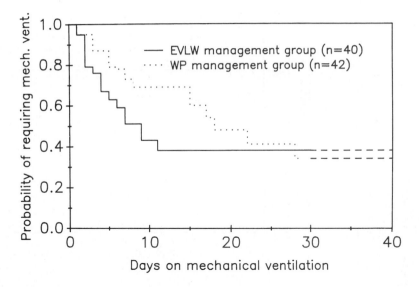

Figure 18–10
Kaplan-Meier-type plot of days on mechanical ventilation for 82 patients from both management groups (see Fig. 18–9). Data are the estimates of the probability of still requiring mechanical ventilation as a function of time. Values for patients who died on mechanical ventilation were treated as censored observations. Patients in the group managed with fluid restriction (*solid line*) had a significantly shorter median requirement for mechanical ventilation. (From Mitchell JP, Schuller D, Calandrino FS, et al: Improved outcome based on fluid management in critically ill patients requiring pulmonary artery catheterization. Am Rev Respir Dis 145(5):990–998, 1992. With permission.)

nary arterial pressure, right ventricular compromise, or hypoxemia refractory to other measures.

PROGNOSIS

The outcome for an individual patient with ARDS is difficult to predict. General scoring systems provide an estimate of the probability of mortality upon admission to the ICU (Schuster, 1992). A specific scoring system for ARDS has been developed (Murray et al, 1988); however, its predictive accuracy has not been validated. The number of acquired organ system failures is often the most important prognostic indicator for patients requiring intensive care, including patients with ARDS. In addition, liver failure in association with ARDS carries a particularly poor prognosis.

For most of the two decades since ARDS was first reported, mortality seemed to remain relatively constant at 60 to 70% (Rinaldo, 1990). Later reports, however, suggest that mortality rates may be falling to about 40% (Milberg et al, 1995; Schuster, 1995) (Fig. 18–11). The explanation for this apparent improvement in patient outcomes is not clear, but the decrease may be the result of differences in patient populations, reduced use

of corticosteroids in early ARDS, greater use of corticosteroids in late ARDS, greater attention to fluid management, improved hemodynamic and nutritional support, improved antibiotics for nosocomial infection, changes in ventilator support strategies, or benefits of protocol-driven management learned from clinical trials.

More specific predictors of outcome for patients with ARDS have been sought from measurements of various serum and lung lavage factors. The concentrations of von Willebrand factor antigen in serum, of neutrophil activating factor-1/interleukin-8 in airspace lavage fluid, and of procollagen peptide in BAL fluid correlate with outcomes or progression in some but not all studies (Clark et al, 1995; Miller et al, 1992; Rubin et al, 1990).

The integrity of the epithelial barrier in relation to resolution of alveolar edema also appears to be a determinant of outcome in patients with ARDS (Matthay and Wiener-Kronish, 1990). Similarly, the change in the PaO_2/FIO_2 ratio following initial treatment of ARDS can discriminate between survivors and nonsurvivors (Bone et al, 1989a). At the present time, none of these markers has been validated as an accurate method for predicting outcome in the individual ARDS patient. Not surprisingly, patients who develop

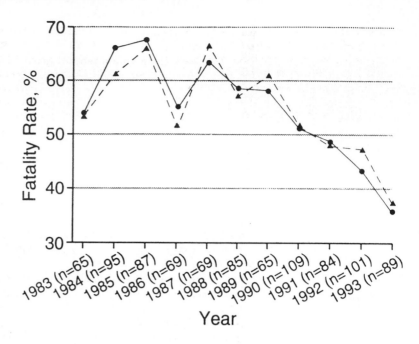

Figure 18–11
Crude (*solid line*) and adjusted (*dashed line*) fatality rates for ARDS patients from Harborview Medical Center, 1983–1993. Rates are adjusted for ARDS risk group, age, and gender. (From Milberg JA, Davis R, Steinberg KP, et al: Improved survival of patients with acute respiratory distress syndrome (ARDS): 1983–1993. JAMA 273(4):306–309, 1995. Copyright 1995, American Medical Association. With permission.)

fibrosis have a poorer outcome than patients who do not (Martin et al, 1995; Meduri, 1995).

The long-term functional outlook for survivors of ARDS is generally good (McHugh et al, 1994). Long-term abnormalities in pulmonary function are more common if lung function is impaired for more than a few days after the onset of ARDS. Most of the improvement in pulmonary function and perceived health occurs in the first 3 months following an episode of ARDS (McHugh et al, 1994). The best predictors of long-term pulmonary impairment in survivors seem to be persistence of impaired lung function for more than 3 days after the onset of ARDS and physiologic indices of the severity of ARDS (e.g., maximal pulmonary artery pressures, lowest static thoracic compliance, and maximal level of PEEP).

REFERENCES

Abraham E, Park YC, Covington P, et al: Liposomal prostaglandin E1 in acute respiratory distress syndrome: A placebo-controlled, randomized, double-blind, multicenter clinical trial. Crit Care Med 24:10–15, 1996.

Albert RK: A critique of the ACCP Consensus Conference on mechanical ventilation. J Intensive Care Med 10:200–206, 1995.

Allen JN, Pacht ER, Gadek JE, et al: Acute eosinophilic pneumonia as a reversible cause of noninfectious respiratory failure. N Engl J Med 321:569–574, 1989.

Amato MBP, Barbas CSV, Medeiros DM, et al:

Beneficial effects of the "open lung approach" with low distending pressures in acute respiratory distress syndrome: A prospective randomized study on mechanical ventilation. Am J Respir Crit Care Med 152:1835–1846, 1995.

Anzueto A, Baughman R, Guntupalli K, et al: An international randomized, placebo-controlled trial evaluating the safety and efficacy of aerosolized surfactant in patients with sepsis-induced ARDS. Am J Respir Crit Care Med 149:A567, 1994.

Bell RC, Coalson J, Smith JD, et al: Multiorgan failure and infection in adult respiratory distress syndrome. Ann Intern Med 99:293–297, 1983.

Bernard GR, Artigas A, Brigham KL, et al: The American-European Consensus Conference on ARDS. Definitions, mechanisms, relevant outcomes, and clinical trial coordination. Am J Respir Crit Care Med 149(3):818–824, 1994.

Bernard GR, Luce JM, Sprung CL, et al: High-dose corticosteroids in patients with the adult respiratory distress syndrome. N Engl J Med 317(25):1565–1570, 1987.

Berthiaume Y, Broaddus VA, Gropper MA, et al: Alveolar liquid and protein clearance from normal dog lungs. J Appl Physiol 65(2):585–593, 1988.

Bevilacqua MP and Nelson RM: Endothelial-leukocyte adhesion molecules in inflammation and metastasis. Thromb Haemost 70(1):152–154, 1993.

Bombino M, Gattinoni L, Presenti A, et al: The value of portable chest roentgenography in adult respiratory distress syndrome: Comparison with computed tomography. Chest 100:762–769, 1991.

Bone RC: The ARDS lung: New insights from computed tomography. JAMA 269:2134–2135, 1993.

Bone RC, Fisher CJ Jr, Clemmer TP, et al: Early methylprednisolone treatment for septic syndrome and the adult respiratory distress syndrome. Chest 92(6):1032–1036, 1987.

Bone RC, Maunder R, Slotman G, et al: An early test of survival in patients with the adult respiratory distress syndrome. The PaO_2/FIO_2 ratio and its differential response to conventional therapy. Prostaglandin E1 Study Group. Chest 96(4):849–851, 1989a.

Bone RC, Slotman G, Maunder R, et al: Randomized double-blind, multicenter study of prostaglandin E1 in patients with the adult respiratory distress syndrome. Prostaglandin E1 Study Group. Chest 96(1):114–119, 1989b.

Bongard FS, Matthay M, MacKersie RC, et al: Morphologic and physiologic correlates of increased extravascular lung water. Surgery 96(2):395–403, 1984.

Clark JG, Milberg JA, Steinberg KP, et al: Type III procollagen peptide in the adult respiratory distress syndrome. Association of increased peptide levels in bronchoalveolar lavage fluid with increased risk for death [see comments]. Ann Intern Med 122(1):17–23, 1995.

Conrad SA, Eggerstedt JM, Morris VF, et al: Prolonged extra-corporeal support of gas exchange with an intravenacaval oxygenator. Chest 103:158–161, 1993.

Crouch E: Pathobiology of pulmonary fibrosis. Am J Physiol 259:L159–184, 1990.

Dantzker DR, Brook CJ, Dehart P, et al: Ventilation-perfusion distribution in the adult respiratory distress syndrome. Am Rev Respir Dis 120:1039–1052, 1979.

Deby-Dupont G, Lamy M, Faymonville ME, et al: Proteases and antiproteases in the Adult Respiratory Distress Syndrome. In Zapol WM, and Lemaire F (eds): Adult Respiratory Distress Syndrome. New York, Marcel Dekker, 1991, pp 305–352.

Fowler AA, Hamman RF, Good JT, et al: Adult respiratory distress syndrome: Risk with common predispositions. Ann Intern Med 98:593–597, 1983.

Fowler AA, Hamman RF, Zerbe GO, et al: Adult respiratory distress syndrome. Prognosis after onset. Am Rev Respir Dis 132(3):472–478, 1985.

Frostell CG, Blomquist H, Hedenstierna G, et al: Inhaled nitric oxide selectively reverses human hypoxic pulmonary vasoconstriction without causing systemic vasodilation. Anesthesiology 78:427–435, 1993.

Gattinoni L, Presenti A, Torresin A, et al: Adult respiratory distress syndrome profiles by computed tomography. J Thorac Imaging 1(3):25–30, 1986.

Gauger PG, Pranikoff T, Schreiner RJ, et al: Initial experience with partial liquid ventilation in pediatric patients with the acute respiratory distress syndrome. Crit Care Med 24:16–22, 1996.

Hickling KG, Henderson SJ, Jackson R, et al: Low mortality associated with low volume pressure limited ventilation with permissive hypercapnia in severe adult respiratory distress syndrome. Intensive Care Med 16(6):372–377, 1990.

Hickling KG, Walsh J, Henderson S, et al: Low mortality rate in adult respiratory distress syndrome using low-volume, pressure-limited ventilation with permissive hypercapnia: A prospective study. Crit Care Med 22(10):1568–1578, 1994.

Hirschl RB, Pranikoff T, Wise C, et al: Initial experience with partial liquid ventilation in adult patients with the acute respiratory distress syndrome. JAMA 275:383–389, 1996.

Holzapfel L, Robert D, Perrin F, et al: Comparison of high-frequency jet ventilation to conventional ventilation in adults with respiratory distress syndrome. Intensive Care Med 13(2):100–105, 1987.

Hudson LD, Milberg JA, Anardi D, et al: Clinical risks for development of the acute respiratory distress syndrome. Am J Respir Crit Care Med 151(2):293–301, 1995.

Jones R, Reid LM, Zapol WM, et al: Pulmonary vascular pathology: Human and experimental studies. In Zapol WM, and Falke KJ (eds): Lung Biology in Health and Diseases. New York, Marcel Dekker, 1992, pp 23–160.

Kaplan JD, Calandrino FS, Schuster DP, et al: A positron emission tomographic comparison of pulmonary vascular permeability during the adult respiratory distress syndrome and pneumonia. Am Rev Respir Dis 143(1):150–154, 1991.

Kollef MH and Schuster DP: The acute respiratory distress syndrome. N Engl J Med 332(1):27–37, 1995.

Lamm WJ, Graham MM, Albert RK, et al: Mechanism by which the prone position improves oxygenation in acute lung injury. Am J Respir Crit Care Med 150:184–193, 1994.

Leach CL, Fuhrman BP, Morin FC, et al: Perfluorocarbon-associated gas exchange (partial liquid ventilation) in respiratory distress syndrome: A prospective, randomized, controlled study. Crit Care Med 21(9):1270–1278, 1993.

Leeper KV Jr: Diagnosis and treatment of pulmonary infections in adult respiratory distress syndrome. New Horizons 1: 550–562, 1993.

Lewandowski K, Metz J, Deutschmann C, et al: Incidence, severity, and mortality of acute respiratory failure in Berlin, Germany. Am J Respir Crit Care Med 151:1121–1125, 1995.

McDonald JA: Idiopathic pulmonary fibrosis: A paradigm for lung injury and repair. Chest 99:87S–93S, 1991.

McHugh LG, Milberg JA, Whitcomb ME, et al: Recovery of function in survivors of the acute respiratory distress syndrome. Am J Respir Crit Care Med 150(1):90–94, 1994.

MacIntyre NR: Building consensus on the use of mechanical ventilation. Chest 104:334–335, 1993.

Marcy TW and Marini JJ: Inverse ratio ventilation in

ARDS. Rationale and implementation. Chest 100:494–504, 1991.

Marinelli WA, Henke CA, Harmon KR, et al: Mechanisms of alveolar fibrosis after acute lung injury. Clin Chest Med 11(4):657–672, 1990.

Marinelli WA and Ingbar DH: Diagnosis and management of acute lung injury. Clin Chest Med 15(3):517–546, 1994.

Marini JJ: Lung mechanics in the adult respiratory distress syndrome. Recent conceptual advances and implications for management. Clin Chest Med 11(4):673–690, 1990.

Marini JJ: New options for the ventilatory management of acute lung injury. New Horiz 1(4):489–503, 1993.

Marini J: Tidal volume, PEEP, and barotrauma: An open and shut case? Chest 109:302–304, 1995.

Marini JJ and Kelsen SG: Re-targeting ventilatory objectives in adult respiratory distress syndrome. New treatment prospects—persistent questions. Am Rev Respir Dis 146(1):2–3, 1992.

Martin C, Papazian L, Payan MJ, et al: Pulmonary fibrosis correlates with outcome in adult respiratory distress syndrome. A study in mechanically ventilated patients. Chest 107(1):196–200, 1995.

Matamis D, Lemaire F, Harf A, et al: Total respiratory pressure-volume curves in the adult respiratory distress syndrome. Chest 86(1):58–66, 1984.

Matthay MA: Resolution of pulmonary edema: Mechanisms of liquid, protein, and cellular clearance from the lung. Clin Chest Med 6:521–545, 1985.

Matthay MA, Berthiaume Y, Staub NC, et al: Long-term clearance of liquid and protein from the lungs of unanesthetized sheep. J Appl Physiol 59:928–934, 1985.

Matthay MA and Wiener-Kronish JP: Intact epithelial barrier function is critical for the resolution of alveolar edema in humans. Am Rev Respir Dis 142(6):1250–1257, 1990.

Meduri GU: Pulmonary fibroproliferation and death in patients with late ARDS. Chest 107:5–6, 1995.

Meduri GU, Chinn AJ, Leeper KV, et al: Corticosteroid rescue treatment of progressive fibroproliferation in late ARDS—patterns of response and predictors of outcome. Chest 105:1516–1527, 1994a.

Meduri GU, Mauldin GL, Wunderink RG, et al: Causes of fever and pulmonary densities in patients with clinical manifestations of ventilator-associated pneumonia. Chest 106(1):221–235, 1994b.

Mercat A, Graini L, Teboul JL, et al: Cardiorespiratory effects of pressure-controlled ventilation with and without inverse ratio in the adult respiratory distress syndrome [see comments]. Chest 104(3):871–875, 1993.

Meyrick B: Pathology of the adult respiratory distress syndrome. Crit Care Clin 2(3):405–428, 1986.

Milberg JA, Davis DR, Steinberg KP, et al: Improved survival of patients with acute respiratory distress syndrome (ARDS): 1983–1993. JAMA 273(4):306–309, 1995.

Miller EJ, Cohen AB, Nagao S, et al: Elevated levels of NAP-1/interleukin-8 are present in the airspaces of patients with the adult respiratory distress syndrome and are associated with increased mortality. Am Rev Respir Dis 146(2):427–432, 1992.

Milne EN, Pistolesi M, Miniati M, et al: The radiologic distinction of cardiogenic and noncardiogenic edema. AJR 144(5):879–894, 1985.

Mitchell JP, Schuller D, Calandrino FS, et al: Improved outcome based on fluid management in critically ill patients requiring pulmonary artery catheterization [see comments]. Am Rev Respir Dis 145(5):990–998, 1992.

Montgomery AB, Stager MA, Carrico CJ, et al: Causes of mortality in patients with the adult respiratory distress syndrome. Am Rev Respir Dis 132(3):485–489, 1985.

Morris AH, Wallace CJ, Menlove RL, et al: Randomized clinical trial of pressure-controlled inverse ratio ventilation and extracorporeal CO_2 removal for adult respiratory distress syndrome. Am J Respir Crit Care Med 149(2):295–305, 1994.

Murray JF, Matthay MA, Luce JM, et al: An expanded definition of the adult respiratory distress syndrome. Am Rev Respir Dis 138(3):720–723, 1988.

Pepe PE, Potkin RT, Reus DH, et al: Clinical predictors of the adult respiratory distress syndrome. Am J Surg 144:124–130, 1982.

Puybasset L, Rouby JJ, Mourgeon E, et al: Factors influencing cardiopulmonary effects of inhaled nitric oxide in acute respiratory failure. Am J Respir Crit Care Med 152(1):318–328, 1995.

Ravenscraft SA, Burke WC, Nahum A, et al: Tracheal gas insufflation augments CO_2 clearance during mechanical ventilation. Am Rev Respir Dis 148:345–351, 1993.

Rinaldo JE: The prognosis of the adult respiratory distress syndrome: Inappropriate pessimism? Chest 90:470–471, 1990.

Rossaint R, Falke Kjaulf, Slama K, et al: Inhaled nitric oxide for the adult respiratory distress syndrome. N Engl J Med 328(6):399–405, 1993.

Roupie E, Dambrosio M, Servillo G, et al: Titration of tidal volume and induced hypercapnia in acute respiratory distress syndrome. Am J Respir Crit Care Med 152(1):121–128, 1995.

Rubin DB, Wiener-Kronish JP, Murray JF, et al: Elevated von Willebrand factor antigen is an early plasma predictor of acute lung injury in nonpulmonary sepsis syndrome. J Clin Invest 86(2):474–480, 1990.

Sandiford P, Province MA, Schuster DP, et al: Distribution of regional density and vascular permeability in the adult respiratory distress syndrome. Am J Respir Crit Care Med 151(3):737–742, 1995.

Schuster DP: A physiologic approach to initiating,

maintaining, and withdrawing mechanical ventilatory support during acute respiratory failure. Am J Med 88(3):268–278, 1990.

Schuster DP: Predicting outcome after ICU admission. The art and science of assessing risk. Chest 102:1861–1870, 1992.

Schuster DP: What is acute lung injury? What is ARDS? Chest 107(6):1721–1726, 1995.

Schuster DP and Kollef M: The acute respiratory distress syndrome. Disease-a-Month 42:5–64, 1996.

Seidenfeld JJ, Pohl DF, Bell RC, et al: Incidence, site, and outcome of infections in patients with the adult respiratory distress syndrome. Am Rev Respir Dis 134(1):12–6, 1986.

Sivak ED and Wiedemann HP: Clinical measurement of extravascular lung water. Crit Care Clin 2(3):511–526, 1986.

Sloane PJ, Gee MH, Gottlieb JE, et al: A multicenter registry of patients with acute respiratory distress syndrome. Physiology and outcome. Am Rev Respir Dis 146(2):419–426, 1992.

Slutsky A: Mechanical ventilation (American College of Chest Physicians Consensus Conference). Chest 104:1833–1859, 1993.

Staub NC: Pulmonary edema. Physiol Rev 54:678–721, 1974.

Staub NC: The forces regulating fluid filtration in the lung. Microvasc Res 15:45–55, 1978.

Tharratt RS, Allen RP, Albertson TE, et al: Pressure controlled inverse ratio ventilation in severe adult respiratory failure. Chest 94(4):755–762, 1988.

Tomashefski JF Jr: Pulmonary pathology of the adult respiratory distress syndrome. Clin Chest Med 11(4):593–619, 1990.

Tsuno K, Miura K, Takeya M, et al: Histopathologic pulmonary changes from mechanical ventilation at high peak airway pressures. Am Rev Respir Dis 143:1115–1120, 1991.

Villar J, Winston B, Slutsky AS, et al: Non-conventional techniques of ventilatory support. Crit Care Clin 6:579–603, 1990.

Zapol WM, Snider MT, Hill JD, et al: Extracorporeal membrane oxygenation in severe acute respiratory failure. JAMA 242:2193–2196, 1979.

C H A P T E R

Heart-lung Interactions in Sepsis

Sheldon Magder, M.D.

Management of septic patients has become an increasingly common medical problem over the last few decades. In 1979 the incidence of sepsis was 75 in 100,000 hospital admissions and by 1986 it had increased to 176 in 100,000 (Bone et al, 1989; Parillo, 1993; Rackow and Astiz, 1993). In the United States, the annual incidence was estimated at 400,000 cases in 1990 (Parillo, 1990). The cost of treating patients with sepsis was estimated to be between $5 billion and $10 billion in 1990 (Rackow and Astiz, 1993). A European study found an attack rate of severe sepsis in 9% of intensive care unit (ICU) admissions (Brun-Buisson, 1995). Factors for the increased incidence of sepsis include the increased number of immunocompromised patients and patients with chronic and debilitating disease plus more invasive technologies and the aging population.

The term *sepsis* has been vague and inconsistent in the past, but a consensus has now been reached on the definition (Bone et al, 1989; Bone, 1991; Sibbald et al, 1991; Benjamin et al, 1992; Members of the American College of Chest Physicians/Society of Critical Care Medicine Consensus Conference Committee, 1992). This definition has allowed much more rigor in the analysis of the syndrome and its treatment.

DEFINITIONS

Sepsis is defined as the systemic response to infection (Members of the American College of Chest Physicians/Society of Critical Care Medicine Consensus Conference Committee, 1992). This systemic response is manifested by two or more of the following conditions as a result of infection: temperature higher than 38°C or lower than 36°C; heart rate greater than 90 beats/min; respiratory rate greater than 20 breaths/min or $PaCO_2$ 32 mmHg or less (<4.3 kPa); white blood cell count higher than 12,000 cells/mm³, less than 4000 cells/mm³, or greater than 10% immature (band) forms.

Severe sepsis is defined as sepsis in association with organ dysfunction, hypoperfusion, or hypotension. Hypoperfusion and perfusion abnormalities may include, but are not limited to, lactic acidosis, oliguria, or acute mental status alteration. Examples of organ dysfunction include disseminated intravascular coagulation characterized by fibrin split products level greater than 1:40 or D-dimers greater than 2.0, low platelets, increased prothrombin time (PT) and partial thromboplastin time (PTT); adult respiratory distress syndrome (ARDS) characterized by bilateral pulmonary infiltrate, PaO_2/FiO_2 less than 175, and pulmonary arterial occlusion less than 18 mm Hg; renal dysfunction characterized by elevated serum creatinine levels and urinary sodium greater than 40 mmol/l or increase in serum creatinine level by by 180 μmol/l (2.0 mg/dl); hepatic dysfunction characterized by bilirubin level greater than 35 μmol/l, or alkaline phosphatase, gamma glutamyltransferase (GT), aspartate aminotransferase (AST) levels that are twice normal; and central nervous system dysfunction characterized by Glasgow Coma Scale score of less than 15.

Shock is said to be present when tissue perfusion is inadequate for the metabolic needs of the tissues. This finding usually means hypotension with systolic arterial pressure of less than 90 mm Hg, but it is also considered present if the blood pressure falls by more than 40 mm Hg from baseline.

Another term has been offered, and that is the *Systemic Inflammatory Response Syndrome* (SIRS) (Sibbald et al, 1991; Benjamin et al, 1992; Members of the American College of Chest Physicians/Society of Critical Care Medicine Consensus Conference Committee, 1992). This syndrome has all the criteria of sepsis but applies to patients in whom there is no evidence of an infectious cause. This term has come about from our understanding that an infectious agent triggers the immune response, but infectious agents are not the only agents that can initiate the process.

GENERAL PATHOPHYSIOLOGY OF SEPSIS

Sepsis or SIRS occurs when an inducer turns on an immune cascade. The reader is referred to Chapter 1 for a review of the effects of the immune cascade on lung injury. Inducers include endotoxin, enterotoxin, toxic shock syndrome toxin, mycobacterial cell wall, antibodies to CD 14, and complement products (Parillo, 1990, 1993; Rackow and Astiz, 1993). These inducers lead to the release of mediators of sepsis. There are numerous mediators, and the list keeps growing. Important ones are the cytokines such as tumor necrosis factor; interleukin-1, -2, -6, -8;

platelet activating factor; endorphins; nitric oxide (NO); arachidonic acid metabolism products, including prostaglandins, leukotrienes, lipoxgenase, and cyclooxygenase; the C5a fragment of complement; kinins; and coagulation products such as thrombin. These inducers activate plasma cells, monocytes and macrophages, endothelial cells, neutrophils, and vascular smooth muscle to produce endogenous mediators of sepsis and further amplify the process. These mediators then affect various organ systems. Myocardial contractility is depressed, and the heart dilates. There is a generalized loss of vascular tone, loss of response to vasopressors, impaired endothelial function, leukocyte aggregation, and, very importantly, increased capillary permeability. There is also generalized organ dysfunction, which is possibly related to the inadequate matching of flow to metabolic needs and possibly related to metabolic derangements associated with the actions of the various mediators.

Presently, there are active research efforts into the mechanisms behind the vascular abnormalities in sepsis, which include increased capillary permeability (Brigham et al, 1979; Kubes and Granger, 1992; Kurose et al, 1993; Kurose et al, 1995), loss of vascular tone (Borland et al, 1993), and loss of response to vasopressors (Datta et al, 1996; Fleming et al, 1991; Gray et al, 1991; Szabo, 1995). These abnormalities are related to both endothelial dysfunction and disorders of vascular smooth muscle. An important factor is an increase in the presence of adhesion molecules on both the endothelium and neutrophils, resulting in attachment of neutrophils to the endothelium and the release of their toxic contents (Kurose et al, 1993, 1995). This process leads to increased capillary permeability and decreased function of the endothelium. It can also result in less production of factors that are important to normal regulation of vascular tone and can produce abnormalities in the coagulation system (Suffredini et al, 1989; Parillo, 1993).

An important endothelial product that is altered in sepsis is NO (Busse et al, 1993). This small volatile molecule is an important regulator of smooth muscle tone (Busse and Mulsch, 1990). NO also inhibits the production of adhesion molecules and thereby inhibits neutrophil aggregation and platelet aggregation. The concentration of NO is increased in blood during sepsis (Stoclet et al, 1993; Mitaka et al, 1994), and blocking the enzyme responsible for its production reverses the loss of vascular responsiveness (Julou-Schaeffer et al, 1990; Gray et al, 1991; Szabo, 1995) and restores the blood pressure (Thiemermann and Vane, 1990; Nava et al, 1992; Pastor et al, 1994) (see Chapter 15). It is not clear whether the increased NO is from the increased endothelial production or from the induction of nitric oxide synthase (NOS) in vascular smooth muscle and macrophages (Hom et al, 1995; Szabo, 1995). In isolated muscle strips and cultured cells, cytokines such as tumor necrosis factor decrease the production of the constitutive, endothelial form of the enzyme (NOS-III) (Aoki et al, 1989; Myers et al, 1992; Parker et al, 1993). *In vivo* it is possible that endothelial NO production is increased by the presence of other factors, such as an elevation in the cofactor tetrahydrobiopterin, which raise the activity of NOS (Rosenkranz-Weiss et al, 1994). Other direct effects on the endothelium may occur via increases in intracellular calcium. There appears to be a decrease in receptor function on both endothelial cells and vascular smooth muscle, meaning less response to catecholamines (Parker et al, 1991; Parker and Adams, 1993; Parker et al, 1994).

In rats and mice there is an increase in inducible nitric oxide synthase (NOS-II) in vascular smooth muscle, which leads to vasodilation in areas where there should not be vasodilation. Vasodilation may then result in a mismatch between metabolic needs and flow and produce the shunt-like phenomena observed in sepsis. This may explain the common observation of increased venous oxygen content in sepsis (Wright et al, 1971). It is still not clear whether inducible NOS is an important part of the pathophysiology in humans or animals of higher order than rats. We failed to find evidence of NOS-II protein or mRNA in our porcine mode of sepsis (Javeshghani et al, 1996). It has also never been documented in human sepsis. The concentration of NO is also much lower in human studies than in rat models.

Besides dilators, there is an increase in production of substances that constrict. In particular, sepsis is associated with an increase in endothelin production that is most likely from the endothelium (Sugiura et al, 1989; Voerman et al, 1992; Hirata et al, 1993; Mitaka et al, 1993, 1994; Morise et al, 1994; Lundblad and Giercksky, 1995). This production seems to play a role in the pulmonary hypertension in sepsis and may counteract the dilating effect of increased NO production (Owada et al, 1994).

Cardiopulmonary interactions play a prominent part in the clinical manifestation of sepsis. As noted earlier, the definition of sepsis includes tachycardia, tachypnea, and hypotension (Members of the American College of Chest Physicians/ Society of Critical Care Medicine Consensus Conference Committee, 1992). Prominent fea-

tures of the typical septic syndrome include greater cardiac output, pulmonary hypertension, hyperpnea, hypoxemia, and lactic acidosis (MacLean et al, 1967). In the following discussion, the pathophysiology of these signs is reviewed based on changes in circulatory function, gas exchange abnormalities, and respiratory pump disorders.

CIRCULATORY ABNORMALITIES

Circulatory disorders play a major part in the clinical presentation of the sepsis syndrome. The characteristic observations include hypotension and increased cardiac output, which imply decreased systemic vascular resistance. To understand the mechanisms for the higher cardiac output, one must first review the mechanisms involved in the normal control of cardiac output. The reader is also referred to Chapters 4 and 5 for additional discussion of the determinants of cardiac output.

Arterial pressure is often viewed as a major determinant of cardiac output (Berne and Levy, 1983). This view is based on Poiseuille's Law and is reflected in the equation for systemic vascular resistance (SVR), which states that SVR is equal to the difference between arterial pressure and right atrial pressure divided by cardiac output. The fallacy of this approach, however, is quite apparent in the hemodynamics of sepsis. In sepsis, cardiac output rises with a fall in arterial pressure. The argument is often made that cardiac output is high in sepsis because arterial resistance is low and the ventricle is unloaded. At the same time that the systemic pressure is decreased in sepsis, the pulmonary pressure is usually increased (Shoemaker et al, 1993). Thus, the load on the right heart is elevated (Suffredini et al, 1989). Furthermore, for there to be an increase in cardiac output there must also be an increase in return of blood to the heart. The blood must come from somewhere. The only way a decrease in arterial pressure can result in an increase in cardiac output is by producing a decrease in right atrial pressure (Guyton et al, 1955b; Guyton et al, 1973; Magder, 1992). In sepsis, the right atrial pressure is usually normal or elevated (MacLean et al, 1967). What, then, are the factors that control the return of blood to the heart and thus control cardiac output?

A helpful analogy for understanding the return of blood to the heart is that of water in a bathtub. Consider a bathtub with a large surface area that is filled, the plug in the drain is removed, and the tap filling the tub is turned off (Fig. 19–1). Initially, the water level does not change

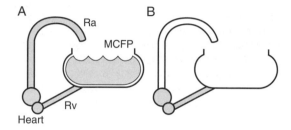

Figure 19-1
Bathtub and water analogy of the circulation. *(A)*
The tub is filled with water and is draining through a
pipe, which represents the resistance to venous return
(Rv). The blood is pumped from the heart through
the aorta and the arterial resistance *(Ra)*. *(B)* In this
example, the tub drains from the bottom and
therefore can completely empty.

very much, whether the tap is turned on or not.
The large surface area of the tub, relative to the
size of the drain, provides a large reservoir of fluid.
The drainage of the tub is determined by the
height of the water above the drain, resistance in
the pipe from the tub, and pressure at the end of
the pipe.

Similarly, in the body, small venules and
veins provide a large reservoir of blood; it is estimated that 70% of the total blood volume is in
this region (Guyton et al, 1973). The height of
water in the bathtub is analogous to the pressure
in the veins. In the tub, the height of water is
determined by the surface area of the tub and
the volume filling the tub. Similarly, the pressure
distending the small veins and venules depends
on their compliance and the volume filling them
(Guyton et al, 1955a, 1955b). Guyton called this
pressure the *mean circulatory filling pressure*
(MCFP). The pipe draining the tub is analogous
to the larger veins, and the pressure at the downstream end of the pipe is analogous to the pressure
in the right atrium. The primary role of the heart
in this model is to control right atrial pressure.
When the heart is very effective, right atrial pressure is low and the gradient for flow from the
venules and veins is large. When the heart is
ineffective, the right atrial pressure is higher and
the gradient for resistance to venous return is
decreased. The only way a decrease in arterial
pressure can increase cardiac output is by lowering
right atrial pressure.

In a standard bathtub, the drain is at the
bottom for the obvious reason that not all the
water would drain out of the tub if the drain were
on the side (see Fig. 19-1). When the drain
opening is on the side of the tub (Fig. 19-2),
water must be added to reach the level of the

opening, but only the water above the drain provides the force for water to flow out the drain.
Similarly, in blood vessels, a volume is necessary
to fill the normal round shape of the vessels, and
it is only the volume above this amount that
distends the vessels and produces the pressure in
them (i.e., MCFP). The volume that stretches the
vessel wall and produces pressure is called *stressed
volume*, and the volume that just fills out the
shape of the vessel but does not lead to stretch of
the wall is called *unstressed volume*. In the normal
relaxed state, approximately 25 to 30% of blood
volume is stressed and the rest is unstressed
(Rothe, 1983a, 1983b; Deschamps and Magder,
1992). The unstressed volume provides a large
reserve that can be recruited when volume is lost
or when MCFP needs to be elevated (Deschamps
and Magder, 1992; Nanas and Magder, 1992;
Deschamps et al, 1994).

There is one more determinant of resistance
to venous return and that is the distribution of
flow in a system with different compliances in
parallel (Caldini et al, 1974; Permutt and Caldini,
1978). In the bathtub analogy, this can be considered as a bathtub and sink sitting side by side
(Fig. 19-3). If they are both filled from a common
pipe that divides into two separate faucets, the
ratio of resistances in the two faucets determines
how much flow goes to each. If the resistance to
the sink is lowered relative to that of the bathtub,
more volume fills the sink. The water level rises,
and the flow out of the sink rises. If the resistance
is lowered to the bathtub, the increase in inflow
has a much smaller effect. There is only a small
change in outflow.

In the body, the splanchnic bed behaves like
a large bathtub (i.e., it has a large compliance),
whereas the extremities are more like a sink and
have a small compliance. Furthermore, in the
body, unlike the bathtub-sink analogy, the total
volume is constant, so that an increase in the

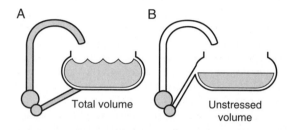

Figure 19-2
(A and *B)* Bathtub and water analogy with the tub
opening on the side. Fluid below the level of the
opening cannot escape. This volume is known as the
unstressed volume.

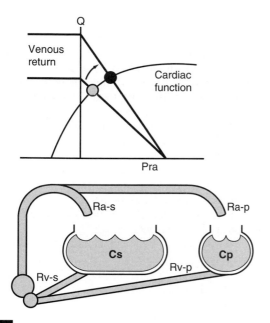

Figure 19–3
The concept of the two-compartment model with an area of large compliance *(Cs)* and parallel with a region of smaller compliance *(Cp)*. This can be compared with the analogy of a bathtub and sink in parallel. The Cs region is fed by an arterial resistance *(Ra-s)* and the peripheral region by another resistance *(Ra-p)*. The ratio of these two resistances determines the distribution of flow between the regions. Each region drains through its own resistance. The Cs region drains through its resistance to venous return *(Rv-s)*, and the Cp region drains through its own resistance (Rv-p).

fractional flow to the splanchnic bed results in a loss of volume in the extremities and a decrease in the flow from those regions. Thus, increased fractional flow to the extremities raises cardiac output and a decrease in fractional flow to this region lowers cardiac output (Caldini et al, 1974).

Resistance to venous return in the steady state must equal cardiac output, which is determined by heart rate, preload, afterload, and contractility. The preload for the right heart is approximated by the mean right atrial pressure, which, as noted earlier, is the outflow pressure of the venous system. The right atrial pressure thus represents the crucial point of interaction between cardiac function and circuit function (i.e., resistance to venous return). Because left heart output equals right heart output, the global function of the heart can be examined from the relationship of cardiac output to right atrial pressure. Guyton (1955a) developed a very useful graphic analysis of the interaction of the heart and circuit by combining the cardiac function curve and re-

sistance to venous return curve into one graph (see Fig. 4–2). Their intersection point is the right atrial pressure.

How then can cardiac output change? As already indicated, resistance to venous return and cardiac output increases if right atrial pressure is lowered by an improvement in cardiac function. However, cardiac output can also increase with a rise in right atrial pressure, which implies a change in circuit function. An important way that cardiac output is regulated is through changes in vascular capacitance (Shoukas and Sagawa, 1973; Sagawa and Eisner, 1975; Rothe, 1983a, 1983b; Deschamps and Magder, 1992; Deschamps and Magder, 1994; Deschamps et al, 1994). Thus, contraction of small veins in the capacitant part of circulation leads to an increase in stressed volume and a decrease in unstressed volume. This increases the MCFP and thus increases the gradient for resistance to venous return. Graphically, this appears as a parallel shift to the right of the resistance to the venous return curve. A decrease in vascular capacitance can occur through activation of the sympathetic nervous system (Deschamps and Magder, 1992) or through the action of pharmacologic agents, such as catecholamines (Mitzner and Goldberg, 1975). An increase in vascular capacitance results in a decrease in MCFP and resistance to venous return. Graphically, this change appears as a left shift of the resistance to venous return curve (Fig. 19–4). This process can occur through the loss of sympathetic tone (Vincent et al, 1987; Manyari et al, 1993); decreased temperature (Green and Jackman, 1979); or action of pharmacologic agents that produce vasodilation such as nitroglycerin (Wang et al, 1995), narcotics (Green et al, 1978), and anesthetic agents.

Vascular volume is often increased clinically by exogenous administration of fluids. Volume can be lost through excessive diuresis, gastrointestinal loss, diaphoresis, or hemorrhage. Changes in volume lead to changes in MCFP and appear graphically on the resistance to venous return curve to be the same as the change in capacitance. Changes in resistance to venous return alter the slope of the resistance to venous return curve (Fig. 19–5). Resistance to venous return can increase with alpha stimulation (Appleton et al, 1985), inhibition of NOS (Wang, 1993; Magder and Kabsele, 1994), and it can decrease with beta-agonists (Green, 1977). Changes in the distribution of flow also alter the slope of the resistance to venous return curve (Caldini et al, 1974), but the changes have to be large to have a major affect on resistance to venous return. Such a change occurs, for example, in exercise when a

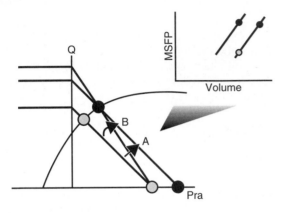

Figure 19–4

An increase in total volume or a decrease in unstressed volume shifts the resistance to venous return curve to the right (point A). The increase in volume moves up the pressure-volume curve shown in the inset, whereas the decrease in unstressed volume results in a parallel shift to the left of the pressure-volume curve and an increase in MCFP. A decrease in resistance to venous return rotates the resistance to venous return curve. This finding would also occur with the redistribution of blood flow to an area of low compliance (i.e., the Cp region in Fig. 19–3). This is represented by arrow B in this figure. (Q = flow; Pra = right atrial pressure.)

large fraction of the blood flow goes to the muscle. This effect could be a significant contributor to the higher cardiac output that occurs in sepsis.

MECHANISMS OF INCREASED CARDIAC OUTPUT IN SEPSIS

What are the possible mechanisms that can produce the high cardiac output that is frequently observed in sepsis? The right atrial pressure is usually elevated or normal in sepsis (MacLean et al, 1967), and therefore changes in cardiac function, including the decrease in left ventricular afterload, cannot explain the elevated cardiac output. It also does not appear that changes in the distribution of flow can explain the rise in cardiac output, because the distribution of flow did not change in one animal study (Magder et al, 1991). Even if there were a redistribution of blood flow to muscle, it can be shown that almost 90% of the blood flow would have to go to the muscle vasculature in order to explain the high outputs in some patients. It is unlikely that changes in venous compliance play a major role, although changes in splanchnic compliance played a small role in one study (Magder and Quinn, 1991).

That leaves stressed volume and resistance to venous return.

A major feature of sepsis is a general loss of vascular tone as represented by a decline in systemic vascular resistance (MacLean et al, 1967). An exception is the pulmonary vasculature in which resistance increases (Shoemaker et al, 1993). The loss of tone even includes the pulmonary and systemic veins (Vanelli et al, 1992). In a porcine model of endotoxemia, we observed a leftward shift of the pressure-volume curve of the vasculature, which implies an increase in vascular capacitance. Sepsis is also associated with increased capillary leak (Kubes and Granger, 1992; Kurose et al, 1993, 1995).

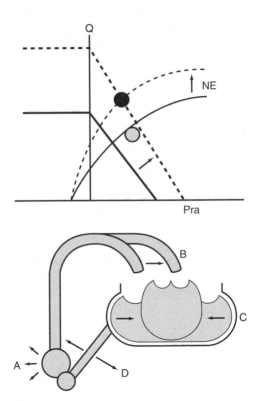

Figure 19–5

The potential hemodynamic effects of norepinephrine. (A) Norepinephrine (NE) can increase cardiac contractility. (B) There is an increase in arterial resistance, which, combined with the increase in cardiac output, leads to an augmentation of arterial pressure. (C) Contraction of small venules and veins leads to a decrease in capacitance (i.e., a decrease in unstressed volume), which increases MCFP. (D) There is a possible decrease in resistance to venous return. The combined results yield an upward shift in the cardiac function curve and a shift to the right with possible increased slope of the resistance to venous return curve. The net effect is increased cardiac output. (Q = flow; Pra = right atrial pressure.)

Based on the increase in capacitance and increase in capillary transduction, one would expect a decrease in stressed vascular volume and MCFP. Standard clinical practice, however, is to give an infusion of volume when hypotension develops in septic patients. This volume compensates for the loss of venous tone and the transudation of fluid, which can lead to an increase in MCFP; this may contribute to an increase in cardiac output (Vanelli et al, 1992). Indeed, we found in our animal studies that when we gave volume to try to maintain the central venous pressure at a constant level, we observed a rise in MCFP even though capacitance increased. When we did not volume-resuscitate the animals, MCFP fell, although not as much as would have been predicted from the increase in capacitance when animals were volume-resuscitated. This finding is most likely because neurohumoral mechanisms, triggered by the more marked hypotension in these animals, helped maintain vascular volume.

The final factor to be considered is venous return. In our animal studies (Vanelli et al, 1992), we failed to find a decrease in resistance to venous return, but the increase in cardiac output was also not very large. When endotoxin was injected into normal human volunteers, there was an almost 40% increase in cardiac output 2 hours after the injection, even without the infusion of volume (Suffredini et al, 1989). Based on the analysis, it is most likely that a decrease in resistance to resistance to venous return plays an important role in the development of this marked rise in cardiac output, which can occur even without an increase in volume.

If resistance to venous return is increased without much change in cardiac function, one would expect a large rise in right atrial pressure. More often in septic patients, however, right atrial pressure does not rise by a large amount, at least in the early stages. This observation suggests that there is an improvement in cardiac function despite the fact that myocardial depressant factors have been identified in sepsis (Parillo et al, 1985; Natanson et al, 1986, 1988; Lee et al, 1988; Natanson et al, 1989; Parker et al, 1990). In the intact organism, the preservation of cardiac function is most likely the result of the presence of circulating inotropic factors that counteract depressant factors. It is unlikely that cardiac output is maintained simply because of the fall in arterial pressure and left ventricular afterload. There is usually a rise in pulmonary artery pressure that increases the load on the right heart. This would not allow the reduced load on the left heart to pass to the right heart. The increase in pulmonary vascular resistance can have an important impact on cardiac output in sepsis and pulmonary hypertension, most likely contributing to the cardiac failure of later stages in sepsis (Parker et al, 1990).

A great deal of attention has been paid to the decrease in cardiac function in sepsis. A characteristic observation is cardiac dilation and ejection fraction decline (Natanson et al, 1986, 1988, 1989; Parker et al, 1990; Parillo, 1990, 1993). Outcome is likely worse in both patients and animals whose hearts do not dilate. The mechanism for depressed cardiac function is not clear, but is not due to a decrease in coronary flow. Rather, a circulating myocardial depressant factor or factors are responsible. The specific substance has not been identified. An increased level of NO, resulting from cytokine activation, has been proposed as a possible mechanism. NO decreases the contraction of isolated myocytes (Brigham et al, 1979; Brady et al, 1993; Notarius et al, 1994). Finkel and coworkers (1992) showed that NOS inhibitors reverse the contractile depressions seen in isolated guinea pig papillary muscles that were exposed to tumor necrosis factor alpha (TNFα), interleukin (IL)-6 and IL-2. In contrast, when NOS is inhibited, cardiac function is often worse. Absence of NO had no effect on isolated rat papillary muscle in a study by Weyrich and coworkers (1994) except when high doses of catecholamines were added. The decrease in cardiac function observed *in vitro* must be compensated for by counter-regulatory mechanisms *in vivo*. Most commonly in sepsis, cardiac output is elevated and not lowered except in the late phases. Persistence of a low cardiac output with high cardiac filling pressures is a grave prognostic sign (Parker et al, 1987; Metrangolo et al, 1995). In our studies, the cardiac function curve was depressed in animals without volume resuscitation. This observation suggests that volume resuscitation had an indirect effect by preventing the release of substances that have a negative inotropic effect. Cohen and coworkers (1996) also found that fluid resuscitation improved cardiac function and that the increase in stroke work with volume resuscitation was associated with the increase in myocardial oxygen consumption and coronary flow.

THERAPEUTIC IMPLICATIONS

What are the therapeutic implications of the analysis presented? The first therapeutic maneuver in the hypotensive septic patient should be volume infusion of between 1 and 2 liters of crystalloid. A higher quantity is often not helpful and possibly is harmful. Volume works by increasing the preload of the heart (Guyton et al, 1954). This then increases myocardial sarcomere length and leads to a greater output through the Frank-Starling relationship. A limit to the filling of the heart exists, which is determined by the pericardium or the cytoskeleton of a heart without a pericardium (Holt et al, 1960; Bishop et al, 1964). Once this limit is reached, right atrial pressure rises without a change in sarcomere length and without a change in cardiac output (Magder et al, 1992). This mechanism is represented by the flat portion of the cardiac function curve. The increase in right atrial pressure leads to greater left heart pressures and greater transudation of fluid in the lungs. Increased pressure in the wall of the heart can also lead to an impediment to coronary flow. Furthermore, increased right atrial pressure leads to increased systemic venous pressures and consequently to increased capillary pressures and transudation of fluid in the systemic circulation. The right atrial pressure then drops, and further volume infusions result in more peripheral edema. This situation can sometimes lead to extremely large infusions of volume (Hayes et al, 1994).

A very helpful therapeutic maneuver in the management of sepsis is the administration of adrenergic drugs. Dopamine remains one of the most popular agents (Parillo, 1993) because it has strong beta and alpha properties (Goldberg, 1972). In our unit we have favored norepinephrine. The properties of dopamine change with the dose, and these are not always predictable in a given patient. Therefore, patients receive varying levels of alpha- and beta-agonists without clearly predictable results. Furthermore, dopamine is often used in doses above 10 μg/kg per minute, in which case the alpha properties predominate, and then it acts much like norepinephrine (Goldberg, 1972). The reader is referred to Chapter 15 for additional review of adrenergic agents in sepsis.

To thereby understand the potential role of norepinephrine, it is necessary to return to the analysis of hemodynamics in sepsis (see Fig. 19–5). The most evident clinical problem is hypotension. An alpha-agonist obviously helps increase peripheral resistance and restore blood pressure. However, norepinephrine usually also produces an increase in cardiac output (Hussain et al, 1988; Hannemann et al, 1995). Although not as potent as its alpha properties, norepinephrine has important beta-agonist effects, which increase contractility. When the blood pressure is not low, or cardiac function is poor, the beta-agonist effect is often counteracted by the rise in left ventricular afterload. This rise is usually not a major factor in sepsis because the peripheral resistance is very

low and cardiac function is much better than in cardiogenic shock. An improvement in cardiac function means that the same cardiac output can be produced at a lessened right atrial pressure, which thus lowers venous pressures and the tendency for capillary leak.

Norepinephrine also has an important effect on venous tone, which helps restore cardiac output (see Fig. 19–5). Norepinephrine causes a decrease in vascular capacitance, which means that there is a decrease in unstressed volume and therefore an increase in stressed volume without a change in venous compliance (Mehta et al, 1996). Norepinephrine thus produces an "autotransfusion." The advantage of autotransfusion over volume infusion is that it can be removed without diuresis. Stressed volume is primarily in small veins and venules. It is possible to have a contraction of these vessels without a contraction of the downstream veins, which determine resistance to venous return. In fact there may even be a tendency for resistance to venous return to decrease with norepinephrine, because beta-agonists tend to decrease resistance to venous return (Green, 1977; Mehta et al, 1994).

If norepinephrine acts by producing an effective volume transfusion, why not just give more volume? There are some important differences that need to be considered. Giving volume raises blood pressure by raising cardiac output. This increases the pressures throughout the vasculatures, including capillaries (Fig. 19–6). This mechanism results in increased fluid exudation, especially in septic patients in whom increased capillary permeability is an important part of the pathophysi-

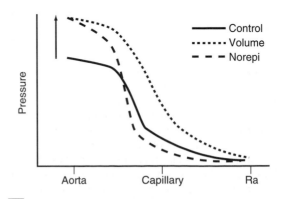

Figure 19–6
Theoretical pressure contour lines for the circulation. Increasing blood pressure by giving volume raises pressure throughout the system and raises capillary pressures. An increase in arterial pressure produced by norepinephrine can potentially maintain or even reduce capillary pressure and thus can reduce the hydrostatic forces for filtration in the capillaries.

ology. In contrast, the rise in blood pressure with norepinephrine is associated with rise in arteriolar resistance, and therefore capillary pressures should stay the same or decrease, assuming no increase in resistance to venous return.

Concern is often raised that norepinephrine will decrease renal perfusion and therefore worsen renal function. This concern arises from use of norepinephrine in cardiogenic shock in which systemic resistance is already high, and adding a vasoconstrictor makes matters worse. The situation is very different in sepsis; the presence of a widespread decrease in vascular resistance means that flow is increased to metabolically inactive areas. The general rise in vascular tone thus allows greater perfusion of the kidneys. Norepinephrine can then increase blood flow and glomerular filtration rate when given in sepsis (Schaer et al, 1985; Desjars et al, 1989).

Because oxygen consumption is elevated in sepsis and tissue extraction of oxygen is impaired, it is often considered appropriate to increase cardiac output further in sepsis (Shoemaker et al, 1988; Tuchschmidt et al, 1992; Metrangolo et al, 1995). The previous discussion explains how norepinephrine helps, but another possibility is to give a drug with prominent beta-agonist properties, such as dobutamine (Berne and Levy, 1983; Ruffolo and Messick, 1985). It should be appreciated, however, that the negative enantiomer of dobutamine also has alpha-agonist properties. Indeed, dobutamine has been successfully given in sepsis (Shoemaker et al, 1986; Vincent et al, 1987; Kilbourn et al, 1994; Hannemann et al, 1995). It must be given cautiously. Unlike norepinephrine, dobutamine does not have a major effect on vascular capacitance or arterial tone. The rise in blood pressure, or at least its maintenance, is thus dependent upon a rise in cardiac output. If the patient does not have initially an adequate stressed volume, or the heart does not respond to the dobutamine, there can be a further fall in blood pressure and potentially serious consequences. Therefore, before administration of dobutamine, the clinician should make sure that volume resuscitation has been adequate. It is often prudent to have some norepinephrine ready (Vincent et al, 1987). Subsequent studies have failed to find a benefit to survival from increased oxygen delivery (Hayes et al, 1994).

RESPIRATORY ABNORMALITIES IN SEPSIS AND THEIR EFFECTS ON THE CIRCULATION

Patients with septic shock frequently have to be intubated because gas exchange abnormalities and demands on respiratory muscles lead to respiratory failure (Hussain et al, 1985b; Hussain et al, 1986). When patients are subsequently on a ventilator, the positive-pressure ventilation can have important implications for hemodynamic status. As discussed earlier, septic patients require an adequate volume to maintain an adequate mean systemic pressure to sustain the increased cardiac output. An increase in intrathoracic pressure means that the central venous pressure must be higher relative to atmosphere to maintain the same transmural filling pressure in the heart. MCFP must be higher to maintain the gradient for resistance to venous return (Fessler et al, 1991; Fessler et al, 1992). The higher MCFP means, in turn, that the capillary pressures that are upstream from this region will be higher, and the forces favoring capillary filtration will be higher. Edema will thereby increase. Positive intrathoracic pressures indicate that the veins will collapse when they enter the thorax at a positive value rather than at zero (Fessler et al, 1992). This occurrence limits the maximal resistance to venous return and cardiac output. In addition, if large transpulmonary pressures are utilized to ventilate the patient, the pressures increase the load on the right ventricle (Scharf et al, 1979), which depresses the cardiac function curve and leads to a further rise in right-sided pressures.

Hypoxemia is another frequent problem in sepsis. The main causes of hypoxemia are ventilation-perfusion mismatch and shunt. In sepsis, these are most likely due to pulmonary congestion. A primary cause of the pulmonary edema is increased capillary leak, which is a generalized feature of sepsis. As discussed earlier, this leak is due to a number of factors including the attachment and activation of neutrophils to the endothelium and the release of their toxic substances (Kubes and Granger, 1992; Kurose et al, 1993).

There are also direct effects on the permeability of the endothelium because of release of cytokines. Increased capillary permeability is defined as fluid filtration being greater at any given capillary pressure. Capillary leak is made worse because the concentration of albumin is decreased in sepsis, which lowers intravascular oncotic pressure. This adds a further factor to the increased net capillary filtration. The cardiac dysfunction associated with sepsis results in higher cardiac filling pressures than normal for any given cardiac output, leading to higher pulmonary capillary pressures (Parker et al, 1987; Parillo, 1993).

Because of these factors, fluids must be administered cautiously in sepsis. As discussed earlier, volume resuscitation is important for raising cardiac output and restoring blood pressure, but vasopressors can reduce the need for fluid. If a vasoconstricting drug such as norepinephrine is given the drug also improves cardiac function and allows the same cardiac output at lower cardiac filling pressures. When cardiac function is very depressed, it can be useful to give a drug that has stronger beta-agonist properties, such as dobutamine, but the blood pressure must be monitored very carefully. If cardiac output does not rise there may be a further fall in blood pressure due to dobutamine-mediated vasodilation in peripheral vessels.

Typically, in sepsis, the mixed venous oxygen content is high, but when depression of cardiac function becomes more marked, the mixed venous oxygen function falls. If a large shunt fraction is present, the fall in mixed venous oxygen contributes to a worsening of the arterial oxygenation. It may then be necessary to increase cardiac output, which leads to a higher mixed venous oxygen content and an improved arterial oxygen saturation (Shoemaker et al, 1986).

SEPSIS AND THE VENTILATORY PUMP

Characteristic findings in sepsis are tachypnea and respiratory alkalosis. These signs are caused by the direct effect of endotoxin or cytokines on respiratory centers (Hussain et al, 1991). Sepsis is also associated with metabolic acidosis, which increases respiratory drive. Increased ventilation requires increased respiratory muscle work, which in turn requires increased blood flow to respiratory muscles (Hussain et al, 1985a; Hussain et al, 1986) (Fig. 19–7). Thus at a time when hypotension is present, tissue perfusion is compromised, and oxygen extraction by tissues is impaired (Wright et al, 1971), the energy demands of the respiratory muscles are increased. Initially, vasodilation of the vasculature of the respiratory muscles allows respiratory muscle blood flow to increase (Hussain et al, 1985a; Hussain et al, 1986), but when the blood pressure decreases substantially, there is not enough driving pressure to sustain blood flow, and respiratory muscle failure occurs (Hussain et al, 1985). Increased carbon dioxide levels and worsening hypoxia lead to worsening acidosis, and death occurs unless ventilation is supported artificially. Maintenance of arterial pressure can help respiratory muscle blood flow and prevent respiratory muscle failure (Hussain et al, 1985a, 1985b). Respiratory muscle failure is probably the major cause of death in patients who are not ventilated.

The increase in ventilatory effort combined

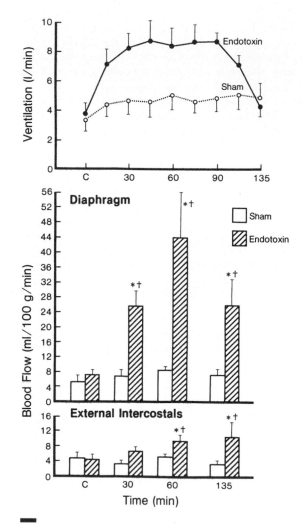

Figure 19–7
Results in animals treated with endotoxin. (*Upper chart*) Mean changes in minute ventilation in endotoxin-treated animals compared with the sham group. (*Middle chart*) Increase in blood flow to the diaphragm over time in the two groups of animals. (*Bottom chart*) Increase in external intercostal blood flow. Ventilation almost doubled with endotoxemia, resulting in a marked increase in diaphragmatic and intercostal blood flow. However, after 2 hours, the ventilation decreased and the animals died if the experiment continued. (From Hussain SNA, and Roussos C: Distribution of respiratory muscle and organ blood flow during endotoxic shock in dogs. J Appl Physiol 59:1802, 1985. With permission.)

with altered lung mechanics (i.e., increased airway resistance and decreased compliance from pulmonary congestion) also has important implications for cardiac function. Increased negative pleural pressure swings with inspiration raise the inspiratory filling of the right ventricle and raise the afterload on the left ventricle. This process can result in a considerable increase in the left atrial transmural pressure and consequently in pulmonary capillary transmural pressure (Magder et al, 1983). When combined with increased capillary permeability and decreased intravascular oncotic pressures, it leads to worsening of pulmonary edema. Possibly as a result, the condition of severely septic patients often cannot be stabilized until the ventilation is totally controlled with paralysis and mechanical means.

Besides the direct hemodynamic effects of increased respiratory activity, there are important indirect effects. Increased muscle activity leads to increased activity in afferent neurons, which leads to a further rise in the drive for ventilation (Hussain et al, 1990; Teitelbaum et al, 1992) as well as a generalized rise in the sympathetic tone (Hussain et al, 1991b). The latter results in renal vasoconstriction, which can contribute to the worsening of renal function associated with sepsis. Placing the patient on a ventilator removes the respiratory muscle work, results in decreased metabolite accumulation in the respiratory muscles, and should produce decreased reflex vasoconstriction.

CONCLUSIONS

Sepsis has major interactive effects on the pulmonary and systemic vascular systems, which worsen the clinical picture. The management of sepsis requires enough volume to maintain adequate cardiovascular function, but not so much that it worsens pulmonary function. Sepsis also requires close observation of the respiratory status because control of the ventilatory system is important for maintenance of both gas exchange and stable hemodynamic function.

REFERENCES

Aoki N, Siegfried M, and Lefer AM: Anti-EDRF effect of tumor necrosis factor in isolated, perfused cat carotid arteries. Am J Physiol 256:H1509, 1989.

Appleton C, Olajos M, Morkin E, and Goldman S: Alpha-1 adrenergic control of the venous circulation in intact dogs. J Pharmacol Exp Ther 233:729, 1985.

Benjamin E, Leibowitz AB, Oropello J, and Iberti TJ: Systemic hypoxic and inflammatory syndrome: An alternative designation for "sepsis syndrome." Crit Care Med 20:680, 1992.

Berne RM and Levy MN: The cardiovascular system. In Berne RM, Levy MN (eds): Physiology. St. Louis, CV Mosby Company, 1983, p 439.

Bishop VS, Stone HL, and Guyton AC: Cardiac function curves in conscious dogs. Am J Physiol 207(3):677, 1964.

Bone RC: The pathogenesis of sepsis. Ann Intern Med 115:457, 1991.

Bone RC, Fisher CJ, Clemmer TP, et al: Sepsis syndrome: A valid clinical entity. Crit Care Med 17:389, 1989.

Borland C, Cox Y, and Higenbottam T: Measurement of exhaled nitric oxide (NO) production in man. Thorax 48:1160, 1993.

Brady AJB, Warren JB, Poole-Wilson PA, et al: Nitric oxide attenuates cardiac myocyte contraction. Am J Physiol 265:H176, 1993.

Brigham KL, Bowers RE, and Haynes J: Increased sheep lung vascular permeability caused by *Escherichia coli* endotoxin. Circ Res 45:292, 1979.

Brun-Buisson C: Incidence, risk factors, and outcome of severe sepsis and septic shock in adults. A multicenter, prospective study in intensive care units. JAMA 274:968, 1995.

Busse R and Mulsch A: Induction of nitric oxide synthase by cytokines in vascular smooth muscle cells. FEBS Letter 275:87, 1990.

Busse R, Mulsch A, Fleming I, and Hecker M: Mechanisms of nitric oxide release from the vascular endothelium. Circulation 87:v–18, 1993.

Caldini P, Permutt S, Waddell JA, and Riley RL: Effect of epinephrine on pressure, flow, and volume relationships in the systemic circulation of dogs. Circ Res 34:606, 1974.

Cohen RI, Huberfeld S, Genovese J, et al: A comparison between the acute effects of nitric oxide synthase inhibition and fluid resuscitation on myocardial function and metabolism in endotoxemic dogs. J Crit Care 9:27, 1996.

Datta P and Magder S: Circuit response to norepinephrine with and without L-NAME in porcine endotoxemia (abstr). Int Care Med 22(3):S381, 1996.

Deschamps A, Fournier A, and Magder S: The influence of neuropeptide Y on regional vascular capacitance in dogs. Am J Physiol 266:H165, 1994.

Deschamps A and Magder S: Baroreflex control of regional capacitance and blood flow distribution with or without alpha adrenergic blockade. J Appl Physiol 263:H1755, 1992.

Deschamps A and Magder S: Effects of heat stress on vascular capacitance. Am J Physiol 266:H2122, 1994.

Desjars P, Pinaud M, Bugnon D, and Tasseau F: Norepinephrine therapy has no deleterious renal effects in human septic shock. Crit Care Med 17:426, 1989.

Fessler HE, Brower RG, Wise RA, and Permutt S: Effects of positive end-expiratory pressure on the gradient for venous return. Am Rev Respir Dis 143:19, 1991.

Fessler HE, Brower RG, Wise RA, and Permutt S: Effects of positive end-expiratory pressure on the gradient for venous return. Am Rev Respir Dis 146:4, 1992.

Finkel MS, Oddis CV, Jacob TD, et al: Negative inotropic effects of cytokines on the heart mediated by nitric oxide. Science 257:397, 1992.

Fleming I, Julou-Schaeffer G, Gray GA, et al: Evidence that an L-arginine/nitric oxide dependent elevation of tissue cyclic GMP content is involved in depression of vascular reactivity by endotoxin. Br J Pharmacol 103:1047, 1991.

Goldberg LI: Cardiovascular and renal actions of dopamine: Potential clinical applications. Pharmacol Rev 24:1, 1972.

Gray GA, Schott C, Julou-Schaeffer G, et al: The effect of inhibitors of the L-arginine/nitric oxide pathway on endotoxin-induced loss of vascular responsiveness in anaesthetized rats. Br J Pharmacol 103:1218, 1991.

Green JF: Mechanism of action of isoproterenol on venous return. Am J Physiol 232(2):H152, 1977.

Green JF and Jackman AP: Mechanism of the increased vascular capacity produced by mild hypothermia in the dog. Circ Res 44:411, 1979.

Green JF, Jackman AP, and Krohn KA: Mechanism of morphine-induced shifts in blood volume between extracorporeal reservoir and the systemic circulation of the dog under conditions of constant blood flow and vena caval pressures. Circ Res 42(4):479, 1978.

Guyton AC: Determination of cardiac output by equating venous return curves with cardiac response curves. Physiol Rev. 35:123, 1955a.

Guyton AC, Jones CE, and Coleman TG: Circulatory physiology: Cardiac output and its regulation. In Guyton AC (ed), Philadelphia, WB Saunders, 1973.

Guyton A, Lindsey AW, and Gilluly JJ: The limits of right ventricular compensation following acute increase in pulmonary circulatory resistance. Circ Res II:326, 1954.

Guyton AC, Lindsey AW, and Kaufman BN: Effect of mean circulatory filling pressure and other peripheral circulatory factors on cardiac output. Am J Physiol 180:463, 1955b.

Hannemann L, Reinhart K, Grenzer O, et al: Comparison of dopamine to dobutamine and norepinephrine for oxygen delivery and uptake in septic shock. Crit Care Med 23:1962, 1995.

Hayes M, Timmins AC, Yau EHS, et al: Elevation of systemic oxygen delivery in the treatment of critically ill patients. N Engl J Med 330:1717, 1994.

Hirata Y, Mitaka C, Emori T, et al: Plasma endothelins in sepsis syndrome. JAMA 270:2182, 1993.

Holt JP, Rhode EA, and Kines H: Pericardial and ventricular pressure. Circ Res VIII:1171, 1960.

Hom GJ, Grant SK, Wolfe G, et al: Lipopolysaccharide-induced hypotension and vascular hyporeactivity in the rat: Tissue analysis of nitric oxide synthase mRNA and protein expression in the presence and absence of dexamethason, N^G-monomethyl-L-arginine or indomethacin. J Pharmacol Exp Ther 272:452, 1995.

Hussain SNA, Chatillon A, Comtois A, et al: Chemical activation of thin-fiber phrenic afferents: The cardiovascular responses. J Appl Physiol 70:159, 1991a.

Hussain SNA, Graham R, Rutledge F, Roussos C: Respiratory muscle energetics during endotoxic shock in dogs. J Appl Physiol 60:486, 1986.

Hussain SNA and Magder S: Respiratory muscle function in shock and infection. Semin Respir Med 12:287, 1991b.

Hussain S, Magder S, Chatillon A, and Roussos C: Chemical activation of thin-fiber phrenic afferents: The respiratory responses. J Appl Physiol 69(3):1002, 1990.

Hussain SNA and Roussos C: Distribution of respiratory muscle and organ blood flow during endotoxic shock in dogs. J Appl Physiol 59:1802, 1985a.

Hussain SNA, Rutledge F, Magder S, and Roussos C: Effects of norepinephrine and fluid infusion on selective blood distribution in septic shock. J Crit Care 3:32, 1988.

Hussain SNA, Simkus G, and Roussos C: Respiratory muscle fatigue: A cause of ventilatory failure in septic shock. J Appl Physiol 58:2033, 1985b.

Javeshghani D, Mehta S, and Magder S: Failure to detect inducible nitric oxide in a porcine model of hyperdynamic sepsis (abstr.). Circulation, 1996, in press.

Julou-Schaeffer G, Gray GA, Fleming I, et al: Loss of vascular responsiveness induced by endotoxin involves L-arginine pathway. Am J Physiol 259:H1038, 1990.

Kilbourn RG, Cromeens DM, Chelley FD, and Griffith OW: N^G-methyl-L-arginine, an inhibitor of nitric oxide formation, acts synergistically with dobutamine to improve cardiovascular performance in endotoxemic dogs. Crit Care Med 22:1835, 1994.

Kubes P and Granger DN: Nitric oxide modulates microvascular permeability. Am J Physiol 31:H611, 1992.

Kurose I, Kubes P, Wolf R, et al: Inhibition of nitric oxide production: Mechanisms of vascular albumin leakage. Circ Res 73:164, 1993.

Kurose I, Wolf R, Grisham MB, et al: Microvascular responses to inhibition of nitric oxide production: Role of active oxidants. Circ Res 76:30, 1995.

Lee K, Van der Zee H, Dziuban SWJ, et al: Left ventricular function during chronic endotoxemia in swine. Am J Physiol H324:H330, 1988.

Lundblad R and Giercksky K: Effect of volume support, antibiotic therapy, and monoclonal antiendotoxin antibodies on mortality rate and blood concentrations of endothelin and other mediators in fulminant intra-abdominal sepsis in rats. Crit Care Med 23:1382, 1995.

MacLean LD, Mulligan WG, McLean APH, and Duff JH: Patterns of septic shock in man—a detailed study of 56 patients. Ann Surg 166:543, 1967.

Magder S: Shock Physiology. In Pinsky MR, and

Dhainault JF (eds): Physiological Foundations of Critical Care Medicine. Baltimore, Williams & Wilkins, 1992, p 140.

Magder SA, Georgiadis G, and Tuck C: Respiratory variations in right atrial pressure predict response to fluid challenge. J Crit Care 7:76, 1992.

Magder S and Kabsele K: Nitric oxide and venous return. Clin Invest Med 17:A34, 1994.

Magder SA, Lichtenstein S, and Adelman AG: Effects of negative pleural pressure on left ventricular hemodynamics. Am J Cardiol 52(5):588, 1983.

Magder S and Quinn R: Endotoxin and the mechanical properties of the canine peripheral circulation. J Crit Care 6:81, 1991.

Magder S and Vanelli G: Circuit factors in the high cardiac output of sepsis. J Crit Care 11:155–166, 1996.

Manyari DE, Wang Z, Cohen J, and Tyberg JV: Assessment of human splanchnic venous volume-pressure relation using radionuclide plethysmography. Circulation 87:1142, 1993.

Mehta S, Levy RD, Datta P, et al: Hemodynamics and nitric oxide production via expired gas analysis during endotoxemia in pigs (abstr.). Am J Respir Crit Care Med 149:A647, 1994.

Mehta S, Levy RD, Rastegarpanh M, et al: Increased cardiac output and decreased resistance are associated with increased nitric oxide excretion in expired gas during porcine endotoxemia. Clin Invest Med 17:A101, 1994.

Members of the American College of Chest Physicians/Society of Critical Care Medicine Consensus Conference Committee: Definitions for sepsis and organ failure and guidelines for the use of innovative therapies in sepsis. Crit Care Med 20:864, 1992.

Metrangolo L, Fiorillo M, Friedman G, et al: Early hemodynamic course of septic shock. Crit Care Med 23:1971, 1995.

Mitaka C, Hirata Y, Ichikawa K, et al: Effects of TNF-α on hemodynamic changes and circulating endothelium-derived vasoactive factors in dogs. Am J Physiol 267:1530, 1994.

Mitaka C, Hirata Y, Makita K, and Nagura T: Endothelin-1 and atrial natriuretic peptide in septic shock. Am Heart J 126:466, 1993.

Mitzner W and Goldberg H: Effect of epinephrine on resistive and compliant properties of the canine vasculature. J Appl Physiol 39(2):272, 1975.

Morise Z, Ueda M, Aiura K, et al: Pathophysiologic role of endothelin-1 in renal function in rats with endotoxin shock. Surgery 115:199, 1994.

Myers PR, Wright TF, Tanner MA, and Adams HR: EDRF and nitric oxide production in cultured endothelial cells: Direct inhibition by *E. coli* endotoxin. Am J Physiol 262:H710, 1992.

Nanas S and Magder S: Adaptations of the peripheral circulation to PEEP. Am Rev Respir Dis 146:688, 1992.

Natanson C, Danner RL, Elin RJ, et al: Role of endotoxemia in cardiovascular dysfunction and mortality. J Clin Invest 83:243, 1989.

Natanson C, Danner RL, Fink MP, et al: Cardiovascular performance with E. coli challenges in a canine model of human sepsis. Am J Physiol 254:H558, 1988.

Natanson C, Fink MP, Ballantyne HK, et al: Gram-negative bacteremia produces both severe systolic and diastolic cardiac dysfunction in a canine model that stimulates human septic shock. J Clin Invest 78:259, 1986.

Nava E, Palmer RMJ, and Moncada S: The role of nitric oxide in endotoxic shock: Effects of N^G-monomethyl-L-arginine. J Cardiovasc Pharmacol 20:S132, 1992.

Notarius CF, MacLean LD, Rhode B, and Magder S: Exerise capacity and energy expenditure of morbidly obese and previously obese subjects (abstr.). Int J Obesity 19(Suppl. 4):S134, 1995.

Owada A, Tomita K, Terada Y, et al: Endothelin (ET)-3 stimulates cyclic guanosine 3',5'-monophosphate production via ET$_B$ receptor by producing nitric oxide in isolated rat glomerulus, and in cultured rat mesangial cells. J Clin Invest 93:556, 1994.

Parillo JE: Septic shock in humans: Advances in the understanding of pathogenesis, cardiovascular dysfunction, and therapy. Ann Intern Med 113:227, 1990.

Parillo JE: Pathogenetic mechanisms of septic shock. N Engl J Med 328:1471, 1993.

Parillo JE, Burch C, Shelhamer JH, et al: A circulating myocardial depressant substance in humans with septic shock. Septic shock patients with a reduced ejection fraction have a circulating factor that depresses in vitro myocardial cell performance. J Clin Invest 76:1539, 1985.

Parker JL and Adams HR: Selective inhibition of endothelium-dependent vasodilator capacity by Escherichia coli endotoxemia. Circ Res 72:539, 1993.

Parker JL, Keller RS, DeFily DV, et al: Coronary vascular smooth muscle function in E. coli endotoxemia in dogs. Am J Physiol 260:H832, 1991.

Parker JL, Keller RS, DiFily DV, et al: Coronary vascular smooth muscle function in E. coli endotoxemia in dogs. Am J Physiol 76:361, 1994.

Parker MM, McCarthy KE, Ognibene FP, and Parillo JE: Right ventricular dysfunction and dilatation, similar to left ventricular changes, characterize the cardiac depression of septic shock in humans. Chest 97:126, 1990.

Parker MM, Shelhamer JH, Natanson C, et al: Serial cardiovascular variables in survivors and nonsurvivors of human septic shock: Heart rate as an early predictor of prognosis. Crit Care Med 15:923, 1987.

Pastor C, Teisseire B, Vicaut E, and Payen D: Effects of L-arginine and L-nitro-arginine treatment on blood pressure and cardiac output in a rabbit endotoxin shock model. Crit Care Med 22:465, 1994.

Permutt S and Caldini P: Regulation of cardiac output by the circuit: Venous return. In Boan J,

Noordergraaf A, Raines J (eds): Cardiovascular System Dynamics. Cambridge, MA, MIT Press, 1978, p 465.

Rackow EC and Astiz ME: Mechanisms and management of septic shock. Crit Care Clin 9:219, 1993.

Rosenkranz-Weiss P, Sessa WC, Milstien S, and Kaufman S: Regulation of nitric oxide synthesis by proinflammatory cytokines in human umbilical vein endothelial cells. J Clin Invest 93:2236, 1994.

Rothe C: Venous system: Physiology of the capacitance vessels. In Shepherd JT, and Abboud FM (eds): Handbook of Physiology. Bethesda, American Physiological Society, 1983a, p 397.

Rothe CF: Reflex control of veins and vascular capacitance. Physiol Rev 63(4):1281, 1983b.

Ruffolo RR Jr and Messick K: Effects of dopamine, (±)-dobutamine and the (+) and (−)-enantiomers of dobutamine on cardiac function in pithed rats. J Pharmacol Exp Ther 235:558, 1985.

Sagawa K and Eisner A: Static pressure-flow relation in the total systemic vascular bed of the dog and its modification by the baroreceptor reflex. Circ Res 36:406, 1975.

Schaer GL, Fink MP, and Parrillo JE: Norepinephrine alone versus norepinephrine plus low-dose dopamine: Enhanced renal blood flow with combination pressor therapy. Crit Care Med 13:492, 1985.

Scharf SM, Brown R, Tow DE, and Parisi AF: Cardiac effects of increased lung volume and decreased pleural pressure. J Appl Physiol 47:257, 1979.

Shoemaker WC, Appel PL, and Bishop MH: Temporal patterns of blood volume, hemodynamics, and oxygen transport in pathogenesis and therapy of postoperative adult respiratory distress syndrome. New Horiz 1:522, 1993.

Shoemaker WC, Appel PL, and Kram HB: Hemodynamic and oxygen transport effects of dobutamine in critically ill general surgical patients. Crit Care Med 14:1032, 1986.

Shoemaker WC, Appel P, Kram HB, et al: Prospective trial of "supranormal" values of survivors as therapeutic goals and high risk surgical patients. Chest 94:1176, 1988.

Shoukas AA and Sagawa K: Control of total systemic vascular capacity by the carotid sinus baroreceptor reflex. Circ Res 33:22, 1973.

Sibbald WJ, Marshall J, Christou NV, et al: "Sepsis"—clarity of existing terminology ... or more confusion? Crit Care Med 19:996, 1991.

Stoclet J, Fleming I, and Gray G: Nitric oxide and endotoxemia. Circulation 87:v–77, 1993.

Suffredini AF, Fromm FE, Parker MM, et al: The cardiovascular response of normal humans to the administration of endotoxin. N Engl J Med 321(5):280, 1989.

Sugiura M, Inagami T, and Kon V: Endotoxin stimulates endothelin-release in vivo and in vitro as determined by radioimmunoassay. Biochem Biophys Res Commun 161(3):1220, 1989.

Szabo C: Alterations in nitric oxide production in various forms of circulatory shock. New Horiz 3:2, 1995.

Teitelbaum JS, Magder SA, Roussos C, and Hussain SNA: Effects of diaphragmatic ischemia on the inspiratory motor drive. J Appl Physiol 72:447, 1992.

Thiemermann C and Vane J: Inhibition of nitric oxide synthesis reduces the hypotension induced by bacterial lipopolysaccharides in the rat in vivo. Eur J Pharmacol 182:591, 1990.

Tuchschmidt J, Fried J, and Astiz M: Elevation of cardiac output and oxygen delivery improves outcome in septic shock. Chest 102:216, 1992.

Vincent JL, Van der Linden P, Domb M, et al: Dopamine compared with dobutamine in experimental septic shock: Relevance of fluid administration. Anesth Analg 66:565, 1987.

Voerman HJ, Stehouwer CDA, van Kamp GJ, et al: Plasma endothelin levels are increased during septic shock. Crit Care Med 20:1097, 1992.

Wang SY, Manyari DE, Scott-Douglas N, et al: Splanchnic venous pressure-volume relation during experimental acute ischemic heart failure. Differential effects of hydralazine, enalaprilat, and nitroglycerin. Circulation 91:1205, 1995.

Wang Y: Vascular pharmacodynamics of N^G-nitro-L-arginine methyl ester in vitro and in vivo. J Pharmacol Exp Ther 267:1091, 1993.

Weyrich AS, Ma X, Buerke M, et al: Physiological concentrations of nitric oxide do not elicit an acute negative inotropic effect in unstimulated cardiac muscle. Circ Res 75:692, 1994.

Wright CJ, Duff JH, McLean APH, and MacLean LD: Regional capillary blood flow and oxygen uptake in severe sepsis. Surg Gynecol Obstet 132:637, 1971.

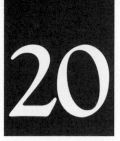
Community-acquired Pneumonia

George A. Sarosi, M.D.

Philip C. Johnson, M.D.

Infections of the pulmonary parenchyma, or pneumonia, are still a common cause of illness leading to hospitalization and frequently to periods of treatment in an intensive care unit (ICU) setting. By convention, pneumonias are divided into community-acquired pneumonia (CAP), nosocomial pneumonia, and pneumonia in immunocompromised hosts.

CAP is any lower respiratory tract infection (LRI) that is either present on admission or develops within the first 72 hours of hospitalization and is the subject of this chapter. Nosocomial pneumonias, LRIs that develop in the hospital after 72 hours of hospital stay, and pneumonias that occur in compromised hosts, are discussed in Chapter 21.

CLINICAL PROBLEM

Pneumonia, or LRI, refers to a condition in a patient with fever, symptoms of pulmonary involvement (cough, shortness of breath, pleuritic chest pain), and abnormal chest radiograph.

Although infections of the pulmonary parenchyma represent the etiology for most patients presenting with the aforementioned constellation of signs and symptoms, a large number of noninfectious nosologic entities may occur with the same clinical picture.

PATHOGENESIS OF LOWER RESPIRATORY TRACT INFECTION

NORMAL HOST DEFENSES

To understand why the lower respiratory tract is so often the site of an infectious process, remember that the tracheobronchial tree and the terminal bronchioles, along with the alveolar sacs, are in constant contact with the outside world. To fulfill its main function, oxygenation of partially desaturated venous blood, the entire surface of the lung is exposed constantly to the ambient air that we inhale. This ambient air often contains droplets from the expectorated secretions of other individuals, which act as vehicles for the transmis-

Table 20–1
Pulmonary Defense Mechanism

Upper Airway

Nasal turbinates
Nasal hairs
Epiglottis

Conducting Airways

Ciliary action
Mucous blanket
Acute angulation of the bronchi
IgA

Alveoli

IgG (subclasses IgG2 and 4)
Complement and properdin system
Transferrin and lactoferrin
Alveolar macrophages
Granulocytes

sion of infecting agents such as bacteria or viruses. Furthermore, inhaled air often mixes with aspirated material and is heavily laden with potentially infectious organisms from the oropharynx.

To protect its main function of gas exchange, the respiratory system evolved a series of protective mechanisms to purify the inhaled air and prevent inhaled infectious agents from reaching the terminal air spaces (Newhouse et al, 1976). These are listed in Table 20–1.

The first component of this protective mechanism consists of the nose and the nasal turbinates (Proctor and Wagner, 1967), epiglottis, and larynx, all of which serve to stop larger inhaled particles. After passing through the larynx, the inhaled air must pass over sharply angled branches of the trachea and bronchi, causing precipitation of many inhaled particles on the mucous surface of these branch points (Hoffman and Billingham, 1975).

After precipitation of these particles on the mucous surfaces, ciliary action moves this mucous blanket upward (Luchsinger et al, 1968), and coughing eventually expels the infected material from the airways. Despite its considerable efficiency, these nonspecific defense mechanisms are not foolproof, and a certain number of infectious particles reach the alveolar sacs, where the next layer of protection comes into action.

Surfactant lining the alveoli, along with opsonizing IgG immunoglobulins, components of the complement and properdin system, and transferrin all have their role in eliminating infecting particles (Toews, 1986). Even with the considerable efficiency of these alveolar lining compounds, a few (or occasionally many more) microorgan-

isms get through and reach the surface of the alveolus, where they are normally picked up by roving alveolar macrophages that are assisted in their phagocytic role by the presence of many classes of opsonic material. When the resident population of alveolar macrophages is overwhelmed, an inflammatory reaction is initiated and acts as a chemotactic stimulus, leading to the appearance of polymorphonuclear phagocytes (PMNs) that usually finish the process. Thus, among healthy individuals, the well-developed defense mechanisms of the respiratory tract are usually adequate to prevent infections from becoming established in the air exchange areas of the lungs (Reynolds, 1983).

ALTERATION IN NORMAL HOST DEFENSES

The normally efficient defense system may be overwhelmed by many different mechanisms. Alterations in the anatomy and function may occur along any of the components of the defense system (Table 20–2). The mechanical barriers of the nose, epiglottis, and larynx may be circumvented by endotracheal intubation or tracheostomy, leading to a potential conduit that allows deposits of infecting particles directly into the conducting airways.

Because intact cilia have an important role in removing particles trapped in the mucous blanket, any process that alters normal ciliary function may lead to an accumulation of secretions. Examples are immotile cilia syndrome, infections that

Table 20–2
Alterations in Pulmonary Defenses

Site	Nature of Alteration
Upper airways	Tracheostomy
	Tracheal intubation
Conducting airways	
Ciliary action	Smoking
	Immotile cilia syndrome
Mucous blanket	Cystic fibrosis
	Reactive airways disease
IgA	Congenital deficiency
	Breakdown by bacterial proteases
Alveoli	
IgG	Hypogammaglobulinemia seen with clonal B cell neoplasms
Alveolar macrophages and granulocytes	Cytotoxic chemotherapy

destroy cilia-bearing cells, or chronic irritation by cigarette smoke, which immobilizes cilia and leads to squamous cell metaplasia and the loss of cilia-bearing cells (Afzelius, 1981).

Loss of mucosal IgA, either due to the congenital absence of the immunoglobulin or its rapid removal by bacterial proteases, leads to colonization of the lower respiratory tract by potentially pathogenic microorganisms (Tomassi, 1983), whereas the development of iron deficiency leads to the loss of transferrin and lactoferrin, resulting in the loss of host defenses against certain gram-negative bacteria.

Absent or greatly decreased levels of IgG and its subclasses, which are usually the result of B cell proliferative diseases (e.g., myeloma and chronic lymphocytic leukemia), lead to the loss of opsonization. This results in the development of severe sinopulmonary infections, especially by the encapsulated bacteria *Streptococcus pneumoniae* and *Haemophilus influenzae* (Reynolds, 1988). Deficiency of various components of the complement system, especially of C3 and C5, also leads to frequent infections (Toews, 1986).

Properly functioning granulocytes are essential to successful handling of most LRIs. Alterations in the normal function or the migration of these phagocytic cells may result in the development of poor inflammatory reaction and may lead to serious, life-threatening infection, with gram-positive cocci and gram-negative bacteria, as well as with *Aspergillus* species (Malech and Gallin, 1987). Except for rare cases of intrinsic defects, which are seldom seen in adult populations, the most common cause of granulocyte dysfunction in daily clinical practice is the result of cytotoxic chemotherapy.

Similarly, intact alveolar macrophages are essential to proper handling of intracellular infections (Nathan, 1987; Nathan et al, 1980), especially tuberculosis, various fungal illnesses, and *Pneumocystis carinii* infection. Once again, the usual cause of such macrophage dysfunction is the administration of cytotoxic drug therapy.

Since the advent of the worldwide epidemic of the acquired immunodeficiency syndrome (AIDS), destruction of helper T lymphocytes by the human immunodeficiency virus (HIV) has become a common cause of alveolar macrophage dysfunction (Young et al, 1985). This is frequently encountered in daily clinical practice, even exceeding in frequency macrophage dysfunction due to cytotoxic drug therapy in many cities.

ACQUISITION OF THE INFECTION

CAP may be acquired by several different means. The three main avenues of infection are (1) mi-

croaspiration of oropharyngeal contents (Finegold, 1988); (2) inhalation of the infecting organism from droplets produced by expectoration of lower respiratory secretions by other infected individuals (Wells et al, 1948); and (3) inhalation of the microorganism from an infectious aerosol in the environment (Sawyer et al, 1987).

Pulmonary parenchymal infection (pneumonia) may occur during the course of an infection elsewhere. Hematogenous spread of the infecting organism may involve the lung; however, the pathophysiology and epidemiology of these infections are markedly different from those of the more common CAPs.

Microaspiration occurs in all of us, especially during sleep. As long as the quantity of aspirated material is small and the normal tracheal defense mechanism is not altered by disease or cigarette smoke, most of the aspirated material is caught by the mucous blanket and with ciliary motion moves cephalad to be expectorated. Occasionally, the small amount that reaches the alveoli is easily taken care of by macrophages, thus ending the threat of self-perpetuating LRIs.

Any alteration in the mucous blanket or of the ciliary apparatus interferes with effective clearing, and larger amounts of aspirated material may then reach the alveoli, where they may overwhelm the ability of alveolar macrophages to contain the infection, leading to the establishment of pneumonia. Common causes of altered ciliary action are the various viral infections that are cytotoxic (Little et al, 1978) and cigarette smoking, which may either destroy the cilia-bearing columnar epithelium leading to squamous metaplasia, or, early on, paralyze ciliary action (Afzelius, 1981).

Inhalation of infecting microorganisms occurs when an infected individual forcibly expels respiratory secretions laden with potential pathogens. Sneezing, coughing, and spitting all may produce droplets that carry infectious agents such as *Mycobacterium tuberculosis* and *Mycoplasma pneumoniae*. After drying of these droplets, the organisms become airborne and may be inhaled. Following inhalation, some of the microorganisms may escape the nonspecific defenses and reach the alveoli, where they may cause pneumonia in nonimmune individuals.

Various infectious agents may be encountered from environmental sources. The endemic mycoses are encountered characteristically when the sites of their growth are disturbed, such as with construction or digging, creating the infectious aerosol (Davies, 1986; Klein et al, 1986; Werner et al, 1972). Accidental exposure to zoonosis should be considered.

EPIDEMIOLOGY

After it is ascertained that the patient has pneumonia, a careful search for clinical clues must be initiated. The presence of an underlying condition that may lead to an alteration of the patient's sensorium, such as alcohol abuse, diabetes treated with insulin, or history of seizure disorders, should make one suspicious of aspiration of oropharyngeal contents, in which case the pulmonary infiltrate may be due to *Staphylococcus pneumoniae* or to the numerous anaerobic organisms that are common inhabitants of the mouth and oropharynx (Bartlett and Finegold, 1974). A history of heavy smoking and chronic bronchitis frequently underlies *S. pneumoniae* as well as *Haemophilus influenzae* and *Branhamella catarrhalis* LRIs.

During the fall/winter/spring influenza season, it is important to know what, if any, influenza viruses have been isolated in the community, and the patient's influenza vaccination history needs to be elicited. In general, LRIs caused by the influenza virus have a characteristic history of arthralgia and myalgia combined with a slow and hesitant onset of the illness. When respiratory symptoms occur 7 to 10 days after the onset of these prodromal symptoms, and the patient appears to have taken a sudden turn for the worse, superinfection with *Staphylococcus aureus* should be considered along with *S. pneumoniae* as the etiologic agent (Louria et al, 1959).

A history of a similar illness among relatives or friends in a younger subject who is complaining of severe headache and photophobia suggests M. *pneumoniae* (Murray et al, 1975), *Chlamydia pneumoniae* (Saikku et al, 1985), or *C. psittaci* infection.

Recent travel by the patient to Arizona or California is helpful to focus attention on *Coccidioides immitis* (Stevens, 1995), especially if other individuals also develop the disease, or if arthralgias and myalgias accompany the respiratory illness. Similarly, the presence of erythema nodosum in such patients almost certainly establishes the fungal etiology of the infiltrate. A similar symptom complex after a caving expedition or after clearing up an abandoned chicken coop should suggest histoplasmosis (Sarosi, 1971), whereas a recent trip to wooded areas, especially along rivers, in both the upper Midwest and the Alabama/Arkansas area, should strongly suggest blastomycosis (Klein et al, 1986).

Although numerically small, when humans become infected with an organism commonly seen in domestic or wild animals or birds, a careful epidemiologic history is indispensable. Exposure to ill psittacine birds or turkeys is usually in the background for *C. psittaci*, whereas contact with parturient cats may be uncovered to suggest *C. burnetii* infection (Langley et al, 1988). Hunting and skinning rabbits is suggestive of exposure to *Francisella tularensis* (Olsen, 1975), whereas exposure to sick wildlife in the Southeast United States should suggest infection with *Yersinia pestis* (Kaufmann et al, 1980).

INITIAL EVALUATION

PHYSICAL EXAMINATION

In addition to careful epidemiologic and exposure history, a complete and directed physical examination is very helpful. Examination of the skin should precede everything else. Jaundice, although uncommon, may indicate severe hepatic involvement, such as in miliary tuberculosis, Q fever, or psittacosis, or is the result of severe congestion of the liver due to extensive pulmonary disease, as seen in severe pneumococcal or H. *influenzae* pneumonia. Crops of vesicles on the face and trunk should suggest chickenpox and its serious pulmonary complication, varicella pneumonia (Schlossberg and Littman, 1988).

Erythema multiforme frequently accompanies mycoplasmal infections and is not uncommon with any of the fungal pneumonias (Murray et al, 1975; Sarosi, 1971). Painful, raised, red-to-violaceous nodules, which are usually seen over the pretibial areas and other extensor surfaces, should suggest erythema nodosum. These lesions are frequently seen in the various endemic mycoses (Drutz and Catanzaro, 1978; Klein et al, 1986; Miller et al, 1982), tuberculosis, and rarely in syphilis. Red-to-purple subcutaneous nodules that lead to ulceration are frequently noted in the various fungal infections, whereas painful necrotic skin lesions on an erythematous base are noted in *Pseudomonas* or other gram-negative rod pneumonias (Crane and Komshian, 1988).

The presence of multiple spider telangiectasias, as well as palmar erythema, with or without the presence of jaundice, strongly suggests underlying serious liver disease, which is most commonly caused by alcohol abuse. In such patients, special care must be taken to rule out aspiration and to expect other alcohol-related complications. Conjunctival infection is observed in the various viral and chlamydial pneumonias along with mycoplasmal infections. Bullous lesions on the tympanic membranes are found in M. *pneumoniae* pneumonia (Murray et al, 1975). Multiple painful ulcerating lesions in the mouth are noted occasionally in mycoplasmal infections (Stevens-

Johnson syndrome) (Murray et al, 1975), whereas painful ulcers with raised rolled edges that are in the mouth, on the glans penis, or in the perirectal area should suggest either histoplasmosis (Goodwin and Des Prez, 1978) or blastomycosis (Sarosi and Davies, 1979). Crusted blood in the mouth or on the lips is the result of hemoptysis and is frequent in tuberculosis and in necrotizing gram-negative rod pneumonia, especially after gross aspiration of oropharyngeal and gastric contents. The presence of clubbing (pulmonary osteoarthropathy), although quite rare in the modern era, when present, should suggest a long-standing pulmonary process, which is most often associated with anaerobic lung abscesses or tuberculosis. Diffuse lymphadenopathy should bring to mind the AIDS-related complex (ARC) with its propensity to predispose patients to both tuberculosis (Fertel and Pitchenik, 1989) and to pneumonia caused by encapsulated organisms (Polsky et al, 1986). Similarly, B cell neoplasms with their associated IgG deficiency predispose the patient to infection by the same encapsulated microorganisms (Coonrod, 1989).

Auscultation of the heart frequently reveals a systolic flow murmur, which is usually the result of the febrile state and increased cardiac output. The presence of a significant murmur (i.e., either aortic insufficiency or mitral stenosis) or the worsening state or a previously noted murmur of mitral insufficiency suggests the presence of infective endocarditis. This is usually caused by bacteremic pneumonia owing to S. pneumoniae but is occasionally found with other agents, such as Q fever and S. aureus. When infective endocarditis is suspected, a careful search should commence for its distant manifestations, such as Roth's spots or splinter hemorrhages.

Hepatomegaly is rare, unless it is the result of severe hepatic congestion that may complicate extensive pneumococcal pneumonia. Rarely, hepatic enlargement accompanies disseminated tuberculosis, Q fever, and C. psittaci infections. Splenomegaly, with or without accompanying hepatomegaly, is found in infections that involve the reticuloendothelial system, such as disseminated tuberculosis and progressive disseminated histoplasmosis.

As a general rule, the initial laboratory evaluation only helps to point the clinician in the right direction. Seldom is the original admission laboratory battery diagnostic. The white blood cell count (WBC) may be elevated with a marked shift to the left in bacterial pneumonia, but occasionally in the presence of overwhelming pneumococcal infection, the WBC may be quite depressed, often under 3000 cells/mm³, albeit with a marked left shift (Austrian and Gold, 1964). A normal or low WBC may be the rule with either influenza or mycoplasma LRIs, with or without neutrophilic preponderance. A low serum sodium level may be seen in a number of different pneumonias, not just in legionellosis, which was originally suggested. Elevated alkaline phosphatase levels are noted occasionally, especially in Q fever, tuberculosis, and occasionally in legionellosis. Frank hemolytic anemia may be observed in mycoplasmal infections, and high-titer cold agglutinins are also suggestive of M. pneumoniae infections. A cold agglutinin titer by itself is not diagnostic of Mycoplasma infection. It is seen frequently in other respiratory infections.

RADIOGRAPHIC EVALUATION

Even though the careful evaluation of the posteroanterior chest radiograph, along with a lateral view, is an important initial test, and although it often helps to narrow the multiple differential diagnostic considerations, it is almost never sufficiently specific to establish the microbiologic etiology of the disease. Nevertheless, the careful viewing of the admission chest radiograph is one of the most important early diagnostic tests.

Lobar or segmental consolidation is usually associated with S. pneumoniae (Coonrod, 1989) (Fig. 20–1), and identical radiographs could be expected in H. influenzae (Quinones et al, 1989) (Fig. 20–2) and Klebsiella pneumoniae (Crane and Komshian, 1988) infections as well. Although less common, legionella, tularemia, and blastomycosis may also produce a similar lobar or segmental picture, and further differentiation can only be made with recovery of the infecting agent (Fig. 20–3). Patchy infiltrates, usually peribronchial in location, are seen in Mycoplasma infection (Murray et al, 1975) (Fig. 20–4) and chlamydial pneumonias (Saikku et al, 1985). Frequently, pneumococcal pneumonia presents with a similar radiographic picture, not at all like the more characteristic lobar or segmental infiltrate (Coonrod, 1989).

Nodules can be characterized as large (>2 cm in diameter), small (between 0.5 and 2 cm in diameter), and miliary (<0.5 cm in diameter). Large nodules are seen in some of the fungal infections (e.g., cryptococcal and coccidioidomycotic pulmonary infections), and in staphylococcal disease, often with cavitation. Rarely, the encapsulated microorganisms S. pneumoniae and H. influenzae produce a "round pneumonia" picture (Hershey and Panaro, 1988); putrid or anaerobic lung abscesses often have a large (occasionally multiple) nodule, frequently with a discernible air-

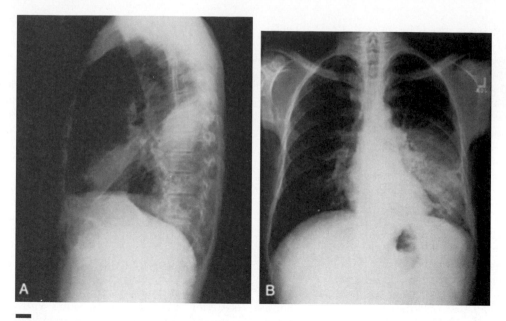

Figure 20–1
Admission chest radiographs of a patient with bacteremic *S. pneumoniae*. Note the involvement of the left lower lobe.

fluid level (Finegold, 1988). Smaller nodules are seen in the endemic mycoses, especially in histoplasmosis (Goodwin and Des Prez, 1978), in varicella pneumonia (Schlossberg and Littman, 1988), and early during the course of staphylococcal pneumonia. Miliary nodules (or millet seed–sized lesions) are classically associated with disseminated tuberculosis, but progressive disseminated histoplasmosis can appear identical to tuberculosis in every respect radiographically (and clinically) (Goodwin and Des Prez, 1978).

INITIAL MICROBIOLOGIC EVALUATION

Traditionally, sputum smears with Gram's stain were used to identify pneumococci and then to type them with the Quellung process to determine which antiserum should be given to a patient. A pneumonia that had the characteristic sputum smear was called "typical," whereas a pneumonia that had a sputum smear that did not show the expected pneumococci was called "atypical." The main problem with the examination of the spu-

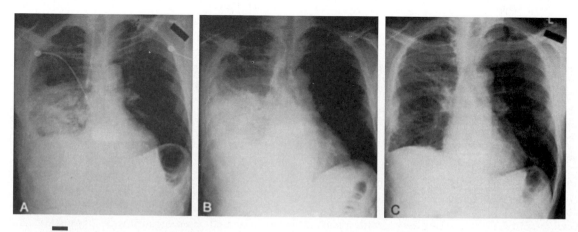

Figure 20–2
Bacteremic *H. influenzae* pneumonia. (A) On admission. Note the dense infiltrate and small pleural effusion. (B) Three days later, the patient is better despite enlarged effusion. (C) Marked improvement is readily apparent after 18 days of antibiotic treatment.

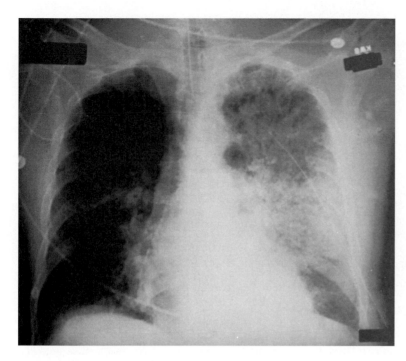

Figure 20–3
Fatal pneumonia was caused by *Legionella pneumophila*. There is extensive involvement of the entire left lung.

tum smear is that it is always contaminated with oropharyngeal content during the process of expectoration. Because pneumococci are common inhabitants of the oropharynx, it is to be expected that the sputum will be mixed with pneumococcal organisms from the pharynx and the mouth. To avoid overdiagnosis, only sputum, not sputum mixed with saliva, should be examined. Any respiratory secretions that have more than 10 squamous epithelial cells or less than 25 PMNs per lower power field should be discarded because it is obvious that it is heavily contaminated with saliva (except in granulocytopenic patients) (Washington, 1988).

In the modern era of diagnosis, microorganisms seen on such a "good" sputum specimen are accepted as probable cause of LRI but should not be accepted as definite proof of etiology. When care is taken to evaluate only good-quality sputum, useful *preliminary* information may be gained. When the slide is teaming with encapsulated lancet-shaped diplococci, pneumococcal pneumonia is a likely diagnosis. Similarly, when slender gram-negative coccobacilli are seen, *H. influenzae* should be considered: plump, large gram-negative rods are likely to be Enterobacteriaceae, whereas large, plump gram-positive cocci are most likely to be *S. aureus*. Good-quality sputum smears are

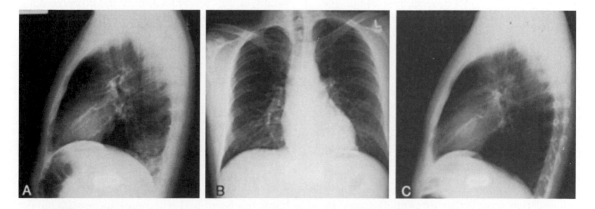

Figure 20–4
Mycoplasma pneumoniae pneumonia. (A) Admission lateral radiograph. (B) PA radiograph showing left lower lobe infiltrate. (C) Complete clearance after 6 days of therapy.

now quite rare, because sputum is seldom collected by knowledgeable physicians. What has contributed a great deal to the uncertainty of sputum smear evaluation is the fact that most examinations are now *ordered*, and the resultant saliva is not a useful specimen! Sputum is a body fluid that needs careful handling, collection, and examination.

Moreover, experience in the last 20 years or so resulted in the recognition of many other respiratory pathogens (previously all grouped together as "atypical" pneumonia agents), in which the sputum smear evaluation cannot be expected to provide a diagnostic clue. Because many large series characterizing atypical pneumonias represent the majority of patients, the sputum smear has lost some of its previous importance (Table 20–3).

INITIAL CULTURE EVALUATION

Sputum culture is one of the most commonly ordered laboratory tests. Although it is relatively easy to perform, it is exceedingly difficult to interpret. Because both S. *pneumoniae* and H. *influenzae* are frequent residents of the oropharynx, growth of these organisms from sputum may truly represent the infecting organism, or alternatively, may just represent contamination from pharyngeal material (Mackowiak, 1982). Heavy growth in pure culture from the original sputum, although not constituting definite proof, is certainly highly suggestive, especially if a concomitant Gram's smear confirms that the material is sputum and not saliva.

Recovery of Legionellaceae, M. *pneumoniae*, and the various species of *Chlamydia* can always be accepted as proof of etiology, and this recovery applies to all the endemic mycoses as well as to the zoonoses (e.g., Q fever, tularemia, and plague), because none of these organisms is thought to cause colonization only. Because many of these organisms require special culture media, the laboratory should be alerted to these organisms when they are suspected (Washington, 1988).

Blood cultures are extremely helpful in establishing the microbiologic etiology of CAP. Recovery of the pneumococcus H. *influenzae* or any other bacteria is proof of etiology. Unfortunately, the frequency of a positive blood culture result is usually low, ranging from 15 to 25%. Just how many blood cultures one should obtain before initiating treatment is unclear. Most experts recommend two sets. When intracellular organisms are suspected, the lysis-centrifugation system (DuPont isolator) should be used to enhance the chance of recovery. If an episode of LRI is accompanied by an accumulation of fluid that can be reached, such as pleural effusion or joint effusion, the material should be aspirated and cultured. Such material may be the only source of the infecting organism (Fig. 20–5).

Invasive attempts to obtain respiratory secretions are available. Transtracheal aspiration (TTA), bronchoalveolar lavage (BAL), transbronchial or percutaneous lung biopsy, or open lung biopsy can be attempted, but their exact role is difficult to define in the diagnosis of CAP (Bartlett, 1988).

Transtracheal Aspiration

Although TTA aspiration is an excellent method to obtain respiratory secretions, it is no longer used in routine clinical practice. When it is, aspirated material may be processed as regular sputum. As a general rule, TTA is not helpful in patients with established chronic obstructive pulmonary disease (COPD), because their airways usually contain large numbers of S. *pneumoniae* and H. *influenzae*. Recovery of these two agents, therefore, may not represent the infecting organism, but rather shows colonization of the tracheobronchial tree. TTA should not be performed in patients who cannot cooperate or in those who have coagulopathy (prolonged prothrombin time or a platelet count below 100,000 μl). Prior antibiotic therapy is a relative contraindication. Unless the patient is suspected of having developed a secondary bacterial infection, the results cannot be relied on. Hypoxemia (arterial PO_2 under 60 mm Hg) that cannot be corrected with supplemental oxygen is also a strong contraindication. Material obtained by TTA should be processed in the same manner as expectorated sputum. In addition, the material obtained should also be cultured anaerobically, which is a procedure that cannot be done on expectorated sputum. In general, most experts recommend that TTA not be performed routinely owing to the high incidence of complications.

Bronchoscopy

Bronchoscopy by flexible fiberoptic bronchoscope is seldom needed in the initial evaluation of CAP. Bronchoscopy has its main utility in evaluating patients with nosocomial LRIs, especially when empiric antibiotic therapy has failed to produce the expected improvement. To avoid contamination by oropharyngeal organisms, the shielded brush has been used with some success (Wimberley et al, 1979). It is generally used in nosocomial pneumonias, especially in immunosuppressed patients.

Table 20-3
Rank Order of Recognized Pathogens in Large Series (Over 100 Patients) of Community-acquired Pneumonia

Reference	Year	Decade	No. of Patients	Recognized Organisms						Undiagnosed (%)
				First (%)		Second (%)		Third (%)		
Bath	1964	60s	141	S. pneumoniae	(44)	H. influenzae	(22)	Viruses	?	38
Fekety	1971	60s	100	S. pneumoniae	(62)	Viruses	(12)	Mycoplasma	(3)	34
Sullivan	1972	60s	292	S. pneumoniae	(62)	Gram negative	(20)	Viruses	(11)	43
Dorff	1973	60s	148	S. pneumoniae	(53)	S. aureus	(7)	Klebsiella	(6)	17
Moore	1977	70s	144	S. pneumoniae	(47)	H. influenzae	(46)	S. aureus	(14)	13
MacFarlane	1982	80s	127	S. pneumoniae	(76)	Legionella	(15)	Chlamydia psittaci	(6)	3
Marrie	1985	80s	138	Aspiration	(15)	S. pneumoniae	(9)	H. influenzae	(9)	44
Berntsson	1985	?	127	S. pneumoniae	(54)	Mycoplasma	(14)	Influenza A	(12)	21
Holmberg	1987	80s	147	S. pneumoniae	(39)	H. influenzae	(5)	Mycoplasma	(5)	29
Research Comm.	1987	80s	453	S. pneumoniae	(42)	Mycoplasma	(10)	Influenza A	(7)	33
Aubertin	1987	80s	274	S. pneumoniae	(12)	Legionella	(11)	Mycoplasma	(9)	49
Marrie	1987	80s	301	Aspiration	(11)	S. pneumoniae	(9)	H. influenzae	(6)	37
Woodhead	1987	80s	236	S. pneumoniae	(36)	Viruses	(13)	H. influenzae	(10)	45
Levy	1988	80s	116	S. pneumoniae	(26)	H. influenzae	(12)	Tuberculosis	(10)	35
Marrie	1989	80s	719	S. pneumoniae	(9)	Aspiration	(7)	Mycoplasma	(6)	
								Influenza A	(6)	47
Woodhead	1991	80s	106	S. pneumoniae	(17)	H. influenzae	(4)	No agent identified more than once		74
Bates	1992	80s	154	Legionella	(10)	Gram-negative	(8)	C. pneumoniae	(8)	50
Moine	1994	80s	132	S. pneumoniae	(33)	H. influenzae	(11)	Gram-negative	(11)	28
Mundy	1995	90s	164	S. pneumoniae	(15)	Aspiration*	(14)	H. influenzae	(8)	34

*Approximation. Immunosuppressed and immunocompetent patients and non–HIV-infected patients with this diagnosis were not distinguished.

457

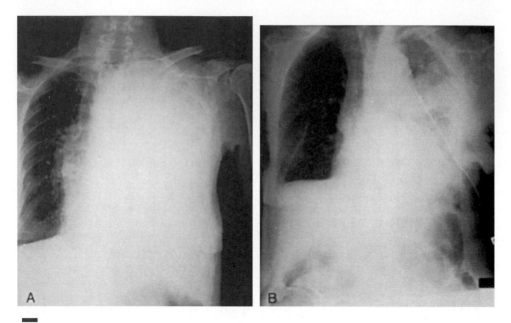

Figure 20–5
S. pneumoniae empyema. (A) On admission. (B) After chest tube placement. Note the underlying infiltrate.

Transbronchial biopsy may be performed when a diffuse process is suspected. Its main use has been in immunosuppressed patients and in patients with pneumonias complicating AIDS. Contraindications to transbronchial biopsy include established pulmonary hypertension, severe hypoxemia not correctable by supplemental oxygen administration, and severe coagulopathy (Bartlett, 1988). In patients who have a severe coagulopathy, segmental BAL may be used. This technique is especially helpful in pneumonias complicating AIDS, in which P. carinii or cytomegalovirus (CMV) are easily recovered with this technique (Murray et al, 1987). BAL is seldom needed in CAP.

Percutaneous Needle Biopsy

Percutaneous needle biopsy is a useful adjunct to diagnosis, especially when the infiltrate in question is localized to the periphery of the lung, is 1 cm or larger, and is readily observed in two projections. Since the availability of the smaller gauge needles ("skinny needles"), the previously, prohibitively high complication rate has been moderated. This technique is especially good in evaluating peripheral cavitary lesions in which, in addition to the solid core of infiltrate, fluid can also be aspirated (Fishman, 1986).

Open Lung Biopsy

Open lung biopsy is seldom indicated in the evaluation of CAP. This is the most definitive procedure, however, especially when material for histopathologic evaluation is needed. Although this procedure is the most invasive of the available diagnostic tests, modern anesthesia and postoperative care have reduced its mortality rate to under 1% and have kept the rate of serious complications to an acceptably low level (Fishman, 1986).

Usually open lung biopsy is done only as a last resort when TTA, bronchoscopy with brushings, and BAL studies have failed to establish a diagnosis, and when the patient is deteriorating rapidly. Frequently, however, a patient's condition gets worse so rapidly that the usual stepwise progression from least invasive to more invasive tests takes too long. Some experts, therefore, advocate early intervention with open lung biopsy to circumvent further delays.

Although the majority of hospitalized patients can be treated on general medical wards, more severely ill patients require admission to the ICU. Certain clinical and laboratory features of CAP are predictive of a more severe illness and an increase in the risk of death from pneumonia. Table 20–4 outlines the most common of these clinical and laboratory features (British Thoracic Society, 1993). We consider transfer or admission of patients to the ICU when intubation and ven-

Table 20–4
Clinical Features and Laboratory Values Associated With an Increased Risk of Death in Patients With Community-acquired Pneumonia

Clinical Features

Hypotension (systolic <90 mm Hg, diastolic <60 mm Hg)
Tachypnea of over 30/min
Age over 60 years
Comorbid conditions
Decreased mental state

Laboratory and Radiographic Findings

Elevated creatinine
Diminished serum albumin (under 3.5 g/dl)
Hypoxemia PO_2 60 mm Hg or less on room air
Leukocytosis of 20,000/mm³ or more
Leukopenia of 4000/mm³ or less
Positive blood culture result
Multilobar infiltrate of chest radiograph
New-onset atrial fibrillation

Adapted from British Thoracic Society: Guidelines for the management of community-acquired pneumonia in adults admitted to hospital. Br J Hosp Med 49:346–350, 1993.

tilator management are imminent. Decreasing blood pressure, shock, and difficulty in maintaining adequate arterial blood PO_2 above 60 mm Hg in our opinion must lead to immediate transfer to the ICU.

INITIATION OF THERAPY

Once the initial assessment is completed and the admission chest radiograph confirms the presence of an infiltrate, treatment may be initiated. A firm diagnosis is seldom possible initially, although a strong suspicion may be present. Except for rare cases when the diagnosis is clear, therefore, initial treatment is by definition empiric.

A generation ago, choosing initial empiric therapy was simple. Because the most frequently recognized etiologic agent was S. pneumoniae, initial therapy consisted of penicillin, given either intravenously or intramuscularly (Mufson, 1990). Except under special circumstances, such as during influenza A outbreaks, when superinfection with S. aureus was recognized to be common during the 1960s and early 1970s (Schwarzmann et al, 1971), S. pneumoniae was overwhelmingly the most common bacterial pathogen, and H. influenzae emerged as a distant second. The emergence of H. influenzae and the rarity of S. aureus changed the nature of initial empiric therapy.

Ampicillin replaced penicillin G as the agent of choice. It provided adequate coverage for S. pneumoniae and certainly was adequate for H. influenzae.

This rather comfortable approach to CAP changed overnight when a large outbreak caused by a heretofore unrecognized respiratory pathogen occurred in Philadelphia in 1976. Subsequently recognized to be caused by Legionella pneumophila (Fraser et al, 1977), the outbreak changed the complacent approach to empiric therapy using only cell wall–active antibiotics, occasionally supplemented by aminoglycosides. Isolation and further study of L. pneumophila showed that it was sensitive to erythromycin, and a review of the Philadelphia experience confirmed this agent as the drug of choice (Tsai et al, 1979). Subsequent prospective experience in Los Angeles and Burlington, Vermont confirmed the efficacy of erythromycin (Keys, 1987).

Even before the recognition of Legionella as an important pathogen, it should have been obvious that β-lactam antibiotics *alone* were not adequate for the treatment of CAP. Long recognized as an important respiratory pathogen, M. pneumoniae clearly did not respond to cell wall–active antibiotics and required erythromycin (Murray et al, 1975). Fortunately, because this organism did not usually lead to severe illness, not a great deal of harm was caused by the stubborn adherence to the customary use of β-lactam antibiotics as the sole agents for the treatment of CAP. Studies during the mid-1980s in Finland (Saikku et al, 1985) and in Seattle, Washington (Grayston et al, 1986) documented the existence of a new pulmonary pathogen, Chlamydia pneumoniae, earlier known as PWAR. Subsequent studies by many other investigators have confirmed this agent as a relatively frequent cause of CAP (Grayston et al, 1989; Sundeloff et al, 1993). Although generally thought of as a disease seen in young, otherwise healthy adults, it is also a common cause of pneumonia among hospitalized patients and is frequent among the severely ill elderly as well (Bates, 1992). Treatment should be with either a tetracycline or macrolide agent.

The role of Enterobacteriaceae in CAP is still controversial. Although these organisms represent only a small percentage of etiologic agents in many series of CAP, they appear to be more common in some other series, especially among more severely ill patients treated in an ICU setting (Pachon et al, 1990; Bates et al, 1992; Moine et al, 1994; Mundy et al, 1995). The role of Pseudomonas aeruginosa is even more difficult to determine with certainty (Almiral, 1995). Although this organism is generally an uncommon cause of CAP, it may be present in certain subpopulations of patients, such as those with cystic fibrosis and bronchiectasis.

The issue of antibiotic resistance among common pathogens causing CAP began with the recognition of the rising incidence of β-lactamase production of *H. influenzae* reaching 40% in some series in the 1980s (Quinones et al, 1989). This widespread resistance necessitated the shift from penicillin G and ampicillin as the mainstays of empiric therapy of CAP to either antibiotics containing a β-lactamase inhibitor or a second- or third-generation cephalosporin.

The alarming rise in the frequency of penicillin- and cephalosporin-resistant isolates of *S. pneumoniae* has led to serious concern about the role of these agents in the initial empiric treatment of CAP. Pneumococcal meningitis caused by even moderately resistant *S. pneumoniae* minimum inhibitory concentration (MIC 0.12 mg/ml to 2.0 mg/ml) should no longer be treated with penicillin G. This observation has led to the recommendation that all patients with suspected pneumococcal meningitis be treated with either ceftriaxone or cefotaxime. Most worrisome are the occasional reports of therapeutic failures with these agents when the meningitis was caused by pneumococcal strains with high MICs to even these agents (John, 1994).

Although the potential risk for failure of penicillin G (or ampicillin) and cephalosporin therapy for patients with *S. pneumoniae*–caused CAP is considerable, large studies have not shown an increase in mortality among patients whose CAP was caused by resistant pneumococci (Pallares et al, 1995). This seemingly paradoxical response is most likely due to the fact that the high doses of penicillin G (150,000–200,000 units/kg body weight) provided blood levels that were high enough to deal with moderate to high (≤ 2 mg/ml) levels of penicillin G resistance. From published data it appears that when penicillin G resistance exceeds 2 mg/ml, and resistance to cephalosporins is under 2 mg/ml, cephalosporins may be used safely. It is not yet clear whether even higher levels of resistance may be overcome

Table 20–5
Recommended Initial Treatment for Hospitalized Patients with Community-acquired Pneumonia

Second- or third-generation cephalosporin
or
β-lactam/β-lactamase inhibitor
plus
macrolide (add rifampin if *Legionella* is suspected)

Table 20–6
Recommended Initial Treatment for Patients with Community-acquired Pneumonia Hospitalized in the Intensive Care Unit

Third-generation cephalosporin with anti-pseudomonal activity
or
imipenem/cilastatin
plus
macrolide (add rifampin if *Legionella* is suspected)

by increased doses of these agents. Although data are not yet available, it seems prudent to use vancomycin in areas where there is a high incidence of penicillin G and cephalosporin resistance. This practice emphasizes the importance of knowing the current profile of antibiotic resistance in any given locale or in individual hospitals.

SPECIFIC RECOMMENDATIONS

Because it is clear that CAP is caused by many potential organisms, empiric initial therapy should cover most possibilities (Niederman et al, 1993). Table 20–5 outlines the recommended *empiric* therapy for hospitalized patients with CAP. These recommendations are slightly different from the American Thoracic Society recommendations that advocate the use of a macrolide in *all* patients in addition to an extended-spectrum cephalosporin or a β-lactamase inhibitor, because we do not think that it is *ever* safe to assume that the etiologic agent is the pneumococcus alone. Experience has shown that the various common etiologic agents may produce illnesses that are indistinguishable (Marrie, 1994).

Table 20–6 shows our recommendations for patients admitted to the ICU. These recommendations are identical to those of the American Thoracic Society (Niederman, 1993). They take into consideration the fact that gram-negative bacilli may play a significant etiologic role in patients requiring ICU care. Anti-pseudomonal cephalosporins should be reserved for those patients who are likely to be infected with this organism, such as those with known bronchiectasis or cystic fibrosis.

REFERENCES

Afzelius BA: Immotile cilia syndrome and ciliary abnormalities induced by infection and injury. Am Rev Respir Dis 124:107–109, 1981.

Almiral J, Mesalles E, Klamburg J, et al: Prognostic factors of pneumonia requiring admission to the intensive care unit. Chest 107:511–516, 1995.

Aubertin J, Dabis F, and Fleurette J: Prevalence of Legionellosis among adults: A study of community-acquired pneumonia in France. Infection 15:328–331, 1987.

Austrian R, and Gold J: Pneumococcal bacteremia with especial reference to bacteremic pneumococcal pneumonia. Ann Intern Med 60:759–776, 1964.

Bartlett JG: Diagnostic accuracy of transtracheal aspiration bacteriologic studies. Am Rev Respir Dis 115:777–782, 1977.

Bartlett JG: Invasive diagnostic techniques in pulmonary infections. In Pennington JE (ed.): Diagnosis and Management, 2nd ed. New York, Raven Press, 1988, pp 69–96.

Bartlett JG, and Finegold SM: Anaerobic infections of the lung and pleural space. Am Rev Respir Dis 110:56–77, 1974.

Bates JH, Campbell GD, Barron AL, et al: Microbial etiology of acute pneumonia in hospitalized patients. Chest 101:1005–1012, 1992.

Bath JC Jr, Boissard GPB, Calder MA, and Moffat MAJ: Pneumonia in hospital practice in Edinburgh 1960–62. Br J Dis Chest 58:1–16, 1964.

Berntsson E, Blomberg J, Lagergard T, and Trollfors B: Etiology of community-acquired pneumonia in patients requiring hospitalization. Eur J Clin Microbiol 4:268–272, 1985.

British Thoracic Society: Guidelines for the management of community-acquired pneumonia in adults admitted to hospital. Br J Hosp Med 49:346–350, 1993.

Coonrod JD: Pneumococcal pneumonia. Semin Respir Infect 4:4–11, 1989.

Crane LR, and Komshian S: Gram-negative bacillary pneumonias in respiratory infections. In Pennington JE (ed): Diagnosis and Management, 2nd ed. New York, Raven Press, 1988, pp 314–340.

Davies SF: Serodiagnosis of histoplasmosis. Semin Respir Infect 1:9–15, 1986.

Dorff GF, Rytel MW, Farmer SG, and Scanlon G: Etiologies and characteristic features of pneumonias in a municipal hospital. Am J Med Sci 266:349–358, 1973.

Drutz DJ, and Catanzaro A: Coccidioidomycosis: State of the art. Am Rev Respir Dis 117:559–585, 727–771, 1978.

Fekety FR Jr, Caldwell J, Gump D, et al: Bacteria, viruses and mycoplasmas in acute pneumonia in adults. Am Rev Respir Dis 104:499–507, 1971.

Fertel D, and Pitchenik AE: Tuberculosis in acquired immunodeficiency syndrome. Semin Respir Infect 4:198–204, 1989.

Finegold SM: Aspiration pneumonia lung abscess and empyema. In Pennington JE (ed): Respiratory Infections: Diagnosis and Management, 2nd ed. New York, Raven Press, 1988.

Fishman JA: Diagnostic approach to pneumonia in the immunocompromised host. Semin Respir Infect 1:133–144, 1986.

Fraser DW, Tsai TR, and Orenstein W: Legionnaires' disease: Description of an epidemic of pneumonia. N Engl J Med 297:1189–1197, 1977.

Goodwin RA Jr, and Des Prez RM: Histoplasmosis: State of the art. Am Rev Respir Dis 117:929–956, 1978.

Grayston JT, Kuo CC, Wang SP, and Altman J: A new Chlamydia psittaci strain, TWAR, isolated in acute respiratory tract infections. N Engl J Med 315:161–168, 1986.

Grayston JT, Mordhorst C, Bruu A-L, et al: Countrywide epidemics of Chlamydia pneumoniae, TRIN, TWAR, in Scandinavia, 1981–83. J Infect Dis 159:1111–1114, 1989.

Hershey CO, and Panaro V: Round pneumonia in adults. Arch Intern Med 148:1155–1157, 1988.

Hoffman RA, and Billingham J: Effect of altered G levels on deposition of particulates in the human respiratory tract. J Appl Physiol 38:955–960, 1975.

Holmberg H: Aetiology of community-acquired pneumonia in hospital treated patients. Scand J Infect Dis 19:491–501, 1987.

John CC: Treatment failure with use of a third-generation cephalosporin for penicillin-resistant pneumococcal meningitis: Case report and review. Clin Infect Dis 18:188–192, 1994.

Kaufmann AF, Boyce JM, and Aartone WJ: Trends in human plague in the United States. J Infect Dis 141:522–524, 1980.

Keys TF: Therapeutic considerations in the treatment of legionella infections. Semin Respir Infect 2:270–273, 1987.

Klein BS, Vergeront JM, and Davis JP: Epidemiologic aspects of blastomycosis, the enigmatic systemic mycosis. Semin Respir Infect 1:29–39, 1986.

Langley JM, Marrie TJ, Covert A, et al: Poker players' pneumonia: An urban outbreak of Q fever following exposure to a parturient cat. N Engl J Med 319:354–356, 1988.

Levy M, Dromer F, Brion N, et al: Community acquired pneumonia—importance of initial noninvasive bacteriologic and radiographic investigations. Chest 93:4348, 1988.

Little JW, Hall WJ, Douglas RG Jr, et al: Airway hyperactivity and peripheral airway dysfunction in influenza A infection. Am Rev Respir Dis 118:295–303, 1978.

Louria DB, Blumenfeld HL, Ellis JT, et al: Studies on influenza in the pandemic of 1957–58. II: Pulmonary complications of influenza. J Clin Invest 38:313–365, 1959.

Luchsinger PC, LaGarde B, and Kilfeather JE: Particle clearance from the human tracheobronchial tree. Am Rev Respir Dis 97:1046–1050, 1968.

MacFarlane JT, Finch RG, Ward MJ, and MacRae AD: Hospital study of adult community-acquired pneumonia. Lancet 2:255–258, 1982.

Mackowiak PA: The normal microbial flora. N Engl J Med 307:83–86, 1982.

Malech HL, and Gallin JI: Current concepts in

immunology: Neutrophils in human diseases. N Engl J Med 317:687–694, 1987.

Marrie TJ: Community-acquired pneumonia. Clin Infect Dis 18:501–513, 1994.

Marrie TJ, Durant H, and Yates L: Community-acquired pneumonia requiring hospitalization: 5-year prospective study. Rev Infect Dis 11:586–599, 1989.

Marrie TJ, Grayston JT, Wang S-P, and Kuo C-C: Pneumonia associated with the TWAR strain of chlamydia. Ann Intern Med 106:507–511, 1987.

Marrie TJ, Haldane EV, Faulkner RS, et al: Community-acquired pneumonia requiring hospitalization: Is it different in the elderly? J Am Geriatr Soc 33:671–680, 1985.

Miller DD, Davies SF, and Sarosi GA: Erythema nodosum and blastomycosis. Arch Intern Med 142:1839, 1982.

Moine P, Vercken J-B, Cheuret S et al: Severe community-acquired pneumonia. Etiology, epidemiology and prognosis factors. Chest 105:1487–1495, 1994.

Moore MA, Merson MH, Charache P, and Shepard RH: The characteristics and mortality of outpatient-acquired pneumonia. Johns Hopkins Med J 140:9–14, 1977.

Mufson MA: Streptococcus pneumoniae. In Mandell GL, Douglas RG Jr, and Bennett JE (eds): Principles and Practice of Infectious Diseases, 3rd ed. New York, Churchill Livingstone, 1990, p 1547.

Mundy LM, Auwaerter PG, Oldach D, et al: Community-acquired pneumonia: Impact of immune status. Am J Respir Crit Care Med 152:1309–1312, 1995.

Murray HW, Masur H, Senterfit LB, and Roberts RB: The protean manifestations of Mycoplasma pneumoniae infection in adults. Am J Med 58:229–242, 1975.

Nathan CF: Secretory products of macrophages. J Clin Invest 79:319–326, 1987.

Nathan CF, Murray HW, and Cohn ZA: The macrophage as an effector cell. N Engl J Med 303:622–626, 1980.

Newhouse M, Sanchis J, and Bienestock J: Lung disease mechanisms. N Engl J Med 295:990–998, 1976.

Niederman MS, Bass JB, Campbell GD, et al: Guidelines for the initial management of adults with community-acquired pneumonia: Diagnosis, assessment of severity, and initial antimicrobial therapy. Am Rev Respir Dis 148:1418–1426, 1993.

Olsen PF: Tularemia. In Hubbert WT, McCulloch WF, and Schnurrenberger PR (eds): Diseases Transmitted from Animals to Man. Springfield, IL, Charles C Thomas, 1975, pp 191–223.

Pachon J, Prados MD, Capote F, et al: Severe community-acquired pneumonia. Etiology, prognosis and treatment. Am Rev Respir Dis 142:369–373, 1990.

Pallares R, Linares J, Vadillo M, et al: Resistance to penicillin and cephalosporin and mortality from severe pneumococcal pneumonia in Barcelona, Spain. N Engl J Med 333:474–480, 1995.

Polsky B, Gold JWM, Whimey E, et al: Bacterial pneumonia in patients with the acquired immunodeficiency syndrome. Ann Intern Med 10:438–441, 1986.

Proctor DF, and Wagner HN: Mucociliary particle clearance in the human nose. In Davis CN (ed): Inhaled Particles and Vapours, Vol 2. London, Pergamon Press, 1967, pp 25–33.

Quinones CA, Memom MA, and Sarosi GA: Bacteremic Haemophilus influenzae pneumonia in the adult. Semin Respir Infect 4:12–18, 1989.

Research Committee of the British Thoracic Society and the Public Health Laboratory Service: Community-acquired pneumonia in adults in British hospitals in 1982–1983: A survey of aetiology, mortality, prognostic factors and outcome. Q J Med 62:195–220, 1987.

Reynolds HY: Lung inflammation: Role of endogenous chemotactic factors that attract polymorphonuclear granulocytes. Am Rev Respir Dis 127:516–525, 1983.

Reynolds HY: Immunoglobulin G and its function in the human respiratory tract. Mayo Clin Proc 63:161–174, 1988.

Saikku P, Wang SP, Kleemola M, et al: An epidemic of mild pneumonia due to an unusual strain of Chlamydia psittaci. J Infect Dis 151:832–839, 1985.

Sarosi GA: Histoplasmosis outbreaks: Their patterns. In Balows A (ed): Histoplasmosis. Springfield, IL, Charles C Thomas, 1971, pp 123–128.

Sarosi GA, and Davies SF: Blastomycosis: State of the art. Am Rev Respir Dis 120:911–938, 1979.

Sawyer LA, Fishbein DB, and McDade JE: Q fever: Current concepts. Rev Infect Dis 9:935–946, 1987.

Schlossberg D, and Littman M: Varicella pneumonia. Arch Intern Med 148:1630–1632, 1988.

Schwarzmann SW, Adler JL, Sullivan RJ, and Marine WM: Bacterial pneumonia during the Hong Kong influenza epidemic of 1968–69. Arch Intern Med 127:1037–1041, 1971.

Stevens DA: Coccidioidomycosis. N Engl J Med 332:1077–1082, 1995.

Sullivan RJ Jr, Dowdle WR, Marine WM, and Heierholzer JC: Adult pneumonia in a general hospital: Etiology and host risk factors. Arch Intern Med 129:935–942, 1972.

Sundeloff B, Gnarpe J, Gnarpe H, et al: Chlamydia pneumoniae in Swedish patients. Scand J Infect Dis 25:429–433, 1993.

Toews GB: Determinants of bacterial clearance form the lower respiratory tract. Semin Respir Infect 1:68–78, 1986.

Tomassi TB Jr: Mechanism of immune regulation at mucosal surfaces. Rev Infect Dis 5:5784–5792, 1983.

Tsai TR, Finn DR, and Plikaytis BD: Legionnaires' disease: Clinical features of the epidemic in Philadelphia. Ann Intern Med 90:509–517, 1979.

Washington JA II: Noninvasive diagnostic techniques for lower respiratory infections. In Pennington JE (ed): Respiratory Infections: Diagnosis and Management. New York, Raven Press, 1988, pp 52–68.

Wells WF, Ratcliff HL, and Crumb C: On the mechanics of droplet nuclei infection. Am J Hygiene 47:11–28, 1948.

Werner SB, Pappagianis D, Heindl I, and Mickel A: An epidemic of coccidioidomycosis among archeology students in northern California. N Engl J Med 286:507–512, 1972.

Wimberley NW, Faling J, and Bartlett JG: A fiberoptic bronchoscopy technique to obtain uncontaminated lower airway secretions for bacterial culture. Am Rev Respir Dis 119:337–343, 1979.

Woodhead MA, Arrowsmith J, Chamberlain-Webber R, et al: The value of routine microbial investigation in community-acquired pneumonia. Respir Med 85:313–317, 1991.

Woodhead MA, MacFarlane JT, McCracken JS, et al: Prospective study of the aetiology and outcome of pneumonia in the community. Lancet 1:671–674, 1987.

Young KR, Rankin JA, Negal GP, et al: Bronchoalveolar cells and proteins in patients with the acquired immunodeficiency syndrome—an immunologic analysis. Ann Intern Med 103:522–533, 1985.

CHAPTER

Hospital-acquired Pneumonia and Pneumonia in the Immunosuppressed Host

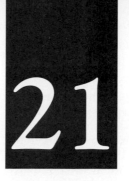

Philip C. Johnson, M.D.

George A. Sarosi, M.D.

Host defenses against respiratory pathogens are altered in a number of clinical situations, which include routine medical care, antimalignancy care, transplanted allograft care, and, most recently, care after acquisition of retrovirus infections. Pulmonary infections in these settings are the major cause of mortality. Pneumonia is a predictable occurrence with a varied spectrum of causative agents. Diagnosis and treatment can be complicated by factors that are absent in the management of community-acquired pulmonary infections. An understanding of the epidemiology and pathogenesis of these infections is required for proper diagnosis, treatment, and prevention of these increasingly common infections.

HOSPITAL-ACQUIRED PNEUMONIA

Hospital-acquired pneumonia differs from community-acquired pneumonia because by definition it is not incubating when a patient is admitted to the hospital. By convention, any pneumonia that becomes apparent after 48 hours of admission excluding any infection incubating at the time is classified as hospital-acquired pneumonia (American Thoracic Society, 1995). Pneumonia is the third most common hospital-acquired pneumonia after urinary tract infections and surgical wound infections (Gross et al, 1980) and consists of between 10 and 20% of all hospital infections (La-Force, 1981). Pneumonia is the most important hospital-acquired infection due to its high rate of mortality. Among the hospital-acquired infections, pneumonia is the most difficult to diagnose and results in the largest economic loss (Simmons and Wong, 1982; Toews, 1986).

EPIDEMIOLOGY

The Centers for Disease Control (CDC) National Hospital Acquired Infection Surveillance System in 1984 estimated that 0.6% of patients discharged from hospitals in the United States acquired pneumonia (Simmons and Wong, 1982). This represents 15% of all nosocomial infections and the most common cause of death due to nosocomial infections (Fagon et al, 1988). Rates of pulmonary infection differ depending on the setting within the hospital and the patient composition. Infection rates were four times higher in patients on surgical services than in patients admitted to a medical service in an earlier national survey (Haley et al, 1985). Approximately one half of all patients with hospital-acquired pneumonia are surgical patients (Eickhoff, 1980). The incidence of hospital-acquired pneumonias is higher in large teaching hospitals (0.7%) compared with smaller teaching hospitals (0.5%) and nonteaching hospitals (0.4%) (Horan et al, 1986). Infection rates in patients admitted to an intensive care unit (ICU) during their hospital stay are reported as high as 10% (Horan et al, 1986). Up to 25% of patients on mechanical ventilation develop pneumonia (Craven and Steger, 1996). The mortality rate in patients with hospital-acquired pneumonia has been estimated to be up to 50%, depending on the setting (Haley et al, 1985).

RISK FACTORS

Several risk factors have been recognized to be associated with hospital-acquired pneumonia (American Thoracic Society, 1995; Craven et al, 1984; Driks et al, 1987; Hooten et al, 1981). These include the following:

1. Preoperative markers of underlying disease severity. Garibaldi and colleagues demonstrated in a study of 520 postoperative patients that the hospital-acquired pneumonia was associated with low serum albumin levels, a history of smoking, and a high American Society of Anesthesiologist preanesthesia physical status classification (Garibaldi et al, 1981). This early study has been confirmed by others (Hanson et al, 1992; Konrad et al, 1991).
2. Age. As documented by several studies, rates of hospital-acquired pneumonia increase in persons over 40 years of age (Garibaldi et al, 1981). This is due to increased comorbidity among the elderly and age-associated immune factors (American Thoracic Society, 1995).
3. Sex. Men are more likely to develop hospital-acquired pneumonia than women. In some studies, sex as a risk factor is more important than age (Garibaldi et al, 1981; Konrad, 1991). The reasons for this are not clear and may be related to other independent variables, such as cigarette smoking and underlying illness.
4. Duration of hospitalization. Whether this

factor is related to greater period at risk, severity of underlying illness, or effect of acquisition of gram-negative bacilli colonizing the oropharynx with a longer hospital stay is not clear from the studies done to date; however, the length of hospitalization is an important risk factor identified in several studies (Garibaldi et al, 1981).
5. Site of surgical procedure. Thoracic and abdominal surgical procedures have the highest risk of associated hospital-acquired pneumonia (Garibaldi et al, 1981; Joshi et al, 1992). In Garibaldi's series, 41 of 102 patients (40%) undergoing thoracic surgery, 35 of 201 (17%) undergoing upper abdominal procedures, and 11 of 208 (5%) undergoing lower abdominal surgery developed hospital-acquired pneumonia (Garibaldi et al, 1981). The duration of each procedure was also a factor in the acquisition of pneumonia, with longer procedures exhibiting the highest rates of pulmonary infections (Garibaldi et al, 1981).
6. Reduced gastric acidity. In a study among intubated and ventilated patients in an ICU setting, patients who received H_2 blockers and antacids to prevent gastrointestinal bleeding had higher rates of hospital-acquired pneumonia than patients who were treated with sucralfate, which has no effect on gastric pH *per se* (Driks et al, 1987; Gaynes et al, 1991).
7. Immunosuppressed state. Patients with immunosuppression because of treatment with corticosteroids, treatment to prevent allograft rejection, or treatment with antineoplastic agents are at the highest risk for development of hospital-acquired pneumonia (Garibaldi et al, 1981).
8. Ventilator support. Patients who are mechanically ventilated are 21 times more likely to develop hospital-acquired pneumonia compared with patients who are not (Carlon et al, 1987; Cross and Roup, 1981; Dekker et al, 1987; Gaynes, 1991; Reynolds, 1983; Simmons and Wong, 1982). Endotracheal intubation bypasses the normal defense mechanisms of the upper respiratory tract, allows the potential inhalation of contaminated aerosols, and facilitates aspiration in critically ill patients.

PATHOGENESIS

Three main methods exist in developing hospital-acquired pneumonia: (1) aspiration of oropharyn-

Table 21–1
Etiologic Pathogens and Modes of Transmission of Primary Nosocomial Pneumonia

Etiology	Mode of Transmission
Bacteria	
Pseudomonas aeruginosa	A, V, B
Staphylococcus aereus	A, P, B
Klebsiella pneumonia	A, V, B
Enterobacteriaceae	A, V, B
Escherichia coli	A, V, B
Streptococcus pneumoniae	A, V
Haemophilus influenzae	A, V
Serratia marcescens	A, V, B
Legionella	H
Anaerobic organisms	A
Viruses	
Respiratory syncytial virus	P
Influenza virus	P
Parainfluenza	P
Fungi	
Aspergillus	H
Candida	B
Mycobacteria	
Tuberculosis	P, V

A = aspiration of oropharyngeal secretion; V = ventilation devices; B = blood-borne; P = person-to-person spread; H = hospital environment

geal sections and direct inoculation into airways of intubated patients by hospital personnel; (2) inspiration of contaminated air from other infected patients, other sources of contamination in the hospital, or infected aerosols generated by ventilatory devices; and (3) hematogenous spread of organisms to the lung from indwelling venous catheters, septic foci, or translocation of bacteria from the gastrointestinal mucosa. Table 21–1 lists the major organisms causing hospital-acquired pneumonia and the various ways in which these organisms are acquired. Each of these aspects in the pathogenesis of hospital-acquired pneumonia is discussed in detail.

Aspiration of Oropharyngeal Secretions

The most common cause of bacterial hospital-acquired pneumonia is the aspiration of contaminated oropharyngeal contents (Craven et al, 1986). Small amounts of oropharyngeal secretions are aspirated by up to 45% of normal persons during sleep (Huxley et al, 1978). In hospitalized patients, the opportunities for aspiration are numerous due to the underlying disease of the pa-

tient (especially dysphagia due to neurologic or esophageal disorders), use of sedatives, treatment with antimicrobials that alter normal host flora, oropharyngeal or nasotracheal intubation, and nasogastric feeding. An example of how these factors are related to aspiration was demonstrated in the studies by Craven that have clearly shown an increased incidence of aspiration pneumonia in ventilator-dependent patients with intracranial pressure-monitoring devices (Craven et al, 1986). The factors responsible for aspiration pneumonia included the depressed state of consciousness of the patient and the observation that hospital personnel often avoided chest physiotherapy and frequent suctioning of pulmonary secretions in patients with increased intracranial pressures (Craven et al, 1986).

The oropharynx of healthy persons has several defense mechanisms to decrease the number of harmful bacteria that are able to get through to the upper airways. These defense mechanisms include lactoferrin, lysozyme, and secretory IgA in saliva; mechanical abrasion by the tongue; bacterial interference by nonpathogenic flora; and mucociliary clearance (Murphy and Florman, 1983; Reynolds, 1983). All of these defense mechanisms may be altered by illness or by mechanical factors in the hospitalized patient. In addition, adherence of gram-negative bacilli to the oropharyngeal mucosa of hospitalized patients may be increased. Cellular fibronectin, a surface glycoprotein, promotes the binding of gram-positive organisms to mucosal surfaces in the oropharynx under normal circumstances. Woods and colleagues have shown that increased levels of salivary protease in patients, caused presumably by the stress of the illness, may be associated with a loss of fibronectin in the oropharynx (Woods et al, 1981). This loss may decrease the numbers of gram-positive aerobes and organisms and may allow repopulation of the oropharynx with gram-negative bacilli.

Johanson has demonstrated the role of oropharyngeal colonization with bacterial respiratory pathogens as it is related to the occurrence of lower respiratory tract infections (Johanson et al, 1969). Within several days after hospitalization, a patient's normal oropharyngeal flora changes from predominantly gram-positive aerobes and anaerobes to aerobic gram-negative bacilli (Johanson et al, 1969). Colonization results from ascension of gram-negative bacilli from the gastrointestinal tract (Johanson et al, 1972; 1979). This colonization is clearly related to the development of pneumonia. Hospital-acquired pneumonia has been shown to occur in 23% of patients colonized with gram-negative bacilli versus 3% of patients not colonized (Johanson et al, 1972). Several factors assist in this change of respiratory flora, including antibiotic pressure that selects gram-negative bacilli in the hospital setting (Philip and Spencer, 1974) and antacids and H_2 blockers that increase gastric pH, allowing a several thousandfold increase in gram-negative aerobes in the stomach, pharynx, and sputum (Donowitz et al, 1986; Driks et al, 1987). The stomach serves as a reservoir for these organisms. Strategies to decrease the level of gram-negative bacilli have been used with success in preventing hospital-acquired pneumonia in patients who are granulocytopenic as a result of cancer chemotherapy (Dekker et al, 1987; Karp et al, 1987).

Intubated patients are at increased risk for aspiration and have the highest rates of hospital-acquired pneumonia. Aspiration occurs even though most endotracheal tubes have soft inflatable balloons that occlude the space between the tube and trachea. Secretions can pool above these subglottic cuffs and then become aspirated with leak or distention of the airways caused by tracheomalacia or changes in caliber of the airways observed with breathing and coughing. Subglottic secretion aspiration can be accomplished by the use of a special endotracheal tube with a suction port located above the cuff. Suction of these secretions has reduced incidence of some types of hospital-acquired pneumonia in intubated patients (American Thoracic Society, 1995; Mahul et al, 1992; Valles et al, 1995). To avoid gastric distention, most intubated patients also have nasogastric tubes placed and connected to low suction. The nasogastric tube passes through the upper and lower esophageal sphincters. This position inadvertently assists in the passage of gastric contents into the esophagus and oropharynx. Whether a greater degree of aspiration may occur in the presence of gastric distention without a nasogastric tube is not clear.

Another source of hospital-acquired pneumonia may be the frequent suctioning of intubated patients. Although, in general, frequent suctioning of oropharyngeal secretion reduces the rate of pneumonia, it also provides an opportunity to introduce pathogens directly into the bronchi. The act of suctioning an intubated patient breaks a normally closed system between the respirator and the patient. During suctioning, bacteria may be passed from one patient to another by hand contact with hospital personnel (Simmons and Wong, 1982). Contaminated secretions and aerosols can also be introduced in the system. Thus, it is recommended not to suction patients routinely, but rather to do so only when it is necessary to remove secretions (Simmons and Wong, 1982). Closed-sheath suction catheters have been

designed to avoid this problem (Carlon et al, 1987), but they do not alter the overall incidence of pneumonia (American Thoracic Society, 1995). The encouragement of aseptic technique during suctioning by hospital personnel is worth re-emphasizing. The overall effect of new suction systems and stricter hand washing rules on reducing hospital-acquired pneumonia is not clear and must still be studied.

Inspiration of Contaminated Air

The inspiration of contaminated air can occur in the hospital setting in three major ways: (1) passage of respiratory pathogens between patients by aerosols or direct contact; (2) contamination of the air as a result of the hospital environment; and (3) acquisition of respiratory pathogens as a result of mechanical ventilation devices and other devices used in the diagnosis and treatment of pulmonary disease. Each of these is considered separately, because each has different implications for the prevention of hospital-acquired pneumonia.

Person-to-person Spread in the Hospital

Viral agents, such as respiratory syncytial virus (RSV), influenza A and B, and parainfluenza virus, have all been shown to pass from person to person in hospitals, especially among patients who are young, old, or debilitated (Hall, 1981; Hall et al, 1975; Kapila et al, 1977; Meibalane et al, 1977; Simmons and Wong, 1982; Valenti et al, 1978, 1980). The occurrence of these viral outbreaks closely reflects the virus' activity in the community (Simmons and Wong, 1982). Tuberculosis should also be considered as a cause of hospital-acquired pulmonary infection. These diseases have additional importance not only for hospitalized patients but also for hospital personnel, who are at risk.

RSV, which causes bronchiolitis and pneumonia in infants, is passed mainly via person-to-person contact among hospital personnel and their patients rather than by exposure to respiratory secretions (Hall, 1981). RSV is the leading cause of hospital-acquired respiratory infection in infancy (Hall, 1981). Peaks of activity occur in the late fall and early spring (Hall, 1981). The highest morbidity and mortality from RSV occur in critically ill neonates, neonates with congenital heart defects, and immunocompromised patients (Hall, 1981; Hall et al, 1975, 1983, 1986; MacDonald et al, 1982). Rarely, immunocompromised adults are affected (Garvie and Gray, 1980). Glove and gown isolation precautions, rather than respiratory isolation, reduced hospital-acquired transmission of RSV in one study (Leclair et al, 1987). In another study, however, the benefits of these precautions were not as clear, perhaps owing to decreased adherence to the precautions by hospital personnel (Hall, 1981). The recognition of RSV infection has increased in importance now that ribovirin has been shown to be effective treatment for this virus (Hall et al, 1983).

Influenza A virus has caused recognized hospital-acquired outbreaks in both hospital and nursing home settings (Horman et al, 1986; Kapila et al, 1977; Patriarca et al, 1985). Unlike RSV, influenza A is passed primarily by respiratory secretions. Annual immunization of persons over 65 years of age or those with chronic diseases is an important preventive strategy (Patriarca et al, 1985). Amantadine has been given effectively for the prevention of influenza A in nonvaccinated individuals and is recommended for susceptible people in nursing homes during outbreaks in the community (Arden et al, 1988; O'Donoghue et al, 1973). Ribovirin has been used experimentally for treatment (Knight et al, 1981). At least one parainfluenza outbreak has been described in the hospital setting (Boyce et al, 1985). Other viruses that occasionally cause hospital-acquired pneumonia are measles and enterovirus (Boyce et al, 1985).

Contamination of the Air in the Hospital

Legionella pneumophila and *Aspergillus* species are two etiologic agents of hospital-acquired pneumonia caused by a contaminated hospital environment. *L. pneumophila* has been cultured from cooling towers, hot water tanks, and shower heads in hospitals where hospital-acquired outbreaks of *Legionella* pneumonia have occurred (Arnow et al, 1982; Muder et al, 1983). In one study by Yu and associates, almost 15% of the hospital-acquired pneumonias in one hospital were caused by *L. pneumophila* (Muder et al, 1983). Low levels of free chlorine were thought to be the cause for the contaminated water in another outbreak of *Legionella* pneumonia associated with tap-water–filled respiratory devices (Arnow et al, 1982). Current strategies to prevent *Legionella* outbreaks include hyperchlorination of water supplies and raising the temperature of water to 60°C in hot water lines (Helms et al, 1988). Unfortunately, hyperchlorination also leads to deterioration of water pipes in the hospital; thus, improved methods of control are clearly needed (Helms et al, 1988).

Aspergillus has been implicated as a hospital-acquired pathogen among immunosuppressed patients in hospitals that are undergoing renovation or those that are near construction sites where soil is disturbed (Arnow et al, 1978). *Aspergillus* lives in soil, and the disturbance and aerolization of infected soil are necessary for the production of the disease. Thus, potted plants are not allowed in the rooms of patients with immunosuppression (Muckelmann et al, 1981).

Mechanical Ventilation Devices

Contaminated respiratory care equipment is an established cause of hospital-acquired pneumonia primarily the result of gram-negative bacilli (Craven et al, 1982, 1984a,b, 1986; Harris et al, 1973; LaForce, 1981; Malecka-Griggs and Reinhardt, 1983; Reinarz et al, 1965; Rhame et al, 1986; Simmons and Wong, 1982). The source of these gram-negative bacilli has been shown to be oropharyngeal flora, which are colonized by these same organisms. The primary source of gram-negative bacilli colonizing the oropharynx is usually the gastrointestinal tract. Evidence for the relationship between respiratory equipment and acquisition of hospital-acquired pneumonia is suggested by the finding that the highest numbers of gram-negative bacilli are along the course of ventilator tubing located closest to the patient (Craven et al, 1984a). A temporary reduction of contamination and subsequent hospital-acquired gram-negative pneumonia may be achieved by the use of inhaled aminoglycosides (Feeley et al, 1975; Klastersky et al, 1974; Levine et al, 1973). Respiratory care equipment serves as both a reservoir for colonizing organisms and as a generator of aerosols that allow these organisms to reach the terminal airways.

Reinarz was the first investigator to show that contaminated reservoir nebulizers in ventilator circuits generated aerosols, which resulted in necrotizing gram-negative bacillary pneumonia (Reinarz et al, 1965). These nebulizers were replaced by cascade humidifiers in newer ventilators. The problem of hospital-acquired gram-negative bacillary pneumonia was thus reduced but was not eliminated. Craven and associates later demonstrated that hospital-acquired pneumonia was related to the condensate in respirator tubing and medication nebulizers (Craven et al, 1984a,b). In the case of respirator tubing, warm humidified air condensed in the respirator tubing as it cooled along its course. Condensate was produced at a rate of 30 ml/hour in some cases (Craven et al, 1984b). This condensate then became a reservoir for gram-negative bacilli, including *Pseudomonas*, *Actinobacter*, *Klebsiella*, and *Serratia* (Craven et al, 1984b). *Pseudomonas* particularly thrives in warm, moist environments. It is thought that while turning or suctioning the patient or raising the bedrail, this condensate occasionally is delivered in a bolus fashion directly into the lungs (Craven et al, 1982).

In other studies, these same investigators showed that there was no difference in infection rates in patients who had the ventilator tubing changed every 48 hours compared with those who had the tubing changed every 24 hours. This study has been confirmed by a subsequent study in which rates of pneumonia were compared when the tubing was changed every 48 hours or left in place (Dreyfuss et al, 1991). These results are explained by the rapid rate of colonization of the tubing with organisms (Craven et al, 1982). Medication nebulizers were also shown to become contaminated early, presumably from the condensate in the adjacent tubing (Craven et al, 1984b). These nebulizers further increase the risk of hospital-acquired pneumonia by generating an infectious aerosol. Rhame and coworkers have demonstrated that cascade humidifiers can also generate aerosols (Rhame et al, 1986). Whether these aerosols are sufficient to cause hospital-acquired pneumonia must still be shown (Rhame et al, 1986).

Gram-positive organisms including *Streptococcus pneumoniae* and *Staphylococcus aureus* have also been isolated in about one fourth of the time from respiratory therapy equipment (Craven et al, 1984b). At least one case of hospital-acquired transmission of *S. pneumonia* was apparently caused by a contaminated Y joint in a respiratory mask used in a resuscitation device (Mehtar et al, 1986). This case demonstrates the potential of sources of hospital-acquired pneumonia associated with respiratory devices and the fact that any part of the system can serve as a source of infection.

Hematogenous Spread

The third and least common cause of hospital-acquired pneumonia is hematogenous or lymphatic spread of the organisms to the lung from contaminated intravenous catheters, urinary tract, surgical wounds, and abscesses. The most important organism associated with intravenous catheters is *S. aureus*. *Candida albicans* may also be associated with the spread from infected catheters to the lung. Gram-negative bacilli can cause hospital-acquired pneumonia by hematogenous spread from indwelling catheters. The radiographic appearance of these hematogenously spread pneumonias is that of multiple nodular densities.

DIAGNOSIS

The clinical diagnosis of hospital-acquired pneumonia is difficult. A Gram's stain of expectorated sputum as a useful aid in presumptive diagnosis is completely dependent on the quality of the specimen examined. In the case of hospital-acquired pneumonia, this problem is compounded by the fact that the oropharynx of hospitalized patients is frequently colonized by gram-negative bacilli (Johanson et al, 1969, 1979; Schwartz et al, 1978). These organisms are usually considered pathogens. Therefore, obtaining a representative sputum specimen that is not contaminated by colonizing organisms is rare. Sputum cultures are difficult to interpret even under the best of circumstances (see Chapter 20). In addition to this problem of accurate diagnosis are underlying illnesses that clinically resemble pneumonia in hospitalized patients and the urgency of making a correct diagnosis in critically ill patients. An ICU patient with hospital-acquired pneumonia can ill afford to have antimicrobials incorrectly withheld on the assumption that the organisms observed on a Gram's stain of respiratory secretions represent colonization. Patients also can ill afford to have antimicrobials given incorrectly, which results in further oropharyngeal colonization with even more resistant bacteria.

The diagnosis of hospital-acquired bacterial pneumonia, like that of community-acquired bacterial pneumonia, is based on the presence of certain findings. These findings include fever, increase in cough and sputum production, new infiltrate on chest radiographs, leukocytosis, reduction in normal arterial P_{O_2}, sputum Gram's stain with more than 25 polymorphonuclear leukocytes (PMNs) and less than 10 squamous epithelial cells per low power field, and sputum culture growing a predominant organism. Hospitalized patients may have other hospital-acquired or community-acquired infections or conditions causing fever, congestive heart failure, pulmonary embolism, postoperative atelectasis, or tracheitis. All of these conditions can be confused with hospital-acquired pneumonia. Intubated patients in an ICU setting are particularly difficult to evaluate for the presence of hospital-acquired pneumonia because of the higher rates of bacterial colonization, recurrent aspiration, and atelectasis.

How can a clinician accurately diagnose hospital-acquired pneumonia? This question has been the subject of several studies (Courcol et al, 1984; Fagon et al, 1989; Salata et al, 1987; Schmid et al, 1979). The basic assumption of these studies is that appropriate specimens of sputum or transtracheal aspirates can be identified, and colonizers can be distinguished from pathogens by specific techniques. Early reports on the utility of quantitative sputum cultures to separate colonizing bacteria from pathogens that cause pneumonia have been questioned by investigators. They found an overlap in the numbers of gram-negative bacilli between patients who had pneumonia and those who were colonized (Bartlett and Feingold, 1978; Bartlett et al, 1978; Johanson et al, 1972).

Counterimmunoelectrophoresis of sputum to diagnose pneumococcal pneumonia has been reported as useful but has not yet been validated (Schmid et al, 1979). Others have suggested that alveolar macrophages (Courcol et al, 1984) and elastin fibers in sputum smears are associated with a noncontaminated specimen and necrotizing pneumonia, respectively (Salata et al, 1987). The observation of elastin fibers involves the preparation of a 10% potassium hydroxide (KOH) smear of respiratory secretions. In a study of 51 intubated patients with pulmonary infection or colonization, Salata and associates reported detecting elastin fibers in 11 of 21 patients (52%) with pneumonia versus 2 of 22 patients (9%) with colonization (Salata et al, 1987). These investigators also found that quantitative sputum cultures and the number of PMNs and bacteria on Gram's stain were associated with pneumonia (Salata et al, 1987). It remains to be seen if criteria can be developed for evaluating respiratory secretions that can eventually overcome the numerous difficulties arising when an attempt is made to diagnose the etiology of hospital-acquired pneumonia.

Transtracheal aspiration has been advocated in the past as the best method of obtaining a noncontaminated specimen in patients who are not intubated. This procedure is relatively simple to perform. Because of the high rate of complication, it is not frequently used. Because of this potential complication, bronchoscopy with sterile bronchial brushings, with and without the addition of quantitative cultures, has also been used to evaluate hospital acquired pneumonia (Fagon et al, 1989).

Sterile brushings are obtained by passing a sheathed brush through the bronchoscope, which is exposed as the brush is extended into the terminal airway for sampling. Bronchoalveolar lavage may also be helpful in some settings, specifically for the diagnosis of viral processes, but the lavage fluid is subject to contamination caused by passing the bronchoscope through the oropharynx. Percutaneous lung aspiration, transbronchial lung biopsy, and open lung biopsy are also useful in critical situations.

Certain organisms are clearly pathogens rather than upper airway colonizers. These organisms include viruses, such as RSV, influenza A and B, and parainfluenza; and bacteria, such as *L. pneumophila* and mycobacteria. When bacterial pathogens, except *Legionella*, are isolated, it is impossible to be certain whether these organisms are colonizers or pathogens, unless they are isolated concomitantly from blood cultures or from other normally sterile sites. Because positive blood culture results occur in only 8 to 20% of hospital-acquired pneumonias (American Thoracic Society, 1995), this differentiation is still a vexing clinical problem. The low percentage of positive results on blood cultures may be due to the frequent use of antimicrobials in the most common hospital-acquired pneumonia—the case in the intubated patient in the ICU. Furthermore, patients with positive blood culture results and severe hospital-acquired pneumonia have additional infections half the time (American Thoracic Society, 1995).

When a hospital-acquired pneumonia is suspected, one must empirically cover the resident flora applying all available information, including a Gram's stain and culture of respiratory secretions until further microbiologic information is available. Knowledge of the susceptibilities of local hospital-acquired pathogens is essential, especially because of the emergence of multiple resistant gram-negative organisms. Despite rapid diagnostic methods and early initiation of empiric therapy, the diagnosis of hospital-acquired pneumonias is still difficult to make. In an autopsy series of patients dying in ICUs, pathologic evidence of hospital-acquired pneumonia was undiagnosed in 30% (Andrews et al, 1981).

TREATMENT

Once the clinical diagnosis of hospital-acquired pneumonia is suspected, empiric treatment must be initiated. The number of antimicrobial agents is large and the choices are increasing each year. There are many factors that should determine the selection of a treatment regimen. Some of these factors include

1. Clinical setting. Certain organisms are associated with specific clinical situations. Is the patient aspirated or intubated? Can hematogenous spread from an known source be a factor? Is there an outbreak of viral pneumonia in the community at present?
2. Susceptibility of organisms in a specific hospital. Some hospitals have a background of multiple resistant *S. aureus* or gram-negative bacilli with unusual but predictable susceptibilities.

3. Information from Gram's stain and culture of respiratory secretions. Are there multiple gram-positive and gram-negative organisms? Is there a fungus present?
4. Patient factors. Is the patient immunosuppressed? Are there any other concurrent infections that may be related? Is the patient allergic to any medications or are there any potential toxicities of antimicrobials that should be specifically avoided (e.g., nephrotoxicity from aminoglycosides in an elderly patient)?
5. Cost and availability of antimicrobials in a specific hospital. Given the numerous choices of antimicrobials, many hospitals are now limiting the availability of antibiotics on their formularies in an effort to contain costs.

These factors make it difficult to give any one or a series of recommendations to cover the usual clinical situations. Some general principles are helpful, however, in choosing therapy.

Many empiric regimens include aminoglycosides. This has some merit because resistance patterns to the β-lactam antibiotics by gram-negative bacilli are difficult to predict. Aminoglycosides, however, have proved synergy with β-lactam antibiotics in only two specific situations (i.e., in the treatment of *Pseudomonas aeruginosa* bacteremia in the neutropenic patient and in the treatment of the patient with enterococcal bacteremia) (Love et al, 1980; Mandell et al, 1970). Although there is some belief that aminoglycosides may discourage the development of bacterial resistance in patients with gram-negative bacillary pneumonia, the levels achieved by intravenous aminoglycosides in respiratory secretions are low (Pennington, 1981). Therefore, if aminoglycosides are given for treatment in hospital-acquired pneumonia, they should be given in combination with other agents. They need to cover for anaerobic bacteria, specifically *Bacteroides fragilis* and *B. melaninogenicus*, which are usually resistant to penicillins. These are a frequent concern in patients who have aspirated. Agents that cover these anaerobes include clindamycin, metronidazole, ticarcillin/clavulanic acid, ampicillin/sulbactam, piperacillin/tazabactam, some second-generation and third-generation cephalosporins, and imipenem/cilastatin.

In hospitals with multiple resistant *S. aureus*, vancomycin is the empiric drug of choice until susceptibilities are known. Vancomycin has adequate antimicrobial coverage for gram-positive organisms, including gram-positive anaerobes, but does not cover *Bacteroides*. The CDC has recommended that because of the emergence of *S. aureus* and enterococci resistant to vancomycin, the use of vancomycin be limited.

Coverage for *Haemophilus influenzae* is important when the Gram's stain result suggests that this organism may be present in the respiratory flora. Approximately 23% of *H. influenzae* are β-lactamase producers in pediatric patients, and a somewhat smaller but rising percentage is found among adult patients (Doern et al, 1988). Second-generation and third-generation cephalosporins and ampicillin/sulbactam are resistant to the action of this β-lactamase. These should be used instead of ampicillin until it is known whether the organism produces β-lactamase.

PREVENTION

Measures to prevent hospital-acquired pneumonia have been outlined in several reports (American Thoracic Society, 1995; Maki, 1989; Simmons and Wong, 1982). In general, the recommendations protect patients who are at the highest risk of hospital-acquired pneumonia, safeguard equipment and procedures that are at risk for causing the development of hospital-acquired infection, and reduce the opportunity for person-to-person spread of pathogens. The Centers for Disease Control (CDC) studies have demonstrated that almost a quarter of hospital-acquired pneumonias may be prevented (Haley et al, 1985).

Postsurgical patients, especially those who have undergone upper abdominal or thoracic procedures, constitute one group in which specific preventive measures exist (Garibaldi et al, 1981). Preoperative evaluations to identify and optimize treatment of pre-existing lung infections, chronic obstructive pulmonary diseases, or smoking habits have helped these efforts. Any measure that improves or eliminates these risk factors also decreases the chance for the development of hospital-acquired pneumonia.

Antimicrobial prophylaxis is given once, at the time of surgery, when the patient is at greatest risk for infection. Continued antimicrobial "prophylaxis" for more than 3 days has been shown to encourage the development of resistant flora. Instead, incentive respirometers are used to encourage the patient to breathe deeply postoperatively to reduce the likelihood of atelectasis. Pain relief is necessary so that the patient is able to cough and mobilize upper airway secretions, but is not so excessive as to cause depression of the gag reflex, which may lead to aspiration. Early mobilization of the patient is also useful. The practice of admitting the patient to the hospital on the day of elective surgery and early discharge with home care, if necessary, may also help to reduce hospital-acquired pneumonia.

Patients should be maintained in semi-upright positions to prevent gastrointestinal reflux and aspiration. In selected patients, sucralfate should be used rather than antacids or H_2 blockers to prevent stress ulceration. (Hospital Infection Control Practices Advisory Committee, 1994)

To reduce the risk of infection as a result of mechanical factors, all solutions given by a nebulizer should be sterile, and the nebulizer must be cleaned and dried after each treatment (Simmons and Wong, 1982). Respiratory tubing and connection devices are now disposable. They may be kept functional for 48 hours or longer without difficulty. Changing tubing every 48 hours rather than every 24 hours is estimated to save $30 million annually without increasing the risk of hospital-acquired pneumonia (Craven et al, 1982). New systems that reduce the amount of condensated fluid are now available (Maki, 1989; Stange and Bygdeman, 1980). Routine suctioning of patients on ventilators should be avoided, and when it is performed, sterile and disposable equipment should be utilized.

These procedural changes have been more effective in decreasing the incidence of hospital-acquired pneumonia than all measures aimed to encourage hospital personnel to wash their hands between patients and to use proper sterile techniques. Hand washing is nevertheless important, especially in preventing the spread of viruses. Maki has shown that hand washing with an antiseptic solution can reduce rates of hospital-acquired pneumonia (Maki, 1982). Unfortunately, this simple procedure is performed between handling patients less than half the time by caregivers (Maki and Heck, 1982). Surprisingly, physicians are the worst offenders (Albert and Condie, 1981). Educational efforts to encourage hand washing usually change the behavior of hospital personnel for a short time only and must be reinforced continually.

Proper nutrition support is necessary for many patients who are intubated and severely ill. In one study of patients who suffered abdominal trauma, those who received total parenteral alimentation had higher rates of hospital-acquired pneumonia than those who had enteral alimentation (Moore et al, 1989). These results raised the question of whether bacteria translocate across the intestinal mucosa and cause infection. Those with enteral feedings preserved their mucosa better than those with parenteral alimentation.

The aforementioned measures to avoid exposure to *Aspergillus* and to prevent outbreaks owing to *L. pneumophila* are examples of situations in which once the pathogenesis of infection was understood, appropriate preventive strategies were developed. For prevention of RSV infection, the institution of contact isolation procedures and cohorting hospital personnel is recommended (Hall and Douglas, 1981; Snydman et al, 1988). Influenza vaccine and amantadine are both effective preventive strategies for influenza A, and vaccine prevents influenza B. Preventive measures for tuberculosis are well described. A routine system of surveillance for hospital-acquired pulmonary infections should be practiced in all hospitals. Such procedures are reviewed routinely and are approved by hospital accreditation committees. These procedures should lower the incidence of hospital-acquired pneumonia in the United States.

Preventive measures that have been tried unsuccessfully include selective pulmonary decontamination with prophylactic antibiotics. The administration of polymyxin and aminoglycoside antibiotics via a respirator has been tried. (Feeley et al, 1975; Klastersky et al, 1974; Levine et al, 1978). This method temporarily reduces colonization but results ultimately in microbial resistance (Klastersky et al, 1974).

Further studies are needed to better understand the pathogenesis of hospital-acquired pneumonia and to design effective and economical preventive strategies. Much progress has been made in the last few decades, but the emergence of resistant organisms, identification of new pathogens, and development of new techniques that alter host defenses ensure that hospital-acquired respiratory infections continue to be a major clinical problem well into the next century.

PNEUMONIA IN IMMUNOSUPPRESSED HOSTS

The epidemiology, diagnosis, and treatment of immunosuppressed patients with pulmonary infections is of particular interest to the critical care physician. Lung infections constitute the major cause of morbidity in these patients. Diagnosis is hindered by the usual problems encountered in the diagnosis of community-acquired pneumonia and hospital-acquired pneumonia plus the factors of impaired host inflammatory response, presence of different and sometimes multiple etiologic agents, and urgency of initiating proper therapy. An understanding of the epidemiology and pathogenesis of these infections offers some guidance in the management of patients. Specifically considered are granulocytopenic patients, organ transplant recipients, and acquired immunodeficiency syndrome (AIDS) patients to demonstrate the problems encountered in different groups of immunosuppressed hosts with respiratory infections.

PATIENTS WITH GRANULOCYTOPENIA

Granulocytopenia is the expected result of aggressive cytotoxic chemotherapy used to treat malignancy. During the period of bone marrow suppression, patients are at high risk for all types of infections, including pneumonia. The diagnosis of pulmonary infections in these patients is complicated by the absence of granulocytes and presence of impaired inflammatory response. This often results in the lack of infiltrates on the chest radiograph and small amounts of sputum production in the face of overwhelming pneumonia. Among patients with acute myelogenous leukemia, pneumonia occurs in approximately 80%. Half of the patients with pneumonia die (Sickles et al, 1973).

Infection in granulocytopenic patients is correlated directly with the absolute granulocyte count. Patients with absolute granulocyte counts less than 500 are severely granulocytopenic, and counts less than 100 place the patient at most risk (Bodey et al, 1966). In patients with acute myelogenous leukemia, the period of greatest risk may last for several weeks during the induction phase of therapy. These patients are hospitalized; thus, factors that cause the colonizaiton of the upper airways with gram-negative bacilli (see earlier) are also present. In addition, granulocytopenia renders patients susceptible to infections with S. aureus and fungi due to the presence of intravenous lines and frequent use of antimicrobials. The list of organisms that often cause pneumonia in patients with granulocytopenia is shown in Table 21–2.

Therapeutic Approach

Empiric broad-spectrum therapy should be initiated without delay once blood, urine, and, if possible, sputum cultures are obtained. Although empiric therapy is designed to cover all infections, it is relevant particularly to the treatment of pulmonary infections.

![]

Table 21–2
Usual Causes of Pneumonia in Granulocytopenic Patients

Pseudomonas aeruginosa	Aspergillus species
Klebsiella pneumoniae	Phycomycetes
Escherichia coli	Candida
Staphylococcus aureus	

The absence of sputum production, inherent problems of obtaining a representative sputum specimen, and frequent lack of infiltrates on chest radiographs all make pulmonary infections exceedingly difficult to diagnose at times. Invasive procedures (transtracheal aspirate, bronchoalveolar lavage, and bronchial brushing) assume increasing importance, although thrombocytopenia, which is frequently present, increases the likelihood of bleeding during these procedures.

Several empiric treatment regimens have been studied (EORTC International Antimicrobial Therapy Cooperative Group, 1987; Pizzo, 1989; Pizzo et al, 1982). All provide coverage for bacterial pathogens shown in Table 21–2. Combinations of a broad-spectrum β-lactam antibiotic covering S. aureus and Pseudomonas aeruginosa, and an aminoglycoside; two broad-spectrum β-lactam antibiotics; or a β-lactam and a monobactam antibiotic have been given. The new carbepenem, imipenem/cilastatin, may have further value in the empiric treatment of these patients. In hospital settings in which multiple resistant S. aureus occur, vancomycin is usually substituted for one of the β-lactam antibiotics. The additional benefit of a regimen with vancomycin is coverage of S. epidermidis, which is commonly resistant to β-lactams. Although this organism is a rare cause of pneumonia, it may be associated with bacteremia.

Problems with empiric therapy occur when the patient's condition does not improve rapidly. Options then are the addition of antibiotics, such as erythromycin and trimethoprim/sulfamethoxazole (TMP/SMX), initiation of antifungal therapy, and continuation of the initial antimicrobial therapy.

The expected duration of granulocytopenia also has a bearing on further diagnostic or therapeutic maneuvers. When the bone marrow is recovering and the absolute granulocyte count is increasing, no change in therapy may be necessary. In contrast, if the granulocyte count is continuing to fall, transbronchial biopsy or open lung biopsy is warranted. The empiric addition of trimethoprim/sulfamethoxazole and erythromycin should be considered if Pneumoceptis carinii or L. pneumophila are suspected.

Pizzo has demonstrated increased survival of granulocytopenic patients. Amphotericin B was empirically added to the therapeutic regimen in patients who remained febrile for 7 days in the presence of broad-spectrum antibiotics (Pizzo et al, 1982; 1989). Amphotericin B should then be continued until granulocytopenia resolves or it appears clinically that such treatment is not helpful.

Granulocyte transfusions in the febrile granulocytopenic patient remain controversial. In general, this approach is reserved for granulocytopenic patients with known bacterial infections who do not respond to antimicrobial therapy (Winston et al, 1982). The benefit of granulocyte transfusions is short-lived and may cause hypersensitivity reactions. A review by Wright and associates showed severe respiratory complications when granulocyte transfusions were given with amphotericin B. Acute respiratory deterioration occurred in 7 of 22 patients (64%) who received both therapies concomitantly versus 2 of 35 patients (6%) who received granulocyte transfusions alone (Wright et al, 1981). Most physicians prescribe colony stimulating factors to increase the white blood count if the patient is to be neutropenic for a long period. There is no evidence yet that this practice decreases the mortality from pulmonary infections. Granulocyte colony stimulating factor use is contraindicated in patients with leukemia.

Prevention

Several preventive strategies have been studied in granulocytopenic patients (Dekker et al, 1987; Henry, 1985; Karp et al, 1987; Levine et al, 1973; Pizzo, 1989; Rodriguez et al, 1978). Some of these have been very costly for example, total protective isolation rooms (Levine et al, 1973; Rodriguez et al, 1978). As yet no approach has had a significant impact on reducing infections in these patients (Henry, 1985). Studies included quinolone drugs prophylactically to sterilize the aerobic flora in the gastrointestinal tract (Dekker et al, 1987; Karp et al, 1987), fluconazole to prevent fungal infection (Winston et al, 1993), passive immunization with intravenous immunoglobulin (Pizzo, 1989), biologic response modifiers such as granulocyte-colony stimulating factor (G-CSF) and granulocyte-macrophage-colony stimulating factor (GM-CSF) (Pizzo, 1989). Although none of these studies has specifically examined the prevention of pneumonia by decreasing gastrointestinal colonization, by improving the opsonization of encapsulated bacteria, and by restoring granulocyte number and function, prevention of pneumonia is likely to occur. The future may bring the combination of several strategies to prevent these infections, modify the immunosuppressive effects of granulocytopenia, and rapidly restore the patient's immune function.

TRANSPLANT RECIPIENTS

Pneumonia is a serious complication of the immunosuppressive therapy that is used to prevent allograft rejection in recipients of organ and bone marrow transplantation. In one autopsy series of 116 renal transplant recipients, 43 died of pulmonary infections, and pneumonia was the leading cause of death (Scroggs et al, 1987). In lung transplant patients, the prevalence of pulmonary infections is over 60% (Dauber et al, 1990, Mauer et al, 1992). In another large series of bone marrow transplant recipients, interstitial pneumonitis was the primary cause or contributing cause of death in 84% (Weiner et al, 1986). Pneumonia due to a wide range of pathogens is also the leading cause of morbidity in these patients. Cytomegalovirus (CMV), the most common infectious complication of organ transplantation, has a 50% mortality if there is pulmonary involvement (Peterson et al, 1980).

The etiology and onset of pulmonary infections in the transplant recipient follow a fairly predictable pattern. Knowledge of this sequence of events is useful clinically and aids the diagnosis, treatment, and prevention of these infections.

Epidemiology

The major etiologic agents and the expected onset of pneumonia in solid organ transplant recipients are shown in Table 21–3. During the first 2 weeks after the transplant, the usual postoperative hospital-acquired pneumonias are prevalent. The patients have not received immunosuppressive therapy long enough to allow for most of the opportunistic pathogens to gain a foothold.

Most pulmonary infections in solid organ transplant recipients occur within 1 to 6 months after the transplant has been made. This is the time when the patient is most severely immunosuppressed and when high-dose treatment for acute rejection with glucocorticoids, antilympho-

---

Table 21–3
General Etiology and Timing of Pulmonary Infections in Transplant Recipients

Etiology	Timing Post-transplant
Cytomegalovirus	1–6 months
Herpes simplex virus	0–2 months
Pneumocystis carinii	1–4 months
Legionella pneumophila	1 month on
Nocardiosis	1–6 months
Mycobacterium tuberculosis	3 months on
Histoplasma capsulatum	2 months on
Aspergillosis	1–6 months
Cryptococcus neoformans	3 months on
Candida	1–4 months
Bacterial pneumonias	0–1 month, 6 months on

cyte preparations, and additional immunosuppressants usually occurs (Munda et al, 1978; Peterson et al, 1981; Ramsey et al, 1980). This is also the usual time for CMV infection, which not only causes pneumonia by itself but also predisposes the patient to pulmonary infections caused by *P. carinii*, bacteria, and fungi. Six months after transplantation, the patient becomes less susceptible to *P. carinii* and more susceptible to bacteria, mycobacteria, and fungi infections.

Pathogenesis

Transplant recipients may develop pulmonary infections caused by organisms encountered in normal hosts. They are also at risk for reactivating dormant pathogens that may later cause pneumonia. These pathogens include CMV, varicella-zoster virus, herpes simplex virus, *P. carinii*, tuberculosis, *Histoplasma*, and *Cryptococcus*. Transplant recipients are also the "sentinel chickens" for organisms in the community and in the hospital. Examples have been seen with outbreaks of *Asper-*

gillus, L. pneumophila, and influenza A (Rubin et al, 1981).

The immunosuppressive regimen has an important role in the patient's susceptibility to pulmonary infection. In one randomized study of 224 renal transplant recipients, 96% of patients receiving cyclosporine immunosuppression were free of pneumonia during the first year, whereas only 91% of patients treated with azathioprine and antilymphocyte globulin were free of pneumonia, which is a significant difference (Hesse et al, 1986). Among bone marrow transplant recipients, methotrexate and methotrexate plus irradiation treatments were associated with increased risk of interstitial pneumonitis compared with the risk in patients receiving cyclosporine (Weiner et al, 1986).

In lung transplantation there are specific risk factors for pneumonia that occur as a result of the surgery. During transplantation there may be injury to the airway mucosa, disruption of the mucociliary clearance at the airway anastomosis, denervation that impairs the cough reflux, and

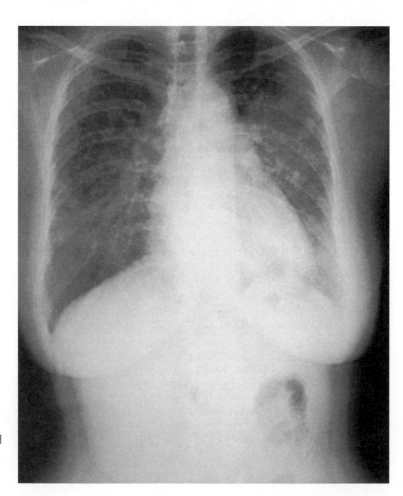

Figure 21–1
Chest radiograph of a patient 3 months after renal transplantation with a 3-day history of hypoxia and fever. Bronchoalveolar lavage revealed *Pneumocystis carinii*, and viral cultures grew cytomegalovirus.

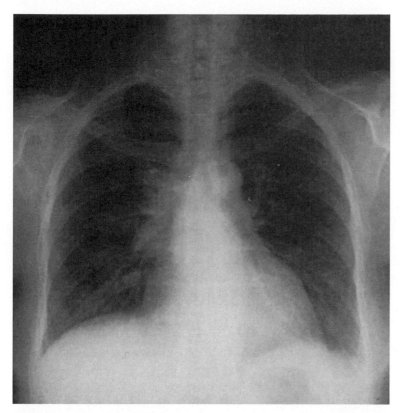

Figure 21–2
Chest radiograph of a patient 5 months after renal transplantation with a history of hypoxia and fever. Bronchoalveolar lavage grew *Legionella pneumophila* and cytomegalovirus.

interruption of the lymphatic drainage (Dauber et al, 1990). Organisms that colonize the donor can be passed in the immediate postoperative period. Later rejection can be associated with bacterial pneumonia (Nickolson et al, 1994).

Diagnosis

The diagnosis of pulmonary infections in transplant recipients must be rapid and all-encompassing, particularly in patients with diffuse interstitial infiltrates on chest radiographs. The causes of these pulmonary infections may be multiple. Characteristic chest radiograph appearances are not helpful (Figs. 21–1 to 21–3). In addition, several antimicrobial agents used in treating these infections can interact with cyclosporine, the mainstay of current antirejection therapy (Dieperink and Moller, 1982). Thus, early diagnosis must be specific to limit and avoid undesirable drug interactions.

Sputum Gram's stain and culture studies are usually not helpful in transplant recipients because of the lack of cell-mediated immunity and the subsequent meager inflammatory response to the causative organisms. Immediate bronchoscopy with sterile brushings and bronchoalveolar lavage constitutes a reasonable approach to the rapid diagnosis of pulmonary infections in transplant recipients. Among 54 renal transplant recipients who had bronchoscopy for diffuse interstitial pneumonia, we identified the causative agent or agents within 24 hours in one half of the cases. CMV was subsequently shown to be the etiologic agent in three quarters of the remaining patients (Johnson et al, 1990). Closed and open pulmonary biopsy and lung aspiration have also been done in some centers with success.

Not all febrile organ transplant recipients with infiltrates on chest radiographs have pulmonary infections. Diffuse interstitial infiltrate, hypoxia, and fever may also occur in the setting of (1) graft-versus-host disease in bone marrow transplantation, (2) rejection in heart transplantation, and (3) result of antilymphocyte preparations in the treatment of rejection.

Treatment

When considering the treatment of pulmonary infections in transplant recipients, it is important to consider possible drug interactions with cyclosporine, which is primarily metabolized by the hepatic cytochrome 450 enzyme system. These interactions fit three general categories:

1. Antimicrobials that downregulate the

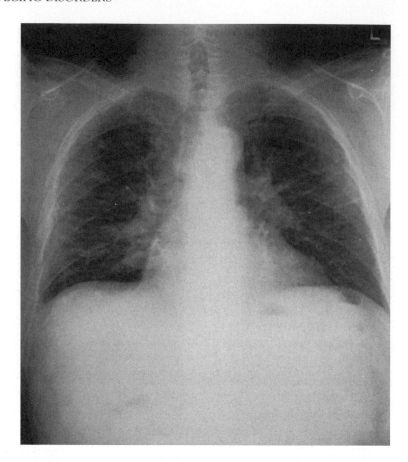

Figure 21–3
Chest radiograph of a patient 4 months after renal transplantation with a 1-week history of fever, chills, and hypoxia. Bronchoalveolar lavage grew influenza virus A (H3N2) and cytomegalovirus.

hepatic cytochrome p450 enzyme system may result in increased cyclosporine blood levels and a potential for cyclosporine toxicity or overimmunosuppression. These antimicrobials include erythromycin, clarithromycin, and antifungal agents, such as ketoconazole and itraconazole (Dieperink and Moller, 1982; Jensen et al, 1987).

2. Antimicrobials that upregulate the cytochrome p450 system may result in decreased cyclosporine blood levels and a potential for rejection. The main cause of this interaction is rifampin (Van Buren et al, 1992).

3. Antimicrobials that exhibit synergistic or enhanced nephrotoxicity in combination with cyclosporine that include TMP/SMX (Thompson et al, 1983) and amphotericin B (Kennedy et al, 1983).

Because these antimicrobial agents are administered frequently in the treatment of pulmonary infections in the transplant recipient, they must be used cautiously and discontinued if they are inappropriate to treat the likely cause of the pneumonia. Our approach is to start a combination of TMP/SMX and erythromycin empirically for renal allograft recipients with diffuse interstitial infiltrates and fever. Rapid processing of respiratory secretions allows omitting TMP/SMX when *P. carinii* is not identified, and erythromycin if *L. pneumophila* is not observed by direct fluorescent antibody smears. When culture of respiratory secretions identifies other pathogens, such as bacteria or fungi, antibiotic coverage may be changed accordingly. The current treatment of CMV requires lowering or stopping immunosuppression treatment and ensuring good nutrition and supportive care.

Ganciclovir, an antiviral agent similar to acyclovir but with better *in vitro* activity against CMV, appears to have good activity when used in CMV chorioretinitis, but this drug has not proved to be effective in the treatment of CMV pneumonia. This dichotomy of response is most likely occurring because pneumonia is a relatively late event in CMV infection and because the histopathologic changes in the lung may not be due to destruction by the organism itself but rather to the host's response to infection. If this were true, all antiviral therapies that are started late in the course of disease would be ineffective.

Prevention

Several strategies have prevented pulmonary infections in transplant recipients (Lichenstein and MacGregor, 1983; MacDonald et al, 1982; Pettersson et al, 1985; Snydman et al, 1987). To prevent *P. carinni* infections, prophylaxis with TMP/SMX during the first 2 weeks to 4 months after transplant has been effective (Maki et al, 1985). Acyclovir prophylaxis given to renal transplant recipients is effective in preventing herpes simplex virus infection during the first 6 months (Pettersson et al, 1985). Influenza A vaccine is effective in renal transplant recipients after the transplant. Intravenous immune serum globulin has been effective in preventing CMV infections in bone marrow and renal transplant recipients who are seronegative before transplant and who receive allografts from seropositive donors (Snydman et al, 1987). The concept of pre-emptive treatment with ganciclovir and immune globulin in at-risk patients has been advocated (Rubin, 1991). Screening for tuberculin skin test reactivity is included in most pretransplant evaluations, because patients are at approximately 12 times greater risk of developing tuberculosis after transplant than normal hosts (Lichenstein and Mac-Gregor, 1983). Because some patients with chronic renal failure are anergic, this strategy is not always successful in preventing tuberculosis in renal allograft recipients.

PATIENTS WITH AIDS

Respiratory infections are the major cause of life-threatening infections complicating infections with the human immunodeficiency virus (HIV) (Murray et al, 1984; Selik et al, 1987; Stover et al, 1985). Pulmonary infections may establish the diagnosis of AIDS and are usually the first manifestation of AIDS. We must include the causes of pulmonary infection associated with HIV infection in the differential diagnosis of community-acquired pneumonia. We must also consider everyone with risk factors for HIV to be potentially immunosuppressed unless HIV infection is excluded by testing. HIV-infected patients may present with the usual causes of community-acquired pneumonia, or they may have pulmonary infections caused by organisms that occur only in compromised hosts.

Epidemiology

The various causes of pulmonary infections in patients with AIDS are shown in Table 21–4. Patients with AIDS may have more than one

Table 21–4
Pulmonary Infections in Patients With Acquired Immunodeficiency Syndrome

> *Pneumocystis carinii*
> *Mycobacterium tuberculosis*
> *Mycobacterium avium intracellulare*
> *Mycobacterium kansasii*
> *Histoplasma capsulatum*
> *Cryptococcus neoformans*
> Coccidioidomycosis
> Blastomycetes dermatitis
> Aspergillosis
> Nocardiosis
> Influenza
> Cytomegalovirus
> Human immunodeficiency virus (lymphocytic interstitial pneumonitis)
> *Streptococcus pneumoniae*
> *Haemophilus influenzae*
> *Staphylococcus aureus*
> *Legionella pneumoniae*
> *Pseudomonas aeruginosa*

pulmonary infection at the same time. In a series of pneumonia cases in patients with AIDS in which fiberoptic bronchoscopy was performed, 15% had more than one possible etiologic agent suspected of causing pneumonia (Broaddus et al, 1985). *P. carinii* pneumonia (PCP) is the most important pulmonary infection in patients with AIDS. It is estimated that 65% of patients with AIDS develop PCP at some time during the illness (Hopewell, 1988). Thus, the CDC is now recommending prophylaxis of PCP with TMP/SMX in patients infected with HIV who have a CD4 lymphocyte count of less than 200 (Centers for Disease Control, 1987).

It is useful to consider when the various pulmonary infections occur during the course of HIV infection. Routine bacterial pathogenic infections, tuberculosis, histoplasmosis, cryptococcosis, and coccidioidomycosis all occur early in HIV-infected patients. Although routine bacterial pneumonias do not define AIDS, disseminated histoplasmosis, cryptococcosis, and coccidioidomycosis are all included in the case definition of AIDS established by the CDC for patients infected with HIV (Centers for Disease Control, 1989a,b). PCP, atypical mycobacteria including *Mycobacterium avium intracellulare* (MAI) complex, and viruses including CMV all occur after the patient has been severely immunosuppressed for some time.

Pathogenesis

The normal pulmonary defense mechanisms are altered in HIV infection (Beck and Shellito,

1989). The total extent of this alteration is just beginning to be defined. Along with the other alterations in cell-mediated immunity found in patients with AIDS, we now know that HIV directly infects pulmonary alveolar macrophages (Beck and Shellito, 1989). These alterations help to explain the frequency of infections with organisms that are usually seen in patients with deficient cell-mediated immunity, in organ transplant recipients, and in patients undergoing chemotherapy for hematologic neoplasms.

Diagnosis

Although it is tempting to treat all AIDS patients with pneumonia for PCP and forego establishing a definitive diagnosis, this practice is potentially dangerous. Most HIV-infected patients present with fever, tachypnea, and hypoxemia along with diffuse interstitial infiltrates on the chest radiograph, without appreciable sputum production or peripheral leukocytosis. All attempts at a definitive diagnosis should be made for several reasons. In 15% of the cases, more than one pulmonary pathogen is found (Broaddus et al, 1985). In the HIV-infected patient, diagnosis of disseminated tuberculosis; histoplasmosis; cryptococcosis; and PCP, MAI, or CMV establishes the diagnosis of AIDS (Broaddus et al, 1985).

Tuberculosis may present with an unusual appearance in HIV-infected patients, and these individuals may be contagious to family members and the public (Hopewell, 1989). Patients receiving prophylaxis for PCP with inhaled pentamidine are now known to present with irregular upper lobe presentations of PCP (Montgomery, 1989). Pulmonary infections caused by *Mycobacteria, Nocardia,* fungi, and PCP require permanent suppressive therapy after the initial treatment of pneumonia. If patients receive suppressive therapy, relapses occur in approximately 25%. The treatments for these infections are varied, toxic, and expensive and should not be undertaken haphazardly. Moreover, the usual organisms causing community-acquired pneumonia may also infect HIV-infected patients.

Community-acquired pneumonia may respond to routine antibacterial therapy and does not require suppressive therapy. Furthermore, noninfectious causes of pulmonary infiltrates can mimic pulmonary infections in patients with AIDS. These noninfectious causes include B cell lymphoma and Kaposi's sarcoma (Luce and Clement, 1989; Ognibene et al, 1985). All of these are reasons why an initial attempt for an accurate diagnosis should be made.

Pulmonary secretions obtained by either ex-

pectorated sputum or bronchoalveolar lavage are needed for diagnosis. Mycobacteria, bacteria, and PCP are not difficult to identify with this approach, because the number or organisms seen microscopically is high. Bronchoalveolar lavage alone is diagnostic for most pulmonary infections in patients with AIDS (Coleman et al, 1983). Hadley and Ng at the San Francisco General Hospital have established a team approach to collect and quickly analyze expectorated sputum from patients with AIDS. Using Giemsa and toluidine blue stains on induced samples of expectorated sputum that has been liquefied with dithiothreitol and concentrated, they have been able to diagnose PCP with a sensitivity of 75% and a negative predictive value of 63% (Hadley and Ng, 1989).

We believe that all HIV-infected patients with a pulmonary process and a compatible clinical and radiologic picture should be treated empirically for PCP at the same time. We also advocate that aggressive diagnostic steps be initiated, beginning with induced sputum specimen collection. We recommend quick diagnostic bronchoscopy if the patient fails to improve on empiric therapy.

Another alternative to bronchoscopy may be transthoracic lung aspiration with a skinny needle (Wallace, 1985). This is a very sensitive diagnostic technique, however, and it is complicated by a high incidence of pneumothorax (Wallace et al, 1985). All of these approaches may result in a savings of time and money in these critically ill patients. It is unusual that an open lung biopsy is needed to make a diagnosis in these patients.

Results of ancillary tests, such as the finding of a high lactate dehydrogenase level, may offer a clue to the diagnosis of PCP and progressive disseminated histoplasmosis (Kagawa et al, 1988; Zaman and White, 1988). The serum cryptococcal antigen level is elevated in more than 95% of patients with cryptococcal disease (Chuck and Sande, 1989). Bone marrow biopsy may be particularly helpful in the diagnosis of mycobacterial and fungal infections (Johnson et al, 1989). Although routinely recommended for all HIV-infected individuals, a tuberculin skin test with appropriate controls is frequently nonreactive in these patients (Centers for Disease Control, 1989a). Lysis centrifugation blood cultures are useful in recovering fungi and mycobacteria (Kiehn et al, 1983). Serologic diagnosis of *H. capsulatum* is very useful and is positive only in approximately one half of the patient population (Johnson et al, 1989). Antigen testing for *Histoplasma capsulatum* antigen is highly sensitive and specific in the urine and blood (Wheat et al, 1992).

Treatment

The regimen for transplant recipients (i.e., TMP/SMX and erythromycin) in general is also a reasonable empiric therapy for diffuse interstitial pneumonitis in the patient with HIV infection. With identification of other organisms, therapy may be changed accordingly. Standard regimens for PCP include TMP/SMX (15 mg/kg per day TMP and 75 mg/kg per day SMX) given either intravenously or orally every 6 hours (Montgomery, 1989). For a 70-kg adult this is the equivalent of three single-strength TMP/SMX tablets or three 5-ml intravenous ampules given every 6 hours (Montgomery, 1989). Alternatively, pentamidine may be given over 2 hours at a dose of 4 mg/kg per day (Montgomery, 1989). Therapy is continued for 14 to 21 days, and then prophylactic treatment is administered. Corticosteroids have been shown to reduce mortality in patients with severe hypoxia (PO_2 <60 mm Hg) (Bozzette et al, 1990). Oral agents for mild PCP include TMP/SMX, dapsone/trimethoprim, and atovaquone.

Amphotericin B is the mainstay of therapy for treatment of severe progressive disseminated histoplasmosis, coccidioidomycosis, and cryptococcosis (Johnson et al, 1989). Fluconazole is effective for isolated pulmonary cryptococcosis (Saag et al, 1992) and for coccidioidomycosis. Itraconazole is effective induction therapy for mild to moderate progressive disseminated histoplasmosis. Continued suppression is recommended to prevent relapses with these infections (Chuck and Sande, 1989).

The appropriate treatment of mycobacterial infections in the patient with AIDS is fairly straightforward. In adult patients with either pulmonary or disseminated tuberculosis, isoniazid (INH), rifampin, and pyrazinamide are given. Pyrazinamide should be given for the first 2 months, and the other medications should be given for a total of at least 9 months. If the results of cultures remain positive for more than 3 months into therapy, treatment is continued until the cultures have been clear for 6 months (Hopewell, 1989; Jones et al, 1994). Relapse rates are approximately 5%, and maintenance treatment is not needed (Small et al, 1991).

The regimen for direct-observed therapy in patients who are noncompliant includes up to five drugs (American Thoracic Society, 1994). If the organism is likely to be resistant to INH, a fourth agent, usually ethambutol, is added until drug sensitivity test results become available. When the organism is fully sensitive, ethambutol is stopped along with pyrazinamide; with resistant organisms, all agents are continued until the end of therapy. Treatment for M. *kansasii* infection includes INH, rifampin, and ethambutol for at least 15 months after culture conversion (MacDonell and Glassroth, 1989). Some strains are resistant to INH at a level of 1 μg/ml, and thus INH should be discontinued (MacDonell and Glassroth, 1989). For MAI (*Mycobacterium avium-intracellulare*), clarithromycin and ethambutol are the most effective agents.

Prevention

Several strategies have been effective in preventing certain pulmonary infections in HIV-infected adults. PCP can be prevented by either TMP/SMX at a dose of one double-strength tablet daily or aerosolized pentamidine at a dose of 300 mg every 4 weeks by Respirgard II jet nebulizer (Centers for Disease Control, 1995). Prophylaxis is started when the patient is at highest risk for PCP, usually when the total CD4 lymphocyte count is less than 200/mm³ (Centers for Disease Control, 1989). Pentamidine is usually preferred because of the high percentage of patients with AIDS who have allergic reactions to TMP/SMX. Other possible preventive regimens include dapsone, dapsone plus trimethoprim, dapsone plus primethamine, and pyramethamine-sulfadoxine (Centers for Disease Control, 1995).

Although many patients infected with HIV are anergic when tested against common skin test antigens, it is recommended that all HIV-infected patients be given a Mantoux skin test with 5 units of tuberculin purified protein derivative and controls (Centers for Disease Control, 1995). Patients with a greater than 5-mm reaction should be considered to have tuberculosis and should be given INH prophylaxis for at least 12 months (Centers for Disease Control, 1995). Studies are underway to determine the appropriateness and effectiveness of oral azoles for prevention of histoplasmosis and coccidioidomycosis in highly endemic areas.

To prevent bacterial pneumonias in children and adults, immunization with conjugated *Haemophilus influenzae* type b capsular vaccine and pneumococcal polysaccharide vaccine has been recommended (Chaisson, 1989). To prevent influenza, annual influenza immunization is also recommended. The efficacy of these immunization regimens is not established, because many HIV-infected patients do not respond adequately to the vaccines. There is concern that vaccines stimulate HIV production (Centers for Disease Control, 1995).

REFERENCES

Albert RK and Condie F: Handwashing patterns in medical intensive care units. N Engl J Med 304:1465–1466, 1981.

American Thoracic Society: Treatment of tuberculosis and tuberculosis infection in adults and children. Am J Respir Crit Care Med 149:1359–1374, 1994.

American Thoracic Society: Hospital-acquired pneumonia in adults: Diagnosis, assessment of severity, initial antimicrobial therapy, and preventative strategies. Official Statement of the American Thoracic Society, 1995. Am J Respir Crit Care Med 153:1711–1715, 1996.

Andrews CP, Coalson JJ, Smith SD, et al: Diagnosis of nosocomial bacterial pneumonia in acute diffuse lung injury. Chest 80:254–258, 1981.

Arden NH, Patriarca PA, Fasano MB, et al: The roles of vaccination and amantadine prophylaxis in controlling an outbreak of influenza A (H3N2) in a nursing home. Arch Intern Med 148:865–868, 1988.

Arnow PM, Anderson RL, Mainous PD, et al: Pulmonary aspergillosis during hospital renovation. Am Rev Respir Dis 118:49–53, 1978.

Arnow PM, Chou T, Weil D, et al: Nosocomial legionnaire's disease caused by aerosolyzed tap water from respiratory devices. J Infect Dis 146:460–467, 1982.

Bartlett JG, Faling LJ, and Willey S: Quantitative tracheal bacteriologic and cytologic studies in patients with long-term tracheostomies. Chest 74:635–639, 1978.

Bartlett JG and Finegold SM: Bacteriology of expectorated sputum with quantitative culture and wash technique compared to transtracheal aspirates. Am Rev Respir Dis 117:1019–1027, 1978.

Beck JM and Shellito J: Effects of human immunodeficiency virus on pulmonary host defenses. Semin Respir Infect 4:75–84, 1989.

Bodey GP, Buckley M, Sathe YS, et al: Quantitative relationship between circulating leukocytes and infection in patients with acute leukemia. Ann Intern Med 64:328–340, 1966.

Boyce JM, White RL, Spruill EY, et al: Cost-effective application of the Centers for Disease Control guideline for prevention of nosocomial pneumonia. Am J Infect Control 13:228–232, 1985.

Bozette SA, Sattler FR, Chiu J, et al: A controlled trial of early adjunctive treatment with corticosteroids for Pneumocystis carinii pneumonia in the acquired immunodeficiency syndrome. N Engl J Med 323:1451–1456, 1990.

Broaddus C, Dake MD, Steelberg MS, et al: Bronchoalveolar lavage and transbronchial biopsy for the diagnosis of pulmonary infections in the acquired immunodeficiency syndrome. Ann Intern Med 102:747–752, 1985.

Carlon GC, Fox SJ, and Ackerman NJ: Evaluation of a closed-tracheal suction system. Crit Care Med 15:522–525, 1987.

Centers for Disease Control: Revision of the CDC surveillance case definition of acquired immunodeficiency syndrome. JAMA 258:1143–1154, 1987.

Centers for Disease Control: Advisory Committee for Elimination of Tuberculosis: Tuberculosis and human immunodeficiency virus infection. MMWR 38:236–250, 1989a.

Centers for Disease Control: Guidelines for prophylaxis against Pneumocystis carinii pneumonia for persons infected with human immunodeficiency virus. MMWR 38:1–9, 1989b.

Centers for Disease Control: USPHS/IDSA guidelines for the prevention of opportunistic infections in persons infected with human immunodeficiency virus: A summary. MMWR 44:4–10, 1995.

Chaisson RE: Bacterial pneumonia in patients with human immunodeficiency virus infection. Semin Respir Infect 4:133–138, 1989.

Chuck SL and Sande MA: Infections with Cryptococcal neoformans in the acquired immunodeficiency syndrome. N Engl J Med 321:794–799, 1989.

Coleman DL, Dodek PM, Luce JM, et al: Diagnostic utility of fiberoptic bronchoscopy in patients with Pneumocystis carinii pneumonia and the acquired immunodeficiency syndrome. Am Rev Respir Dis 128:795–799, 1983.

Courcol RJ, Damien JM, Ramon P, et al: Presence of alveolar macrophages as a criterion for determining the suitability of sputum specimens for bacterial culture. Eur J Clin Microbiol Infect Dis 3:122–125, 1984.

Craven DE, Connolly MG, Lichtenberg DA, et al: Contamination of mechanical ventilator with tubing changes every 24 or 48 hours. N Engl J Med 306:1505–1509, 1982.

Craven DE, Goularte TA, and Make BJ: Contaminated condensate in mechanical ventilation circuits: A risk factor for nosocomial pneumonia? Am Rev Respir Dis 129:625–628, 1984a.

Craven DE, Kunches LM, Kilinsky V, et al: Risk factors for pneumonia and fatality in patients receiving continuous mechanical ventilation. Am Rev Respir Dis 133:792–796, 1986.

Craven DE, Lichtenberg DA, Goularte TA, et al: Contaminated medication nebulizers in mechanical ventilator circuits: Source of bacterial aerosols. Am J Med 77:834–838, 1984b.

Craven DE and Steger KA: Nosocomial pneumonia in mechanically ventilated adult patients: Epidemiology and prevention in 1996. Semin Respir Dis 11:32–53, 1996.

Cross AS and Roup B: Role of respiratory assistance devices in endemic nosocomial pneumonia. Am J Med 70:681–685, 1981.

Dauber JH, Paradis IL, and Dummer JS: Infectious complications in pulmonary allograft recipients. Clin Chest Med 11:291–308, 1990.

Dekker AW, Rozenberg-Arska M, and Verhoff J:

Infection prophylaxis in acute leukemia: A comparison of ciprofloxacin with trimethoprim-sulfamethoxazole. Ann Intern Med 106:7–12, 1987.

Dieperink H and Moller J: Ketoconazole and cyclosporine (Letter). Lancet ii:1217, 1982.

Doern GV, Jergensen JH, Thornsberry C, et al: National collaborative study of the prevalence of antimicrobial resistance among clinical isolates of *Haemophilus influenzae*. Antimicrob Agents Chemother 32:964–971, 1988.

Donowitz LG, Page MC, Mileur BL, et al: Alteration of normal gastric flora in critical care patients receiving antacid and cimetidine therapy. Infect Control 7:23–26, 1986.

Dreyfuss DK, Djedaini P, Weber P, et al: Prospective study of nosocomial pneumonia and of patient and circuit colonization during mechanical ventilation with circuit changes every 48 hours versus no change. Am Rev Respir Dis 143:738–743, 1991.

Driks MR, Craven DE, Celli BR, et al: Nosocomial pneumonia in intubated patients given sucralfate as compared with antacids or histamine type 2 blockers: The role of gastric colonization. N Engl J Med 317:1376–1382, 1987.

Eickhoff TC: Pulmonary infections in surgical patients. Surg Clin North Am 60:175–183, 1980.

EORTC International Antimicrobial Therapy Cooperative Group: Ceftazidime combined with a short or long course of amikacin for empirical therapy of gram-negative bacteremia in cancer patients with granulocytopenia. N Engl J Med 317:1692–1698, 1987.

Fagon JY, Chastre J, Domart Y, et al: Nosocomial pneumonia in patients receiving continuous mechanical ventilation: Prospective analysis of 52 episodes with use of a protected specimen brush and quantitative culture techniques. Am Rev Respir Dis 139:877–884, 1989.

Feeley TW, DuMoulin GC, Hedley-Whyte J, et al: Aerosol polymyxin and pneumonia in seriously ill patients. N Engl J Med 293:471–475, 1975.

Garibaldi RA, Britt MR, Coleman ML, et al: Risk factors for postoperative pneumonia. Am J Med 70:677–680, 1981.

Garvie DG and Gray J: Outbreak of respiratory syncytial virus infection in the elderly. Br Med J 281:1253–1254, 1980.

Gaynes R, Bizek B, Mowry-Hanley J, et al: Risk factors for nosocomial pneumonia after coronary artery bypass graft operations. Ann Thorac Surg 51:215–218, 1991.

Gross PA, Neu HC, Aswapokee P, et al: Deaths from nosocomial infections: Experience in a university hospital and a community hospital. Am J Med 68:219–223, 1980.

Hadley WK and Ng VL: Organization of microbiology laboratory services for the diagnosis of pulmonary infections in patients with human immunodeficiency virus infection. Semin Respir Infect 4:85–92, 1989.

Haley RW, Culver DH, White JW, et al: The nationwide nosocomial infection rate: A new need for vital statistics. Am J Epidemiol 121:159–167, 1985.

Hall CB: Nosocomial viral respiratory infections: Perennial weeds on pediatric wards. Am J Med 70:670–676, 1981.

Hall CB and Douglas RG Jr: Nosocomial respiratory syncytial viral infections: Should gowns and masks be used? Am J Dis Child 135:512–515, 1981.

Hall CB, Douglas RG Jr, Geiman JM, et al: Nosocomial respiratory syncytial virus infections. N Engl J Med 293:1343–1346, 1975.

Hall CB, McBride JT, Walsh EE, et al: Aerosolized ribavirin treatment of infants with respiratory syncytial viral infection: A randomized double-blind study. N Engl J Med 308:1443–1447, 1983.

Hall CB, Powell KR, MacDonald NE, et al: Respiratory syncytial viral infection in children with compromised immune function. N Engl J Med 315:77–81, 1986.

Hanson LC, Weber DJ, Rutala WA, et al: Risk factors for nosocomial pneumonia in the elderly. Am J Med 92:161–166, 1992.

Harris TM, Raman TK, Richards WJ, et al: An evaluation of bacterial contamination of ventilator humidifying system. Chest 63:922–925, 1973.

Helms CM, Massonari M, Wenzel RP, et al: Legionnaire's disease associated with a hospital water system (a five year report on continuous hyperchlorination). JAMA 259:2423–2427, 1988.

Henry SA: Chemoprophylaxis of bacterial infections in granulocytopenic patient. In Brown AE and Armstrong D (eds): Infectious Complications of Neoplastic Disease: Controversies in Management. New York, Yorke Medical Books, 1985, pp 303–316.

Hesse WJ, Fryd DS, Chatterjee SN, et al: Pulmonary infections: The Minnesota randomized prospective trial of cyclosporine vs azathioprine-antilymphocyte globulin for immunosuppression in renal allograft recipients. Arch Surg 121:1056–1060, 1986.

Hooten TM, Haley RW, Culver DH, et al: The joint association of multiple risk factors with the occurrence of nosocomial infection. Am J Med 70:960–966, 1981.

Hopewell PC: Diagnosis of *Pneumocystis carinii* pneumonia. In Sande MA and Volberding PA (eds): Medical Management of AIDS. Philadelphia, WB Saunders, 1988, pp 169–179.

Hopewell PC: Tuberculosis and human immunodeficiency virus infection. Semin Respir Infect 4:111–122, 1989.

Horan TC, White JW, Jarvis WR, et al: Nosocomial infection surveillance. MMWR 35W [Suppl]:17SS–29SS, 1986.

Horman JT, Stetler HC, Israel E, et al: An outbreak of influenza A in a nursing home. Am J Public Health 76:501–504, 1986.

Hospital Infection Control Practices Advisory

Committee. Infect Control Hosp Epidemiology 15:587, 1994.

Huxley EJ, Viroslav J, Gray WR, et al: Pharyngeal aspiration in normal adults and patients with depressed consciousness. Am J Med 64:564–568, 1978.

Jensen CWB, Flechner SM, Van Buren CT, et al: Exacerbation of cyclosporine toxicity by concomitant administration of erythromycin. Transplantation 43:263–270, 1987.

Johanson WG Jr, Pierce AK, and Sanford JP: Changing pharyngeal bacterial flora of hospitalized patients. N Engl J Med 281:1137–1140, 1969.

Johanson WG Jr, Pierce AK, Sanford JP, et al: Nosocomial respiratory infections with gram-negative bacilli: The significance of colonization of the respiratory tract. Ann Intern Med 77:701–706, 1972.

Johanson WG Jr, Woods DE, and Chaudhuri T: Association of respiratory tract colonization with adherence of gram-negative bacilli to epithelial cells. J Infect Dis 139:667–673, 1979.

Johnson PC, Hamill RJ, and Sarosi GA: Clinical review: Progressive disseminated histoplasmosis in the AIDS patient. Semin Respir Infect 4:139–146, 1989.

Johnson PC, Hogg K, and Sarosi GA: Rapid diagnosis of diffuse pulmonary infections in solid organ transplant recipients. Semin Respir Infect 5:2–9, 1990.

Jones BE, Otaya M, Antoniskis, et al: A prospective evaluation of antituberculosis therapy in patients with human immunodeficiency virus infection. Am J Respir Crit Care Med 150:1499–1502, 1994.

Joshi HN, Localio AR, and Hamory BH: A predictive risk index for nosocomial pneumonia in the intensive care unit. Am J Med 93:135–142, 1992.

Kagawa FT, Kirsch CM, Yenokida GG, et al: Serum lactate dehydrogenase activity in patients with AIDS and Pneumocystis carinii pneumonia: An adjunct to diagnosis. Chest 94:1031–1033, 1988.

Kapila R, Lintz DI, Tecson FT, et al: A nosocomial outbreak of influenza A. Chest 71:576–579, 1977.

Karp JE, Merez WG, Hendricksen C, et al: Oral norfloxacin for prevention of gram-negative bacterial infections in patients with acute leukemia and granulocytopenia. Ann Intern Med 106:1–6, 1987.

Kennedy MS, Degg HJ, Siegel M, et al: Acute renal toxicity with combined use of amphotericin B and cyclosporine after marrow transplantation. Transplantation 35:211–215, 1983.

Kiehn T, Wong B, Edwards FF, et al: Comparative recovery of bacteria and yeast from lysis centrifugation and a conventional blood culture system. J Clin Microbiol 18:300–304, 1983.

Klastersky J, Huysmans E, Weerts D, et al: Endotracheally administered gentamicin for the prevention of infections of the respiratory tract in patients with tracheostomy: A double-blind study. Chest 65:650–654, 1974.

Konrad F, Wiedeck H, Kilian J, et al: Risk factors in nosocomial pneumonia in intensive care patients: A prospective study to identify high-risk patients. Anaesthetist 49:483–490, 1991.

Knight V, McClung HW, Wilson SZ, et al: Ribovirin small-particle aerosol treatment of influenza. Lancet ii:945–949, 1981.

LaForce FM: Hospital acquired gram-negative rod pneumonias: An overview. Am J Med 70:664–669, 1981.

Leclair JM, Freeman J, Sullivan BF, et al: Prevention of nosocomial respiratory syncytial virus infections through compliance with glove and gown precautions. N Engl J Med 317:329–334, 1987.

Levine AS, Siegel SE, Schrieber AD, et al: Protected environments: A prospective controlled study of their utility in the therapy of acute leukemia and lymphoma. N Engl J Med 288:477–483, 1973.

Levine BA, Petroff PA, Slade CL, et al: Prospective trials of dexamethasone and aerosolized gentamicin in the treatment of inhalation injury in the burned patient. J Trauma 18:188–193, 1978.

Lichenstein IH and MacGregor RR: Mycobacterial infections in renal transplant recipients: Report of five cases and review of the literature. Rev Infect Dis 5:216–226, 1983.

Love LJ, Schimpff SC, Schriffer CA, et al: Improved prognosis for granulocytopenic patients with gram-negative bacteremia. Am J Med 68:643–648, 1980.

Luce JM and Clement MJ: Pulmonary diagnostic evaluation in patients suspected of having an HIV-related disease. Semin Respir Infect 4:93–101, 1989.

MacDonald NE, Hall CB, Suffin SC, et al: Respiratory syncytial viral infection in infants with congenital heart disease. N Engl J Med 307:397–400, 1982.

MacDonell KB and Glassroth J: Mycobacterium avium complex and other nontuberculous mycobacteria in patients with HIV infection. Semin Respir Infect 4:123–132, 1989.

Mahul PC, Auboyer RJ, Ros A, et al: Prevention of nosocomial pneumonia in intubated patients: Respective role of mechanical subglottic secretions drainage and stress ulcer prophylaxis. Intensive Care Med 18:20–25, 1992.

Maki DG: Risk factors for nosocomial infection in intensive care. Arch Intern Med 149:30–34, 1989.

Maki DG and Heck TJ: Antiseptic-containing handwashing agents reduce nosocomial infections—a prospective study (Abstract 699). Abstracts of the Twenty-second Interscience Conference on Antimicrobial Agents and Chemotherapy, Miami Beach, 1982.

Maki DG, Karreman E, Glass N, et al: Controlled double-blind study of TMP/SMZ prophylaxis in renal transplantation (RT): TMP/SMZ toxicity and interaction with cyclosporine A (CSA). In Program and Abstracts 25th Interscience

Conference on Antimicrobial Agents and Chemotherapy, Minneapolis, 1985.

Malecka-Griggs B and Reinhardt DJ: Direct dilution sampling, quantitation and microbial assessment of open-system ventilation circuits in intensive care units. J Clin Microbiol 17:870–877, 1983.

Mandell GL, Kaye D, Levison ME, et al: Enterococcal endocarditis: An analysis of 38 patients observed at the New York Hospital–Cornell Medical Center. Arch Intern Med 125:258–264, 1970.

Mauer JR, Tullis ED, Grossman RF, et al: Infectious complications following isolated lung transplantation. Chest 101:1056–1059, 1992.

Mehtar S, Drabu YJ, Vijeratnam S, et al: Cross infection with *Streptococcus pneumoniae* through a resuscitaire. Br Med J 292:25–26, 1986.

Meibalane R, Sedmak GV, Sasidharan PS, et al: Outbreak of influenza in a neonatal intensive care unit. J Pediatr 91:974–976, 1977.

Montgomery AB: *Pneumocystis carinii* pneumonia in patients with the acquired immunodeficiency syndrome: Pathophysiology, therapy and prevention. Semin Respir Infect 4:102–110, 1989.

Moore FA, Moore EE, Jones TN, et al: TEN versus TPN following major abdominal trauma: Reduced septic mortality. J Trauma 29:916–923, 1989.

Muckelmann R, Kunkel G, Staib R, et al: Respirationsallergien verursacht durck Aspergillus-Arten aus der Topferde von Zimmerpflanzen. Prax Pneumol 8:343–350, 1981.

Muder RR, Yu VL, McClure JK, et al: Nosocomial legionnaires' disease uncovered in a prospective pneumonia study. JAMA 249:3184–3188, 1983.

Munda R, Alexander JW, First MR, et al: Pulmonary infections in renal transplant recipients. Ann Surg 187:126–133, 1978.

Murphy S and Florman AL: Lung defenses against infection: A clinical correlation. Pediatrics 72:1–15, 1983.

Murray JF, Felton CP, Garay SM, et al: Pulmonary complications of the acquired immunodeficiency syndrome: Report at National Heart, Lung and Blood Institute workshop. N Engl J Med 310:1682–1688, 1984.

Nicholson V and Johnson PC: Infectious complications in solid organ transplant recipients. Surg Clin North Am 74:5:1223–1245, 1994.

O'Donoghue JM, Ray CG, Terry DW Jr, et al: Prevention of nosocomial influenza infection with amantadine. Am J Epidemiol 97:276–282, 1973.

Ognibene FP, Steis RG, Macher AM, et al: Kaposi's sarcoma causing pulmonary infiltrates and respiratory failure in the acquired immunodeficiency syndrome. Ann Intern Med 102:471–475, 1985.

Patriarca PA, Weber JA, Parker RA, et al: Efficacy of influenza vaccine in nursing homes: Reduction in illness and complications during an influenza A (H3N2) epidemic. JAMA 253:1136–1139, 1985.

Pennington JE: Penetration of antibiotics into respiratory secretions. Rev Infect Dis 3:67–73, 1981.

Peterson PK, Balfour HH, Fryd DS, et al: Fever in renal transplant recipients: Causes, prognostic significance and changing patterns at the University of Minnesota hospital. Am J Med 71:345–351, 1981.

Peterson PK, Balfour HH, Marker SC, et al: Cytomegalovirus disease in renal allograft recipients: A prospective study of the clinical features, risk factors and impact on renal transplantation. Medicine 59:283, 1980.

Pettersson E, Hovi T, Ahonen J, et al: Prophylactic oral acyclovir after renal transplantation. Transplantation 39:279–281, 1985.

Philip JR and Spencer RC: Secondary respiratory infections in hospital patients: Effect of antimicrobial agents and environment. Br Med J 2:359–362, 1974.

Pizzo PA: Empirical therapy and prevention of infection in the immunocompromised host. In Mandell GL, Douglas RG Jr, and Bennett JE (eds): Principles and Practice of Infectious Diseases, 3rd ed. New York, Churchill Livingstone, 1989, pp 2303–2312.

Pizzo PA, Robichaud KS, Gill FA, et al: Empiric antibiotic and antifungal therapy for cancer patients with prolonged fever and granulocytopenia. Am J Med 72:101–111, 1982.

Ramsey PG, Rubin RH, Tolkoff-Rubin NE, et al: The renal transplant patient with fever and pulmonary infiltrates: Etiology, clinical manifestations, and management. Medicine 59(3):206–222, 1980.

Reinarz JA, Pierce AK, Mays BB, et al: The potential role of inhalation therapy equipment in nosocomial pulmonary infections. J Clin Invest 44:831–839, 1965.

Reynolds HY: Normal and defective respiratory host defenses. In Pennington JE (ed): Respiratory Infections: Diagnosis and Management. New York, Raven Press, 1983.

Rhame FS, Streifel A, McComb C, et al: Bubbling humidifiers produce microaerosols which can carry bacteria. Infect Control 7:403–407, 1986.

Rodriguez V, Bodey GP, Freireich EJ, et al: Randomized trial of protected environment-prophylactic antibiotics in 145 adults with acute leukemia. Medicine 57:253–266, 1978.

Rubin RH: Pre-emptive therapy in immunocompromised hosts. N Engl J Med 324:1057–1059, 1991.

Rubin RH, Wolfson JS, Cosimi AB, et al: Infection in the renal transplant recipient. Am J Med 70:405–411, 1981.

Saag MS, Powderly WG, Cloud GA, et al and the Mycosis Study Group and the AIDS Clinical Trials Group: Comparison of amphotericin B with fluconazole in the treatment of acute AIDS-associated cryptococcal meningitis. N Engl J Med 326:83–89, 1992.

Salata RA, Lederman MM, Shales DM, et al: Diagnosis of nosocomial pneumonia in intubated, intensive care patients. Am Rev Respir Dis 135:426–432, 1987.

Schmid RE, Anhalt JP, Wold AD, et al: Sputum

counterimmunoelectrophoresis in the diagnosis of pneumococcal pneumonia. Am Rev Respir Dis 119:345–348, 1979.

Schwartz SN, Dowling JN, Benkovic C, et al: Sources of gram-negative bacilli colonizing the tracheae of intubated patients. J Infect Dis 138:227–231, 1978.

Scroggs MW, Wolfe JA, Bollinger RR, et al: Causes of death in renal transplant recipients: A review of autopsy findings from 1966 through 1985. Arch Pathol Lab Med 111:983–987, 1987.

Selik RM, Starcher ET, and Curran JW: Opportunistic diseases reported in AIDS patients: Frequencies, associations and trends. AIDS 1:175–182, 1987.

Sickles EA, Young VM, Greene WH, et al: Pneumonia in acute leukemia. Ann Intern Med 79:528–535, 1973.

Simmons BP and Wong ES: Guidelines for prevention of nosocomial pneumonia. Infect Control 3:327–333, 1982.

Small PM, Schecter GF, Goodman PC, et al: Treatment of tuberculosis in patients with advanced human immunodeficiency virus infection. N Engl J Med 324:289–294, 1991.

Snydman DR, Greer C, Meissner HC, et al: Prevention of nosocomial transmission of respiratory syncytial virus in a newborn nursery. Infect Control Hosp Epidemiol 9:105–108, 1988.

Snydman DR, Werner BG, Heinze-Lacey B, et al: Use of cytomegalovirus immunoglobulin to prevent cytomegalovirus disease in renal transplant recipients. N Engl J Med 317:1049–1054, 1987.

Stange K and Bygdeman RP: Do moisture exchangers prevent patient contamination of ventilators? Acta Anaesthesiol Scand 24:487–490, 1980.

Stover DE, White DA, Romano PA, et al: Spectrum of pulmonary diseases associated with the acquired immunodeficiency syndrome. Am J Med 78:429–437, 1985.

Thompson JF, Chalmers DHK, Hunnisett AGW, et al: Nephrotoxicity of trimethoprim and cotrimoxazole in renal allograft recipients treated with cyclosporine. Transplantation 36:204–206, 1983.

Toews GB: Southwestern internal medicine conference: Nosocomial pneumonia. Am J Med Sci 291:355–366, 1986.

Valenti WM, Hall CB, Douglas RG Jr, et al: Nosocomial viral infections. I: Epidemiology and significance. Infect Control Hosp Epidemiol 1:33–37, 1980.

Valenti WM, Trudell RG, and Bentley DW: Factors predisposing to oropharyngeal colonization with gram-negative bacilli in the aged. N Engl J Med 298:1108–1111, 1978.

Valles J, Artigas A, Rello J, et al: Continuous aspiration of subglottic secretions in preventing ventilator-associated pneumonia. Ann Intern Med 122:179–186, 1995.

Van Buren D, Wideman CA, Reid M, et al: The antagonistic effect of rifampin upon cyclosporine bioavailability. Transplant Proc 16:1642–1645, 1984.

Wallace JM, Batra P, Gong H, et al: Percutaneous needle lung aspiration for diagnosing pneumonitis in the patient with acquired immunodeficiency syndrome (AIDS). Am Rev Respir Dis 131:389–392, 1985.

Weiner RS, Bortin MM, Gale RP, et al: Interstitial pneumonitis after bone marrow transplantation: Assessment of risk factors. Ann Intern Med 104:168–175, 1986.

Winston DJ, Ho WG, and Cole RP: Therapeutic granulocyte transfusions for documented infections: A controlled trial in ninety-five infectious granulocytomenic episodes. Ann Intern Med 97:509–515, 1982.

Woods DE, Straus DC, Johanson WG Jr, et al: Role of salivary protease activity in adherence of gram-negative bacilli to mammalian buccal epithelial cells in vivo. J Clin Invest 68:1435–1440, 1981.

Wright DG, Robichaud KJ, Pizzo PA, et al: Lethal pulmonary reactions associated with the combined use of amphotericin B and leukocyte transfusions. N Engl J Med 304:1186–1189, 1981.

Zaman MK and White DA: Serum lactate dehydrogenase levels and Pneumocystis carinii pneumonia. Am Rev Respir Dis 137:796–800, 1988.

Deep Venous Thrombosis and Pulmonary Embolism

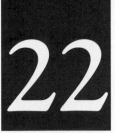

Gilbert E. D'Alonzo, D.O.

Every physician involved in patient care encounters patients at risk for venous thromboembolism. Despite our ability to diagnose and treat this problem, there continues to be unacceptably high morbidity and mortality associated with its underdiagnosis and improper treatment. Recognizing patients at risk for deep venous thrombosis is essential if we are to reduce the overall impact that this disease has on patients in our care.

Many of the deaths that occur from thromboembolic disease are in patients for whom the diagnosis was not considered and therapy was never administered. There is evidence to suggest that deep venous thrombosis occurs in more than 5 million patients each year. More than 500,000 people eventually develop pulmonary thromboemboli, which is a primary cause of death or contributing cause of death in more than 100,000 patients annually in the United States (Dalen and Alpert, 1975). If pulmonary embolism is diagnosed and patients survive for more than 1 hour, mortality is less than 10%; however, if the diagnosis of pulmonary embolism is missed, mortality is fourfold to sixfold greater (Dalen and Alpert, 1975; Urokinase Trial, 1973).

The presence of concomitant diseases, some of which are characterized by many of the clinical features of pulmonary embolism and deep venous thrombosis, compound the difficulty of diagnosing venous thromboembolism (Rubinstein et al, 1988; Sandler and Martin, 1989). The clinician must be aware of the multiple and complex clinical manifestations of venous thromboembolism, maintaining a keen level of suspicion. The best approach to this problem, however, is the development of protocols that enhance awareness for and prophylaxis of deep venous thrombosis in patients who are at high risk.

VENOUS THROMBOSIS AND THE HYPERCOAGULABLE STATE

Venous thrombosis is an inevitable precursor of pulmonary thromboembolism, and a clear understanding of its pathophysiology is necessary. If venous thrombosis is prevented, pulmonary embolism does not occur. To prevent venous thrombosis embolism, one must understand the hypercoagulable state.

Various clinical conditions, diseases, and laboratory markers have been associated with an apparent patient predisposition for the development of deep venous thrombosis. Many of these risk factors have been associated with one or more of the classic thrombogenic alterations that have been recognized as being responsible for the development of the hypercoagulable state. Clinical conditions and diseases associated with venostasis, vascular injury, or enhanced blood viscosity increase the risk for deep venous thrombosis (Virchow 1862). More than one factor generally is present in patients with deep venous thrombosis, and it is thought that risk factors are cumulative in enhancing thrombogenic potential (Cogo et al, 1994; Wheeler et al, 1982). Immobilization, obesity, surgical and nonsurgical trauma, congestive heart failure, and previous thromboembolic disease are additional risk factors or at least coexisting factors associated with thromboembolism. Uncommon disorders such as Behçet's syndrome (Chajek et al, 1973), systemic lupus erythematosus (Mueh et al, 1980), polycythemia vera (Parker and Smith, 1958), homocystinuria (Harker et al, 1974; Mudd et al, 1985; Rees and Rodgers, 1993), and paroxysmal nocturnal hemoglobinuria (Rosse and Ware, 1995; Sirchia and Lewis, 1975) have all been associated with venous thromboembolism. Immobilization is often associated with trauma, malignancy, and cardiopulmonary disease (Cogo et al, 1994; Ibarra Pérez et al, 1988; Kierkegaard et al, 1987).

The length of immobilization (Gibbs, 1957), as well as the increasing age of the patient (Cogo et al, 1994), seems to increase the frequency of deep venous thrombosis. Elderly patients have venous dilatation (Gibbs, 1957) and reduced fibrinolytic response (Robertson et al, 1972), as compared with younger patients. Low vascular fibrinolytic activity has been associated with obesity (Almer and Janzon, 1975). Thromboembolic risk after surgical or nonsurgical trauma appears to be related to the severity, site, and extent of the trauma, length of surgery, immobilization factors, age of the patient, and previous thromboembolic episodes (Hull et al, 1986a). The posttraumatic setting is the paradigm for the hypercoagulable state. In a rigorous prospective study performed at a regional trauma center, noninvasive lower extremity venous studies were performed in more than 700 patients and venography in nearly 350 (Greets et al, 1994). Fifty-eight percent had lower extremity deep venous thrombosis; for 18% it was proximal in location. For this particular study, multivariate analysis revealed five independent risk factors for thrombosis, including older age, need for blood transfusions, need for surgery, fracture of long bones or bones of the pelvis, and spinal cord injury.

Most postoperative thrombosis develops in the calf (Bauer, 1940; Kakkar et al, 1969b) and eventually extends proximally before pulmonary thromboembolism occurs. Isolated calf thrombosis is often asymptomatic (Kakkar et al, 1970), contributing to a delay in diagnosis. It is not until the clot extends proximally (Kakkar et al, 1969b; Langerstedt et al, 1985; Philbrick and Becker, 1988) that it becomes clinically important and dangerous (Moser and LeMoine, 1981; Sevitt and Gallagher, 1959). Untreated or undertreated calf vein thrombosis has a 20 to 30% risk of proximal extension, which usually occurs soon after the calf thrombosis forms (Hirsh, 1992). In a study in which pulmonary embolism was found at autopsy as the cause of death, 24% of cases had undergone surgery a mean period of 7 days before the fatal embolic event (Sandler and Martin, 1989).

Among patients with heart disease, chronic cardiac failure is associated with a frighteningly high incidence of deep venous thrombosis, with pulmonary embolism found at autopsy in more than 50% of cases (Anderson and Hull, 1950).

Reducing the length of immobility and administering prophylactic anticoagulant therapy have dramatically lowered the incidence of clinically recognized thromboembolic disease in cardiac patients (Anderson and Hull, 1950; Warlow et al, 1974).

Like cardiac patients, those with malignancies are at increased risk for the development of thromboembolic disease (Anlyan et al, 1956; Hirsh, 1977; Kakkar et al, 1970; NIH Consensus Conference, 1986; Nordstrom et al, 1994; Pineo et al, 1974). More than 100 years ago, Trousseau (1882) described recurrent migratory venous thrombosis of both superficial and deep veins in patients with visceral malignancies (Lieberman et al, 1961; Rickles and Edwards, 1983; Sack et al, 1977). Isolated deep venous thrombosis, however, is a more common presentation associated with cancer. It has been recognized in patients with occult cancer (Aderka et al, 1986; Gore et al, 1982; Nordstrom et al, 1994; Prandoni et al, 1992b). Venous thrombosis may occur weeks or even months before the diagnosis of malignancy and when recognized is difficult to treat.

The incidence of thromboembolic disease during pregnancy is seven times greater than in age-matched nonpregnant women (Inman and Vessay, 1978; McDevitt and Smith, 1969). Approximately two thirds of embolic events are recognized in the immediate postpartum period (Henderson et al, 1972). Lower extremity venous compression (Ikard et al, 1971), venous dilation (Goodrich and Wood, 1964), thrombocytosis, increased platelet adhesiveness (Wright, 1942; Yggi, 1969), and decreased fibrinolytic activity have all been identified in the third trimester and during labor (Bonnar et al, 1969; Yggi, 1969). The release of tissue thromboplastin seems to occur during placental separation (Yggi, 1969). Furthermore, the incidence of fatal pulmonary thromboembolism after a cesarean section is nine times greater than after an uncomplicated vaginal delivery. Thromboembolic risk is higher in women who use oral contraceptives (Gerstman et al, 1991; Goodrich and Wood, 1964; Jeffcoate et al, 1968; Vessey and Doll, 1969), and the risk appears to be related to the dosage of the estrogen component rather than the progesterone (Inman et al, 1970). Low-dose estrogen contraception reduces the thromboembolic risk but does not negate it (Gerstman et al, 1991; Helmrich et al, 1987).

A new group of patients has been identified who carry a mutation of factor V that destroys an activated protein C cleavage site (factor V Leiden), enhancing thrombosis risk (Bertina et al, 1994). Five percent of the general population may be affected, and thus this mechanism may account for a high percentage of patients with recurrent deep venous thromboses (Koster et al, 1993; Sun et al, 1994). In regard to factor V Leiden and oral contraceptives, Vandenbroucke and colleagues (1994) studied 155 women ages 15 to 49 years in whom deep venous thrombosis developed. They compared this group with age-matched controls. The risk of thrombosis was increased fourfold among oral contraceptive users compared with controls. In addition, the risk of thrombosis was increased eightfold in carriers of the factor V Leiden mutation compared with noncarriers. The combination of oral contraceptive therapy and inheritance of this mutation increased the risk by more than thirtyfold. Oral contraceptive therapy should be avoided in patients who have the factor V Leiden mutation as well as in patients who have additional risk factors such as obesity, immobilization, and recent surgery or trauma.

A number of other laboratory abnormalities are correlated with an increased incidence of thrombosis development. These abnormalities are either inherited or acquired; they may be related to a variety of disease states or clinical conditions. The most clearly recognized inherited hypercoagulable states are those with either qualitative or quantitative deficiencies of plasma proteins involved as natural anticoagulants or of those in the fibrinogen/fibrinolytic pathways. Deficient factors include antithrombin III (AT III), protein C, protein S, and protein C substrate (activated protein C); abnormalities of factors in the plasma fibrinolytic system also occur, such as in plasminogen, plasminogen activator, and even fibrinogen itself.

Families have been described with inherited AT-III deficiency and a history of thromboembolic events. Inheritance occurs in an autosomal dominant pattern (Carvalho and Ellman, 1976; Demers et al, 1992; Egeberg, 1965; Johansson et al, 1978b). Clinical manifestations include thrombosis of the deep venous system, including the legs and other sites like the mesenteric veins, as well as pulmonary embolism. For many patients the syndrome begins and is recognized in the first decade of life and increases in intensity and prevalence with age. In others, a predisposing state, such as the initiation of oral contraceptive therapy (Sagar et al, 1976), pregnancy, or trauma (Owen and Bowie, 1982), helps to initiate the thromboembolic episode. Heparin therapy itself lowers plasma AT-III levels (Marciniak and Gockerman, 1977). When screening for AT-III deficiency, plasma levels are best measured at a time distant from the acute thromboembolic event when the patient is not on anticoagulant therapy.

Protein C deficiency is also an inherited autosomal dominant condition and is similar in many respects to AT-III deficiency clinically (Brockmans et al, 1983; Griffin et al, 1981). Thromboembolic events usually begin before the age of 20 years and increase in frequency with age. Although deep venous thrombosis and pulmonary embolism are responsible for the majority of clinical manifestations, cerebral vein and mesenteric vein thrombosis have been reported. Most patients with protein C deficiency are heterozygotes with protein C levels of 50% of normal (Miletich, 1990). A subset of patients have been identified who carry a factor V mutation that destroys activated protein C and enhances thromboembolism risk.

Warfarin-induced skin necrosis is a complication that can occur in patients with heterozygous protein C deficiency (McGehec et al, 1984). Truncal and extremity purpuric skin lesions develop within the first few days or weeks of warfarin therapy and can proceed to full-thickness skin necrosis. Intravascular fibrin thrombi occluding the skin vasculature can be found on biopsy. Warfarin-induced skin necrosis is the result of the development of a hypercoagulable state caused by an immediate depression of protein C levels early during warfarin therapy in the presence of near-normal or relatively higher levels of coagulation factors IX, X, and prothrombin, all of which have much longer plasma half lives than protein C.

Protein S functions as a cofactor in the activation of protein C. Families have been reported whose members have recurrent episodes of venous thromboembolic phenomena associated with deficiency of plasma protein S (Comp and Esmon, 1984; Engesser et al, 1987; McGehec et al, 1984). Like protein C and AT-III deficiency, these patients can manifest complex and unusual deep venous thrombotic states with pulmonary embolic episodes. This condition is inherited by an autosomal dominant pattern with heterozygotes having about 50% of normal total protein S levels.

Acquired protein C and S deficiencies have been described in patients with liver disease, disseminated intravascular coagulopathy, trauma, and various other high-risk conditions previously mentioned, such as pregnancy (Comp et al, 1986; D'Angelo et al, 1986, 1988; Mannucci and Vigano, 1982; Vigano-D'Angelo et al, 1987). In fact, decreases in protein S levels have been reported in patients infected with the human immunodeficiency virus (Stahl et al, 1993), which most likely places them at additional risk for thrombotic disease.

Perhaps the most common acquired hypercoagulable state involves the presence of a lupus-type inhibitor or anticoagulant (LAC) (Alarcon-Segovia et al, 1989; Petri et al, 1987). The presence of LAC can prolong the activated partial thromboplastin time (APTT). LAC is generally considered to be targeted against anionic phospholipids. Anticardiolipin antibodies (ACA) are antibodies detected by immunologic assays using cardiolipin as the antigen (Triplett, 1993). LAC and ACA occur in 30% and 40% of patients with systemic lupus erythematosus, respectively, and also occur in patients with other rheumatic disorders, lymphoproliferative diseases, acquired immunodeficiency disease syndrome (AIDS), and various acute infections (Love and Santoro, 1990). They can also occur in individuals with no known disease at all (Fields et al, 1989).

The presence of LAC and ACA is associated with enhanced thrombotic tendency, rather than bleeding. Furthermore, LAC and ACA have been associated with recurrent fetal loss and thrombocytopenia, and all of these manifestations have been referred to as the *antiphospholipid antibody syndrome* (Harris et al, 1986). Both the arterial and venous circulations are at risk for recurrent thrombotic events; however, in a given patient either one system or the other usually predominates (Khamashta et al, 1995; Rosove and Brewer, 1992). Lupus anticoagulant or anticardiolipin antibodies can be detected by blood testing.

Patients receiving heparin by any route of administration can develop thrombocytopenia, which seems to be an immune-mediated reaction (Bell and Royall, 1980). Up to 20% of patients who develop thrombocytopenia may subsequently develop a morbid, severe thrombotic diathesis (Warkentin and Kelton, 1989; 1990; 1991). Thrombocytopenia often occurs 5 to 10 days after initiation of heparin, but the time relationship to heparin administration can be remote and even complex. Arterial and venous thromboses involving medium and large vessels can cause devastating conditions, including lower limb ischemia, mesenteric and renal ischemia, and even coronary vessel occlusion. Pre-existing vascular damage, such as at the site of an arterial graft (Makhoul and McCann, 1986), may be a predisposing factor. Of the various laboratory studies used to diagnose heparin-induced thrombocytopenia (HIT), the best test is heparin-dependent release of ^{14}C-serotonin from washed normal platelets in the presence of the patient's plasma (Warkentin and Kelton, 1990). When suspected, heparin should be immediately stopped and an alternative intervention employed. If heparin is continued and HIT is allowed to persist, morbidity is high, with major sequelae including limb amputation, neurologic defects, and even death (Aster, 1995).

The presence of abnormal fibrinogen can predispose patients to thrombosis (Martinez, 1991). These variant fibrinogens have been detected by abnormalities in the thrombin time and reptilase time, which are prolonged. The mechanisms by which abnormal fibrinogens lead to increased thrombosis remain unknown. Impaired release of fibrinopeptides A and B from the molecule by thrombin, which is a step required for conversion of fibrinogen to fibrin, abnormal binding of plasminogen to fibrin, and abnormal resistance to lysis by plasmin have all been identified. Both arterial and venous thrombosis have been identified. In contrast, abnormalities in the fibrinolytic system have been described (Heijboer et al, 1990; Johansson et al, 1978a). Decreased levels of plasminogen and abnormalities in the plasminogen molecule have been identified. Other abnormalities of the fibrinolytic system have been reported and include high plasma levels of plasminogen activator inhibitor and low plasma levels or impaired release of tissue-type plasminogen activator (Lijnen and Collen, 1989). These conditions are rare and difficult to diagnose.

DETECTION OF LOWER EXTREMITY VENOUS THROMBOSIS

Clinically important emboli arise mainly from thrombi in the deep veins of the lower extremities (Havig, 1977; Hull et al, 1981a; Sevitt and Gallagher, 1961). Some patients have emboli coming from the pelvis, right side of the heart, and upper extremity veins. With the increased use of central venous catheters, a higher incidence of subclavian and internal jugular vein thrombosis has been identified (Donayre et al, 1986; Horatlaset et al, 1988; Monreal et al, 1991; Warden et al, 1973). Rarely, veins that drain into the internal iliac system, such as the prostatic and uterine veins, may be responsible for emboli, but normally these emboli are small because the vessels themselves are small in comparison with those of the central deep venous system. Right ventricular infarction or any condition with severe right ventricular or right atrial dilation can predispose a patient to pulmonary emboli because of the formation of intracardiac thrombi. Renal vein thrombosis should be considered in patients with hematuria and flank pain.

From autopsy studies, a large percentage of cases, almost one third, were found to have clinically important thromboemboli. The most proximal location of the deep venous clot was found below the knee (Havig, 1977). It is thought that in many of these cases, the thrombosis in the lower extremities extended up into the proximal deep venous system of the knee or thigh before being released and embolized to the lung.

The clinical diagnosis of acute deep venous thrombosis of the lower extremities is both insensitive and nonspecific (Cranley et al, 1976; Haeger, 1969). It is insensitive because thrombosis often is present but the clinical manifestations are absent. Erythema, pain, and swelling are often not found because the phlebitic component to the thrombotic process is not present or is clinically insignificant, often because venous blood flow is not completely obstructed. In those patients with absent or minor symptoms, dangerous venous thrombosis can still be present. The triad of leg pain, erythema, and swelling is nonspecific because these classic symptoms of thrombophlebitis when present may not be caused by venous thrombosis. When the classic symptoms and signs are present, only 45% of patients have thrombosis proved by venography (Gallus et al, 1976). The eventual diagnosis in those patients who fail to show evidence of thrombosis include disorders of the muscles, cutaneous tissues, joints, lymphatics, bones, and nerves. Objective studies for the diagnosis of deep venous thrombosis can be divided into invasive and noninvasive studies. Each test has its own advantages and disadvantages, with the specific tests chosen depending chiefly on the patient and the question being asked but also on available technologic resources and expertise.

VENOGRAPHY

Contrast venography is the standard method for the diagnosis of venous thrombosis. Venography can demonstrate graphically the presence and extent of filling defects when thrombosis is present. Considerable expertise is necessary not only to perform the test but also to interpret the results (Rabinov and Paulin, 1972). Interpretation can be difficult if technical components of the test prevent an optimal study from being obtained. Interpretation is difficult, particularly when small, nonocclusive thrombi are present. At times, the venous system is not visualized satisfactorily, and this nonvisualization may be due to thrombosis or technical problems. Such problems include an inadequate quantity of contrast material, flow-mixing effects within the vasculature, or increased calf muscle tension that interferes with vascular contrast filling. Ninety percent accuracy for the diagnosis of deep venous thrombosis has been reported with contrast venography (Bounameaux et al, 1993; Sandler et al, 1984; Sauerbrei et al, 1981). Studies have demonstrated contrast venography to be cost-effective (Hull et al, 1981b) in certain clinical situations, particularly those for the diagnosis of deep venous thrombosis in symptomatic patients requiring confirmation when recurrent disease is suspected or, postoperatively, when hip surgery patients are suspected to have thrombosis and noninvasive diagnostic measures cannot be relied upon (Hillner et al, 1992; Paiement et al, 1988).

Contrast venography occasionally may induce minor venous thrombi (Albrechtson and Olsson, 1976) or reactions ranging from discomfort to hypersensitivity. Repetitive contrast venograms are impractical, and the procedure is expensive (Bettman and Paulin, 1977).

IMPEDANCE PLETHYSMOGRAPHY

Impedance plethysmography (IPG) has undergone rigorous testing using methodologically acceptable study design (Hull et al, 1983b; 1985a; 1976). This technique measures blood volume changes of the calf indirectly through alteration in the electrical resistance of the leg to detect the venous thrombosis. Inflation of a thigh cuff causes temporary venous occlusion; venous volume response in the calf is measured during cuff inflation and release. Normally, there is a progressive increase in blood volume of the calf and thigh vasculature that eventually plateaus, followed by a rapid runoff once the cuff occlusion is released. Deep vein thrombosis in the popliteal, femoral, and iliac veins interferes with the normal pressure-volume relationships in the deep venous system, usually preventing normal venous capacitance and obstructing blood outflow. This decrease in capacitance and outflow is shown by a reduced volume increase during cuff inflation and a slow runoff during cuff release. Often, a clear separation of response between patients with deep venous thrombosis and normal individuals is observed (Hull et al, 1976; Wheeler et al, 1974).

IPG is considered to be both sensitive and specific for the diagnosis of symptomatic proximal leg deep venous thrombosis (Hull et al, 1976; Wheeler et al, 1975). It is insensitive to thrombosis of the calf veins. Initial studies showed the specificity of IPG, as it correlates with contrast venography, to range between 83 and 100% (Hirsh et al, 1981a; White et al, 1989). A review of multiple studies (Wheeler et al, 1994), separating patients who were symptomatic from those who were asymptomatic for lower extremity deep venous thrombosis, showed even higher specificities, ranging between 94 and 97%, respectively. Many of the asymptomatic patients had IPG performed as part of a surveillance of high-risk patients following hip replacement surgery. Correlation with abnormal venography (sensitivity) has been reported to range between 83 and 100% (Hull et al, 1984; White et al, 1989).

The high sensitivity of IPG for proximal nonocclusive thrombi has been questioned. In a small retrospective study, the sensitivity for IPG for proximal thrombotic disease was 66% (Anderson et al, 1993a). More importantly, in a larger prospective study the sensitivity for proximal disease is reported to be 65% (Ginsburg et al, 1994). This reduced sensitivity was believed to be due to the high frequency of proximal thrombi confined to the popliteal veins (Kearon and Hirsh, 1994) or to a change or shift in the demographics of the patient population studied (Ginsberg et al, 1994) as compared with the older, larger classic studies. In other words, an increase in the number of patients studied who had clinical disease with small nonocclusive clots mainly can explain the discrepancy in sensitivities between earlier and later studies. Contrast venography technique may also be improving to the point that disease is being detected earlier and small thrombi previously missed are being recognized, thereby affecting IPG diagnostic sensitivity. When we review a study that took into account the data from multiple studies (Wheeler et al, 1994), and when we distinguish symptomatic from asymptomatic patients, the diagnostic sensitivity of IPG falls from 90 to 29%, respectively.

False-positive IPG results can occur from unrecognized leg muscle contraction (Biland et al, 1979), which is a problem that can be reduced when the test is performed by an experienced technician. Improper positioning and fitting of the electrodes and cuff, increased central venous pressure, decreased arterial filling, and presence of a large proximal pelvic mass can also cause a false-positive IPG result. A false-negative IPG result can occur when the thrombus is a small, nonocclusive proximal clot. Long-standing proximal disease may be difficult to identify because of the formation of collateral vascular channels or clot recanalization.

A positive IPG result in a patient with clinically suspected venous thromboembolism and without confounding features establishes the diagnosis of deep venous thrombosis. A normal study result excludes the diagnosis of extensive and occlusive proximal deep venous thrombosis. IPG does not confirm a diagnosis of calf vein thrombosis, a condition that does not have to be treated with anticoagulant therapy if the results of repeated IPG studies remain negative. If there is a suspicion for more proximal disease developing, which can occur by popliteal extension of clot from the calf vein thrombosis in 20 to 30% of patients, it generally is during the first 7 days of presentation and can be detected by performing serial IPG testing over a 2-week period (Huisman et al, 1986, 1989a; Hull et al, 1985a). Serial IPG testing can thus be used strategically in patients with adequate cardiopulmonary reserves and nondiagnostic lung scans to identify a group who will eventually develop proximal vein thrombosis and require treatment. This sequential or serial noninvasive testing process can avoid the need for angiography and for some patients, the need for treatment (Hull et al, 1994).

Hull and colleagues (1990a) followed pregnant women with suspected deep vein thrombosis in whom anticoagulant therapy was withheld because serial IPG test results remained negative over 14 days. None of the patients who had anticoagulation therapy withheld developed thromboembolic disease during 3 months of follow-up. Other larger studies in nonpregnant patients have shown similar findings (Huisman et al, 1988; Wheeler et al, 1982).

When the results of these studies are pooled, patients suspected of having thromboembolic disease with negative serial IPG study results have a 1 to 2% risk of having an acute thromboembolic event despite not having received anticoagulant therapy, and the risk for a fatal event is nearly nonexistent. These outcome results are similar to those that are achieved when anticoagulation is used for patients with documented thromboembolic disease (Hull et al, 1994).

The frequency of repeated IPGs can range from four to six studies performed over a 10- to 14-day period. Therefore, if the reports of a lower sensitivity of IPG testing prove to be accurate, the probability of an adverse clinical outcome as a result of undiagnosed disease in acute presentations may still be extremely low.

Serial IPG measurements seem to be helpful in the follow-up of patients with proven deep venous disease to re-establish a "baseline" reference for comparative use in those patients with recurrent symptoms (Huisman et al, 1988).

ULTRASOUND TECHNIQUES

Duplex ultrasound examination is now considered the primary imaging test for patients suspected of having deep vein thrombosis (Pearson et al, 1995; Talbot, 1982). Unlike IPG, which is a hemodynamic test, ultrasound imaging can directly visualize thrombosis noninvasively and assess the deep venous system of the lower extremity for patency, blood flow, and thrombosis (Flanagan et al, 1985; Lensing et al, 1989). Furthermore, when a Doppler component is added, thrombi can be identified by their noncompressibility and by absent or altered flow sounds (Polak, 1991). Like IPG, ultrasonography is helpful mainly in the diagnosis of femoral and popliteal clots. There is a question as to how useful it is for diagnosis of calf and iliac thrombi. An analysis of 15 studies (Becker et al, 1989) evaluated duplex sonography for its ability to help diagnose lower extremity venous thrombosis, comparing results with this technique with those of contrast venography. Sensitivity and specificity varied in those studies from 78 to 100%. For femoral and popliteal disease, however, the mean sensitivity and specificity were 96% and 99%, respectively.

At our institution, duplex ultrasonography and venography were compared in more than 225 consecutive patients suspected of having deep vein thrombosis (Comerota et al, 1988). Ultrasonography had a sensitivity of 99% and specificity of 100% for proximal leg thrombosis and a sensitivity of 70% for calf thrombosis. Like IPG testing, however, lower sensitivities have been reported for asymptomatic patients with deep vein thrombosis (Davidson et al, 1992; Lensing et al, 1994; Wells et al, 1995). Pooled results from several studies revealed a 50 to 76% sensitivity for proximal deep vein thrombosis, but duplex ultrasonography remained highly specific (96 to 98%) (Comerota et al, 1993; Lensing et al, 1994). The results in any individual hospital are dependent on the expertise of the technician. Small nonocclusive clots may explain these results, and venography may be the only reliable test for the diagnosis of deep vein thrombosis in these high-risk asymptomatic patients if a diagnosis is highly suspected and immediately needed.

Serial duplex ultrasonography measurements, like IPG, have been found to be a good diagnostic approach for patients suspected of having deep venous thrombosis when the initial test was found to be nondiagnostic (Cronan et al, 1988; Heijboer et al, 1993). Because of its enhanced ability to evaluate the popliteal vein, it most likely has an important role in the diagnosis of suspected progressive deep venous disease. In patients with repeatedly normal results, prevalence of thromboembolism over a 6-month follow-up period was acceptably low (Heijboer et al, 1993).

ADDITIONAL DIAGNOSTIC METHODS

It would be extremely helpful to have a blood test that could help to diagnose the presence of venous thromboembolic disease. A large number of tests have been investigated, without success. Measurement of plasma deoxyribonucleic acid (DNA) (Vargo, et al, 1990) initially showed some promise, but it is not available to most clinicians and seems to lack specificity and sensitivity. Because of these problems, it has not yet been tested prospectively for a suitable role in the diagnostic algorithm of venous thromboembolism.

The level of D-dimer, a specific derivative of cross-linked fibrin that can be found in the plasma of patients with thromboembolism, has shown particular promise. A plasma D-dimer level below 500 µg/l has been shown to statistically rule out the diagnosis of pulmonary embolism (Bounameaux et al, 1991) in a group of patients with nondiagnostic lung scans. This test can be done rapidly (Dale et al, 1994). The sensitivity and negative predictive value has been reported at 98%. Unfortunately, the positive predictive value and specificity is 44% and 39%, respectively (Bounameaux et al, 1991; 1992; 1994). These preclude it from use as a test for diagnosing thromboembolism. Goldhaber and colleagues (1993) have found similar results.

A technique that labels thrombin protein (Pollak et al, 1975), red blood cells (Leclerc et al, 1988), or platelets (Fenech et al, 1980), employing radionuclide venography (Bentley and Kakkar, 1979), can be utilized to locate thrombus in the deep venous system. A similar technique employing radiolabeled monoclonal antibodies (Alavi et al, 1990; Peters et al, 1986) to cross-linked fibrin also shows promise. Computer-assisted tomography and magnetic resonance venography have both been tried as diagnostic tools for deep vein thrombosis, but both techniques have high cost and are not always available. These tools may have definite advantages in exceptional situations. For example, they may be helpful in imaging thrombosis in the deep veins of the abdomen and pelvis (Bauer and Flyn, 1988; Orron et al, 1992; Vogelzang, 1991) or extensive disease in the iliofemoral veins or vena cava (Carpenter et al, 1993; Evans et al, 1993; Spritzer et al, 1993).

PRACTICAL APPROACH TO THE DIAGNOSIS OF DEEP VENOUS THROMBOSIS

Because there are numerous tests that can be employed, several approaches can be taken to establish a diagnosis of deep venous thrombosis before treatment is initiated. If contrast venography is the only available diagnostic test, it should be performed when disease is suspected. Noninvasive tests often make venography unnecessary, and duplex ultrasonography is the diagnostic test of choice (Fig. 22–1).

If results of duplex ultrasonography are positive and conditions known to cause false-positive results are absent, a diagnosis of deep venous thrombosis can be made and anticoagulant therapy initiated. An unexpectedly high prevalence of silent pulmonary emboli exist in patients with deep venous thrombosis (Huisman et al 1989b; Moser et al, 1994). If the initial noninvasive study result is negative, duplex ultrasonography can be repeated in a serial fashion over a 2-week period in an effort to detect extending deep vein thrombosis, or contrast venography can be employed. Because contrast venography is invasive and

costly, serial duplex ultrasonography is generally used.

Because thrombus extension occurs in only a few patients with calf vein thrombosis, it is possible to delay treatment and perform serial noninvasive tests to look for thrombosis extension. It has been proposed that impedance plethysmography or duplex ultrasonography be repeated at 5 and 10 days after the initial study (Dalen, 1993). If the noninvasive test result becomes positive, a diagnosis of clinically significant deep venous thrombosis can be made and anticoagulant therapy instituted. In contrast, if the study results remain negative, anticoagulation can be avoided. Screening of asymptomatic patients among selected patient groups is unsatisfactory with noninvasive testing, and venography should be performed if a strong clinical suspicion for disease exists. This particular recommendation is most significant for patients following orthopedic surgery. Pregnant and nonpregnant patients have had anticoagulant therapy held while serial noninvasive testing (to rule out lower extremity deep venous thrombosis) was being performed, with good results.

A particularly difficult problem is diagnosis of an acute thrombotic disease in a portion of the deep venous system previously involved with thrombosis. Recurrent deep venous thrombosis presents unique diagnostic challenges. One study has provided a practical approach to this problem (Hull et al, 1983a). A diagnostic algorithm for acute recurrent deep venous thrombosis is shown in Figure 22–2. It is helpful to have the results of previous noninvasive tests available to expedite the process of diagnosing acute recurrent deep venous thrombosis. A negative test result pre-

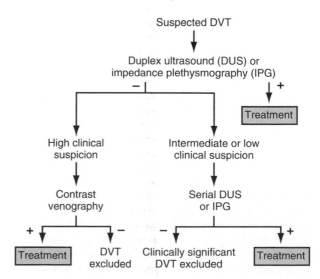

Figure 22–1

Approach to the diagnosis of acute lower extremity deep venous thrombosis (DVT).

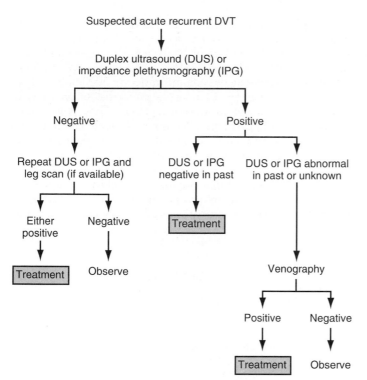

Figure 22–2
Approach to the patient with suspected acute but recurrent DVT.

viously performed with a positive test result currently is diagnostic of acute recurrent disease. A negative test result in an individual suspected of having an acute recurrence should signal the need to have serial noninvasive studies performed for 3 days. If the results are still negative, the diagnosis of acute recurrent deep vein thrombosis is excluded and anticoagulant therapy is not needed. If the study result becomes positive, however, a diagnosis of recurrent disease is made and therapy can be initiated.

Venography should be done in patients (1) known to have a higher likelihood for either false-positive or false-negative results (2) with previously abnormal noninvasive lower extremity testing, and (3) with a noninvasive test result that is positive and the results of a previous study are unknown. Occasionally, results of venography are indeterminate, often because of non- or poorly visualized femoral or iliac veins. In this setting, anticoagulant therapy should be administered, but if the femoral and iliac veins are well visualized the patient should undergo serial noninvasive testing for 3 days. A negative result eliminates the need for therapy. The majority of patients suspected of having deep vein thrombosis can be managed adequately with noninvasive tests when the clinical probability of disease is incorporated into the decision-making process. Discord between the results of noninvasive testing and the

clinical suspicion for deep venous disease requires venography for diagnosis.

PREVENTION OF VENOUS THROMBOEMBOLISM

Prophylactic maneuvers in patients who are at risk for venous thromboembolism are necessary, because most patients who die from pulmonary embolism die rapidly, without the opportunity of receiving therapy. Efficacy, safety, ease of administering and monitoring, and various cost issues are all essential elements when an ideal preventative method is being considered. For venous thromboembolism, pharmacologic and mechanical methods are used, often as combined intervention, in a variety of clinical settings. Low-dose subcutaneous heparin and warfarin have been given as the principal pharmacologic preventative interventions, with some patients receiving intravenous dextran. Aspirin and other antiplatelet agents have no role in preventing venous thrombosis. Low-molecular-weight heparin has been added selectively to this medication armamentarium.

Over the last decade, various mechanical methods have been developed and, in the proper setting, may be applied for the prevention of deep venous thrombosis. Intermittent sequential pneumatic compression devices applied to the lower extremities and graded-compression stockings can be used with or without pharmacologic intervention in this prophylactic process.

The general approach to prophylaxis is to employ the simplest method, which is usually a single modality in the patient at low or medium risk and combined modalities or very special interventions for the patient at higher risk. A strategy for the prevention of deep venous thrombosis according to risk category is shown in Table 22–1 (Clagett and Reisch, 1988; Hull et al, 1986a; Hyers et al, 1995; Imperiale and Speroff, 1994; NIH Consensus Conference, 1986).

Low-dose subcutaneous heparin, administered

at doses of 10,000 to 15,000 units per day in two divided doses has been given as the most frequent method of prophylaxis in both medical and surgical patients. For low- or moderate-risk patients, subcutaneous administration of 5000 units of heparin every 12 hours is preferable to an every-8-hour administration regimen. These lower doses of heparin are effective only before the initiation of intravascular coagulation. Less AT-III activity is necessary to stop coagulation before it is initiated than at a stage when thrombin has already formed. Surgical patients should receive heparin several hours preoperatively, which is continued until the patients are fully ambulatory. Low-dose

Table 22–1

Incidence of Thromboembolic Events After Surgery or Trauma or With Certain Medical Conditions and Recommended Deep Venous Thrombosis (DVT) Prophylaxis

Risk Group and Thromboembolic Incidence		Recommendation
Low Risk		
Under 40 years old		Early ambulation
Minor surgery (<60 min duration)		and
Bedridden, uncomplicated		Graduated-compression stockings (GCS)
Medical patients, pregnancy		
Incidence (%)		
Distal DVT	2–6	
Proximal DVT	0.4–1	
Pulmonary embolism (PE)	0.2–1	
Fatal PE	0.002	
*Moderate Risk**		
Over 40 years old		Early ambulation
Abdominal, pelvic, thoracic surgery		and
Myocardial infarction, cardiomyopathy,		Low-dose heparin (LDH)
previous thromboembolism		or
Incidence (%)		Low-molecular-weight heparin (LMWH)
Distal DVT	8–40	or
Proximal DVT	1–8	Intermittent pneumatic compression (IPC)†
PE	1–8	
Fatal PE	0.1–0.4	
*High Risk**		
Elderly		IPC and LDH
Extended surgery duration		or
Hip and major knee surgery		LMWH and early ambulation
Fractured hip		
Extensive trauma including soft-tissue injury		
and multiple fractures‡		
Stroke		
Incidence (%)		For elective hip and major knee surgery, use
Distal DVT	40–80	low-dose warfarin or adjusted-dose heparin
Proximal DVT	10–20	or LMWH and IPC with early ambulation
PE	5–10	
Fatal PE	1–5	

*Risk is increased further by the following factors: Obesity, prolonged bedrest, estrogens, and venous varicosities.
†IPC is the prophylactic method of choice for neurosurgery, ophthalmologic surgery, certain urologic procedures or when the bleeding risk is considered to be high.
‡Consider early placement of vena cava filter.

heparin has been proved to be efficacious in reducing the frequency of venous thrombosis in patients recovering from myocardial infarction and various general surgeries, and for most patients in intensive care units.

Less success has been noted in patients who undergo major orthopedic surgery, including femoral fracture repair and reconstructive operations of the hips and knees. Heparin is inadequate after prostate surgery and cystectomy. Although low-dose heparin has been shown to reduce the incidence of venous thromboembolism in these patients (Collins et al, 1988), the degree of protection is not sufficient when compared with results found in general surgical patients (Prevention . . . International Trial, 1995). Patients who have had ophthalmologic surgery or neurosurgery should not receive low-dose heparin (Council on Thrombosis, 1977).

Low-molecular-weight heparins (LMWH) are the most recently introduced preparations. These agents have distinct advantages over the conventional unfractionated heparins (Hirsh and Fuster, 1994a). They have a much greater antithrombotic than anticoagulant effect and thus appear to produce less bleeding for an equivalent antithrombotic effect than unfractionated heparin (Levine et al, 1991; Kakkar et al, 1993). In addition, they have a longer half life. LMWH has proven effectiveness at preventing venous thromboembolism in patients undergoing elective general surgery (Bergvist et al, 1986; Caen, 1988; European Fraxiparin Study Group, 1988; Kakkar and Murray, 1985; Kakkar et al, 1993; Koller et al, 1988; Pezzuoli et al, 1990) and elective hip and knee surgery (Anderson et al, 1993b; Colwell et al, 1994; Dechavanne et al, 1989; Erikkson et al, 1988, 1991; Leclerc et al, 1992; Levine et al, 1991; Planes et al, 1988, 1991; Spiro et al, 1994; Turpie, 1991; Turpie et al, 1986), and for those patients who have suffered a thrombotic stroke (Turpie et al, 1987; 1992) and spinal cord injury (Green et al, 1990). When compared with dextran 70 or warfarin, LMWHs have been shown to be more effective in patients having either hip or knee implant surgery (Danish Enoxaparin Study Group, 1991; Hull et al, 1993).

Dextran's ability to protect against pulmonary embolism is about the same as that of low-dose heparin (Bonnar and Walsh, 1972; Bonnar et al, 1973; Carter and Eban, 1973; Heparin, 1974; Kline et al, 1975). It is an acceptable alternative to warfarin therapy, with a lower risk of bleeding (Clagett and Reisch, 1988). In particular, dextran is effective at reducing the incidence of postoperative venous thrombosis in the patient undergoing orthopedic surgery (Ahlberg et al, 1968; Evarts

and Feli, 1971). With the use of dextran, however, there is an increased incidence of congestive heart failure and renal failure, anaphylactoid reactions, and difficulty in cross-matching blood.

Warfarin can be administered in low doses as a prophylactic agent in patients at high risk for developing venous thromboembolism. Such patients include those who have undergone total hip or knee replacement (Amstutz et al, 1989; Francis et al, 1983), surgery for a fractured hip (Savitt and Gallagher, 1961), and general surgery (Taberner et al, 1978). Warfarin has not been widely accepted as a prophylactic agent, for the most part, because of the perception of an increased risk of bleeding and the need for laboratory monitoring. A very-low-dose warfarin intervention (1 mg daily for 6 weeks, adjusted to an INR of 1.3 to 1.9) has been shown to reduce thromboembolic risk in breast cancer patients who are receiving chemotherapy (Levine et al, 1994).

Intermittent sequential pneumatic compression of the legs and plantar foot compression devices, often initiated immediately after the patient is placed on the operating room table, have been shown to effectively reduce the incidence of venous thromboembolism (Hull et al, 1986a; Mittlemann et al, 1982; Nicolaides et al, 1980). These devices are effective prophylaxis for deep venous thrombosis in intermediate-risk patient undergoing general surgery (Borow et al, 1981; Butson 1981; Caprini et al, 1983, 1988; Clark et al, 1974; Colditz et al, 1986), major knee and hip surgery (Harris et al, 1976; Hartman et al, 1982; Hull et al, 1979, 1990c), open urologic procedures (Coe et al, 1978; Salzman et al, 1980), and gynecologic surgery (Clark-Pearson et al, 1984). They also have a substantial role in patients having ophthalmic and neurologic surgery (Black et al, 1986; Skillman et al, 1978; Turpie et al, 1979). For patients, whether medical or surgical, who have a substantial risk of bleeding from pharmacologic prophylaxis, these devices are the prophylaxis of choice. Plantar foot compression devices are attractive because they do not interfere with the lower extremity surgical field, and for some patients they may be more comfortable than sequential compression leg devices (Bradley et al, 1993; Santori et al, 1994). These devices are generally well accepted by the patient and can be removed easily for physical therapy and ambulation.

Some of the failures reported with the use of these devices in preventing lower extremity venous thrombosis may be due to either improper application or reluctance on the part of the patient to wear them regularly (Comerota et al,

1992). Furthermore, it has been suggested that a duplex ultrasound or an IPG examination of the lower extremity be performed in any patient in whom deep venous thrombosis may be suspected, before applying one of these devices.

Graded compression elastic stockings can improve lower extremity venous return and provide a safe, simple, and inexpensive method for preventing deep venous thrombosis when fitted and worn properly (Borow and Goldson, 1981; Burnard and Layer, 1986; Noyes et al, 1987). A meta-analysis has shown that these stockings, when worn in moderate-risk surgical patients, can account for a 68% risk reduction in the incidence of postoperative deep vein thrombosis (Wells et al, 1994). The stockings, when used in combination with heparin (Borow and Goldson, 1983; Torngren, 1980; Willie-Jorgensen et al, 1985), intravenous dextran (Berquist and Lindblad, 1984), and even intermittent sequential pneumatic compression (Hartman et al, 1982; Nicolaides et al, 1983; Scurr et al, 1987) have been shown to enhance the effectiveness of preventing deep venous thrombosis during surgery.

PATHOPHYSIOLOGY OF PULMONARY EMBOLISM

When a deep venous thrombosis embolizes to the lung, the process affects not only the pulmonary circulation but also lung tissue and right- and left-heart function. The degree of cardiopulmonary compromise seems to be correlated with the extent of embolic occlusion and the degree of antecedent cardiopulmonary disease.

RESPIRATORY PATHOPHYSIOLOGY

Pulmonary gas-exchange abnormalities that occur with pulmonary emboli are often complex and multifactorial from a pathophysiologic standpoint (D'Alonzo and Dantzker, 1984). The type and degree of abnormal gas-exchange are influenced by the size of the embolized vessels, completeness of occlusion, degree of underlying cardiopulmonary disease, and time period that has elapsed since embolism has occurred.

Nearly every form of abnormal gas exchange has been described (D'Alonzo et al, 1983; Huet et al, 1985; Manier et al, 1985; Santolicandro et al, 1995; Severinghaus and Stupfel, 1957; Wilson et al, 1971). The fall in oxygen and the hypoxemia and hypercapnia that generally occur are best explained, however, by the presence of ventilation-perfusion inequality and low mixed venous oxygen saturation (Santolicandro et al, 1995).

Lung units with low ventilation-perfusion ratios predominate because of overperfusion of unembolized regions of the lung (Dantzker et al, 1978). Shunt may occur as atelectasis develops in lung tissue beyond the embolic obstruction, and, once reperfusion occurs, lung tissue becomes further compromised with edema and hemorrhage (Caldini, 1965; Wilson et al, 1971). Hemorrhagic atelectasis has been shown to be the result of the loss of surfactant (Chernick et al, 1966), which occurs when the pulmonary artery blood flow is occluded. Regional pulmonary hypoperfusion causes alveolar hypocapnia, which may induce bronchiolar constriction and pneumoconstriction, leading to further atelectasis (the air-shift phenomenon) (Levy and Simmons, 1974). Furthermore, when a pulmonary embolism occurs, there is the transient release of various humoral mediators from blood products, which can promote pneumoconstriction and loss of surfactant, causing atelectasis (Levy and Simmons, 1974, 1975; Wilson et al, 1971). In certain patients, pulmonary edema has been shown to play a role in the development of hypoxemia.

The development of acute pulmonary hypertension and right ventricular overload and failure may induce an intracardiac shunt through a patent foramen ovale (Moorthy and Lasasso, 1974; Moorthy et al, 1978). This mechanism must be taken seriously, because a significant percentage of the normal population has the potential for developing a patent foramen ovale.

The abnormal gas exchange induced by ventilation-perfusion inequality and shunt is usually accentuated by the development of mixed-venous hypoxemia resulting from reduced cardiac output. This may be a particularly significant mechanism in patients with pre-existing heart disease (McIntyre and Sasahara, 1971; 1973).

The majority of patients who develop abnormal parenchymal infiltrates on chest radiographs after pulmonary embolism and hemoptysis have pulmonary hemorrhage. Occasionally, pulmonary infarction and death of lung tissue distal to the vascular obstruction can occur. Lung infarction is infrequent because the lung has multiple oxygen supplies (Butler et al, 1989; Tsao et al, 1982). The bronchial circulation, pulmonary arterial circulation, alveolar oxygen, and back-perfusion from the pulmonary venous side of the circulation all contribute to lung tissue oxygenation. The majority of lung tissue ischemia and infarction occurs in the periphery of the lung, where the bronchial circulation is minimal to nonexistent and other tissue oxygenation mechanisms can be impaired during the acute embolic period. This factor probably explains why lung infarctions are more likely to occur with small peripheral emboli than with large central clots (Dalen et al, 1977). Infarction is also more likely in the presence of left ventricular failure or chronic obstructive lung disease, two clinical states that potentially compromise the oxygen supply to the lungs (Dalen et al, 1977; Moser, 1990).

HEMODYNAMIC PATHOPHYSIOLOGY

The hemodynamic compromise that occurs with acute pulmonary embolism is correlated with the extent of vascular obstruction and degree of previous cardiopulmonary disease (Dexter and Smith, 1964; McIntyre and Sasahara, 1971, 1973; Nelson and Smith, 1959; Parmley et al, 1962). With pulmonary embolism, there is increased resistance to blood flow through the lungs, and if the cardiac output remains constant or increases, pulmonary arterial pressure rises. The maintenance of blood flow through the pulmonary vascular bed depends on the ability of the right ventricle to pump against this additional afterload. In previously normal persons, significant pulmonary hypertension usually does not occur until 50% of the vascular bed is occluded. With more than 50% occlusion, severe pulmonary hypertension results and right ventricular work increases. Because the right ventricle is not equipped to pump against a higher pressure and perform high-intensity work for an extended period, there are limits to the ability of the right ventricle to compensate for embolic occlusion. In patients without previous cardiopulmonary disease, the maximal mean arterial pressure that can be developed and maintained is approximately 40 mm Hg (Dexter and Smith, 1964; McIntyre and Sasahara, 1973; Miller and Sutton, 1970). If this pressure load is excluded, right ventricular failure, acute cor pulmonale, and shock generally develop. In patients with cardiopulmonary disease who already have an impaired vascular reserve capacity, a relatively smaller amount of vascular occlusion results in greater pulmonary arterial hypertension and more serious right ventricular dysfunction. The mean pulmonary arterial pressure in these patients may exceed the highest values observed in patients free of previous disease, suggesting the presence of pre-existing right ventricular hypertrophy.

As the right ventricle fails, its volume increases; this alteration can have a direct effect on left ventricular function (Taylor et al, 1967) by shifting the intraventricular septum. Any fall in systemic arterial pressure may lead to right ventricular ischemia, causing a further decline in cardiac output and death due to arrhythmia or right ventricular collapse (Dalen et al, 1967; Dexter

and Smith, 1964; Vlahakes et al, 1981). As the right ventricle fails and flow through the pulmonary vascular bed decreases, pulmonary arterial pressure often falls, although pulmonary vascular resistance remains elevated. Therefore, pulmonary arterial pressure is a potentially misleading marker of the severity of embolic obstruction under these circumstances.

NATURAL HISTORY

The clinical course of deep venous thrombosis can be a complex and dynamic process. When thrombi remain confined to calf veins, as defined by serial negative noninvasive testing, withholding treatment appears to be safe, with very low recurrence rates of proximal thrombosis (Huisman et al, 1986). Symptomatic calf vein thrombosis, however, may have a significant recurrence rate unless both acute and long-term anticoagulation therapy are initiated, first with heparin and subsequently with warfarin (Langerstedt et al, 1985). Noninvasive studies suggest that for most adequately treated patients proximal vein thrombosis disappears over a period of 12 months. Huisman and colleagues (1988) demonstrated that 65% of patients with initially positive IPG study results returned to normal within 3 months. At the end of 12 months over 90% of patients with such results have normalized. In most patients in whom IPG normalizes, recurrence of the venous thrombotic problem is less likely (Huisman et al, 1988; Jay et al, 1984).

Normalization of the IPG can be misleading, however, because the test is performed in the supine position. Venous hypertension may still be present in the standing position and may lead to the post-thrombotic syndrome. Lower extremity venous hypertension is the result of residual venous obstruction, often incomplete or partial in character, and deep vein valvular incompetence. The venous obstruction is generally incomplete because of the process of recanalization and endothelialization of thrombus. Resting venous pressure may normalize with recanalization, but with ambulation, pressure rises. In the presence of valvular incompetence, the post-thrombotic syndrome develops. Valvular incompetence and venous flow reflux have been reported to increase in frequency and intensity from the time of the initial diagnosis of acute deep vein thrombosis (Markel et al, 1992). Using duplex ultrasonography, the Markel and colleagues' study reported that at the time of initial diagnosis, 14% of patients have valvular reflux; the incidence increased to 40% and 66% at 1 month and 1 year, respectively. Valvular reflux appears to be both more common and severe in patients with more occlusive thrombosis.

Following an acute pulmonary embolism, the process of vascular restoration and healing begins with an initial goal of restoring vascular luminal patency. With impact into the pulmonary circulation, the thrombus fragments and reshapes and the fibrinolytic process begins. Clot fibrinolysis and organization occur over several days to weeks, and restoration of blood flow to the occluded segment often returns, at least in part, quickly. Complete clearing of the clot can be variable from patient to patient in terms of rate and completeness. The process, depending on clot organization, is slower than fibrinolysis, and involves endothelialization and clot incorporation into the vessel wall. Recanalization of the clot and endothelial scarring or "web" formation can also occur.

Several studies have demonstrated that, at 6 to 8 days after the acute embolic event, only minor angiographic or lung scan evidence of resolution is present in most patients (Dalen et al, 1969; Tow and Wagner, 1969). In the National Institutes of Health thrombolytic trials, when heparin was administered and both angiography and perfusion lung scanning were used to track the clot resolution process, most emboli resolved rather rapidly during the first 2 weeks after the embolic event (Urokinase, 1973; 1974). At 5 days after starting heparin, 36% of the perfusion lung scan defects had resolved; at 14 days, 52% had resolved; at 3 months, 73% had resolved; and at 1 year, 76% had resolved. Prediletto and co-workers (1990) found similar resolution rates. Rarely, a patient can demonstrate marked resolution of a large emboli in as little as 2 days (Fred et al, 1966a), with further progressive resolution over 6 weeks (Dalen et al, 1969; Tow and Wagner, 1969). Clot resolution may be delayed in patients with cardiopulmonary disease. In general, both the ventilation-perfusion lung scan and the pulmonary angiogram results are likely to remain positive for weeks to months after the acute event.

A small number of patients with pulmonary embolism have persistent unresolved thrombus. Many of these patients fail to express the typical symptoms and signs of acute embolic disease at any time. This group of patients tends to develop chronic pulmonary hypertension, and it is actually the signs and symptoms of cor pulmonale that lead to the diagnosis (Benotti et al, 1983; Moser et al, 1983). This syndrome may occur in less than 2% of patients with acute pulmonary embolism. The syndrome is most likely the result of multiple recurrent embolic episodes that remain clinically unrecognized and hence untreated (Par-

askos et al, 1973; DeSoyza and Murphy, 1972). Primary pulmonary hypertension and recurrent thromboembolic pulmonary hypertension are similar clinically. The perfusion lung scan is the most important diagnostic tool in distinguishing these forms of pulmonary hypertension (D'Alonzo et al, 1984). For primary pulmonary hypertension the perfusion lung scan is generally normal or near normal, showing, at worst, minor, bilateral, nonspecific perfusion defects. The perfusion scan in recurrent thromboembolic disease, by contrast, demonstrates multiple segmental or lobar defects (D'Alonzo et al, 1984; Fishman et al, 1983).

DIAGNOSIS OF PULMONARY EMBOLISM

The clinical signs and symptoms of acute pulmonary embolism are nonspecific and insensitive, but they often raise the initial suspicion and guide the physician to more appropriate diagnostic studies. A high index of suspicion is essential for the diagnosis of pulmonary embolism to be made in most patients.

The pre-embolic cardiopulmonary status and the extent of embolization are the two most important factors that influence the clinical picture at presentation (Bell et al, 1977). Dyspnea and chest discomfort are common, and more than one half of all patients have cough and excessive anxiety. Syncope or near-syncope and a sensation of impending doom or serious anxiety are generally associated with massive pulmonary embolism. The duration and intensity of dyspnea seem to be related to the extent of embolization (Bell et al, 1977). Two types of chest discomfort commonly occur: dull chest heaviness, tightness, or pleuritic chest pain. Hemoptysis and pleuritic chest pain are more likely to occur after a submassive embolic event. Table 22–2 shows the frequency of symptoms observed in patients with angiographically proven pulmonary embolism. It has been said that if a patient does not have dyspnea or chest discomfort, especially with an absence of tachypnea, the diagnosis of pulmonary embolism is unlikely (Stein et al, 1981).

Although numerous signs of pulmonary embolism have been described, tachypnea is the only consistent physical finding (Table 22–3). Tachycardia, which often is said to occur commonly, is present only about 40% of the time, and the heart rate rarely exceeds 120 beats per minute (Bell et al, 1977). Tachypnea and tachycardia may be only transient, and persistent and more severe tachypnea and tachycardia have been associated with a massive pulmonary embolic event. On ausculta-

Table 22–2
Symptoms in Patients With Angiographically Diagnosed Acute Pulmonary Embolism

Symptom	Total Percent (N = 328)	Percent with Massive Embolism (N = 197)	Percent with Submassive Embolism (N = 130)
Chest pain	88	85	89
Pleuritic	74	64	85
Nonpleuritic	14	6	8
Dyspnea	85	85	82
Apprehension	59	65	50
Cough	53	53	52
Hemoptysis	30	23	40
Syncope	13	20	6

*Adapted from Bell WR, Simon TL, De Mets DL: The clinical features of submassive and massive pulmonary emboli. Am J Med 62:355–360, 1977.

tion of the lungs, crackles can be heard but wheezing is uncommon. Transient fever occurs approximately 40% of the time, with temperatures generally below 102°F.

With more severe embolic events or submassive events in patients with pre-existing cardiopulmonary disease, the signs of right ventricular strain and failure may be identified. An augmented pulmonic component to the second heart sound, right ventricular diastolic gallop, systolic murmur heard over the pulmonic area, and prominent jugular venous pulse A wave generally indicate serious and worrisome right ventricular strain and dysfunction. Protracted hypotension and even shock can be seen with massive pulmonary embolism; cyanosis is seen only with cardiovascular collapse.

Standard laboratory tests enhance the clinician's suspicion that a pulmonary embolic event has occurred. Most of the electrocardiographic

and chest radiographic findings associated with pulmonary embolism are nonspecific and are difficult to separate from abnormalities found in other acute or pre-existing cardiopulmonary diseases (Urokinase, 1973). Table 22–4 shows the common electrocardiographic abnormalities found in pulmonary embolism, but the electrocardiogram (ECG) shows only sinus tachycardia in a significant percentage of cases. The ECG is most useful for ruling out acute myocardial infarction and pericarditis, which are two conditions that may mimic pulmonary embolism.

Like the ECG, the chest radiograph can be normal in patients with pulmonary embolism, although nonspecific abnormalities are generally found (Table 22–5) (Kelly and Elliot, 1974; Urokinase, 1973). The PIOPED trial found 12% of patients with normal chest radiographs (Worsley et al, 1993). Parenchymal abnormalities such as tissue consolidation and atelectasis are common;

Table 22–3
Physical Findings in Patients With Angiographically Diagnosed Acute Pulmonary Embolism*

Sign	Total Percent (N = 327)	Percent with Massive Embolism (N = 197)	Percent with Submassive Embolism (N = 130)
Tachypnea	92	95	87
Crackles	58	57	60
Increased S_2P†	53	58	45
Tachycardia	44	48	38
Fever	43	43	42
Diaphoresis	36	42	27
Gallop	34	39	25
Phlebitis	32	36	26
Edema	24	28	28
Cyanosis	19	25	9

*Adapted from Bell WR, Simon TL, De Mets DL: The clinical features of submassive and massive pulmonary emboli. Am J Med 62:355–360, 1977.
†S_2P = pulmonic component of the second heart sound.

Table 22–4
Electrocardiographic Findings in Patients With Acute Pulmonary Embolism (N = 132)*

Finding	Percent of Patients
Sinus tachycardia	43
T-wave inversion	40
ST segment depression	33
Low voltage in frontal plane	16
Left axis deviation	12
$S_1Q_3T_3$ pattern	11
ST segment elevation	11
Right bundle branch block	11
Premature ventricular contractions	9
P-pulmonale	4
Right axis deviation	5
Atrial fibrillation	3

*Adapted from the Urokinase Pulmonary Embolism Trial: A Cooperative Study. Circulation 47[Suppl II]:1–108, 1973. By permission of the American Heart Association, Inc.

the abnormalities are multiple and pleural-based and are found more commonly in the lower and middle lung fields. Elevation of the hemidiaphragm is a relatively frequent finding.

Hypoxemia is a common finding in patients with pulmonary embolism; however, when several studies were reviewed (McIntyre and Sasahara, 1973; Stanek et al, 1978; Wilson et al, 1971), the arterial PO_2 while breathing air was reported by higher than 90 mm Hg and 80 mm Hg, in 6%

Table 22–5
Chest Radiographic Findings in Patients With Acute Pulmonary Embolism (N = 128)*

Finding	Number of Patients	Percent of Patients
Lung parenchyma		
Consolidation	53	41
Atelectasis	26	20
Pleural effusion	36	28
Diaphragm elevation	52	41
Pulmonary vessels		
Distention of proximal pulmonary arteries	30	23
Focal oligemia	19	15
Heart		
Left ventricular enlargement	21	16
Right ventricular enlargement	7	5

*Adapted from the Urokinase Pulmonary Embolism Trial: A Cooperative Study. Circulation 47[Suppl II]:1–108, 1973. By permission of the American Heart Association, Inc.

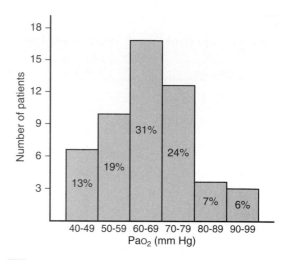

Figure 22–3
Arterial PO_2 values from 54 patients with angiographically proven acute pulmonary embolism and without a history of cardiopulmonary disease. (Redrawn from Dantzker DR, Bower JS: Alterations in gas exchange following pulmonary thromboembolism [Review]. Chest 81:495–501, 1982. With permission.)

and 13% of patients, respectively (Fig. 22–3). The calculated alveolar-arterial oxygen gradient in those patients, however, was widened. An arterial PO_2 value of less than 50 mm Hg may generally indicate that a massive pulmonary embolic event has occurred. One study reporting the results of 64 patients angiographically documented to have acute pulmonary embolism revealed three patients who had a normal alveolar-arterial oxygen gradients (Overton and Bocka, 1988).

A normal alveolar-arterial oxygen gradient may be helpful in reducing the need for lung scanning (McFarland and Imperiale, 1994). In 57 patients without a history of venous thromboembolism and a normal gradient, the risk of pulmonary embolism was less than 2%. In patients with previous thromboembolic disease, however, a normal alveolar-arterial oxygen gradient was not as helpful. In addition to an increased alveolar-arterial gradient, hypocapnia is a common finding in patients without a history of cardiopulmonary disease. In fact, even patients who have an existing hypercapnia resulting from underlying lung disease show a reduction in the arterial PCO_2 after pulmonary embolism (Lippman and Fein, 1981), although the value may still be high. To complicate matters further, an occasional patient has been found to increase the arterial PCO_2 after pulmonary embolism (Bouchama et al, 1988; Goldberg et al, 1984).

Table 22–6
Causes of Abnormal Regional Pulmonary Perfusion on Nuclear Lung Scanning

Intraluminal occlusion
  Embolic clots
  Fat emboli
  Tumor emboli
  Vascular stenosis
  Vasculitis
  Parasites
  Fungi

Extraluminal compression
  Tumor
  Adenopathy
  Vascular structures

Increased pulmonary vascular resistance
  Congestive heart failure
  Pneumonia

Regional hypoxia with reflex vasoconstriction
  Reactive airways disease
  Mucous plugging
  Airway foreign body

LUNG SCANNING

Ventilation-perfusion lung scanning, because it is relatively noninvasive, has become the initial screening procedure for the majority of patients suspected of having pulmonary embolisms. Pulmonary embolism is one of many diseases or distrubances associated with perfusion defects (Table 22–6). A completely normal result on a perfusion scan taken from six views excludes the diagnosis of pulmonary embolism, and further diagnostic testing is generally not necessary (Caride et al, 1976; Hull et al, 1990b; Kelley et al, 1991; Kipper et al, 1982; Nielsen et al, 1977). When perfusion defects are present, however, the distribution and extent of these defects and the means by which they are related to the vascular anatomy of the lung must be considered. Because most clinically significant pulmonary emboli are large, segmental or lobar perfusion defects have more significance than subsegmental defects. Pulmonary emboli are usually multiple, so that the finding of multiple perfusion defects should be considered more suggestive of the diagnosis. Once the perfusion scan is reviewed, the ventilation lung scan and chest radiograph can be integrated into the process to enhance diagnostic specificity. If a perfusion defect corresponds with a chest radiographic abnormality or an area of absent ventilation, then its specificity for diagnosing pulmonary embolism is reduced.

Diseases that cause regional hypoventilation, such as chronic obstructive lung disease and pneumonia, also cause concomitant reflex hypoxic vasoconstriction, which can produce a perfusion defect on lung scanning. An area with both decreased or absent ventilation and perfusion—in the presence of a normal chest radiograph—generally is presumed to represent a disease other than pulmonary embolism (Moser et al, 1971). In contrast, an area with normal ventilation and absent perfusion (a mismatched defect) is presumed to represent a pulmonary embolism. These simple concepts, however, do not hold up consistently. Because vascular and ventilatory compartments are in close proximity, and because most disease processes involve both compartments, it is difficult to conceive of an pathologic process that always limits itself to one compartment or the other.

A number of investigators have developed criteria based on the size and number of perfusion defects, chest radiographic findings in the areas of the defects, and distribution of ventilation in the corresponding areas, in an effort to establish criteria for high, low, intermediate, and indeterminate probabilities for pulmonary embolism (Table 22–7) (Alderson et al, 1976; Biello et al, 1979; NcNeil, 1974, 1976, 1980; Webber et al, 1990). A normal perfusion scan essentially eliminates the diagnosis of pulmonary embolism (Kelley et al, 1991), and withholding anticoagulation therapy has been shown to be safe (Hull et al, 1990; Hull and Raskob, 1991). Only rarely have nonobstructing pulmonary emboli been reported to be present at the time of a negative result on a perfusion lung scan (Brandstetter et al, 1987; Gutnick, 1983). Likewise, it is reasonable to conclude that a high-probability scan, defined as one with multiple lobar or segmental perfusion defects in the presence of normal ventilation, has a high sensitivity to detect a pulmonary embolism (Alderson et al, 1976; Biello, 1979, 1987; Cheely et al, 1981; Hull et al, 1985b; Hull and Raskob, 1991), provided certain known causes of false-positive scintigraphy, as previously outlined, are excluded.

The majority of ventilation-perfusion lung scans, however, fall between normal and high-probability for pulmonary embolism (PIOPED, 1990). These so-called low-probability, intermediate-probability, and indeterminate scan results are often found in patients with pulmonary embolisms. In fact, it has been suggested that 20 to 40% of patients with a low-probability scan have pulmonary embolism (Hull et al, 1983c; Hull et al, 1985b; Hull and Raskob, 1991; PIOPED, 1990). Additional studies are, therefore, usually needed to confirm the presence of either pulmonary embolism or lower extremity thrombosis for an abnormal lung scan that has not been interpreted as high-probability.

Table 22–7
Ventilation (V̇)-Perfusion (Q̇) Lung Scan Criteria for the Diagnosis of Acute Pulmonary Embolism According to Biello*

Probability of Embolism	Lung Scan Result†	Number of Patients in Category	Frequency of Embolism (%)
None	Normal perfusion	0	0
Low	Small V̇/Q̇ mismatches	19	0
	Focal V̇/Q̇ matches with normal chest radiograph	21	4.8
	Q defects less than chest radiograph abnormalities	13	7.7
Intermediate	Diffuse, obstructive lung disease	5	20
	Perfusion defects with equal-sized corresponding chest radiograph abnormalities	44	27
	Single moderate V̇/Q̇ mismatch with normal chest radiograph	3	33
High	Perfusion defects greater than corresponding chest radiograph abnormalities	15	87
	One or more large, or two or more moderate, V̇/Q̇ mismatches with normal chest radiograph	26	92

*Adapted from Biello DR, Mattar AR, McKnight RC, et al: Ventilation-perfusion studies in suspected pulmonary embolism. AJR Am J Roentgenol 133:1033–1037, 1979. Used by permission.
†Small = <25% of a lung segment; moderate = 25% to 75% of a lung segment; large = >75% of a lung segment.

Additional studies may not always be necessary, based on the results of outcome analysis. Untreated patients without a history of cardiopulmonary disease and with low-probability lung scan results are unlikely to experience significant morbidity and mortality as an outcome of pulmonary embolic disease during a 6- to 12-month period following the lung scan (Kahn et al, 1989; Lee et al, 1985; Smith et al, 1987). Although a low-probability scan result does not exclude embolism as a diagnosis, studies that use clinical outcome as the end point suggest that the risk of having a significant embolic event during the immediate follow-up period is relatively low. In contrast, in patients with inadequate cardiopulmonary reserves and a low-probability scan results there is a risk for serious morbidity and mortality from recurrent pulmonary embolism. These patients should undergo further studies to rule out or diagnose pulmonary embolism.

The results of the largest study that focused on the value of ventilation-perfusion lung scan in the diagnosis of pulmonary embolism have been published. The Prospective Investigation Of Pulmonary Embolism Diagnosis (PIOPED) trial involved multiple centers and was sponsored by the National Heart, Lung, and Blood Institute to determine the accuracy of lung ventilation-perfusion scanning in the diagnosis of pulmonary embolism (PIOPED Investigators, 1990) (Table 22–8). In the 755 patients who had angiography, the overall prevalence of pulmonary embolism was 33%. Almost every patient who was diagnosed as having pulmonary embolism had an abnormal result on the scan; five patients had a near-normal or normal scan result as did most patients without emboli (sensitivity 98%; specificity 10%). On angiography, if a patient did not have a pulmonary embolism, that patient had a normal-, low-, or indeterminate-probability scan result, with only 14 patients having a high-probability result. Of the 116 patients with a high-probability scan result and a interpretable angiogram, 102 had a pulmonary embolism, yielding a positive predictive value of 88%. Sensitivity of the high-probability scan is 41%, which means that many patients who had a scan interpretation other than high-probability also had an angiographically proven pulmonary embolism. Only 3% of patients with a high-probability scan result had a negative angiogram reading.

Specificity of the high-probability scan was 97%, but in patients with a history of pulmonary embolism, the positive predictive value was only 74%, as compared with 91% for patients without such a history. The percentage of patients having a positive pulmonary angiogram for emboli was lower in the intermediate-, low-, and near-normal lung scan categories (33%, 16%, and 9%, respectively). Importantly, patients with low- and near-normal ventilation-perfusion (V̇/Q̇) lung scan results can have a significant incidence of pulmonary embolism, as determined by angiography. In the entire study, only 21 patients showed a normal appearance on ventilation-perfusion lung scan.

Table 22–8

Ventilation (V̇)-Perfusion (Q̇) Lung Scan Criteria for the Diagnosis of Acute Pulmonary Embolism According to the Prospective Investigation of Pulmonary Embolism Diagnosis Trial (PIOPED)*

Probability of Embolism	Description of Findings
Normal	Normal perfusion
Low	Nonsegmental perfusion defects
	Single moderate subsegmental perfusion defect with normal chest radiograph (ventilation results irrelevant)
	Perfusion defect less than chest radiograph defect
	V̇/Q̇ matches ≤50% of the lung, ≤75% of the lung zone; with a normal chest radiograph
	More than three small perfusion defects regardless of chest radiograph or ventilation results
	Three or fewer small perfusion defects with corresponding chest radiograph abnormalities
Intermediate or indeterminate	Any findings not defined as either of low or high probability
High	Two or more large perfusion defects with normal chest radiograph and ventilation
	Two or more large perfusion defects greater than corresponding ventilation or chest radiograph abnormalities
	Two or more moderate and one large mismatched perfusion defects with normal chest radiograph
	Four or more moderate mismatched perfusion defects with normal chest radiograph

*From PIOPED Investigators: Value of ventilation/perfusion scan in acute pulmonary embolism: Results of the prospective investigation of pulmonary embolism diagnosis (PIOPED). JAMA 263:2753–2759, 1990. Used by permission.

The PIOPED group was comprised of investigators who are considered experts in the field of pulmonary thromboembolism. Their assessment as to the clinical probability of pulmonary embolism was found to improve the sensitivity and specificity of the V̇/Q̇ scan (Table 22–9). When embolism was strongly suspected, regardless of the lung scan result, the clinicians were correct 68% of the time, and when the probability was considered low, they were correct 91% of the time. The pretest clinical assessment by an expert, therefore, was more valuable for excluding pulmonary embolism than for identifying the presence of this condition. This should strongly influence the clinical approach to patients who have low-probability and near-normal lung scan results. This concept of using the clinician's assessment to enhance the predictive value of nondiagnostic scans has been confirmed by other investigators (Hull et al, 1983c; 1985a).

PULMONARY ANGIOGRAPHY

Two pulmonary angiographic findings are considered diagnostic for the presence of emboli in a

Table 22–9

Relationship Between a Clinically-derived Assessment of the Probability for Pulmonary Embolism and Lung Scan Results From the PIOPED Study*

| Scan Category | No. of Patients With Embolism/No. of Patients (%) | | | |
	CP of 80–100%	CP of 20–79%	CP of 0–19%	All Probabilities
High	28/29 (96)	70/80 (88)	5/9 (56)	103/118 (87)
Intermediate	27/41 (66)	66/236 (28)	11/68 (16)	104/345 (30)
Low	6/15 (40)	30/191 (16)	4/90 (4)	40/296 (14)
Near-normal or normal	0/5 (0)	4/62 (6)	1/61 (2)	5/128 (4)
Total	61/90 (68)	170/569 (30)	21/228 (9)	252/887 (28)

*From the PIOPED Investigators: Value of the ventilation/perfusion scan in acute pulmonary embolism: Results of the Prospective Investigation of Pulmonary Embolism Diagnosis (PIOPED). JAMA 263:2753–2759, 1990.

CP = clinical probability

pulmonary vessel (Dalen et al, 1971). The abrupt cutoff of a major vessel because of obstruction by an impacted clot and a filling defect caused by a clot with incomplete obstruction of a pulmonary artery are important angiographic findings diagnostic of pulmonary embolism. The performance of pulmonary angiography is generally safe for the majority of patients who require this intervention. In one study, which reviewed more than 4200 angiograms, the incidence of serious morbidity was less than 2% and the mortality was less than 0.01% (Goodman, 1984). Cardiopulmonary arrest, heart and pulmonary artery perforation, arrhythmia, vascular intimal dissection, and allergy to contrast media have all been described, although experienced professionals can reduce dramatically the incidence of significant morbidity and mortality from this procedure. Fatalities are more likely to occur in patients who are critically ill with serious pulmonary hypertension and clinical manifestations of cor pulmonale. For these reasons, angiography should be performed only when less invasive procedures do not confirm or exclude the diagnosis.

Pulmonary angiography is highly specific and sensitive for the diagnosis of pulmonary embolism (Alexander et al, 1966; Bell and Simon, 1976, Fred et al, 1966b), and patients with negative study results have an extremely low risk of subsequent pulmonary embolism (Kelley et al, 1991; Novelline et al, 1978). Equivocal angiograms do occur 5 to 15% of the time, and lack of interpretive agreement has been reported in up to 6% of cases (Bell and Simon, 1976; Urokinase-Streptokinase, 1974).

It may be better to perform pulmonary angiography from an arm approach, because this allows for better hemostasis during concurrent heparin and subsequent thrombolytic therapy. This route also reduces the potential for lower extremity deep venous system clot dislodgement. In high-risk patients for angiographic complications, the perfusion lung scan can be helpful in directing where a more limited contrast volume ejection should occur. With the use of nonionic contrast media and smaller ejection volumes, the incidence of cardiovascular instability is reduced.

Patients many times are unable to undergo pulmonary angiography because of hemodynamic or renal instability, which is often related to the primary illness. New techniques including digital subtraction angiography (Goodman and Brant-Zawadski, 1982; Ludwig et al, 1983; Misttretta, 1981; Pond et al, 1983) and contrast-enhanced magnetic resonance angiography (Loubeyre et al, 1994) have been utilized in patients with severe pulmonary hypertension or renal insufficiency,

wherein the risk for right ventricular collapse and renal failure are high.

DIAGNOSTIC EVALUATION

For each patient, the diagnostic evaluation of pulmonary embolism must be individualized. Clinicians must consider the immediacy of need for diagnosis, stability of the patient's condition, and degree of risk of the planned therapeutic interventions (Fig. 22–4). Because almost all thromboemboli originate in the deep veins of the legs, the combined approach of a V̇/Q̇ scan and a noninvasive assessment for deep vein thrombosis, such as duplex ultrasonography, has replaced pulmonary angiogram as the diagnostic method of choice. In those patients with a nondiagnostic lung scan result and a noninvasive lower extremity study that suggests deep venous thrombosis, the pulmonary angiogram is no longer necessary (Fig. 22–5) (Hull et al, 1989; Oudker et al, 1993; Stein et al, 1993, 1995). If the patient's condition is unstable, especially with manifestations of right ventricular failure or persistent severe hypoxemia while inspiring 100% oxygen, the diagnosis of pulmonary embolism must be established without delay. For these patients, pulmonary angiography should be considered as the initial diagnostic study.

TREATMENT OF VENOUS THROMBOEMBOLISM

Proper treatment is necessary to reduce the incidence of lower extremity post-thrombotic syndromes and chronic thromboembolic-induced pulmonary hypertension (Hirsh et al, 1981b; Hirsh and Hull, 1986). Supportive care continues to be the first step in the management of pulmonary embolism and usually includes the supplemental administration of oxygen and intravenous fluids to maintain right ventricular function. Occasionally, vasoactive agents and antiarrhythmics are necessary. Generally, heparin therapy is initiated based on the suspicion for pulmonary embolism, even before a definitive diagnosis has been made. The patient remains on heparin as the course of the diagnostic algorithm is followed. Therapies that should be considered include pharmacologic, surgical, and combination interventions.

HEPARINS

Heparinization is the treatment of choice for most patients with venous thromboembolic disease. Heparin acts by changing the conformity of a naturally occurring inhibitor, AT III so that the

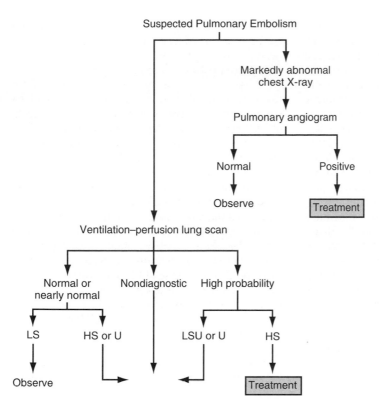

Figure 22–4
Approach to diagnosing acute pulmonary embolism in patients with apparent clinical stability.

inhibitor quickly combines with and inactivates certain clotting proteases, thrombin, and factor Xa. Mortality is reduced when heparin is used for the treatment of pulmonary thromboembolism (Barritt and Jordan, 1960; Kanis, 1974; Kernohan and Todd, 1966). Heparin can be administered by continuous intravenous infusion, intermittent intravenous bolus injection, or subcutaneous in-

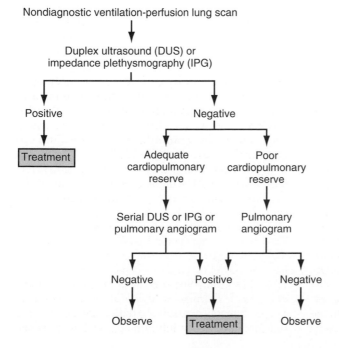

Figure 22–5
Diagnostic approach for acute pulmonary embolism in patients whose ventilation-perfusion lung scan results are other than normal or are of high probability.

jection. Regardless of the route, a minimal level of anticoagulation must be quickly achieved and maintained to ensure an antithrombotic state and prevent recurrent embolization.

Heparin therapy is usually initiated as an intravenous bolus, followed by a continuous intravenous infusion. Generally, 5000 units are administered initially as a bolus intravenously, but starting doses as high as 20,000 units have been suggested (Moser, 1994). Another method is to adjust the bolus to the patient's weight, similar to that of the hourly dosage. Following the initial bolus, the intravenous infusion of heparin is adjusted to keep the APTT, which is measured about every 6 hours, between 1.5 and 2.5 times control (Basu et al, 1972; Hirsh, 1991; Hyers et al, 1995) (blood heparin level at 0.2 to 0.4 units/ ml) (Brill-Edwards et al, 1993; Hirsh, 1991; Hyers et al, 1995). Studies have shown that the risk of recurrent thromboembolism is 15 times greater in patients with an APTT less than 1.5 times control for at least 24 hours after starting heparin compared with patients with a value greater than 1.5 times control (Basu et al, 1972; Hull et al, 1986b; Wessler and Gitel, 1979).

Previous standardized heparin protocols have been shown to be inadequate for many patients (Cruickshank et al, 1991; Raschke et al, 1993; Wheeler et al, 1988). More aggressive anticoagulation protocols with heparin based on standardized nomograms have been developed, which are dependent on weight (Raschke et al, 1993) or altered slightly by the risk of bleeding (Elliott et al, 1994; Hull et al, 1992b) and adjusted by subsequent APTT values. These weight-based nomogram protocols have been found to be easy to use, quickly achieving and maintaining the anticoagulated state while minimizing recurrent thromboembolic events and major bleeding. These protocols recommend an hourly infusion dosage ranging from 1250 units/hour to 1650 units/hour, or 30,000 to 40,000 units every 24 hours. When adjusted subcutaneous heparin therapy is given, an effective anticoagulant response is generally not achieved unless a high starting dose, approximately 17,500 units, is administered (Pini et al, 1990). The dose of heparin is then adjusted to a level that provides a therapeutic anticoagulant response 6 hours after each twice-daily subcutaneous administration.

Adjusted subcutaneous heparin therapy was compared with continuous intravenous heparin therapy by performing a meta-analysis of eight studies and nearly 1000 patients with deep vein thrombosis. These studies assessed the overall risk for clot extension and recurrence of venous thromboembolism and found that twice-daily sub-cutaneous therapy was more effective than the continuous intravenous route and probably can be used to simplify and facilitate home therapy for selected patients (Hommes et al, 1992).

Heparin usually is initiated and continued for the first 5 to 10 days. Warfarin therapy can be started concomitantly with a 4- to 5-day overlap of the two anticoagulants (Hyers et al, 1995). After the second day of warfarin therapy, the prothrombin time should be monitored daily and the dose of warfarin adjusted to obtain an INR of 2 to 3 (Hirsh and Pollen, 1994). A 5-day course of heparin was compared with a 10-day course, in which warfarin was begun on the fifth day, and the frequency of recurrent thromboembolism and major bleeding problems was similar between groups. There was perhaps a greater cost savings with the shorter course of heparin therapy because of the earlier patient discharge from the hospital (Hull, et al, 1990d). This shorter course of heparin therapy can be recommended for most patients; however, it may not be appropriate for patients with major thromboembolic disease.

Heparin therapy is the treatment of choice for pregnant patients (Ginsberg and Hirsh, 1995; Ginsberg et al, 1989). Adjusted subcutaneous administration of heparin is the long-term regimen of choice for pregnant patients and for patients in whom careful monitoring is not practical.

Heparin requirements are generally highest in the first few days after a thromboembolic event (Hirsh et al, 1976, 1995; Hirsh and Fuster, 1994; Simon et al, 1978). Blood levels, therefore, should be monitored very closely during that time. Resistance to heparin therapy is unusual, but if recognized, it should raise the possibility of a congenital deficiency of AT III, a severe liver disease, or a substantial ongoing thrombotic process. The platelet count should be checked every 2 to 3 days while heparin is being administered, because the drug can induce thrombocytopenia and paradoxical arterial thrombosis (Bell and Royale, 1980; Bell et al, 1976). When heparin is being administered by continuous intravenous infusion, the APTT can vary considerably. There is a known circadian rhythm in the anticoagulant effect of heparin (Decousus et al, 1985); therefore, the APTT can vary in a predictable manner over each 24-hour period.

Bleeding is the major risk of heparin therapy. Fatal hemorrhage occurs 1 to 2% of the time, and major hemorrhage requiring a transfusion occurs in 5 to 20% of patients (Glazier and Crowell, 1976; Jick et al, 1968; Levine et al, 1995a,b; Mant et al, 1977; Salzman et al, 1975; Urokinase Trial, 1973). Several controlled studies have suggested that the continuous infusion approach with heparin causes fewer bleeding complications than intermittent intravenous bolus therapy (Glazier and Crowell, 1976; Mant et al, 1977; Salzman et al, 1975; Wilson and Lampman, 1979). This lower bleeding incidence, however, may be related to a reduced total daily dose of heparin with the continuous infusion technique. Other factors may increase the bleeding risk, such as serious concurrent illness (Jick et al, 1968; Morabia, 1986), chronic alcohol use (Walker and Jick, 1980), aspirin use (Yett et al, 1978), and age (Jick et al, 1968). Mentioned previously was thrombocytopenia and arterial thrombosis, and when patients receiving heparin therapy have a decreased platelet count below 100,000/mm^3 (Bell et al, 1976; Engelberg, 1975; King and Kelton, 1984; Warkantin and Kelton, 1989, 1991), heparin should be discontinued because of a higher risk of these complications. Additional complications of heparin include osteoporosis, alopecia, hypersensitivity reactions, hyperkalemia, and hypoaldosteronism (Oster et al, 1995).

If heparin therapy has to be discontinued, an inferior vena cava filter should be considered. For patients with disturbed platelet function while on heparin therapy, danaparoid, a unique heparinoid, may be given as a temporary anticoagulant until a therapeutic warfarin level can be achieved (Hull et al, 1982a). Danaparoid has almost no physiologic effect on platelet function and it has low cross-reactivity with heparin-induced antibodies against platelets (deValk et al, 1995). Danaparoid may prevent the need for an inferior vena caval filter.

Low-Molecular-Weight Heparins

LMWHs like standard unfractionated heparins, bind with AT III and cause an anticoagulant effect. Because this complex has a higher affinity for factor Xa than for thrombin, it does not affect the APTT (Hirsh and Fuster, 1994a; Green et al, 1994). Preparations of LMWH are fragments of standard heparin produced commercially by controlled depolymerization, which are processes that yield heparin chains with mean molecular weights of about 4000 to 6000. These LMWH agents have been considered theoretically superior to standard heparins for several reasons. They have a very high bioavailability following subcutaneous injection, a longer serum half life, and a more predictable anticoagulant response. They may cause fewer hemorrhagic complications. Their anticoagulant effect is highly predictable. These properties allow LMWHs to be administered only once or twice daily and without laboratory monitoring.

A meta-analysis assessed the relative efficacy and safety of LMWH versus unfractionated heparin for the initial treatment of deep vein thrombosis (Lensing et al, 1995). This analysis included 10 studies and showed that when LMWH dose was adjusted for body weight, it was more effective and safer than standard heparin. Two studies have used symptomatic recurrent thromboembolism as the efficacy measure (Hull et al, 1992a; Prandoni et al, 1992a). Another study assessed the prevention of the extension of an existing lower extremity thrombus (Thery et al, 1992). LMWH is at least as safe and perhaps more effective than continuous intravenous heparin monitored for appropriate anticoagulant effect. When LMWH is used, warfarin therapy should be instituted in the same fashion as described for standard unfractionated heparin, unless LMWH therapy will be continued for the long term.

Although LMWHs have not yet recovered regulatory approval for the treatment of thromboembolism in the United States, they are used for this purpose in many countries throughout the world. These new heparins will likely provide distinct advantages for many patients, affording shorter hospital stays for what appears to be effective and safe therapy that can be provided at home without the need for laboratory monitoring. Two studies have confirmed the efficacy and safety of LMWH therapy for proximal deep vein thrombosis at home (Koopman et al, 1996; Levine et al, 1996).

WARFARIN

Warfarin inhibits the liver synthesis of vitamin K–dependent clotting factors (II, VII, IX and X) (Hirsh and Fuster 1994b). In addition, warfarin inhibits the action of protein C, a vitamin K–dependent protein with anticoagulant and fibrinolytic actions. It takes several days for warfarin to become effective because time is required for the clearance of clotting factors already present in the plasma. This lag time varies from patient to patient; therefore, it is important to institute warfarin early and to overlap it with heparin for several days (Hyers et al, 1995). Early initiation of warfarin within the first 24 to 48 hours of heparin therapy usually results in a total duration of heparin of 7 days or approximately 5 days for the warfarin to take full anticoagulant effect (Gallus et al, 1986; Hull et al, 1990d). The prothrombin time and the International Normalized Ratio (INR) should be monitored daily, and heparin should be discontinued once these values are within therapeutic range for 2 days. When the clinical condition and anticoagulation effect have stabilized, the prothrombin time and INR need to be monitored only periodically, perhaps weekly or biweekly, for the duration of warfarin therapy.

Warfarin requires a minimal level of anticoagulation to achieve and maintain an antithrombotic state. Warfarin therapy is usually adjusted with the prothrombin time, which can be reported with reference to an INR in an effort to eliminate differences between laboratories in test results caused by thromboplastins with different sensitivities. The INR is determined by calculating the prothrombin time ratio (a patient's prothrombin time divided by a reference normal prothrombin time) to a coefficient power known as the International Sensitivity Index (ISI). The ISI relates the sensitivity of monitoring warfarin with the thromboplastin being used to the sensitivity of an international reference preparation of thromboplastin that is assigned an ISI of 1.0 (Hirsh and Pollen, 1994). An INR of 2 to 3 is recommended for the treatment of venous thromboembolic disease (Hyers et al, 1995).

Most patients require warfarin for 3 to 6 months (Research Committee, 1992; Schulman et al, 1995), generally 3 months (Hyers et al, 1995). Patients who have persistent hypercoagulability, however, such as those with certain malignancies; AT III deficiency; protein C or protein S deficiency; and the presence of lupus anticoagulant, may need lifetime anticoagulation (Hyers et al, 1995). Symptomatic calf vein thrombosis without proximal extension or pulmonary embolism should be treated with anticoagulation for 3 months (Hyers et al, 1995; Langerstedt et al, 1985). If anticoagulation cannot be given, serial noninvasive lower extremity venous studies should be performed to assess for proximal extension of thrombus. When warfarin cannot be used, prophylactic subcutaneous low-dose heparin should not be considered. Adjusted subcutaneous heparin to prolong the activated partial thromboplastin time to 1.5 times the control or higher at the mid-dosing interval can be considered (Hyers et al, 1995; Hull et al, 1982b) as can subcutaneous LMWH therapy.

Numerous medications and foods may influence the metabolism of warfarin, by either interfering with protein binding or altering drug clearance. Allopurinol, amiodarone, cimetidine, quinidine, and trimethoprim-sulfamethoxazole can all potentiate the effects of warfarin (Wells et al, 1994), whereas its effect can be inhibited or reduced by barbiturates, oral contraceptives, and corticosteroids. Eating leafy green vegetables can also reduce the effectiveness of warfarin therapy.

Like heparin, warfarin's major complication is hemorrhage (Levine et al, 1995b). The incidence of bleeding increases with age and with the duration and intensity of treatment. Bleeding risk is reduced, without a change in efficacy, when the therapeutic range of warfarin is reduced from an INR of 3.0 to 4.5 to an INR of 2.0 to 3.0. An INR above 3 is not necessary in the management of venous thromboembolic disease, with rare exception (Hyers et al, 1995). If clinically significant bleeding occurs, warfarin should be discontinued. Vitamin K should be administered and the clinician should anticipate a reversal of warfarin's anticoagulant effect within 36 hours. Severe bleeding should be managed with the immediate infusion of fresh frozen plasma. If the patient requires surgery, warfarin should be discontinued, but it may take as long as 5 days for the INR to decrease to less than 1.2, which is a safe level for surgery. If the original INR was 3 or higher, the period of time for the INR to normalize may take considerably longer (White et al, 1995).

Skin necrosis is a rare and unpredictable complication of warfarin therapy. It is likely to occur within the first few days or weeks of the initiation of warfarin, often in obese middle-aged women (Brooks and Blais, 1991; Flood et al, 1943). This life-threatening necrotic process commonly involves the buttocks, breasts, thighs, and dorsum of the feet. Malignancy and low protein C levels, either inherently or iatrogenically, place the patient at additional risk for this syndrome. Early skin necrosis may look like subcutaneous hemorrhage, which is a benign condition that responds to stopping warfarin therapy. Concomitant heparin therapy during the initiation of warfarin reduces the incidence of skin necrosis. Once necrosis occurs, surgical management is often necessary.

Warfarin is generally contraindicated during pregnancy. Warfarin crosses the placenta and can cause spontaneous abortion and teratogenicity (Hall et al, 1980; Stevenson et al, 1980). Teratogenic effects are most likely to occur during the sixth through twelfth weeks of gestation, and it is possible that warfarin may be safe during the initial 4 to 6 weeks of pregnancy (Ginsberg and Hirsh, 1995). Heparinization is the best form of anticoagulation during pregnancy (Ginsberg et al, 1989), and there has been an increased interest in using LMWH (Ginsberg and Hirsh, 1995). Warfarin can be given in the postpartum period, even to nursing mothers, because the warfarin metabolite found in breast milk has no anticoagulant effect (Ginsberg and Hirsh, 1995; McKenna et al, 1983).

THROMBOLYTIC THERAPY

Streptokinase, urokinase, and tissue plasminogen activator are three thrombolytic agents available for the treatment of venous thromboembolism. These agents lyse clots, and they have been proposed as the treatment of choice in selected patients with pulmonary embolism and deep venous thrombosis of the lower extremities. Although a 1992 description of newer methods make thrombolytic therapy safer, easier to administer and monitor, and more economical (Goldhaber, 1992a), its place in therapy of thrombolic disease remains controversial.

Streptokinase, followed by urokinase, represented the first two thrombolytic agents available, both being enzymes that activate the natural endogenous fibrinolytic system. By forming a complex with plasminogen in the blood, streptokinase forms an activated complex that converts uncomplexed plasminogen to plasmin by proteolytic cleavage. Subsequent lysis of clot occurs, breaking down fibrin, fibrinogen, and various other clotting factors to soluble peptides. In contrast, urokinase directly activates plasminogen to plasmin. Tissue plasminogen activator lyses thrombus fibrin selectively with minimal systemic fibrinogenolysis. Despite this relative selectivity, tissue plasminogen activator appears to cause as much bleeding as streptokinase and urokinase (Goldhaber et al, 1986).

Thrombolytic therapy has been shown to accelerate the lysis of pulmonary emboli to a greater degree than heparin (Urokinase, 1973; 1974). Although survival appears to be similar among patients on thrombolytic therapy and heparin, this has not been definitively shown because most studies do not and cannot use death as a primary end point. Because of the low mortality of patients treated with heparin and warfarin alone, the identification of a reduction in mortality with thrombolytic therapy is extremely difficult to demonstrate. To show a 50% reduction in mortality in patients who were treated with thrombolytic agents compared with heparin, nearly 1000 patients are required in each treatment group (Anderson and Levine, 1992).

Because thrombolytics enhance clot lysis in the first 48 hours after a documented pulmonary embolism, these therapies have intuitively been considered for major pulmonary embolism, especially if it is complicated by severe hemodynamic or gas exchange instability (Marder, 1979; Thrombolytic Therapy, 1980; Urokinase, 1973, 1974). Patients who have submassive embolic events and underlying cardiac and pulmonary disease and persistent physiologic instability may be considered as candidates for thrombolysis.

Both intravenous and intrapulmonary infusions of tissue plasminogen activator have been used in the treatment of acute massive pulmonary embolism (Verstraete et al, 1988). A 2-hour infusion of tissue plasminogen activator followed by heparin has been shown to improve right ventricular function and lung perfusion when compared with anticoagulation alone (Dalla-Volta et al, 1992; Goldhaber et al, 1993). Nearly complete clot lysis has been achieved within a 2- to 6-hour period following tissue plasminogen activator infusion (Goldhaber et al, 1986). When lung scan reperfusion is evaluated at 48 hours, results with all of these thrombolytic agents are nearly identical. The rapidity of action and completeness of clot lysis should not be surprising for the tissue plasminogen activator because the entire dose is administered by 2 hours, whereas those patients who receive urokinase or streptokinase have only received a fraction of the 24- to 48-hour infusion.

A novel 2-hour dosing regimen of urokinase, when compared with a 2-hour infusion of tissue plasminogen activator, demonstrated similar efficacy and safety with each treatment regimen (Goldhaber et al, 1992b). The 2-hour urokinase regimen "compressed" the typically 24-hour dose as a bolus over 10 minutes followed by a 110-minute infusion. Patients receiving urokinase did not experience a pyretic response because they were pretreated with hydrocortisone, diphenhydramine, and acetaminophen. The patients who received tissue plasminogen activator did not undergo any pretreatment regimen. Bolus regimens of any thrombolytic therapy are likely to produce accelerated thrombolysis; therefore, this form of dosage administration may be optimal for patients in whom a minimal drug delivery time has advantages, such as those with life-threatening massive pulmonary thromboembolism (Diehl et al, 1992). In addition, repeated bolus administrations may have an advantage in patients with extensive deep venous thrombosis of the lower extremities (Goldhaber et al, 1994).

Thrombolytic therapy has been compared with heparin therapy in the management of acute deep venous thrombosis (Arnesen et al, 1982; Elliot et al, 1979; Kakkar et al, 1969a; Marder et al, 1977). There may be certain advantages with thrombolytic therapy. Patients who have acute symptomatology and those with excessive iliofemoral and popliteal thrombosis generally have better results with thrombolytic therapy. Even though thrombolytic therapy seems to have advantages over heparin in the initial management of acute deep venous thrombosis, the higher incidence of bleeding, including intracranial hemorrhage, has indicated caution in the use of thrombolytic therapy (Levine et al, 1995a). Thrombolytic therapy is also expensive. Nonetheless, proponents of this form of therapy for deep vein thrombosis claim that these issues do not preclude the potential reduction in morbidity and overall long-term expense that is associated with the post-thrombotic syndromes (O'Donnell et al, 1977).

An additional benefit of thrombolytic therapy is prevention of chronic venous insufficiency and eventual development of lower extremity syndromes. Patients who receive thrombolytic therapy are more likely to eventually have normal valve function and venograms, as compared with patients who receive heparin alone (Arnesen et al, 1982; Common et al, 1976; Elliot et al, 1979; Johansson et al, 1979).

Potential causes for thrombolytic therapy failure include inadequate fibrinolytic responses and problems with patient selection. Premature termination of therapy and failure of the thrombolytic agent to make sufficient contact with the clot are likely causes for inadequate fibrinolytic response. Furthermore, patients selected for this form of therapy often have the most extensive thrombotic disease, a factor that obviously influences eventual outcome.

At times, thrombosis fills the entire vessel, making it difficult for the thrombolytic agent to adequately reach and affect the clot. Older occlusive thrombi are particularly difficult to lyse by systemic infusion. Unfortunately, it is at times difficult to accurately predict the age of the thrombus from the patient's symptoms. Failure of the thrombolytic agent to achieve or maintain a fibrinolytic response for a long enough period of time must also be considered. Monitoring for complete clot lysis, as an end point, is rarely performed, and therapy is often stopped before this goal has been accomplished. At our own institution, 33% of 28 prospectively evaluated patients had thrombolytic therapy terminated before complete clot dissolution occurred.

It is generally easier to follow or monitor response to therapy for lower extremity thrombosis than it is for pulmonary embolism. Lower extremity thrombolytic response can be followed by duplex ultrasonography (every 12 to 24 hours). Once dissolution of clot occurs, therapy can be stopped, but if the process is slow extended lytic therapy should be considered. Duration of therapy, however, is a factor that must be considered for risk of complications, such as bleeding. Thrombolytic therapy, therefore, should be discontinued if no benefit is demonstrated after 24 or, perhaps at the most, 48 hours. At this time, the ideal method for monitoring response requires further study.

Thrombolytic agents are generally administered by a standard-dose, constant intravenous infusion protocol after heparin has been stopped. Streptokinase is given in a dosage of 100,000 to 150,000 units/hour after a priming dose of 250,000 units administered over 30 minutes. Urokinase is initially administered as a loading dose of 4400 units/kg over 30 minutes. Maintenance therapy with urokinase is 2200 units/kg per hour. The length of therapy for either agent has not been clearly established, although available information suggests that pulmonary embolism should be treated for 12 to 24 hours with urokinase or 24 to 48 hours with streptokinase. Deep venous thrombosis may be treated for 48 to 72 hours with streptokinase or 24 to 48 hours with urokinase. Tissue plasminogen activator is generally administered by intravenous infusion over 2 hours at a cumulative dose of 100 mg. A bolus dosage regimen has been tried, however, using 0.6 mg/kg of ideal body weight over 2 minutes intravenously, while heparin is being administered concurrently (Levine et al, 1990a, b). This regimen is different than that which is done with other forms of thrombolytic therapy, such as streptokinase and urokinase, wherein heparin generally is discontinued but reinstituted following the thrombolytic infusion, once the thrombin time or APTT returns to near normal. This usually occurs about 4 hours after thrombolytic therapy infusion.

Thrombolytic therapy is generally administered peripherally, by an intravenous infusion. Catheter-directed thrombolysis, however, with or without clot manipulation, may be helpful for patients who cannot tolerate or who fail the general systemic approach. When the catheter tip is positioned into and past the clot for local lytic therapy, patients with massive pulmonary emboli who are receiving streptokinase infusion and experiencing hemodynamic instability can potentially became more hemodynamically stable (Brady et al, 1992; Essop et al, 1992). A form of local thrombolytic therapy has been given successfully in the treatment of pulmonary embolism in which the thrombotic focus was the right atrium (Proano et al, 1988). In addition, infusions of lower doses of thrombolytic agents through a properly positioned pulmonary artery catheter in proximity to the embolic obstruction have been reported to be successful at reducing the risks associated with systemic thrombolytic therapy (Ambrose et al, 1985; Gonzalez-Juanatery et al, 1992; Hirsh et al, 1967; Leeper et al, 1988).

Locally infused thrombolytic therapy can be considered for deep vein thrombosis of the lower extremity, especially if previous systemic thrombolytic therapy has failed and the patient suffers from extensive iliofemoral thrombosis. Because this intervention does not prevent propagation of the deep venous thrombosis, a prophylactic vena caval filter and eventually an administration of heparin must be considered. Local catheter manipulation of the clot with thrombolytic therapy for patients with extensive iliofemoral venous thrombosis should also be considered, because the problem often leads to complex post-thrombotic lower limb syndromes, often with permanent functional impairment and occasionally amputation. If this more aggressive approach fails, contemporary venous thrombectomy has been shown to help some patients (Comerota et al, 1994; Molina et al, 1992). This more aggressive local lytic therapy, with or without thrombectomy, has a considerable degree of therapeutic attractiveness, but its complete role and outcome in this subset of rather complex patients needs to be further defined.

Contraindications to thrombolytic therapy are often present in patients with massive pulmonary embolism or extensive iliofemoral thrombosis. Active internal bleeding or cerebral vascular accident or other active intracranial processes occurring within 2 months of the consideration of thrombolytic therapy are absolute contraindications for this type of intervention. Recent gastrointestinal hemorrhage, substantial systemic diastolic hypertension (above 100 mm Hg), trauma, and surgical biopsy within 10 days are additional concerns when thrombolytic therapy is being considered. In an effort to avoid surgical embolectomy, thrombolytic therapy has been given successfully during pregnancy (Fagher et al, 1990; Hall et al, 1972). If the patient had received a catheter or needle puncture into a noncompressible vessel, thrombolytic therapy should be withheld or cautiously administered.

The incidence of both fatal and nonfatal recurrent pulmonary emboli after thrombolytic therapy appeared to be similar to the incidence associated with heparin when the results of 15 comparative studies were analyzed (Rogers and Lutcher, 1990; 1991). Approximately 4.5% and 0.5% of patients were noted to develop nonfatal and fatal emboli, respectively, with streptokinase and heparin therapies. Hemorrhage is the most common of all the complications associated with thrombolytic therapy. Major hemorrhage has been reported to occur in between 6 and 30% of patients being treated for deep venous thrombosis— a threefold greater incidence than with heparin therapy (Fennerty et al, 1989). Patients being treated with thrombolytic therapy for pulmonary emboli have been reported to have serious bleeding from thrombolytics occurring in between 6 and 45%. The risk of bleeding can be reduced by optimally using noninvasive diagnostic testing and avoiding large-vessel needle punctures, including catheterizations (Stein et al, 1994). The discontinuation of thrombolytic therapy, the appropriate application of pressure dressings, and the administration of fresh frozen plasma are often effective in controlling serious hemorrhage.

VENA CAVAL PROCEDURES

Vena caval interruption is generally reserved for patients who (1) had an acute pulmonary embolism and have a major contraindication to anticoagulation; (2) have documented recurrent pulmonary embolism despite appropriate anticoagulation; (3) require a surgical embolectomy or pulmonary thromboendarterectomy, because anticoagulation is difficult to use postoperatively; (4) have sustained a massive embolism and are at risk of dying with a recurrent clot; (5) have a large free-floating vena caval thrombus; (6) have chronic thromboembolic disease and pulmonary hypertension; and (7) have developed paradoxical emboli to the arterial circuit via a patent foramen ovale (Hyers et al, 1995).

The vena caval filter is usually placed transvenously, without general anesthesia, utilizing either a Greenfield filter (Greenfield, 1984; Greenfield et al, 1971, 1973, 1977; Kanter and Moser, 1988) or a bird's nest–like filter (Martin et al, 1990; Roehm, 1984; Roehm et al, 1988). Clinically determined recurrent pulmonary emboli are exceedingly rare after filter placement, and serious filter-related complications are uncommon (Becker et al, 1992). If not contraindicated, anticoagulation therapy should be used in conjunction with vena caval filters (Hyers et al, 1995).

EMBOLECTOMY

Embolectomy should be considered in a patient with acute massive pulmonary embolism (Clarke and Abrams, 1986; Gray et al, 1988; Mattox et al, 1982; Miller et al, 1977; Meyer et al, 1991), ideally documented by angiography, who has a persistent hemodynamic instability despite optimal medical therapy or an absolute contraindication to anticoagulation. Generally, the patient has signs of an acute cor pulmonale and a low cardiac output. Often the patient has received anticoagulation and thrombolytic therapy and the systemic blood pressure remains low, as does urinary output. Hypoxemia despite high concentrations of inspired oxygen is generally the rule rather than the exception in this setting.

An uncontrolled study compared embolectomy with thrombolytic therapy in patients with cardiovascular instability, including shock, after massive pulmonary embolism and showed comparable survival results (Gulba et al, 1994). Patients who sustained a cardiac arrest before the operation have the highest mortality rate, as do patients with preoperative cardiopulmonary disease (Clarke and Abrams, 1986; Greenfield, 1984; Meyer et al, 1991).

A different type of open-chest pulmonary vascular procedure is performed for patients with chronic recurrent thromboembolic pulmonary hypertension and cor pulmonale (Chitwood et al, 1984; Daily et al, 1980; Sabiston et al, 1977). Thromboendarterectomy has been shown to provide remarkable symptomatic relief and hemodynamic improvement in carefully selected patients. This complex surgical procedure is not widely available.

PRACTICAL APPROACH TO THE TREATMENT OF PULMONARY EMBOLISM

An approach to the management of pulmonary embolism is shown in Figure 22–6 (Kinasewitz and George, 1984). Individualization to the patient's clinical condition should guide this approach. For the majority of patients diagnosed to have pulmonary embolism, heparinization is the treatment of choice. Thrombolytic therapy is reserved for patients who have had a massive pulmonary embolic event and continue to display

shock, severe hypoxemia, or both. Long-term anticoagulation, generally for a minimum of 3 to 6 months, is administered in the form of warfarin or adjusted-dose subcutaneous heparin.

An inferior vena caval filter is indicated when (1) anticoagulation is either contraindicated or failed, (2) risk of recurrent embolization is high and would likely lead to death, and (3) a lower extremity clot needs to be manipulated by a catheter. Embolectomy, generally by the open-chest approach, performed during cardiopulmonary bypass surgery, is reserved for that unusual patient who has had a massive pulmonary embolism and in whom anticoagulation therapy either is ineffective or complicating the clinical course. Thromboendarterectomy, a procedure different from embolectomy, is reserved for patients with cor pulmonale secondary to recurrent pulmonary embolic disease. This procedure can be curative, and patients are normally anticoagulated for life and protected by an inferior vena caval filter placement.

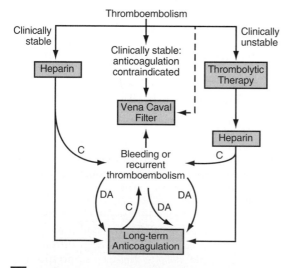

Figure 22–6
Management of acute pulmonary embolism. C = complications; DA = dosage adjustment. (Redrawn from Kinasewitz GT, George RB: Chest 86:106–111, 1984. With permission.)

REFERENCES

Aderka D, Brown A, Zelikovski A, et al: Idiopathic deep vein thrombosis in an apparently healthy patient as a premonitory sign of occult cancer. Cancer 57:1846–1849, 1986.

Ahlberg A, Nylander G, Robertson B, et al: Dextran in prophylaxis of thrombosis in fractures of the hip. Acta Chir Scand 387[Suppl]:83–85, 1968.

Alarcon-Segovia D, Deleze M, Oria CV, et al: Antiphospholipid antibodies and the antiphospholipid syndrome in systemic lupus erythematosus: A prospective analysis on 500 consecutive patients. Medicine (Baltimore) 68:353–365, 1989.

Alavi A, Palevsky H, Gupta N, et al: Radiolabeled antifibrin antibody in the detection of venous thrombosis: Preliminary results. Radiology 175:79–85, 1990.

Albrechtson V and Olsson CO: Thrombotic side effects of lower limb phlebography. Lancet 1:723–725, 1976.

Alderson PO, Rujanavech N, Secker-Walker RH, et al: The role of ¹³³Xe ventilation studies in the scintigraphic detection of pulmonary embolism. Radiology 120:633–640, 1976.

Alexander JR, Gonzalez DA, Fred HL: Angiographic studies in cardiorespiratory diseases. JAMA 198:575–578, 1966.

Almer L-O and Janzon L: Low vascular fibrinolytic activity in obesity. Thromb Res 6:171–175, 1975.

Ambrose JE, Venditto M, and Dickerson WH: Local fibrinolysis for the treatment of massive pulmonary embolism: Efficacy of streptokinase infusion through pulmonary arterial catheter. J Am Osteopath Assoc 85:105–109, 1985.

Amstutz HC, Fiscia DA, Dorcy F, et al: Warfarin prophylaxis to prevent mortality from pulmonary embolism after total hip replacement. J Bone Joint Surg 71A:321–326, 1989.

Anderson DR, Lensing AW, Wells PS, et al: Limitations of impedance plethysmography in the diagnosis of clinically suspected deep-vein thrombosis. Ann Intern Med 118:25–30, 1993a.

Anderson DR and Levine MN: Thrombolytic therapy for the treatment of acute pulmonary embolism. Can Med Assoc J 146:13–17, 1992.

Anderson DR, O'Brien BJ, Levine MN, et al: Efficacy and cost of low-molecular weight heparin compared with standard heparin for the prevention of deep vein thrombosis after total hip arthroplasty. Ann Intern Med 119:1105–1112, 1993b.

Anderson GM and Hull E: The effect of dicumarol upon the mortality and incidence of thromboembolic complications in congestive heart failure. Am Heart J 39:697–702, 1950.

Anlyan WG, Shingleton WW, and DeLaughter GD: Significance of idiopathic venous thrombosis and hidden cancer. JAMA 161:964–966, 1956.

Arnesen H, Hoiseth A, Ly B: Streptokinase or heparin in the treatment of deep vein thrombosis. Acta Med Scand 211:65–68, 1982.

Aster R: Heparin-induced thrombocytopenia and thrombosis. N Engl J Med 332:1334–1337, 1995.

Atik M: Dextran 40 and Dextran 70: A review. Arch Surg 94:664–672, 1967.

Barritt DW and Jordan SC: Anticoagulant drugs in treatment of pulmonary embolism. Lancet 1:1309–1312, 1960.

Basu D, Gallus A, Hirsh J, et al: A prospective study of the value of monitoring heparin treatment with the activated partial thromboplastin time. N Engl J Med 287:324–327, 1972.

Bauer AR Jr and Flynn RR: Computed tomography diagnosis of venous thrombosis of the lower extremities and pelvis with contrast material. Surg Gynecol Obstet 167:12–15, 1988.

Bauer G: Avenographic study of thrombo-embolic problems. Acta Chir Scand 84[Suppl 61]:1–75, 1940.

Becker DM, Phillbrick JT, and Abbitt PL: Real-time ultrasonography for the diagnosis of lower extremity deep venous thrombosis. The wave of the future? Arch Intern Med 149:1731–1734, 1989.

Becker DM, Phillbrick JT, and Selby JB: Inferior vena cava filters: Indications, safety, effectiveness. Arch Intern Med 152:1985–1994, 1992.

Bell WR and Royall RM: Heparin-induced thrombocytopenia: A comparison of three preparations. N Engl J Med 303:902–907, 1980.

Bell WR and Simon TL: A comparative analysis of pulmonary perfusion scans with pulmonary angiograms. Am Heart J 92:700–706, 1976.

Bell WR, Simon TL, and DeMets DL: The clinical features of submassive and massive pulmonary emboli. Am J Med 62:355–360, 1977.

Bell WR, Tomasulo PA, Alving BM, et al: Thrombocytopenia occurring during the administration of heparin. A prospective study in 52 patients. Ann Intern Med 85:155–160, 1976.

Benotti JR, Ockene IS, Alpert JS, et al: The clinical profile of unresolved pulmonary embolism. Chest 84:669–678, 1983.

Bentley PG and Kakkar VV: Radionuclide venography for the demonstration of the proximal deep venous system. Br J Surg 66:687–690, 1979.

Berqvist D, Burmark US, Frisell J, et al: Low molecular weight heparin once daily compared with conventional low-dose heparin twice daily. A prospective double-blind multi-centre trial on prevention of postoperative thrombosis. Br J Surg 73:204–208, 1986.

Berqvist D and Lindblad B: The thromboprophylactic effect of graded elastic compression stockings in combination with dextran 70. Arch Surg 119:1329–1331, 1984.

Bertina RM, Koeleman BP, Koster T, et al: Mutation in blood coagulation factor V associated with resistance to activated protein C. Nature 369:64–67, 1994.

Bettmann MA and Paulin S: Leg phlebography. The incidence, nature and modification of undesirable side effects. Radiology 122:101–104, 1977.

Biello DR: Radiological (scintigraphic) evaluation of patients with suspected pulmonary embolism. JAMA 257:3257–3259, 1987.

Biello DR, Mattar AG, McKnight RC, et al: Ventilation-perfusion studies in suspected pulmonary embolism. AJR Am J Roentgenol 133:1033–1037, 1979.

Biland L, Hull R, Hirsh J, et al: The use of electromyograph to detect muscle contraction responsible for false-positive impedance plethysmographic results. Thromb Res 14:811–816, 1979.

Black PM, Crowell RM, and Abbott WM: External pneumatic calf compression reduces deep venous thrombosis in patients with ruptured intracranial aneurysms. Neurosurgery 18:25–28, 1986.

Bonnar J, McNicol GP, and Douglas AS: Fibrinolytic enzyme system and pregnancy. Br Med J 3:387–389, 1969.

Bonnar J and Walsh JJ: Prevention of thrombosis after pelvic surgery by British dextran 70. Lancet 1:614–616, 1972.

Bonnar J, Walsh JJ, and Haddon M: Thromboembolism following radical surgery for carcinoma: Prevention by dextran 70 infusion during and immediately after operation. IVth International Congress on Thrombosis and Haemostasis, Vienna, 1973, p 278A.

Borow M and Goldson H: Postoperative venous thrombosis: Evaluation of five methods of treatment. Am J Surg 141:245–251, 1981.

Borow M and Goldson HJ: Prevention of postoperative deep venous thrombosis and pulmonary emboli with combined modalities. Ann Surg 49:599–605, 1983.

Bouchama A, Curely W, Al-Dossary S, et al:

Refractory hypercapnia complicating massive pulmonary embolism. Am Rev Respir Dis 138:466–468, 1988.

Bounameaux H, Cirafici P, deMoerloose P, et al: Measurement of D-dimer in plasma as a diagnostic aid in suspected pulmonary embolism. Lancet 337:196–200, 1991.

Bounameaux H, Couson F, Didier D, et al: Variability of interpretation of contrast venography for screening of postoperative venous thrombosis influences results of a thrombo-prophylactic study (abstr). Thromb Haemost 69:618, 1993.

Bounameaux H, de Moerloose P, Perrier A, et al: Plasma measurement of D-dimer as diagnostic aid in suspected venous thromboembolism: An overview. Thromb Haemost 71:1–6, 1994.

Bounameaux H, Khabiri E, Huber O, et al: Value of liquid crystal contact thermography and plasma levels of D-dimer for screening of deep venous thrombosis following general abdominal surgery. Thromb Haemost 67:603–606, 1992.

Bradley JG, Krugener GH, and Jager JH: The effectiveness of intermittent plantar venous compression in prevention of deep venous thrombosis after total hip arthroplasty. J Arthroplasty 8:57–61, 1993.

Brady AJB, Crake T, and Oakley CM: Simultaneous mechanical clot fragmentation and pharmacologic thrombolysis in acute massive pulmonary embolism. Am J Cardiol 70:836, 1992.

Brandstetter RD, Naccarato E, Sperber RJ, et al: Normal lung perfusion scan with extensive thromboembolic disease. Chest 92:565–566, 1987.

Brill-Edwards P, Ginsberg JS, Johnston M, et al: Establishing a therapeutic range for heparin therapy. Ann Intern Med 119:104–109, 1993.

Brockmans AW, Veltkamp JJ, and Bertina RM: Congenital protein C deficiency and venous thromboembolism. A study of three Dutch families. N Engl J Med 309:340–344, 1983.

Brooks LW and Blais FX: Coumarin-induced skin necrosis. JAMA 91:601–605, 1991.

Burnand KG and Layer GT: Graduated elastic stockings. Br Med J (Clin Res) 293:224–225, 1986.

Butler J, Kowalski TF, Willoughly S, et al: Preventing infarctions after pulmonary artery occlusion (abstr). Clin Res 37:163A, 1989.

Butson ARC: Intermittent pneumatic calf compression for prevention of deep venous thrombosis in general abdominal surgery. Am J Surg 142:525–527, 1981.

Caen JP: A randomized double-blind study between a low molecular heparin Kabi 2165 and standard heparin in the prevention of deep vein thrombosis in general surgery. A French multicenter trial. Thromb Haemost 59:216–220, 1988.

Caldini P: Pulmonary hemodynamics and arterial oxygen saturation in pulmonary embolism. J Appl Physiol 20:184–190, 1965.

Caprini JA, Chucker JL, Zuckerman L, et al: Thrombosis prophylaxis using external compression. Surg Gynecol Obstet 156:599–604, 1983.

Caprini JA, Scurr JH, and Hasty JH: Role of compression modalities in a prophylactic program for deep vein thrombosis. Sem Thromb Hemostast 14[Suppl]:77–87, 1988.

Caride VJ, Puri S, Slavin JD, et al: The usefulness of the posterior oblique views in perfusion lung imaging. Radiology 121:669–671, 1976.

Carpenter JP, Holland GA, Baum RA, et al: Magnetic resonance venography for the detection of deep venous thrombosis: Comparison with contrast venography and duplex Doppler ultrasonography. J Vasc Surg 18:734–741, 1993.

Carter AE and Eban R: The prevention of postoperative deep venous thrombosis with Dextran 70. Br J Surg 60:681–683, 1973.

Carvalho A and Ellman L: Hereditary antithrombin III deficiency. Effect of anti-thrombin III deficiency on platelet function. Am J Med 61:179–183, 1976.

Chajek T and Fainaru M: Behcet's disease with decreased fibrinolysis and superior vena caval occlusion. Br Med J 1:782–783, 1973.

Cheely R, McCartney WH, Perry JR, et al: The role of noninvasive tests versus pulmonary angiography in the diagnosis of pulmonary embolism. Am J Med 70:17–22, 1981.

Chernick V, Hodson WA, and Greenfield LJ: Effect of chronic pulmonary artery ligation on pulmonary mechanics and surfactant. J Appl Physiol 21:1315–1320, 1966.

Chitwood WR Jr, Sabiston DC Jr, and Wechsler AS: Surgical treatment of chronic unresolved pulmonary embolism. Clin Chest Med 5:507–536, 1984.

Clagett GP and Reisch JS: Prevention of venous thromboembolism in general surgical patients. Results of a meta-analysis. Ann Surg 208:227–240, 1988.

Clark WB, MacGregor AB, Prescott RJ, et al: Pneumatic compression of the calf and postoperative deep-vein thrombosis. Lancet 2:5, 1974.

Clarke DB and Abrams LD: Pulmonary embolectomy: A 25 year experience. J Thorac Cardiovasc Surg 92:442, 1986.

Clark-Pearson DL, Synan IS, Hinshaw WM, et al: Prevention of postoperative venous thromboembolism by external pneumatic calf compression in patients with gynecologic malignancy. Obstet Gynecol 63:92–98, 1984.

Coe NP, Collins REC, Klein LA, et al: Prevention of deep vein thrombosis in urological patients: A controlled, randomized trial of low dose heparin and external pneumatic compression boots. Surgery 83:230–234, 1978.

Cogo A, Bernardi E, Prandoni P, et al: Acquired risk factors for deep-vein thrombosis in symptomatic outpatients. Arch Intern Med 154:164–168, 1994.

Colditz GA, Tuden RL, and Oster G: Rates of venous

thrombosis after general surgery: Combined results of randomized clinical trials. Lancet 2:143–146, 1986.

Collins R, Scrimgeour A, Yusuf S, et al: Reduction of fatal pulmonary embolism and venous thrombosis by preoperative administration of subcutaneous heparin. N Engl J Med 318:1162–1173, 1988.

Colwell CW Jr, Spiro TE, Trowbridge AA, et al: Use of enoxaparin, a low-molecular-weight heparin, and unfractionated heparin for the prevention of deep venous thrombosis after elective hip replacement: A clinical trial comparing the efficacy and safety. J Bone Joint Surg 76A:3–14, 1994.

Comerota AJ, Aldridge SC, Cohen G, et al: A strategy of aggressive regional therapy for acute iliofemoral thrombosis with contemporary venous thrombectomy or catheter-directed thrombolysis. J Vasc Surg 20:244–254, 1994.

Comerota AJ, Katz ML, Grossi RJ, et al: The comparative value of noninvasive testing for diagnosis and surveillance of deep vein thrombosis. J Vasc Surg 7(L):40, 1988.

Comerota SJ, Katz ML, and Hashemi HA: Venous duplex imaging for the diagnosis of acute deep venous thrombosis. Haemostasis 23:61–71, 1993.

Comerota AJ, Katz ML, and White JV: Why does prophylaxis with external pneumatic compression fail? Am J Surg 164:265–268, 1992.

Common HH, Seaman AJ, Rosch J, et al: Deep vein thrombosis treated with streptokinase or heparin: Follow-up of a randomized study. Angiology 27:645–654, 1976.

Comp PC and Esmon CT: Recurrent venous thromboembolism in patients with a partial deficiency of protein S. N Engl J Med 311:1524–1529, 1984.

Comp PC, Thurnau GR, Welsh J, et al: Functional and immunologic protein S levels are decreased during pregnancy. Blood 68:881–885, 1986.

Comroe JH, VanLingen B, Stroud RC, et al: Reflex and direct cardiopulmonary effects of 5-OH-tryptamine (serotonin): Their possible role in pulmonary embolism and coronary thrombosis. Am J Physiol 173:379–386, 1966.

Council on Thrombosis, American Heart Association: Prevention of venous thromboembolism in surgical patients by low dose heparin. Circulation 55:423A–426A, 1977.

Cranley JJ, Canos AJ, and Sull WI: The diagnosis of deep venous thrombosis: Fallibility of clinical symptoms and signs. Arch Surg 111:34–36, 1976.

Cronan JJ, Dorfman GS, and Grusmark J: Lower-extremity deep venous thrombosis: Further experience with and refinements of US assessment. Radiology 168:101–107, 1988.

Cruickshank MK, Levine MN, Hirsh J, et al: A standard heparin nomogram for the management of heparin therapy. Arch Intern Med 151:333–337, 1991.

Daily PO, Johnston GG, Simmons CJ, et al: Surgical management of chronic pulmonary embolism: Surgical treatment and late results. J Thorac Cardiovasc Surg 79:523–531, 1980.

Dale S, Godstad GO, Brosstad F, et al: Comparison of three D-Dimer assays for the diagnosis of DVT: ELISA, latex and immunofiltration assay (nycoCard D-Dimer). Thromb Haemost 71(3):270–274, 1994.

Dalen JE: When can treatment be withheld in patients with suspected pulmonary embolism? 153:1415–1418, 1993.

Dalen JE and Alpert JS: Natural history of pulmonary embolism. In Sasahara AA, Sonnenblick EH, Lesch M (eds): Pulmonary Embolism. New York, Grune & Stratton, 1975, pp 77–88.

Dalen JE, Banas JS, Brooks HL, et al: Resolution rate of acute pulmonary embolism in man. N Engl J Med 280:1194–1199, 1969.

Dalen JE, Brooks HL, Johnson LW, et al: Pulmonary angiography in acute pulmonary embolism: Indications, techniques, and results in 367 patients. Am Heart J 81:175–185, 1971.

Dalen JE, Haffajee CI, Alpert JS, et al: Pulmonary embolism, pulmonary hemorrhage, and pulmonary infarction. N Engl J Med 296:1431–1435, 1977.

Dalla-Volta S, Pella A, Santolicardro A, et al: PAINS 2: Alteplase combined with heparin vs. heparin in the treatment of acute pulmonary embolism. Plasminogen activator Italian multicenter study 2. J Am Coll Cardiol 20:520–526, 1992.

D'Alonzo GE, Bower JS, and Dantzker DR: Differentiation of patients with primary and thromboembolic pulmonary hypertension. Chest 85:457–461, 1984.

D'Alonzo GE, Bower JS, DeHart P, et al: The mechanism of abnormal gas exchange in acute massive pulmonary embolism. Am Rev Respir Dis 128:170–172, 1983.

D'Alonzo GE and Dantzker DR: Gas exchange alterations following pulmonary thromboembolism. Clin Chest Med 5:411–419, 1984.

D'Angelo SV, Comp PC, Esmon CT, et al: Relationship between protein C antigen and anticoagulant activity during oral anticoagulation and in selected disease states. J Clin Invest 77:416–425, 1986.

D'Angelo A, Vigano-D'Angelo SV, Esmon CT, et al: Acquired deficiencies of protein S. J Clin Invest 81:1445–1454, 1988.

Danish Enoxaparin Study Group: Low-molecular-weight heparin (Enoxaparin) vs dextran 70. The prevention of post operative deep vein thrombosis after total hip replacement. Arch Intern Med 151:1621–1624, 1991.

Dantzker DR, Wagner PD, Thornabene VM, et al: Gas exchange after pulmonary thromboembolism in dogs. Circ Res 42:92–103, 1978.

Davidson BI, Elliott CG, and Lensing AWA: Low accuracy of color Doppler ultrasound in the detection of proximal leg vein thrombosis in asymptomatic high-risk patients. Ann Intern Med 117:735–738, 1992.

Dechavanne M, Ville D, Berruyer M, et al: Randomized trial of a low-molecular weight heparin (Kabi 2165) versus adjusted-dose subcutaneous standard heparin in the prophylaxis of deep vein thrombosis after elective hip surgery. Haemostasis 19:5–12, 1989.

Decousus H-A, Croze M, Levi FH, et al: Circadian changes in anticoagulant effect of heparin infused at constant rate. Br Med J 290:341–344, 1985.

Demers C, Ginsberg JS, Hirsh J, et al: Thrombosis in antithrombin III deficiency. Report of a large kindred and literature review. Ann Intern Med 116:754–761, 1992.

DeSoyza NDB and Murphy ML: Persistent postembolic pulmonary hypertension. Chest 62:665–668, 1972.

deValk HW, Banga JD, Wester JWJ, et al: Comparing subcutaneous danaparoid with intravenous heparin for the treatment of venous thromboembolism. Ann Intern Med 123:1–9, 1995.

Dexter L and Smith GT: Quantitative studies of pulmonary embolism. Am J Med Sci 247:641–648, 1964.

Diehl J, Meyer G, Igual J, et al: Effectiveness and safety of bolus administration of alteplase in massive pulmonary emboli. Am J Cardiol 70:1477–1480, 1992.

Donayre CE, White GH, Mehringer SM, et al: Pathogenesis determines late morbidity of axillosubclavian vein thrombosis. Am J Surg 152:179–184, 1986.

Egeberg O: Inherited antithrombin deficiency causing thrombophilia. Thromb Diath Haemorrh 13:516–530, 1965.

Elliott CG, Hiltunen SJ, Suchyta M, et al: Physician-guided treatment compared with a heparin protocol for deep vein thrombosis. Arch Intern Med 154:999–1004, 1994.

Elliott MS, Immelman EJ, Jeffery P, et al: A comparative randomized trial of heparin versus streptokinase in the treatment of acute proximal venous thrombosis: An interim report of a prospective trial. Br J Surg 66:838–843, 1979.

Engelberg H: The clinical use of heparin. Curr Ther Res 18:34–44, 1975.

Engesser L, Broekmans A, Briét E, et al: Hereditary protein S deficiency: Clinical manifestations. Ann Intern Med 106:677–682, 1987.

Erikkson BI, Zachrissan BE, Teger-Nilsson AC, et al: Thrombosis prophylaxis with low molecular weight heparin in total hip replacement. Br J Surg 75:1053–1057, 1988.

Erikkson BI, Kalebo P, Anthmyr BA, et al: Prevention of deep vein thrombosis and pulmonary embolism after total hip replacement: comparison of low-molecular weight heparin and unfractionated heparin. J Bone Joint Surg 73A:484–493, 1991.

Essop MR, Middlemost S, Skoularigis J, et al: Simultaneous clot fragmentation and pharmacologic thrombolysis in acute massive pulmonary embolism. Am J Cardiol 69:427, 1992.

European Fraxiparin Study Group: Comparison of low molecular weight heparin and unfractionated heparin for the prevention of deep vein thrombosis in patients undergoing abdominal surgery. Br J Surg 75:1058–1063, 1988.

Evans AJ, Sostman HD, Knelson MH, et al: Detection of deep venous thrombosis: Prospective comparison of MR imaging with contrast venography. AJR Roentgenol 161:131–139, 1993.

Evarts CM and Feli EJ: Prevention of thromboembolic disease after elective surgery of the hip. J Bone Joint Surg 53A:1271–1280, 1971.

Fagher B, Ahigren M, and Åstedt B: Acute massive pulmonary embolism treated with streptokinase during labor and the early puerperium. Acta Obstet Gynecol Scand 69:659–662, 1990.

Fenech A, Dendy PP, Hussey JK, et al: Indium-111 labelled platelets in diagnosis of leg-vein thrombosis: Preliminary findings. Br Med J 280:1571–1573, 1980.

Fennerty AG, Levine MN, and Hirsh J: Hemorrhagic complications of thrombolytic therapy in the treatment of myocardial infarction and venous thromboembolism. Chest 95:885–975, 1989.

Fields RA, Toubbeh H, Searles RP, et al: The prevalence of anticardiolipin antibodies in a healthy elderly population and its association with antinuclear antibodies. J Rheumatol 16:223–225, 1989.

Fischer HW, Spataro RF, and Rosenberg PM: Medical and economic considerations in using a new contrast medium. Arch Intern Med 146:1717–1721, 1986.

Fishman AJ, Moser KM, and Fedullo PF: Perfusion lung scans vs. pulmonary angiography in evaluation of suspected primary pulmonary hypertension. Chest 84:679–683, 1983.

Flanagan LD, Sullivan ED, and Cronley JJ: Venous imaging of the extremities using real-time B-mode ultrasound. In Bergan JJ, Yao JST (eds): Surgery of the Veins. New York, Grune & Stratton, 1985, pp 89–98.

Flood EP, Redish MH, Bociek S, et al: Thrombophlebitis migrans disseminata: Report of a case in which gangrene of breast occurred (observations on therapeutic use of Dicumarol). N Y State J Med 43:1121–1124, 1943.

Francis CW, Marder VJ, Evarts CM, et al: Two step warfarin therapy: Prevention of postoperative venous thrombosis without excessive bleeding. JAMA 249:374–378, 1983.

Fred HL, Axelrad M, Lewis JM, et al: Rapid resolution of pulmonary thromboemboli in man. JAMA 196:1137–1139, 1966a.

Fred HL, Burdine JA, Gonzales DA, et al: Arteriographic assessment of lung scanning in the diagnosis of pulmonary thromboembolism. N Engl J Med 275:1025–1032, 1966b.

Gallus AS, Hirsh J, Hull R, et al: Diagnosis of venous thromboembolism. Semin Thromb Hemost 2:203–231, 1976.

Gallus A, Jackaman J, Tillett J, et al: Safety and efficacy of warfarin started early after submassive venous thrombosis or pulmonary embolism. Lancet 2:1293–1296, 1986.

Gerstman BB, Piper JM, Tomita DK, et al: Oral contraceptive estrogen dose and the risk of deep venous thromboembolic disease. Am J Epidemiol 133:32–37, 1991.

Gibbs NM: Venous thrombosis of the lower limbs with particular reference to bed-rest. Br J Surg 45:209–236, 1957.

Ginsberg JS and Hirsh J: Use of antithrombotic agents during pregnancy. Chest 108:305S–311S, 1995.

Ginsberg JS, Kowalachuck G, Hirsh J, et al: Heparin therapy during pregnancy. Risks to fetus and mother. Arch Intern Med 149:2233–2236, 1989.

Ginsberg JS, Wells PS, Hirsh J, et al: Reevaluation of the sensitivity of impedance plethysmography for the detection of deep vein thrombosis. Arch Intern Med 154:1930–1933, 1994.

Glazier RL and Crowell EB: Randomized prospective trial of continuous versus intermittent heparin therapy. JAMA 236:1365–1367, 1976.

Goldberg SK, Lipschutz JB, Fein AM, et al: Hypercapnia implicating massive pulmonary embolism. Crit Care Med 12:686–688, 1984.

Goldhaber SZ: Evolving concepts in thrombolytic therapy for pulmonary embolism. Chest 101:183S–185S, 1992a.

Goldhaber SZ, Haire WD, Feldstein ML, et al: Alteplase vs. heparin in acute pulmonary embolism: Randomized trial assessing right ventricular function and pulmonary perfusion. Lancet 341:507–511, 1993.

Goldhaber SZ, Kessler CM, Heit JA, et al: Recombinant tissue type plasminogen activator versus a novel dosing regimen of urokinase in acute pulmonary embolism. A randomized controlled multicenter trial. J Am Coll Cardiol 20:24–30, 1992b.

Goldhaber SZ, Polak JF, Feldstein ML, et al: Efficacy and safety of repeated boluses of urokinase in the treatment of deep venous thrombosis. Am J Cardiol 73:75–79, 1994.

Goldhaber SZ, Simmons GR, Elliott G, et al: Quantitative plasma D-Dimer levels among patients undergoing pulmonary angiography for suspected pulmonary embolism. JAMA 270:2819–2822, 1993.

Goldhaber SZ, Vaughan DE, and Markis JE: Acute pulmonary embolism treated with tissue plasminogen activator. Lancet 2:886–889, 1986.

Gonzalez-Juanatey JR, Valdes J, Amaro A, et al: Treatment of massive pulmonary thromboembolism with low intrapulmonary dosages of urokinase. Chest 102:341–346, 1992.

Goodman PC: Pulmonary angiography. Clin Chest Med 5:465–477, 1984.

Goodman PC and Brant-Zawadski M: Digital subtraction pulmonary angiography. AJR Am J Roentgenol 139:305–309, 1982.

Goodrich SM and Wood JE: Peripheral venous distensibility and velocity of venous blood flow during pregnancy or during oral contraceptive therapy. Am J Obstet Gynecol 90:740–746, 1964.

Gore JM, Appelbaum JS, Greene HL, et al: Occult cancer in patients with acute pulmonary embolism. Ann Intern Med 96:556–560, 1982.

Gray HH, Morgan JM, Paneth M, et al: Pulmonary embolectomy for acute massive pulmonary embolism: An analysis of 71 cases. Br Heart J 60:196–200, 1988.

Green D, Hirsh J, Heit J, et al: Low molecular weight heparin: A critical analysis of clinical trials. Pharmacol Rev 10:89–109, 1994.

Green D, Lee MY, Lim AC, et al: Prevention of thromboembolism after spinal cord injury using low-molecular-weight heparin. Ann Intern Med 113:571–574, 1990.

Greenfield LJ: Vena caval interruption and pulmonary embolectomy. Clin Chest Med 5:495–505, 1984.

Greenfield LJ, Bruce TA, Nichols NB: Transvenous pulmonary embolectomy by catheter device. Ann Surg 174:881–886, 1971.

Greenfield LJ and Langham MR: Surgical approaches to thromboembolism. Br J Surg 71:968–970, 1984.

Greenfield LJ, McCurdy JR, Brown PP, et al: A new intracaval filter permitting continued flow and resolution of emboli. Surgery 73:599–606, 1973.

Greenfield LJ, Zocco JJ, Wilk J, et al: Clinical experience with the Kim-Ray Greenfield vena caval filter. Ann Surg 185:692–698, 1977.

Greets WH, Code KE, Jay RM, et al: A prospective study of venous thromboembolism after major surgery. N Engl J Med 331:1601–1606, 1994.

Griffin JH, Evatt B, Zimmerman TS, et al: Deficiency of protein C in congenital thrombotic disease. J Clin Invest 68:1370–1373, 1981.

Gulba DC, Schmid C, Borst H, et al: Medical compared with surgical treatment for massive pulmonary embolism. Lancet 343:576–577, 1994.

Gutnick LM: Pulmonary embolus with a normal ventilation perfusion lung scan: Case report. S D J Med 36:17–19, 1983.

Haeger K: Problems of acute deep-vein thrombosis. The interpretations of signs and symptoms. Angiology 20:219–223, 1969.

Hall JG, Pauli RM, and Wilson KM: Maternal and fetal sequelae of anticoagulation during pregnancy. Am J Med 68:122–140, 1980.

Hall RJC, Young C, Sutton GC, et al: Treatment of acute massive pulmonary embolism by streptokinase during labour and delivery. Br Med J 4:647–649, 1972.

Hampson WGJ, Lucas HK, Harris PC, et al: Failure of low-dose heparin to prevent deep-vein thrombosis after hip replacement arthroplasty. Lancet 2:795–800, 1974.

Harker LA, Slichter SJ, Scott CR, et al: Homocystinemia. N Engl J Med 291:537–543, 1974.

Harris EN, Chan JKH, Asherton RA, et al: Thrombosis, recurrent fetal loss, and thrombocytopenia. Predictive value of the anticardiolipin antibody test. Arch Intern Med 146:2153–2156, 1986.

Harris WH, Raines JK, Athanasoulis C, et al: External

pneumatic compression versus warfarin in reducing thrombosis in high-risk hip patients. In Madden JL, Hune M (eds): Venous Thromboembolism: Prevention and Treatment. New York, Appleton-Century-Crofts, 1976, p 51.

Hartman JT, Pugh JL, Smith RD, et al: Cyclic sequential compression of the lower limb in prevention of deep venous thrombosis. J Bone Joint Surg 64:1059–1062, 1982.

Havig O: Deep vein thrombosis and pulmonary embolism. Acta Chir Scand 478[Suppl]:1–120, 1977.

Heijboer H, Brandjes DPM, Baller HR, et al: Deficiencies of coagulation-inhibiting and fibrinolytic proteins in outpatients with deep-vein thrombosis. N Engl J Med 323:1512–1516, 1990.

Heijboer H, Büller HR, Lensing AWA, et al: A comparison of real-time compression ultrasonography with impedance plethysmography for the diagnosis of deep-vein thrombosis in symptomatic outpatients. N Engl J Med 329:1365–1369, 1993.

Helmrich SP, Rosenberg L, Kaufman DW, et al: Venous thromboembolism in relation to oral contraceptive use. Obstet Gynecol 69:91–95, 1987.

Henderson SR, Lund CJ, and Creasman WT: Antepartum pulmonary embolism. Am J Obstet Gynecol 1112:476–486, 1972.

Heparin versus dextran for the prevention of deep-vein thrombosis. A multi-unit controlled trial. Lancet 2:118–120, 1974.

Hillner BE, Philbrick JT, and Becker DM: Optimal management of suspected lower-extremity deep vein thrombosis. Arch Intern Med 152:165–172, 1992.

Hirsh J: Hypercoagulability. Semin Hematol 14:409–425, 1977.

Hirsh J: Heparin. N Engl J Med 324:1565–1574, 1991.

Hirsh J: Antithrombotic therapy in deep vein thrombosis and pulmonary embolism. Am Heart J 123:1115–1122, 1992.

Hirsh J and Fuster V: Guide to anticoagulant therapy. Part 1: Heparin. Circulation 89:1449–1468, 1994a.

Hirsh J and Fuster V: Guide to anticoagulant therapy. Part 2: Oral anticoagulants. Circulation 89:1469–1480, 1994b.

Hirsh J, Genton E, and Hull R: Diagnosis of venous thrombosis. In Venous Thromboembolism. New York, Grune & Stratton, 1981a, pp 73–81.

Hirsh J, Genton E, and Hull R: Treatment of venous thromboembolism. In Venous Thromboembolism. New York, Grune & Stratton, 1981b, pp 122–144.

Hirsh J, Hale GS, McDonald IG, et al: Resolution of acute massive pulmonary embolism after pulmonary artery infusion of streptokinase. Lancet 2:593–597, 1967.

Hirsh J and Hull RD: Treatment of venous thromboembolism. Chest 89:426S–433S, 1986.

Hirsh J and Pollen L: The International Normalized Ratio. A guide to understanding and correcting its problems. Arch Intern Med 154:282–288, 1994.

Hirsh J, Raschke R, Warkentin TE, et al: Heparin: Mechanism of action, pharmacokinetics, dosing considerations, monitoring, efficacy and safety. Chest 108:258S–275S, 1995.

Hirsh J, VanAken WG, Gallus AS, et al: Heparin kinetics in venous thrombosis and pulmonary embolism. Circulation 53:691–695, 1976.

Hommes DW, Bura A, Mazzolai L, et al: Subcutaneous heparin compared with continuous intravenous heparin administration in the initial treatment of deep vein thrombosis. A meta-analysis. Ann Intern Med 116:279–284, 1992.

Horattas MC, Wright DJ, Fenton AH, et al: Changing concepts of deep venous thrombosis of the upper extremity—report of a series and review of the literature. Surgery 104:561–567, 1988.

Huet Y, Lemaire F, Brun-Buisson C, et al: Hypoxemia in acute pulmonary embolism. Chest 88:829–836, 1985.

Huisman MV, Büller HR, ten Cate JW, et al: Serial impedance plethysmography for suspected deep venous thrombosis in outpatients. N Engl J Med 314:823–834, 1986.

Huisman MV, Büller HR, ten Cate JW, et al: Utility of impedance plethysmography in the diagnosis of recurrent deep-vein thrombosis. Arch Intern Med 148:681–683, 1988.

Huisman MV, Büller HR, ten Cate JW, et al: Management of clinically suspected acute venous thrombosis in outpatients with serial impedance plethysmography in a community hospital setting. Arch Intern Med 149:511–513, 1989a.

Huisman MV, Büller HR, ten Cate JW, et al: Unexpected high prevalence of silent pulmonary embolism in patients with deep venous thrombosis. Chest 95:498–502, 1989b.

Hull RD, Carter CJ, Jay RM, et al: The diagnosis of acute, recurrent, deep vein thrombosis: A diagnostic challenge. Circulation 67:901–906, 1983a.

Hull RD, Carter CJ, Turpie AGG, et al: A randomized trial of diagnostic strategies for symptomatic deep vein thrombosis. Thromb Hemost 50:160, 1983b.

Hull RD, Delmore TJ, Carter C, et al: Adjusted subcutaneous heparin versus warfarin sodium in the long-term treatment of venous thrombosis. N Engl J Med 306:189–194, 1982a.

Hull R, Delmore TJ, Hirsh J, et al: Effectiveness of intermittent pulsatile elastic stocking for prevention of calf and thigh vein thrombosis in patients undergoing knee surgery. Thromb Res 16:37–45, 1979.

Hull RD, Hirsh J, Carter CJ, et al: Pulmonary angiography, ventilation lung scanning, and venography for clinically suspected pulmonary embolism with abnormal perfusion lung scan. Ann Intern Med 98:891–899, 1983c.

Hull RD, Hirsh J, Carter CJ, et al: Diagnostic efficacy of impedance plethysmography for clinically suspected deep vein thrombosis: A randomized trial. Ann Intern Med 102:21–28, 1985a.

Hull RD, Hirsh J, Carter CJ, et al: Diagnostic value of ventilation-perfusion lung scanning in patients with suspected pulmonary embolism. Chest 88:819–828, 1985b.

Hull RD, Hirsh J, Jay R, et al: Different intensities of oral anticoagulant therapy in the treatment of proximal vein thrombosis. N Engl J Med 307:1676–1681, 1982b.

Hull RD, Hirsh J, Sackett DL, et al: Replacement of venography in suspected venous thrombosis by impedance plethysmography and ^{125}I-fibrinogen leg scanning. Ann Intern Med 94:12–15, 1981a.

Hull RD, Hirsh J, Sackett DL, et al: Cost effectiveness of clinical diagnosis, venography, and noninvasive testing in patients with symptomatic deep-vein thrombosis. N Engl J Med 304:1561–1567, 1981b.

Hull RD and Raskob GE: Low-probability lung scan findings: A need for change. Ann Intern Med 114:142–143, 1991.

Hull RD, Raskob GE, and Carter CJ: Serial impedance plethysmography in pregnant patients with clinically suspected deep-vein thrombosis: clinical validity of negative findings. Ann Intern Med 112:663–667, 1990a.

Hull RD, Raskob GE, Coates G, et al: A new noninvasive management strategy for patients with suspected pulmonary embolism. Arch Intern Med 149:2549–2555, 1989.

Hull RD, Raskob GE, Coates G, et al: Clinical validity of a normal perfusion lung scan in patients with suspected pulmonary embolism. Chest 97:23–26, 1990b.

Hull RD, Raskob GE, Gent M, et al: Effectiveness of intermittent pneumatic leg compression for preventing deep vein thrombosis after total hip replacement. JAMA 263:2313–2317, 1990c.

Hull RD, Raskob GE, Ginsberg JS, et al: A noninvasive strategy for the treatment of patients with suspected pulmonary embolism. Arch Intern Med 154:289–297, 1994.

Hull RD, Raskob GE, and Hirsh J: Prophylaxis of venous thromboembolism. An overview. Chest 89:374S–383S, 1986a.

Hull RD, Raskob GE, Hirsh J, et al: Continuous intravenous heparin compared with intermittent subcutaneous heparin in the initial treatment of proximal vein thrombosis. N Engl J Med 315:1109, 1986b.

Hull RD, Raskob GE, LeClere JR, et al: The diagnosis of clinically suspected venous thrombosis. Clin Chest Med 5:439–456, 1984.

Hull RD, Raskob GE, Pineo GF, et al: Subcutaneous low-molecular-weight heparin compared with continuous intravenous heparin in the treatment of proximal-vein thrombosis. N Engl J Med 326:975–982, 1992a.

Hull RD, Raskob G, Pineo G, et al: A comparison of subcutaneous low-molecular-weight heparin with warfarin sodium prophylaxis against deep-vein thrombosis after hip or knee implantation. N Engl J Med 329:1370–1376, 1993.

Hull RD, Raskob GE, Rosenbloom D, et al: Heparin for 5 days as compared with 10 days in the initial treatment of proximal venous thrombosis. N Engl J Med 322:1260–1264, 1990d.

Hull RD, Raskob GE, Rosenbloom D, et al: Optimal therapeutic level of heparin therapy in patients with venous thrombosis. Arch Intern Med 152:1589–1595, 1992b.

Hull RD, VanAken WG, Hirsh J, et al: Impedance plethysmography using the occlusive cuff technique in the diagnosis of venous thrombosis. Circulation 53:696–700, 1976.

Hyers TM, Hull RD, and Weg JG: Antithrombotic therapy for venous thromboembolic disease. Chest 108:335S–351S, 1995.

Ibarra-Pérez C, Lau-Cortés E, Colmenero-Zubiate S, et al: Prevalence and prevention of deep venous thrombosis of the lower extremities in high-risk pulmonary patients. Angiology 39:505–513, 1988.

Ikard RW, Ueland K, and Folse R: Lower limb venous dynamics in pregnant women. Surg Gynecol Obstet 132:483–488, 1971.

Imperiale TF and Speroff T: A meta-analysis of methods to prevent venous thromboembolism following total hip replacement. JAMA 271:1780–1785, 1994.

Inman W and Vessey MP: Investigation of deaths from pulmonary, coronary, and cerebral thrombosis and embolism in women of childbearing age. Br Med J 2:193–196, 1978.

Inman WHW, Vessey WP, Westerholm B, et al: Thromboembolic disease and the steroidal content of oral contraceptives. A report to the committee on safety of drugs. Br Med J 2:203–209, 1970.

International multi-centre trial on the prevention of fatal postoperative pulmonary embolism by low doses of heparin. Lancet 2:45–51, 1975.

Jay R, Hull R, Carter C, et al: Outcome of abnormal impedance plethysmography results in patients with proximal-vein thrombosis: Frequency of return to normal. Thromb Res 36:259–263, 1984.

Jeffcoate TNA, Miller J, Roos RF, et al: Puerperal thromboembolism in relation to the inhibition of lactation by estrogen therapy. Br Med J 4:19–25, 1968.

Jick H, Slone D, Borda IT, et al: Efficacy and toxicity of heparin in relation to age and sex. N Engl J Med 279:284–286, 1968.

Johansson L, Hedner U, and Nilsson IM: A family with thromboembolic disease associated with deficient fibrinolytic activity in vessel wall. Acta Med Scand 203:477–480, 1978a.

Johansson L, Hedner U, and Nilsson IM: Familial antithrombin III deficiency as pathogenesis of deep vein thrombosis. Acta Med Scand 204:491–495, 1978b.

Johansson L, Nylander G, Hedner U, et al: Comparison of streptokinase with heparin: Late results in the treatment of deep venous thrombosis. Acta Med Scand 206:93–98, 1979.

Kahn D, Bushnell DL, Dean R, et al: Clinical outcome of patients with a "low probability" of pulmonary embolism on ventilation-perfusion lung scan. Arch Intern Med 149:377–379, 1989.

Kakkar VV, Cohen AT, Edmonson RA, et al: Low molecular weight versus standard heparin for prevention of venous thromboembolism after major abdominal surgery. Lancet 341:259–265, 1993.

Kakkar VV, Flanc C, Howe CT, et al: Treatment of deep vein thrombosis: A trial of heparin, streptokinase and arvin. Br Med J 1:806–810, 1969a.

Kakkar VV, Howe CT, Flanc C, et al: Natural history of postoperative deep-vein thrombosis. Lancet 2:230–232, 1969b.

Kakkar VV, Howe CT, Nicolaides AN, et al: Deep vein thrombosis of the legs. Is there a high risk group? Am J Surg 120:527–530, 1970.

Kakkar VV and Murray WJG: Efficacy and safety of low-molecular-weight heparin (CY216) in preventing postoperative venous thromboembolism: A cooperative study. Br J Surg 72:786–791, 1985.

Kanis JA: Heparin in the treatment of pulmonary thromboembolism. Thromb Diath Haemorrh 32:519–527, 1974.

Kanter B and Moser KM: The Greenfield vena cava filter. Chest 93:170–175, 1988.

Kasper W, Meinertz T, Hankel B, et al: Echocardiographic findings in patients with proved pulmonary embolism. Am Heart J 112:1284–1290, 1986.

Kearon C and Hirsh J: Factors influencing the reported sensitivity and specificity of impedance plethysmography for proximal deep vein thrombosis. Thromb Haemost 72:652–658, 1994.

Kelly MJ and Elliot LP: The radiographic evaluation of the patient with suspected pulmonary thromboembolic disease. Med Clin North Am 59:3–36, 1974.

Kelley MA, Carson JL, Palevsky HI, et al: Diagnosing pulmonary embolism: New facts and strategies. Ann Intern Med 114:300–306, 1991.

Kernohan RJ and Todd C: Heparin therapy in thromboembolic disease. Lancet 1:621–623, 1966.

Khamashta M, Cuadrado M, Mujic F, et al: The management of thrombosis in the antiphospholipid-antibody syndrome. N Engl J Med 332:393–398, 1995.

Kierkegaard A, Norgren L, Olsson C, et al: Incidence of deep vein thrombosis in bedridden non-surgical patients. Acta Med Scand 222:409–414, 1987.

Kinasewitz GT and George RB: Management of thromboembolism. Anticoagulants, thrombolytics or surgical intervention? Chest 86:106–111, 1984.

King DJ and Kelton JG: Heparin-associated thrombocytopenia. Ann Intern Med 100:535–540, 1984.

Kipper MS, Moser KM, Kortman KE, et al: Long-term followup of patients with suspected pulmonary embolism and a normal lung scan. Chest 82:411–415, 1982.

Kline A, Hughes LE, Campbell H, et al: Dextran 70 in prophylaxis of thromboembolic disease after surgery: A clinically oriented randomized double-blind trial. Br Med J 2:109–112, 1975.

Koller M, Schock U, Buchmann P, et al: Low molecular weight heparin (Kabi 2165) as thromboprophylaxis in elective visceral surgery. Thromb Haemost 59:216–220, 1988.

Koopman MMW, Prandoni P, Piovella F, et al: Treatment of venous thrombosis with intravenous unfractionated heparin administered in the hospital as compared with subcutaneous low-molecular-weight heparin administered at home. N Engl J Med 334:682–687, 1996.

Koster T, Rosendaal FR, de Ronde H, et al: Venous thrombosis due to poor anticoagulant response to activated protein C: Leiden thrombophilia study. Lancet 342:1503–1506, 1993.

Langerstedt CI, Olsson C-G, Fagher BO, et al: Need for long-term anticoagulant treatment in symptomatic calf-vein thrombosis. Lancet 2:515–518, 1985.

Leclerc JR, Geerts WH, Desjardins L, et al: Prevention of deep-vein thrombosis after major knee surgery—a randomized, double-blind trial comparing a low molecular weight heparin fragment (enoxaparin) to placebo. Thromb Haemost 67:417–423, 1992.

Leclerc JR, Wolfson C, Arzoumanian A, et al: Technetium-99m red blood cell venography in patients with clinically suspected deep vein thrombosis: A retrospective study. J Nucl Med 29:1498–1506, 1988.

Lee ME, Biello DR, Kumar B, et al: "Low-probability" ventilation-perfusion scintigrams: Clinical outcomes in 99 patients. Radiology 156:497–500, 1985.

Leeper KV, Popovich J, Lesser BA, et al: Treatment of massive acute pulmonary embolism: The use of low doses of intrapulmonary arterial streptokinase combined with full doses of systemic heparin. Chest 93:234–240, 1988.

Lensing AWA, Hirsh J, and Büller HR: Diagnosis of venous thrombosis. In Colman RW, Hirsh J, Marder VJ, et al (eds): Hemostasis and Thrombosis: Basic Principles and Clinical Practice, 3rd ed. Philadelphia, JB Lippincott, 1994, pp 1297–1321.

Lensing AWA, Prandoni P, Brandjes D, et al: Detection of deep-vein thrombosis by real-time B-mode ultrasonography. N Engl J Med 320:342–345, 1989.

Lensing AWA, Prins MH, Davidson BL, et al: Treatment of deep venous thrombosis with low-molecular-weight heparins. A meta-analysis. Arch Intern Med 155:601–607, 1995.

Levine MN, Gent M, Hirsh J, et al: A comparison of low-molecular-weight heparin administered primarily at home with unfractionated heparin administered in the hospital for proximal deep-vein thrombosis. N Engl J Med 334:677–681, 1996.

Levine MN, Goldhaber SZ, Gore JM, et al: Hemorrhagic complications of thrombolytic therapy in the treatment of myocardial infarction and venous thromboembolism. Chest 108:291S–301S, 1995a.

Levine M, Hirsh J, Gent M: Double-blind randomized trial of very-low-dose warfarin for prevention of thromboembolism in stage IV breast cancer. Lancet 343:886–889, 1994.

Levine MN, Hirsh J, Gent M, et al: Prevention of deep vein thrombosis after elective hip surgery: A randomized trial comparing low-molecular-weight heparin with standard unfractionated heparin. Ann Intern Med 114:545–551, 1991.

Levine M, Hirsh J, Weitz J, et al: A randomized trial of a single bolus dosage regimen of recombinant tissue plasminogen activator in patients with acute pulmonary embolism. Chest 98:1473–1479, 1990a.

Levine MN, Raskob G, Landefeld S, et al: Hemorrhage complications of long-term anticoagulant therapy. Chest 108:276S–290S, 1995b.

Levine MN, Weitz J, Turpie AGG, et al: A new short infusion dosage regimen of recombinant tissue plasminogen activator in patients with thromboembolic disease. Chest 97:168S–171S, 1990b.

Levy SE and Simmons DH: Redistribution of alveolar ventilation following pulmonary thromboembolism in the dog. J Appl Physiol 36:60–68, 1974.

Levy SE and Simmons DH: Mechanism of arterial hypoxemia following pulmonary thromboembolism in dogs. J Appl Physiol 39:41–46, 1975.

Lieberman JS, Borrero J, Urdaneta E, et al: Thrombophlebitis and cancer. JAMA 177:542–545, 1961.

Lijnen HR and Collen D: Review: Congenital and acquired deficiencies of components of the fibrinolytic system and their relationship to bleeding and thrombosis. Fibrinolysis 3:67–78, 1989.

Lippmann M and Fein A: Pulmonary embolism in the patient with chronic obstructive pulmonary disease. Chest 79:39–42, 1981.

Loubeyre P, Revel D, Douek P, et al: Dynamic contrast-enhanced MR angiography of pulmonary embolism: Comparison with pulmonary angiograph. AJR Am J Roentgenol 162:1035–1039, 1994.

Love PE and Santoro SA: Antiphospholipid antibodies: Anticardiolipin and the lupus anticoagulant in systemic lupus erythematosus (SLE) and in non-SLE disorders. Ann Intern Med 112:682–692, 1990.

Ludwig JW, Verhoeven LAJ, Kersbergen JJ, et al: Digital subtraction angiography of the pulmonary arteries for the diagnosis of pulmonary embolism. Radiology 147:639–645, 1983.

McDevitt E and Smith B: Thrombophlebitis during pregnancy and the puerperium. In Sherry S, Bronkhouse KM, Genton E, et al (eds): Thrombosis. Washington, DC, National Academy of Science, 1969, p 55.

McFarland MJ and Imperiale TF: Use of the alveolar-arterial oxygen gradient in the diagnosis of pulmonary embolism. Am J Med 96:57–62, 1994.

McGehec WG, Klotz TA, Epstein DJ, et al: Coumarin necrosis associated with hereditary protein C deficiency. Ann Intern Med 101:59–60, 1984.

McIntyre KM and Sasahara AA: The hemodynamic response to pulmonary embolism in patients without prior cardiopulmonary disease. Am J Cardiol 28:288–294, 1971.

McIntyre KM and Sasahara AA: Determinants of cardiovascular responses to pulmonary embolism. In Moser KM and Stein M (eds): Pulmonary Thromboembolism. Chicago, YearBook Medical Publishers, 1973, pp 144–159.

McKenna R, Cole ER, Vasan M: Is warfarin sodium contraindicated in the lactating mother? J Pediatr 103:325–327, 1983.

McNeil BJ: A diagnostic strategy using ventilation-perfusion studies in patients suspected for pulmonary embolism. J Nucl Med 17:613–616, 1976.

McNeil BJ: Ventilation-perfusion studies and the diagnosis of pulmonary embolism: Concise communication. J Nucl Med 21:319–323, 1980.

McNeil BL, Holman BI, and Adelstein SJ: The scintigraphic definition of pulmonary embolism. JAMA 227:753–756, 1974.

Makhoul RG and McCann RL: Heparin associated thrombocytopenia and thrombosis. A serious clinical problem and potential solution. J Vasc Surg 4:522–528, 1986.

Manier G, Castaing Y, and Guenard H: Determinants of hypoxemia during acute phase of pulmonary embolism in humans. Am Rev Respir Dis 132:332–338, 1985.

Mannucci PM and Vigano S: Deficiencies of protein C, an inhibitor of blood coagulation. Lancet 2:463–467, 1982.

Mant MJ, Thong KL, Birtwhistle RV, et al: Hemorrhagic complications of heparin therapy. Lancet 1:1133–1135, 1977.

Marciniak E and Gockerman JP: Heparin induced decrease in circulatory antithrombin III. Lancet 2:581–584, 1977.

Marder VJ: The use of thrombolytic agents: Choice of patient, drug administration, laboratory monitoring. Ann Intern Med 90:802–808, 1979.

Marder VJ, Soulen RL, Atichartakarn V, et al: Quantitative venographic assessment of deep vein thrombosis in the evaluation of streptokinase and heparin therapy. J Lab Clin Med 89:1018–1029, 1977.

Markel A, Manzo R, Bergelin R, et al: Valvular reflux after deep vein thrombosis: Incidence and time of occurrence. J Vasc Surg 15:377–384, 1992.

Martin B, Martyak TE, Soughton TL, et al: Experience with the Gianturco-Roehm bird's nest vena cava filter. Am J Cardiol 66:1275–1277, 1990.

Martinez J: Quantitative and qualitative disorders of fibrinogen. In Hoffman R, Benz EJ Jr, Shattil SL, et al (eds): Hematology: Basic Principles and Practices. New York, Churchill Livingstone, 1991, pp 1342–1354.

Mattox KL, Feldtman RW, Beall AC Jr, et al: Pulmonary embolectomy for acute massive pulmonary embolism. Ann Surg 195:726–730, 1982.

Meyer G, Tamisier D, Sors H, et al: Pulmonary embolectomy: A 20-year experience at one center. Ann Thorac Surg 51:232–236, 1991.

Miletich JP: Laboratory diagnosis of protein C deficiency. Semin Thromb Hemost 16:169–176, 1990.

Miller GAH, Hall RJC, and Paneth M: Pulmonary embolectomy, heparin, and streptokinase—their place in the treatment of acute massive pulmonary embolism. Am Heart J 93:568–574, 1977.

Miller GAH and Sutton GC: Acute massive pulmonary embolism. Clinical and hemodynamic findings in 23 patients studied by cardiac catheterization and pulmonary arteriography. Br Heart J 32:518–523, 1970.

Misttretta CA: Digital videoangiography. Diagn Imaging 3:14–25, 1981.

Mittleman JS, Edwards WS, and McDonald JB: Effectiveness of leg compression in preventing venous stasis. Am J Surg 14:611–613, 1982.

Molina JE, Hunter DW, and Yedlicka JW: Thrombolytic therapy for iliofemoral venous thrombosis. Vasc Surg 26:630–637, 1992.

Monreal M, Lafoz E, Ruiz J, et al: Upper-extremity deep venous thrombosis and pulmonary embolism. A prospective study. Chest 99:280–283, 1991.

Moorthy SS and Losasso AM: Patency of the foramen ovale in the critically ill patients. Anesthesiology 41:405–407, 1974.

Moorthy SS, Losasso AM, and Gibbs PS: Acquired right to left intracardiac shunt in severe hypoxemia. Crit Care Med 6:28–31, 1978.

Morabia A: Heparin doses and major bleeding. Lancet 1:1276–1279, 1986.

Moser KM: Venous thromboembolism. Am Rev Respir Dis 141:235–249, 1990.

Moser KM: Treating pulmonary embolism: Who, when, and how? J Respir Dis 15:122–127, 1994.

Moser KM, Fedullo PF, Littejohn JK, et al: Frequent asymptomatic pulmonary embolism in patients with deep venous thrombosis. JAMA 271:223–225, 1994.

Moser KM, Guisan M, Cuomo A, et al: Differentiation of pulmonary vascular from parenchymal diseases by ventilation-perfusion scintiphotography. Ann Intern Med 75:597–605, 1971.

Moser KM and LeMoine JR: Is embolic risk conditioned by location of deep venous thrombosis? Ann Intern Med 94:439–444, 1981.

Moser KM, Spragg RG, Utley J, et al: Chronic thrombotic obstruction of major pulmonary arteries. Ann Intern Med 99:299–305, 1983.

Mueh J, Herbst K, and Rapaport S: Thrombosis in patients with the lupus anticoagulant. Ann Intern Med 92:156–159, 1980.

Mudd SH, Skovby F, Levy HL, et al: The natural history of homocystinuria due to cystathionine beta-synthase deficiency. Am J Hum Genet 37:1–37, 1985.

Nelson JR and Smith JR: The pathologic physiology of pulmonary embolism: A physiologic discussion of the vascular reactions following pulmonary arterial obstruction by emboli of varying size. Am Heart J 58:916–932, 1959.

Nicolaides AN, Fernandes JF, and Pollock AV: Intermittent sequential pneumatic compression of the legs in the prevention of venous stasis and postoperative deep venous thrombosis. Surgery 87:69–77, 1980.

Nicolaides AN, Miles C, Hoare M, et al: Intermittent sequential pneumatic compression of the legs and thromboembolism-deterrent stockings in the prevention of postoperative deep venous thrombosis. Surgery 94:21–25, 1983.

Nielsen PE, Kirchner PT, and Gerber FH: Oblique views in lung perfusion scanning. Clinical utility and limitations. J Nucl Med 18:967–972, 1977.

NIH Consensus Conference: Prevention of venous thrombosis and pulmonary embolism. JAMA 256:744–749, 1986.

Nordstrom M, Lindbland B, Anderson H, et al: Deep venous thrombosis and occult malignancy: An epidemiological study. Br Med J 308:891–894, 1994.

Novelline RA, Baltarowich OH, Athanasoulis CA, et al: The clinical course of patients with suspected pulmonary embolism and a negative pulmonary arteriogram. Radiology 126:561–567, 1978.

Noyes LD, Rice JC, and Kerstein MD: Hemodynamic assessment of high-compression hosiery in chronic venous disease. Surgery 102:813–815, 1987.

O'Donnell TF, Browse NL, Burnard KG, et al: The socioeconomic effects of ilio-femoral venous thrombosis. J Surg Res 22:483–488, 1977.

Orren DE, Gornish M, and Bar-Ziv J: Computed tomography. In Kim D, Orron DE (eds): Peripheral Vascular Imaging and Intervention. St. Louis, Mosby-YearBook, 1992, pp 183–200.

Oster JR, Singer I, Fishman LM, et al: Heparin-induced aldosterone suppression and hyperkalemia. Am J Med 98:575–586, 1995.

Oudker KM, van Beck EJR, van Putten WLJ, et al: Cost-effectiveness analysis of various strategies in the diagnostic management of pulmonary embolism. Arch Intern Med 153:947–954, 1993.

Overton DT and Bocka JJ: The alveolar-arterial oxygen gradient in patients with documented pulmonary embolism. Arch Intern Med 148:1617–1619, 1988.

Owen CA and Bowie EJW: Predisposing factors in thrombosis. In Kwaan HC, Bowie EJW (eds):

Thrombosis. Philadelphia, WB Saunders, 1982, pp 29–56.

Paiement G, Wessinger SJ, Waltman AC, et al: Surveillance of deep vein thrombosis in asymptomatic total hip replacement patients: Impedance phlebography and fibrinogen scanning versus roentgenographic phlebography. Am J Surg 155:400–404, 1988.

Paraskos JA, Adelstein SJ, Smith RE, et al: Late prognosis of acute pulmonary embolism. N Engl J Med 289:55–58, 1973.

Parker BM and Smith JR: Pulmonary embolism and infarction. Am J Med 24:402–427, 1958.

Parmley LF, North RL, and Ott BS: Hemodynamic alterations of acute pulmonary thromboembolism. Circ Res 11:450–465, 1962.

Pearson SD, Polak JL, Cartwright S, et al: A critical pathway to evaluate suspected deep vein thrombosis. Arch Intern Med 155:1773–1778, 1995.

Peters AM, Lavender JP, Needham SG, et al: Imaging thrombus with radio labeled monoclonal antibody to platelets. Br Med J 293:1527–1527, 1986.

Petri M, Rheinschmidt M, Whiting-O'Keeke Q, et al: The frequency of lupus anticoagulant in systemic lupus erythematosus. Ann Intern Med 106:524–531, 1987.

Pezzuoli G, Neri Serneri GG, Settembrini PG, et al: Effectiveness and safety of the low-molecular-weight heparin CY 126 in the prevention of fatal pulmonary embolism and thromboembolic death in general surgery. Haemostasis 20[Suppl]:193–204, 1990.

Philbrick JT and Becker DM: Calf deep venous thrombosis. A wolf in sheep's clothing. Arch Intern Med 148:2131–2138, 1988.

Pineo GF, Brain MC, Gallus AS, et al: Tumors, mucous production, and hypercoagulability. Ann N Y Acad Sci 230:262–270, 1974.

Pini M, Pattachini C, Quintavella R, et al: Subcutaneous vs. intravenous heparin in the treatment of deep venous thrombosis: A randomized clinical trial. Thromb Haemost 64:222–226, 1990.

PIOPED investigators: Value of the ventilation/perfusion scan in acute pulmonary embolism: Results of the perspective investigation of pulmonary embolism diagnosis (PIOPED). JAMA 263:2753–2759, 1990.

Planes A, Vochelle N, Mazas F, et al: Prevention of postoperative venous thrombosis: A randomized trial comparing unfractionated heparin with low molecular weight heparin in patients undergoing total hip replacement. Thromb Haemost 60:407–410, 1988.

Planes A, Vochelle M, Fagola M, et al: Efficacy and safety of a perioperative enoxaparin regimen in total hip replacement under various anesthesias. Am J Surg 161:525–531, 1991.

Polak JF: Doppler ultrasound of the deep leg veins. Chest 99:165S–172S, 1991.

Pollak EW, Webber MM, Victery W, et al: Radioisotope detection of venous thrombosis: Venous scan vs. fibrinogen uptake test. Arch Surg 110:613–616, 1975.

Pond GD, Ovitt TW, and Capp MP: Comparison of conventional pulmonary angiography with intravenous digital subtraction angiography for pulmonary embolic disease. Radiology 147:345–350, 1983.

Prandoni P, Lensing AW, Büller HR, et al: Comparison of subcutaneous low-molecular-weight heparin with intravenous standard heparin in proximal deep-vein thrombosis. Lancet 339:441–445, 1992a.

Prandoni P, Lensing A, Büller H, et al: Deep vein thrombosis and the incidence of subsequent symptomatic cancer. N Engl J Med 327:1128–1133, 1992b.

Prediletto R, Paoletti P, Fornai E, et al: Natural course of treated pulmonary embolism. Evaluation by perfusion lung scintigraphy, gas exchange and chest roentgenogram. Chest 97:554–561, 1990.

Prevention of fatal postoperative pulmonary embolism by low doses of heparin: An international multicenter trial. Lancet 2:45–51, 1975.

Proano M, Frye RL, Johnson CM, et al: Successful treatment of pulmonary embolism and associated mobile right atrial thrombus with use of a central thrombolytic infusion. Mayo Clin Proc 63:1181–1185, 1988.

Rabinov K and Paulin S: Roentgen diagnosis of venous thrombosis in the leg. Arch Surg 104:134–144, 1972.

Raschke RA, Reilly BM, Guidry GR, et al: The weight-based heparin dosing nomogram compared with a "standard care" nomogram. A randomized controlled trial. Ann Intern Med 119:874–881, 1993.

Rees DM and Rodgers GM: Homocystinemia: Association of ametabolic disorder with vascular disease and thrombosis. Thromb Res 71:337–359, 1993.

Research Committee of the British Thoracic Society: Optimum duration of anticoagulation for deep-vein thrombosis and pulmonary embolism. Lancet 340:873–876, 1992.

Rickles F and Edwards R: Activation of blood coagulation in cancer: Trousseau's syndrome revisited. Blood 62:14–31, 1983.

Robertson BR, Pandolfi M, and Nilsson IM: "Fibrinolytic capacity" in healthy volunteers at different ages as studied by standardized venous occlusion of arms and legs. Acta Med Scand 191:199–202, 1972.

Roehm JOF: The bird's nest filter: A new percutaneous transcatheter inferior vena cava filter. J Vasc Surg 1:498–501, 1984.

Roehm JOF, Johnsrude IS, Barth MH, et al: The bird's nest inferior vena cava filter: Progress report. Radiology 168:745–749, 1988.

Rogers LQ and Lutcher CL: Streptokinase therapy for deep vein thrombosis: A comprehensive review of the English literature. Am J Med 88:389–395, 1990.

Rogers LQ and Lutcher CL: Streptokinase therapy

and break away pulmonary emboli—the reply. Am J Med 90:412, 1991.

Rosove MH and Brewer P: Antiphospholipid thrombosis: Clinical course after the first thrombotic event in 70 patients. Ann Intern Med 117:303–308, 1992.

Rosse W and Ware R: The molecular basis of paroxysmal nocturnal hemoglobinuria. Blood 86:3277–3286, 1995.

Rubinstein I, Murray D, and Hoffstein V: Fatal pulmonary emboli in hospitalized patients. An autopsy study. Arch Intern Med 148:1425–1426, 1988.

Sabiston DC Jr, Wolfe WG, Oldham HN, et al: Surgical management of chronic pulmonary embolism. Ann Surg 185:699–712, 1977.

Sack GH, Levin J, Bell W: Trousseau's syndrome and other manifestations of disseminated coagulopathy in patients with neoplasms: Clinical, pathophysiologic, and therapeutic features. Medicine (Baltimore) 56:1–37, 1977.

Sagar S, Stamatakis JD, Thomas DP, et al: Oral contraceptives, antithrombin III activity, and postoperative deep vein thrombosis. Lancet 1:509–511, 1976.

Salzman EW, Harris WH, and De Sanctis RW: Anticoagulation for prevention of thromboembolism following fracture of the hip. N Engl J Med 275:122–130, 1966.

Salzman EW, Ploetz J, Bettmann M, et al: Intraoperative external pneumatic calf compression to afford long-term prophylaxis against deep vein thrombosis in urological patients. Surgery 87:239–242, 1980.

Salzman EW, Shapiro RM, Deykin D, et al: Management of heparin therapy: Controlled prospective trial. N Engl J Med 292:1046–1050, 1975.

Sandler DA and Martin JF: Autopsy proven pulmonary embolism in hospital patients: Are we detecting enough deep vein thrombosis? J Royal Soc Med 82:203–205, 1989.

Sandler DA, Martin JF, Duncan JS, et al: Diagnosis of deep-vein thrombosis: Comparison of clinical evaluation, ultrasound, plethysmography and venoscan with x-ray venogram. Lancet 2:716–719, 1984.

Santolicandro A, Prediletto R, Fornai E, et al: Mechanisms of hypoxemia and hypocapnia in pulmonary embolism. Am J Respir Crit Care Med 152:336–347, 1995.

Santori FS, Vitullo A, Stopponi M, et al: Prophylaxis against deep-vein thrombosis in total hip replacement. J Bone Joint Surg 76B:579–583, 1994.

Sauerbrei E, Thomson JG, McLachlan MS, et al: Observer variation in lower limb venography. J Can Assoc Radiol 31:28–29, 1981.

Schulman S, Rhedia A, Lindmarker P, et al: A comparison of six weeks with six months of oral coagulant therapy after a first episode of venous thromboembolism. N Engl J Med 332:1661–1665, 1995.

Scurr JH, Coleridge-Smith PD, and Hasty JH: Regimen for improved effectiveness of intermittent pneumatic compression in deep venous thrombosis prophylaxis. Surgery 102:816–820, 1987.

Severinghaus JW and Stupfel M: Alveolar dead space as an index of distribution of blood flow in pulmonary capillaries. J Appl Physiol 10:335–348, 1957.

Sevitt S and Gallagher NG: Prevention of venous thrombosis and pulmonary embolism in injured patients. Trial of anticoagulant prophylaxis with phenidione in middle-aged and elderly patients with fractured necks of femur. Lancet 2:981–989, 1959.

Sevitt S and Gallagher NG: Venous thrombosis and pulmonary embolism: A clinicopathologic study in injured and burned patients. Br J Surg 48:475–482, 1961.

Simon TL, Hyers TM, Gaston JD, et al: Heparin pharmacokinetics: Increased requirements in pulmonary embolism. Br J Haematol 39:111–120, 1978.

Sirchia G and Lewis SM: Paroxysmal nocturnal hemoglobinuria. Clin Haematol 4:199–229, 1975.

Skillman JJ, Collins REC, Coe NP, et al: Prevention of deep vein thrombosis in neurosurgical patients: A controlled, randomized trial of external pneumatic compression boots. Surgery 83:354–358, 1978.

Smith R, Maher JM, Miller RI, et al: Clinical outcomes of patients with suspected pulmonary embolism and low-probability aerosol-perfusion scintigrams. Radiology 164:731–733, 1987.

Spiro TE, Johnson GJ, Christie MG, et al: Efficacy and safety of enoxaparin to prevent deep venous thrombosis after hip replacement surgery. Ann Intern Med 121:81–89, 1994.

Spritzer CE, Norconk JJ Jr, Softman HD, et al: Detection of deep venous thrombosis by magnetic resonance imaging. Chest 104:54–60, 1993.

Stahl CP, Wideman CS, Spira TJ, et al: Protein S deficiency in men with long-term human immunodeficiency virus infection. Blood 81:1801–1807, 1993.

Stanek V, Riedel M, and Widimsky J: Hemodynamic monitoring in acute pulmonary embolism. Bull Eur Physiopathol Respir 14:561–572, 1978.

Stein PD, Hull RD, and Pineo G: Strategy that includes serial noninvasive leg tests for diagnosis of thromboembolic disease in patients with suspected acute pulmonary embolism based on data from PIOPED. Arch Intern Med 156:2101–2104, 1995.

Stein PD, Hull RD, and Raskob G: Risks for major bleeding from thrombolytic therapy in patients with acute pulmonary embolism. Ann Intern Med 121:313–317, 1994.

Stein PD, Hull RD, Saltzman HA, et al: Strategy for diagnosis of patients with suspected acute pulmonary embolism. Chest 103:1553–1559, 1993.

Stein PD, Willis PW, and DeMets DL: History and

physical examination in acute pulmonary embolism in patients without preexisting cardiac or pulmonary disease. Am J Cardiol 47:218–223, 1981.

Stevenson RE, Burton DM, Ferlanto GJ, et al: Hazards of oral anticoagulants during pregnancy. JAMA 243:1549–1551, 1980.

Sun X, Evatt B, and Griffin JH: Blood coagulation factor Va abnormality associated with resistance to activated protein C in venous thrombophilia. Blood 83:3120–3125, 1994.

Taberner DA, Poller L, Burslem RW, et al: Oral anticoagulants controlled by the British comparative thromboplastin versus low-dose heparin in prophylaxis of deep-vein thrombosis. Br Med J 1:272–274, 1978.

Talbot SR: Use of real-time imaging in identifying deep venous obstruction: A preliminary report. Brit 6:41–42, 1982.

Taylor RR, Covell JW, Sonnenblick EH, et al: Dependence of ventricular distensibility on filing of the opposite ventricle. Am J Physiol 213:711–718, 1967.

Thery C, Simmoneau G, Meyer G, et al: Randomized trial of subcutaneous low-molecular-weight heparin CY 216 (Fraxiparine) with intravenous unfractionated heparin in the curative treatment of submassive pulmonary embolism: A dose-ranging study. Circulation 85:1380, 1992.

Thrombolytic Therapy in Thrombosis: A National Institute of Health Consensus Development Conference. Ann Intern Med 93:141–144, 1980.

Torngren S: Low-dose heparin and compression stocking in the prevention of postoperative deep venous thrombosis. Br J Surg 67:482–484, 1980.

Tow DE and Wagner HN: Recovery of pulmonary arterial blood flow in patients with pulmonary embolism. N Engl J Med 276:1053–1054, 1969.

Triplett DA: Antiphospholipid antibodies and thrombosis. Arch Pathol Lab Med 117:78–88, 1993.

Trousseau A: Lectures on Clinical Medicine Delivered at the Hotel Dieu, Paris, London. The New Sydenham Society, 1882, pp 282–332.

Tsao MS, Schraufnagel D, and Wong NS: Pathogenesis of pulmonary infarction. Am J Med 72:599–608, 1982.

Turpie AGG: Efficacy of a postoperative regimen of enoxaparin in deep vein thrombosis prophylaxis. Am J Surg 161:532–536, 1991.

Turpie AGG, Delmore T, Hirsh J, et al: Prevention of venous thrombosis by intermittent sequential calf compression in patients with intracranial disease. Thromb Res 15:611–616, 1979.

Turpie AGG, Gent M, Cote R, et al: A low-molecular-weight heparinoid compared with unfractionated heparin in the prevention of deep vein thrombosis in patients with acute ischemic stroke. Ann Intern Med 117:353–357, 1992.

Turpie AGG, Levine MN, Hirsh J, et al: A double-blind randomized trial of ORG-10172 low molecular weight heparinoid in the prevention of deep vein thrombosis in thrombotic stroke. Lancet 1:523–526, 1987.

Turpie AGG, Levine MN, Hirsh J, et al: A randomized controlled trial of a low-molecular weight heparin (Enoxaparin) to prevent deep-vein thrombosis in patients undergoing elective hip surgery. N Engl J Med 315:925–929, 1986.

Urokinase Pulmonary Embolism Trial: A cooperative study. Circulation 47[Suppl II]:1–108, 1973.

Urokinase-Streptokinase Pulmonary Embolism Trial, Phase 2 results: A cooperative study. JAMA 229:1606–1613, 1974.

Vandenbrouke JP, Koster T, Briët E, et al: Increased risk of venous thrombosis in oral-contraceptive users who are carriers of factor V Leiden mutation. Lancet 344:1453–1457, 1994.

Vargo JS, Becker DM, Philbrick JT, et al: Plasma DNA. A simple, rapid test for aiding the diagnosis of pulmonary embolism. Chest 97:63–68, 1990.

Verstraete M, Miller GAH, Bounameaux H, et al: Intravenous and intrapulmonary recombinant tissue-type plasminogen activator in the treatment of acute massive pulmonary embolism. Circulation 77:353–360, 1988.

Vessey MP and Doll R: Investigation of relation between use of oral contraceptives and thromboembolic disease. A further report. Br Med J 2:651–657, 1969.

Vigano-D'Angelo SV, D'Angelo A, et al: Protein S deficiency occurs in nephrotic syndrome. Ann Intern Med 107:42–47, 1987.

Virchow RLK: Gesammelte Abhandlungen zur Wissenschaftlichen, Vol IV: Thrombose und Emboli. Berlin: G. Hamm-Grotesche Buchhandlung, 1862, p 219.

Vlahakes GJ, Turley K, and Hoffman JIE: The pathophysiology of failure in acute right ventricular hypertension. Hemodynamic and biochemical correlations. Circulation 63:87–95, 1981.

Vogelzang RL: Computed tomography and magnetic resonance imaging of venous disorders. In Bergan JJ, Yao JST (eds): Venous Disorders. Philadelphia, WB Saunders, 1991, pp 91–122.

Walker AM and Jick H: Predictors of bleeding during heparin therapy. JAMA 244:1209–1212, 1980.

Warden GD, Wilmore DW, and Pruitt BA: Central venous thrombosis: A hazard of medical progress. J Trauma 13:620–625, 1973.

Warkentin T and Kelton J: Heparin and platelets. Hematol Oncol Clin North Am 4:242–254, 1990.

Warkentin T and Kelton J: Heparin induced thrombocytopenia. Prog Hemost Thromb 10:1–34, 1991.

Warkentin TE and Kelton JG: Heparin-induced thrombocytopenia. Ann Rev Med 31:44, 1989.

Warlow C, Beattie AG, Terry G, et al: A double-blind trial of low doses of subcutaneous heparin in the prevention of deep vein thrombosis after myocardial infarction. Lancet 2:934–936, 1974.

Webber MM, Gomes AS, Roe D, et al: Comparison of

Biello, McNiel, and PIOPED criteria for the diagnosis of pulmonary emboli on lung scans. AJR Am J Roentgenol 154:975–981, 1990.

Wells PS, Holbrook AM, Crowther NR, et al: Interaction of warfarin with drugs and food. Ann Intern Med 121:676–683, 1994.

Wells PS, Davidson BL, Prins MH, et al: Accuracy of ultrasound for the diagnosis of deep venous thrombosis in asymptomatic patients after orthopedic surgery. Ann Intern Med 122:47–53, 1995.

Wells PS, Lensing AW, and Hirsh J: Graduated compression stockings in the prevention of postoperative venous thromboembolism: A meta-analysis. Arch Intern Med 154:67–72, 1994.

Wessler S and Gitel SN: Heparin: New concepts relevant to clinical use. Blood 53:525–544, 1979.

Wheeler AP, Jaquiss RDB, and Newman JW: Physician practices in the treatment of pulmonary embolism and deep venous thrombosis. Arch Intern Med 148:1321–1325, 1988.

Wheeler HB, Anderson FH, Cardullo PA, et al: Suspected deep vein thrombosis: Management by impedance plethysmography. Arch Surg 117:1206–1209, 1982.

Wheeler HB, Hirsh J, Wells P, et al: Diagnostic tests for deep vein thrombosis: Clinical usefulness depends on probability of disease. Arch Intern Med 154:1921–1928, 1994.

Wheeler HB, O'Donnell JA, Anderson FA Jr, et al: Occlusive impedance phlebography: A diagnostic procedure for venous thrombosis and pulmonary embolism. Prog Cardiovasc Dis 17:199–205, 1974.

Wheeler HB, O'Donnell JA, Anderson FA, et al: Bedside screening for venous thrombosis using occlusive impedance phlebography. Angiology 26:199–210, 1975.

White RH, McGaham JP, Daschback MM, et al: Diagnosis of deep-vein thrombosis using duplex ultrasound. Ann Intern Med 111:297–304, 1989.

White RH, McKittrick T, Hutchinson R, et al: Temporary discontinuation of warfarin therapy: Changes in the international normalized ratio. Ann Intern Med 122:40–42, 1995.

Willie-Jorgensen P, Thorup J, Fisher A, et al: Heparin with and without graded compression stockings in the prevention of thromboembolic complications of major abdominal surgery: A randomized trial. Br J Surg 72:577–582, 1985.

Wilson JE III, Pierce AK, Johnson RL, et al: Hypoxemia in pulmonary embolism: A clinical study. J Clin Invest 50:481–491, 1971.

Wilson JR and Lampman J: Heparin therapy: A randomized prospective study. Am Heart J 97:155–158, 1979.

Worsley DF, Alavi A, Aronchick JM, et al: Chest radiographic findings in patients with acute pulmonary embolism: Observations from the PIOPED study. Radiology 189:133–136, 1993.

Wright HP: Changes in the adhesiveness of blood platelets following parturition and surgical operations. J Pathol Bacteriol 54:461–468, 1942.

Yett HS, Sbillman JJ, and Salzman EW: The hazards of aspirin and heparin. N Engl J Med 298:1092, 1978.

Yggi J: Changes in blood coagulation and fibrinolysis during the puerperium. Am J Obstet Gynecol 104:2–18, 1969.

Status Asthmaticus

Tahir Ahmed, M.D.

Alejandro D. Chediak, M.D.

Physicians universally cite reversible airways narrowing as the distinguishing clinical feature of asthma. The notion that asthmatic airway narrowing will eventually subside given proper therapy is comforting but serves to promote a sense of complacency toward a potentially lethal illness. The deadly nature of asthma was recently highlighted by the sudden and unexpected death from acute severe asthma of our colleague, Dr. Douglas Onorato. The deceased was a lifelong asthmatic, fully trained in pulmonary diseases with research experience in asthma. Dr. Onorato's academic career was noted for investigations that explored novel means by which to manage acute life-threatening attacks of asthma. That a clinician-scientist specializing in asthma can succumb to this reversible airways disease serves to illustrate the limitations and uncertainties of asthma management. In addition, this tragedy underscores the observation that mortality rates from asthma have been on the rise for several decades.

Basic and clinical research has expanded our understanding of asthma's pathogenesis and has provided new strategies to diagnose, prevent, and manage patients. Although the impact of this knowledge on morbidity and mortality from asthma will likely not be apparent for years, we may use these evolving concepts in hopes of improving outcomes for our patients with asthma (Sheffer, 1991). Nowhere is the information gained from asthma research of greater potential benefit than in the prevention and management of acute, life-threatening attacks of asthma. In this chapter we provide a timely, concise, yet comprehensive review of the most devastating manifestation of acute asthma—status asthmaticus.

DEFINITIONS

The definition of asthma has been controversial primarily because of extreme heterogeneity of this disease. Several groups have proposed various definitions of asthma primarily in terms of function. Attendees of the Ciba Foundation Guest Symposium (1959) suggested that "Asthma refers to the condition of subjects with widespread narrowing of the bronchial airways, which changes in severity over short periods of time either spontaneously or under treatment, and is not due to cardiovascular disease. The clinical characteristics are breathlessness, which may be paroxysmal or persistent, wheezing, and in most cases relieved by bronchodilator drugs." The committee on diagnostic standards of the American Thoracic Society (1962) modified this definition and suggested that "Asthma is a disease characterized by an increased responsiveness of trachea and bronchi to a variety of stimuli and manifested by widespread narrowing of the airways that changes in severity either spontaneously or as a result of therapy." The term *asthma* is not appropriate for the bronchial narrowing that results solely from widespread bronchial infection (e.g., acute or chronic bronchitis), from destructive disease of the lung (e.g., pulmonary emphysema), or from cardiovascular disorders. Asthma may occur in patients with other bronchopulmonary or cardiovascular diseases, but in these instances the airway obstruction is not causally related to these diseases. Committees of the American Thoracic Society and Allergy Foundation of America have further modified the definition on this same basic theme (Spector, 1982).

Status asthmaticus is the critical clinical expression of bronchial asthma, because its advanced gas exchange defects are life-threatening. The clinical state is essentially defined pharmacologically as an episode of asthma unrelieved by the usual bronchodilator therapy. Status asthmaticus is a clinical paradox; that is, by definition, asthma is a reversible obstructive airway disease, but status asthmaticus is refractory to bronchodilator therapy. Refractoriness to therapy is transient in nature. This initial refractoriness is the major criterion for diagnosis of the condition that ultimately does respond to treatment. Because the therapy is far more complex than that required to manage chronic asthma or acute episodic attacks, and especially because status asthmaticus is a life-threatening condition associated with increased mortality, immediate hospitalization of the patient is essential.

The American Thoracic Society has defined status asthmaticus as an acute asthmatic attack in which the degree of airway obstruction is severe from the beginning or increases in severity and is not relieved by the usual treatment (Busey et al, 1968; Heurich et al, 1978). This definition distinguishes the life-threatening acute attack of status asthmaticus from chronic asthma, in which asthmatic individuals wheeze chronically despite therapy. The term *status asthmaticus* also emphasizes the functional state of the patient and incorporates the concept of disabling acute respiratory insufficiency caused by marked airway obstruction sustained for 24 hours or longer, and of potential reversibility with appropriate therapy.

Status asthmaticus varies widely in its severity, from the ambulatory patient seen in the emergency room with an acute attack to the patient in the intensive care unit who is intubated and on controlled mechanical ventilation. The latter is in the most severe form of the disease, culminating in ventilatory failure. This advanced stage reflects a refractoriness to or failure of pharmacologic therapy and is invariably associated with respiratory acidosis. Although an attack of status asthmaticus may develop acutely, it ordinarily builds up over time. Often a patient finds that for several days the asthma is getting worse despite the usual maintenance therapy. Finally, the patient presents to the physician or emergency room. If treatment with aminophylline and sympathomimetic agents fails to break the attack, or if they help only temporarily, hospitalization is required. Asthmatic patients must be made aware that it is essential to seek help quickly if they are not responding to their usual therapeutic regimen. Appropriate therapy in the early stages of an attack can often prevent status asthmaticus, subsequent hospitalization, and mortality.

EPIDEMIOLOGY

INCIDENCE

Asthma affects approximately 3 to 6% of the population (Speizer, 1978). Asthma is prevalent at all ages and in both sexes. Those patients who develop asthma in adult life have predominantly intrinsic-type disease, which tends to be resistant to the usual form of therapy. Status asthmaticus is more common in this group than in patients with extrinsic asthma. Because of classification problems in medical records, it is extremely difficult to obtain reliable figures about the incidence of status asthmaticus.

Asthma is commonly viewed as a health problem of greater importance. An increasing rate of hospital admission for asthma has been observed with an increasing percentage of patients who required intubation and cardiopulmonary resuscitation, (Buist and Vollmer, 1990; Gergen and Weiss, 1990; Weiss et al, 1993; Weiss and Wagener, 1990). This finding is particularly true in the younger age groups, and a substantial increase in the number of hospital admissions and emergency room visits due to childhood asthma has been observed (Anderson, 1989; Gergen and

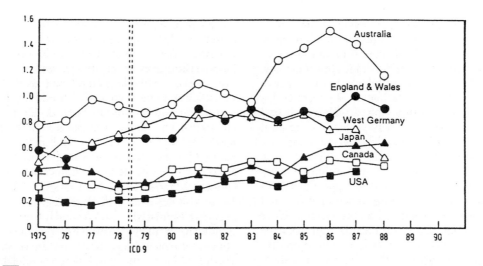

Figure 23-1
Mortality from asthma (rate per 100,000) in 5- to 34-year-old subjects in Australia, England and Wales, West Germany, Japan, Canada, and the United States. (From Sears MR: International trends in asthma mortality. Allergy Proc 12:155–158, 1991. With permission.)

Weiss, 1990). Asthma prevalence has risen in many parts of the world (Erzen et al, 1995; Fleming and Crombie, 1987; Gergen et al, 1988; Haahtela et al, 1990; Vollmer et al, 1992; Weitzman et al, 1992). In some countries the greater prevalence is not associated with a concomitant increase in disease severity (Erzen et al, 1995; Vollmer et al, 1992; Weitzman et al, 1992). Some epidemiologic studies have suggested that increases in asthma prevalence and disease severity may be due to unrelated factors, including disease diagnosis labeling (Carmen and Landall, 1990); changes in practice pattern or service utilization (Keistinen et al, 1993; Vollmer et al, 1992, 1994); and nonstandardized criteria of disease severity (International Consensus Report, 1992). In epidemiologic studies, asthma severity has been assessed in terms of administration data, such as absence from work or school, health-care service utilization and mortality (Aronow, 1988; Vollmer et al, 1994). Insurance data from Manitoba Health showed that the prevalence of physician-diagnosed asthma approximately doubled from 1980 to 1990, but no increase in severity of asthma was detected (Erzen et al, 1995). The higher prevalence was real and only partially explained by unrelated epidemiologic factors as mentioned.

MORBIDITY AND MORTALITY

Asthma-associated mortality is reported to have risen in the United States and throughout the world in both children and adults, especially in those aged 5 to 34 years (Sears, 1991; Weiss et al,

1993) (Fig. 23–1). Although asthma morbidity and mortality appear to be rising, the trend is not uniform (Weiss and Wagener, 1990; Wilkins and Yang, 1993). In part, the increase in asthma mortality can be explained by an increase in asthma prevalence with little or no change in the severity of the disease (Erzen et al, 1995; Vollmer et al, 1992; Weitzman et al, 1992). Fewer than one person per 100,000 dies from this disease; thus, the case fatality rate is extremely low (Ogilvie, 1962; Weiss et al, 1993). Long-term survival among community patients with asthma, but no other lung disease, was not significantly different from expected survival. Patients 35 years or older who had asthma associated with chronic obstructive pulmonary disease, however, did have worse-than-expected survival rates (Silverstein et al, 1994).

Of those patients admitted to a hospital in status asthmaticus, approximately 70 to 80% are managed with relative ease (Crompton and Grant, 1975). The remaining patients are critically ill and are at significant risk of dying, during or as a result of the status asthmaticus episode. It appears that the patients most at risk of dying after entering the hospital in status asthmaticus are those who require intubation. In a review of published work, a total of 149 patients required intubation, generally for increasing hypoventilation (Santiago and Klaustermeyer, 1980; Scoggin et al, 1977). The mortality was 12.1% for intubated and 1 to 2.4% for nonintubated patients in status asthmaticus.

Marquette and coworkers (1992) reviewed

the natural history of very severe asthma. In a retrospective study, they found that of all patients requiring mechanical ventilation in four hospitals in France, the in-hospital mortality rate was 16.5% and the post-hospital mortality rate was 10.1%. Patients over the age of 40 years had a greater risk of mortality (Fig. 23–2). Havill and coworkers (1989) also observed that post-hospital mortality in a 2-year follow-up was 5% in asthmatics who were hospitalized in an intensive care unit in New Zealand. Increase in asthma severity may be a contributing factor to the increase in asthma mortality. Data from a national hospital discharge survey conducted in the United States by the National Center for Health Statistics have shown the prevalence of asthma admissions requiring intubation or cardiopulmonary resuscitation to be 0.5% for the years 1984 to 1987. This represented an increase from 0.11% from the period from 1979 to 1983 (Gergen and Weiss, 1990).

INCREASING ASTHMA MORTALITY

Mortality for asthma has increased in most developed countries over the last 30 years, and hospital admissions, especially of children, have climbed rapidly (Mitchell, 1988; 1989). Some of these countries experienced an epidemic of deaths from asthma in the mid-1960s (Inman and Adelstein, 1969) (Fig. 23–3). An increase in asthma mortal-

ity has been reported in New Zealand (Jackson et al, 1982), England and Wales (Burney, 1986), Canada (Bates and Baker-Anderson, 1987), France (Bousquet et al, 1987), and the United States (Sly, 1984). Hospital admissions for asthma in children have increased 6.6-fold in England and Wales and ten-fold in New Zealand (Mitchell, 1985). The increases in asthma morbidity and mortality appear to be real and not easily explained by the changes in International Classification of Diseases (ICD) coding or death certification (Aronow, 1988; International Consensus, 1992; Vollmer et al, 1994). These findings have occurred against the background of an apparent improvement in the treatment of asthma, development of newer drugs, substantial increase in the sale of asthma drugs, and better understanding of the pathogenesis of asthma. This paradox of improved treatment and greater mortality and morbidity raises the possibility that true changes in the prevalence and severity of disease have occurred, and leads one to question the overall effectiveness of current management of asthma.

Robin (1988) raised an important question: "Is our current management contributing to the increase in asthma mortality?" The reasons for these statistical observations in asthma epidemiology are not clear. Various explanations have included (1) massive undertreatment; (2) changes in the ICD coding; (3) increased prevalence of asthma; (4) improved diagnostic capability; (5)

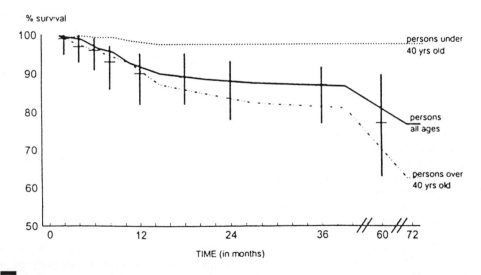

Figure 23–2
Probability of survival (and 95% CI) in patients discharged from the intensive care unit owing to a near-fatal asthma exacerbation. (From Marquette CH, Saulnier F, Leroy O, et al: Long-term prognosis of near-fatal asthma: A 6-year follow-up study of 145 asthmatic patients who underwent mechanical ventilation for a near fatal attack of asthma. Am Rev Respir Dis 146:76–81, 1992. With permission.)

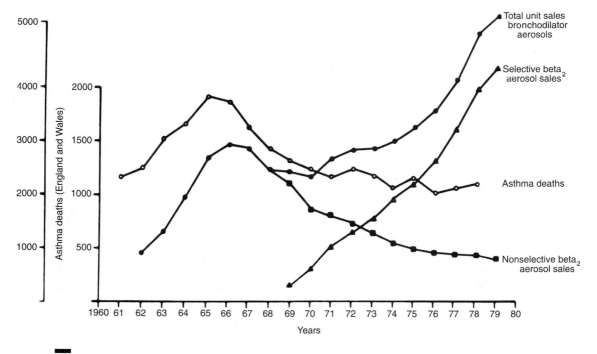

Figure 23–3

Relationship between increased asthma deaths and nonselective beta-agonist aerosol sales in England and Wales in the 60s. (From Clark TJH, and Godfrey S [eds]: Asthma, 2nd ed. London, Chapman & Hall, 1983. With permission.)

shift in the age distribution; (6) increased severity of the disease; (7) increased use of self-medication with over-the-counter drugs; and (8) changes in management including the increased use of multiple drugs. Greater reliance on beta-agonist inhalers may play a part in the higher mortality, and frequent use of these medications has been associated with a greater risk of fatal and near-fatal asthma attacks even after adjustment for severity of illness (Burgess et al, 1994; Spitzer et al, 1992).

Death from asthma, however, is still a rare event. In the United States, death rates reached a nadir in 1977, and since that time, there has been a progressive rise in the total death rate (deaths per 100,000 population) from asthma, which approximately doubled from 0.6 in 1977 to 1.1 in 1984. The increase in the death rate is most dramatic in the older age group, but no age group is spared (Robin, 1988). In 1985, there were 4800 asthma deaths in the United States (Buist, 1988). Death rates for asthma in the United States are still among the lowest in developed countries. This raises the question of whether there is widespread underreporting of asthma deaths in the United States. It is quite possible that there may be fairly extensive false-positive and false-negative reporting of asthma deaths. Certainly, more information is needed be-

fore any credible answer can be given to the question of whether asthma mortality is really rising in the United States.

To address the question of increased asthma mortality, the American Academy of Allergy and Immunology and the American Thoracic Society have established an asthma mortality task force. A workshop was held in November, 1986, to bring together epidemiologists, pathologists, clinicians, pharmacologists, and behavioralists from academia, clinical medicine, and industry to review the evidence relating to asthma mortality. The proceedings of the workshop were published in September, 1987 (Sheffer and Buist, 1987). The recommendations of the workshop need to be put into effect aggressively for education of health professionals and lay public.

FENOTEROL EXPERIENCE

Three case-controlled studies from New Zealand suggested that unsupervised self-administration of fenoterol by inhalation increases the risk of death from asthma (Crane et al, 1989; Grainger et al, 1991; Pearce et al, 1990). Although it remains a controversial issue, the consistency and magnitude of the findings strongly suggest that the risk is unlikely to be related to chance alone. The risk was especially high in patients with chronic severe asthma, with an approximately ten-fold relative risk in the subgroup with the most severe asthma. Following publication of the epidemiologic studies, the New Zealand Department of Health in 1990 severely restricted the availability of fenoterol by withdrawing it from the Drug Tariff. These regulatory actions effectively removed fenoterol from the market in New Zealand, and allowed an experiment in prevention to be undertaken. These regulatory actions were associated with a sudden and marked reduction in asthma mortality trends, thus providing further evidence for a causative role of fenoterol in the epidemic of asthma deaths in New Zealand (Beasley et al, 1995; Pearce et al, 1995). Data on time trends should be assessed with considerable caution, however, because time trends in asthma deaths can be affected by many different factors. Nevertheless, the New Zealand time trends are consistent with other epidemiologic evidence indicating a major role of fenoterol in the second New Zealand asthma mortality epidemic.

SOCIOECONOMIC AND ENVIRONMENTAL FACTORS

Asthma does not affect everyone equally. In particular, asthma is especially likely to occur in a setting of poverty (Coultas et al, 1994; McWhorter et al, 1989; Schwartz et al, 1990; Weiss et al, 1992). Many components of poverty may contribute to the increased risk, including poor access to appropriate and high-quality health care, lack of care continuity, decreased likelihood of treatment with anti-inflammatory drugs, poor housing with high levels of antigen and pollutant exposure, poor system of social support, and low levels of education (Buist and Vollmer, 1994; Lang and Polansky, 1994; Malveaux, 1989; Weitzman et al, 1990). The growing morbidity and mortality rates may also reflect greater exposure to outdoor pollutants and indoor aeroallergens, including dust mites, cat dander, cockroach antigen, and molds in poor inner-city households (Call et al, 1992; Chilmonczyk et al, 1993; Infante-Rivard, 1993; O'Hallaren et al, 1991; Schwartz et al, 1993). In a study by Lang and Polansky, fatal asthma was found significantly more commonly in census tracts with higher percentages of blacks, Hispanics, women, and people living below the poverty level (Lang and Polansky, 1994). Their report provides further confirmation that in the United States deaths from asthma are disproportionately common in minority groups and inner cities. Are race and ethnic background important risk factors or surrogate markers for poverty? Similar findings have been reported by Wissow and coworkers (1988), who studied race and poverty as they were related to death from asthma among Medicare recipients in Maryland and by Marder and coworkers (1992), who looked at death from asthma in Chicago from 1980 to 1988.

In the United States during the 1980s the asthma mortality rate among blacks aged 5 to 34 years was three to five times higher than the rate among whites (Weiss and Wagener, 1990), whereas the hospitalization rate was two to three times higher in nonwhite children (Gergen and Weiss, 1990). Small area analyses of asthma hospitalization rates and mortality in New York City, Chicago, and Boston have demonstrated that asthma morbidity and mortality are concentrated in inner-city neighborhoods characterized by poverty and large minority populations (Carr et al, 1992; Gottlieb et al, 1995; Marder et al, 1992). This trend is especially prominent in children, in whom prevalence of asthma is approximately 50% higher among black children, hospitalization 15% more frequent, and asthma deaths 350 to 600% more frequent (Evans, 1992; Gerstman et al, 1993). Thus, collectively these studies indicate that high mortality rates are reported in the poor inner-city neighborhoods of large industrial cities, such as New York, Philadelphia, and Chicago, but not in the rural states (Mississippi, Louisiana, and West Virginia) with the highest poverty rates. In contrast to cities, rural areas have both a low prevalence of asthma and a lower incidence of severe asthma. This phenomenon has also been observed in Africa, where the prevalence of asthma increases among people who migrate from rural to urban areas. Thus, the aspects of asthma morbidity and mortality linked to "urban poverty" need to be characterized more carefully.

ECONOMIC IMPACT OF ASTHMA

Asthma, being a common illness, is estimated to affect approximately 12 to 15 million persons in the United States, resulting in 2 to 3 million emergency room visits and 0.5 to 1 million hospitalizations (National Center for Health Statistics, 1984; Graves, 1992). One important component of morbidity caused by asthma in the United States is its economic impact. An accurate study of the total cost of asthma care can provide insight into how health care resources are distributed and can lay the groundwork for further policy decisions that can redirect financial resources toward this disease more effectively. In 1990, the cost of illness related to asthma was estimated to be $6.2 billion (1995 estimate is $10 billion). The value of reduced productivity due to loss of school days and missed work represented the largest single indirect cost in 1990, approaching $2.6 billion. Because of inefficient preventive care, 43% of economic impact was associated with emergency room use and hospitalization costs, which can be greatly reduced (Weiss et al, 1992). The potential savings from the shift from more expensive hospital/emergency room care to less expensive preventive ambulatory care is readily apparent. If the costs of asthma are to be reduced, therefore, future efforts to direct health policy toward improvement in asthma care must emphasize improvement in effectiveness of primary preventive care in the ambulatory setting. By using a vigorous medical regimen and an intensive educational program, reduced hospital use among adult asthmatics who had previously required repeated readmissions for severe asthma exacerbation has been clearly demonstrated (Mayo et al, 1990). Cost-effective preventive care is especially important for high-risk patients with asthma who required intubation and mechanical ventilation. An asthma management program after discharge from the hospital can effectively reduce the total cost from over $40,000 to $5000 and inpatient costs from approximately $40,000 to $2000. This finding suggests that "active intervention," including patient education, specialist care, regular outpatient visits, and access to an emergency call service, can significantly reduce the cost of asthma care and morbidity in the high-risk patient.

NEAR-FATAL ASTHMA

Some patients with asthma are at a particularly high risk of dying of this disease. The patients at high risk for near-fatal attacks of asthma include (1) those with unexpected episodes of severe overwhelming asthma; (2) those with chronic progressive worsening of asthma symptoms requiring long-term oral steroid use; and (3) those in neither of these categories but with extremely poor control of asthma in the months before a near-fatal or fatal attack (McFadden, 1991; Molfino et al, 1991; Molfino and Slutsky, 1994; O'Hollaren et al, 1991).

PRECIPITATING FACTORS

As with other aspects of severe asthma, surprisingly few data indicate the precipitating factors and pathogenesis of a life-threatening attack. The stimuli most often associated with fatal or near-fatal airway narrowing are profound emotional upsets, environmental allergens, air pollutants, use of beta-blockers, and ingestion of aspirin and other nonsteroidal anti-inflammatory agents in sensitive patients (Benatar, 1986; McFadden, 1991). The mechanism by which fatal and near-fatal attacks develop is not yet known, but it is likely that the essential ingredients consist of the degree of airway lability, severity of pre-existing airway obstruction, magnitude of the stimulus applied, and patient's ability to respond to extreme airway narrowing.

SUDDEN ASPHYXIC ASTHMA

The deaths from asthma can be divided into two groups. Most deaths follow a period of unstable and deteriorating control of asthma, and pathologic examination of the lung shows an intense inflammatory response with eosinophils and widespread mucous plugging (Barnes, 1994; Strunk, 1993). This finding suggests that therapeutic intervention is possible. A minority of patients, however, die from asthma attacks that progress from minimal symptoms to respiratory arrest within 1 to 2 hours; this condition is termed *sudden asphyxic asthma* (Barnes, 1994a; Wasserfallen et al, 1990). In several retrospective surveys, 10 to 25% of deaths from asthma were estimated to have occurred within 3 hours after onset of an attack. Pathologic examination showed little inflammation and empty airways, indicating extreme airway narrowing. Very little is known of the acute onset of fatal asthma except that its immunohistologic feature differs from that of slow-onset fatal asthma, and there is relative paucity of eosinophils in the submucosa (Sur et al, 1993).

PROFILE OF A FATALITY-PRONE ASTHMA PATIENT

The only accepted criterion in predicting which patient is likely to develop status asthmaticus is a history of an episode of status asthmaticus. Approximately 50% of the patients who have been in status asthmaticus suffer another episode in a 2-year period. About one third of patients who do have more than one attack during a 2-year follow-up suffer four or more attacks. It is not known what determines the risk of repeated episodes in these patients. About 80% of patients who die with status asthmaticus have had asthma for more than 5 years, and about one half have had asthma for less than 10 years. Most patients who die with status asthmaticus have asthma that started after age 40 years. Thus, prognosis for patients whose asthma begin at age 40 or older is worse than that for those whose asthma begins before age 40, because the condition is more likely to terminate in status asthmaticus.

The identification of patients at high risk for a fatal attack of asthma continues to be a difficult problem and challenge for physicians. If high-risk patients are identifiable, appropriate and timely intervention can reduce their risk of hospitalization and sudden death. Retrospective analysis has highlighted several clinical characteristics of patients who die of asthma (Strunk, 1989) (Table 23–1). These include (1) severe asthma; (2) poor compliance with therapy and problems with self-management; (3) denial of disease; (4) delay in seeking or delivering medical help; (5) poor family support system; (6) instability of airway function; (7) psychological factors; (8) recurrent emergency room visits and/or hospitalization; (9) previous occurrences of life-threatening attacks; and (10) poor medical care (Boulet et al, 1991; Molfino and Slutsky, 1994). A history of a near-fatal attack that required hospitalization and mechanical ventilation is the strongest single predictor of subsequent death from asthma. This observation suggests that studies of patients who have near-fatal attacks of asthma may be useful in identifying risk factors for death from asthma. Indeed, in a survey in Australia and Canada the clinical characteristics of patients who had near-fatal attacks were similar to those of patients who died (Campbell et al, 1994; Kikuchi et al, 1994).

Undertreatment rather than overtreatment is the most important factor for an asthmatic at risk. The widely accepted view that many deaths from asthma are due to inadequate or delayed treatment and are, therefore, potentially preventable is supported by the fact that death rates from asthma in different countries are related to availability of adequate health care. The increased death rate from asthma among blacks in the United States and South Africa may reflect variations in the availability and quality of medical care for patients of differing socioeconomic status (Benatar, 1986).

Table 23–1
Profile of a High-risk Patient

1. Severe asthma
2. Poor compliance with therapy
3. Denial of disease
4. Poor family support system
5. Instability of airway function
6. Psychological factors
7. Poor medical care
8. Recurrent severe attacks
9. Recurrent ER visits/hospitalizations

EXTREMELY HIGH-RISK PATIENTS

There are two groups of patients who are especially prone to near-fatal attacks and who may remain unidentified. These patients have abnormal response to airway narrowing that places them at risk for respiratory failure. Some patients are unable to sense the presence of even marked airway obstruction and have no symptoms until the respiratory reserve is virtually exhausted (Boulet et al, 1991; McFadden, 1991; Molfino et al, 1991; Molfino and Statsky, 1994). Thus, when they report breathlessness and wheezing, they may be close to death. Others have observed a blunted hypoxic ventilatory drive, and patients do not respond to the development of bronchial narrowing with hyperventilation, which is so characteristic of an acute attack (Barnes, 1994a; Gibson, 1995; Kikuchi et al, 1994). Hence, alveolar hypoventilation can rapidly develop, even with a moderate degree of obstruction. Perception of dyspnea during resistive loading was significantly decreased in patients with a history of near-fatal asthma, as compared with normal subjects and patients with asthma of similar severity but no previous history of such attacks (Kikuchi et al, 1994). Kikuchi and coworkers also found a significant reduction in hypoxic, but not hypercapnic, respiratory drive in patients with near-fatal asthma; this observation is consistent with previous reports of a reduced hypoxic drive in patients with asthma who had near-fatal attacks (Barnes, 1994a; Hutchison and Olinsky, 1981; Town and Allan, 1989).

Results of studies have important implications for the prevention of death from asthma. Asthma patients who have impaired perception of dyspnea should be monitored closely and a history of a near-fatal attack taken as a warning that a life-threatening attack may occur again. Thus, the majority of asthma deaths are preceded by unexpected rapid and severe deterioration and may occur outside the hospital. Molfino and coworkers (1991) have suggested that near-fatal episodes are the result of severe asphyxia rather than cardiac arrhythmias, and they have suggested that undertreatment rather than overtreatment may contribute to an increase in asthma mortality. The majority of deaths are preventable and result from a failure of the physician, the patient, or both to recognize the seriousness of the episode.

PATHOLOGY

The general pathologic features of asthma have been known for about a century. Osler (1892) listed spasm of bronchial smooth muscles and swelling of bronchial mucous membranes associated with exudative bronchiolitis as the major theories of the cause of asthma. The classic descriptions of the pathology of asthma have been derived mostly from patients dying with status asthmaticus (Hidling, 1943; Houston et al, 1953; Thurlbeck and Hogg, 1988). These changes are a result of the end stage of the disease and must represent extreme derangements.

POSTMORTEM PATHOLOGY

The gross appearance of the lungs in patients dying of status asthmaticus is characteristic. The lungs are greatly overdistended, with evidence of air trapping. Areas of atelectasis are apparent in about one half of the cases. The airways may be occluded by plugs of mucus, which make it difficult to fix the distended lung. The plugs are so tenacious that it may be difficult to remove them even with forceps. Although the lungs are grossly distended because of air trapping and mucous plugging, true emphysema is uncommon. Subpleural apical bronchiectasis has been reported in 15 to 20% of cases; the pathogenesis of these lesions remains controversial. Right ventricular hypertrophy has been found in 10% of patients dying in status asthmaticus, and it usually occurs in those who have bronchiectasis.

Airway Mucous Plugs

Necropsy of those dying in status asthmaticus has demonstrated a widespread occurrence of tenacious mucous plugs occluding medium- and small-sized bronchi (Dunhill, 1960). There is remarkably little difference in the necropsy findings following fatal asthma compared with findings in individuals with a history of chronic asthma but suffering an accidental death or requiring lung resection (Sobonya, 1984). Reid has shown that heterogeneity exists, however. Not all cases of acute fatal asthma show mucous plugging of the airways at necropsy, and in these cases there may be overwhelming bronchoconstriction (Reid, 1987).

Similar observations have been made by others, demonstrating empty airways in sudden asphyxic asthma, indicating extreme airway narrowing (Wasserfallen et al, 1990) and paucity of eosinophils (Sur et al, 1993). The mucoid exudate can form a cast of the airways that may be coughed up as Curschmann's spirals. These plugs contain whorls of shed airway epithelium and compact clusters of columnar cells known as *creola bodies*, many eosinophils, and released eosinophil granules forming Charcot-Leyden crystals. As noted by Dunhill (1960), these mucous plugs have both basophilic and eosinophilic components. The basophilic component is periodic acid Schiff–positive and is probably mucus, whereas the eosinophilic component is thought to be a proteinaceous exudate from the bronchi. Histochemically, the airway plugs in asthma consist of a mixture of proteinaceous, inflammatory exudate together with mucus in which lie desquamated aggregates of surface epithelial cells, lymphocytes, and eosinophils. The cellular elements are often arranged in concentric layers, suggestive of repetitious inflammatory cycles superimposed on an ongoing chronic process rather than one associated with a single acute terminal event.

Epithelium

The epithelial layer shows various changes including goblet cell metaplasia, extensive sloughing of epithelium into the airway plugs, and thickened basement membrane. The damage and shedding of airway surface epithelium is prominent, both in fatal asthma and in transmission electron microscopic biopsy specimens from stable asthmatics (Dunhill, 1960; Jeffery, 1994; Laitinen et al, 1985). Epithelial sloughing may be an indirect effect of airway edema or may be due to damage caused by the release of highly toxic and charged eosinophil granular proteins, including major basic protein or eosinophil cationic protein and eosinophil peroxidase. In areas from which epithelial cells are lost, the basal cells and basal laminae often appear to remain intact without thickening, suggesting that it is the attachment of superficial epithelial cells to both basal cells and basal laminae that is in some way compromised (Montefort et al, 1992).

Loss of epithelial integrity is likely to have several interacting effects in the pathogenesis of severe asthma, including (1) reduced threshold to stimulation of intraepithelial nerve fibers; (2) enhanced access of allergen to antigen-presenting cells (dendritic cells; lymphocyte) or mast cells; (3) loss of epithelial-derived relaxant factors; and (4) loss of neutral endopeptidases, which are responsible for the inactivation of proinflammatory peptides such as substance P. The thickened basement membrane is not diagnostic of asthma and has been described in bronchiectasis and chronic bronchitis, but thickening is usually more severe in asthma (Dunhill et al, 1969; McCarter and Vasquez, 1966).

By light microscopy an approximate twofold thickening of the reticular layer underlying the basal lamina has been observed. In asthma the thickening is from increased collagen and increased amount of IgG, IgA, and fibrinogen. The application of transmission electron microscopy to the study of the human bronchial mucosa has shown that its underlying layer consists of at least two morphologically distinct layers: a basal lamina of approximately 80 μ thickness and a thicker reticular lamina. It is the reticular and not the basal lamina that becomes thickened in asthma (Jeffery et al, 1992). The term *subepithelial fibrosis*, has been introduced to describe the thickening of the reticular lamina, and immunohistochemical studies have shown it to be comprised predominantly of collagen types III and V and fibronectin (Roche et al, 1989).

An immunohistochemical and electron microscopic study (Brewster et al, 1990) of bronchial biopsies from asthmatic patients has provided evidence that α-actin containing myofibroblasts within the subepithelial connective tissue may be responsible for the production of increased extracellular matrix adjacent to the true basal lamina. There is a heavy infiltration of airways with eosinophils, especially in the subepithelial layer, which is a characteristic finding in status asthmaticus (Houston et al, 1953; McCarter and Vasquez, 1966). In some cases of fatal asthma, however, no eosinophil infiltrates were demonstrated (Sur et al, 1993).

Submucosal Glands

There is moderate enlargement of bronchial submucosal glands. The hypertrophy of these submucosal glands is not as great as that in chronic bronchitis (Dunhill, 1960; Takizawa and Thurlbeck, 1971). Goblet cells of the surface epithelium and mucous and serous acini of the submucosal glands are the two major sources of airway mucus. In larger bronchi of individuals dying in status asthmaticus, there is a significant enlargement of the mass of mucous-secreting submucosal glands, similar to that in chronic bronchitis. In asthma a normal serous-to-mucus acinar ratio is reported, whereas in chronic bronchitis there is a relative reduction of serous acini. No mucosubstance unique to asthma has been identified; there may be interaction of mucous glycoproteins with lipid and/or serum proteins, which may cause significant thickening and contribute to the particular tenacity of airway secretions in fatal asthma.

Airway Smooth Muscle

The thickness of airway smooth muscle is increased two- to three-fold in patients dying of status asthmaticus (Heard and Hossain, 1973). The percentage of bronchial wall occupied by bronchial smooth muscle shows a striking rise in status asthmaticus. This rise occurs in the absence of the medial hypertrophy of adjacent muscular pulmonary arteries, which characterizes chronic obstructive pulmonary disease (COPD). An increase in the number of muscle cells (hyperplasia) rather than an increase in their size (hypertrophy) may be responsible for thickening of airway muscle. The increase in muscle is relatively greater in the medium-size airway.

Although the greater muscle mass is an obvious part of the pathology of airways in patients dying of status asthmaticus, one quantitative study of asthmatic patients dying of other causes demonstrated no significant increase in airway smooth muscle (Sobonya, 1984). A 1993 postmortem study showed that the airway wall is thicker in cases of fatal asthma than in cases of nonfatal asthma and cases without asthma (Carroll et al, 1993). This increase in thickness involves the inner and outer airway wall areas. Increased areas of smooth muscle, mucous gland, and cartilage all contribute to the thickening. Structural changes were observed in both large and small airways in fatal asthma, but they were mainly confined to the small airways in nonfatal asthma. Other studies of fatal asthma cases have reported increased areas of inner airway wall (James et al, 1989), smooth muscle (Dunhill et al, 1969; Heard and Hossain, 1973), and mucous glands (Dunhill et al, 1969). Saetta and coworkers (1991) found that the subepithelial wall area of membranous bronchioles was significantly greater in nonfatal cases of asthma than in controls.

Bronchial Vasculature

Dilation, bronchial vasculature, congestion, and wall edema are features of fatal asthma. The greater thickness of the bronchial wall that occurs in asthma is unlikely to be accounted for by the greater muscle thickness and mucous glands alone. It may also be caused by bronchial vasodilation and mucosal edema. The contribution of these vasculature changes to airflow limitation, however, is not well understood.

The data obtained at autopsy suggest that airway obstruction in asthma is associated with (1) mucous hypersecretion leading to plugging of the airway lumen; (2) increased and probably abnormal airway smooth muscle; and (3) increased airway wall thickness due to exudative inflammatory reaction, greater muscle, vascular congestion and dilation, and enlarged mucous glands. It is, however, impossible to appreciate the relative importance of each of these three abnormalities.

ANTEMORTEM PATHOLOGY

Pathologic changes during an asthmatic attack have not been studied for obvious reasons, but it is assumed that lesions are qualitatively similar but quantitatively different from postmortem changes in status asthmaticus. Bronchial eosinophilia, mucous hypersecretion, and rarely mucous plugging are undoubtedly present, but response to bronchodilators suggests that abnormal muscle constriction is an important cause of airway obstruction.

Considerable abnormalities have been detected in the lungs of patients with stable asthma who underwent biopsies or died of unrelated causes (Dunhill, 1971; Glynn and Michaels, 1960; Laitinen et al, 1985; Salvato, 1968; Sobonya, 1984). Mucous plugging has been described at autopsy in apparently asymptomatic asthmatics (Dunhill, 1971). Bronchial eosinophilia, squamous metaplasia of the epithelium, basement membrane thickening, edema, and chronic inflammation have also been described (Glynn and Michaels, 1960; Salvato, 1968; Sobonya, 1984). Changes in mucous-secreting apparatus are less clear and less pronounced than those in chronic bronchitis. An increase in goblet cells is more characteristic of asthma, and it has been suggested that goblet-cell secretions are predominantly acid glycoprotein in asthma, rather than neutral glycoprotein as in chronic bronchitis (Salvato, 1968).

Of particular interest is the electron microscopic study by Laitinen and associates (1985) that showed marked epithelial destruction, especially ciliated cells, in the bronchi. Epithelial nerve endings were also found to be, remarkably, exposed to bronchoconstrictive stimuli.

Cellular Infiltrate

Together with the structural changes already described, there is marked cellular infiltration of the airway wall in fatal asthma (Azzawi et al, 1989; Dunhill, 1960; Reid et al, 1989), which may also involve the wall of adjacent pulmonary arteries (Saetta et al, 1991). The inflammatory cell infiltrate characteristically includes lymphocytes, mononuclear cells, and eosinophils (Azzawi et al, 1990; Jeffery, 1994). Using monoclonal antibodies, it has been suggested that cellular infiltrate in fatal asthma predominantly consists of T lymphocytes (CD3+, CD4+, and CD25+) and activated eosinophils (Azzawi et al, 1990).

In stable atopic asthma, total mast cell count, identified by electron microscopy, shows a tendency for higher mast cell numbers (Jeffrey et al, 1992; Laitinen, 1993). Studies of lung tissue obtained at postmortem examination have shown a reduction of airway and lung mast cells (Heard et al, 1989). These changes are most likely due to widespread mast cell degranulation in a fatal attack rather than to a reduction in number of mast cells. The description of localization and release of the cytokines IL-4 in pulmonary mast cells (Bradding et al, 1992) has provided the mast cells with a renewed prominent role in the pathogenesis of asthma.

PATHOGENESIS

Pathogenesis of asthma is complex, and there is more evidence that a complicated series of immunologic, inflammatory, biochemical, and cellular events plays a pivotal role. These events, in a yet poorly understood sequence, affect airway smooth muscle, epithelial function, mucociliary transport, and pulmonary and bronchial macro- and microcirculations to produce the syndrome of an asthmatic attack. A broad spectrum of immunologic and inflammatory mechanisms is potentially involved in the pathogenesis of asthma in general and status asthmaticus in particular, as indicated by pathologic findings and by heightened appreciation of the multitude of proinflammatory events that are mediated by diverse cell types. Therefore, it is appropriate to expand the traditional view of asthma as an IgE-mediated mast cell disease to include newly described inflammatory and biochemical pathways that may contribute to the pathogenesis of asthma.

IMMUNOLOGIC MECHANISMS

Asthmatic patients are usually classified into two main groups: those with extrinsic and those with intrinsic asthma. Extrinsic asthma is characterized by childhood onset, seasonal variation, and well-defined history of allergy to various inhaled allergens. In contrast, intrinsic asthma usually begins in adulthood, tends to be perennial, and is often more severe than extrinsic asthma. By definition, in intrinsic asthma an allergic etiology cannot be demonstrated by either skin or inhalation tests. This conceptual division has been questioned, however, and it has been suggested that asthma is almost always associated with some type of IgE-related reaction and, therefore, has an allergic basis (Burrows et al, 1989). Failure to detect an allergic etiology may be related to the limitation of the battery of aeroallergens used to assess atopic status.

Most of the immunologic and biochemical knowledge in bronchial asthma is related to allergic asthma. This involves an interaction between inhaled allergens and specific IgE antibodies, which are fixed to circulating basophils and pulmonary mast cells (Austen, 1973; Ishizaka, 1988). Mast cells, bearing IgE antibody, are present on the mucosal surface of both the upper and lower respiratory tract as well as in the perivascular connective tissue. The membrane of these cells is ruffled and possesses 50 to 500,000 receptors for the Fc portion of IgE antibody. IgE molecules are comprised of two heavy and two light chains linked by disulfide bridges, with a total molecular weight of 190,000. Papain digests IgE into three fragments, two of which (Fab) bind to the specific antigen and (Fc) one of which binds to the specific receptor on the mast cell surface. Each mast cell possesses several hundred metachromatically staining granules. Degranulation of these cells is initiated by the bridging of a pair of cell-bound IgE molecules by the specific antigen. Activation begins immediately upon bridging, and secretion is complete within minutes. Bridging of IgE molecules somehow induces bridging of mast cell IgE receptors, which in turn initiates a sequence of membrane and intracellular events leading to selective secretion of newly formed and preformed mediators of diverse structure and function. In addition, mast cells may be degranulated by nonimmunologic stimuli such as enzymes, ionophores, polycationic amines and proteins, radiocontrast media, opiates, and hypoxia. IgE receptors have also been found on a number of the other cell types, including alveolar macrophages, eosinophils, lymphocytes, and platelets (Joseph et al, 1983). The affinity of Fc receptors for IgE on these cell types, however, is different from that of mast cells and basophils, in which the Fc types exhibit a low-affinity IgE receptor.

It is currently believed that these low-affinity receptors bind very few single monomeric IgE molecules and that the major triggering mechanism involves IgE-immune complexes. The IgE-immune complex is formed by the binding of many IgE molecules to an antigen with antigenic sites. The simultaneous binding of the multiple IgE-Fc sites to low-affinity receptors forms an avid association of antigen with the cell and serves to bridge or to hold in proximity two or more IgE receptors. This bridging event is the first step in the activation of many types of inflammatory cells and in the release of chemical mediators from cells like macrophages, eosinophils, and platelets (Ishizaka, 1988; Rocklin and Findlay, 1985).

Between the bridging event and the mediator release, many interrelated biochemical changes occur in the cell membrane and intracellularly, including methylation of membrane phospholip-

ids, changes in cyclic adenosine monophosphate (AMP), influx of extracellular calcium (Ca^{++}), and mobilization of intracellular Ca^{++}. Phosphatidylinositol (PI) turnover also plays an important role in signal transduction and Ca^{++} mobilization (Grandordy and Barnes, 1987). Stimulus-secretion coupling that leads to mast cell degranulation and mediator release is controlled by multiple signaling pathways. Breakdown of inositol phospholipids leads to formation of inositol triphosphate (IP_3) and diacylglycerol, two important secondary messengers (Berridge, 1987). IP_3 by binding to IP_3 receptors on the endoplasmic reticulum, can cause internal release of Ca^{++} in various cell types, including mast cells. IP_3 can also degranulate permeated mast cells and cause histamine release, thus underscoring the importance of this second messenger in the regulation of mediator release (Ahmed et al, 1994; Tasaka et al, 1987). Diacylglycerol activates protein kinase C in the presence of Ca^{++} and acts as an alternative second messenger leading to mast cell degranulation and mediator release (Penner et al, 1988; Penner, 1988). Heterogeneity of allergic airway responses may be related to differential activation of these secondary messengers (Ahmed et al, 1996).

Degranulation of cells and mediator release may be modulated at several steps by endogenous or exogenous agents. Agents capable of stimulating adenylate cyclase, such as β-adrenergic agonists and prostaglandin E_1, increase tissue concentrations of cyclic 3'-3' AMP and inhibit mediator generation and/or release. Phosphodiesterase inhibitors such as a aminophylline also increase cyclic AMP and block mediator release. Conversely, imidazole (which stimulates phosphodiesterase activity), alpha-adrenergic agents, and $PGF_{2\alpha}$ lower the tissue concentration of cyclic AMP, which enhances the mediator release. Thus, there appears to be an inverse relationship between tissue concentrations of cyclic AMP and the degree of mediator release observed. Cholinergic stimulation of sensitized lung fragments with acetylcholine or carbachol results in enhancement of IgE-dependent release of chemical mediators. This effect is not associated with a decrease in cyclic AMP, but is associated with an increase in cyclic guanidine monophosphate (GMP). The opposing effects of cyclic AMP and cyclic GMP on modulating IgE-dependent mediator generation and release have also been observed in other tissues and cells and are thought to represent competitive effects upon a putative protein kinase, which may regulate the state of cytoskeletal (microtubule) assembly. Colchicine, an agent that binds to the microtubular subunit protein to prevent microtubular assembly and function, inhibits the release of histamine and appears to be acting on the Ca-dependent release phase of the reaction in leukocytes. The finding that agents that chelate calcium ions, alter cyclic nucleotide concentration, or inhibit microtubular assembly all act in the later phases of the release reaction is compatible with the evidence that there is an integral relationship between calcium ion flux, relative concentrations of cyclic nucleotide, and microtubular assembly and function.

CELLULAR INFLAMMATORY RESPONSE

Manifestation of the asthmatic response may conveniently be divided into three stages: a rapid spasmogenic phase, a late sustained phase, and a subacute-chronic inflammatory phase. The immediate response to inhaled allergen has been conventionally associated with activation of pulmonary mast cells and release of histamine and other spasmogenic mediators (Austen, 1973). Studies have indicated that IgE-dependent activation of alveolar macrophages and platelets may also be involved (Joseph et al., 1983). The release of chemotactic factors may lead to the recruitment of other inflammatory cells, including neutrophils, eosinophils, lymphocytes, and monocytes (Kay, 1986). Activation of these cell types may be involved in the late-phase response and bronchial hyperreactivity. Thus, no single cell type can be responsible for all of the manifestations of bronchial asthma, and diversity and interaction of inflammatory cells and mediators are likely to be involved (Fig. 23–4).

Mast Cells

These are widely distributed throughout the human respiratory tract. Mast cells from different sources and even from different locations within a given tissue may exhibit a marked heterogeneity in their morphologic, histochemical, and functional properties (Dvorak et al, 1983). Two distinct types of mast cells ("mucosal" and "connective tissue") may be identified and provide a particularly striking example of mast cell heterogeneity within a single species. The mucosal mast cell is much more common in human lung than in the connective tissue mast cell, and it is widely distributed throughout the lung parenchyma. Based upon neutral protease content, mast cells are also classified into T-type (tryptase-positive, chymase-negative) and TC-type (tryptase-positive, chymase-positive).

Mast cells possess within their granules a variety of amines, peptides, proteins, and complex polysaccharides with bronchospastic, vasoactive, and chemotactic properties, as well as various active enzymes and proteoglycans. Mast cell activation leads to the release of these preformed (stored) granular elements as well as to the generation of other (unstored) bronchospastic, vasoactive, and chemotactic substances (Austen, 1973). Some unstored mediators are generated directly by activated mast cells, whereas others are dependent upon the effect of mast cell products on other cells or on constituents of the local microenvironment.

The relevance of mast cell mediators to asthma has been derived from studies of pathophysiologic changes induced by the individual mediator and from identification of the mediators in tissue or biologic fluids of patients experiencing asthma. These mediators not only possess the ability to induce immediate tissue responses, such as acute and delayed changes in pulmonary functions, but may also mediate a prolonged inflammatory response. The fact that IgE and mast cells are relevant to prolonged inflammatory events has been documented by the passive transfer of delayed inflammatory responses in skin with isolated IgE and by the dependence upon IgE antibody for similar delayed alterations in pulmonary mechanics following antigen challenge. In the lung, these late responses are prevented by pretreatment with cromolyn sodium, supporting the central role of mast cells. Mast cells and basophils can also store a number of cytokines, including interleukin-4 (IL-4), IL-5, and IL-6, and tumor necrosis factor-alpha (TNFα) (Bradding et al, 1994; Gordon et al, 1990). Although the total number of mucosal mast cells was similar in asthmatics and controls, the number of mast cells staining positive for IL-4 and TNFα was elevated in asthmatics. Mast cell–derived IL-4 and IL-5 may play a role in eosinophil recruitment, whereas IL-4 may contribute to T-cell maturation.

Basophils

Despite remarkable similarities in mediator content and responses to stimuli, mammalian mast cells and basophils are clearly not identical. Nevertheless, the two cells do exhibit a number of striking similarities. Basophils may represent the circulating precursor of mast cells. This hypothesis is without definitive evidence, however, and the current view is that basophils represent terminally differentiated granulocytes and not circulating mast cells (Dvorak et al, 1983; Galli and Lichtenstein, 1988). Basophils can be recruited into the tissues during various inflammatory, immunologic, and pathologic responses. Like mast cells,

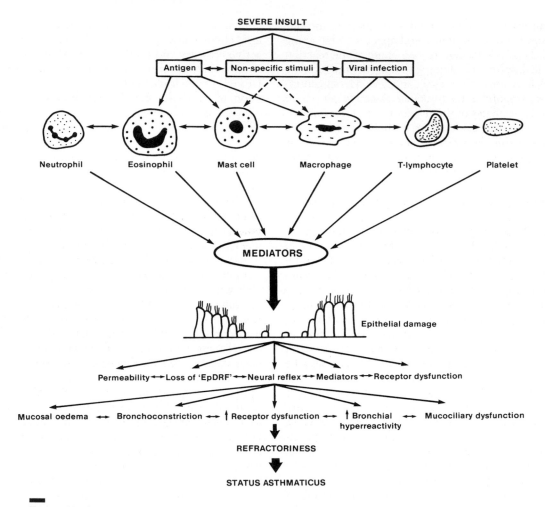

Figure 23–4
A theoretical model of pathogenesis of asthma. A complex interaction of various inflammatory cells and chemical mediators leads to refractoriness and status asthmaticus.

basophils secrete various mediators in immunologic and nonimmunologic reactions; however, there are some well-established differences. For example, the lung mast cells produce equivalent amounts of LTC_4 and PGD_2, whereas basophils generate LTC_4 only. There are also differences between the two cell types in terms of drugs affecting the mediator release.

Eosinophils

The connection between asthma and eosinophils is fundamental, regardless of an allergic component of the disease. The eosinophil is characterized by its distinctive granules, as shown by their staining properties and their unique electron microscopic appearance. The major components of the eosinophils include surface receptors for im-

munoglobulins and complement, Charcot-Leyden crystal protein in the cell membrane with lysophospholipase activity, and a series of cationic proteins localized to the granules. There are also numerous enzymes, including those able to generate platelet activating factor (PAF), LTC_4, PGE_2, and oxygen-derived radicals (Slifman et al, 1988). The granular components include eosinophilic cationic protein (ECP), eosinophilic protein X, eosinophilic peroxidase, major basic protein (MBP), and arylsulfatase B. Some of these proteins possess cytotoxic activity and cause mast cell and basophil degranulation. Eosinophils also have the capacity to elaborate cytokines and chemokines, including transforming growth factor-alpha (TGFα), TGFβ, TNFα, IL-1, IL-3, IL-5, IL-6, IL-8, and granulocyte-macrophage colony stimulating factor (GM-CSF). The secretion of these mediators and cytokines may enable them to participate in the pathogenesis and propagation of asthmatic inflammatory response.

Eosinophils are nondividing granular cells that arise in the bone marrow. Eosinophil differentiation, like that of all leukocytes, is influenced by cytokines. Of the cytokines secreted by activated T lymphocytes, IL-3, IL-5, and GM-CSF promote maturation, activation, and prolonged survival of the eosinophils (Lopez et al, 1986; Rothenberg et al, 1988). IL-5 specifically acts on eosinophils and may be the most important cytokine for eosinophil differentiation and survival (Lopez et al, 1988; Walsh et al, 1990). Other potent eosinophil chemoattractants include PAF, IL-2, RANTES, monocyte chemoattractant protein-3 (MCP-3), and lymphocyte chemotactic factor (LCF). The LCF protein exerts its activity by binding to CD4 molecules, so that, in addition to affecting T lymphocytes, it also specifically acts on eosinophils, which are CD4 expressing cells (Rand et al, 1991; Resnick and Weller, 1993). Adhesion molecules also play an important role in selective eosinophil migration to airway mucosa.

Strong circumstantial evidence exists suggesting that eosinophils are important proinflammatory cells in the pathogenesis of asthmatic reaction. Generally, the blood eosinophil count correlates with the degree of bronchial hyperresponsiveness, and large numbers of activated eosinophils are seen in the bronchial mucosa of patients with fatal asthma (Bousquet et al, 1990). Disease severity correlates with degree of blood eosinophilia (Burrows et al, 1980). Various pharmacologic agents used for the treatment of asthma, like β-agonists, theophylline, steroid, and cromolyn sodium have been shown to decrease circulating eosinophils and serum levels of ECP (Dahl et al, 1988). Thus, eosinophils may play a major pathophysiologic role in asthma, as well as in refractoriness to therapy in status asthmaticus.

Neutrophils

Because inflammatory changes in the lung are a central feature of asthma, it is tempting to speculate that airway hyperresponsiveness is associated with inflammatory events and hence leukocyte recruitment. Neutrophil granules release a number of products that may have an important role in airway hyperresponsiveness and refractoriness seen in status asthmaticus. These granules contain (1) acid hydrolases; (2) serine proteases; (3) antibacterial enzymes; and (4) other products, including cationic proteins. In addition to granule contents, de novo synthesis of mediators by neutrophils may occur. This synthesis includes the production of superoxide anions and arachidonic acid metabolites, especially LTB_4 and thromboxane A_2.

Although neutrophils have been related to airway hyperresponsiveness in animal models of asthma, their role in human asthma is not clear. Abnormal neutrophil function has been observed in the peripheral blood of asthmatics, which can be inhibited by cromolyn sodium, suggesting that mast cell–derived mediators can activate neutrophils (Moqbel et al, 1986). Neutrophils may play a significant role in the late asthmatic response rather than the acute response; in addition, widespread inflammatory changes have been observed in the lungs of patients dying of asthma (Ford-Hutchinson, 1988). Whether neutrophils participate in the functional alterations associated with asthma remains unknown. The frequent recovery of neutrophils from bronchoalveolar lava (BAL) fluid of asthmatic patients, the presence of neutrophils in pathologic sections of asthmatic airways, and the ability of neutrophils to alter airway function together suggest that they may indeed have a role in the exacerbation of severe asthma.

Lymphocytes

T and B lymphocytes normally appear on the pulmonary mucosal surfaces and in the alveolar spaces, yet their regulatory role in asthma is not clearly known. In addition to their role in the regulation of IgE production by B lymphocytes, T lymphocytes can release a number of factors including interleukins that may modulate the activity of other cells within the lung, in particular, mast cells, basophils, and eosinophils. Such factors may be released either spontaneously from the lymphocytes following activation through IgE receptors, or following activation of the lymphocytes by other released mediators such as arachidonic acid metabolites or neuropeptides (Ford-Hutchinson, 1988). A defect in cell-mediated immunity in both intrinsic and extrinsic asthma has been suggested (Engel et al, 1984). Similarly, a number of theories have been advanced to explain possible defects in the regulation of IgE production in asthma and other atopic diseases including defective suppressor T-cell function, overactivity of B-cell IgE synthesis, elaboration of factors released by subsets of T cells that may enhance IgE synthesis, and failure to suppress IgE production (Josephs, 1984). Similarly, changes in lymphocyte ratio exhibiting loss of circulating helper T cells and gain in activated T cells has also been observed following inhalation of antigen by allergic but not by nonallergic subjects (Gerblich et al, 1984).

T lymphocytes not only recruit other cells, such as eosinophils by secreting IL-5, they also promote local and systemic synthesis of IgE through the production of IL-4 (Del Prete et al, 1988). Lymphocytes with such functional activities are termed T-helper 2 (Th2), whereas the T cells that secrete interferon-γ or IL-2 or both are termed T-helper 1 (Th1) and are involved in the delayed hypersensitivity reaction. Th2 cells have been detected in the lungs of atopic asthmatics (Robinson et al, 1992), and these cells bear steroid-sensitive γδ T-cell receptor for antigen on their surface (Spinozzi et al, 1995; 1996). T lymphocytes can directly recognize and respond to processed antigen, and cytokine products of activated T cells have the propensity to sustain asthmatic inflammation regardless of the presence or absence of any antibodies, including IgE. CD4 T cells are clearly an important source of IL-5, IL-4, IL-3, and GM-CSF and may be an important source of chemokines, such as RANTES and MCP3. These agents enhance eosinophil survival, maturation, activation, and migration.

Immunocytochemical studies of bronchial biopsy samples taken from patients with asthma have shown that activated (CD25+) T cells can be detected in the bronchial mucosa, and their numbers can be correlated with the numbers of activated eosinophils and with disease severity (Azzawi et al, 1990; Bentley et al, 1992). Elevated serum concentrations of IL-5, and activated CD4 but not CD8 T lymphocytes, were detected in the peripheral blood of patients with severe asthma (Corrigan and Kay, 1990; Corrigan et al, 1988; 1993). An increased number of CD4 T lymphocytes in the BAL fluid of patients with mild asthma has also been observed to correlate with disease severity and BAL eosinophilia (Robinson et al, 1993a; Walker et al, 1991). It has been suggested that T lymphocytes are involved in the selective recruitment to airway mucosa and activation of eosinophils, via the release of cytokines such as IL-4, IL-5, IL-3, and GM-CSF. Support of this hypothesis has come from the demonstration in bronchial mucosal biopsy samples of mRNA transcripts for IL-5, which are known to be involved in promoting eosinophil differentiation and activation (Hamid et al, 1991). Over a wide range of asthma severity, the percentage of cells in the BAL fluid from atopic asthmatics, expressing mRNA encoding for IL-5, IL-4, and IL-3, can be correlated with the severity of asthma symptoms (Robinson et al, 1993c). Therapy with oral prednisolone resulted in clinical improvement and reduction in the percentage of cells expressing IL-5 and IL-4, as well as reduction in serum concentrations of IL-5 (Corrigan et al, 1993).

These studies provide strong evidence in support of T-cell activation and cytokine secretion in severe asthma, and they also suggest that glucocorticosteroids may exert their antiasthma effect, at least partly, by reducing the synthesis of cytokines by these cells (Robinson et al, 1992; 1993b). The proliferation of lung γδ T cells in allergic asthma and their *in vitro* and *in vivo* apoptotic death after corticosteroid treatment show not only that γδ T cells are involved in the pathogenesis of asthma, but that they may be one of the cellular components on which steroids exert their effect (Spinozzi et al, 1995; 1996). The reduced steroid-receptor binding affinity on T cells, which is a relevant feature in steroid-resistant asthma, can be induced in normal lymphocytes after *in vitro* IL-2 and IL-4 incubation (Sher et al, 1994). Steroid-resistant asthma may be the end result of poorly controlled ongoing T-cell activation, which is refractory to steroid-induced apoptosis.

Macrophages

The role of mononuclear phagocytes as antigen processing and presenting cells is well established. A role for macrophages in the pathogenesis of asthma and type 1 hypersensitivity reaction is being pursued with great interest. This role is based upon the demonstration of low-affinity Fc receptors, release of β-glucuronidase from these cells following challenge with antigen or anti-IgE, and synthesis and release of LTB_4 and other arachidonic acid products upon stimulation (Fels et al, 1982; Joseph et al, 1983; MacDermot and Fuller, 1988). These cells may also play a role in the metabolism of leukotrienes, and drugs like steroids have been shown to inhibit synthesis of LTD_4 and thromboxane. The number of IgE receptors on macrophages is increased in asthmatics, and these cells show enhanced exocytosis in response to antigen challenge *in vitro* (Joseph et al, 1983). IgE-dependent activation of macrophages was also demonstrated to result in the release of IL-1, which has proinflammatory actions, including enhancement of leukocyte adhesion to vascular endothelium. These cells may also play an important role in resolution of inflammation. Because macrophages can manifest many different functional phenotypes, it is possible that airways of asthmatics may contain macrophages that are both contributing to and limiting the inflammatory response.

PROINFLAMMATORY MEDIATORS: CYTOKINES

Cytokines are peptide mediators, released from the inflammatory cells, that are important in signaling between the cells. Cytokines may determine the type and duration of an inflammatory response. It now seems increasingly likely that cytokines play a major role in the inflammation of asthma (Barnes, 1994; 1995a). Growing recognition exists that glucocorticosteroids may suppress asthmatic inflammation by inhibiting the production and effects of cytokines in the airways. Many cytokines including IL-1, IL-2, IL-3, IL-4, and IL-5 have been implicated in asthma, although their precise role *in vivo* is difficult to assess.

Interleukin-1

IL-1 activates T cells to express IL-2, but it has many other proinflammatory effects. There is evidence for increased production of IL-1 in the asthmatic airway, possibly contributing to airway hyperresponsiveness (Mattoli et al, 1991).

Interleukin-2

IL-2 is produced by Th1 lymphocytes and acts as an autocrine growth factor. On stimulation with IL-1, IL-2 synthesis is induced along with IL-2 receptors. In acute asthma, an increase in the number of circulating T cells expressing IL-2 receptors has been reported (Corrigan and Kay, 1990), but this has not been confirmed by others (Brown et al, 1991).

Interleukin-3

IL-3 is produced by T lymphocytes and by mast cells. It may be important for development of mast cells and basophils and promotes eosinophil survival.

Interleukin-4

IL-4 is derived from Th2-type T cells, but there is also evidence for its expression in mast cells of asthmatic patients (Bradding et al, 1992). IL-4 plays a critical role in the switching of B lymphocytes to produce IgE and may be of critical importance in the development of atopy (Sur et al, 1995). IL-4 has many other actions and may increase expression of the adhesion molecules VCAM-1 in endothelial cells, which may be involved in eosinophil adhesion in the bronchial circulation (Schleimer et al, 1992).

Interleukin-5

IL-5 is of particular interest in the pathophysiology of asthma, because it is associated with eosin-

ophilic inflammation. IL-5 is produced by Th2-type lymphocytes, and there is evidence for increased expression in T cells in the asthmatic airways (Hamid et al, 1991). Endobronchial allergen challenge results in IL-5 mRNA expression in eosinophils and an increase in IL-5 concentrations in BAL (Brodie et al, 1992; Ohnishi et al, 1993; Sedgewick et al, 1991). Elevated IL-5 levels in BAL have also been observed from symptomatic, but not from asymptomatic, asthmatics (Ohnishi et al, 1993), especially those with BAL eosinophilia (Sur et al, 1995). IL-5 is important in the terminal differentiation, survival, and activation of eosinophils (Ohnishi et al, 1993). A monoclonal antibody to IL-5 inhibits antigen-induced airway hyperresponsiveness (AHR) and eosinophil influx into the airways in guinea pig and monkey models of asthma (Mauser et al, 1995; Van Oosterhoot et al, 1993).

Interleukin-6

IL-6 is produced by many different activated cells and may be involved in acute-phase reactions. Evidence exists for increased release of IL-6 from alveolar macrophages after antigen challenge in the patient with asthma (Gosset et al, 1991), and perhaps it acts as a proinflammatory factor along with other cytokines.

Chemokines

The scope for a potential role for basophil secretory products in allergic and asthmatic inflammation has been greatly widened, owing to the discovery of a novel class of small cytokine peptides that are part of a growing supergene family. All members of this family are chemoattractants and are termed *chemokines*. To date, at least 16 human chemokines have been identified by cloning or biochemical purification followed by amino acid sequencing. All have four conserved cysteine residues that form characteristic disulfide bonds. Members of the family include IL-8 (neutrophil activating protein-1), platelet factor-4 (PF-4), β-thromboglobulin (βTG), macrophage inflammatory protein-1α (MIP1α) and macrophage chemoattractant protein (MCP-1), MCP-2, and MCP-3. Two subfamilies have been recognized, based on protein structure. The C-X-C family (IL-8, PF-4, and βTG), whose genes are located on chromosome 4 in humans, and the CC family (MIP and RANTES) whose genes are located on chromosome 17. IL-8 and RANTES are potent chemoattractants for neutrophils and eosinophils, whereas MCP-1 induces exocytosis of human basophils. MCP-1, MCP-3, RANTES, and MIP-1α may represent the major histamine-releasing factor species produced by mononuclear cells. Thus, these chemokines have the capacity to recruit and activate neutrophils, eosinophils, and basophils at sites of allergic and asthmatic inflammation through IgE-independent mechanisms (Schall, 1991). In the laboratory, production of chemokines and GM-CSF was demonstrated in the nasal secretions during allergen-induced late nasal responses, which was prevented by topical beclomethasone (Sim et al, 1995).

GM-CSF

GM-CSF is produced by several airway cells, including macrophages, eosinophils, T cells, and epithelial cells. There is evidence for increased expression of GM-CSF in the epithelial cells, T cells, and eosinophils of asthmatic patients (Brown et al, 1991) and increased circulating concentrations have been detected in patients with acute severe asthma (Nakamura et al, 1993). GM-CSF has multiple proinflammatory effects, including priming and extended survival of eosinophils.

Adhesion Molecules

Three major groups of adhesion molecules have been implicated in leukocyte migration: (1) the *immunoglobulin superfamily*, including intercellular adhesion molecule 1 (ICAM-1), vascular cell adhesion molecule 1 (VCAM-1), and platelet-endothelial cell adhesion molecule (PECAM); (2) the *integrins*, including leukocyte function associated antigen 1 (LFA-1), Mac-1, and very late antigen-4 (VLA-4); and (3) the *selectins*, including E-selectin, P-selectin, and L-selectin. Leukocyte migration is initiated by an interaction between receptors on the cell surface with their ligands on the surface of vascular endothelial cells (Bentley et al, 1993).

Like neutrophils, eosinophils can bind to endothelium via L-, P-, and E-selectins. Selectins mediate the initial weak tethering of leukocytes to the endothelial cell surface. Eosinophil β_2-integrins such as LFA-1 and Mac-1, like neutrophils, probably mediate firm adhesion of these cells to endothelium and subsequent transmigration by binding to immunoglobulin-like molecules such as ICAM-1 and VCAM-1 on the endothelium (Cushley and Holgate, 1985; Lansing et al, 1993). Eosinophils, but not neutrophils, express the β_1-integrin VLA-4, which is a ligand for VCAM-1 expressed on the surface of stimulated endothelial cells. Eosinophils may also use VLA-4 for binding to tissue fibronectin, which prolongs

their survival *in vitro*, possibly by inducing autocrine secretion of IL-3. IL-3 and IL-5 upregulate the eosinophil adhesion to unstimulated endothelial cells (Bochner et al, 1991; Walsh et al, 1990), whereas IL-4 enhances the expression of VCAM-1 on endothelial cells, with enhanced VLA-4/VCAM-1–dependent adhesion of eosinophils but not neutrophils to endothelium (Schleimer et al, 1992). Increased eosinophil adhesion to VCAM-1 and ICAM-1 has been observed in patients with more labile asthma, suggesting a relationship with ongoing inflammation in the airways (Håkansson et al, 1995).

Such mechanisms may offer a possible explanation for the selective recruitment of eosinophils in asthmatic inflammatory response. There is also evidence to suggest that VCAM-1 is expressed on bronchial mucosal endothelial cells after antigen challenge (Bentley et al, 1993), thus further supporting the role of adhesion molecule in asthmatic inflammation. Animal studies of allergic bronchoconstriction in monkeys have demonstrated that monoclonal antibody to ELAM-1 (E-selectin) and not ICAM-1 inhibits late-phase bronchoconstriction and neutrophil influx (Gundel et al, 1991). In the sheep model, monoclonal antibody to α_4-β_1 integrin (VLA-4) inhibited the late-phase reactions (Abraham et al, 1994).

Increasing evidence exists that adhesion molecules are important in inflammatory/allergic airway disease (Montefort et al, 1993). Circulating forms of these adhesion molecules have been discovered, although their origin, fate, and formation are not clearly known. Circulating ICAM-1 and E-selectins, but not VCAM-1, levels were significantly raised in acute asthma compared with stable asthma and normal control (Montefort et al, 1994). The elevated concentrations of ICAM-1 and E-selectin in acute asthma may reflect the extensive inflammatory response occurring in the airways during acute exacerbations of the disease and may form the rational basis of therapeutic intervention (Wein and Bochner, 1993).

Cytokines and Asthma

Cytokines play an important role in the perpetuation of inflammatory response in asthma, although the precise role of each cytokine is not clearly known. Cytokines are fundamentally important in the production of specific IgE by B lymphocytes, and IL-4 plays a crucial role in the switching of B cells from IgG to IgE production; but other cytokines, including TNFα and IL-6, may also be important (Barnes, 1994b). Cytokines may enhance or suppress the ability of macrophages to act as antigen-presenting cells, and alveolar macrophages may also be an important source of "first-wave" cytokines like IL-1, TNFα, and IL-6. These cytokines may then act on epithelial cells to release a "second wave" of cytokines, including GM-CSF, IL-8, and RANTES, which then amplify the inflammatory response and lead to an influx of secondary cells, such as eosinophils. Eosinophils themselves may release multiple cytokines. Cytokines may also increase the expression of adhesion molecules, such as ICAM-1, and may switch on the gene transcription of an inducible form of nitric oxide synthetase (iNOS), which is expressed in asthmatic but not in normal epithelium (Barnes and Belvisi, 1993). Mast cells also have the capacity to produce several cytokines that may perpetuate the inflammatory response (Bradding et al, 1994). Thus, multiple inflammatory cells activated in asthma release multiple cytokines, which perpetuate the inflammatory response by acting in an autocrine manner and by recruiting and interacting with other inflammatory cells (Fig. 23–5).

Growth Factors

Other inflammatory cytokines that may also play a role in asthmatic inflammation include TNFα, interferon, and various growth factors, such as platelet-derived growth factor, fibroblast growth factor, epithelial growth factor, transforming growth factor-β, and insulin-like growth factor. Although the role of individual growth factors in the pathogenesis of asthma is not yet known, it is likely that they are important in the structural modeling that occurs in chronic asthma, which

may lead to irreversible airway narrowing in some patients with severe asthma (Barnes, 1994b).

BIOCHEMICAL MEDIATORS

A number of chemical mediators, such as histamine, slow reacting substance of anaphylaxis (leukotrienes), eosinophil chemotactic factor (ECF), neutrophil chemotactic factor (NCF), PAF, ECP, MBP, serotonin, bradykinin, prostaglandins, neurokinins, and tachykinin, have been implicated in the early- and late-phase alterations of pulmonary mechanics, inflammatory response, airway edema, and changes in mucociliary transport and host defense observed during airway anaphylaxis (Fig. 23–6). Histamine, ECF, and PAF are considered to be "primary mediators." Histamine and ECF are stored preformed, whereas leukotrienes and PAF are generated immediately before release. The prostaglandins and bradykinins are considered to be secondary mediators. Although much remains to be clarified, the understanding of target cell activation, discovery of chemical structure of various mediators and interaction of various mediators, and rapidly developing knowledge about their *in vitro* and *in vivo* biologic activity provide a framework for comprehension of complex processes that occur in asthma. The functions of various mast cell mediators are summarized in Table 23–2. No single mediator can be responsible for all the features of asthma. There may be important interactions between the mediators, leading to a "priming" effect, causing magnification and perpetuation of response. This is especially important for actions of cytokines.

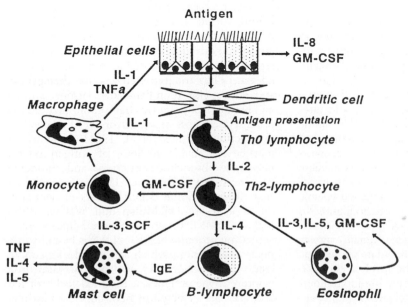

Figure 23–5

Cytokine network in asthma. Cytokines are produced by every cell involved in asthmatic inflammation and cause multiple inflammatory effects by activating other cells, which themselves release cytokines. (IL = interleukin; TNF$_\alpha$ = tumor necrosis factor-α; GM-CSF = granulocyte-macrophage colony stimulating factor; SCF = stem cell factor.) (From Barnes PJ: Cyclic nucleotides and phosphodiesterases and airway function. Eur Respir J 8:457–462, 1995a. With permission.)

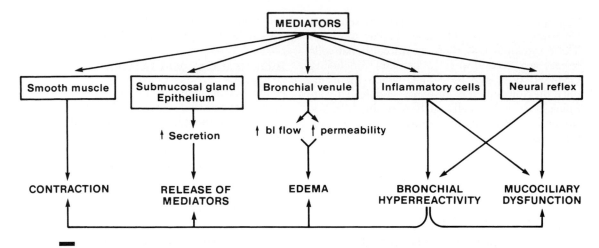

Figure 23–6
Multiple actions of chemical mediators on various target cells in the airway. (Modified from Barnes PJ, Rodger IW, and Thompson NC [eds]: Asthma: Basic Mechanism and Clinical Management. London, Academic Press, 1988. With permission.)

Histamine

Histamine airway responses can mimic many of the symptoms of anaphylaxis. The majority of histamine in the lung is stored in mast cells and to some extent in the basophils. Histamine release from the mast cells and basophils can be induced by a variety of antigenic and nonantigenic stimuli. Histamine has various potent effects on the airways and cardiovascular system, especially the microvasculature. H_1-blockers can inhibit acute antigen-induced bronchoconstriction in animals without an effect on late-phase bronchoconstriction (Abraham and Perruchoud, 1986), whereas they are generally ineffective in subjects with induced or spontaneous asthmatic episodes. Thus, in human asthma histamine may contribute to acute-phase bronchoconstriction, yet it has a minimal role in the late-phase or prolonged inflammatory phase associated with status asthmaticus. Histamine concentrations are elevated in the BAL fluid of asthmatics, both at rest and after allergen challenge (Lui et al, 1991). Histamine has multiple effects on the airways, which are mediated by three types of histamine receptors (H_1, H_2, and H_3 receptors). H_1 receptors mediate airway smooth muscle contraction and airway microvascular leak, contributing to mucosal edema. H_2 receptors, which mediate bronchodilation in many species (Ahmed et al, 1980), have not been convincingly demonstrated in human airway smooth muscle. H_3 receptors modulate cholinergic neurotransmissions both at the level of parasympathetic ganglia and at post-ganglionic cholinergic nerves; they inhibit the release of neuropeptides from sensory nerves (Barnes, 1991). Despite the fact that histamine airway responses mimic many of the pathophysiologic features of asthma, antihistamine has been disappointing in the treatment of asthma.

Leukotrienes

Leukotrienes (LT) are derived from the 5-lipoxygenase (5-LO) pathway of arachidonic acid metabolism. Leukotrienes (LTC_4, LTD_4, LTE_4, and LTB_4) are newly formed mediators. Lung tissue as a whole, as well as relevant cells such as mast cells, neutrophils, basophils, eosinophils, and alveolar macrophages, are capable of forming and releasing various leukotrienes. LTC_4 and LTD_4 are potent mediators, which are capable of causing airway smooth muscle contraction, mucous hypersecretion, mucociliary dysfunction, and mucosal edema. LTB_4 can alter microvascular permeability and is a major proinflammatory agent. Animal and human studies in vivo have confirmed the role of these mediators in antigen-induced mucociliary dysfunction (Ahmed et al, 1981). Leukotrienes may be the major mediator of antigen-induced late-phase bronchoconstriction and bronchial hyperreactivity (Abraham, 1987). Several drugs that directly inhibit 5-LO have been developed for clinical use (McMillan and Walker, 1992), including MK886, which blocks 5-lipoxygenase-activating protein (FLAP). FLAP is bound to the nuclear membrane, which acts as a docking molecule for cytosolic 5-LO, and is a necessary step before enzyme activation. Elevated levels of leukotrienes are detected in BAL fluid from asthma-

Table 23–2
Mediators of Allergic Airway Disease

Mediator	Source	Effect
Histamine	Mast cells and basophils, preformed	Bronchial smooth muscle contraction Vascular permeability Mucous secretion (weak)
Leukotrienes (LTB$_4$, LTC$_4$, LTD$_4$, LTE$_4$)	Mast cells, neutrophils, alveolar macrophages (?) newly formed	Bronchial smooth muscle contraction Vascular permeability Mucous secretion Chemotactic activity
Eosinophil chemotactic factor of anaphylaxis (ECF)	Mast cells and basophils; preformed	Attraction of eosinophils
Eosinophilic cationic protein (ECP)	Eosinophils	Ciliostatic
Major basic protein (MBP)	Eosinophils	Epithelial damage
Neutrophil chemotactic factor (NCF)	Mast cells and basophils; preformed	Attraction of neutrophils
Platelet-activating factor (PAF)	Mast cells and basophils; newly formed	Aggregation of platelets; eosinophil chemotaxis
Prostaglandins	Pulmonary endothelial cells (?) Basophils (?), mast cells (?) Newly formed, secondary mediators	PGF$_2$—smooth muscle constriction PGE$_1$ and E$_2$—smooth muscle relaxation release of other mediators
Cytokines	Inflammatory cells, mast cell Lymphocytes	Multiple proinflammatory actions Chemotaxis
Neurokinins	NANC* system	Bronchoconstriction Proinflammatory Mucous hypersecretion Microvascular permeability
Nitric oxide	Inflammatory cells, endothelial cells Macrophages, epithelial cells	Neurotransmitter Proinflammatory
Adenosine	Epithelial cells	Smooth muscle contraction
Bradykinin	Endothelial cells	Sensory nerve stimulation
Endothelin	Endo/epithelial cells	Vasoconstriction Cell growth
Oxygen radicals	Inflammatory cells	Proinflammatory Bronchial hyperreactivity

*NANC = nonadrenergic noncholinergic

tics after allergen challenge, and elevated LTE$_4$ levels are found in the urine of asthmatics during exacerbations and after allergen challenge (Taylor et al, 1989; Wenzel et al, 1990).

Increasing evidence exists that leukotrienes may play an important role in the pathophysiology of asthma (Arm and Lee, 1993). LTB$_4$ is chemotactic for neutrophils, and it may be relevant to exacerbations of asthma. The role of leukotriene antagonists in chronic asthma still remains to be defined. The therapeutic potential of these drugs in the management of severe asthma is unknown. Because the LTE$_4$ level is elevated in acute asthma, it is possible that these agents may be helpful in the therapy of severe asthma.

Prostaglandins and Thromboxanes

Prostaglandins and thromboxanes are the products of arachidonic acid metabolism via the cyclooxygenase pathway. These are potent mediators and have varied effects on airway and vascular smooth muscle, microvascular permeability, inflammation, and platelet aggregation. These are not the primary mediators of asthma, however, and their modulating role, if any, is controversial.

Platelet Activating Factor

A large amount of interest has been generated for PAF as the mediator of asthma and airway hyperresponsiveness. PAF is a newly formed lipid mediator (Benveniste, 1974), and human alveolar macrophages and eosinophils are extremely good sources of PAF. A number of other cell types have also been shown to release PAF, including neutrophils, platelets, and endothelial cells (Page, 1988). PAF is a very potent mediator and can cause bronchoconstriction in animals and humans (Cuss et al, 1986). PAF can also cause mucociliary dysfunction and marked inflammatory response. PAF is capable of activating a wide range of inflammatory cells *in vitro*, including platelets, neutrophils, macrophages, monocytes, and eosinophils. In particular, it is a very potent inducer of neutrophils and eosinophil chemotaxis (Page, 1988). PAF can elicit various mediators from these inflammatory cells, including eosinophil-rich inflammatory response in lungs following local or systemic administration (Page, 1988). One of the most striking effects of PAF has been to cause prolonged increases in airway hyperreactivity (Cuss et al, 1986), which can be prevented by administration of cromolyn sodium, ketotifen, and specific PAF-receptor antagonists. PAF antagonists can inhibit antigen-induced bronchoconstrictor responses in sheep and humans (Abraham et al, 1989; Guinot et al, 1987), further underscoring the importance of this mediator in the pathophysiology of asthma. PAF antagonists, however, have been disappointing in asthmatics. The role of PAF and its antagonists in severe asthma, during exacerbation, has not yet been explored.

Eosinophilic Proteins

During an asthmatic attack, eosinophils accumulate in the bronchial wall as well as in the airway lumen. They release various proteins that are capable of causing tissue damage. For example, MBP has been shown to cause ciliostasis and damage to the respiratory epithelium. ECP is even damaging to the tissues. In fact, a correlation between ECP and cell injury has been suggested by the lung tissues from those who died of asthma (Dahl et al, 1988). In all cases in which ECP immunoreactivity was restricted to eosinophils with no immunoreactivity in the extracellular space, no cellular injury was observed. In cases with signs of ECP degranulation, however, the extracellular ECP was seen in or near necrotic areas (Dahl et al, 1988).

Nitric Oxide (NO)

NO is increasingly recognized to play an important pathophysiologic role in airway disease (Barnes and Belvisi, 1993). Although NO acts as the neurotransmitter of bronchodilator nerves in human airways, and it mediates endothelium-derived vasodilation, it may also act as an inflammatory mediator. NO is synthesized from L-arginine by the action of NO synthetase (NOS), and several molecular forms of NOS have been characterized. Constitutive calcium-dependent (cNOS) forms of the enzyme are expressed in endothelial cells and neurons, whereas inducible forms of enzymes (iNOS) may be induced by inflammatory cytokines in macrophages, other inflammatory cells, and epithelial cells of asthmatics. An increased amount of exhaled NO has been detected in asthmatics during late phase and disease activity, which is suppressed by steroids (Kharitonov et al, 1995; Yates et al, 1995). Corticosteroids inhibit the expression of iNOS but not cNOS.

Neurotransmitters

Autonomic nerves regulate many aspects of airway function including airway smooth muscle tone, secretion, blood flow, microvascular permeability, and neurogenic inflammation. Abundant evidence now exists that neural control of airways may be abnormal in asthma and that neurogenic mechanisms may contribute to the pathophysiology and symptoms of asthma (Barnes et al, 1991). In addition to cholinergic and adrenergic neural pathways, nonadrenergic noncholinergic (NANC) mechanisms are also present in the airways. Although neuropeptides may mediate many of the NANC effects in the airways, it has been recognized that NO may also function as an NANC transmitter. Thus, neurogenic inflammation due to the release of neuropeptides from sensory nerves may be relevant to severe asthma. Various abnormalities in airway control have been described in asthma, including a defect in NANC-bronchodilator nerves. Many neuropeptides, which have potent effects on many aspects of airway function, have now been identified in human airways. These include substance P, neurokinin A, and calcitonin gene-related peptide. Release of neuropeptides from airway sensory nerves is involved in various models of AHR. Their role in asthma is unknown, although a relationship between acute exacerbations of asthma and low plasma concentrations of vasoactive intestinal polypeptide (VIP) and elevated levels of substance P and neuropeptides has been observed (Cardell et al, 1994).

Other Mediators

The role of less well known mediators like adenosine (Church et al, 1988); bradykinin (Fuller and

Barnes, 1988); and neuropeptides, including VIP, substance P, and other neurokinins (Barnes, 1988), in the pathophysiology of asthma is not clear at present. Many of these mediators can cause bronchoconstriction either directly or indirectly via vagal stimulation; they can also cause mucous hypersecretion, induce inflammation, and increased microvascular permeability. Because the actions of some of these mediators can be blocked by cromolyn sodium, these mediators may act via secondary mediator release from mast cells or other cell types. The role of oxygen radicals and endothelins has also been proposed in the pathogenesis of asthma.

OXYGEN-DERIVED FREE RADICALS | Many inflammatory cells produce oxygen-derived free radicals, such as superoxide anions. These may play an important role in perpetuating asthmatic inflammation. Oxygen-derived free radicals may contribute to the epithelial damage in asthma and has been implicated in AHR in animal models of asthma (Lansing et al, 1993).

ADENOSINE | Adenosine causes a potent bronchoconstriction in asthmatics, and its effects are probably mediated via an A_2 receptor (Cushley and Holgate, 1985). Theophylline at therapeutic concentrations blocks adenosine receptors, which may contribute to its antiasthmatic effect.

ENDOTHELIN | Endothelin-1 (ET-1) is a potent constrictor of airways and vascular smooth muscles. It is expressed in airway epithelial cells in asthma, and elevated concentrations of ET-1 have been detected in BAL fluid of asthmatic patients (Barnes, 1994c). Endothelin expression is upregulated in bronchial epithelial cells of symptomatic asthmatics, and exposure of epithelial cells from asymptomatic subjects to histamine and IL-1 induces endothelin synthesis and release (Ackerman et al, 1995). ET-1 stimulates fibroblasts and airway smooth muscle cell growth, and thus it may have a role in hypertrophy of airway smooth muscle and basement membrane, which is a hallmark of chronic asthma.

BRADYKININ | The role of bradykinin in asthma may be that of an activator of sensory nerves, producing symptoms such as cough and chest tightness. Bradykinin also causes plasma exudation from bronchial vessels, stimulates airway secretions, and serves as a potent bronchial vasodilator. These effects are mediated via bradykinin-B_2 (BK_2). Autoradiographic studies show that BK_2 is widely distributed in animal and human airways (Mak and Barnes, 1991).

TRYPTASE | The role of mast cell serine proteases, like tryptase and chymase in the pathogenesis of asthma, is not well understood. Tryptase is resistant to inhibition by endogenous protease inhibitors, such as α_1 protease inhibitor and secretory leukocyte protease inhibitor. The abundance of this enzyme in mast cells, in conjunction with its ability to inactivate VIP and to potentiate histamine-induced airway smooth muscle contraction in vitro, has led to the suggestion that tryptase may play a role in AHR. Thus, in the sheep model of allergic bronchoconstriction, a tryptase inhibitor attenuated antigen-induced AHR (Clark et al, 1995). Whether tryptase plays a role in airway inflammatory response associated with acute severe asthma is not known at present.

AIRWAY HYPERREACTIVITY

Increased bronchial reactivity is a characteristic feature of bronchial asthma (Boushey et al, 1980). Several mechanisms have been proposed for bronchial hyperreactivity including (1) altered receptor function; (2) chemical mediators; (3) inflammation; (4) loss of epithelium-derived relaxant factors; (5) intrinsic abnormality of airway smooth muscle; (6) late-phase reaction; (7) hypoxia; and (8) viral infection.

Altered Receptor Function

Because β receptors represent the most important endogenous bronchodilator system in human airways, it is attractive to suppose that β-adrenergic function may be abnormal in asthma. Szentivany (1968) proposed a generalized impairment of β-receptor function as being of pathogenetic importance in asthma. A number of earlier studies observed diminished cardiovascular and metabolic responses to isoprenaline in asthmatic subjects. These observations were supported by decreased adenylate cyclase activation by β-agonists and decreased β-receptor density in lymphocytes or leukocytes of asthmatics. The β-receptor defect has been related in some asthmatics to circulatory autoantibody (Venten et al, 1980). A defect in potentiation of adenylyl cyclase has been proposed, which may be correlated with AHR (Dooper et al, 1995). The alternative hypothesis, proposed by Conolly and Greenacre (1976), was that the reduced β-receptor function was a result of prolonged exposure to β-agonists, thus causing a downregulation of β-receptors. These investigators found a marked depression of cyclic AMP response to isoproterenol in lymphocytes of asthmatics using β-adrenergic drugs, but not in those using nonadrenergic drugs. Radioligand studies on lymphocyte cell-membrane from asthmatic subjects have shown a 40% loss of β-receptor density after 3 to 5 weeks of oral terbutaline therapy (Hui et al, 1987). It was also observed that receptor density was restored by steroids. The controversy over these two opposing points, however, continues because of lack of controlled investigations in untreated subjects.

A pivotal issue, which has not been addressed so far, is whether or not human airways smooth muscle β2-receptors undergo desensitization with β2-agonists. Turki and coworkers (1995) demonstrated that administration of inhaled β2-agonists results in substantial downregulation of β2-receptors on epithelial cells and alveolar macrophages obtained via BAL. Result of clinical studies have also suggested that the β-receptor downregulation is more likely to occur on mast cells than on airway smooth muscle (O'Connor et al, 1992).

ALPHA-ADRENERGIC RECEPTORS | The role of α-adrenergic receptors in regulating airway caliber is controversial (Kaliner et al, 1982). A generalized abnormality of α-adrenergic receptor function in asthma has been proposed, and pupillary, cutaneous, and metabolic responses are enhanced in atopic asthmatics (Henderson et al, 1979). The evidence remains inconclusive, because α2-receptor responses were normal from patients with asthma.

MUSCARINIC RECEPTORS | Cholinergic hyperreactivity is a cardinal feature of asthma. Furthermore, cholinergic activity appears to be excessive in other organ systems in asthmatics, suggesting a generalized disturbance in parasympathetic tone (Kaliner et al, 1982). Several mechanisms (including increased vagal tone, increased acetylcholine release, and abnormal muscarinic receptor system) have been proposed, without much evidence, for cholinergic hyperreactivity in asthma. The presence of inhibitory presynaptic muscarinic receptors of M2-subtype has been demonstrated in the airway of animals and humans (Minette and Barnes, 1988; Patel et al, 1995), and it has been proposed that there may be a suppression of inhibitory muscarinic receptors in asthma, contributing to airway hyperreactivity (Ayala and Ahmed, 1989). These prejunctional autoreceptors inhibit acetylcholine release and may serve to limit vagal bronchoconstriction. The loss of normal feedback inhibition of acetylcholine due to a defect in muscarinic autoreceptors may result in exaggerated cholinergic reflexes in asthma. The mechanism of defective M2-autoreceptors in asthma is not known, but it is possible that M2-receptors may be more susceptible to damage by oxidants

or other inflammatory mediators. Studies have shown that viral infection, MBP, and allergen exposure result in a loss of autoreceptor function (Jacoby and Fryer, 1990), which may account for the increase in cholinergic tone in acute severe asthma.

HISTAMINE RECEPTORS | Airway effects of histamine are primarily mediated by H1 and H2 receptors (Eyre, 1977), whereas the role of H3 receptors, at present, is not clear. Stimulation of H1 receptors causes contraction of airway smooth muscle whereas H2-receptor stimulation causes relaxation (Ahmed et al, 1980). Functional suppression of H2 receptors has been observed in experimental models of allergic asthma (Ahmed et al, 1983b). This H2-receptor defect is observed in pulmonary and extrapulmonary sites such as skin and pulmonary and systemic vasculature (Ahmed and King, 1986). Human data are controversial, and no clear suppression of H2 receptors in the airways of asthmatic subjects has been observed, although lymphocyte (Beer et al, 1982) and gastric H2-receptor function is markedly suppressed in allergic asthmatics (Gonzalez and Ahmed, 1986). H2-receptor stimulation also mediates the feedback regulation of histamine release from mast cells *in vitro* (Lichtenstein and Gillespie, 1975). Thus, it is possible that suppressed H2 receptors in asthma on the one hand may cause enhanced release of histamine and on the other hand may potentiate the bronchoconstrictor effects of histamine. Their exact role in asthma, however, is unclear. H3 receptors have also been identified in airways. H3 receptors modulate neurotransmission as well as histamine release from airway mast cells (Ichinose and Barnes, 1990). The regulatory role of H2 or H3 receptors in human asthma, however, is not clear.

Role of Chemical Mediators

Chemical mediators play a major role in the development of bronchial hyperreactivity. Various chemical mediators and cytokines released from different cell types are the end result of the cascade resulting from allergic-inflammatory response. All of these mediators either alone or in combination are capable of causing bronchial hyperreactivity; however, the exact mechanism remains unknown. Leukotrienes and PAF may cause β-receptor dysfunction. These mediators can also perpetuate the inflammatory response and cause bronchoconstriction, mucociliary dysfunction, epithelial damage, and mucosal edema, culminating in bronchial hyperreactivity (see Fig. 23–6). Great interest has been generated in leukotrienes as the mediators of bronchial hyperreactivity.

Inflammation

Growing evidence now exists that airway inflammation plays a critical role in the pathogenesis of asthma and bronchial hyperreactivity. Experimental studies have provided convincing evidence of a close relationship between the amount of airway inflammation and bronchial hyperresponsiveness (Chung, 1986). Most of the stimuli that are known to increase airway responsiveness have been shown to cause airway inflammation. These stimuli include allergens, ozone, viral upper respiratory tract infections, and toluene diisocyanate. Different stimuli may trigger various types of inflammatory responses; thus, ozone stimulates an increase in neutrophils in bronchoalveolar lavage. Allergen, in contrast, is characterized by predominantly eosinophilic inflammation. Several cell types, as mentioned earlier, may be evidenced in this inflammatory response including mast cells, eosinophils, neutrophils, basophils, lymphocytes, and alveolar macrophages (see Fig. 23–4). These activated inflammatory cells can cause mediator release, leading to airway hyperresponsiveness.

Role of Epithelium

The epithelial layer probably acts as an important protective barrier; however, only in the 1980s has its role in bronchial hyperreactivity become obvious (Fedan et al, 1988; Hogg and Eggleston, 1984). Various chemical mediators can increase epithelial permeability, and eosinophilic products like eosinophilic basic proteins can cause epithelial damage. Loss of the epithelial barrier may cause enhanced bronchial reactivity due to (1) increased epithelial permeability and mucosal/submucosal edema; (2) loss of epithelium-derived relaxant factor (EpDRF) (Flavahan et al, 1985); (3) exposure of sensory nerve endings; and (4) release of chemical mediators like LTB_4 or 15-HETE.

Abnormal Airway Smooth Muscles

A fundamental defect may exist in the cellular processes that govern contraction of asthmatic airway smooth muscle. Two different theories, which are not mutually exclusive, have been proposed. The first (Stephens, 1988) is related to an alteration in the electrical excitability (conduction abnormality) of airway smooth muscle cells. The second theory proposes that the excitation-contraction-coupling-uncoupling process is disturbed in some way, resulting in an abnormality of Ca^{++} regulation by airway smooth muscle (Middleton, 1980; Triggle, 1983). Because of poor correlation of in vitro and in vivo data on airway smooth muscle contractility and inconsistency of available data, it is difficult to draw firm conclusion regarding the importance of an intrinsic defect in asthmatic airway smooth muscle. AHR in asthma may be due to the limitation of relaxation with deep inspiration (Skloot et al, 1995).

Late-phase Reaction

Late-phase reactions are of pathophysiologic importance, and a prolonged increase in nonspecific airway hyperresponsiveness has been observed after such reactions. The mechanism and biochemical and cellular basis of late-phase responses is not clear. Cellular inflammation (especially eosinophils) plays a major role in the development of the late response (O'Byrne et al, 1987). There is also increasing evidence that arachidonic acid metabolites of the lipoxygenase pathway and PAF may be the biochemical mediators of this response (Abraham et al, 1989; Cuss et al, 1986; Guinot, 1987; Page, 1988).

The clinical importance of late-phase reaction is not clear. It has been suggested that late-phase reactions and associated airway hyperresponsiveness may be related to worsening of clinical symptomatology. There is no evidence that status asthmaticus is more common in late responders, however. Late-phase reactions have also been observed after nonimmunologic reactions like exercise-induced bronchoconstriction. Investigators (Lemanske et al, 1989) demonstrated that after experimentally induced viral upper respiratory tract infection eight of ten acute responders developed late-phase response. Whether such conversion predisposes these patients to development of status asthmaticus is not known.

Hypoxia

During an asthma attack, severe hypoxemia may develop because of bronchoconstriction and abnormalities of gas exchange. Alterations in oxygen tension may stimulate or inhibit various enzyme systems, resulting in abnormal production of various mediators, including toxic oxygen radicals. Thus, alveolar hypoxia has been suggested to stimulate production of leukotrienes, causing pulmonary vasoconstriction (Ahmed and Oliver, 1983c). The effects of changes in oxygen tension on airway smooth muscle have been appreciated only in the 1980s. It has been shown that short-term alveolar hypoxia can increase nonspecific bronchial reactivity to histamine and carbachol in conscious sheep (Ahmed and Marchette, 1985). Hypoxia-induced enhancement of bronchial reactivity was prevented by pretreatment with cromolyn sodium, suggesting a central role of mast cell mediators. Further work has suggested that leukotrienes may be the putative mediator of hypoxia-induced bronchial hyperreactivity (D'Brot and Ahmed, 1988). Studies in human subjects have also shown enhanced airway reactivity after exposure to a hypoxic gas mixture. Although hypoxia is the result of pathophysiologic processes occurring in the lung during an asthmatic attack, by enhancing bronchial hyperreactivity it may lower the threshold and thus perpetuate bronchoconstriction.

Viral Infection

Epidemiologic data demonstrate that viral infections are the most important trigger for an acute asthma exacerbation. Studies of volunteers experimentally infected with viruses suggest that combining viral infections and allergen exposures may be a high risk for AHR and allergic airway inflammation. The precise mechanisms for this association have yet to be determined. *In vitro* studies have demonstrated that viruses can induce the secretion of a wide range of cytokines from several different cell types in the lower airways. Viral infection typically stimulate T cells to produce Th1-type cytokines such as IFNα and IL-2. Some viruses may enhance allergic inflammation by stimulating Th2-type responses, leading to secretion of IL-4, IL-5, and other cytokines that potentiate allergic responses (Gern and Busse, 1995). Viral infections have also been shown to increase the acute response and increase the probability of late response (Lemanske et al, 1989). Thus, viral infections not only increased AHR but can change the patterns of airway response to that associated with severe exacerbation of asthma (Cheung et al, 1995). Bacterial infections seem to play a minor role in asthma exacerbations, although *Mycoplasma pneumoniae* and *Chlamydia pneumoniae* have been implicated (Allegra et al, 1994).

REFRACTORINESS OF STATUS ASTHMATICUS

Various stimuli may trigger an attack, and all may culminate in the refractoriness to bronchodilator therapy so characteristic of status asthmaticus. These initiating factors include allergen exposure, viral respiratory tract infection, air pollutant and toxins exposure, cold air, and temperature and humidity changes.

Refractoriness to therapy in status asthmaticus is a complex phenomenon, and its exact mechanism is not clear (Bouhuys, 1978). It can be explained in part by pathologic changes in the lungs that limit the access of drugs to effector cells. Because of the extreme nature of an asthmatic attack, it is likely that all those processes that contribute to the development of airway hyperresponsiveness may play a role in the development of refractoriness, including (1) receptor dysfunction, (2) chemical mediators, (3) airway inflammation, (4) damaged epithelium, and (5) abnormal muscles (Table 23–3). The relative role of each of these factors is not clear, and in all likelihood an interaction of these factors plays an important role in the induction of refractoriness. A defect in β-receptor function (Szentivany, 1968) inherent to the asthmatic state and/or induced tachyphylaxis of β receptors may explain the relative lack of response to β-adrenergic drugs often observed in status asthmaticus. β-receptor, H_2-histamine receptor, and PGE_1 receptor dysfunction, however, can also be caused by acute viral infections (Busse et al, 1979). Similarly, chemical mediators like PAF can induce refractoriness to the bronchodilator action of isoproterenol in animals.

On a multifactorial basis it is possible that no matter what the initiating event may be, a massive insult to an inherently abnormal muscle may cause massive release of chemical mediators (including histamine, leukotriene, PAF, eosinophilic proteins, kinins) and may overwhelm the protective mechanisms by simultaneously causing a further suppression of various receptor systems (including β-adrenergic, H_2-histamine, M_2-muscarinic). Severe inflammatory response (including neutrophils, eosinophils, cytokines) may further perpetuate the chemical response and receptor dysfunction. Chemical mediators like eosinophilic basic protein may damage the protective epithe-

---

Table 23–3
Factors Contributing to Refractoriness of Status Asthmaticus

1. Receptor dysfunction
2. Chemical mediators
3. Airway inflammation
4. Damaged airway epithelium
5. Enhanced airway hyperreactivity
6. Abnormal airway smooth muscle
7. Mucosal edema
8. Mucous plugging

lial barrier, thus potentially damaging the EpDRF and exposing the irritant receptors to injurious actions of chemical mediators including neurokinins. These events, along with markedly abnormal mucociliary transport and mucous plugging, may interfere with the action of β-adrenergic agonists and culminate in refractoriness to therapy and the syndrome of status asthmaticus (see Figs. 23–4 and 23–6). Glucocorticosteroids form the basis of therapy of status asthmaticus and restore the responsiveness to β-agonists. The exact mechanism of action of steroids in asthma is not well known. Their varied and multiple sites of action, however, are not inconsistent with the multifactorial basis of refractoriness of status asthmaticus.

PATHOPHYSIOLOGY

The pathophysiology of asthma is complex and is primarily mediated by the effects of various inflammatory mediators on airway smooth muscle and vascular smooth muscle, microvascular permeability, and mucociliary transport. In addition, the secondary effects of bronchoconstriction, pulmonary hyperinflation, and severe gas-exchange abnormalities can cause marked cardiovascular dysfunction, which is so characteristic of status asthmaticus.

PULMONARY MECHANICS

Dynamic Mechanics

The major physiologic change in asthma is obstruction to airflow, especially during expiration. This is manifested by increased airway resistance and decreased forced expired volume in 1 second (FEV_1), FEV_1 as % of forced vital capacity, maximal midexpiratory flow rates (MMFR), and peak expiratory flow rates (PEFR). These changes are accompanied by a decrease in vital capacity and an increase in functional residual capacity and total lung capacity. Airway closure at normal lung volume may play an important role in the pathophysiology of status asthmaticus. Closure not only contributes to increased airway resistance, decreased MMFR, and vital capacity, but also requires the patient to breathe at a higher lung volume to keep the airways open. This airway closure in asthmatic lungs is seen at higher-than-normal transpulmonary or distending pressures, and the more severe the attack, the higher the transpulmonary pressure at which the airways close. Thus, the asthmatic patient must have a very negative pleural pressure during the acute attack to achieve airway patency (Fig. 23–7),

which results in a very high lung volume. The higher the airway closing pressure, the higher the lung volumes must be to keep the airways open for ventilation and gas exchange. These changes result in tremendously increased work of breathing, as observed clinically by the patient's use of accessory muscles for respiration.

Pride, Permutt, and Riley (1967) studied the airway closure in severe asthma. These investigators measured the relationship between expiratory flow and alveolar pressure relative to mouth pressure in a group of volunteers. In normal individuals at high lung volume, with increasing effort the expiratory flow is markedly elevated up to 600 l/min. Hence, there is no tendency at high lung volumes for any flow limitation, because flow continues to increase as the driving pressure increases. In contrast, at high lung volumes asthmatic subjects showed marked expiratory flow limitation with increasing expiratory effort (Fig. 23–8). In most subjects, airflow is limited at 200 l/min or less; further increases in effort and thus in driving pressure have no influence on airflow whatsoever. In an extremely severe attack, the plateau of airflow may even be found close to total lung capacity. It is this limitation of airflow caused by airway collapse that requires an asthmatic patient during an acute attack to breathe at high lung volume.

Obtaining complete pressure-flow curves at different lung volumes is extremely tedious. A more practical way to analyze the factors determining maximal expiratory flow is to plot maximal flow against lung recoil. This approach emphasizes the important role of lung recoil pressure in determining maximal expiratory flow, acting both as a component of the effective maximal driving pressure from alveoli to the flow-limiting segments and as a determinant of airway caliber. The plots of maximal expiratory flow against lung recoil pressure indicate that the cause of reduction in maximal flow is a drop conductance of intrapulmonary airways on forced expiration. The whole maximal flow–static recoil curve is displaced to the right toward the higher values of lung recoil pressure at lower maximal flows, reflecting premature or near-total airway closure.

Static Mechanics

A slight lowering of lung elastic recoil pressure during an asthmatic attack has been reported in several studies. Measurement of the shape of the pressure-volume curve of the lung confirms that lungs are slightly more compliant as the curve is shifted to the left. These changes, although similar to those in aging or mild emphysema, are reversible. In the majority of asthmatic patients,

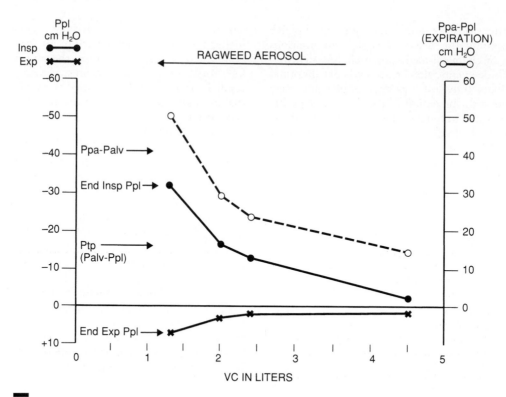

Figure 23–7

Relationship between pleural pressure (Ppl), pulmonary arterial pressure (Ppa) and vital capacity (VC) during antigen-induced bronchoconstriction. Pulmonary artery pressure relative to pleural pressure (Ppa-Ppl) measured at end expiration is shown as an interrupted line, whereas pleural pressure during inspiration (•—•) and expiration (x—x) is shown as a solid line. (From Permutt S: Relation between pulmonary arterial pressure and pleural pressure during the acute asthmatic attack. Chest 63:25S–28S, 1973b. With permission.)

however, static lung compliance (measured over the tidal volume range) remains normal, implying that the alterations in elastic properties of lung are subtle.

Lung Volume

Hyperinflation is a consistent finding during an acute asthmatic attack and is manifested by increases in function residual capacity, residual volume, and even total lung capacity (Woolcock and Read, 1966). The rise in lung volume is perhaps multifactorial (Martin et al, 1980; Peress et al, 1976). Although gas trapping and airway closure certainly contribute to the increase in lung volume, other factors, such as a reversible loss of lung recoil, may also be involved. Furthermore, because of increased inspiratory muscle activity, chest wall compliance may also be altered (Martin et al, 1980). Peress and coworkers (1976) have demonstrated that increased total lung capacity during an acute attack is not only associated with

an acute reversible loss of elastic recoil of lung, but also is accompanied by changes in pressure-volume characteristics of the chest wall.

GAS EXCHANGE

Ventilation-perfusion Inequality

Distribution of ventilation is very uneven during an asthmatic attack. This finding can be shown by single-breath nitrogen test, multiple-breath nitrogen wash-out test, frequency dependence of compliance, and density dependence of maximal expiratory flow-volume curves. This uneven distribution of ventilation leads inevitably to ventilation/perfusion ($\dot{V}/\dot{Q}$) mismatching and arterial hypoxemia unless pulmonary blood flow shows corresponding changes. Perfusion lung scans do show regional abnormalities in pulmonary blood flow, caused by either active vasoconstriction due to mediators or passive obstruction from the increased alveolar pressure and distention. Redistribution of regional blood flow, however, is not

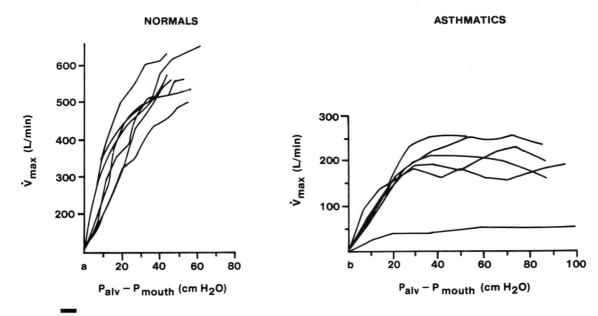

Figure 23–8
Isovolume pressure-flow curves in normals and patients with bronchial asthma. The relationship between the driving pressure (*Palv-Pmouth*) and the maximal expiratory flow (*Vmax*) is altered in asthma, as indicated by plateauing of expiratory flow at high volume. (Modified from Pride NB, Permutt S, Riley RL, et al: Determinants of maximal expiratory flow from the lung. J Appl Physiol 23:646–662, 1967. With permission.)

sufficient to compensate for the uneven ventilation, and a gross insufficiency of pulmonary gas exchange develops, resulting in a wide alveolar-arterial oxygen (O_2) gradient.

Although physiologic dead space is moderately increased, so that high ventilation results in low $PaCO_2$, the $\dot{V}/\dot{Q}$ imbalance is the major factor impairing efficiency of pulmonary gas exchange during an asthmatic attack. Despite gross $\dot{V}/\dot{Q}$ mismatching, an increase in anatomic shunt (i.e., $\dot{V}/\dot{Q}$ ratio of zero) is unusual. The probable explanation is that alveoli beyond occluded airways receive some collateral ventilation. Employing a multiple inert gas technique, a bimodal distribution of $\dot{V}/\dot{Q}$ ratios has been shown even in asymptomatic asthmatics (Wagner et al, 1978). The majority of blood flow was observed going to areas with normal $\dot{V}/\dot{Q}$ ratio (close to 1.0) with a second peak of very poorly ventilated units with $\dot{V}/\dot{Q}$ ratio around 0.1 or less. As much as 25% of cardiac output may be perfusing these poorly ventilated units. Furthermore, no evidence exists that these poorly ventilated units would collapse with 100% O_2 and become the site of an anatomic shunt. The most likely explanation for these findings is that the areas of low $\dot{V}/\dot{Q}$ ratios are receiving collateral ventilation and fail to collapse with 100% O_2. Wagner and coworkers (1978) also showed that the observed degree of $\dot{V}/\dot{Q}$ mis-

matching completely explained the arterial hypoxemia and that there is no true diffusion abnormality.

Diffusion

Diffusing capacity is normal or increased in mild attacks of asthma (Ohman et al, 1973; Weitzman and Wilson, 1974). During severe attacks of asthma, diffusion abnormalities may be artifactual because of abnormally increased alveolar volume, airway obstruction, and $\dot{V}/\dot{Q}$ mismatching.

Arterial Blood Gases

The inevitable result of $\dot{V}/\dot{Q}$ mismatching during an asthmatic attack is hypoxemia (McFadden and Lyons, 1968). As airway obstruction and $\dot{V}/\dot{Q}$ mismatching worsen, the A-aO_2 difference widens, resulting in increasing hypoxemia (Fig. 23–9). Uneven ventilation also impairs the efficiency of the lungs in excreting carbon dioxide (CO_2)—is generally low, and only when airway obstruction is very severe does the $PaCO_2$ rise (Fig. 23–10). Because hypoxemia is due to low $\dot{V}/\dot{Q}$ ratio and not to true shunting, it can be corrected readily by modest increases in inspired O_2 concentration ($\dot{V}$alabhji, 1968). Following bronchodilator therapy with β-agonists, $\dot{V}/\dot{Q}$ mismatching may

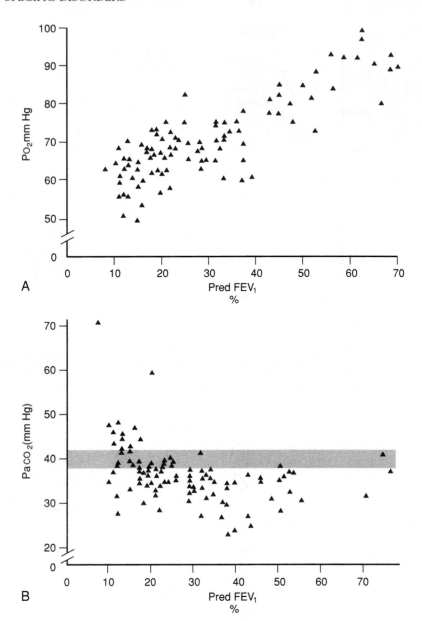

worsen in the presence of clinical and pulmonary function improvement. This occurrence may reflect increased cardiac output and pulmonary blood flow to areas with low V̇/Q̇ ratios, resulting in worsening of arterial hypoxemia.

MUCOCILIARY TRANSPORT

Research has revealed marked pathophysiologic changes in mucociliary transport in allergic bronchial asthma (Wanner, 1983). Mucociliary transport has been found to be depressed in experimental as well as human asthma, and during acute antigen-induced bronchoconstriction a further reduction in mucociliary transport was observed.

The duration of this acute dysfunction is quite remarkable. In allergic sheep, the inhalation of specific antigen impairs mucociliary function for up to 2 days, and impairment of mucociliary transport is not related to short-term alteration in airway function (Allegra et al, 1983). The observation that cromolyn sodium, which is a mast cell membrane stabilizing agent, prevented this impairment suggests that mucociliary dysfunction is related to chemical mediators released during airway anaphylaxis (Mezey et al, 1978). Histamine has been shown to stimulate mucociliary transport and therefore is unlikely to be involved in antigen-induced depression of mucociliary transport. There is evidence to support the belief

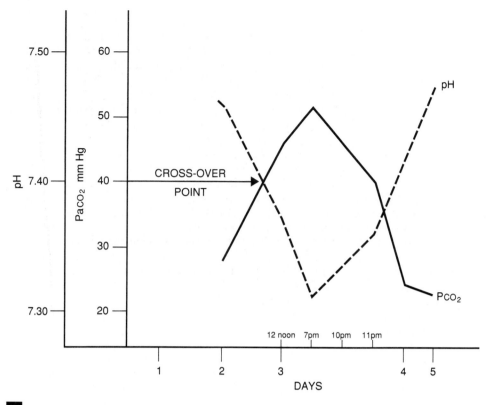

Figure 23–10
$PaCO_2$ and pH in a patient with status asthmaticus. Initial respiratory alkalosis and hypocapnia progressing to normal $PaCO_2$–pH relationship as a prelude to frank respiratory alkalosis. Patient recovered after intubation and mechanical ventilation. (From Weiss EB, and Faling LJ: Clinical significance of $PaCO_2$ during status asthmaticus: The cross over point. Ann Allergy 26:545–555 1968. With permission.)

that leukotrienes may play an important role in the mediation of allergic mucociliary dysfunction. Pretreatment with the specific leukotriene antagonists prevented the expected decrease in antigen-induced mucociliary transport (Ahmed et al, 1981).

These alterations in mucociliary transport may result from changes in ciliary activity, in quality and quantity of mucus and periciliary fluid, or a combination thereof. An insufficient number of cilia or a primary disturbance of ciliary motility does not appear to be the major factor. In ciliated respiratory tract cells of allergic sheep, antigen-increased ciliary beat frequency and antigen-induced ciliostimulation were blocked by cromolyn sodium and specific antagonist of slow reacting substance of anaphylaxis; they were not blocked by H_1- and H_2-histamine receptor blocking agents (Maurer et al, 1982). LTC_4, LTD_4, PGE_1, and PGE_2 all cause dose-dependent increases in ciliary beat frequency, whereas histamine-stimulated cilia cause increases only at relatively high doses

(Wanner et al, 1983). Ciliostimulation by inflammatory stimuli may not translate into enhanced mucociliary function (Seybold et al, 1989).

Alterations in respiratory secretions (mucus, periciliary fluid) are perhaps more likely to cause allergic mucociliary dysfunction. Changes in the quantity and biochemical composition of respiratory secretions, including glycoproteins and electrolytes, have been reported in asthma. Increases in glycoprotein secretion and changes in water transport have been observed in tracheal tissue from allergic sheep and in IgE-sensitized human airway fragments (Phipps et al, 1983). Glycoproteins seem to determine the rheologic properties of mucus to a great extent. Several chemical mediators including histamine and cyclooxygenase and lipoxygenase products have been implicated, with leukotrienes being the most potent. On the basis of these studies (Maurer et al, 1982; Wanner et al, 1983; Seybold et al, 1989; Phipps et al, 1983), it appears that chemical mediators exert their deleterious effect by altering the quantity and rheologic properties of airway secretions. The abnormal physicochemical properties may selectively affect the ciliary activity and thus depress the mucociliary transport.

The abnormal mucociliary transport certainly may contribute to the physiologic abnormalities in airway function. Cough and residual airway dysfunction found in patients with asthma in remission are partially related to the presence of excessive mucus in the peripheral airways. The abnormalities of peripheral airway function are not reversed or only partially reversed by administration of bronchodilators, suggesting the presence of excessive airway mucus or mucosal edema rather than increased bronchomotor tone. The postmortem findings of widespread mucous plugging in the airway of those who die in status asthmaticus have long been considered to represent the major cause of death. In these cases, the contribution of mucous plugs to increase airway resistance is understandable. We have aspirated a bronchial mucous plug obstructing the whole left bronchial tree in a patient with status asthmaticus (Fig. 23–11). The patient obviously did not respond to medical therapy until the mucous plug was removed with a fiberoptic bronchoscope. Mucociliary dysfunction in asthma may predispose asthmatics to respiratory infections by delaying removal of inhaled infectious agents, creating a favorable milieu for growth of infectious agents in

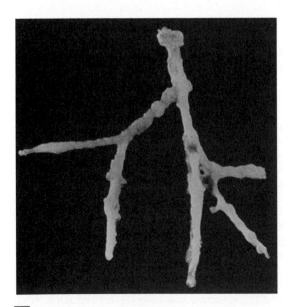

Figure 23–11
Large mucous plug obstructing the left bronchial tree of a patient in status asthmaticus. The plug was removed by bronchoscopic aspiration.

pooled secretions, damaging epithelium facilitating attachment of bacteria to the airway, and inhibiting the effect on mucus on cellular defense mechanisms (Whiteside et al, 1984; Woodside et al, 1983).

CARDIOVASCULAR FUNCTION

During an attack of acute asthma, important pathophysiologic changes occur in the pulmonary circulation, bronchial circulation, and cardiac function. Many of these changes result from the secondary mechanical effects of bronchoconstriction and hyperinflation. The effect of hypoxemia and hypercapnia, however, and the direct action of various chemical mediators on heart, vascular smooth muscle, and microvascular permeability certainly contribute to the cardiovascular dysfunction.

Pulmonary Circulation

Although clinical evidence of abnormalities of the pulmonary circulation and right heart are uncommon in asthma, electrocardiographic changes are frequently found (Ahonen, 1979). Resting pulmonary arterial pressure has been repeatedly reported to be within the normal range in stable asthma. The published data in acute asthmatic attacks are conflicting, with either elevated or normal pulmonary arterial and right ventricular pressures (Helander et al, 1962; Zimmerman, 1951). The pulmonary circulation may be altered in bronchial asthma by (1) mechanical effects, (2) alveolar hypoxia, and (3) chemical mediators.

Marked hyperinflation and increased mean alveolar pressure observed in asthma can be expected to increase resistance to blood flow because of compression of the small intra-alveolar vessels. Thus, pulmonary artery pressure rises in relation to this increased alveolar pressure to maintain the pulmonary blood flow. Permutt (1973a, 1973b) found that the pulmonary artery pressure relative to pleural pressure, measured at end expiration, was markedly elevated during an asthmatic attack (see Fig. 23–7). The difference between pulmonary artery pressure and end-expiratory pleural pressure increased from 15 cm H_2O before an attack to nearly 50 cm H_2O during. This increase was closely related to the increase in lung elastic recoil pressure at end inspiration. Permutt (1973a, 1973b) suggested that the degree of negative pleural pressure produced during inspiration determines how large a lung volume at which the patient breathes (i.e., the larger the lung volume, the greater is the pressure in the alveoli in relation to pleural pressure—transpulmonary pressure—

and the greater the pulmonary artery pressure has to be to propel the blood through the lungs). By subtracting the alveolar pressure from the pulmonary artery pressure most of the elevation in pulmonary artery pressure is accounted for. Based upon these findings, Permutt (1973a, 1973b) implied that the changes in lung mechanics were a major factor contributing to the rise in pulmonary arterial pressure and right ventricular work.

Effects of alveolar hypoxia and chemical mediators released during airway anaphylaxis on the pulmonary circulation are poorly understood. Alveolar hypoxia results in pulmonary vasoconstriction possibly via release of SRS-A (Ahmed and Oliver, 1983). In two studies, however, hypoxia associated with allergic bronchoconstriction did not increase pulmonary vascular resistance in either sheep or dogs with experimental allergic asthma (Cohn et al, 1978; Kung et al, 1980). Furthermore, in allergic sheep antigen challenge not only blunted but also reversed the hypoxic pulmonary vasoconstriction. To explain this effect, it was postulated that a vasodilator chemical mediator released during airway anaphylaxis masked the expected hypoxic pulmonary vasoconstriction. Pretreatment with prostaglandin synthetase inhibitors. (indomethacin and aspirin) unmasked the hypoxic pulmonary vasoconstriction, suggesting the release of vasodilator prostaglandins during airway anaphylaxis.

For obvious reasons, the information available in asthmatics during spontaneous or induced attacks is limited and controversial. The appearance of cor pulmonale and right ventricular hypertrophy, however, both clinically and at autopsy, is rare. The studies of Permutt (1973a, 1973b) have suggested development of acute pulmonary hypertension related entirely to mechanical effects. In contrast, Helander and coworkers (1962) observed a small increase in pulmonary artery pressure without a significant increase in pulmonary vascular resistance. No information on the effect of prostaglandin synthetase inhibition on human pulmonary circulation during an acute asthmatic episode is available.

Bronchial Circulation

Despite the fact that airway inflammation has for a long time been considered an important feature in the pathophysiology of asthma, very little attention has been paid to the secondary effects of the inflammation on the macro- and microcirculation of the tracheobronchial tree. The mechanical effects of bronchoconstriction and pulmonary hyperinflation, changes in vascular smooth muscle tone by the chemical mediators, alteration in microvascular permeability, and development of mucosal and airway wall edema can potentially contribute to the pathophysiology of an asthmatic attack (Wanner, 1989; Persson, 1988). Furthermore, changes in bronchial circulation may interfere with the clearance of various mediators and thus may perpetuate bronchoconstriction. In addition, pharmacologic agents used for the treatment of asthma may also affect various aspects of macro- and microvascular changes of tracheobronchial circulation. Unfortunately, the techniques that are used to obtain information on bronchial circulation are only now being applied in humans. Thus, current knowledge is still in its infancy and is obtained from animal experiments.

In the allergic sheep model, inhalation challenge with the specific antigen produced a dual increase in total bronchial blood flow, which temporally corresponded to the immediate- and late-phase bronchoconstrictor responses but was not the consequence of bronchoconstriction (Long et al, 1988). Inhibition of mediator release with cromolyn sodium blocked the effects of antigen. Various receptor antagonists, including antihistamine, failed to block the antigen-induced "immediate" increase in total bronchial blood flow. In contrast, a cyclooxygenase inhibitor markedly attenuated the bronchovascular response, without reducing the bronchoconstrictor response. Thus, a vasodilator cyclooxygenase product (e.g., prostacyclin) appears to be the putative mediator of the bronchial hyperemia observed immediately after antigen challenge in allergic sheep. The putative mediator of the late-phase increase in bronchial blood flow is not yet clearly known. The chemical mediators are also capable of causing increased microvascular permeability and mucosal airway wall edema.

Intratracheal instillation of antigen in intact allergic sheep leads to tracheal mucosal hyperemia and narrowing of the tracheal lumen (Csete et al, 1991). During an infusion of the vasodilator nitroglycerin, antigen failed to alter airway perfusion or tracheal volume. An infusion of vasopressin, a vasoconstrictor, prevented antigen-induced tracheal mucosal hyperemia and prolonged tracheal narrowing. Vasopressin and nitroglycerin had no effect on the contractile responses of tracheal smooth muscle to antigen in vitro. It seems that vasomotion per se may modify antigen-induced airway smooth muscle contraction.

Results of several investigations have suggested that airway wall hyperemia reduces airway caliber. In peripheral airways of sheep, we observed a rise in airway resistance after topical application of nitroglycerin. Pretreatment with a vasoconstrictor blocked nitroglycerin-induced bronchial narrowing but had no effect on bronchoconstriction produced after topically applied carbachol (Csete et al, 1990). Exercise-induced asthma may be prevented by pretreatment with the potent vasoconstrictor and α-adrenergic agonist, methoxamine (Dinh-Xuan et al, 1989). This suggests that vascular engorgement plays a role in that type of asthma. In asthmatics, methoxamine pretreatment can either blunt or enhance histamine-induced bronchial narrowing. This observation prompted the notion that methoxamine reduces histamine-induced airflow obstruction in asthmatics in whom airway narrowing is primarily caused by bronchial edema (Phan-Puibaraud et al, 1995). Because resistance and radius are not linearly related, airway mucosal vasodilation and edema may have only modest effects on the resistance of airways with relatively greater resting caliber.

The clinical significance of increased bronchial mucosal blood flow, increased microvascular permeability, and mucosal and airway wall edema is not clear. These changes may (1) contribute to bronchoconstriction, (2) interfere with clearance of mediators and thus may perpetuate bronchoconstriction, and (3) interfere with access of pharmacologic agents to their site of action, partially contributing to refractoriness to therapy.

Cardiac Function

Right Ventricle

The previously described acute changes in pulmonary circulation are likely to exert right ventricular strain. At full inspiration, the pressure on the outer surface of the heart may be around −30 cm H_2O (see Fig. 23–7). Thus, the right ventricle has to generate an additional pressure of more than 30 cm H_2O to pump blood through small pulmonary vessels that have been compressed because of pulmonary hyperinflation. The tension the right ventricle has to develop to overcome the forces impeding right ventricular ejection is a function of the pressure surrounding the intra-alveolar pulmonary vessels relative to the pressure on the outside of the right ventricle (Gunstone, 1971). Thus, the greater the lung inflation, the greater the transpulmonary pressure, and the greater the load on the right ventricle. The right ventricle has to do less work at end expiration than it does during inspiration, but the difference is small because lung volume is still very high. In an acute attack, therefore, the right ventricle must generate a greater pressure during expiration because alveolar pressure is still high. The net result of these changes is to increase right ventricular strain and increase tension required by the right ventricle to

pump blood through the lung. Electrocardiographically, this effect may be manifested by p-pulmonale and right axis deviation (Gelb et al, 1979).

Left Ventricle

Direct assessment of left ventricular function during an acute asthmatic attack has been limited. Theoretically, the large negative pleural pressure oscillations during inspiration in an asthmatic attack may be expected to impede the emptying of blood from the left ventricle. Studies in dogs with inspiratory obstruction (simulated Mueller maneuver) demonstrated that increased negative pleural pressure was accompanied by a greater rise in systolic volume than diastolic volume, resulting in decreased ejection fraction of the left ventricle during this inspiratory obstruction. The increased inspiratory load placed on the left ventricle by the increased negative pleural pressure during an asthmatic attack can have a similar effect and may be the major cause of pulsus paradoxus in severe asthma (Jardin et al, 1982; Rebuck and Pengelly, 1973). This response is borne out by an observed correlation between the pulsus paradoxus and severity of an asthmatic attack, and it is not unexpected because a greater negative pleural pressure is associated with a larger lung volume and more severe attack of asthma.

In an echocardiographic study of nine patients in status asthmaticus, a competition between the right and left ventricles for the pericardial space was observed during inspiration (Jardin et al, 1982). This effect was suggested by a reduced left ventricular cross-sectional area at end systole (−24%) and end diastole (−32%), a leftward septal motion, and an increased right ventricular end-diastolic/systolic diameter (+40%). In addition to the ventricular competition, the study also suggested that increased impedance to right ventricle ejection was another factor results of reducing left ventricular preload, thus reducing the left ventricular stroke output during inspiration.

Another report described acute, rapidly reversible, left ventricular dysfunction with ejection fractions of 11 to 34% in three patients with status asthmaticus. Profound hypoxemia and hypotension, acidemia, and myocardial depressor effect of histamine released during anaphylaxis were postulated to explain this phenomena (Levin et al, 1995).

◼ CLINICAL FEATURES

SYMPTOMS AND SIGNS

Patients with status asthmaticus may resemble other patients with severe asthma (Table 23–4).

■
Table 23–4
Clinical Features of Impending Status Asthmaticus

1. Increased frequency of wheezes
2. Large diurnal shifts in peak flow
3. Purulent, tenacious sputum
4. Behavioral alterations (anxiety, insomnia)
5. Progressive dyspnea
6. Refractoriness to therapy
7. Multiple drug regimen

If the condition is identified early and managed aggressively, the progression from acute asthma to status asthmaticus may be aborted. When status asthmaticus occurs, however, patients are diaphoretic, anxious, and often too breathless to give a complete history. A previous history of asthma requiring hospitalization, asthma attacks occurring at increasingly frequent intervals, severe attacks lasting more than 24 hours, and current use of corticosteroids should alert the physician to a diagnosis of status asthmaticus and the need for hospitalization and intensive care.

Patients show intensely labored breathing characterized by the use of accessory muscles of respiration and intercostal retraction, indicating severe impairment of pulmonary functions. Although dyspnea and wheezing are the major sign and symptom, they are poorly related to the pulmonary function impairment in severe asthma. It is important for the physician to be aware that wheezes may be absent on auscultation in a severe case of asthma. Absence of wheezing indicates very severe airway obstruction, so that the patient is unable to generate sufficient airflow to produce sounds (McFadden et al, 1973). An increase in pulsus paradoxus, which is a sign associated with hyperinflation and airway obstruction, is almost always present (Rebuck and Pengelly, 1973). Cyanosis may be difficult to detect; it is a late unreliable sign of hypoxemia. Confusion and loss of consciousness, at times with papilledema, accompanying severe hypoxemia and hypercapnia are preterminal occurrences in many patients with profound respiratory failure resulting from status asthmaticus. These findings are generally associated with fatigue and exhaustion. Many patients report failure of therapy either at home or in the emergency room, which is one of the defining characteristics of status asthmaticus.

LABORATORY INVESTIGATION

Pulmonary Function Studies

During a very severe attack, patients may be too sick to perform pulmonary function tests. Spirometry is bound to reveal decreased forced vital capacity, FEV_1, and PEFR. Orthopneic patients usually have an FEV_1 under 800 ml. Physiologic measurements of lung volume and airway resistance are not feasible as a routine bedside procedure in status asthmaticus but chest radiograph may reveal marked hyperinflation. Emphysema does not account for pulmonary hyperinflation in asthma because asthma pulmonary hyperinflation is readily reversible. Chest overinflation in asthma has been associated with the development of positive intrathoracic pressure at end inspiration (intrinsic PEEP). Arterial blood gases reveal hypoxemia, but $PaCO_2$ and pH levels are variable, depending upon the severity of disease. In milder attacks there is evidence of respiratory alkalosis, whereas extremely severe cases are associated with respiratory acidosis. Hypercarbia in acute asthma is usually seen when the FEV_1 is below 20% of the predicted normal value (McFadden and Lyons, 1968).

Chest Radiographs

Chest radiography invariably reveals evidence of hyperinflation, which at times is associated with pneumomediastinum, pneumothorax, segmental atelectasis due to mucous plugging, or pneumonia.

Electrocardiogram

Electrocardiographic abnormalities, which tend to be rapidly reversible with successful treatment, are common in severe asthma (Ahonen, 1979). They include sinus tachycardia, right axis deviation, clockwise rotation, partial right bundle branch block, ST-T abnormalities, p-pulmonale, and right ventricular strain (Edmunds and Godfrey, 1981; Gelb et al, 1979). P-pulmonale is seen with greater frequency when hypercarbia ($PaCO_2 \geq 45$ mmHg) and acidemia (pH ≤ 7.37) coincided with status asthmaticus (Gelb et al, 1979). There may be occasional premature atrial and ventricular contractions. Reversible inferior lead T-wave abnormalities have also been observed and appear to be related to the severity of the attack (Efthimiou et al, 1991).

Blood Tests

Blood and sputum eosinophilia findings are helpful in differentiating asthma from other causes of obstructive airway disease. Eosinopenia has been used to assess the efficacy of glucocorticosteroids. Asthma exacerbations may occur without sputum eosinophilia however (Turner et al, 1995). There may be increases in hematocrit and blood urea nitrogen levels due to dehydration and neutrophilia associated with pulmonary infection. These tests may be important for therapeutic purposes but are of no help in grading severity of asthma. Electrolyte abnormalities have been observed in some cases of severe status asthmaticus, especially hyponatremia, which is attributed to inappropriate secretion of antidiuretic hormone (Baker et al, 1976).

ASSESSMENT OF SEVERITY

Clinical features of asthma may be misleading and potentially hazardous to the life of the patient, because severity of asthma may be underestimated. Various methods have been used to grade severity, either in the prodromal stage or during an acute attack (Busey et al, 1968; Fischl et al, 1981; Franklin, 1974; Georg, 1981; McFadden et al, 1973). Clinical grading of severity is based primarily upon subjective clinical history and presentation. Grading is a helpful guide for patient education, early diagnosis, and intervention. This must be combined, however, with objective testing of pulmonary functions and arterial blood gases to determine functional stage of status asthmaticus (Table 23–5). The objective assessment helps to determine the true role of airway obstruction in status asthmaticus and ensures that therapy is lessening it. Simple measurements of FEV_1 or PEFR obtained on a spirogram are quite helpful. As shown in Table 23–4, FEV_1 is variable and depends upon the severity of disease. In milder attacks, FEV_1 may be close to 1 liter, with slightly decreased PaO_2 and $PaCO_2$ (stage II). Worsening of airway obstruction is associated with a further decrease in FEV_1, PEFR, and $PaCO_2$ (stage III). In extreme cases, it is generally not possible to measure pulmonary functions; PaO_2 is markedly reduced, and there may be a rise of $PaCO_2$ with development of respiratory acidosis (stages IV and

V) (see Figs. 23–9 and 23–10). Stages III, IV, and V can be considered very severe, and most patients are in stage III when seen in the emergency room.

One clinical sign that is related closely to the functional stage and thus to airway obstruction is the magnitude of pulsus paradoxus (Rebuck and Pengelly, 1973; Rebuck and Read, 1971) (Fig. 23–12). The magnitude of pulsus paradoxus has also been correlated with the increase in $PaCO_2$. In view of the relationship between airflow obstruction and $PaCO_2$, it is important to know the $PaCO_2$ during an episode of severe asthma. As asthma increases in severity the $PaCO_2$ falls owing to hyperventilation, only to climb again with rising airway obstruction (see Fig. 23–10) (Weiss and Faling, 1968). Therefore, an elevated $PaCO_2$ or a $PaCO_2$ rising from its nadir is an important and valuable sign of severe asthma (stages IV and V). The $PaCO_2$ is of far less use, being poorly correlated with severity and particularly dependent upon the degree of $\dot{V}/\dot{Q}$ mismatching. Patients with near-fatal asthma, however, may have reduced chemosensitivity to hypoxia and blunted perception of dyspnea, which are features that can facilitate hypercarbia. (Kikuchi et al, 1994). Hypercapnic patients have greater airway obstruction, higher respiratory rate, and pulsus paradoxus (Mountain and Sahn, 1988). With appropriate therapy most patients with hypercapnia recover rapidly, and mechanical ventilation usually can be avoided. Close monitoring of these patients is required, however, until the acute asthmatic episode has resolved.

A predictive index using a combination of factors has been described by Fischl and coworkers (1981). The factors are pulse rate higher than 120 per min, respiratory rate higher than 30 per min, pulsus paradoxus greater than 18 mm Hg, PEFR less than 120 liters per min, and use of accessory

Table 23–5
Functional Staging of Status Asthmaticus: Assessment of Severity

| Stage | Objective Tests | | |
	FEV_1 (ml)	$PaCO_2$	PaO_2
V (Respiratory acidosis)	Usually not possible	Elevated	Usually low
IV (Marked hypoxemia)	Usually not possible	Normal	Low
III (Severe obstruction)	FEV_1 300–800*	Normal or elevated	Normal or low
II (Moderate obstruction)	FEV_1 800*	Normal or low	Normal
I (Little or no asthma)	FEV_1 near normal*	Usually not done	Usually not done

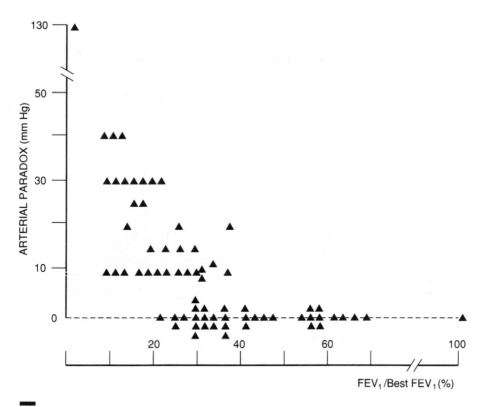

Figure 23–12
Degree of pulsus paradoxus plotted against FEV$_1$ (forced expired volume in one second) on admission. FEV$_1$ is expressed as a percentage of the best FEV$_1$ ever recorded in each patient. (From Rebuck AS, and Read J: Assessment and management of severe asthma. Am J Med 51:788–798, 1971. With permission. Copyright 1971 by Excerpta Medica Inc.)

muscles, and wheezing. The index ranges from 0 to 7 and increases with the severity of symptoms. An index of 4 or higher was 95% accurate in predicting the risk of relapse and 96% accurate in predicting the need for hospitalization. Others, however, have been unable to substantiate these findings (Centor et al, 1984; Rose et al, 1984). Nonetheless, patients with moderate to severe airflow obstruction who demonstrate a poor response to initial therapy (i.e., PEFR increased by <10%) or asthmatics whose condition deteriorates despite therapy in the emergency room should be admitted for ongoing therapy in a unit that can provide frequent clinical assessment and prompt treatment. The duration of treatment in an emergency room can exceed 2 hours. This length of time permits the assessment of response to systemic glucocorticosteroids (Corbridge and Hall, 1995). In one study, the asthma relapse rate after emergency room treatment declined from 50 to 4% if the length of initial therapy and assessment approached 6 hours (Kelsen et al, 1978).

MANAGEMENT

CLINICAL MANAGEMENT

Once the assessment of severity has been made, therapy can be started immediately and adjusted to the needs of the individual patient. Treatment requirements are determined not only by initial assessment of severity but also by subsequent response. Of patients with severe asthma, some may respond rapidly and others poorly to initial therapy. The aim should be to have the patient reach stage II as soon as possible (Busey et al, 1968; Fitzgerald and Hargreave, 1989; Franklin, 1974; Georg, 1981).

General Principles

The following therapeutic modalities may be needed in various combinations for the individual patient with a usual case of status asthmaticus.

Bronchodilators

Most clinicians start treatment with a combination of bronchodilators (inhaled and/or parenteral) supplemented with corticosteroids. Commonly used bronchodilators include aminophylline, β-agonists, and anticholinergic agents. Aminophylline is administered as an intravenous (IV) loading dose followed by a continuous IV infusion. Intravenous aminophylline, however, increased toxicity but not efficacy of inhaled β-agonist in a study of patients with acute severe asthma (FEV_1 <30% predicted) (Rodrigo and Rodrigo, 1994). Once the refractoriness of the bronchospasm has been established, many use IV aminophylline as adjunctive therapy. The experimental data to support this strategy are lacking. The role of nebulized ipratropium bromide, as an anticholinergic bronchodilator, in status asthmaticus awaits further study, but its addition to conventional bronchodilator therapy in patients with recalcitrant asthma may enhance benefit. Because inhaled ipratropium bromide may provoke bronchospasm in chronic airflow obstruction (Connolly, 1982), its use must be carefully monitored. Anticholinergic bronchodilators are the drugs of choice for bronchospasm induced by blockade of β-adrenergic receptors (Grieco and Pierson, 1971).

Aerosol delivery of bronchodilators may be achieved by jet nebulization or metered-dose inhalers (MDI). In nonintubated patients, jet nebulization and properly used MDI drug combined with a spacing device appear to be equally efficacious at relieving asthmatic bronchial obstruction (Idris et al, 1993; Jasper et al, 1987; Newhouse and Fuller, 1993). Jet nebulizers, although generally easier to use, are more expensive than MDIs.

In mechanically ventilated patients, many machine and host factors may affect aerosol drug delivery to the airways (Diot et al, 1995). In general, higher drug dosages are required to achieve a physiologic effect in intubated patients (Corbridge and Hall, 1995; Manthous et al, 1993). In one study, 9 mg (100 puffs) of albuterol delivered by MDI to intubated patients with airflow obstruction had no demonstrable beneficial or adverse effect, whereas 2.5 mg of nebulized albuterol significantly reduced inspiratory flow resistive pressure (Manthous et al, 1993). By using a lung model (Diot et al, 1995), it was concluded that both nebulizers and MDIs with a spacer can effectively deliver aerosolized medications, but the setup and technique may significantly alter drug deposition. Respiratory therapy personnel should be familiar with the equipment and proper techniques needed for optimal delivery of aerosolized medications to intubated patients.

Corticosteroids

All patients with status asthmaticus require corticosteroids in addition to, not as a substitute for, bronchodilators. Patients within stages III, IV, and V asthma should be given "sufficient" doses of corticosteroids (Haskell et al, 1983). In status asthmaticus, overtreatment with steroids is safer than no treatment or undertreatment. There is no evidence that giving steroids *per se* causes steroid dependency, and if it appears that steroids may have been unnecessary, the treatment can be tapered or discontinued rapidly after the airway obstruction clears. Unless there is a relative contraindication, such as diabetes or peptic ulcer, the initial dose should be high enough that a substantial improvement occurs. Hydrocortisone or methylprednisolone should be given parenterally, either as intermittent injections or continuous infusions. Improvement usually occurs rapidly, and patients are in stage III or better within 24 hours. Once improvement has occurred, steroids are tapered as long as the patient can be maintained in stage I.

Oxygen Therapy

Because most patients in status asthmaticus are hypoxic, supplemental O_2 should be given soon after determining arterial blood gas composition. Considering that CO_2 narcosis is rare in asthma, O_2 can be started empirically even if $PaCO_2$ is raised. It is generally preferable to start with 28% Ventimask O_2 (or 2–3 l/min via a nasal cannula) and check that $PaCO_2$ has not risen before proceeding to a higher concentration of O_2.

Chest Physical Therapy

Other than bronchodilator aerosol therapy with a side-arm nebulizer, the role of chest physiotherapy in management of status asthmaticus is limited. Postural drainage, chest percussion and vibration, and assisted cough have little place in the initial management. They may be detrimental. After the acute crisis is over, chest physiotherapy may be of some help if the patient has a productive cough and subsegmental or segmental atelectasis due to mucous plugging.

Fluids

Patients may suffer from fluid deprivation because of difficulty in swallowing food and liquids and from loss of water vapors because of excessive minute ventilation. It has been suggested, without good scientific evidence, that fluid replacement is beneficial for loosening the thick, tenacious sputum. Because of altered mechanical forces, the extravascular lung water may be increased with routine fluid (Stalcup and Mellins, 1977). Theoretically, this increased lung water can worsen $\dot{V}/\dot{Q}$ mismatching. The thick, tenacious sputum and mucous plugs are perhaps related to chemical mediators, not to dehydration.

Antibiotics

Antibiotics are indicated in the presence of bacterial infection. Asthmatic flare-ups are more often associated with viral than with bacterial infections, however, and in any event it may be difficult to recognize infection in asthma. Large numbers of eosinophils in the sputum may cause it to appear misleadingly purulent in the absence of infection. In a dangerously ill patient, however, it may be safer to use a broad-spectrum antibiotic when there is reason to suspect bacterial infection. In one study, viruses were implicated in 9% of patients with acute asthma, whereas intracellular bacteria were detected by serologic testing in 11%. In seven of eight such cases, C. pneumoniae was identified as the pathogen (Allegra et al, 1994). Hahn and coworkers (1991) showed a dose-response relationship between C. pneumoniae antibody titers level and prevalence of wheezes in acute respiratory tract infections; 21% of these cases subsequently developed asthma, suggesting a pathogenic role for C. pneumoniae respiratory tract infection and asthma. Further studies are needed to define the role of airway infections with C. pneumoniae and other respiratory tract pathogens in the development or course of asthma.

Sedation

Sedation in any form should not be given in stages III, IV, and V. No evidence exists that tranquilizers and sedatives *per se* are useful in aborting or treating an attack of status asthmaticus. They may be beneficial in patients receiving mechanical ventilation, however.

Miscellaneous

Cough suppressants (especially those with codeine) should be avoided unless nonproductive cough is disturbing the patient's rest and sleep. Several other remedies, reported to be mucokinetic and mucolytic (including iodides, acetylcysteine, and other mucolytic agents), that show some efficacy *in vitro* have been given but are ineffective clinically.

Special Situations

Special therapeutic considerations need to be given to the treatment of acute severe asthma in the elderly, children, and pregnant women.

Asthma in the Elderly

Acute, life-threatening attacks of asthma do occur as frequently in the elderly as in young asthmatics. The increase in the asthma death rate noted in the 1980s was largely explained by the accelerated death rate in elderly asthmatic patients (Evans et al, 1987). Older patients with asthma usually wait longer before hospital admission for severe acute attacks than do younger patients with asthma (Petheram et al, 1982), perhaps because of a blunted perception of dyspnea (Connolly et al, 1992). Cough, asthma requiring systemic glucocorticosteroids, and clinical course suggestive of chronic bronchitis are features more common in elderly patients with bronchial asthma than in younger patients. The response to inhaled β-agonist, but not to anticholinergic therapy, declines with age, so that older asthmatics tend to require continued inhaled β-sympathomimetics to control wheezes. This may help explain the higher death rates in elderly asthmatics (Ullah et al, 1981). At comparable serum levels of theophylline, individuals over 75 years of age harbor a 16-fold greater risk of life-threatening adverse consequences than those below 25 years (Shannon and Lovejoy, 1990). Given the increasing frequency of bronchospasm, delay in seeking physician advice, refractoriness to β-agonist and diminished threshold for toxicity, it is not surprising that elderly asthmatics are dying at rates exceeding those of younger patients with bronchial asthma.

The clinical signs of tachycardia, pulsus paradoxus, and even wheezing may all occur in a patient with left ventricular failure. The problem may be further compounded by the coexistence of both conditions. Hence, the differential diagnosis of wheezing in the elderly requires good clinical acumen. Furthermore, high-dose steroid therapy may precipitate cardiac failure. Thus, hemodynamic monitoring with a Swan-Ganz catheter may be advisable in such patients.

Elderly patients are also more susceptible than younger ones to developing steroid psychosis when treated with high doses of corticosteroids. Psychosis requires rapid lowering of steroids and optimal use of inhaled and parenteral bronchodilators.

Asthma in Children

The general principles of therapy of status asthmaticus in children are no different from those in adults. Dosages for infants and children of commonly prescribed antiasthmatic agents can be found in Table 23–6. The handheld, inhaled bronchodilator agents can be given at the same doses generally administered to adult asthmatics (Newhouse, 1993). β_2-agonists are the mainstay of treatment in the emergency room and are administered either as aerosols or parenterally. Intravenous theophylline and steroids can be added as indicated. Supplemental O_2 should be given judiciously, as guided by measurements of oxyhemoglobin saturation or arterial blood gases. The patient should be closely monitored in the intensive care unit if the attack is severe enough. There is a tendency among parents and family practitioners to use sedating antihistamines and other cough medications to calm a child. It is important to note that the condition of these patients can deteriorate rapidly, and true severity of disease may be underestimated because of central effects of antihistamine drugs. After discharge,

education of the child, family, teachers, and pediatrician or family physician is of utmost importance to prevent relapse and institute an effective maintenance program.

Asthma in Pregnancy

The goals of therapy in a pregnant patient are similar to those in a nonpregnant patient. It is important to stress that control of asthma is essential so that the risk of life-threatening episodes of status asthmaticus and morbidity and mortality may be lowered for the mother and the fetus. The therapeutic agents must not be harmful for the mother or teratogenic for the fetus. Asthma certainly is not a contraindication for pregnancy. Statistics show that in 33% of patients, pregnancy has no effect on the disease state; 28% of patients improve, and in 35% of patients asthma is worse (Schatz et al, 1988). Beta-agonists, theophyllines, and steroids can all be given safely during an

▬
Table 23–6
Inhaled and Parenteral Drugs for Use in Infants and Children With Acute Severe Asthma

Agent	Dose	Route	Frequency	FDA Approval
Epinephrine	0.01 ml/kg; max of 0.3 ml	SQ	Every 20 min × 3	Yes
Isoproterenol	0.1 μ/kg/min increase by 0.1 μ/kg q 15 min to max of 0.8 μ/kg/min	IV	Continuous	No
Terbutaline	0.005–0.01 ml/kg; max of 0.3 ml	SQ	Every 2–4 hours	≥12 years age
	Load 10 μ/kg, then 0.25 μ/kg/min to max of 20 μ/min	IV	Continuous every 10 minutes	≥12 years age
	0.01–0.03 ml/kg in 2 ml saline, max = 1 ml	Aerosol	Every 4–6 hours	≥12 years age
Metaproterenol	0.25–0.5 mg/kg in 2 ml saline; max = 15 mg	Aerosol	Every 4–6 hours	≥12 years age
Albuterol	0.1–0.15 mg/kg in 2 ml saline; max = 2.5 mg	Aerosol	Every 4–6 hours	≥4 yrs age
Atropine sulfate	0.015 ml/kg in 2 ml saline	Aerosol	Every 6 hours	≥6 years age
Ipratropium bromide	250 μg in 2 ml saline	Aerosol	Every 6 hours	No
Hydrocortisone	Load 5–7 mg/kg; maintenance 2–4 mg/kg/day	IV	Every 6 hours	Yes
Methylprednisolone	Load 1–2 mg/kg; maintenance 0.5–1 mg/kg	IV	Every 6 hours	Yes
Theophylline	Loading dose 0–6 mg/kg Infusion 0.8–1.2 mg/kg/hr to sustain adequate serum levels	IV	Continuous	Yes

From Brugman SM and Larson GL: Childhood asthma: Wheezing in infants and small children. Seminars in Respiratory and Critical Care Medicine. 15:147–160, 1994.

acute attack. Similarly, inhaled steroids and cromolyn sodium are considered safe as preventive
therapy of asthma. Exacerbations of asthma during
labor and delivery can be effectively treated with
parenteral steroids and other bronchodilators.
Aerosolized β-agonists are preferred, because systemic bronchodilators may delay labor, because
of their direct effect on uterine smooth muscle.
Systemic β-agonists should be given with caution
because postpartum pulmonary edema has been
reported in association with preventive therapy
for premature labor with terbutaline (Lapinsky et
al, 1995; Rogge et al, 1979). If a cesarean section
is indicated, epidural or spinal anesthesia is recommended in relatively stable cases, whereas patients in severe respiratory distress may be given
general anesthesia (preferably halothane).

Management of a Refractory Case

Most patients in status asthmaticus respond to
medical therapy with bronchodilators and corticosteroids, as outlined in the previous section. Occasionally, however, a patient may be refractory to
such therapy, requiring additional measures including mechanical ventilation and bronchial lavage. Such measures must be undertaken *in addition to* and not as a substitute for medical therapy.

Mechanical Ventilation

The aim of controlled mechanical ventilation is
to (1) relieve the exhausted patient of the increased work of breathing; (2) improve the gas
exchange; and (3) remove secretions. Patients
with status asthmaticus requiring mechanical ventilation are rare, however, and its use generally
indicates inappropriate therapy, such as sedatives,
or failure of conventional medical therapy. Less
than 1% of the patients in status asthmaticus
require mechanical ventilation. Usually, ventilation is short-term (24–72 hours on the respirator),
thus giving time for medical therapy to become
effective. It is a procedure associated with an
appreciable mortality in patients with status asthmaticus (10–20%), but evidence suggests that
over 80% of high-risk patients in status asthmaticus can be effectively rescued by mechanical
ventilation (Darioli & Parret, 1984; Westerman
et al, 1979; Williams et al, 1992).

No simple criteria can be given as absolute
guidelines for instituting mechanical ventilation
in status asthmaticus, except coma and apnea.
Other criteria for starting ventilation include (1)
rising PaCO₂ and severe hypoxemia; (2) severe
tachycardia (heart rate over 140/min); (3) marked
pulsus paradoxus; (4) onset of arrhythmias; and

(5) declining level of consciousness and exhaustion. These must always be related to the total
clinical picture, however. Mechanical ventilation
is best performed with semi-elective endotracheal
(nasal or oral) intubation and a volume-cycled
respirator. Traditionally, the required tidal volume
is 10 to 12 ml/kg, at a relatively slow rate of 10
to 14 min. The assist mode is preferred; however,
in some patients completely controlled mechanical ventilation may be needed. Expiration should
occupy over 60% of the cycle, which can be
achieved by delivering a relatively fast inspiration.
The high inspiratory flow rates may require a
higher airway inflation pressure limit (i.e., 50–80
cm H₂O). Ventilator management should be individualized, however, taking into account the peak
inflation pressure, mean airway pressure, intrinsic
PEEP, and hemodynamic parameters. Most exhausted patients requiring mechanical ventilation
are placed on the ventilator; pain, restlessness,
and initial discomfort can be controlled with sedatives and analgesics. The patients can usually be
intubated for about 1 to 2 weeks before tracheostomy is contemplated, which is rarely needed.

Pulmonary hyperinflation with associated risk
of barotrauma, hypoxia, and cardiovascular complications is the major factor implicated in the
high mortality in status asthmaticus patients requiring mechanical ventilation (Williams et al,
1992). Mechanical ventilation in status asthmaticus should be used for the correction of hypoxemia with hyperoxic gas mixture without attempting to restore an adequate alveolar ventilation
(Darioli and Perret, 1984).

Nonmassive respiratory acidosis (PaCO₂ ≤80
mm Hg, pH ≥7.15) is reversible and has minor
physiologic effects (Feihl and Perret, 1994). The
pH can be corrected by supplemental bicarbonate
infusion (Menitove and Goldring, 1983). Darioli
and Perret reported improved outcome in ventilated asthmatics when peak inspiratory pressure
(PIP) was kept at or below 50 cm H₂O. Others
have demonstrated that thoracic gas volume at
end inspiration (V_EI) (Fig 23–13), an index of
dynamic hyperinflation, but not the PIP is predictive of ventilator-associated cardiopulmonary
complications in severe airflow limitation from
asthma (Williams et al, 1992). They reasoned that
in severe airway narrowing, pressure measured at
the mouth is not representative of alveolar pressure and overdistention. In their series of mechanically ventilated asthmatic patients, no deaths
were recorded, and ventilator-associated complications such as barotrauma and hypotension were
seen only when V_EI was 1.4 liters or more. Ventilatory parameters, airway pressures, or arterial
blood gas values were similar between mechani-

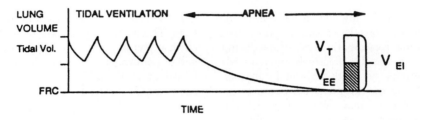

Figure 23–13

Schematic representation of the measurement of VEI during a period of apnea, following steady state tidal ventilation. VEE = end-expiratory lung volume above functional residual capacity at the end of tidal expiration (i.e., the trapped gas volume). VEI = end-inspiratory lung volume. VT = tidal volume. (From Williams TJ, Tuxen DV, Scheinkestel CD, et al: Risk factors for morbidity in mechanically ventilated patients with acute severe asthma. Am Rev Respir Dis 146:607–615, 1992. With permission.)

cally ventilated asthmatics with and without complications. The technique needed to measure V_{EI} usually requires heavy sedation and neuromuscular paralysis, so it is not suitable for all ventilated asthmatics.

Helium-oxygen Mixtures

Mixtures of 60 to 80% helium, plus O_2 have been shown to improve alveolar ventilation and respiratory acidemia while decreasing PIP in ventilated asthmatics with severe airflow limitation and respiratory acidemia (Gluck et al, 1990). The presumed mechanisms by which helium-O_2 mixture exerts its beneficial effect involves elimination of premature ventilator recycling by reducing PIP for a given tidal volume and inspiratory flow rate and enhanced diffusivity for CO_2. The mean duration of time to achieve maximal decline in PIP after introduction of the helium-O_2 mixture was only 2.5 minutes, whereas significant improvement in PaO_2 was seen within 20 minutes of helium-O_2 ventilation. The mean magnitude of reduction in PaO_2 and PIP were 35.7 mm Hg and 32.7 cm H_2O, respectively; these values were both statistically and clinically significant (Fig. 23–14). In one trial of helium-O_2 breathing in nonintubated patients with acute severe asthma, pulsus paradoxus decreased and peak expiratory flow improved after 15 minutes of therapy with a mixture of 80% helium and 20% O_2 (Manthous et al, 1995). Patients presenting with shorter duration of symptoms may receive the greatest benefit from this treatment strategy (Kass and Castriotta, 1995).

Bronchial Lavage

Bronchial lavage for status asthmaticus can be done effectively with flexible fiberoptic bronchos-

copy (Kovnat, 1978; Lang et al, 1991). Lavage can be achieved using local anesthesia in patients refractory to conventional medical therapy or in intubated patients on controlled mechanical ventilation. There is a risk of worsening bronchospasm with this procedure. Lavage can be performed in large volume–controlled fashion (unilateral). Small volumes of fluid can simply be injected through a fiberoptic bronchoscope. To remove mucous plugs, the volume-controlled lavage is probably not necessary. When "plugs" are aspirated, the patient is more likely to have benefitted from the lavage. In status asthmaticus, instillation of 5% N-acetyl-L-cysteine through a fiberoptic bronchoscope has been utilized to alleviate life-threatening bronchial obstruction caused by inspissated mucus (Donaldson et al, 1978). Because N-acetyl-L-cysteine may provoke bronchospasm, it should be given with great caution and in combination with a bronchodilator. There are no controlled studies that demonstrate the clinical benefit of such therapy, however.

The evidence supporting the benefits of bronchial lavage remain largely unproved, and the procedure should be done rarely and with caution. Furthermore, insertion of a bronchoscope into an asthmatic airway increases airway resistance, whereas lavage may transiently produce hypoxemia and worsen $\dot{V}/\dot{Q}$ matching. The major indication of bronchial lavage in status asthmaticus is when major volume loss is radiographically apparent and is unresponsive to conservative measures.

Sedation and Paralysis

The necessity to control breathing pattern during mechanical ventilation of patients with status asthmaticus mandates sedatives and, at times, neuromuscular blockade to produce muscle paralysis. Some investigators advocate routine pharma-

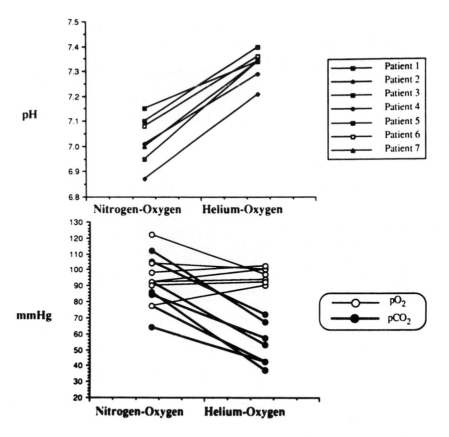

Figure 23–14

Effect of helium-oxygen ventilation on arterial carbon dioxide tension and pH in asthmatics with severe airflow obstruction and respiratory acidemia. (From Gluck EH, Onorato DJ, and Castriotta R: Helium-oxygen mixtures in intubated patients with status asthmaticus and respiratory acidosis. Chest 98:693–698, 1990. With permission.)

cologic paralysis with neuromuscular blocking agents for all such cases. This approach permits the clinician to control ventilator parameters in such a manner to minimize dynamic hyperinflation. Neuromuscular paralysis may also diminish production of CO_2 and O_2 consumption from exhausted respiratory muscles. When this approach is made, it is important to ensure adequate sedation and amnesia for the duration of paralysis. Parenteral benzodiazepines of short to intermediate duration given as a continuous infusion are well suited for this purpose, because the duration of assisted ventilation in status asthmaticus is generally brief. We use lorazepam (half life of 10–20 hours) at doses of 0.5 to 5 mg/hour or midazolam (half life 1–4 hours) infused at 1 to 10 mg/hour when sedating ventilated asthmatics. Benzodiazepines may be given in combination with opiates to produce sedation and eliminate pain.

The enthusiasm for sustained neuromuscular blockade in patients with status asthmaticus requiring mechanical ventilation must be tempered

with the knowledge that prolonged neuromuscular weakness may result from this strategy and complicate eventual weaning from respirator support (Douglass et al, 1992; Griffin et al, 1992). Two distinct patterns of neuromuscular dysfunction have emerged: (1) persistent blockade of the neuromuscular junction; and (2) acute myopathy. The former is often observed in patients with renal failure and is presumably due to drug accumulation or effects of active metabolites, whereas the latter is more prevalent in those receiving concomitant glucocorticosteroids. Prolonged weakness after neuromuscular blockade has been described following administration of pancuronium, vecuronium, or atracurium. At large doses, atracurium may cause release of histamine, and thus it should be administered with caution in status asthmaticus. Regardless of the neuromuscular blocking agent, intermittent discontinuation of the agent to assess the necessity for continuing the agent and monitoring the degree of blockade are prudent. Temporary discontinuation of the neuromuscular blocking drug and the "train-of-four" method to assess the neuromuscular junction are the strategies commonly used (Jones, 1980).

Miscellaneous

Rarely, the derangements of respiratory physiology cannot be adequately temporized with the interventions previously described, and extraordinary rescue methods are warranted. One such strategy involved "general inhaled anesthesia" to relax airways and facilitate ventilation (Roy et al, 1992). Halothane, enflurane, ketamine, and isoflurane have all been administered as bronchodilators in status asthmaticus (Echeverria et al, 1986; O'Rourke et al, 1982; Robertson et al, 1985; Schwartz, 1984). Improved indices of respiratory resistance and reduction in dynamic hyperinflation and intrinsic PEEP were demonstrated after isoflurane in three cases of refractory respiratory failure from status asthmaticus (Maltais et al, 1994). Halothane may produce encephalopathy from bromide poisoning, but in one case was superior to enflurane.

Magnesium sulfate ($MgSO_4$) has also been given in the management of acute asthma (Okayama et al, 1987; Schiermeyer and Finkelstein, 1994). In milder attacks, 0.5 mmol/min $MgSO_4$ infused over 20 minutes improved respiratory resistance and FEV_1 by 71% and 118%, respectively, whereas 2 g of $MgSO_4$ IV over 2 minutes reversed mild, acute respiratory acidemia and impending respiratory collapse. Rapid infusion of $MgSO_4$ may produce hypotension, and thus it should be avoided in hemodynamically unstable patients.

Venovenous partial bypass with extracorporeal membrane oxygenation (ECMO) and filtering of CO_2 has been utilized to reduce hypercarbia in status asthmaticus (Shapiro et al, 1993). This technique permits control of respiratory acidemia and obviates the need to raise minute ventilation and the risk of barotrauma. Because hypercapnia is generally well tolerated, extracorporeal life support is seldom needed in status asthmaticus.

PHARMACOLOGIC PRINCIPLES

Beta-Adrenergic Agents

Beta-adrenergic agonists, in addition to relaxing airway smooth muscle, inhibit release of mast cell mediators and stimulate mucociliary transport (Tattersfield, 1983; Webb-Johnson, 1977a, 1977b). Beta-agonists act directly on β receptors. Work with radioligand studies has helped to clarify their mode of action (Sibley, 1985; Swillens,

1980). The membrane β-receptor complex consists of three components, all of which exist in an active and inactive form: the β-receptor, the transducer (diguanine nucleotide regulatory protein), and the catalyst (adenylate cyclase). Beta-adrenergic receptors have a characteristic structure associated with G-protein-coupled receptors of seven hydrophobic stretches. These are 20 to 25 amino acids linked with intervening hydrophilic sections in the form of an alpha helix, such that the hydrophilic portions are exposed alternately, intracellularly, and extracellularly. An amino (N)-terminal end is exposed extracellularly, whereas a carboxy (C)-terminal portion is situated within the cytoplasm of the cell. To date, three human β-adrenergic receptors have been cloned and termed β_1 to β_3. β_1 receptors are 54% homologous with β_2 receptors. $Beta_3$ receptors have not been identified in human lungs and appear to be important in the regulation of metabolic rate (Barnes, 1995c).

Stimulation of β receptors by an agonist causes a transient sequential change of each from the inactive to the active form. The agonist-receptor complex stimulates the transducer, which when activated stimulates adenylate cyclase. Activation of adenylate cyclase catalyzes the intracellular conversion of adenosine triphosphate (ATP) to cyclic 3,5-AMP. The concentration of cyclic 3,5-AMP is determined by the relative activity of adenylate cyclase and the phosphodiesterase enzymes that metabolize cyclic 3,5-AMP. Intracellular cyclic 3,5-AMP is responsible for activation of specific protein kinases, which in the case of airway smooth muscle reduce phosphorylation of myosin light chain. This causes a reduction in the calcium-dependent coupling of actin and myosin, inducing relaxation of airway smooth muscle.

$Beta_1$ receptors are found predominantly in the heart and β_2 receptors predominantly in the airway smooth muscle. Beta receptors are widely distributed in human airways and alveoli, and their distribution has been studied by autoradiography (Carstairs et al, 1985). The greatest density of β receptors is on airway epithelium, alveolar walls, and submucosal glands, and lesser density is on airway and vascular smooth muscle. The β receptors on airway and vascular smooth muscle and on airway epithelium appear to be entirely β_2 receptors, whereas both β_1 and β_2 receptors are present on submucosal glands and alveolar walls.

Epinephrine is the classic β-agonist, and it is a powerful bronchodilator. Because it acts on α receptors as well as on β receptors, it can have undesirable side effects. For many years it was the primary therapy for acute asthma attacks in children and young adults. Because of its short duration of action and availability of specific β_2-agonists, however, the role of epinephrine (except in children) is now limited. Agonists with high β_2-receptor affinity include (1) β_2-selective catecholamines (isoetharine, metaproterenol, and rimiterol); and (2) noncatecholamine β_2-selective agonists (albuterol [salbutamol], pirbuterol, terbutaline, fenoterol, formoterol, and salmeterol). Isoetharine, metaproterenol, albuterol, pirbuterol, terbutaline, and salmeterol are available in this country and have been most widely used. Isoproterenol is a potent β-agonist with equivalent affinity for β_1 and β_2 receptors. At least *in vitro* isoproterenol is more potent than the selective β_2-agonists in relaxing tracheal smooth muscle.

Figure 23–15 shows the structure of several sympathomimetic amines with relatively shorter duration of action. The relative selectivity of the β_2-agonists is a function of the size of the substituent on the nitrogen atom. Norepinephrine, which is predominantly an α-agonist, has no nitrogen substituent. Epinephrine has a single methyl group and possesses both α- and β-adrenergic activity. An increase in the size of the nitrogen substitution to an isopropyl group abolishes α-adrenergic activity and produces high, equal affinity for β_1 and β_2 receptors. An additional methyl group gives the tertiary butyl compounds (terbutaline and albuterol), which have a higher affinity for β_2 than β_1 receptors. None is totally β_2-receptor-specific.

The refinement of β-adrenergic drugs as bronchodilators has been to create compounds with greater β_2 selectivity and a prolonged duration of action. Isoproterenol has typically the short half life of catecholamines, whereas prolonged duration of activity in the newer compounds has been achieved by altering the catechol nucleus either by changes at the three-hydroxyl group or by moving the four-hydroxyl to the five position on the ring. The elimination half life of terbutaline is about 4 hours, whereas estimates for albuterol have varied from 3 to 6 hours. Two new β_2-agonists, bitolterol and procaterol, have unique features. Bitolterol is an inactive "pro-drug," which after aerosolization undergoes esterase hydrolysis in the bronchial mucosa to the active drug colterol (Kass and Mingo, 1980). The drug not only has greater duration of action but also a lower risk of cardiac side effects. Procaterol is

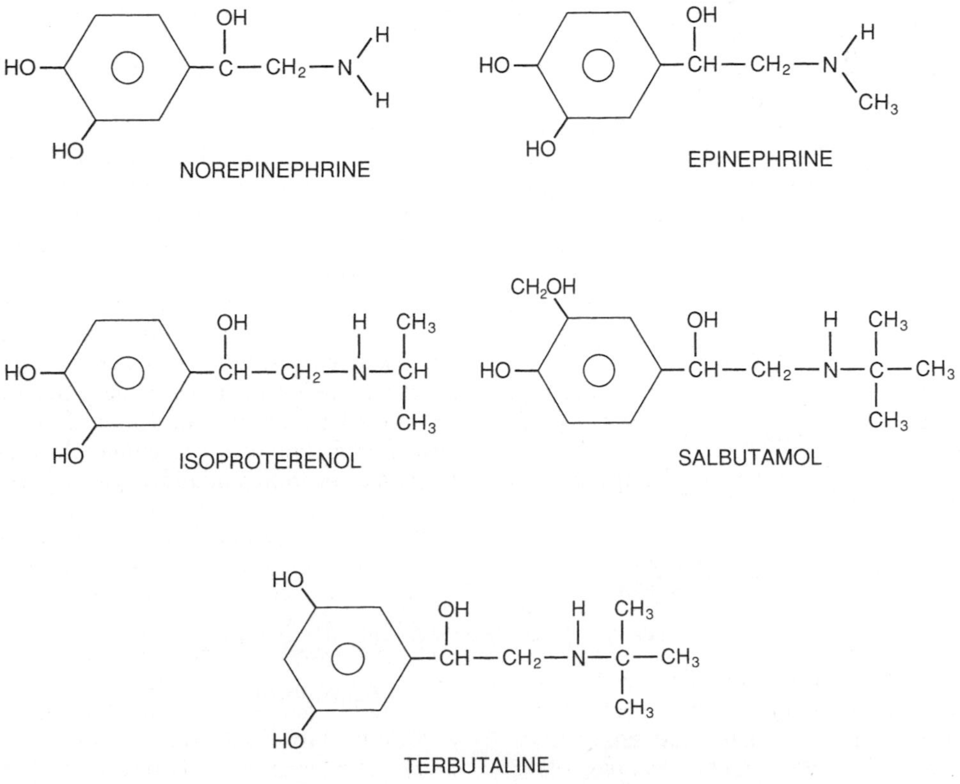

Figure 23–15
Chemical structure of catecholamines.

more potent than isoproterenol. It can be given by inhaled or oral route, and it is a longer acting β_2-agonist (Zanetti et al, 1982). Formoterol and salmeterol are β_2-agonists that produce bronchodilation of relatively longer duration (Fig. 23–16). Compared with shorter action albuterol, both drugs are more lipophilic, which is a feature that has been used to explain, in part, their duration of action. Formoterol and salmeterol also display a higher affinity, selectively, and potency than shorter acting β_2-agonists (Linden et al, 1996). In asthmatics, inhaled salmeterol and formoterol produce bronchorelaxation of slightly slower onset (4 minutes for albuterol versus 10 and 11 minutes for salmeterol and formoterol, respectively) but longer duration than inhaled albuterol (Ullman and Svedmyr, 1988). Because of their slow onset of action, high affinity, rapid downregulation of β_2 receptors (Bhagat et al, 1995), and potential side effects, these agents have limited use in status asthmaticus.

The catecholamines isoproterenol, rimiterol, and isoetharine have a rapid onset of action, producing near maximal bronchodilation within 5 minutes of inhalation. They also have a short duration of action, varying from 1/2 to 2 hours, depending upon dose. Metaproterenol and β_2-agonists such as albuterol, terbutaline, pirbuterol, salmeterol, and fenoterol cause a slower onset of bronchodilation with maximal effect by 15 minutes. The duration of bronchodilation with these agents is considerably longer (i.e., 4–12 hours) and is a function of dose and potency. Overall, there appears to be little difference between albuterol, terbutaline, pirbuterol, and fenoterol. The intensity and duration of action of a particular β-agonist aerosol depend upon the length of time over which optimal concentration of the drug remains at the receptor site, and thus depends upon (1) dosage of inhaled drug; (2) potency; and (3) rate of elimination. The potency, onset of action, and duration of action of various β_2-agonists are summarized in Table 23–7.

β_2-agonists drugs can be given orally, subcutaneously (epinephrine, terbutaline), slowly by IV infusion, or by the aerosol route. The aerosol route, because of its lower cardiac and systemic side effects, is preferable. The presence of mucous plugs in acute asthma may interfere with drug delivery via aerosol route, giving some theoretical advantages for the parenteral route, especially in children and younger adults (Appel et al, 1989). Because acute asthma may be associated with considerable tachycardia, it is advisable to use a β_2-agonist (metaproterenol, isoetharine, or albuterol) initially as an aerosol and to reserve the parenteral route for patients who are unable to use a nebulizer or who fail to respond, or children. Comparison of the nebulized and parenteral modes shows that the nebulized β-agonists produce a similar degree of bronchodilatation with fewer side effects. Of the noncatecholamine β_2-agonists, most of the clinical experience is with albuterol and terbutaline, which have been widely used throughout the world. Cooke and coworkers (1979) gave 0.5% albuterol (5–10 mg) by inhalation for 3 minutes to 276 patients and repeated the dose every 2 to 4 hours. Most patients responded rapidly. Although β-agonists can alter cardiac rhythm, serious arrhythmias are uncommon. Arrhythmias occur mostly in older patients with underlying coronary artery disease (Barnes, 1995c).

Theophylline

Theophylline relaxes bronchial smooth muscle probably by inhibiting phosphodiesterase (PDE). Inhibition of PDE with slow degradation of cyclic AMP results in increased tissue concentration of cyclic AMP. Because both β-agonists and theophylline increase intracellular cyclic AMP, it was anticipated that given together they would have synergistic effects; however, the majority of clinical studies failed to confirm this. Theophylline is a nonselective inhibitor of PDE, and several families of PDE are now recognized. Isoenzymes of PDE may be differentially expressed in distinct

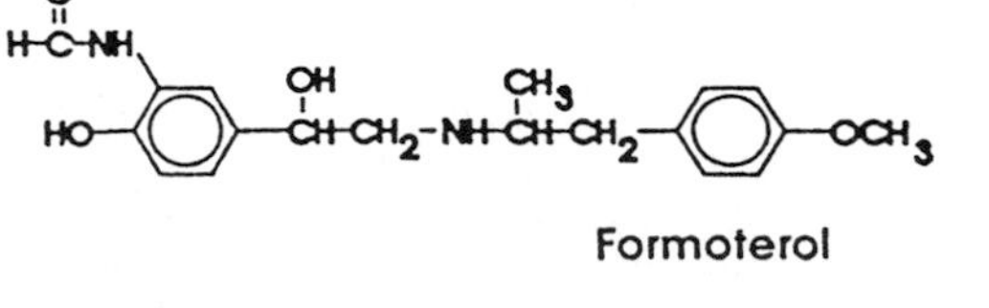

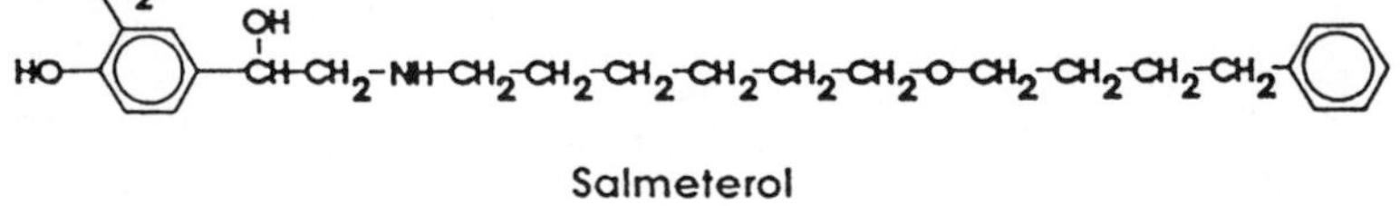

Figure 23–16
Structure of long acting β-symphathomimetics.

Table 23–7
Sympathomimetic Bronchodilators

Drug	β_1-Action	β_2-Action	Onset	Duration of Action
Epinephrine	+ + + +	+	+	Rapid	Short (2–3 hours)
Isoproterenol	+ + + +	+ + + +	Rapid	Short (2–3 hours)
Rimeterol	(+)	+ + + +	Rapid	Short (2–3 hours)
Isoetharine	+ (+)	+ + +	Rapid	Short (2.5–3 hours)
Metaproterenol	+ +	+ + +	Rapid	Medium (4–5 hours)
Albuterol	+ (+)	+ + + +	Rapid	Medium (4–5 hours)
Pirbuterol	+ (+)	+ + + +	Rapid	Medium (4–5 hours)
Terbutaline	+ +	+ + +	Medium	Medium (4–5 hours)
Fenoterol	+ (+)	+ + + +	Medium	Medium (5–6 hours)
Salmeterol	+ (+)	+ + + +	Slow	Longer (12 hours)
Formoterol	+ (+)	+ + + +	Slow	Longer (12 hours)

cell lines, PDE III is relevant to airway smooth muscle relaxation, whereas inflammatory cells appear to be influenced predominantly by PDE IV. At present we lack data to comment on the role of selective PDE subtype inhibition in acute asthma.

Other proposed mechanisms by which theophylline may exert beneficial effects in asthma included adenosine receptor antagonism, interference with inflammatory mediators (PGEs, tumor necrosis factor), effect on T cells, enhanced adrenaline release from the adrenal medulla, and inhibition of calcium mobilization in airway smooth muscle (Banner et al, 1995; Barnes, 1995a; Barnes and Pauwels, 1994; Djukanovic et al, 1995; Rabe et al, 1995). Apart from theophylline's effect on relaxing airway smooth muscle, it

has also been shown to possess anti-inflammatory effects (Table 23–8). Many of the proposed actions of the theophyllines occur at serum levels that are within the therapeutic range for clinical use.

Aminophylline is usually given as a loading dose (IV) over 10 to 20 minutes, followed by a maintenance infusion. Therapeutic blood level range is at a plasma concentration of 10 to 20 mg/l. The initial loading dose can be calculated with reasonable accuracy from the estimated distribution volume. If this is taken as half the body weight, a blood concentration of 10 mg/l requires a dose of 5 mg/kg. The maintenance dose is more difficult to calculate, however, and necessitates estimation of theophylline levels.

Mitenko and Ogilvie (1973) recommended

Table 23–8
Anti-inflammatory Effects of Theophylline

In Vitro	
Mast cells	Decreased mediator release
Macrophages	Decreased release of reactive oxygen species
Monocytes	Decreased cytokine release
Eosinophils	Decreased basic protein release
	Increased/decreased release of reactive oxygen species
T lymphocytes	Decreased proliferation
	Decreased cytokine release
Neutrophils	Decreased release of reactive oxygen species
In Vivo	
Experimental animals	Decreased late response to allergen (guinea pigs)
	Decreased airway responsiveness to allergen and PAF (guinea pigs, sheep)
	Decreased airway inflammation after endotoxin and allergen (guinea pigs, rats)
Asthmatic patients	Inhibition of late response to allergen
	Decreased CD8 cells in peripheral blood
	Decreased T lymphocytes in airways

PAF = platelet activating factor
Adapted from Barnes PJ and Pauwels RA: Theophylline in the management of asthma: Time for reappraisal? Eur Resp J 7:579–591, 1994.

an initial IV loading dose of aminophylline of 5.6 mg/kg, given over 20 minutes, followed by an IV infusion of 0.9 mg/kg per hour. This scheme has been widely employed but has met with some criticism. It is based on studies of nine asthmatics and was aimed at producing a plasma theophylline concentration of about 10 mg/l. Later it became apparent that with such a dose many older and some acutely ill patients reach plasma concentrations over 20 mg/l, which may produce adverse side effects. Older patients should receive a 25% lower infusion rate, and patients with congestive cardiac failure and liver disease a 50% lower rate. If a patient has previously been taking oral theophylline, the loading dose should be reduced.

An estimation of plasma theophylline must be made approximately 20 to 24 hours after starting therapy. The average plasma half life of intravenous theophylline is about 4.5 hours. It is lower in children and smokers and is prolonged in patients with hepatic cirrhosis or congestive cardiac failure. Other drugs may also interfere with plasma levels of theophylline. Erythromycin and cimetidine decrease theophylline clearance, whereas phenobarbitone and diphenylhydantoin increase it. At serum concentration above 20 mg/l, theophylline has the potential for a wide range of side effects. These include nausea, vomiting, headache, diarrhea, irritability, insomnia, cardiac arrhythmias, and seizures. Measurements of serum theophylline levels can avoid this and assure safety. Allergic reactions to aminophylline such as urticaria and exfoliative dermatitis have been reported and are presumably due to the ethylenediamine component.

Corticosteroids

A generally accepted mechanism of action of corticosteroids is via changes in deoxyribonucleic acid (DNA)-dependent, ribonucleic acid (RNA)-mediated protein synthesis. How this action ultimately interferes with the pathogenesis of bronchial asthma is unclear. In vitro studies suggest that corticosteroids inhibit anaphylactic histamine release, increase the sensitivity of β-adrenergic receptors, suppress H_1-histamine receptors, modify cyclic AMP metabolism, give an anti-inflammatory effect, suppress cytokine production, and alter prostaglandin synthesis (Ahmed et al, 1983a; Morris, 1985). They have little effect on immediate hypersensitivity but suppress the late response. Experiments in sheep, however, demonstrated that if sufficient time (3 hours) was allowed between administration and antigen challenge, both early and late responses were attenuated (Delehunt et al, 1984).

In severe asthma, glucocorticosteroids cause clinical improvement and reduction in the percentage of cells expressing IL-4 and IL-5, as well as reduction in the serum concentration of IL-5 (Robinson et al, 1992; 1993b). These studies provide strong evidence in support of anti-inflammatory action of glucocorticosteroids and suggest that, in part, these agents exert their antiasthma effect by reducing synthesis of cytokines. In vitro and in vivo apoptotic death of γδ T cells after glucocorticosteroid therapy in asthma suggests that these may be one of the target cells on which steroids exert their effect (Spinozzi et al, 1995).

Two studies, one conducted by the Medical Research Council (1956) and the other by Pierson and coworkers (1974), form the basis of corticosteroid therapy in acute asthma. These studies demonstrated that, compared with placebo, corticosteroids were effective in status asthmaticus, but they required time to act (Haskell et al, 1983). These observations were confirmed by other studies (Fanta et al, 1983; Harrison et al, 1986).

The rate of onset of corticosteroid action is not clearly known and is dependent upon the disease severity. The earliest response to IV hydrocortisone or methylprednisolone was found approximately 1 to 2 hours after administration, with peak effect at 4 to 6 hours. Refractoriness to bronchodilators in status asthmaticus can be reversed by high doses of parenteral steroids, resulting in both improved FEV_1 and arterial PO_2 (Figs. 23–17 and 23–18) (Ellul-Micallef et al, 1974; Ellul-Micallef and Fenech, 1974, 1975; Pierson et al, 1974).

In a study of patients with acute severe asthma who failed to respond to parenteral aminophylline and inhaled salbutamol, addition of intravenous hydrocortisone was associated with significant bronchodilation and reduction in pulse rate by 6 to 8 hours after the start of corticosteroid treatment (Collins et al, 1975). In chronic stable asthma, however, the restoration of β-adrenergic responsiveness by corticosteroids was identifiable as early as 60 minutes following a single IV dose of 40 mg of prednisolone, and the maximal effect was achieved between 5 to 8 hours (see Fig. 23–17) (Ellul-Micallef and Fenech, 1974; 1975). Corticosteroids appear to act on both large and small airways and improve gas exchange.

In children with acute severe asthma, the addition of glucocorticosteroids to standard bronchodilators resulted in greater improvement in PaO_2 after 24 hours of treatment than bronchodilators alone (see Fig. 23–18) (Pierson et al, 1974). In adult patients, however, improvement of PaO_2 generally lags behind the improvement of airflow.

The optimal dose of corticosteroids is not

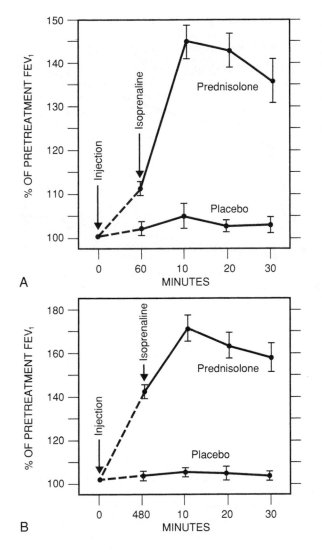

Figure 23–17
Restoration of beta-adrenergic responsiveness in asthma with corticosteroids. Changes in FEV_1 are seen after 200 µg of inhaled isoproterenol at 1 hour (A) and 8 hours (B) after a single intravenous injection of 40 mg prednisolone or placebo. (From Ellul-Micallef R and Fenech FF: Intravenous prednisolone in chronic bronchial asthma. Thorax 30:312–315, 1974. With permission.)

well established. The dose of hydrocortisone recommended has varied from 100 mg to 1000 mg within 24 hours. High plasma cortisol levels can be achieved with IV hydrocortisone at a dose of 4 mg/kg administered every 4 to 6 hours (Collins et al, 1975). This dose is aimed at keeping the serum cortisol level above 1 mg/l, which has been suggested to be necessary for a satisfactory clinical response. Higher doses of corticosteroids have not been found to offer any additional advantage in controlled studies (Tanaka et al, 1982). Corticosteroids can be administered by intermittent injection (every 4–6 hours) or by continuous infusion. Total daily dose of hydrocortisone can be much reduced while maintaining adequate plasma levels, if the treatment is given by a loading dose followed by a continuous infusion rather than by intermittent injections (Collins et al, 1975). To maintain adequate and uniform blood levels after the initial bolus, both aminophylline and steroids can be administered as a continuous infusion. The infusion rate and concentration of the drugs can be adjusted as determined by the individual patient's requirement. The duration of high-dose steroid therapy should be guided by the clinical response and evaluated for each patient. The dose of corticosteroids should be tapered gradually, and rapid withdrawal should be discouraged to avoid relapse, especially in older patients and in those with associated bronchial infection.

Steroid-resistant Asthma

Clinical practice illustrates that asthmatics may have differential responses to glucocorticosteroids, and a subset of asthmatics with steroid resistance have been described (Barnes and Adcock, 1995). Reduced steroid responsiveness may arise by vari-

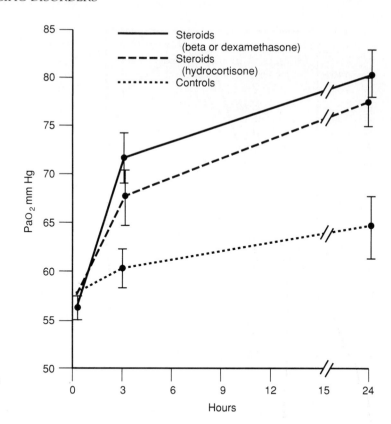

Figure 23–18
Changes in arterial oxygen tension (PaO₂) in children with acute asthma treated by bronchodilators alone (control) or by bronchodilators and corticosteroids. (From Pierson WE, Bier CW, and Kelly VC: A double-blind trial of corticosteroid therapy in status asthmaticus. Pediatrics 54:282–288, 1974. With permission.)

ous mechanisms. *Primary resistance* refers to an intrinsic abnormality in response. *Secondary resistance* denotes reduced responsiveness when a mechanism that increases steroid requirement can be identified (Table 23–9). Primary resistance may be familial or acquired (i.e., multiple myeloma) and is characterized by high serum levels of cortisol in the absence of the clinical stigma of Cushing's syndrome. Hypertension and hyperandrogenism dominate the clinical manifestation of familial glucocorticosteroid resistance. A point

mutation in the steroid-binding domain of the glucocorticosteroid receptor was detected in one family afflicted with this disorder (Hurley et al, 1991).

Various studies have identified glucocorticosteroid resistance in several cell lines of steroid resistant asthmatics *in vitro* (Barnes and Adcock, 1995). Cytokines (e.g., IL-2 to IL-4) liberated in asthmatic inflammation may activate transcription factor, which forms complexes with the glucocorticosteroid receptor, thus decreasing density (Sher et al, 1994). In this manner, asthmatic inflammation *per se* may produce a temporary state of relative glucocorticosteroid resistance. The degree to which this phenomena occurs in acute severe asthma remains speculative. Once inflammation is arrested with higher doses of glucocorticosteroids, however, steroid responsiveness improves.

Table 23–9
Extrinsic Factors That Increase Requirements of Glucocorticosteroids

Pharmacologic agents that enhance hepatic
    metabolism
    Rifampin
    Carbamazepine
    Agents that activate P-450 enzymes
Downregulation of glucocorticosteroid
    reception density
    High doses of β-sympathomimetics
    Viral infection
    Any drug that increases cyclic AMP
    Systemic glucocorticosteroids

Anticholinergic Agents

The role of anticholinergic agents including atropine and ipratropium bromide for the treatment of asthma is controversial, and the drugs are currently not approved by the FDA for its treatment. More than 300 studies have been conducted with ipratropium bromide in patients with asthma, and the majority of these studies were conducted in stable asthmatics. These studies were reviewed by Schleuter (1986), and in most ipratropium bromide was not superior to β-agonists. The peak effect of ipratropium bromide is achieved in about 60 minutes, which is less rapid than that of β-agonists. A combination of β-agonists and ipratropium bromide may have a synergistic effect. The aim of combination therapy is to provide rapid bronchodilation with β$_2$-agonists and prolonged bronchodilatation with anticholinergic agents. There is limited information available on ipratropium bromide in acute asthma. The addition of ipratropium bromide to a β-agonist resulted in greater bronchodilation than did a β-agonist alone (Beck et al, 1985; Reisman et al, 1988). The results are difficult to interpret, however, because of concomitant therapy with steroids and xanthines.

PREVENTION

As mentioned in the epidemiology section, the relapse rate in status asthmaticus is over 50% in the first 2 years. Appropriate measures must therefore be taken upon discharge to prevent future attacks (Strunk, 1989). These include a maintenance therapeutic regimen and patient education for drug compliance and for seeking medical help early (Table 23–10). Prophylaxis can be achieved in many cases by prompt use of oral corticosteroids during the early evolution of an attack. It is always safer to overtreat during the early prodromal stage than to treat a potentially life-threatening episode of status asthmaticus.

In most detailed and well-planned evaluations of deaths in patients with asthma, avoidable factors were identified in the events that led to 82% of deaths (Benatar, 1986). In only 11% of patients deaths were considered unavoidable, either because the fatal attack was so sudden and progressed so rapidly that appropriate medical help could not be summoned in time or because there was delay in the arrival of such help. In only a few cases was death attributed to a failure to respond to adequate treatment. Up to 25% of deaths from asthma occur within 30 minutes of onset of attack, and almost 60% of deaths occur within 8 hours, thus underscoring the importance of early treatment (Benatar, 1986).

CONCLUSIONS

It is difficult to avoid the conclusion that improved patient and physician education about asthma is needed. If such education leads to a wider application of objective assessments of the severity of airflow obstruction, aggressive use of prophylactic therapy, early institution of appropriate therapy, and careful monitoring of response, it can have a major impact on mortality and morbidity from asthma. Available evidence suggests that such measures may be effective, as demonstrated by considerably lower morbidity and mortality rates among patients with access to Edinburgh emergency asthma service (Crompton and Giant, 1979).

Socioeconomic and environmental factors clearly indicate that attacks of near-fatal asthma are disproportionately common in minority groups of inner cities living below the poverty level (Lang and Polansky, 1994). Thus, asthma management is not only a public health problem but also a major economic problem. The efforts to direct public health policy toward improved asthma care must emphasize the necessity of aggressive and cost-effective primary preventive care in ambulatory settings. "Active intervention," including patient and family education, specialist care, regular outpatient visits, and access to an emergency call service, significantly reduce the cost of asthma care and morbidity in high-risk patients, (Doan et al, 1996; Mayo et al, 1990).

Table 23–10
Prevention of Status Asthmaticus

1. Identification of high-risk patients
2. Improve patient and family education
3. Improve education of medical and paramedical staff
4. Establish effective maintenance therapy
5. Early detection of increasing airway obstruction
6. Early use of steroids
7. Special planning for high-risk patients
8. A crisis plan for each high-risk patient

REFERENCES

Abraham WM, Sielczak MW, Ahmed A, et al: α$_4$-Integrins mediate antigen-induced late bronchial responses and prolonged airway hyperresponsiveness in sheep. J Clin Invest 93:776–787, 1994.

Abraham WM: The importance of lipoxygenase products of arachidonic acid in allergen-induced late responses. Am Rev Respir Dis 135:S49–S53, 1987.

Abraham WM and Perruchoud A: Allergen-induced late bronchial responses: Physiologic and pharmacologic studies in the allergic sheep. In Kay AB (ed): Asthma Clinical Pharmacology and Therapeutic Progress. London, Blackwell Scientific Publications, 1986, pp 11–22.

Abraham WM, Stevenson J, and Garrido R: A possible role for PAF in allergen-induced late responses: Modification by a selective antagonist. J Appl Physiol 66:2351–2375, 1989.

Ackerman V, Carip S, Bellini A, et al: Constitutive expression of endothelin in bronchial epithelial cells of patients with symptomatic and asymptomatic asthma and modulation by histamine and interleukin-1. J Allergy Clin Immunol 96:618–627, 1995.

Ahmed T, D'Brot J, Abraham WM, et al: Heterogeneity of allergic airway responses in sheep: Differences in signal transduction? Am J Respir Crit Care Med, 154:843–849, 1996.

Ahmed T, Eyre P, Januszkiewicz AJ, et al: The role of H_1 and H_2 receptors in airway reactions to histamine in conscious sheep. J Appl Physiol 49:826–833, 1980.

Ahmed T, Greenblatt DW, Birch S, et al: Abnormal mucociliary transport in allergic patients with antigen-induced bronchospasm: Role of SRS-A. Am Rev Respir Dis 124:110–114, 1981.

Ahmed T and King M: Suppression of pulmonary and systemic vascular histamine H_2-receptors in allergic sheep. J Appl Physiol 60:791–797, 1986.

Ahmed T, King MM, and Krainson JP: Modification of airway histamine receptor function with methylprednisolone succinate. J Allergy Clin Immunol 71:224–229, 1983a.

Ahmed T, Krainson J, and Yerger L: Functional depression of H_2-histamine receptors in sheep with experimental allergic asthma. J Allergy Clin Immunol 72:310–320, 1983b.

Ahmed T and Marchette B: Hypoxia enhances non-specific bronchial reactivity. Am Rev Respir Dis 132:839–844, 1985.

Ahmed T, Mirbahar KB, Oliver W, et al: Characterization of H_1 and H_2 receptor function in pulmonary and systemic circulations of sheep. J Appl Physiol 53:175–184, 1982.

Ahmed T and Oliver W Jr: Does slow reacting substance of anaphylaxis mediate hypoxic pulmonary vasoconstriction? Am Rev Respir Dis 127:566–571, 1983c.

Ahmed T, Syriste T, Mendelssohn R, et al: Heparin prevents antigen-induced airway hyperresponsiveness: Interference with IP_3-mediated mast cell degranulation? J Appl Physiol 76:893–901, 1994.

Ahonen A: Analysis of the changes in ECG during status asthmaticus. Respiration 37:85–90, 1979.

Allegra L, Abraham WM, Chapman GA, et al: Duration of mucociliary dysfunction following antigen challenge in allergic sheep. J Appl Physiol 55:726–730, 1983.

Allegra L, Basi F, Centanni S, et al: Acute exacerbations of asthma in adults: Role of Chlamydia pneumoniae infection. Eur Respir J 7:2165–2168, 1994.

American Thoracic Society Committee on Diagnostic Standards: Definitions and classifications of chronic bronchitis, asthma, and pulmonary emphysema. Am Rev Respir Dis 85:762–766, 1962.

Anderson HR: Increase in hospital admissions for childhood asthma: Trends in referral, severity, and readmissions from 1970–1985 in a health region of the United Kingdom. Thorax 44:614–619, 1989.

Appel D, Karpel JP, and Sherman M: Epinephrine improves expiratory flow rates in patients with asthma who do not respond to inhaled metaproterenol sulfate. J Allergy Clin Immunol 84:90–98, 1989.

Arm JP and Lee TH: Sulphidopeptide leukotrienes in asthma. Clin Sci 84:501–510, 1993.

Aronow DB: Severity-of-illness measurement: applications in quality assurance and utilization review. Med Care 45:339–366, 1988.

Austen KR: A review of immunological, biochemical, and pharmacological factors in the release of chemical mediators from human lung. In Austen KF, and Lichtenstein LM (eds): Asthma—Physiology, Immunopharmacology, and Treatment. New York, Academic Press, 1973, pp 109–122.

Ayala LE and Ahmed T: Is there loss of a protective muscarinic receptor mechanism in asthma? Chest, 96:1285–1291, 1989.

Azzawi M, Bradley B, Jeffery PK, et al: Identification of activated T-lymphocytes and eosinophils in bronchial biopsies in stable chronic asthma. Am Rev Respir Dis 142:1407–1413, 1990.

Azzawi M, Jeffery PK, Frew AJ, et al: Activated eosinophils in bronchi obtained at post-mortem from asthma deaths. J Clin Exp Allergy 19:118–123, 1989.

Baker JW, Yerger S, and Segar WE: Elevated plasma antidiuretic hormone levels in status asthmaticus. Mayo Clin Proc 51:31–34, 1976.

Banner KH, Marchini F, Buschi A, et al: The effect of selective phosphodiesterase inhibitors in comparison with other anti-asthma drugs on allergen-induced eosinophilia in guinea-pig airways. Pulm Pharmacol 8:37–42, 1995.

Barnes PJ: Airway neuropeptides. In Barnes PJ, Rodger IW, and Thomson NC (eds): Asthma: Basic Mechanism and Clinical Management. London, Academic Press, 1988, pp 395–414.

Barnes PJ: Histamine receptors in airways. Agents Actions 33[Suppl]:103–122, 1991.

Barnes PJ: Blunted perception and death from asthma. Editorial. N Engl J Med 330:1383–1384, 1994a.

Barnes PJ: Cytokines as mediator of chronic asthma. Am J Resp Crit Care Med 150:42–49, 1994b.

Barnes PJ: Endothelins and pulmonary disease. J Appl Physiol 77:1051–1059, 1994c.

Barnes PJ: Cyclic nucleotides and phosphodiesterases and airway function. Eur Respir J 8:457–462, 1995a.

Barnes PJ: Inflammatory mediators and neural mechanisms: In Severe Asthma: Pathogenesis and Clinical Management. Szefler SJ, and Leung DYM (eds): Marcel Dekker, 1995b, pp 129–163.

Barnes PJ: State of the art. Beta-adrenergic receptors and their regulation. Am J Respir Crit Care Med 152:838–860, 1995c.

Barnes PJ and Adcock IM: Steroid resistance in asthma. Q J Med 88:455–468, 1995.

Barnes PJ, Baraniuk J, and Belvisi MG: Neuropeptides in the respiratory tract. Am Rev Respir Dis 144:1187–1198; 144:1391–1399, 1991.

Barnes PJ and Belvisi MG: Nitric oxide and lung disease. Thorax 48:1034–1043, 1993.

Barnes PJ, Grandordy BM, Page CP, et al: The effect of platelet activating factor on pulmonary beta-adrenoceptors. Br J Pharmacol 90:709–715, 1987.

Barnes PJ, Greening AP, and Crompton GK: Glucocorticosteroid resistance in asthma. Am J Respir Crit Care Med 152:S125–S142, 1995.

Barnes PJ and Pauwels RA: Theophylline in the management of asthma: Time for reappraisal? Eur Resp J 7:579–591, 1994.

Bates DV, and Baker-Anderson M: Asthma mortality and morbidity in Canada. J Allergy Clin Immunol 80[Suppl]:S395–397, 1987.

Beasley R, Pearce N, Crane J, et al: Withdrawal of Fenoterol and the end of New Zealand asthma mortality epidemic. Int Arch Allergy Immunol 107:325–327, 1995.

Beck R, Robertson C, Galdes-Sebaldt M, et al: Combined salbutamol and ipratropium bromide by inhalation on the treatment of severe acute asthma. J Pediatr 107:605–610, 1985.

Beer DJ, Osband ME, McCaffrey RP, et al: Abnormal histamine induced suppressor-cell function in atopic subjects. N Engl J Med 306:454–458, 1982.

Benatar SR: Fatal asthma. N Engl J Med 314:423–429, 1986.

Bentley AM, Durham SR, Robinson DS, et al: Expression of the endothelial and leucocyte adhesion molecules ICAM-1, E-selectin and VCAM-1 in the bronchial mucosa in steady state and allergen-induced asthma. J Allergy Clin Immunol 92:857–865, 1993.

Bentley AM, Menz G, Storz C, et al: Identification of T-lymphocytes, macrophages and activated eosinophils in bronchial mucosa in intrinsic asthma: Relationship to symptoms and bronchial responsiveness. Am Rev Respir Dis 146:500–506, 1992.

Benveniste J: Platelet activating factor, a new mediator of anaphylaxis and immune complex deposition from rabbit and human basophils. Nature 249:581–582, 1974.

Berridge MI: Inositol triphosphate and diacylglycerol: Two interacting second messengers. Ann Rev Biochem 56:159–193, 1987.

Bhagat R, Kalra S, Swystun VA, et al: Rapid onset of tolerance to the bronchoprotective effect of salmeterol. Chest 108:1235–1239, 1995.

Bochner BS, Luscinskas FW, Gimbrone MAJ, et al: Adhesion of human basophils, eosinophils and neutrophils to IL-1 activated human vascular endothelial cells: Contribution of endothelial cell adhesion molecules. J Exp Med 173:1553–1557, 1991.

Bouhuys A: Pharmacological basis for refractoriness. In Weiss EB (ed): Status Asthmaticus. Baltimore, University Park Press, 1978, pp 49–57.

Boulet LP, Deschesnes F, Turcotte H, et al: Near fatal asthma: Clinical and physiologic features, perception of bronchoconstriction and psychologic profile. J Allergy Clin Immunol 88:838–846, 1991.

Boushey H, Holtzman A, Sheller JR, et al: Bronchial hyperreactivity. Am Rev Respir Dis 121:389–413, 1980.

Bousquet J, Chanez P, Lacoste JY, et al: Eosinophilic inflammation in asthma. N Engl J Med 323:1033–1039, 1990.

Bousquet J, Hatton F, Godard P, et al: Asthma mortality in France. J Allergy Clin Immunol 80 [Suppl]:389–394, 1987.

Bradding P, Feather IH, Howarth PH, et al: Interleukin-4 is localized to and released by human mast cells. J Exp Med 176:1381–1386, 1992.

Bradding P, Roberts JA, Britten KM, et al: Interleukin-4, IL-5, IL-6, and TNF-α in normal and asthmatic airways: Evidence for the human mast cell as a source of these cytokines. Am J Respir Cell Mol Biol 10:471–480, 1994.

Brewster CEP, Howarth PH, Djukanovic R, et al: Myofibroblasts and subepithelial fibrosis in bronchial asthma. Am J Respir Cell Mol Biol 3:507–511, 1990.

Brodie D, Paine MM, and Feinstein GS: Eosinophils express interleukin-5 and granulocyte-macrophage colony stimulating factor mRNA at sites of allergic inflammation in asthmatics. J Clin Invest 90:1414–1424, 1992.

Brown PA, Crompton GK, and Greening AP: Pro-inflammatory cytokines in acute asthma. Lancet 338:590–593, 1991.

Brugman SM and Larson GL: Childhood asthma: wheezing in infants and small children. Semin Respir Crit Care Med 15:147–160, 1994.

Buist AS and Vollmer WM: Reflections on the rise in asthma morbidity and mortality. JAMA 264:1719–1720, 1990.

Buist AS and Vollmer WM: Preventing deaths from asthma (editorial). N Engl J Med 331:1584–1585, 1994.

Buist AS: Is asthma mortality increasing? (editorial). Chest 93:449–450, 1988.

Burgess C, Pearce N, Thiruchelvam R, et al: Prescribed drug therapy and near fatal asthma attacks (Fenoterol). Eur Respir J 7:498–503, 1994.

Burney PG: Asthma mortality in England and Wales: Evidence for a further increase, 1974–1984. Lancet 2:323–326, 1986.

Burrows B, Hasan GM, Barbee RA, et al: Epidemiologic observations on eosinophilia and its relation to respiratory disorders. Am Rev Respir Dis 122:709–719, 1980.

Burrows B, Martinez FD, Halonen M, et al:

Association of asthma with serum IgE levels and skin-test reactivity to allergens. N Engl J Med 320:271–277, 1989.

Busey JF, Fenger EP, Hepper NG, et al: Management of status asthmaticus: A statement by the committee of therapy. Am Rev Respir Dis 97:735–736, 1968.

Busse WW, Cooper W, Warhauser DM, et al: Impairment of isoproterenol, H$_2$-histamine and PGE$_1$ responses of human granulocytes after incubation in vitro with live influenza vaccines. Am Rev Respir Dis 119:561–569, 1979.

Call RS, Smith TF, Morrise E, et al: Risk factors for asthma in inner city children. J Pediatr 121:862–866, 1992.

Campbell DA, McLennon G, Coates JR, et al: A comparison of asthma deaths and near fatal asthma attacks in South Australia. Eur Resp J 7:490–497, 1994.

Cardell LO, Uddman R, and Edvinsson L: Low plasma concentrations of VIP and elevated levels of other neuropeptides during exacerbations of asthma. Eur Respir J 7:2169–2173, 1994.

Carmen PG and Landall LI: Increased paediatric admission with asthma in Western Australia: A problem of diagnosis? Med J Aust 152:23–26, 1990.

Carr W, Zeitel L, and Weiss K: Variations in asthma hospitalizations and deaths in New York City. Am J Public Health 82:59–65, 1992.

Carroll N, Elliott J, Morton A, et al: The structure of large and small airways in nonfatal and fatal asthma. Am Rev Respir Dis 147:405–410, 1993.

Carstairs JR, Nionmo AJ, and Barnes PJ: Autoradiographic visualization of beta-adrenoceptor subtypes in human lung. Am Rev Respir Dis 132:541–547, 1985.

Centor RM, Yarbrough B, and Wood JP: Inability to predict relapse in acute asthma. N Engl J Med 310:577–580, 1984.

Cheung D, Dick EC, Timmers MC, et al: Rhinovirus inhalation causes long-lasting excessive airway narrowing in response to methacholine in asthmatic subjects in vivo. Am J Respir Crit Care Med 152:1490–1496, 1995.

Chilmonczyk BA, Salmun LM, Megathlin KN, et al: Association between exposure to environmental tobacco smoke and exacerbation of asthma in children. N Engl J Med 328:1665–1669, 1993.

Chung KF: Role of inflammation in the hyperreactivity of the airways in asthma. Thorax 41:657–662, 1986.

Church MK, Cushley MJ, and Holgate ST: Adenosine, a positive modulation of asthmatic response. In Barnes PJ, Rodger IW, and Thomson NC (eds): Asthma: Basic Mechanisms and Clinical Management. London, Academic Press, 1988, pp 273–282.

Ciba Foundation Guest Symposium: Terminology definitions and classification of chronic pulmonary emphysema and related conditions. Thorax 14:286, 1959.

Clark JM, Abraham WM, Fishman CE, et al: Tryptase

inhibitors block allergen-induced airway and inflammatory responses in allergic sheep. Am J Respir Crit Care Med 152:2076–2083, 1995.

Cohn MA, Baier H, and Wanner A: Failure of hypoxic pulmonary vasoconstriction in the canine asthma model. Effect of prostaglandin inhibitors. J Clin Invest 61:1463–1470, 1978.

Collins JV, Clark TJH, Brown D, et al: The use of corticosteroids in the treatment of acute asthma. Q J Med 44:259–273, 1975.

Connolly CK: Adverse reaction to ipratropium bromide. Br Med J 5:934–935, 1982.

Connolly MJ, Crawley JJ, Charan NB, et al: Reduced subjective awareness of bronchoconstriction provoked by methacholine in elderly asthmatics and normal subjects as measured on a simple awareness scale. Thorax 47:410–413, 1992.

Conolly ME and Greenacre JK. The lymphocyte beta adrenoreceptor in normal subjects and patients with bronchial asthma: The effects of different forms of treatment on receptor function. J Clin Invest 58:1307–1316, 1976.

Cooke NJ, Crompton GK, and Grant IW: Observations on the management of acute bronchial asthma. Br J Dis Chest 73:157–163, 1979.

Corbridge TC and Hall JB: The assessment and management of adults with status asthmaticus. Am J Respir Crit Care Med 151:1296–1316, 1995.

Corrigan CJ, Haczku A, Gemou-Engesaeth V, et al: CD4 T-lymphocytes activation in asthma is accompanied by increased concentrations of interleukin-5: Effect of glucocorticoid therapy. Am Rev Respir Dis 147:540–547, 1993.

Corrigan CJ, Hartnell A, and Kay AB: T-lymphocytes in acute severe asthma. Lancet 1:1129–1131, 1988.

Corrigan CJ and Kay AB: CD4 T-lymphocyte activation in acute severe asthma: Relationship to disease severity and atopic status. Am Rev Respir Dis 141:970–977, 1990.

Coultas DB, Gong H Jr, Grad R, et al: Respiratory disease in minorities of the United States. Am J Respir Crit Care Med 149[Suppl]:S93–S131, 1994.

Crane J, Pearce NE, Flatt A, et al: Prescribed Fenoterol and death from asthma in New Zealand, 1981–1983: Case control study. Lancet 1:917–922, 1989.

Crompton GK and Grant IW: Edinburgh emergency asthma admission service. Br Med J 4:680–682, 1975.

Csete M, Abraham WM, and Wanner A: Vasomotion influences airflow in peripheral airways. Am Rev Respir Dis 141:1409–1413, 1990.

Csete M, Chediak A, Abraham W, et al: Airway blood flow modifies allergic smooth muscle contraction. Am Rev Respir Dis 84:231–243, 1991.

Cushley MJ and Holgate ST: Adenosine induced bronchoconstriction in asthma: Role of mast cell mediator release. J Allergy Clin Immunol 75:272–278, 1985.

Cuss FM, Dixon CM, and Barnes PJ: Effect of inhaled platelet activating factor on pulmonary function and bronchial responsiveness in man. Lancet 2:189–192, 1986.

D'Brot J and Ahmed T: Hypoxia-induced enhancement of non-specific bronchial reactivity: Role of leukotrienes. J Appl Physiol 65:194–199, 1988.

Dahl R: Comparative studies of inhaled salmeterol with other bronchodilators. Eur Resp Rev 5:138–141, 1995.

Dahl R, Venge P, and Fredens K: Eospinophils. In Barnes PJ, Rodger IW, and Thomson NC (eds): Asthma: Basic Mechanism and Clinical Management. London, Academic Press, 1988, pp 283–304.

Darioli R and Perret C: Mechanical controlled hypoventilation in status asthmaticus. Am Rev Respir Dis 129:385–387, 1984.

Del Prete G, Maggi E, Parronchi P, et al: IL-4 is an essential cofactor for the IgE-synthesis induced in vitro by human T-cell clones and their supernatants. J Immunol 140:4193–4198, 1988.

Delehunt JC, Yerger L, Ahmed T, and Abraham WM: Inhibition of antigen-induced bronchoconstriction by methylprednisolone succinate. J Allergy Clin Immunol 73:479–483, 1984.

Dinh-Xuan AT, Chaussain M, Regnard J, et al: Pretreatment with an inhaled α_1-adrenergic agonist, methoxamine, reduces exercise-induced asthma. Eur Respir J 2:409–414, 1989.

Diot P, Morra L, and Smaldone GC: Albuterol delivery in a model of mechanical ventilation. Comparison of metered-dose inhaler and nebulizer efficiency. Am J Respir Crit Care Med 152:1391–1394, 1995.

Djukanovic R, Finnerty JP, Lee C, et al: The effects of theophylline on mucosal inflammation in asthmatic airways: Biopsy results. Eur Respir J 8:831–833, 1995.

Doan T, Grammer LC, Yarnold PR, et al: An intervention program to reduce the hospitalization cost of asthmatic patients requiring intubation. Ann Allergy Asthma Immunol 76:513–518, 1996.

Dooper MWSM, Timmermans A, Weersink EJM, et al: Defect in potentiation of adenylyl cyclase correlates with bronchial hyperreactivity. J Allergy Clin Immunol 96:628–634, 1995.

Douglass JA, Tuxen DV, Horne M, et al: Myopathy in severe asthma. Am Rev Respir Dis 146:517–519, 1992.

Dunhill MS: The pathology of asthma, with special reference to changes in bronchial mucosa. J Clin Pathol 13:27–33, 1960.

Dunhill MS: Pathology of asthma. In Porter R, and Birch J (eds): Identification of asthma. Proceedings of study group No. 38, Ciba Foundation Symposium. Edinburgh, Churchill Livingstone, 1971.

Dunhill MS, Massarella GR, and Anderson JA: A comparison of the quantitative anatomy of the bronchi in normal subjects, in status asthmaticus, in chronic bronchitis, and in emphysema. Thorax 24:176–179, 1969.

Dvorak AM, Dvorak HF, and Galli S: Ultrastructural criteria for identification of mast cells and basophils in humans, guinea pigs, and mice. Am Rev Respir Dis 128:S49–52, 1983.

Echeverria M, Gelb AW, Wexler HR, et al: Enflurane and halothane in status asthmaticus. Chest 89:152–154, 1986.

Edmunds AT and Godfrey S: Cardiovascular response during severe acute asthma and its treatment in children. Thorax 36:534–540, 1981.

Efthimiou J, Hassan AB, Ormerod O, et al: Reversible T-wave abnormality in severe acute asthma: An electrocardiographic sign of severity. Respir Med 85:195–201, 1991.

Ellul-Micallef R, Borthwick RC, and McHardy GJR: The time course of response to prednisolone in chronic bronchial asthma. Clin Sci 47:105–117, 1974.

Ellul-Micallef R and Fenech FF: Intravenous prednisolone in chronic bronchial asthma. Thorax 30:312–315, 1974.

Ellul-Micallef R and Fenech FF: Effect of intravenous prednisolone in asthmatics with diminished adrenergic responsiveness. Lancet 2:1269–1271, 1975.

Engel P, Huguet J, Sanosa J, et al: T-cell subsets in allergic respiratory disease using monoclonal antibodies. Ann Allergy 53:337–340, 1984.

Erzen D, Roos LL, Manfreda J, et al: Changes in asthma severity in Manitoba. Chest 108:16–23, 1995.

Evans R: Asthma among minority children a growing problem. Chest 101[Suppl]:368S–371S, 1992.

Evans R, Mullaly DI, Wilson RW, et al: National trends in the morbidity and mortality of asthma in the U.S. Prevalence, hospitalization and death from asthma over two decades: 1965–1984. Chest 91[Suppl]:65S–74S, 1987.

Eyre P: Pulmonary histamine H_1 and H_2 receptor studies. In Lichtenstein LM, and Austen, KF (eds): Asthma: Physiology, immunopharmacology and treatment. New York, Academic Press, 1977, pp 169–180.

Fanta CH, Rossing TH, and McFadden ER: Glucocorticoids in acute asthma: A critical control trial. Am J Med 74:845–851, 1983.

Fedan JS, Hay DWP, Farmer SG, et al: Epithelial cells: Modulation of airway smooth muscle reactivity. In Barnes PJ, Rodger IW, and Thomson NC (eds): Asthma: Basic mechanisms and clinical management. London, Academic Press, 1988, pp 143–159.

Feihl F and Perret C: Permissive hypercapnia. Am J Respir Crit Care Med 150:1722–1737, 1994.

Fels AO, Pawlowski NA, Cramer EB, et al: Human alveolar macrophages produce LTB_4. Proc Natl Acad Sci USA 79:7866–7870, 1982.

Fischl MA, Pitchenik A, and Gardner LB: An index

predicting relapse and need for hospitalization in patients with acute bronchial asthma. N Engl J Med 305:783–789, 1981.

Fitzgerald JM and Hargreave FE: The assessment and management of acute life threatening asthma. Chest 95:888–894, 1989.

Flavahan NA, Aarhus L, Rimele TJ, et al: Respiratory epithelium inhibits bronchial smooth muscle tone. J Appl Physiol 58:834–838, 1985.

Fleming DM and Crombie DL: Prevalence of asthma and hayfever in England and Wales. Br Med J 294:279–283, 1987.

Ford-Hutchinson AW: The neutrophil and lymphocytes. In Barnes PJ, Rodger IW, and Thomson NC (eds): Asthma: Basic Mechanisms and Clinical Management. London, Academic Press, 1988, pp 131–142.

Franklin W: Treatment of severe asthma. N Engl J Med 290:1469–1472, 1974.

Fuller RW and Barnes PJ: Kinins. In Barnes PJ, Rodger IW, and Thomson NC (eds): Asthma: Basic Mechanism and Clinical Management. London, Academic Press, 1988, pp 259–272.

Galli SJ and Lichtenstein LM: Biology of mast cells and basophils. In Middleton E, Reed CE, Ellis, EF, et al (eds): Allergy: Principles and Practices. St. Louis, CV Mosby, 1988, pp 106–134.

Gelb AF, Lyons HA, Fairshter RD, et al: P. pulmonale in status asthmaticus. J Allergy Clin Immunol 64:18–22, 1979.

Georg J: The treatment of status asthmaticus. Allergy 36:219–232, 1981.

Gerblich AA, Cambell AE, and Schuyler MR: Changes in T-lymphocyte, sub-population after antigenic bronchial provocation in asthmatics. N Engl J Med 310:1349–1352, 1984.

Gergen PJ, Mullally DI, and Evans R: National survey of prevalence of asthma among children in the United States. Paediatrics 81:1–7, 1988.

Gergen PJ and Weiss KB: Changing patterns of asthma hospitalization among children 1979–1987. JAMA 264:1688–1692, 1990.

Gern JE and Busse WW: The effects of rhinovirus infections on allergic airway responses. Am J Respir Crit Care Med 152[Suppl]:S40–S45, 1995.

Gerstman BB, Bosco LA, and Tonita DK: Trends in the prevalence of asthma hospitalization in the 5 to 14 year old Michigan Medicaid population 1980–1986. J Allergy Clin Immunol 91:838–843, 1993.

Gibson GJ: Perception, personality and respiratory control in life-threatening asthma. Thorax 50[Suppl]:S2–S4, 1995.

Gluck EH, Onorato DJ, and Castriotta R: Helium-oxygen mixtures in intubated patients with status asthmaticus and respiratory acidosis. Chest 98:693–698, 1990.

Glynn AN and Michaels L: Bronchial biopsy in chronic bronchitis and asthma. Thorax 15:142–149, 1960.

Gonzalez H and Ahmed T: Suppression of gastric H_2-receptor mediated function in patients with bronchial asthma and ragweed allergy. Chest 89:491–496, 1986.

Gordon JR, Burd PR, and Galli SJ: Mast cells as a source of multifunctional cytokines. Immunol Today 11:458–467, 1990.

Gosset P, Tsicopoulos A, Wallaert B, et al: Increased secretion of tumor necrosis factor α, and interleukin-6 by alveolar macrophages consecutive to the development of the late asthmatic reaction. J Allergy Clin Immunol 88:561–571, 1991.

Gottlieb DJ, Beiser AS, and O'Connor GT: Poverty, race, and medication use are correlation of asthma hospitalization rates: A small area analysis in Boston. Chest 108:28–35, 1995.

Grainger J, Woodman K, Pearce N, et al: Prescribed Fenoterol and death from asthma in New Zealand, 1981–1987. A further case-control study. Thorax 46:105–111, 1991.

Grandordy BM and Barnes PJ: Phosphoinositide turnover. Am Rev Respir Dis 136[Suppl]:S17–S20, 1987.

Graves EJ: Detailed diagnosis and procedures, National Hospital Discharge Survey, 1990. Vital Health Stat 13:16, 1992.

Grieco MH and Pierson RN: Mechanism of bronchoconstriction due to beta-adrenergic blockade. J Allergy Clin Immunol 48:143–152, 1971.

Griffin D, Fairman N, Coursin D, et al: Acute myopathy during treatment of status asthmaticus with corticosteroids and steroidal muscle relaxants. Chest 102:510–514, 1992.

Guinot P, Brambilla C, Duchier J, et al: Effect on BN 52063, a specific PAF-acether antagonist, on bronchial provocation test to allergens in asthmatic patients. A preliminary study. Prostaglandins 34:723–731, 1987.

Gundel RH, Wegner CD, Torcellini CA, et al: Endothelial leukocyte adhesion molecule-1 mediates antigen-induced acute airway inflammation and late-phase airway obstruction in monkeys. J Clin Invest 88:1407–1411, 1991.

Gunstone RF: Right heart pressures on bronchial asthma. Thorax 26:39–45, 1971.

Haahtela T, Lindholm H, Björksten F, et al: Prevalence of asthma in Finnish young men. Br Med J 301:266–268, 1990.

Hahn DL, Dodge RW, Golubjatnikov R: Association of Chlamydia pneumoniae (strain TWAR) infection with wheezing, asthmatic bronchitis, and adult-onset asthma. JAMA 266:225–230, 1991.

Håkansson L, Björnsson E, Janson C, et al: Increased adhesion to vascular cell adhesion molecule-1 and intercellular adhesion molecule-1 of eosinophils from patients with asthma. J Allergy Clin Immunol 96:941–950, 1995.

Hamid Q, Azzawi M, Ying S, et al: Expression of mRNA for interleukin-5 in mucosal bronchial biopsies from asthma. J Clin Invest 87:1541–1546, 1991.

Harrison BDW, Stokes TC, Hart GJ, et al: Need for

intravenous hydrocortisone in addition to oral prednisolone in patients admitted to hospital with severe asthma without ventilatory failure. Lancet 1:181–184, 1986.

Haskell RJ, Wong BM, and Hansen JE: A double-blind randomized clinical trial of methylprednisolone in status asthmaticus. Arch Intern Med 143:1324–1327, 1983.

Havill JH, Walker L, and Sceats JE: Three hundred admissions to the Waikato Hospital intensive therapy unit: Survival cost, and quality of life after two years. N Z Med J 102:179–181, 1989.

Heard BE and Hossain S: Hyperplasia of bronchial muscle in asthma. J Pathol 110:319–331, 1973.

Heard BE, Nunn AJ, and Kay AB: Mast cells in human lungs. J Pathol 157:59–63, 1989.

Helander E, Lindell SE, Soderholm B, et al: Observations on the pulmonary circulation during induced bronchial asthma. Acta Allergologica 17:112–129, 1962.

Henderson WR, Shelhamer JH, Reingold DB, et al: Alpha-adrenergic hyper-responsiveness in asthma. Analysis of vascular and pupillary responses. N Engl J Med 300:547–642, 1979.

Heurich AD, Huang CT, and Lyons HA: Status Asthmaticus: Definition, criteria for diagnosis, and clinical causes. In Weiss EB (ed): Status Asthmaticus. Baltimore, University Park Press, 1978, pp 3–12.

Hidling AC: The relationship of ciliary insufficiency to death from asthma and other respiratory diseases. Ann Otol Rhinol Laryngol 52:5–19, 1943.

Hoang PT, Pourriat JL, Rathat C, et al: Status asthmaticus. Mechanical ventilation in association with sodium gamma hydroxy-butyrate and pancuronium bromide. Anesth Analg (Paris) 38:43–46, 1981.

Hogg JC and Eggleston PA: Is asthma an epithelial disease? Am Rev Respir Dis 129:207–208, 1984.

Houston JC, DeNevasquez S, and Trounce JR: Clinical and pathological study of fatal cases of status asthmaticus. Thorax 8:207–213, 1953.

Hui KKP, Conolly ME, Tashkin DP: Reversal of human lymphocyte B-adrenoreceptor desensitization by glucocorticoids. Clin Pharmacol Ther 32:566–571, 1987.

Hurley DM, Accili D, Stratakis CA, et al: Point mutation causing a single amino acid substitution in the hormone binding domain of the glucocorticosteroid receptor in familial glucocorticosteroid resistance. J Clin Invest 87:680–686, 1991.

Hutchison AA and Olinsky A: Hypoxic and hypercapnic response in asthmatic subjects with previous respiratory failure. Thorax 36:759–763, 1981.

Ichinose M and Barnes PJ: Histamine H3-receptors modulate antigen-induced bronchoconstriction in guinea pigs. J Allergy Clin Immunol 86:491–495, 1990.

Idris AH, McDermott MF, Raucci JC, et al: Emergency department treatment of severe asthma. Metered-dose inhaler plus holding chamber is equivalent in effectiveness to nebulizer. Chest 103(3):665–672, 1993.

Infante-Rivard C: Childhood asthma and indoor environmental risk factors. Am J Epidemiol 137:834–844, 1993.

Inman WHW and Adelstein AM: Rise and fall of asthma mortality in England and Wales in relation to use of pressurized aerosols. Lancet 2:279–285, 1969.

International consensus report on diagnosis and treatment of asthma. Eur Resp J 5:601–641, 1992.

Ishizaka T: Mechanisms of IgE-mediated hypersensitivity. In Middleton E, Reed CE, Ellis EF, et al (eds): Allergy: Principles and Practices. St. Louis, CV Mosby, 1988, pp 71–93.

Jackson RT, Beaglehole R, Rea HH, et al: Mortality from asthma: A new epidemic in New Zealand. Br Med J 285:771–774, 1982.

Jacoby DB and Fryer AD: Abnormalities in neural control of smooth muscle in virus infected airways. Trends Pharmacol Sci 11:393–395, 1990.

James AL, Paré PD, and Hogg JC: The mechanics of airway narrowing in asthma. Am Rev Respir Dis 132:242–246, 1989.

Jardin F, Farcot JC, Boisante L, et al: Mechanism of paradoxic pulse in bronchial asthma. Circulation 66:887–894, 1982.

Jasper AC, Mohsenifar Z, Kahan S, et al: Cost-benefit comparison of aerosol bronchodilator delivery methods in hospitalized patients. Chest 91(4):614–618, 1987.

Jeffery PK: Structural changes in asthma. In Page C and Black J (eds): Airways and Vascular Remodelling. Orlando, Academic Press, 1994, pp 3–19.

Jeffery PK, Godfrey RW, Adelroth E, et al: Effect of treatment on airway inflammation and thickening of reticular collagen in asthma: A quantitative light and electron microscopy study. Am Rev Respir Dis 145:890–899, 1992.

Jones RJ: Use of the peripheral nerve stimulator. J Am Assoc Nurs Anesth April: 152–154, 1980.

Joseph M, Tonnel AB, Torpier G, et al: Involvement of IgE in the secretory processes of alveolar macrophages from asthmatic patients. J Clin Invest 71:221–230, 1983.

Josephs SH: Immunologic mechanisms in pulmonary disease. Pediatr Clin North Am 31:919–936, 1984.

Kaliner M, Shelhamer JH, Davis PB, et al: Autonomic nervous system abnormalities and allergy. Ann Intern Med 96:349–357, 1982.

Kass I and Mingo TS: Bitolterol mesylate (WIN 32784) aerosol. A new long-acting bronchodilator with reduced chronotropic effects. Chest 78:283–287, 1980.

Kass JE and Castriotta RJ: Heliox therapy in acute severe asthma. Chest 107:757–760, 1995.

Kay AB: Mediators and inflammatory cells in asthma. In Kay AB (ed): Asthma: Clinical Pharmacology and Therapeutic Progress. Oxford, Blackwell Scientific Publications, 1986, pp 1–10.

Keistinen T, Tuuponen T, and Kivelä SL: Asthma related hospital treatment in Finland: 1972–1986. Thorax 48:44–47, 1993.

Kelsen SG, Kelsen DP, Fleeger BF, et al: Emergency room assessment and treatment of patients with acute asthma. Adequacy of the conventional approach. Am J Med 64(4):622–628, 1978.

Kharitonov SA, O'Connor BJ, Evans DJ, et al: Allergen-induced late asthmatic reactions are associated with elevation of exhaled nitric oxide. Am J Respir Crit Care Med 151:1894–1899, 1995.

Kikuchi Y, Okabe S, Tamura G, et al: Chemosensitivity and perception of dyspnea in patients with a history of near fatal asthma. N Engl J Med 330:1329–1334, 1994.

Kovnat D: In Weiss EB (ed): Status Asthmaticus. Baltimore, University Park Press, 1978, pp 293–304.

Kung M, Abraham WM, Greenblatt DW, et al: Modification of hypoxic pulmonary vasoconstriction by antigen challenge in sensitized sheep. J Appl Physiol 49:22–27, 1980.

Laitinen LA, Heino M, Laitinen A, et al: Damage to the airway epithelium and bronchial reactivity in patients with asthma. Am Rev Respir Dis 131:599–606, 1985.

Laitinen LA, Laitinen A, Haahtela T: Airway mucosal inflammation even in patients with newly diagnosed asthma. Am Rev Respir Dis 147:697–704, 1993.

Lang DM, Simon RA, Mathison DA, et al: Safety and possible efficacy of fiberoptic bronchoscopy with lavage in the management of refractory asthma with mucous impaction. Ann Allergy 67:324–330, 1991.

Lang DM and Polansky M: Patterns of asthma mortality in Philadelphia from 1969 to 1991. N Engl J Med 331:1542–1546, 1994.

Lansing MW, Ahnud A, Cortes A, et al: Oxygen radical contributes to antigen-induced airway hyperresponsiveness in conscious sheep. Am Rev Respir Dis 147:321–326, 1993.

Lapinsky SE, Kruczynski K, and Slutsky AS: Critical care in the pregnant patient. Am J Respir Crit Care Med 152:427–455, 1995.

Lemanske RF Jr, Dick EC, Swenson CA, et al: Rhinovirus upper respiratory infection increases airway hyperreactivity and late asthmatic reactions. J Clin Invest 83:1–10, 1989.

Levin GN, Powell C, Bernard SA, et al: Acute, reversible left ventricular dysfunction in status asthmaticus. Chest 107:1469–1473, 1995.

Lichtenstein LM and Gillespie E: The effects of H_1 and H_2 antihistamines on allergic histamine release and its inhibition by histamine. J Pharmacol Exp Ther 192:441–450, 1975.

Linden A, Rabe KF, and Löfdahl CG: Pharmacologic basis for duration of effect: Formoterol and salmeterol versus short-acting β2-adrenoceptor agonists. Lung 174:1–22, 1996.

Long WM, Yerger M, Martinez H, et al: Modification of bronchial blood flow during allergic airway responses. J Appl Physiol 65:272–282, 1988.

Lopez AF, Sanderson CJ, Gamble JR, et al: Recombinant human interleukin-5 is a selective activator of eosinophil function. J Exp Med 167:219–224, 1988.

Lopez AF, Williamson DJ, Gamble JR, et al: Recombinant human granulocyte-macrophage colony stimulating factor stimulates in vitro mature human eosinophil and neutrophil function, surface receptor expression and survival. J Clin Invest 78:1220–1228, 1986.

Lui MC, Hubbard WC, Proud D, et al: Immediate and late inflammatory responses to ragweed antigen challenge of the peripheral airways in allergic asthmatics. Am Rev Respir Dis 144:51–58, 1991.

MacDermot J and Fuller RW: Macrophages. In Barnes PJ, Rodger IW, and Thomson NC (eds): Asthma: Basic Mechanisms and Clinical Management. London, Academic Press, 1988, pp 97–113.

McCarter JH and Vasquez JJ: The bronchial basement membrane in asthma. Arch Pathol 82:328–335, 1966.

McFadden ER Jr: Fatal and near fatal asthma. Editorial. N Engl J Med 324:409–411, 1991.

McFadden ER Jr, Kiser R, and DeGrot WJ: Acute bronchial asthma. Relations between clinical and physiologic manifestations. N Engl J Med 288:221–225, 1973.

McFadden ER Jr and Lyons HA: Arterial blood gas tension in asthma. N Engl J Med 278:1027–1032, 1968.

McMillan RM and Walker ERM: Designing therapeutically effective 5-lipoxygenase inhibitors. Trends Pharmacol Sci 13:323–330, 1992.

McWhorter WM, Polis MA, and Kaslow RA: Occurrence, predictors and consequences of adult asthma in NHANESi and follow up survey. Am Rev Respir Dis 139:721–724, 1989.

Mak JCW and Barnes PJ: Autoradiographic visualization of bradykinin receptors in human and guinea pig lungs. Eur J Pharmacol 194:37–44, 1991.

Maltais F, Sovilj M, Goldberg P, et al: Respiratory mechanics in status asthmaticus. Effects of inhalational anesthesia. Chest 106:1401–1406, 1994.

Malveaux FJ: Asthma care for the indigent. J Allergy Clin Immunol 83:1029–1031, 1989.

Manthous CA, Hall JB, Melmed A, et al: Heliox improves pulsus paradoxus and peak expiratory flow in nonintubated patients with severe asthma. Am J Resp Crit Care Med 151:310–314, 1995.

Manthous CA, Hall JB, Schmidt GA, et al: Metered-dose inhaler versus nebulized albuterol in mechanically ventilated patients. Am Rev Respir Dis 148:1567–1570, 1993.

Marder D, Targonski P, Orris P, et al: Effect of racial and socio-economic factors on asthma mortality in Chicago. Chest 101[Suppl]:426S–429S, 1992.

Marquette CH, Saulnier F, Leroy O, et al: Long-term prognosis of near-fatal asthma: A 6-year follow-up study of 145 asthmatic patients who underwent mechanical ventilation for a near fatal attack of asthma. Am Rev Respir Dis 146:76–81, 1992.

Martin J, Powell E, Shore S, et al: The role of respiratory muscles in the hyperinflation of bronchial asthma. Am Rev Respir Dis 121:441–447, 1980.

Mattoli S, Mattoso VL, Soloperto M, et al: Cellular and biochemical characteristics of bronchoalveolar lavage fluid in symptomatic nonallergic asthma. J Allergy Clin Immunol 84:794–802, 1991.

Maurer DR, Sielczak M, Oliver W Jr, et al: Role of ciliary motility in acute allergic mucociliary dysfunction. J Appl Physiol 52:1018–1023, 1982.

Mauser PJ, Pitman AM, Fernandez X, et al: Effects of an antibody to interleukin-5 in a monkey model of asthma. Am J Respir Crit Care Med 152:467–472, 1995.

Mayo PH, Richman J, and Harris HW: Results of a program to reduce admissions for adult asthma. Ann Intern Med 112:864–871, 1990.

Medical Research Council: Controlled trial of effects of cortisone acetate in status asthmaticus. Lancet 2:803–806, 1956.

Menitove SM and Goldring RM: Combined ventilator and bicarbonate strategy in the management of status asthmaticus. Am J Med 74:898–901, 1983.

Mezey RJ, Cohn MA, Fernandez RJ, et al: Mucociliary transport in allergic patients with antigen-induced bronchospasm. Am Rev Respir Dis 118:677–684, 1978.

Middleton E: Antiasthmatic drug therapy and calcium ions: Review of pathogenesis and role of calcium. J Pharmacol Sci 89:243–251, 1980.

Minette PA and Barnes PJ: Prejunctional inhibitory muscarinic receptors on cholinergic nerves in human and guinea pig airways. J Appl Physiol 64:2532–2537, 1988.

Mitchell EA: International trends in hospital admission rates for asthma. Arch Dis Child 60:376–378, 1985.

Mitchell EA: Is current treatment increasing asthma mortality and morbidity? Editorial. Thorax 44:81–84, 1989.

Mitchell EA and Dawson KP: Why are hospital admissions of children with acute asthma increasing? Eur Respir J 2:470–472, 1988.

Mitenko PA and Ogilvie RI: Rational intravenous doses of theophylline. N Engl J Med 289:600–603, 1973.

Molfino NA, Nannin LJ, Martelli AN, et al: Respiratory arrest in near fatal asthma. N Engl J Med 324:285–288, 1991.

Molfino NA and Slutsky AS: Near fatal asthma. Eur Resp J 7:981–990, 1994.

Montefort S, Holgate ST, and Howarth PH: Leucocyte-endothelial adhesion molecules and their role in bronchial asthma and allergic rhinitis. Eur Resp J 6:1044–1054, 1993.

Montefort S, Lai CKW, Kapahi J, et al: Circulating adhesion molecules in asthma. Am J Respir Crit Care Med 149:1149–1152, 1994.

Montefort S, Roberts JA, Beasley R, et al: The site of disruption of the bronchial epithelium in asthmatic and non-asthmatic subjects. Thorax 47:499–503, 1992.

Moqbel R, Durham SR, Shaw RJ, et al: Enhancement of leukocyte cytotoxity after exercise-induced asthma. Am Rev Respir Dis 133:609–613, 1986.

Morris HG: Mechanism of action and therapeutic role of corticosteroids in asthma. J Allergy Clin Immunol 75:1–13, 1985.

Mountain RD and Sahn SA: Clinical features and outcome in patients with acute asthma presenting with hypercapnia. Am Rev Respir Dis 138:535–539, 1988.

Nakamura Y, Ozaki T, Kamei T, et al: Increased GM-CSF production by mononuclear cells from peripheral blood of patients with bronchial asthma. Am Rev Respir Dis 147:87–91, 1993.

National Center for Health Statistics, 1984: Emergency room visits. DHHS publication no. (PHS) 85-1232. Washington D.C., United States Government Printing Office, December 1984.

Newhouse MT: Are nebulizers obsolete for administering asthma medications to infants and children? Pediatr Pulmonol 15:271–272, 1993.

Newhouse MT and Fuller HD: Rose is a rose is a rose? Aerosol therapy in ventilated patients: Nebulizers versus metered dose inhalers—a continuing controversy. Am Rev Respir Dis 148:1444–1446, 1993.

O'Byrne PM, Dolovich J, and Hargreave FE: Late asthmatic responses. Am Rev Respir Dis 136:740–751, 1987.

O'Connor BJ, Aikman S, and Barnes PJ: Tolerance to the non-bronchodilator effects of inhaled beta-2 agonists in asthma. N Engl J Med 327:1204–1208, 1992.

Ogilvie AG: A study of prognosis in 1000 patients. Thorax 17:183–189, 1962.

O'Hollaren MT, Yunginger JW, Offord KP, et al: Exposure to an aeroallergen as a possible precipitating factor in respiratory arrest in young patients with asthma. N Engl J Med 324:359–363, 1991.

Ohman JL, Schmidt-Nowara W, Lawrence W, et al: The diffusing capacity of asthma. Effect of airflow obstruction. Am Rev Respir Dis 107:932–939, 1973.

Ohnishi T, Collins DS, Sur S, et al: IgE-mediated release of eosinophil viability enhancing activity in the lung in vivo: Identification as IL-5 and association with eosinophil recruitment and degranulation. J Allergy Clin Immunol 62:607–615, 1993a.

Ohnishi T, Kita H, Weiler D, et al: Il-5 is the predominant eosinophils-active cytokine in the antigen-induced pulmonary late-phase reaction. Am Rev Respir Dis 147:901–907, 1993b.

Okayama H, Aikawa T, Okayama M, et al: Bronchodilating effect of intravenous magnesium sulfate in bronchial asthma. JAMA 257:1076–1078, 1987.

O'Rourke PP and Crone RK: Halothane in status asthmaticus. Crit Care Med 10:341–343, 1982.

Osler W: The Principle and Practice of Medicine. New York, Classics of Medicine Library, 1892.

Page CP: Platelet activating factor. In Barnes PJ, Rodger IW, and Thomson NC (eds.): Asthma: Basic Mechanisms and Clinical Management. London, Academic Press, 1988, pp 283–304.

Patel HJ, Barnes PJ, Takahashi T, et al: Evidence of prejunctional muscarinic autoreceptors in human and guinea pig trachea. Am J Respir Crit Care Med 152:872–878, 1995.

Pearce N, Beasley R, Crane J, et al: End of the New Zealand asthma mortality epidemic. Lancet 345:41–44, 1995.

Pearce N, Grainger J, Atkinson M, et al: Case-control study of prescribed Fenoterol and death from asthma in New Zealand, 1977–1981. Thorax 45:170–175, 1990.

Penner R: Multiple signaling pathways control stimulus-secretion coupling in rat peritoneal mast cells. Proc Natl Acad Sci 85:9856–9860, 1988.

Penner R, Matthews G, and Neher E: Regulation of calcium influx by second messengers in rat mast cells. Nature 334:499–504, 1988.

Peress L, Sybrecht G, and Macklem PT: The mechanism of increase in total lung capacity during acute asthma. Am J Med 61:165–169, 1976.

Permutt S: Physiologic changes in the acute asthmatic attack. In Austen KF, and Lichtenstein LM (eds): Asthma—Physiology, Immunopharmacology and Treatment. New York, Academic Press, 1973a, pp 15–27.

Permutt S: Relation between pulmonary arterial pressure and pleural pressure during the acute asthmatic attack. Chest 63:25S–28S, 1973b.

Persson CGA: Bronchial microcirculation. In Barnes PJ, Rodger IW, and Thomson NC (eds): Asthma: Basic Mechanisms and Clinical Management. London, Academic Press, 1988, pp 187–201.

Petheram IS, Jones DA, and Collins JV: Assessment and management of acute asthma in the elderly: A comparison with younger asthmatics. Postgrad Med J 58:149–151, 1982.

Phan-Puibaraud TTC, Regnard J, Monchi M, et al: Effects of pretreatment with inhaled methoxamine on responses to histamine in asthmatic subjects. Eur Resp J 8:40–46, 1995.

Phipps RJ, Denas SM, and Wanner A: Antigen stimulates glycoprotein secretion and alters ion fluxes in sheep trachea. J Appl Physiol 55:1593–1602, 1983.

Pierson WE, Bier CW, and Kelly VC: A double-blind trial of corticosteroid therapy in status asthmaticus. Pediatrics 54:282–288, 1974.

Pisani RJ and Rosenow EC: Pulmonary edema associated with tocolytic therapy. Ann Intern Med 40:714–718, 1989.

Pride NB, Permutt S, Riley RL, et al: Determinants of maximal expiratory flow from the lung. J Appl Physiol 23:646–662, 1967.

Rabe KF, Magnussen H, and Dent G: Theophylline and selective PDE inhibitors as bronchodilators and smooth muscle relaxants. Eur Respir J 8:637–642, 1995.

Rand TH, Cruikshank WW, Center DM, et al: CD4-mediated stimulation of human eosinophils: Lymphocyte chemoattractant factor and other CD4-binding ligands elicit eosinophil migration. J Exp Med 173:1521–1528, 1991.

Rebuck AS and Pengelly LD: Development of pulsus paradoxus in the presence of airway obstruction. N Engl J Med 288:66–69, 1973.

Rebuck AS and Read J: Assessment and management of severe asthma. Am J Med 51:788–798, 1971.

Reid LM: The presence or absence of bronchial mucus in fatal asthma. J Allergy Clin Immunol 80:415–416, 1987.

Reid LM, Gleich GJ, Hogg J, et al: Pathology. In Holgate ST (ed): The role of Inflammatory Processes in Airway Hyperresponsiveness. London, Blackwell Scientific Publications, pp 36–79, 1989.

Reisman J, Galdes-Sebaldt M, Kazim F, et al: Frequent administration by inhalation of salbutamol and ipratropium bromide in the initial management of severe acute asthma in children. J Allergy Clin Immunol 81:16–20, 1988.

Resnick MB and Weller PF: Mechanisms of eosinophil recruitment. Am J Resp Cell Mol Biol 8:349–355, 1993.

Robertson CF, Steedman D, Sinclair CJ, et al: Use of ether in life-threatening acute severe asthma. Lancet 1:187–188, 1985.

Robin ED: Death from bronchial asthma. Chest 93:614–620, 1988.

Robinson DS, Bentley AM, Hartnell A, et al: Activated memory T-helper cells in bronchoalveolar lavage from atopic asthmatics: Relationship to asthma symptoms, lung function and bronchial responsiveness. Thorax 48:26–32, 1993a.

Robinson DS, Hamid Q, Ying S, et al: Predominant "Th2-like" bronchoalveolar T-lymphocyte population in atopic asthma. N Engl J Med 326:298–304, 1992.

Robinson DS, Hamid Q, Ying S, et al: Prednisolone treatment in asthma is associated with modulation of bronchoalveolar lavage cell IL-4, IL-5 and interferon-α cytokine gene expression. Am Rev Respir Dis 148:401–406, 1993b.

Robinson DS, Ying S, Bentley AM, et al: Relationship among numbers of bronchoalveolar lavage cells expressing messenger ribonucleic acid for cytokines, asthma symptoms; and airway methacholine responsiveness in atopic asthma. J Allergy Clin Immunol 92:397–403, 1993c.

Roche WR, Beasley R, Williams JH, et al: Subepithelial fibrosis in the bronchi of asthmatics. Lancet 1:520–523, 1989.

Rocklin RE and Findlay SR: Immunologic mechanisms and recent advances in asthma. In

Weiss ED, Segal MS, and Stein M (eds): Bronchial Asthma, Mechanisms and Therapeutics. Boston, Little, Brown, 1985, pp 41–51.

Rodrigo C and Rodrigo G: Treatment of acute asthma, lack of therapeutic benefit and increase of the toxicity from aminophylline given in addition to high doses of salbutamol delivered by metered dose inhaled with a spacer. Chest 106:1071–1076, 1994.

Rogge R, Young S, and Goodlin R: Post-partum pulmonary edema associated with preventive therapy for premature labor. Lancet 1:1026–1027, 1979.

Romagnani S: Regulation and deregulation of human IgE-synthesis. Immunol Today 11:316–321, 1990.

Rose CC, Murphy JG, and Schwartz JS: Performance of an index predicting the response of patients with acute bronchial asthma to intensive emergency treatment. N Engl J Med 310:573–576, 1984.

Rothenberg ME, Owen WF, Silberstein DS, et al: Human eosinophils have prolonged survival, enhanced functional properties and become hypodense when exposed to human interleukin-3. J Clin Invest 81:1986–1992, 1988.

Roy TM, Pruitt VL, Garner PA, et al: The potential role of anesthesia in status asthmaticus. J Asthma 29:73–77, 1992.

Saetta M, DiStefano A, Rosina C, et al: Quantitative structural analysis of peripheral airways and arteries in sudden fatal asthma. Am Rev Respir Dis 143:138–143, 1991.

Salvato G: Some historical changes in chronic bronchitis and asthma. Thorax 23:168–183, 1968.

Santiago SM Jr and Klaustermeyer WB: Mortality in status asthmaticus: A nine year experience in a respiratory intensive care unit. J Asthma Res 17:75–79, 1980.

Schall TJ: Biology of the RANTES/SIS cytokine family. Cytokine 3:165–183, 1991.

Schatz M, Harden K, Forsythe A, et al: The course of asthma during pregnancy, post partum, and with successive pregnancies: A prospective analysis. J Allergy Clin Immunol 81:509–517, 1988.

Schiermeyer RP and Finkelstein JA: Rapid infusion of magnesium sulfate obviates need for intubation in status asthmaticus. Am J Emerg Med 12:164–166, 1994.

Schleimer RP, Sterbinsky CA, Kaiser J, et al: Interleukin-4 induces adherence of human eosinophils and basophils, but not neutrophils to endothelium: Association with expression of VCAM-1. J Immunol 148:1086–1092, 1992.

Schleuter DP: Ipratropium bromide in asthma: A review of the literature. Am J Med 81[Suppl]:55–60, 1986.

Schwartz J, Gold D, Dockery DW, et al: Predictors of asthma and persistent wheeze in a national sample of children in the United States. Association with social class, perinatal events and race. Am Rev Respir Dis 142:555–562, 1990.

Schwartz J, Slater D, Larson TV, et al: Particulate air pollution and hospital emergency room visits for asthma in Seattle. Am Rev Respir Dis 147:826–831, 1993.

Schwartz SH: Treatment of status asthmaticus: A nine year experience. JAMA 251:2688–2689, 1984.

Scoggin CH, Sahn SA, and Petty TL: Status asthmaticus: A nine year experience. JAMA 238:1158–1162, 1977.

Sears MR: International trends in asthma mortality. Allergy Proc 12:155–158, 1991.

Sedgewick JB, Calhoun WJ, Gleich GJ, et al: Immediate and late airway response of allergic rhinitis patients to segmental antigen challenge. Characterization of eosinophil and mast cell mediators. Am Rev Respir Dis 144:1274–1281, 1991.

Seybold ZV, Mariassy AT, Stroh D, et al: Mucociliary interaction in vitro: Effects of physiologic and inflammatory stimuli. Am Rev Respir Dis 139(4):A229, 1989.

Shannon M and Lovejoy FH Jr: The influence of age vs peak serum concentration on life threatening events after chronic theophylline intoxication. Arch Intern Med 150:2045–2048, 1990.

Shapiro MB, Kleaveland AC, and Bartlett RH: Extracorporeal life support for status asthmaticus. Chest 103:1651–1654, 1993.

Sheffer AL: Guidelines for the diagnosis and management: National Heart, Lung and Blood Institute, national asthma education program expert panel report. J Allergy Clin Immunol 88[Suppl]:425–534, 1991.

Sheffer AL and Buist S (eds): Proceedings of the asthma mortality task force. J Allergy Clin Immunol 80[Suppl 3]:361–514, 1987.

Sher ER, Leung DY, Surs W, et al: Steroid-resistant asthma. Cellular mechanisms contributing to inadequate response to glucocorticoid therapy. J Clin Invest 93:33–39, 1994.

Sibley DR and Lefkowitz RJ: Molecular mechanisms of receptor desensitization using the beta-adrenergic receptor-coupled adenylate cyclase system as a model. Nature 317:124–129, 1985.

Silverstein MD, Reed CE, O'Connell EJ, et al: Long term survival of a cohort of community residents with asthma. N Engl J Med 331:1537–1541, 1994.

Sim TC, Reece LM, Hilsmeier KA, et al: Secretion of chemokines and other cytokines in allergen-induced nasal responses: Inhibition by topical steroid treatment. Am J Respir Crit Care Med 152:927–933, 1995.

Skloot G, Permutt S, and Togias A: Airway hyperresponsiveness in asthma: A problem of limited smooth muscle relaxation with inspiration. J Clin Invest 96:2393–2403, 1995.

Slifman NR, Adolphson CR, and Gleich GL: Eosinophils: Biochemical and cellular aspects. In Middleton E, Reed CE, Ellis EF, et al (eds): Allergy: Principles and Practices. St. Louis, CV Mosby, 1988, pp 179–205.

Sly RMP: Increases in deaths from asthma. Ann Allergy 98:271–275, 1984.

Sobonya RE: Quantitative structural alterations in long-standing allergic asthma. Am Rev Respir Dis 130:289–292, 1984.

Spector SL: Definitions of asthma. ATS News 8:5, 1982.

Speizer FE: Epidemiology and mortality patterns in asthma. In Weiss EB (ed): Status Asthmaticus. Baltimore, University Park Press, 1978, pp 13–18.

Spinozzi F, Agea E, Bistoni O, et al: T lymphocytes bearing the γδ T cell receptor are susceptible to steroid-induced programmed cell death. Scand J Immunol 41:404–408, 1995.

Spinozzi F, Agea E, Bistoni O, et al: Increased allergen-specific, steroid-sensitive γδ T cells in bronchoalveolar lavage fluid from patients with asthma. Ann Intern Med 124:223–227, 1996.

Spitzer WD, Suissa S, Ernest P, et al: The use of β-agonists and the risk of death and near death from asthma. N Engl J Med 326:501–506, 1992.

Stalcup SA and Mellins RB: Mechanical forces producing pulmonary edema in acute asthma. N Engl J Med 279:592–596, 1977.

Stephens NL: Structure of airway smooth muscles. In Barnes PJ, Rodger IW, and Thomson NC (eds): Asthma: Basic Mechanisms and Clinical Management. London, Academic Press, 1988, pp 11–34.

Strunk RC: Identification of the fatality-prone subject with asthma. J Allergy Clin Immunol 83:477–485, 1989.

Strunk RC: Death due to asthma (editorial). Am Rev Respir Dis 148:550–552, 1993.

Sur S, Crotty TB, Kephart GM, et al: Sudden onset fatal asthma: A distinct entity with few eosinophils and relatively more neutrophils in the airway submucosa? Am Rev Respir Dis 148:713–719, 1993.

Sur S, Gleich GJ, Swanson MC, et al: Eosinophilic inflammation is associated with elevation of interleukin-5 in the airways of patients with spontaneous symptomatic asthma. J Allergy Clin Immunol 96:661–668, 1995.

Swillens S and Dumont JE: A unifying model of current concepts and data on adenylate cyclase activation by beta-adrenergic agonists. Life Sci 27:1013–1028, 1980.

Szentivany A: The beta adrenergic theory of atopic abnormality in bronchial asthma. J Allergy 42:203–232, 1968.

Takizawa T and Thurlbeck WM: Muscle and mucus gland size in the major bronchi of patients with chronic bronchitis, asthma, and asthmatic bronchitis. Am Rev Respir Dis 104:331–336, 1971.

Tanaka RM, Santiago SM, Kuhn GJ, et al: Intravenous methylprednisolone in adults in status asthmaticus: Comparison of two dosages. Chest 82:438–440, 1982.

Tasaka K, Mio M, and Okamoto M: The role of intracellular Ca^{++} in the degranulation of skinned mast cells. Agents Actions 20:157–160, 1987.

Tattersfield AE: Autonomic bronchodilators. In Clark TJH, and Godfrey S (eds): Asthma, 2nd ed. London, Chapman & Hall, 1983, pp 301–335.

Taylor GW, Taylor I, Black P, et al: Urinary leukotriene E4 after allergen challenge and in acute asthma and allergic rhinitis. Lancet 1:584–588, 1989.

Thurlbeck WM and Hogg JC: Pathology of asthma. In Middleton E, Reed CE, Ellis EF, et al (eds): Allergy: Principles and Practice. St. Louis, CV Mosby, 1988, pp 1008–1017.

Town GI and Allan C: Ventilatory responses to hypoxia and hypercapnia in asthmatics with previous respiratory failure. Aust N Z J Med 19:426–430, 1989.

Triggle DJ: Calcium, the control of smooth muscle function and bronchial hyperreactivity. J Allergy 38:1–9, 1983.

Turki J, Green SA, Newman KB, et al: Human lung cell β2-adrenergic receptors desensitize in response to in vivo administered β-agonist. Am J Physiol 269:L709–L714, 1995.

Turner MO, Hussack P, Sears MR, et al: Exacerbations of asthma without sputum eosinophilia. Thorax 50:1057–1061, 1995.

Ullah MI, Newman GB, and Saunders KB: Influence of an age on response to ipratropium and salbutamol in asthma. Thorax 36:523–529, 1981.

Ullman A and Svedmyr N: Salmeterol, a new long acting inhaled β2 adrenoceptor agonist: Comparison with salbutamol in adult asthmatic patients. Thorax 43:674–678, 1988.

Valabhji P: Gas exchange in the acute and asymptomatic phases of asthma breathing air and oxygen. Clin Sci 34:431–440, 1968.

Van Oosterhoot AJM, Ladenius ARC, Savelkoul HFJ, et al: Effect of anti-IL-5 and IL-5 in airway hyperreactivity and eosinophils in guinea pigs. Am Rev Respir Dis 147:548–552, 1993.

Venten TC, Fraser CM, and Harrison LC: Auto antibodies to β2 adrenergic receptors: A possible cause of adrenergic hyporesponsiveness in allergic rhinitis and asthma. Sciences 207:1351–1363, 1980.

Vollmer WM, Buist AS, and Osborne ML: Twenty year trends in hospital discharges for asthma among members of a health maintenance organization. J Clin Epidemiol 45:999–1006, 1992.

Vollmer WM, Osborne ML, and Buist AS: Uses and limitations of mortality and health-care utilization statistics in asthma research. Am J Resp Crit Care Med 149[Suppl]:79–87, 1994.

Wagner PD, Dantzker DR, Iacovoni VE, et al: Ventilation perfusion inequality in asymptomatic asthma. Am Rev Respir Dis 118:511–524, 1978.

Walker C, Kaegi MK, Braun P, et al: Activated T-cells and eosinophils in bronchoalveolar lavages from subjects with asthma correlated with disease severity. J Allergy Clin Immunol 88:935–942, 1991.

Walsh GM, Hartnell A, Wardlaw AJ, et al: IL-5 enhances the in vitro adhesion of human eosinophils, but not neutrophils, in a leucocyte integrin (CD11/CD18)-dependent manner. Immunology 71:258–265, 1990.

Wanner A: Allergic mucociliary dysfunction. J Allergy Clin Immunol 72:347–350, 1983.

Wanner A: Circulation of the airway mucosa. J Appl Physiol 67:917–925, 1989.

Wanner A, Maurer D, Abraham WM, et al: Effects of chemical mediators of anaphylaxis on ciliary function. J Allergy Clin Immunol 72:663–667, 1983.

Wasserfallen JB, Schaller MD, Feihl F, et al: Sudden asphyxic asthma: A distinct entity? Am Rev Respir Dis 142:108–111, 1990.

Webb-Johnson D and Andrews JL Jr: Bronchodilator therapy. N Engl J Med 297:476–482, 1977a.

Webb-Johnson D and Andrews JL Jr: Bronchodilator therapy. N Engl J Med 297:759–764, 1977b.

Wein M and Bochner B: Adhesion molecule antagonists: Future therapies for allergic diseases? Eur Respir J 6:1239–1242, 1993.

Weiss EB and Faling LJ: Clinical significance of PaCO$_2$ during status asthmaticus: The cross over point. Ann Allergy 26:545–555, 1968.

Weiss KB, Gergen PJ, and Crain EF: Inner city asthma: The epidemiology of an emerging U.S. public health concern. Chest 101[Suppl]:362S–367S, 1992.

Weiss KB, Gergen PJ, and Hodgson TA: An economic evaluation of asthma in the United States. N Engl J Med 326:862–866, 1992.

Weiss KB, Gergen PJ, and Wagener DK: Breathing better or wheezing worse? The changing epidemiology of asthma morbidity and mortality. Ann Rev Public Health 14:491–513, 1993.

Weiss KB and Wagener DK: Changing patterns of asthma mortality: Identifying target populations at high risk. JAMA 264:1683–1687, 1990.

Weitzman RH and Wilson AF: Diffusing capacity and overall ventilation-perfusion in asthma. Am J Med 57:767–774, 1974.

Weitzman M, Gortmaker SL, and Sobol AM: Racial, social, and environmental risks for childhood asthma. Am J Dis Child 144:1189–1194, 1990.

Weitzman M, Gortmaker SL, Sobol AM, et al: Recent trends in the prevalence and severity of childhood asthma. JAMA 268:2673–2677, 1992.

Wenzel SE, Larsen GL, Johnston K, et al: Elevated levels of leukotriene C4 in bronchoalveolar lavage fluid from atopic asthmatics after endobronchial allergen challenge. Am Rev Respir Dis 142:112–119, 1990.

Westerman DE, Benatar SR, Potgieter PD, et al: Identification of high risk asthmatic patient: Experience with 39 patients undergoing ventilation for status asthmaticus. Am J Med 66:565–572, 1979.

Whiteside M, Lauredo I, Chapman GA, et al: Effect of atropine on tracheal mucociliary clearance and bacterial counts. Bull Eur Physiopath Resp 20:347–351, 1984.

Wilkins K and Yang M: Trends in rates of admissions of hospital and death from asthma among children and young adults in Canada during the 1980's. Can Med Assoc J 148:185–188, 1993.

Williams TJ, Tuxen DV, Scheinkestel CD, et al: Risk factors for morbidity in mechanically ventilated patients with acute severe asthma. Am Rev Respir Dis 146:607–615, 1992.

Wissow LS, Gittelsohn AM, Szklo M, et al: Poverty, race and hospitalization for childhood asthma. Am J Public Health 78:777–782, 1988.

Woodside KH, Denas SM, Smith KL, et al: Inhibition of pulmonary macrophage function by airway mucus. J Appl Physiol 54:94–98, 1983.

Woolcock AJ and Read J: Lung volume in exacerbations of asthma. Am J Med 41:259–273, 1966.

Yates DH, Kharitonov SA, Robbins RA, et al: Effect of a nitric oxide synthase inhibitor and a glucocorticosteroid on exhaled nitric oxide. Am J Respir Crit Care Med 152:892–896, 1995.

Zanetti CU, Rotman HH, and Dresner AJ: Efficacy and duration of action of procaterol, a new bronchodilator. J Clin Pharmacol 22:250–253, 1982.

Zimmerman HA: A study of the pulmonary circulation in man. Dis Chest 20:46–74, 1951.

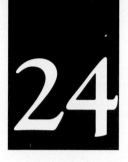

C H A P T E R

Chronic Obstructive Pulmonary Disease

Kenneth I. Berger, M.D.

David M. Rapoport, M.D.

Acute cardiopulmonary failure in patients with chronic obstructive pulmonary disease is commonly encountered in intensive care units. It may account for 15% of all cases of respiratory failure (Pontoppidan et al, 1972). Because acute respiratory failure may occur on a background of chronic respiratory failure, acute respiratory failure in a patient with chronic obstructive lung disease (COPD) is best defined by either a decrease in arterial P_{O_2} or an increase in arterial P_{CO_2} to levels above those that may be expected.

Many precipitating factors for the development of acute cardiopulmonary failure have been described. Although each factor by itself may not be sufficient to cause respiratory failure, each may be sufficient to cause a life-threatening illness in a patient with limited cardiopulmonary reserve due to COPD. Treatment needs to be geared directly at the respiratory failure and at the specific inciting condition. This chapter outlines an approach to the assessment and management of acute cardiopulmonary failure in patients with chronic obstructive pulmonary disease.

PRECIPITATING FACTORS OF CARDIOPULMONARY FAILURE

Cardiorespiratory failure in patients with COPD can be precipitated by numerous factors. These can be divided into three general categories (Table 24–1): (1) worsening lung function, (2) cardiac consequences of worsening lung function, and (3) interaction between other acute diseases and limited cardiopulmonary reserve due to COPD.

WORSENING LUNG FUNCTION

In many patients with cardiopulmonary failure, the inciting cause for respiratory failure is worsening of the baseline obstructive airways dysfunction. Worsening obstruction may be related to bronchospasm or infection. The differentiation between these two causes is often difficult because identification of a pathogenic organism may be complicated by a high rate of airway colonization by bacterial microorganisms (Leeder, 1975;

Table 24–1
Precipitating Etiologies for Cardiorespiratory Failure in Patients With COPD

Worsening lung function
    Bronchospasm
    Infection
Cardiac consequences of worsening lung function
    Cor pulmonale
Interaction between other acute diseases and limited
        cardiopulmonary reserve due to COPD
    Pulmonary embolus
    Congestive heart failure
    Sleep-disordered breathing
        Sleep state–related ventilatory abnormalities
            Alterations in control of breathing
            Alterations in respiratory muscle function
        Obstructive sleep apnea syndrome

Buscho et al, 1978). Although bacterial pathogens such as *Streptococcus pneumoniae* and *Haemophilus influenzae* may be isolated in patients with acute respiratory failure, these organisms can also be found in up to 50% patients with stable COPD (Haas et al, 1977). Therefore, a positive result on culture of airway secretions is not always indicative of acute infection. Microscopic examination of sputum may also be misleading because inflammatory cells may be identified in the absence of an infection. In addition, other infectious causes of acute exacerbations of chronic bronchitis, such as viral pathogens, are not identified by standard microbiologic diagnostic techniques (Gump et al, 1976). Because of these limitations for the diagnosis of acute infection, antimicrobial therapy is often instituted on an empirical basis in combination with treatment for bronchospasm (Anthonisen et al, 1987). The reader is referred to Chapters 20 and 21 for extensive discussion of acute infections in critical care.

CARDIAC CONSEQUENCES OF WORSENING LUNG FUNCTION

Some patients with COPD present to the intensive care unit with cor pulmonale. Cor pulmonale is defined as an alteration of right ventricular function due to pulmonary hypertension that has resulted from a disease affecting the lung parenchyma or its vasculature. Disorders due to primary disease of the left heart are excluded in the definition of cor pulmonale. Numerous reports have demonstrated a high incidence of abnormalities in right ventricular function in patients with COPD. Fishman has shown that right ventricular hypertrophy can be identified at autopsy in approxi-

mately 50% of those with COPD (Fishman, 1976). In a study by Berger and coworkers, noninvasive assessment revealed a decreased right ventricular ejection fraction in 19 of 36 randomly selected patients with COPD (Berger et al, 1978). Even in patients with normal resting right ventricular function, abnormalities in function may be demonstrated during exercise (Matthay et al, 1980; Mahler et al, 1984).

The development of pulmonary hypertension in a subgroup of patients with COPD may be due to either structural changes in the vasculature or hypoxic pulmonary vasoconstriction. Weitzenblum and colleagues followed mean pulmonary artery pressure in 93 patients for a mean duration of 8 years and found that 29% of patients demonstrated a worsening of cardiac function, which was defined as a rise of 5 mm Hg in mean pulmonary artery pressure. In this subgroup of patients, there was a marked worsening of arterial hypoxemia not observed in the other patients, suggesting a role for hypoxemia in the development and progression of pulmonary hypertension (Weitzenblum et al, 1984). Kawakami and coworkers extended these observations in 50 patients and demonstrated that decreased survival was associated with arterial hypoxemia and reduced mixed venous oxygen saturation (Kawakami et al, 1983). Structural and other factors that may contribute to the development of pulmonary hypertension include decreased cross-sectional area of the pulmonary vasculature resulting from loss of capillaries from emphysema; increased cardiac output, blood viscosity, and blood volume; and increased intrathoracic pressures as a consequence of expiratory airflow limitation (Harris et al, 1968; Agarwal et al, 1970; Wright et al, 1983).

Much debate exists about whether chronic obstructive pulmonary disease is associated with a primary abnormality in left ventricular function. There are multiple physiologic mechanisms by which COPD may adversely affect left ventricular function (Wise, 1991). Decreased venous return may occur as a consequence of increased right atrial pressure and/or increased pleural pressure during exhalation. Left ventricular ejection may be decreased through the effects of distention of the right ventricle (ventricular interdependence with bowing of the intraventricular septum). Left ventricular ejection may be decreased through increased left ventricular afterload because of the large negative pleural pressures that occur as a consequence of COPD or direct compression of the left heart by hyperinflated lungs (see Chapter 4).

Despite the potential for abnormalities in left ventricular function, investigators making comprehensive reviews of the literature have suggested that only a minority of patients with COPD have left ventricular dysfunction in the absence of other causes of impairment (Kachel, 1978; Wise, 1991). Although cases of left ventricular dysfunction not related to other causes can be identified, it is unclear if these are of any clinical significance.

INTERACTION BETWEEN OTHER ACUTE DISEASES AND LIMITED CARDIOPULMONARY RESERVE DUE TO COPD

Patients with advanced COPD are susceptible to acute respiratory failure following acute insults from many diseases. Most important among these are thromboembolic disease, congestive heart failure, and sleep-disordered breathing.

Thromboembolic Disease

Pulmonary embolus can precipitate acute cardiopulmonary failure in patients with COPD through either impairment of lung function or increasing pulmonary vascular pressures. Although the precise incidence of pulmonary embolus is unclear, up to 50% of those with COPD have evidence of pulmonary thromboembolic disease at autopsy (Baum and Fisher, 1960; Moser et al, 1981). Patients with COPD may be vulnerable to the development of thromboembolic disease for several reasons, including sedentary lifestyle, secondary polycythemia, and right ventricular mural thrombi that may occur in cor pulmonale. Cordova and colleagues have demonstrated a predisposition to thromboembolic disease in patients with COPD due to increased platelet aggregation and plasma β-thromboglobulin (Cordova et al, 1985).

The importance of diagnosing acute pulmonary embolism in COPD is highlighted by a mortality of approximately 30% for untreated cases (Dalen and Alpert, 1975). Unfortunately, difficulties are frequently encountered by clinicians attempting to diagnose pulmonary embolus. Patients with pulmonary embolus often present with dyspnea and hypoxia, which are nonspecific features that may be attributed to an exacerbation of underlying COPD. Although laboratory diagnosis of pulmonary embolus using noninvasive tests may yield indeterminate results, tests may provide useful data (PIOPED Investigators, 1990). In situations when ventilation-perfusion scans reveal normal perfusion of the lung, the diagnosis of acute pulmonary embolus is virtually excluded. Similarly, the appearance of multiple perfusion

defects in areas where ventilation and chest radiograph results are normal is usually diagnostic of pulmonary embolus. Unfortunately, most patients with COPD demonstrate indeterminate results between these two extremes on ventilation-perfusion scans. For patients with such indeterminate results, noninvasive testing for deep venous thrombosis of the lower extremity should be conducted.

Numerous tests for deep venous thrombosis are available, including venous duplex-Doppler scans (Lensing et al, 1989) and impedance plethysmography (Wheeler et al, 1974). If positive results for deep venous thrombosis are obtained, treatment with anticoagulation needs to be initiated. Serologic measurement of D-dimer has been proposed as an aid in the evaluation of pulmonary embolus; this measurement has a sensitivity of 98% and a specificity of 39% (Bounameaux et al, 1991). Further evaluation of this test, however, particularly in patients with COPD, is needed. Because significant doubt may exist about a diagnosis of pulmonary embolus after completion of all noninvasive tests, pulmonary angiography remains the standard for diagnosis of pulmonary embolus. Although the safety of pulmonary angiography in patients with cor pulmonale has been questioned, data from the PIOPED study have shown that pulmonary angiography is both safe and accurate in patients with COPD (PIOPED Investigators, 1990).

Cardiac Dysfunction and Arrhythmia

Clinical decompensation in patients with stable COPD may also occur as a result of congestive heart failure or cardiac arrhythmia. About 27% of COPD patients die as a result of coronary artery disease rather than the pulmonary disorder, emphasizing that left ventricular failure commonly occurs in patients with COPD (Kuller et al, 1989). This high incidence of ischemic cardiac disease in patients with COPD may be due in part to the common risk factor of cigarette smoking. In addition, coronary artery disease may be exacerbated by the hypoxemia and/or hypercapnia that occurs in patients with pulmonary disorders. During an exacerbation of COPD, left ventricular function may be further compromised by the development of a positive end-expiratory alveolar pressure (auto-PEEP). Although low levels of PEEP may be beneficial to some patients with left ventricular failure (Grace and Greenbaum, 1982), high levels often lead to cardiovascular compromise (Cournand et al, 1948; Braunwald et al, 1957). Chapter 15 deals with effects of PEEP on cardiovascular function in detail.

Cardiac disease manifested by an arrhythmia may also precipitate acute respiratory failure. Both supraventricular and ventricular arrhythmias have been reported in patients with COPD, although approximately 80% of arrhythmias are supraventricular in origin (Sideris et al, 1975). The propensity for arrhythmias may result from the hypoxemia and hypercapnia/acidosis that occur in advanced COPD, as well as from medications such as theophylline preparations and β-adrenergic agonists. In addition, once an arrhythmia develops, gas exchange, hypoxemia, and hypercapnia/acidosis may worsen, thereby further augmenting cardiac irritability.

Sleep-disordered Breathing

Several factors may lead to the development of hypoxemia during sleep, even in normal subjects. Measurement of ventilation during sleep reveals a reduction in total ventilation that is most pronounced during rapid eye movement (REM) sleep (Douglas et al, 1982a). Although some of this reduction may reflect a reduced metabolic rate and a reduced requirement for ventilation (White et al, 1985), there may also be some degree of hypoventilation leading to a mild increase in arterial P_{CO_2}. This intermittent hypoventilation may be severe during periods of frequent eye movements and may result in a 40% reduction in alveolar ventilation with corresponding hypoxemia in some cases, without known pathology (Douglas et al, 1982a,b; Gould et al, 1988). These same factors may be particularly significant in patients with baseline hypoxemia due to COPD (Catterall et al, 1985).

There are several physiologic mechanisms for nocturnal hypoventilation. During non-REM (NREM) sleep, it has been shown that there is an altered set point for carbon dioxide (CO_2) and there are small changes in the ventilatory response to CO_2 (Douglas et al, 1982b). These alterations in the ventilatory response to CO_2 rarely result in significant hypercapnia in a normal individual, but can easily exacerbate preexisting hypercapnia in COPD. In addition, there is a normal two- to threefold increase in the resistance of the upper airway that occurs with sleep (Lopes et al 1983; Hudgel et al, 1984). This presence of a high upper airway resistance has two consequences: (1) it adds to the already elevated total airway resistance in COPD and may exceed the mechanical reserve in patients with severely compromised lungs; and (2) it creates large intrathoracic pressure fluctuations, which couple the movements of the diaphragm and the rib cage. Because in REM sleep rib cage muscle activity

may cease, diaphragmatic function may remain as the sole determinant of ventilation (Johnson and Remmers, 1984). In patients with COPD and flattened diaphragms who depend heavily on their accessory muscles, loss of rib cage muscle activity may result in a precipitous decrease in ventilation in REM.

Patients with COPD may also demonstrate sleep-disordered breathing as a result of the obstructive sleep apnea and hypopnea syndrome (OSAS). The prevalence of OSAS in COPD is currently not known, but this disorder may have a prevalence of 2 to 10% in the general population (Young et al, 1993). In otherwise normal patients with OSAS, only a minority develop chronic hypercapnia due to OSAS. In patients with underlying COPD, however, the additional stress and loading of CO_2 that occurs during periods of apnea may compound a pre-existing state of hypercapnia. In OSAS, a pattern of cyclically frequent oxygen desaturation may be noted during sleep. The presence of OSAS may be suspected based on the presence of typical symptoms of loud snoring and excessive daytime hypersomnolence. The diagnosis of OSAS may then be confirmed with nocturnal polysomnography that reveals periods of apnea despite persistent respiratory efforts.

The importance of diagnosing OSAS in patients with acute respiratory failure is related to the therapeutic strategies employed to improve awake ventilation. In patients treated with noninvasive mechanical ventilatory support, changes in the ventilator settings may be required during sleep if OSAS is suspected. Similarly, in patients intubated for mechanical ventilation, the success of extubation may be influenced by appropriate therapy for OSAS after extubation (see later).

SIGNS AND SYMPTOMS OF CARDIOPULMONARY FAILURE

The clinical presentation of patients with acute cardiopulmonary failure results from the combination of a precipitating etiology for respiratory failure and cardiopulmonary failure itself. This section focuses on clinical signs and symptoms that result from the cardiopulmonary failure itself, because the signs and symptoms are common to all patients with cardiopulmonary failure. Although other presenting signs and symptoms are not discussed, they may provide important clues that aid in identification of the precipitant of an acute episode of respiratory failure.

One of the most prominent complaints of patients with cardiopulmonary failure is worsening dyspnea. Mechanisms contributing to dyspnea in this setting include length-tension inappropriateness of respiratory muscles (Campbell et al, 1961), disturbances in load perception (Killian and Campbell, 1983), respiratory muscle fatigue (Gandevia et al, 1981), increased respiratory drive (Bradley et al, 1979), and increased oxygen cost of breathing (Levison and Cherniack, 1968; see Chapter 6). When dyspnea becomes sufficiently severe, patients may adopt a rapid shallow breathing pattern and may be unable to complete a sentence without gasping for air. As the severity of respiratory distress increases, accessory muscles may be recruited during inspiration and expiration. At that point, intercostal and/or suprasternal retractions may be noticeable.

Mechanisms related to the precipitating factor may also contribute to the dyspnea in patients with acute cardiopulmonary failure. These mechanisms may include worsening dyspnea related to worsening airflow obstruction, dyspnea related to the presence of an acute pneumonic process such as tracheobronchitis or pneumonia, and dyspnea related to congestive heart failure or pulmonary embolus. Physical examination may help distinguish these diseases. The presence of wheezing suggests worsening obstruction, which may be accompanied by fever and purulent sputum if the cardiopulmonary failure is precipitated by an infectious source. When congestive heart failure is present, lung examination may reveal rales, which are indicative of pulmonary vascular congestion. In contrast, a normal result on pulmonary examination may be a clue for the diagnosis of pulmonary embolus.

Hypoxemia is almost invariably present during an episode of cardiopulmonary failure. The mechanisms for hypoxemia in patients with cardiopulmonary failure may be multifactorial and may include ventilation-perfusion mismatch, hypoventilation, and shunt. The most prominent mechanism leading to hypoxemia is ventilation-perfusion mismatch related to the underlying obstructive lung disease. Hypoventilation, which usually contributes minimally to hypoxemia in patients with stable COPD, may worsen acutely during an exacerbation, thereby leading to significant hypoxemia.

Right-to-left shunting of blood may also be a significant factor contributing to the hypoxemia in patients with acute cardiopulmonary failure. Right-to-left shunting of blood can be intrapulmonary, from infectious pneumonia or congestive heart failure, or intracardiac, typically through the atrial septum. Intra-atrial shunts can occur through a congenital atrial septal defect or through a patent foramen ovale, which may be present in up to 35% of otherwise normal people

(Hagen et al, 1984; Davidson et al, 1990). The foramen ovale is kept closed as a result of the normal interatrial pressure gradient (left > right); however, when there is an acute increase in right atrial pressure, as frequently occurs in COPD or hypoxia, right-to-left shunting may result. A hallmark of this condition is a large shunt, marked by persistent hypoxemia despite high FiO_2, which suddenly disappears several hours into treatment. The explanation offered is that the initial elevation of right atrial pressure opening the foramen ovale was in part caused by hypoxic vasoconstriction. Relief of the hypoxemia results in a drop of the atrial pressure with reversal of the interatrial pressure gradient and consequent closing of the patent foramen ovale, correcting the shunt.

Worsening hypercapnia and acidosis are commonly encountered in patients with cardiopulmonary failure. Patients may present with central nervous system signs related to worsening acidosis. These include disorientation, confusion, somnolence, or even coma (Kilburn, 1965). The level of consciousness has been shown to be correlated with the cerebrospinal fluid pH, which is in turn affected by serum pH and PCO_2 (Posner and Plum, 1967).

Worsening hypercapnia in patients with COPD generally occurs in the setting of rapid shallow breathing with an increased minute ventilation, suggesting an increased dead space ventilation. The failure to further increase minute ventilation to correct acidemia is not well understood; the failure may represent respiratory muscle fatigue or decreased respiratory muscle effort to prevent fatigue (Roussos, 1985). In a patient with a depressed level of consciousness, decreased central respiratory drive may account for worsening hypercapnia. In contrast, respiratory muscle fatigue may be suggested by the presence of thoracoabdominal paradox or respiratory alternans (Cohen et al, 1982). Normally both the chest wall and the abdomen move outward during inspiration owing to expansion of the rib cage and descent of the diaphragm. When thoracoabdominal paradox is present, either the chest or abdomen moves inward during inspiration while the other moves outward. Thoracoabdominal paradox occurs when the increased airways resistance causes large intrathoracic negative pressures during inspiration, which couples the movement of the chest and abdomen, with one overpowering the other. Respiratory alternans is a more unusual manifestation of respiratory muscle fatigue wherein inspiration occurs owing to alternating activity of the diaphragm and chest muscles.

Numerous studies have underscored an interplay between cardiac and pulmonary failure. Patients with COPD and pulmonary hypertension and cor pulmonale may present to the intensive care unit with peripheral edema. Asmundsson and Kilburn (1969) prospectively described 176 cases of respiratory failure of which 22% had peripheral edema. Farber and Manfredi have noted that approximately 50% of patients with COPD admitted to their intensive care unit have peripheral edema (Farber and Manfredi, 1991). Subsequently, Kilburn and Dowel described weight loss between 7 and 30 kg during recovery from respiratory failure in 39 patients (Kilburn and Dowel, 1971). The development of peripheral edema may be accompanied by pulmonary edema, which can be expected to adversely affect gas exchange. The pathogenesis of peripheral edema has been thought to arise from the following sequence: pulmonary hypertension, right ventricular failure, venous engorgement, and edema (Braunwald, 1987). Renal and hormonal perturbations have been identified, however, that may account for the development of peripheral edema. These include decreased renal perfusion and/or decreased sodium and water excretion due to hypercapnia and hypoxia (Farber et al, 1982), increased sympathetic tone (Henriksen et al, 1980), and activation of the renin-aldosterone system (Raff and Levy, 1986). It is controversial that a primary abnormality in left ventricular function may account for the development of peripheral and pulmonary edema in patients with COPD.

PHYSIOLOGIC ASSESSMENT

Evaluation of a patient with cardiopulmonary failure should include a detailed history, physical examination, and laboratory evaluation with a focus on defining the severity and etiology of the acute illness. Once respiratory failure is suspected, arterial blood gas analysis is usually performed. Interpretation of the arterial blood gas values may provide valuable insight into the precipitating etiology for respiratory failure in addition to defining the severity of hypercapnia and hypoxia. As a first step, assessment may be made whether the degree of lung disease accounts for observed hypercapnia. Patients with stable COPD and chronic hypercapnia usually have severely reduced airflow on pulmonary function testing as demonstrated by a forced expiratory volume in 1 second that is less than 1 liter (Javaheri et al, 1981). Even patients with lesser degrees of chronic airflow obstruction, however, may develop hypercapnia during an acute exacerbation.

Hypercapnic patients on physical examination usually demonstrate signs of hyperinflation and severe airflow obstruction. They may appear hyperinflated, with increased anteroposterior chest diameters and flattened diaphragms. On auscultation, they may exhibit limited air exchange with a markedly prolonged expiratory phase. If clinical evaluation does not reveal signs of severe obstructive dysfunction, the presence of a coexisting disease process may be suspected. These diseases may include congestive heart failure, infection with pneumonia, or obstructive sleep apnea syndrome, or sedative use.

Assessment of the arterial blood gas values should include evaluation of any observed hypoxemia. The mechanisms responsible for hypoxemia include a combination of hypoventilation, ventilation-perfusion mismatch, and shunt. If hypoventilation with an elevated arterial P_{CO_2} is observed, its effects on the arterial P_{O_2} should be evaluated first. The influence of hypercapnia on producing hypoxemia may be evaluated by calculation of the alveolar to arterial oxygen gradient (A-a gradient). This value is obtained by subtracting the arterial P_{O_2} ($P_{a_{O_2}}$) from the ideal alveolar P_{O_2} ($P_{A_{O_2}}$). The alveolar P_{O_2} is derived using the alveolar gas equation, as follows (Comroe, 1965):

$$P_{A_{O_2}} = F_{I_{O_2}}(P_B - 47) - P_{A_{CO_2}}[F_{I_{O_2}} + \frac{1 - F_{I_{O_2}}}{R}]$$

in which $F_{I_{O_2}}$ equals fraction of oxygen in inspired air, P_B equals barometric pressure, $P_{A_{CO_2}}$ equals mean alveolar P_{CO_2}, which is equal to arterial P_{CO_2}, and R equals respiratory exchange ratio. At sea level with the patient breathing room air and a respiratory exchange ratio of 0.8, this equation can be simplified as follows:

$$P_{A_{O_2}} = 149 - P_{A_{CO_2}} * 1.25$$

The presence of a normal or narrowed A-a gradient suggests that hypercapnia due to hypoventilation is the sole cause of hypoxemia. If the A-a gradient is widened, the observed hypoxemia is the result of either ventilation-perfusion mismatch or right-to-left shunting of blood flow. If the predominant mechanism for hypoxemia is ventilation-perfusion mismatch, administration of low concentrations of supplemental oxygen should correct the hypoxia. Failure to correct hypoxemia with low concentrations of supplemental oxygen should prompt suspicion of an anatomic shunt, which can be confirmed and quantitated from measurement of arterial P_{O_2} after 30 minutes of breathing 100% oxygen (Fig. 24–1).

If a right-to-left shunt is suspected, history, physical examination, and chest radiograph may reveal an alveolar filling process such as pulmonary edema or pneumonia that may account for

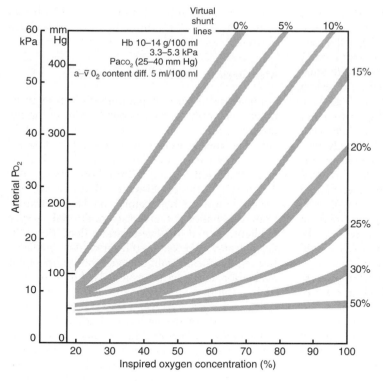

Figure 24–1
Iso-shunt diagram. On coordinates of inspired oxygen concentration (abscissa) and arterial P_{O_2} (ordinate), iso-shunt bands have been drawn to include all values of hemoglobin (*Hb*), Pa_{CO_2} and arterial-mixed venous oxygen content difference (*a-v̄ O_2 content diff*) shown above. (Redrawn from Nunn JF: Applied Respiratory Physiology, 2nd ed. Newton, MA, Butterworth and Heineman, 1993, p 459. With permission.)

the shunt. If no acute lung pathology is evident, an intracardiac shunt through an atrial septal defect or through a patent foramen ovale should be suspected. The presence of a patent foramen ovale may be further suggested by the observation of a rapidly improving anatomic shunt after administration of high concentrations of oxygen sufficient to improve oxygen saturation to levels greater than 90%. The mechanism for a rapid decrease in right-to-left shunt after treatment with oxygen is related to an acute decrease in pulmonary vascular pressures due to relief of hypoxic vasoconstriction.

TREATMENT

Treatment of patients with cardiorespiratory failure should be directed at the precipitating factor; treatment should also address the worsening cardiopulmonary status. Often these goals are addressed simultaneously. For example, treatment for worsening airflow obstruction may also be effective in improving hypercapnia and hypoxemia, although this is not always true. Complications of therapy in patients with severe airflow obstruction may result in major morbidity or even mortality. Complications include barotrauma related to dynamic hyperinflation, cardiovascular collapse due to elevated intrathoracic pressures from dynamic hyperinflation, and worsening hypercapnia and

acidosis due to sedative use. Thus, it is important to consider the risks as well as the benefits of a therapeutic strategy. In many cases, supportive care directed at bringing life-threatening hypoxemia and acidosis to a safe range (not necessarily to a normal range) coupled with therapy of the precipitating factor suffice, and iatrogenic complications are avoided.

Three basic guidelines can be developed for treatment of patients with cardiopulmonary failure.

1. Correct life-threatening hypoxemia and acidosis to a safe range (oxygen saturation greater than 90%, serum pH greater than 7.2)
2. Treat the underlying precipitating disease
3. Avoid complications

Measures to Correct Dyspnea

Increased airflow obstruction during acute exacerbations may cause significant respiratory symptoms. Treatments aimed at relieving bronchoconstriction, airway inflammation, and mucous plugging may be used to improve lung and airway mechanics. The mainstays of therapy include β_2-adrenergic agents, anticholinergic agents, methylxanthines, and corticosteroids (Sherman et al, 1991). Use of these agents in patients with respiratory failure is similar to use in patients with milder exacerbations except that the drugs are usually applied more intensively. Inhaled bronchodilators may be administered every 1 to 2 hours and should be titrated to each individual patient's needs. Theophylline should be dosed to maintain serum levels above 10 µg/ml to achieve a therapeutic effect but below 20 µg/ml to avoid toxicity. Corticosteroids may be given to decrease airway inflammation. In a controlled study performed by Albert and colleagues, significant improvement in airway function was demonstrated in patients treated with corticosteroids compared with function in patients that received placebo (Albert et al, 1980). Because the peak effects of corticosteroids may not occur for up to 9 to 12 hours after administration, corticosteroids should be started on admission to the hospital.

For some patients with COPD and respiratory failure, impaired expectoration of respiratory secretions may result in significant respiratory distress. For this subgroup of patients, it is reasonable to attempt empirical therapy to assist in removal of secretions. Therapeutic modalities include chest percussion and postural drainage. Patients should be encouraged to cough and take deep breaths, inhalation of heated humidified air is also recommended. Unfortunately, it is not known which of these procedures is most efficacious.

A significant group of patients remain tachypneic and dyspneic despite treatment of obstructive disease; they require mechanical ventilatory assistance. The indications for intubation and mechanical ventilation include severe hypoxemia not responsive to supplemental oxygen, hypercapnia with acidosis, inability to expectorate respiratory secretions, and need for airway protection against aspiration (Table 24–2). Strategies for implementing ventilatory assistance may lead to significant improvement in both respiratory rate and patient comfort. In one study, it was shown that a passive increase in tidal volume may lead to significant reductions in respiratory rate through reflexes mediated by stretch and/or irritant receptors (Berger et al, 1996). Although the use of sedatives to alleviate dyspnea is occasionally re-

quired, sedatives should be administered with caution so as to avoid worsening hypercapnia and acidosis.

Measures to Correct Hypoxemia

Clinical evaluation of patients with respiratory failure may provide an etiology for worsening hypoxemia and may suggest appropriate initial therapy. The mechanisms responsible for hypoxemia in patients with cardiopulmonary failure include a combination of hypoventilation, shunt, and ventilation-perfusion mismatch. The effects of hypoventilation on hypoxemia can be determined from calculation of alveolar to arterial oxygen gradient. When hypoventilation does not fully account for hypoxemia (elevated A-a gradient) history, physical examination, and radiographic evaluation may reveal an alveolar filling process, such as infiltrate or pulmonary edema, or pneumothorax, which may account for the hypoxemia. In patients without the presence of acute disease on radiographic evaluation, the presumed mechanism for hypoxemia is alteration in ventilation and perfusion. In this case, low concentrations of oxygen should be sufficient to correct the hypoxemia. If the hypoxemia remains refractory to low concentrations of oxygen, in the presence of a normal chest radiograph, intracardiac right-to-left shunting of blood through a patent foramen ovale should be suspected. In this case, higher concentrations of supplemental oxygen may be required to correct the hypoxemia.

Occasionally a significant elevation of P_{CO_2} occurs during oxygen therapy (Campbell, 1967). The elevation was assumed to occur because of removal of hypoxic ventilatory drive in a patient who already had a reduced ventilatory drive to CO_2. The increase in CO_2 that occurs as a result of oxygen therapy may result from changes in ventilation and perfusion (Aubier et al, 1980). Whatever the mechanism, it is important to correct hypoxemia despite an elevation in P_{CO_2}. Patients should not be left with a significant degree of hypoxemia to avoid acidosis. For those patients with worsening hypoventilation, the ensuing respiratory acidosis can be treated with ventilatory assistance.

Severe hypoxemia may be life-threatening and should be treated to maintain oxyhemoglobin saturation greater than 90%. If possible, treatment should be accomplished while avoiding the risk of oxygen toxicity and worsening hypoventilation and acidosis. These goals can usually be accomplished by increasing the arterial P_{O_2} level to approximately 60 mm Hg but not significantly higher. For patients in whom ventilation-perfu-

---

Table 24–2
Indications for Intubation and Mechanical Ventilation

Hypoxemia despite therapy with supplemental oxygen
Hypercapnia with an associated acidosis
Inability to expectorate respiratory secretions
Airway protection from aspiration

sion mismatch is mostly responsible for hypoxemia, increasing the P_{O_2} level can be achieved with administration of low-flow oxygen via a nasal cannula at 1 to 2 l/min. Alternatively, a Venturi mask can be employed to deliver low concentrations of oxygen (24–28%). For patients with intrapulmonary shunting due to an acute pneumonic process or intracardiac shunting due to a patent foramen ovale, higher concentrations of inspired oxygen are required in accord with the severity of the underlying shunt.

Measures to Correct Hypercapnia and Acidosis

The urgency for treatment of respiratory acidosis depends on the severity of the acidosis and the time period over which it has developed. Often, treatment of the underlying cause coupled with treatment of airflow obstruction suffices, with resolution of the acute increase in P_{CO_2}. If the acidosis is not life-threatening and does not interfere with other therapy, specific therapy is not indicated.

Bicarbonate therapy can correct a life-threatening acidosis in the acute stage. In addition, the increased pH allows other medications, such as bronchodilators, to work in a more beneficial pH range. In some circumstances, bicarbonate therapy may transiently mitigate the effects of severe hypercapnia (permissive hypercapnia, see later). Despite these advantages, therapy with bicarbonate has major drawbacks.

Administration of bicarbonate can be expected to acutely increase CO_2 production through neutralization of bicarbonate, producing carbonic acid, which is then dissociated into water and CO_2 in the presence of carbonic anhydrase. In a patient with limited cardiopulmonary reserve, such as a patient with respiratory failure, this increase in CO_2 production may lead to worsening hypercapnia and acidosis. In addition, although the serum pH improves with bicarbonate therapy, the intracellular acidosis may worsen. In another drawback, as the precipitating condition for respiratory acidosis improves, metabolic alkalosis can develop (Narins et al, 1984). For these reasons, bicarbonate therapy is usually reserved for patients who have life-threatening acidosis despite maximal medical therapy and despite attempts to correct the acidosis through an increased CO_2 excretion during mechanical ventilation.

For patients in whom the risks of bicarbonate therapy are prohibitive, acidosis can be corrected with buffers, such as tris(hydroxymethyl)aminomethane(TRIS)-buffer or carbicarb, that do not increase CO_2 production or increase intracellular acidosis (Conant and Hughs, 1961). The decision to use buffer therapy for life-threatening acidosis should also take into account the expected time until improvement of the underlying disease. For example, bicarbonate therapy may be withheld in a patient with acute asthma while intensive therapy with β-adrenergic agonists is begun. In contrast, a lower threshold for treatment may exist for a patient with fixed airway obstruction from emphysema.

Mechanical ventilatory support to the extent that it augments ventilation is usually effective in treating acidosis but may result in iatrogenic complications. These include pneumothorax, dynamic hyperinflation with the development of auto-PEEP, and cardiovascular collapse due to impaired venous return. These complication can be avoided by adopting a treatment strategy aimed at (1) minimizing airway pressures and dynamic hyperinflation, and (2) improving acidosis to a safe range without necessarily correcting the acidosis to normal (Darioli and Perret, 1984). Dynamic hyperinflation may be minimized by several techniques (Table 24–3), which have in common increasing the time available for exhalation (Tuxen and Lane, 1987). Increasing the time for exhalation can usually be accomplished by slow respiratory rates. High inspiratory flow rates may also be beneficial by shortening inspiratory time and thereby lengthening the time available for exhalation, but the technique carries the risk of raising peak inspiratory airway pressures. Although it may be difficult to decrease respiratory rate in patients with high intact respiratory drives, investigators in one study have suggested that a passive increase in tidal volume may result in a slowing of respiratory frequency through effects on vagal reflexes (Berger et al, 1996). The increase in peak inflation pressures that may result from an increase in tidal volume is not predictable in patients with COPD. Unpredictability is characteristic because the effects of increased tidal volume on airway pressure may be counteracted by the opposing effects of decreased auto-PEEP due to a slowing of respiratory rate. If airway pressures

---

Table 24–3
Ventilatory Strategies to Minimize Airway Pressures and Dynamic Hyperinflation

Decrease tidal volume
Decrease respiratory rate
Decrease inspiratory time (increase inspiratory flow)
Increase expiratory time

cannot be maintained in a safe range (plateau pressure <35 cm H_2O and peak pressure <50 cm H_2O) with this strategy, tidal volume may then be decreased. Because many patients cannot tolerate a decrease in respiratory rate and tidal volume, intravenous sedation may have to be administered. Although this strategy may result in only small increases in minute ventilation, a significant reduction in hypercapnia may result from a combination of a reduced metabolic rate secondary to sedation and the hyperbolic relationship between Pco_2 and alveolar ventilation (Fig. 24–2; see Chapter 2).

In some patients with severe airway obstruction, arterial Pco_2 may remain elevated; this should not be a concern if arterial pH remains above 7.2. Several studies have documented the safety of the strategy of permissive hypercapnia in the setting of severe airflow obstruction (Menitove and Goldring, 1983; Darioli and Perret, 1984). There are three different situations in which this strategy may be useful: (1) during the acute phase when Pco_2 is increasing due to increasing bronchospasm; (2) during the preparation for intervention such as bronchoscopy; and (3) during the extubation of the patient despite persistent hypercapnia (Menitove and Goldring, 1983). For any of these clinical settings, when arterial pH remains severely reduced, buffers such as bicarbonate or TRIS-buffer may be used to raise the serum pH to levels above 7.2. Alternatively, renal compensatory mechanisms result in elevation of serum bicarbonate with a subsequent return of pH toward normal. It is unclear which approach (buffer administration versus waiting for renal compensation) is optimal for treatment of refractory acidemia in patients with acute respiratory failure.

Ventilatory support may be applied with a noninvasive as well as an invasive technique (Garay et al, 1981; Meduri et al, 1989). Noninva-sive ventilation may obviate the need for intubation in select patients. Advantages of using noninvasive ventilation include maintenance of a patient's ability to clear respiratory secretions, eat, and communicate. Infections such as sinusitis and nosocomial pneumonia may be avoided, as may complications related to placement of an endotracheal tube including mucosal ulceration, mucosal edema, and tracheal stenosis. Selection of patients who are appropriate for noninvasive ventilation is critical. Patients with altered mental status, hemodynamic instability, or inability to tolerate the mask should be excluded from receiving noninvasive ventilatory support.

Having selected a patient for noninvasive ventilation, the next decision is choosing an interface between the patient and the ventilator. Nasal masks have frequently been utilized for nocturnal continuous positive airway pressure (CPAP) therapy. They offer less dead space, lower risk of claustrophobia, and lower risk of aspiration when compared with full face masks. Their use in dyspneic patients with acute respiratory failure, however, may be limited by persistent mouth breathing. Mouthpieces offer a third interface. They may, however, require a nose clip to prevent nasal breathing, and it may be difficult to maintain a tight seal around the mouthpiece for prolonged periods of time. Choice of a particular interface should be customized to an individual's needs and comfort.

Selection of a specific device for noninvasive ventilation has implications for its application. The choices of ventilators can be separated into two basic groups: (1) traditional ventilators used in the critical care unit; and (2) bilevel ventilators currently used for nocturnal treatment of sleep apnea. Traditional ventilators offer multiple modes of ventilation including volume and pressure control. These modes may facilitate hyperventilation of the patient, which may be desirable

Figure 24–2
The relationship between arterial Pco_2 and alveolar ventilation is plotted for a CO_2 production of 200 ml/min assuming a stable V_D/V_T of 0.25. For patients with pre-existing hypercapnia, a small increase in alveolar ventilation will result in a significant reduction in Pco_2.

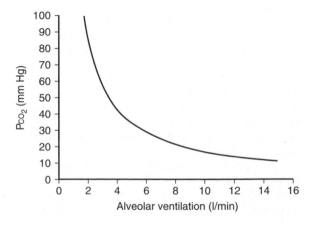

if the patient has significant acidosis. The drawbacks of these devices are that they were designed to operate in a leakproof system. A nasal or face mask commonly leads to problems from leakage of air around the mask. The reaction of the ventilator to leakage is dependent on the specific machine and mode. Whatever the response of the ventilator, significant dyssynchrony between the patient and ventilator may occur. The problems related to leakage can be remedied with a bilevel pressure device, which was initially intended for home care. These devices require a small air leak for proper functioning (Rapoport, 1987). Ventilator modes are limited, however, to spontaneous ventilation with pressure support or controlled ventilation with a pressure-controlled mode.

Strategies for noninvasive ventilation may need to be modified from those for invasive ventilation, which was outlined earlier.

Patients selected for noninvasive ventilation generally have an increased central respiratory drive related to superimposition of acute cardiopulmonary decompensation on a background of chronic disease. Because of the high central respiratory drive, it may not be possible to use a volume-controlled mode of ventilation to alter respiratory rate, inspiratory flow, and tidal volume to decrease dynamic hyperinflation and auto-PEEP. In addition, because maintenance of a normal mental status and intact central drive are prerequisites for therapy with noninvasive ventilation, sedatives cannot be employed to allow patients to adapt to a volume-controlled mode. Therefore, pressure-support ventilation is commonly chosen as the mode of noninvasive ventilation. It may not be possible to decrease the auto-PEEP. The persistent auto-PEEP presents a threshold load to the respiratory muscles and may contribute to the work of breathing, dyspnea, and tachypnea (Smith and Marini, 1988). Although the ventilator may be adjusted to deliver external PEEP to counteract the threshold load associated with auto-PEEP, the adverse hemodynamic effects related to PEEP may not be similarly decreased (Tuxen, 1989; Marini, 1989). Caution must, therefore, be exercised when setting external PEEP on the ventilator.

Noninvasive ventilation can be done in various ways in addition to substituting for invasive total mechanical support. Because of the ease of application of noninvasive ventilation, it may be used intermittently with the hope that benefits will persist between times when noninvasive ventilation is applied. One potential benefit of intermittent noninvasive ventilation is intermittent periods of increased ventilation with a consequent rise in pH that may stimulate renal excretion of excess bicarbonate (Cropp and Dimarco, 1987; Scano et al, 1990). Alternatively, intermittent ventilation may allow for respiratory muscle rest with a subsequent improvement in respiratory muscle function and ventilation (Braun and Marino, 1984; Bach and Alba, 1990; Carrey et al, 1990).

In addition to effects that may result in an improvement in total ventilation, noninvasive ventilation can help prevent the decrease in ventilation that often occurs during sleep (Garay et al, 1981). Because the sleep-associated decrease in ventilation is largely due to an increase in the resistance of the upper airway, CPAP may suffice, even without assisted ventilation, in preventing hypoventilation during sleep. This may be particularly important for patients who already have some degree of obstructive sleep apnea syndrome. If desired, a further increase in ventilation to relieve hypoxemia or hypercapnia can be achieved by adding assisted ventilation to CPAP therapy (Gay et al, 1991).

Measures to Correct an Edematous State

Approximately 20% of patients with COPD and respiratory failure may also have peripheral edema (Asmundsson and Kilburn, 1969). In one study, treatment of patients to relieve hypoxia resulted in water losses of as much as 30 kg (Kilburn and Dowell, 1971). Treatment should begin with optimizing ventilatory function and correcting hypoxemia and hypercapnia toward normal, as described previously. The importance of improving ventilation and hypoxemia is highlighted by patients who do not respond to diuretic or inotropic therapy and who respond only after correction of hypoxemia and hypercapnia. Often, a spontaneous diuresis occurs without the need for specific therapy if the Po_2 and oxygen saturation are increased.

Treatment of the underlying obstructive disease may have effects on cardiac function. Parker and colleagues have shown that pulmonary artery pressure and left ventricular stroke work may decrease with theophylline administration (Parker et al, 1966). Similarly, Matthay and coworkers reported that right ventricular as well as left ventricular function may improve during therapy with theophylline (Matthay et al, 1978). Both of these studies, however, failed to demonstrate beneficial effects on oxygen saturation. The β-adrenergic agonists may lead to pulmonary vasodilation, with a consequent decrease in pulmonary vascular resistance or an increase in myocardial performance due to a direct inotropic effect (Brent et al, 1982; MacNee et al 1983). Accordingly, numerous studies have demonstrated an improvement in right and left ventricular function associated with a decrease in pulmonary vascular resistance after terbutaline administration (Stockley et al, 1977; Teule and Majid, 1980). Despite these potential beneficial effects of theophylline and β-agonists, their use in patients with coexisting left ventricular disease can be associated with the precipitation of angina from an increase in heart rate and myocardial oxygen consumption. Patients therefore must be monitored closely for both beneficial and detrimental effects during therapy of underlying obstructive dysfunction.

Despite the beneficial effects of digitalis on myocardial contractility, its use in patients with cor pulmonale is probably not indicated unless there is coexisting left ventricular dysfunction (Berglund et al, 1963; Green and Smith, 1977). The lack of efficacy of digitalis is probably related to two factors: (1) pulmonary vasoconstriction with a consequent rise in pulmonary vascular resistance (Kim and Aviado, 1961), and (2) decrease in right ventricular preload with a subsequent fall in cardiac output (Sylvester et al, 1983). In addition, digitalis is associated with an increased risk of cardiac arrhythmias in patients already being treated with arrhythmogenic drugs who may also be hypokalemic. For these reasons, routine use of digitalis is not recommended.

Diuretic agents may be prescribed to patients with peripheral edema. The beneficial effects of diuretics are probably confined to patients with either overt pulmonary edema or increased central blood volume (Mathur et al, 1981). Use in patients with only peripheral edema needs to done with caution because hypochloremia, hypokalemia, and metabolic alkalosis may develop. In addition, adverse effects on cardiac output may occur because of a decrease in venous return. Therefore, close monitoring of hemodynamic status and serum electrolytes should be performed during therapy with diuretics.

Vasodilating agents for treatment of cor pulmonale were fueled by their beneficial effects in left ventricular failure. Because the hemodynamic effects of systemic vasodilators are complex, it is difficult to assess their effects in cor pulmonale. For example, the effects of pulmonary vasodilation on pulmonary artery pressure may be offset by an increase in cardiac output. Similarly, reduction in pulmonary artery pressure by agents such as nitroglycerin that decrease venous return may result in reduction in cardiac output. Vasodilators in patients with acute cardiopulmonary failure may be further complicated by the unstable hemodynamic status. For these reasons, vasodilators are not routinely prescribed in patients while they are acutely ill (Michael, 1991).

DISCONTINUATION OF MECHANICAL VENTILATION

Intubation and mechanical ventilation are associated with numerous short- and long-term complications. Withdrawal of mechanical ventilation and extubation should be done as soon as the patient can sustain ventilation without assistance. Discontinuation of support, however, re-exposes the patient to an increased work of breathing that may be difficult to sustain. This effect is particularly true in hyperinflation and alteration in thoracic structure that mechanically interferes with optimal function of the respiratory muscles. The patient may be further stressed by cardiovascular disorders and central ventilatory control abnormalities. Multiple strategies have been proposed for the evaluation of the patient during gradual withdrawal of support, but it is important to avoid prolongation of weaning because of an excessively complex stepwise protocol. Selection of a particular weaning protocol should be a secondary concern to optimizing a patient's cardiopulmonary status, which is often the critical factor determining weaning's success or failure.

The following six questions represent a rational approach to the evaluation of the patient who is a candidate for extubation:

1. Has there been sufficient improvement in the underlying obstructive disease?
2. Has the hypercapnia resolved and if not how should it be approached?
3. Has there been sufficient improvement in the acute illness that precipitated intubation?
4. Are there iatrogenic complications related to the patient's therapy that require correction to maximize the likelihood of successful extubation?
5. Are there any potential problems that may occur after extubation that require assessment and treatment?
6. What is the optimal weaning strategy?

Improvement in Underlying Lung Disease

Liberation of a patient from the ventilator should be timed to coincide with improvement of the acute and underlying diseases. Improvement of the obstructive airways disease may be noted from monitoring of the patient's respiratory status while on the ventilator. A decrease in airways resistance may be inferred from a decrease in peak inspiratory airway pressure. Often, a corresponding decrease in plateau pressures may be noted, indicating a reduction in dynamic hyperinflation and auto-PEEP. In addition, before extubation, hypoxemia due to either shunt or ventilation-perfusion mismatch improves sufficiently that supplemental oxygen can be administered adequately without the ventilator.

Approach to Persistent Hypercapnia

Although clinical improvement is usually accompanied by return of hypercapnia to its baseline value, this is not always true. Clinically it may be difficult to distinguish established chronic hypercapnia from an acute decompensation state from which the patient has not been able to recover. One approach to distinguishing these situations is to normalize arterial PCO_2 and acid-base status using mechanical ventilation before extubation. Although this approach carries the risk of producing significant acidosis after extubation in the patient who is unable to maintain the required ventilation, careful monitoring at the time of extubation identifies acidosis and allows reinstitution of mechanical support. In contrast, some patients show a resetting of PCO_2 in response to the normalization maneuver and are able to maintain eucapnia (Garay et al, 1981). Removing the hypercapnia is beneficial because it optimizes arterial PO_2 (based on the alveolar gas equation), thereby raising the likelihood that a patient will not require therapy with supplemental oxygen. For a patient unable to maintain a normal PCO_2 or whose acute episode has led to a marked progression of disease, it is reasonable to avoid normalizing the PCO_2. A better choice is to correct PCO_2 to a sustainable level. When in doubt, however, our policy has been to allow the patient a trial of a normal PCO_2 level.

Improvement in Acute Precipitating Illness

Since patients with cardiopulmonary failure require intubation and mechanical ventilation because of the added stress of an acute disease on a background of limited cardiopulmonary reserve, improvement of the inciting illness is a prerequisite to an attempt at extubation. Specifically, there should be improvement of abnormal mental status, control of respiratory infection, and reduction of respiratory secretions.

Particular attention must be given to any underlying left ventricular cardiac dysfunction. Positive-pressure ventilation produces a positive intrathoracic pressure, which raises left ventricular end-diastolic pressure relative to aortic pressure, thereby reducing left ventricular afterload (Grace and Greenbaum, 1982)(see Chapters 4 and 15). Upon discontinuation of mechanical ventilation, this positive intrathoracic pressure is replaced by the negative pressure from spontaneous ventilation, which may have the opposite effect and may increase left ventricular afterload (Buda et al, 1979, Scharf et al 1979). The degree to which this influences left ventricular function in the tidal range in patients with COPD, however, has yet to be determined. Thus, removing positive-pressure ventilation may stress cardiac performance (see Chapter 15). Optimization of left ventricular performance through medications and techniques to improve intravascular volume status is essential.

Correction of Iatrogenic Complications

Metabolic alkalosis can occur as a result of aggressive diuretic therapy and can decrease central respiratory drive. Several factors contribute to generation and maintenance of alkalosis, including reduced serum chloride and potassium levels, which prevent renal excretion of bicarbonate. Chloride depletion can be treated with potassium chloride supplementation, which is given until chloride appears in the urine independent of diuretic administration (if this can be achieved).

Persistent sedation and paralysis may also interfere with extubation. Long-lasting fat-soluble agents (barbiturates and benzodiazepines) may be extensively stored in the body, and they take a long time to clear. This mechanism is particularly relevant for patients with either hepatic or renal disease. An increasing body of evidence shows an interaction between paralytic agents and corticosteroids resulting in myopathy and prolonged muscle weakness, which is particularly relevant to asthmatic patients (Gooch et al, 1991; Kupfer et al, 1992). All of these conditions are marked by altered mental status, severe hypoventilation, and decreased or absent ventilatory effort. Frank apneas, however, may or may not be present in the absence of sleep. Persistent paralysis may be confirmed by applying a peripheral nerve stimulator. These findings are in contrast to the severe respiratory distress that characterizes a patient limited by lung function.

Potential Post-extubation Problems

Sleep effects on control of breathing and on the upper airway may also interfere with the removal of mechanical ventilation. It is important to anticipate post-extubation problems, particularly when obstructive or central sleep apnea is suspected. Even in the absence of apnea, removal of the endotracheal tube re-exposes the patient to the normal increase in upper airway resistance related to sleep, which may be exacerbated by post-intubation laryngeal edema. For clinical situations in which central sleep apnea and hypoventilation are suspected (hypercapnia out of proportion to lung disease, severe obesity with a history of snoring, and coexisting neuromuscular disease), evaluation is necessary of spontaneous *unsupported* ventilation during a period of sleep while the patient is intubated. The evaluation allows detection of a regulatory abnormality when there is no possibility of upper airway obstruction due to the presence of the endotracheal tube. Having such an evaluation as a baseline allows the clinician to better interpret hypoventilation and periodic breathing that may occur after extubation and be either obstructive or central in origin.

When sleep-related problems are identified, several approaches to intermediate levels of airway or ventilatory support are available after extubation. Although central apnea and hypoventilation may require ongoing ventilatory support, which may be supplied noninvasively, it is sufficient in cases of obstructive apnea and hypoventilation to apply nocturnal nasal CPAP to combat the increase in upper airway resistance. The determination of an appropriate pressure setting may require monitoring the patient for any apnea, hypopnea, or oxygen desaturation that would prompt an increase in pressure.

Optimal Weaning Strategy

The most important factor to consider in choosing a strategy for discontinuation of mechanical ventilation is to avoid prolongation of weaning and extubation because of a stepwise protocol. Therefore, before initiating a plan for gradual withdrawal of ventilatory support, it is reasonable to assess the patient's ability to breathe spontaneously without support. The trial of spontaneous ventilation can be conducted either with a T-piece or with a small amount of pressure support to counteract the pressure drop due to endotracheal tube resistance (usually about 5 cm H_2O). If spontaneous ventilation cannot be sustained, an evaluation to determine the reason for failure should be undertaken to develop a treatment plan for its correction.

There has been renewed interest in different strategies for the gradual discontinuation of mechanical ventilation (Brochard et al, 1994; Esteban et al, 1995). As with prior experiments, these studies failed to identify the optimal protocol for success. Therefore, choice of a particular

weaning protocol is usually dependent upon the practitioner's experience and comfort with a reliable technique.

REFERENCES

Agarwal JB, Paltoo R, and Palmer WH: Relative viscosity of blood at varying hematocrits in pulmonary circulation. J Appl Physiol 29:866–871, 1970.

Albert RK, Martin TR, and Lewis SW: Controlled clinical trial of methylprednisolone in patients with chronic bronchitis and acute respiratory insufficiency. Ann Intern Med 92:753–758, 1980.

Anthonisen NR, Manfreda J, Warren CPW, et al: Antibiotic therapy in exacerbations of chronic obstructive pulmonary disease. Ann Intern Med 106:196–203, 1987.

Asmundsson T and Kilburn KH: Survival of acute respiratory failure. Ann Intern Med 70:471–485, 1969.

Aubier M, Murciano D, Milic-Emili J, et al: Effects of the administration of O_2 on ventilation and blood gases in patients with chronic obstructive pulmonary disease during acute respiratory failure. Am Rev Respir Dis 122:747–754, 1980.

Bach JR and Alba AS: Management of chronic alveolar hypoventilation by nasal ventilation. Chest 97:52–57, 1990.

Baum GL and Fisher FD: The relationship of fatal pulmonary insufficiency with cor pulmonale, right-sided mural thrombi and pulmonary emboli: A preliminary report. Am J Med Sci 240:609–612, 1960.

Berger HJ, Matthay RA, Loke J, et al: Assessment of cardiac performance with quantitative radionuclide angiography: Right ventricular ejection fraction with reference to findings in chronic obstructive disease. Am J Cardiol 41:897–905, 1978.

Berger KI, Sorkin IB, Norman RG, et al: Mechanism of relief of tachypnea during pressure support ventilation. Chest 109:1320–1327, 1996.

Berglund E, Widimsky J, and Malmberg R: Lack of effect of digitalis in patients with pulmonary disease with and without heart failure. Am J Cardiol 11:477–482, 1963.

Bounameaux H, Cirafici D, DeMoerloose P, et al: Measurement of D-dimer in patients as a diagnostic aid in suspected pulmonary embolism. Lancet 337:196–200, 1991.

Bradley CA, Fleetham JA, and Anthonisen NR: Ventilatory control in patients with hypoxemia due to obstructive lung disease. Am Rev Respir Dis 120:21–30, 1979.

Braun NMT and Marino WD: Effect of daily intermittent rest of the respiratory muscles in patients with severe chronic airflow limitation (CAL). Chest 85:595–596, 1984.

Braunwald E: Edema. In Braunwald E, Isselbacher KJ, Petersdorf RG, et al (eds): Harrison's Principles of Internal Medicine, 11th ed. New York, McGraw-Hill, 1987, p 149.

Braunwald E, Binion JT, Morgan WL, et al: Alterations in central blood volume and cardiac output induced by positive pressure breathing and counteracted by metaraminol (Aramine). Circ Res 5:670–675, 1957.

Brent BN, Mohler D, Berger HJ, et al: Augmentation of right ventricular performance in chronic obstructive pulmonary disease by terbutaline: A combined radionuclide and hemodynamic study. Am J Cardiol 50:313–319, 1982.

Brochard L, Rauss A, Benito S, et al: Comparison of three methods of gradual withdrawal from ventilatory support during weaning from mechanical ventilation. Am J Respir Crit Care Med 150:896–903, 1994.

Buda AS, Pinsky MR, Ingles NB, et al: Effect of intrathoracic pressure on left ventricular performance. N Engl J Med 301:453–459, 1979.

Buscho R, Saxtan D, Shultz P, et al: Infections with viruses and Mycoplasma pneumoniae during exacerbations of chronic bronchitis. J Infect Dis 377:377–383, 1978.

Campbell EJM: The J. Burns Amberson Lecture: The management of acute respiratory failure in chronic bronchitis and emphysema. Am Rev Respir Dis 96:626–639, 1967.

Campbell EJM, Freedman S, Smith PS, et al: The ability of man to detect added elastic loads to breathing. Clin Sci 20:223–231, 1961.

Carrey Z, Gottfried SB, and Levy RD: Ventilatory muscle support in respiratory failure with nasal positive pressure ventilation. Chest 97:150–158, 1990.

Catterall JR, Calverley PMA, MacNee W, et al: Mechanism of transient nocturnal hypoxemia in hypoxic chronic bronchitis and emphysema. J Appl Physiol 59:1698–1703, 1985.

Cohen CA, Zagelbaum G, Gross D, et al: Clinical manifestations of inspiratory muscle fatigue. Am J Med 73:308–316, 1982.

Comroe JH. Alveolar ventilation. In Comroe JH (ed): Physiology of Respiration. Chicago, Year Book Medical Publishers, 1965, p 17.

Conant JS and Hughs RE: The usefulness of THAM in metabolic acidosis. Ann N Y Acad Sci 92:751–754, 1961.

Cordova C, Musca A, Violi F, et al: Platelet hyperfunction in patients with chronic airway obstruction. Eur J Respir Dis 66:9–12, 1985.

Cournand A, Motley HL, Werko L, et al: Physiologic studies of the effect of intermittent positive pressure breathing on cardiac output in man. Am J Physiol 152:162–174, 1948.

Cropp A and Dimarco AF: Effects of intermittent negative pressure ventilation on respiratory muscle function in patients with severe chronic obstructive pulmonary disease. Am Rev Respir Dis 136:1056–1061, 1987.

Dalen JE and Alpert JS: Natural history of pulmonary embolism. Prog Cardiovasc Dis 17:259–270, 1975.

Darioli R and Perret C: Mechanical controlled hypoventilation in status asthmaticus. Am Rev Respir Dis 129:385–387, 1984.

Davidson A, Chandrasekaran K, Guida L, et al: Enhancement of hypoxemia by atrial shunting in cystic fibrosis. Chest 98:543–545, 1990.

Douglas NJ, White DP, Pickett CK, et al: Respiration during sleep in normal man. Thorax 37:840–844, 1982a.

Douglas NJ, White DP, Weil JV, et al: Hypercapnic ventilatory response in sleeping adults. Am Rev Respir Dis 126:758–762, 1982b.

Esteban A, Frutos F, Tobin MJ, et al: A comparison of four methods of weaning patients from mechanical ventilation. Spanish Lung Failure Collaborative Group. N Engl J Med 332:345–350, 1995.

Farber MO and Manfredi F: Sodium and water metabolism in COPD. In Cherniack NS (ed): Chronic Obstructive Pulmonary Disease. Philadelphia, WB Saunders, 1991, p 216.

Farber MO, Roberts LR, Weinberger MH, et al: Abnormalities of sodium and H_2O handling in chronic obstructive lung disease. Arch Intern Med 142:1326–1330, 1982.

Fishman AP: Chronic cor pulmonale. Am Rev Respir Dis 114:775–794, 1976.

Flenley DC: Oxygen therapy in the treatment of COPD. In Cherniack NS (ed): Chronic Obstructive Pulmonary Disease. Philadelphia, WB Saunders, 1991, p 468.

Gandevia SC, Killian KJ, and Campbell EJM: The effect of respiratory muscle fatigue on respiratory sensation. Clin Sci 60:463–466, 1981.

Garay SM, Turino GM, and Goldring RM: Sustained reversal of chronic hypercapnia in patients with alveolar hypoventilation syndromes: Long term maintenance with noninvasive nocturnal mechanical ventilation. Am J Med 70:269–274, 1981.

Gay PC, Patel AM, Viggiano RW, et al: Nocturnal nasal ventilation for treatment of patients with hypercapnic respiratory failure. Mayo Clin Proc 66:695–703, 1991.

Gooch JL, Suchyta MR, Balbierz JM, et al: Prolonged paralysis after treatment with neuromuscular blocking drugs. Crit Car Med 19:1125–1131, 1991.

Gould GA, Gugger M, Molloy J, et al: Breathing pattern and eye movement density during REM sleep in man. Am Rev Respir Dis 138:874–877, 1988.

Grace MP and Greenbaum DM: Cardiac performance in response to PEEP in patients with cardiac dysfunction. Crit Care Med 20:358–360, 1982.

Green LH and Smith TW: The use of digitalis in patients with pulmonary disease. Ann Intern Med 89:459–465, 1977.

Gump DW, Phillips CA, Forsyth BR, et al: Role of infection in chronic bronchitis. Am Rev Respir Dis 113:465–474, 1976.

Haas H, Morris JF, Samson S, et al: Bacterial flora of the respiratory tract in chronic bronchitis:

Comparison of transtracheal, fiber-bronchoscopic and oropharyngeal sampling methods. Am Rev Respir Dis 13:41–47, 1977.

Hagen PT, Scholz DG, and Edwards WD: Incidence and size of patent foramen ovale during the first ten decades of life: An autopsy study of 965 normal hearts. Mayo Clin Proc 59:17–20, 1984.

Harris P, Segel N, Creen I, et al: The influence of airways resistance and alveolar pressure on the pulmonary vascular resistance in chronic bronchitis. Cardiovasc Res 2:84–92, 1968.

Henriksen JH, Christensen NJ, Kok-Jensen A, et al: Increased plasma noradrenaline concentration in patients with chronic obstructive lung disease: Relation to hemodynamics and blood gases. Scand J Clin Lab Invest 40:419–427, 1980.

Hudgel DW, Martin RJ, Johnson B, et al: Mechanics of the respiratory system and breathing pattern during sleep in normal man. J Appl Physiol 56:133–137, 1984.

Javaheri S, Blum J, and Kazemi H: Pattern of breathing and carbon dioxide retention in chronic obstructive lung disease. Am J Med 71:228–234, 1981.

Johnson MW and Remmers JE: Accessory muscle activity during sleep in chronic obstructive pulmonary disease. J Appl Physiol 57:1011–1017, 1984.

Kachel RG: Left ventricular function in chronic obstructive disease. Chest 74:286–290, 1978.

Kawakami Y, Kishi F, Yamamoto H, et al: Relation of oxygen delivery, mixed venous oxygenation, and pulmonary hemodynamics to prognosis in chronic obstructive pulmonary disease. N Engl J Med 308:1045–1049, 1983.

Kilburn KH: Neurologic manifestations of respiratory failure. Arch Intern Med 115:155–160, 1965.

Kilburn KH and Dowell AR: Renal function in respiratory failure. Arch Intern Med 127:754–762, 1971.

Killian KJ and Campbell EJM: Dyspnea and exercise. Ann Rev Physiol 45:465–479, 1983.

Kim YS and Aviado DM: Digitalis and the pulmonary circulation. Am Heart J 62:680–686, 1961.

Kuller L, Ockene J, Townsend M, et al: The epidemiology of pulmonary function and COPD mortality in the multiple risk factor intervention trial. Am Rev Respir Dis 140:S76–81, 1989.

Kupfer JL, Namba T, Kaldawi E, et al: Prolonged weakness after long-term infusion of vecuronium. Ann Intern Med 117:484–486, 1992.

Leeder SR: Role of infection in the cause of chronic bronchitis. J Infect Dis 131:731–742, 1975.

Lensing AW, Pradoni P, Brandjes D, et al: Detection of deep venous thrombosis by real time B-mode ultrasonography. N Engl J Med 320:342–345, 1989.

Levison H and Cherniack RM: Ventilatory cost of exercise in chronic obstructive pulmonary disease. J Appl Physiol 25:21–27, 1968.

Lopes JM, Tabachnik E, Muller NL, et al: Total airway resistance and respiratory muscle activity during sleep. J Appl Physiol 54:773–777, 1983.

MacNee W, Wathen CG, Hannan WJ, et al: Effects of pirbuterol and sodium nitroprusside on pulmonary hemodynamics in hypoxic cor pulmonale. Br Med J 287:1169–1172, 1983.

Mahler DA, Brent BN, Loke J, et al: Right ventricular performance and central circulatory hemodynamics during upright exercise in patients with chronic obstructive pulmonary disease. Am Rev Respir Dis 130:722–729, 1984.

Marini JJ: Should PEEP be used in airflow obstruction. Am Rev Respir Dis 140:1–3, 1989.

Mathur PN, Pugsley SO, Powles ACP, et al: Effects of diuretics on cardiopulmonary performance in severe chronic airflow obstruction. Arch Intern Med 144:2154–2157, 1981.

Matthay RA, Berger HJ, Davies RA, et al: Right and left ventricular exercise performance in chronic obstructive pulmonary disease: Radionuclide assessment. Ann Intern Med 93:234–239, 1980.

Matthay RA, Berger HJ, Loke J, et al: Effects of aminophylline on right and left ventricular performance in chronic obstructive pulmonary disease: Noninvasive assessment by radionuclide angiocardiography. Am J Med 65:903–910, 1978.

Meduri GU, Conoscenti CC, Menashe P, et al: Noninvasive face mask ventilation in patients with acute respiratory failure. Chest 95:865–870, 1989.

Menitove SM and Goldring RM: Combined ventilator and bicarbonate strategy in the management of status asthmaticus. Am J Med 74:898–901, 1983.

Michael JR: Pulmonary vasodilators in the treatment of bronchitis and emphysema. In Cherniack NS (ed): Chronic Obstructive Pulmonary Disease. Philadelphia, WB Saunders, 1991, p 481.

Moser K, Lemoine J, Nachtwey R, et al: Deep venous thrombosis and pulmonary embolism: Frequency in a respiratory intensive care unit. JAMA 246:1422–1424, 1981.

Narins RG, Jones ER, and Dornfeld LP: Alkali therapy of the organic acidoses: A critical assessment of the data and the case for judicious use of sodium bicarbonate. In Narins RG (ed): Controversies in Nephrology and Hypertension. New York, Churchill Livingstone, 1984, p 359.

Nunn JF: Applied Respiratory Physiology, 2nd ed. Newton, MA, Butterworth and Heineman, 1993, p 459.

Parker JO, Kelkar K, and West RO: Hemodynamic effects of aminophylline in cor pulmonale. Circulation 33:17–25, 1966.

PIOPED Investigators: Value of ventilation/perfusion scan in acute pulmonary embolism: Results of the PIOPED. JAMA 263:2753–2759, 1990.

Pontoppidan H, Geffin B, and Lowenstein E: Acute respiratory failure in the adult (part 1). N Engl J Med 287:690–698, 1972.

Posner JB and Plum F: Spinal fluid pH and neurologic symptoms in systemic acidosis. N Engl J Med 277:605–606, 1967.

Raff H and Levy SA: Renin-angiotensin II–aldosterone and ACTH-cortisol control during hypoxemia and exercise in patients with chronic obstructive pulmonary disease. Am Rev Respir Dis 133:396–399, 1986.

Rapoport DM: Techniques for administering nasal CPAP. Respir Management 17:17–21, 1987.

Roussos C: Ventilatory failure and respiratory muscles. In Roussos C, and Macklem PT (eds): The Thorax, Part B. New York, Marcel Dekker, 1985, p 1253.

Scano G, Gigliotti F, Duranti R, et al: Changes in ventilatory muscle function with negative pressure ventilation in patients with severe COPD. Chest 97:322–327, 1990.

Scharf SM, Brown R, Tow DE, and Parisi AF: Cardiac effects of increased lung volume and decreased pleural pressure in man. J Appl Physiol 47:257–262, 1979.

Sherman CB, Osmanski JP, and Hudson LD: Acute exacerbations in COPD patients. In Cherniack NS (ed): Chronic Obstructive Pulmonary Disease. Philadelphia, WB Saunders, 1991.

Sideris D, Katsadoros D, Valianos G, et al: Types of cardiac dysrhythmias in respiratory failure. Am Heart J 89:32–35, 1975.

Smith TC and Marini JJ: Impact of PEEP on lung mechanics and work of breathing in severe airflow obstruction. J Appl Physiol 65:1488–1499, 1988.

Stockley RA, Finnegan P, and Bishop JM: Effect of intravenous terbutaline on arterial blood gas tensions, ventilation, and pulmonary circulation in patients with chronic bronchitis and cor pulmonale. Thorax 32:601–605, 1977.

Sylvester JT, Goldber HS, and Permutt S: The role of the vasculature in the regulation of cardiac output. Clin Chest Med 4:111–126, 1983.

Teule GJJ and Majid PA: Hemodynamic effects of terbutaline in chronic obstructive airways disease. Thorax 35:536–542, 1980.

Tuxen DV: Detrimental effects of positive end-expiratory pressure during controlled mechanical ventilation of patients with severe airflow obstruction. Am Rev Respir Dis 140:5–9, 1989.

Tuxen DV and Lane S: The effects of ventilatory pattern on hyperinflation, airway pressures, and circulation in mechanical ventilation of patients with severe airflow obstruction. Am Rev Respir Dis 136:872–879, 1987.

Weitzenblum E, Sautegeau A, Ehrhart M, et al: Long-term course of pulmonary arterial pressure in chronic obstructive pulmonary disease. Am Rev Respir Dis 130:993–998, 1984.

Wheeler HB, O'Donnell JA, Anderson FA, et al: Occlusive impedance phlebography: A diagnostic procedure for venous thrombosis and pulmonary embolism. Prog Cardiovasc Dis 17:199–205, 1974.

White DP, Weil JV, and Zwillich CK: Metabolic rate and breathing during sleep. J Appl Physiol 59:384–391, 1985.

Wise RA: COPD and the peripheral circulation. In Cherniack NS (ed): Chronic Obstructive Pulmonary Disease. Philadelphia, WB Saunders, 1991, p 167.

Wright JL, Lawson L, Pare PD, et al: The structure and function of the pulmonary vasculature in mild chronic obstructive pulmonary disease: The effect of oxygen and exercise. Am Rev Respir Dis 128:702–707, 1983.

Young T, Palta M, Dempsey J, et al: The occurrence of sleep-disordered breathing among middle-aged adults. N Engl J Med 328:1230–1235, 1993.

CHAPTER 25

Smoke Inhalation Injury

Harly E. Greenberg, M.D.

Jean K. Fleischman, M.D.

More than 5000 fatalities result from fire-related injuries each year in the United States. Most studies estimate that 50 to 70% of these deaths occur as a result of pulmonary complications (Pruitt et al, 1970). Thus, damage to the respiratory tract, largely resulting from inhalation of toxic substances found in smoke, accounts in large part for the morbidity and mortality of fire-related injuries.

Although thermal injury to the respiratory tract occurs in fires, burns are usually confined to the upper airway because of the efficient heat-exchanging capacity of the nasopharynx and oropharynx. Upper airway burns may cause life-threatening airway obstruction. In addition, chemical injury to the upper and lower respiratory tract may occur from inhalation of toxic components of smoke (Cahalane and Demling, 1984). Current evidence suggests that the toxicity of most of these substances results primarily from oxidants in the particulate fraction of smoke, which can damage the lipid component of cell membranes. Strong acids and alkalis may also be created when water-soluble gases in smoke react with water on the mucous membrane surface of the airways, resulting in mucosal ulceration, edema, and bronchospasm. Mucociliary clearance may also be severely impaired, resulting in airway plugging by mucus, soot, and cellular debris. Profound injury and necrosis with sloughing of the airway mucosa also occur, with substantial compromise of pulmonary function. Subsequently, alveolar capillary leak may develop, resulting in further pulmonary compromise (Cahalane and Demling, 1984). Systemic inflammation from burn injury or sepsis may exacerbate the pulmonary injury owing to activation of mediators of inflammation. Sepsis, pneumonia, and adult respiratory distress syndrome may later supervene, further increasing morbidity and mortality.

Much has been learned about the pathophysiology of smoke inhalation injury from animal models. This information has led to improvement in the management of affected patients. However, controlled smoke inhalation studies, with well-characterized gaseous and particulate smoke components, may not fully reflect respiratory damage resulting from household and industrial fires. In such fires, exposure to many different toxic gases may occur, depending on the fuel burned, oxygen available, and combustion method. Furthermore, investigators employing animal models for exposure to different types of smoke have identified somewhat different pathophysiologic processes with each type of smoke.

In this chapter, basic mechanisms of smoke-induced pulmonary injury are presented initially. Subsequently, the clinical features and management of smoke inhalation injury are discussed.

TOXIC COMPONENTS OF THE PRODUCTS OF COMBUSTION

Smoke is comprised of both gaseous and particulate phases. The gas phase contains many toxic substances such as carbon monoxide and cyanide. In addition, many oxidants, in particular, aldehydes, are present in the gas phase of smoke. Burning of plastics and polyvinyl chloride materials releases hydrogen chloride, phosgene, and chlorine. Substances with both short- and long-acting oxidant activity are present. The particulate phase of smoke, which consists of particles 0.1 to 10 μm in diameter, is also potentially injurious because many oxidants found in the gas phase are also adherent to these particles. In addition, heavy metals, which have the potential to produce damaging free radicals, may also be present in the particulate component of smoke (Lalonde, 1994a). Although the nasopharynx removes most particles with a diameter of more than 5 μm, mouth breathing, which frequently occurs during fires as a result of nasopharyngeal irritation, bypasses this protective mechanism. Furthermore, large tidal volumes, which may be necessary particularly if the person is attempting to escape from the fire, increase distal airway and alveolar deposition of particles. These particles may be especially injurious in that they have the propensity to adhere to airway and alveolar epithelium and can result in continued oxidant release and progressive cellular damage. Components of cotton smoke, a well-characterized smoke used in many animal models of smoke inhalation injury, are listed in Table 25–1.

A study in an ovine model compared pulmonary injury resulting from whole cotton smoke with that resulting from particulate-filtered smoke (gaseous phase only) (Lalonde et al, 1994a). Peak carboxyhemoglobin levels were similar after both exposures, indicating similar degrees of gas phase exposure. Tissue samples for pulmonary pathology examination 24 hours after whole smoke exposure were characterized by sloughing and ulceration of

Table 25–1
Toxic Components of Cotton Smoke

Gas Phase	Particulate Phase
Carbon monoxide	Soot particles
Oxidants	Adherent substances
Aldehydes	Heavy metals
Formaldehyde	Stable oxidants
Acrolein	Aldehydes
Hydrogen chloride	Other hydrocarbons
Phosgene	
Chlorine	

From Haponik EF, Summer ER: Respiratory complications in burned patients: pathogenesis and spectrum of inhalation injuries. J Crit Care 2:49–53, 1987.

the airway mucosa and severe submucosal edema and bronchorrhea. Alveolar injury was confined to atelectases, with only minor increases in extravascular lung water. In contrast, no significant airway or alveolar injury was evident after exposure to particle-free smoke. One explanation for these results is that oxidants, which are major toxic components of smoke, require direct and prolonged tissue contact provided by adherent particulate matter to produce epithelial damage. In contrast, oxidant activity in the gas phase is extremely short-lived (Lachocki et al, 1988). Thus, pulmonary damage during the first 24 hours after smoke exposure is primarily a result of compounds delivered to the lung via the particulate phase of smoke.

OXIDANT ACTIVITY AND PULMONARY INJURY FROM SMOKE INHALATION

Mechanisms of lung injury resulting from substances in the particulate phase of smoke remain under investigation. Lipid peroxidation has been found to correlate with cellular injury as well as with alveolar capillary permeability in several lung injury models (Demling and Lalonde, 1990), and this may be one mechanism by which pulmonary injury from smoke inhalation occurs. Such injury may occur from oxidants such as oxygen radicals, which are present in large quantities in smoke released in most household fires. Such oxidants have been demonstrated to remain active for longer than 20 minutes (Lachocki et al, 1989). Furthermore, the systemic inflammatory response to burn injury or infection may release additional oxidants. Release of free iron from ferritin can lead to further oxidant injury owing to damaging hydroxyl radical formation (Cosgrove et al, 1985).

These oxidants may cause epithelial injury by lipid peroxidation, which damages cell membranes.

Oxidants may also deactivate endogenous antiproteases, increasing tissue damage from proteases released as part of the inflammatory process. A number of inflammatory mediators, including prostanoids, leukotrienes, and other chemoattractants and neuropeptides having the capacity to alter bronchovascular tone, bronchial blood flow, and microvascular permeability, may also be activated by oxidants (Lansing et al, 1991). The airway mucosa is particularly vulnerable to oxidant-mediated damage because of its direct exposure to smoke and its particulate components.

Studies of airway lavage fluid from animals exposed to cotton smoke have demonstrated evidence of increased oxidant activity as measured by malondialdehyde levels, a marker of tissue lipid peroxidation (Lalonde et al, 1994b). In these studies, however, markers of lipid peroxidation were not evident in lung parenchymal samples at 24 hours after smoke exposure, suggesting that lipid peroxidation is primarily at the level of airways and not at the alveoli at that interval. Lipid peroxidation and injury to the airways were attenuated in this model by aerosolization of the iron chelator deferoxamine, implicating iron-induced free radical formation in oxidant damage to airway mucosa (Lalonde et al, 1994b).

Antioxidant systems may also be affected by smoke inhalation. Catalase, which is an important antioxidant, may be inactivated by oxidants (Kono and Fridovich, 1982). Catalase levels were noted to be reduced in pulmonary as well as other tissues in a rat smoke inhalation model in association with increased levels of markers of lipid peroxidation (Lalonde et al, 1994c). Histologic findings included severe pulmonary congestion with large areas of atelectasis. Airway edema was prominent, and free fluid was evident in airway lumens. Alveolar flooding was also seen, as was neutrophil sequestration in the lung parenchyma. The extent of lipid peroxidation, as measured by malondialdehyde levels, was found to be correlated with histologic lung changes. Furthermore, a dose-response relationship was evident between the degree of alveolar edema and atelectasis and the amount of smoke exposure (Lalonde et al, 1994c).

In the ovine cotton smoke exposure model, during the first 24 hours after smoke inhalation, the site of injury is predominantly limited to the airways because no increase in alveolar capillary permeability is noted at that interval, as assessed by lung lymph to plasma protein ratio (Demling et al, 1993). This finding is consistent with the clinical course of smoke inhalation injury, in which radiographic evidence of alveolar filling is uncommon during the first 24 hours (Tranbaugh et al, 1983). The increase in lung water seen early after smoke inhalation is probably primarily a consequence of elevated permeability of the bronchial circulation with subsequent bronchorrhea. Any alveolar flooding that occurs during the first 24 hours after smoke injury is likely to be a result of retrograde filling from the airways.

IMPORTANCE OF THE SYSTEMIC INFLAMMATORY RESPONSE IN LUNG INJURY

When the same smoke inhalation injury is combined with a body surface burn in the ovine model, the degree of lung parenchymal peroxidation and decrease in antioxidant defenses is substantially augmented (Tranbaugh et al, 1983). This increase in lung tissue peroxidation in the setting of a concomitant body surface burn is likely to result from activation of a systemic inflammatory response, which produces or activates mediators of inflammation. These inflammatory mediators then deliver oxidant activity to the pulmonary endothelial surface.

The role of the systemic inflammatory response in magnifying pulmonary injury after smoke inhalation has been further elucidated in a rat model of exposure to the oxidant gas phosgene (Ghio et al, 1991). Clinically, exposure to this gas produces a latent period followed by noncardiogenic pulmonary edema. Pulmonary injury is most likely a consequence of oxidant activity after phosgene exposure. The systemic inflammatory response plays an important role in this form of lung injury because mortality after phosgene exposure is significantly attenuated in leukocyte-depleted rats and in animals pretreated with a 5-lipoxygenase inhibitor or colchicine. Furthermore, lung lavage fluid protein concentrations are significantly higher at 24 hours after injury than during the immediate post-injury period. This increase in protein content occurs at a time when neutrophil migration to the lung is increased, as evidenced by higher bronchoalveolar lavage fluid neutrophil counts. Leukocyte depletion, 5-lipoxygenase inhibition, and colchicine pretreatment all prevent neutrophilic influx to the lung by depleting neutrophils, inhibiting production of leukotriene chemoattractants, or impairing neutrophil migration.

Further evidence for the importance of the systemic inflammatory response comes from a rat model of wood and polyvinyl chloride smoke inhalation (Thom et al, 1994). In this model, smoke inhalation alone resulted in tracheobronchitis without alveolar injury. When a similar smoke exposure occurred in the setting of an additional inflammatory process (in this case glycogen-induced peritonitis), however, alveolar injury ensued, as assessed by histologic changes and by increased alveolar capillary permeability to radiolabeled albumin. Control animals, in which glycogen-induced peritonitis was produced without smoke inhalation, did not develop pulmonary injury.

In the rat model of wood and polyvinyl chloride smoke inhalation, bronchoalveolar lavage neutrophil counts, which reflect both airway and alveolar neutrophil infiltration, were similar whether or not peritonitis accompanied smoke exposure. When pulmonary myeloperoxidase activity was assessed as a marker of neutrophil activation, however, only those animals with concomitant glycogen peritonitis demonstrated such evidence of neutrophil activation (Fig. 25–1). Thus, the systemic inflammatory response may activate neutrophils that are subsequently recruited to the pulmonary parenchyma, where they induce alveolar injury. These findings are consistent with clinical studies in which fatal pulmonary injury is seen in fewer than 10% of patients with smoke inhalation alone, whereas in patients with a concomitant body surface burn, mortality can reach 70% (Marchal and Dimick, 1983).

Platelet activating factor (PAF) may have a significant role in modulating oxidant injury after smoke inhalation. PAF not only activates platelets but also activates neutrophils and functions as a chemoattractant. PAF may also regulate production of lipoxygenase products and generation of oxidants by neutrophils (Ikeuchi et al, 1992). In an ovine model, the increase in lung tissue malondialdehyde levels, a marker of lipid peroxidation, which was observed to occur after smoke inhalation, was attenuated by pretreatment with a PAF antagonist (Ikeuchi et al, 1992). One possible explanation for this result is that platelets may interact with neutrophils, increasing their cytotoxic effect and enhancing their adhesion to endothelial cells (Kjellstrom and Risberg, 1985). The PAF antagonist may have limited this interaction.

Thus, smoke inhalation can lead to direct injury to the lung, which is primarily limited to the airway mucosa at least during the early post-injury period. This injury is most likely the result of oxidants present in smoke or production of free radicals and oxidants by recruited neutrophils and other components of the inflammatory response. The systemic inflammatory response, which can

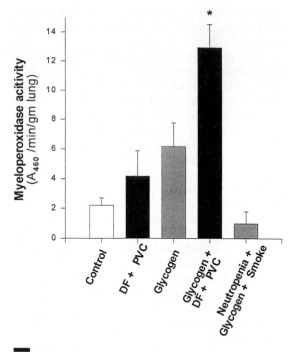

Figure 25–1
Myeloperoxidase activity, an index of neutrophil activation, of lung homogenates obtained 24 hours after smoke exposure in a rat model of smoke inhalation with and without glycogen-induced peritonitis. (DF = Douglas fir wood smoke; PVC = polyvinyl chloride smoke.) * = p<.05, ANOVA. (Modified from Thom S, Mendiguren I, van Winkle T, et al: Smoke inhalation with a concurrent system stress results in lung alveolar injury. Am J Respir Crit Care Med 149:220–226, 1994. With permission.)

be activated by a body surface burn or other form of inflammation, appears to cause concomitant alveolar injury and exacerbates the overall degree of pulmonary inflammation and injury.

EFFECT OF SMOKE INHALATION ON ALVEOLAR MACROPHAGE FUNCTION

Because the inflammatory process plays a major role in pulmonary injury following smoke inhalation, and because pneumonia often complicates the recovery phase, the effect of smoke on the alveolar macrophage, which is an immune cell that plays a crucial role in inflammatory processes and pulmonary defenses, is important to consider. Dysfunctional alveolar macrophages may permit bacterial invasion or may not appropriately control the inflammatory response. Evidence suggests that the alveolar macrophage plays a crucial role in regulating neutrophil activity in addition to other important roles in the inflammatory process (Colatta et al, 1992; Whyte et al, 1993). Uncontrolled neutrophil activation can lead to excessive release of proteases and oxidants, which can increase pulmonary injury. Alternatively, failure of the alveolar macrophage to support neutrophil function can lead to inadequate defenses.

Cotton smoke inhalation in an ovine model has been demonstrated to impair several of these aspects of macrophage function. Phagocytic capacity and the ability of alveolar macrophages to kill ingested bacteria are impaired by smoke (Herlihy et al, 1995). In addition, smoke impairs alveolar macrophage phagocytosis of inactivated or apoptotic neutrophils. Concurrently, smoke decreases the ability of alveolar macrophages to sustain activity of neutrophils and prevent premature neutrophil lysis. Thus, the ability of alveolar macrophages to regulate neutrophil function and to remove bacteria and products of lysed neutrophils is impaired by smoke.

ROLE OF ARACHIDONIC ACID PRODUCTS IN SMOKE INHALATION LUNG INJURY

In a ovine model of exposure to acrolein smoke, a common component of household fire smoke, pulmonary edema and lung lymph fluid have been found to contain high concentrations of arachidonic acid products including leukotriene B_4, C_4, D_4, and E_4, and thromboxane B_2 (Quin et al, 1990; Hales et al, 1992). In the ovine model, noncardiogenic pulmonary edema occurs, as measured by an increase in lung lymph protein flux. Inhibition of both cyclooxygenase and lipoxygenase pathways prevents pulmonary edema formation, whereas selective cyclooxygenase and thromboxane synthase inhibitors are ineffective. These observations suggest that leukotrienes may play a crucial role in lung injury. Leukotrienes may directly alter microvascular permeability, they may contribute to the inflammatory process by increasing secretion of cytokines such as tumor necrosis factor and interleukin-1, or they may function as chemoattractants (Quin et al, 1990).

Specific blockade of thromboxane synthase in the ovine model abolished the rise in pulmonary artery pressure and peak airway pressure observed after smoke exposure, implicating thromboxane B_2 in mediating pulmonary vasoconstriction and bronchoconstriction.

EFFECT OF SMOKE INHALATION ON SURFACTANT

Pulmonary surfactant is produced by type II alveolar epithelial cells and is stored in intracellular lamellar bodies from which it is released to the alveoli. A monolayer is then formed, and a continuous process of degradation and replenishment occurs. This metabolic process produces a series of subfractions of surfactant that have been identified by centrifugation. A progression from heavy to light subfractions occurs as surfactant progresses through this process and is ultimately resorbed by the alveolar epithelium (Gross and Narine, 1989). The synthesis and degradation of surfactant may be disturbed by smoke, thus decreasing alveolar stability.

In a murine model, smoke exposure has been demonstrated to alter the lamellar bodies and cause nearly a doubling of the extracellular surfactant pool (Oulton et al, 1991). These changes were evident by 4 hours after smoke inhalation. Identification of the subfractions of surfactant after smoke exposure demonstrated an increase in the heaviest subfraction (P10), which may result from an increase in surfactant secretion (Oulton et al, 1994). An increase in surfactant secretion is not unique to smoke inhalation, because it has been observed in response to inhalation of various noxious substances such as silica, diesel particles, and ozone (Dethloff et al, 1986; Eskelson et al, 1987; Balis et al, 1988). In addition, substantial increases in the lighter surfactant subtypes (P100, S100) were also observed, suggesting accelerated conversion to or impaired clearance of these subfractions. The accumulation of lighter subfractions may reflect injury to the alveolar type II cell or damage to the alveolar macrophages, because both cells participate in clearance of surfactant (Oulton et al, 1994). Furthermore, changes in the release and degradation and/or uptake of surfactant, or changes in the structure of the P100 subfraction, have been observed. Structural changes in the P100 subfraction may also contribute to impaired clearance. The surface properties of these surfactant subfractions were *not* affected by smoke exposure.

Because smoke induces abnormalities in the surfactant system, exogenous surfactant replacement may be useful in treatment of smoke inhalation injury. Improvement in gas exchange, shunt fraction, static compliance, and surface tension minimum, in lung extracts up to 4 hours after wood smoke exposure, was observed after administration of calf lung surfactant extract (Infasurf). This improvement was not seen after administration of synthetic surfactant (Exosurf) (Nieman et al, 1995b). The difference in efficacy of these agents may be related to the existence of surfactant proteins (which are not present in the synthetic surfactant product) in the calf surfactant extract.

CHANGES IN BRONCHIAL BLOOD FLOW AFTER SMOKE INHALATION INJURY

Bronchoscopic inspection of the airways in both animal models and humans after smoke inhalation almost always demonstrates airway mucosal erythema, hyperemia, and edema with evidence of bronchorrhea. Radioactive microsphere studies have demonstrated increases in bronchial blood flow after smoke inhalation (Ashley et al, 1990). In conjunction, increases in bronchial artery flow, up to eight times above baseline, have been in observed in the ovine model of smoke inhalation (Kramer et al, 1989; Abdi et al, 1990). These increases in bronchial artery flow are much greater than any changes in cardiac output. Radiolabeled microsphere studies have also demonstrated that increases in blood flow are greater in the smaller airways than in the larger bronchi (Abdi et al, 1991).

The elevated bronchial blood flow contributes to the increase in extravascular lung water seen at 24 hours after smoke inhalation. Lung lymph flow and wet-to-dry ratios were 30% less in animals in which the bronchial artery was occluded before smoke exposure (Abdi et al, 1991). The increase in bronchial blood flow after smoke inhalation may be mediated by neuropeptides, because pretreatment of animals with capsaicin, which blocks neuropeptide release, blunted the rise in bronchial blood flow (Traber et al, 1990).

ALTERATION OF PULMONARY VASCULAR RESISTANCE AND MICROVASCULAR PERMEABILITY AFTER SMOKE INHALATION

Increases in extravascular lung water are usually observed 24 hours or later after smoke inhalation injury in humans. This finding cannot be fully explained by factors such as iatrogenic fluid overload or hypoproteinemia. When systematically evaluated in a clinical study of smoke inhalation or burn injury, elevated extravascular lung water was observed, as determined by thermal dilution techniques, despite normal central venous pressure, cardiac index, and serum protein concentration (Herndon et al, 1987). This observation suggests that smoke exposure is associated with increases in pulmonary microvascular permeability and/or increases in pulmonary capillary hydrostatic pressure.

A study of wood smoke inhalation in dogs demonstrated a marked increase in the pressure drop across the pulmonary vasculature, which was primarily due to pulmonary venous vasoconstriction (Nieman et al, 1995a). As a result of this increase in venous resistance, pulmonary vascular hydrostatic pressure is expected to rise. Such an effect would increase pulmonary edema formation if a concomitant rise in microvascular permeability was present. Additionally, the increase in static recoil resulting from impaired surfactant activity decreases pulmonary interstitial pressure, further elevating the transmural pulmonary capillary pressure gradient and heightening the propensity to develop noncardiogenic pulmonary edema. The mechanisms responsible for the increase in pulmonary venous resistance remain unknown. Atelectasis, increased alveolar pressure, increased alveolar surface tension, and hypoxia cannot individually or collectively account for the entirety of the observed elevation in pulmonary venous resistance.

Studies with nitric oxide inhalation in an ovine model of wood smoke exposure further support a role for pulmonary vasoconstriction in response to smoke. Inhaled nitric oxide significantly attenuated the rise in pulmonary arterial pressure occurring up to 48 hours after smoke exposure (Ogura et al, 1994). No changes in extravascular lung water or in protein content of bronchoalveolar lavage fluid were noted, however, indicating that nitric oxide had no effect on the greater pulmonary microvascular permeability after smoke inhalation.

The relative contribution of increased microvascular permeability and pulmonary capillary hydrostatic pressure to the development of pulmonary edema in smoke inhalation was addressed in an ovine model of cotton smoke inhalation (Fig. 25–2). In this model, increased transvascular fluid flux occurred after smoke injury in association with increased capillary hydrostatic pressure and increased microvascular permeability to proteins (Isago et al, 1991). The relative contribution of each of these factors, however, changed with time during the post-exposure period. At 24 hours after smoke exposure, 66% of the rise in total capillary filtration resulted from a rise in microvascular permeability, with elevated capillary hydrostatic pressure contributing 34% of the increase. At 48 hours after inhalation, however, only 25% of the

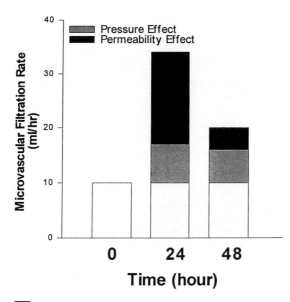

Figure 25–2
Relative contribution of increased capillary pressure
and increased microvascular permeability to total
capillary filtration after smoke inhalation. (Modified
from Isago T, Noshima S, Traber L, et al: Analysis of
pulmonary microvascular permeability after smoke
inhalation. J Appl Physiol 71:1403–1408, 1991.)

increased filtration was caused by increased permeability, with elevated hydrostatic pressure accounting for 75% of the increased permeability. The early increase in microvascular permeability was associated with an increase in plasma levels of conjugated dienes, a marker of oxidant activity resulting from oxygen free radicals. Thus, in the early phase after smoke inhalation injury, a reversible rise in pulmonary microvascular permeability, possibly induced by oxidants, predominates, whereas elevation of capillary hydrostatic pressure plays a greater role during the later phase.

EFFECT OF SMOKE INHALATION ON OXYGEN CONSUMPTION

Smoke inhalation injury has immediate and profound effects on total body oxygen consumption (VO_2). In an ovine model of smoke exposure, a nearly 75% increase in VO_2 occurred during the first 2 hours after smoke inhalation (Demling et al, 1994). The increase in VO_2 may be related to a systemic oxygen debt developed as a result of initially high carboxyhemoglobin levels with compensatory increases in VO_2 during the early post-exposure period. The initiation of both pulmonary and systemic inflammatory responses can

also result in increased metabolic demands reflected in an increased VO_2. Initiation of positive-pressure ventilation during this period had no effect on the VO_2 level, suggesting that increased work of breathing was not a major contributing factor. The level of VO_2 declined somewhat at 4 hours after exposure. A more gradual increase ensued over the next 12 to 24 hours. This late rise in VO_2 was attenuated by positive-pressure ventilation, suggesting that increased work of breathing, resulting from impaired pulmonary mechanics and altered gas exchange, contributes to the delayed rise in oxygen demands.

CLINICAL FEATURES OF SMOKE INHALATION INJURY

The clinical spectrum of injury related to smoke inhalation ranges from mild exacerbations of pre-existing pulmonary conditions, such as asthma or bronchitis, resulting from transient smoke exposure to lethal effects of entrapment in a smoke-filled environment. Because of the wide variation in severity of illness, inconsistent diagnostic criteria, and under-reporting of cases, the precise incidence of smoke inhalational injury is unknown. Pulmonary injury also may occur as a direct result of smoke inhalation or indirectly from the systemic effects of burn injury, further confounding many epidemiologic reports (Clark, 1992).

The 1942 Coconut Grove fire in Boston was probably the most notorious event serving to focus attention on the dangers of smoke inhalation (Aub et al, 1943). Four hundred ninety-one fatalities occurred in that fire. Of the 114 people transported to Massachusetts General Hospital, 75 died within minutes of arrival. Thirty-six of the 39 initial survivors eventually died of respiratory complications, even though they did not have cutaneous burns.

The clinical consequences of smoke inhalation may be a result of systemic injury due to carbon monoxide and cyanide, which cause tissue hypoxia, as well as direct injury to respiratory tissues from chemical components of smoke. In addition, thermal injury may occur, which primarily affects the upper respiratory tract. The anatomic sites of injury along with the accompanying clinical presentation and associated physiologic abnormalities from smoke inhalation injury are summarized in Table 25–2.

TISSUE HYPOXIA

Tissue hypoxia in fire victims may be the result of a critical reduction of the inspired oxygen tension

Table 25–2
Clinical Consequences of Smoke Injury

Anatomic Site of Injury	Clinical Presentation	Principal Physiologic Abnormality
Systemic/neurologic	Confusion/obtundation (early onset)	Tissue asphyxia
Respiratory system		
Conducting airways		
Upper airways	Respiratory distress (early onset)	Airway obstruction
		Alveolar hypoventilation
Tracheobronchial	Respiratory distress (early onset)	Airway obstruction
		Alveolar hypoventilation
		Mild hypoxemia
		Atelectasis
Parenchyma	Respiratory distress (delayed onset)	Hypoxemic respiratory failure
		Pulmonary edema
		Adult respiratory distress syndrome (ARDS)

Modified from Haponik E: Clinical smoke inhalation injury: Pulmonary effects. Occup Med 8:431–468, 1993.

due to displacement of oxygen by smoke and to oxygen consumption during combustion. Inspired oxygen concentrations of less than 15% frequently occur during fires in enclosed areas (Dressler, 1979). This abrupt decrease in inspired oxygen concentration poses particular hazards for patients with underlying cardiopulmonary or cerebrovascular disease.

Toxic elements of smoke such as carbon monoxide (CO) and cyanide (CN) also cause tissue hypoxia by compromising the delivery and utilization of oxygen. The affinity of hemoglobin for CO is 200 times greater than its affinity for oxygen. As a result, marked elevations of carboxyhemoglobin (COHb) levels are common in victims of both fatal and nonfatal fires (Anderson et al, 1981). CO shifts the oxygen-hemoglobin dissociation curve to the left, impairing unloading of oxygen at the tissue level and further decreasing oxygen delivery. CO also binds to other elements in the oxygen transport chain, although with less affinity than hemoglobin.

Symptoms of CO intoxication usually appear after COHb levels exceed 15%; symptoms include neurologic dysfunction, which may progress to permanent cerebral dysfunction (Watanabe and Makino, 1985). Myocardial dysfunction may be observed particularly in the setting of coronary artery disease. CO intoxication of moderate degree can be associated with patchy myocardial necrosis in normal individuals and transmural myocardial infarction in patients with pre-existing coronary artery disease (Scharf et al, 1974). In a report of New York City fire victims, one-third of patients who survived for less than 12 hours after a fire had COHb levels higher than 50% at autopsy, whereas an additional one-third of the fa-

talities had COHb levels of 11 to 49% (Zikira et al, 1972). In the MGM Grand Hotel fire in Las Vegas, smoke inhalation was noted as the cause of death in 79 victims; 42 of these had COHb levels higher than 50% (Birky et al, 1983). Among those succumbing to fires, lower COHb levels have been noted in those victims with advanced age and/or significant coronary artery disease, suggesting impaired ability of such victims to tolerate CO exposure (Anderson et al, 1981).

Both clinical and autopsy data have also demonstrated that hydrogen CN exposure commonly occurs in smoke inhalation victims. Elevated blood CN levels were found in 39 of 53 fire fatalities in one study, although only one specimen was in the lethal range (i.e., >2.0 mg/ml) (Wetherell, 1966). CO and CN may act synergistically to produce a more severe asphyxiant effect in these victims. Synergism may act at the level of the electron transport chain.

DISTRIBUTION, TIMING, AND CLINICAL PATHOPHYSIOLOGY OF SMOKE INHALATION INJURY

The pathophysiology and time course of injury to the respiratory system after smoke inhalation are outlined in Figure 25–3. Severe pharyngeal and laryngeal edema may result from thermal injury to the upper airway and may cause acute upper airway obstruction. Because of the efficient cooling capacity of the upper airways, however, thermal injury to the lungs rarely occurs in smoke inhalation with burn injury. Even when hot air is instilled below the larynx in a dog model, thermal injury to the lower respiratory tract does not occur, indicating that the trachea also possesses great cooling capacity (Moritz et al, 1945). This protective mechanism can be overcome with thermal pulmonary injury by direct inhalation of steam, inhalation exposure in hyperoxic conditions, and aspiration of hot liquids, such as during inhalation of ignited ether during crack cocaine use. In general, however, damage to the lower airways and alveoli is usually a consequence of chemical and not thermal injury.

Most of the irritant gases that may be present in smoke are highly reactive acids or bases that denature or oxidize cellular components after inhalation and hydration. The water solubility of the gas may affect the clinical presentation. Highly water-soluble agents such as ammonias, sulfur dioxide, hydrogen fluoride, and acrolein have a predilection for proximal airway injury. Therefore, their toxicity is more likely to be recognized early in the course of injury. Agents with intermediate or lower water solubility (chlorine, phosgene, nitrogen oxide) produce a more insidious pattern of injury.

Damage to the proximal airways is generally more severe than damage to the distal airways. In fact, distal airway and alveolar injury is unlikely in the absence of proximal airway damage. Ciliated columnar epithelial cells, which line the airway, are particularly susceptible to injury from smoke inhalation. An early increase in permeability of the epithelium usually occurs after smoke exposure, resulting primarily from disruption of intercellular tight junctions (Crapo et al, 1984). Increased permeability of the tracheobronchial epithelium leads to exudation of proteinaceous

fluid and bronchorrhea. Furthermore, increased bronchial blood flow contributes to airway edema formation. Subsequently, desquamation and sloughing of the tracheobronchial epithelium may occur (Lykens et al, 1991). When combined with soot and other airway debris, frank airway obstruction may ensue. Bronchoconstriction may also occur in this setting, further increasing airway resistance. Bronchospasm may be due to release of mediators, such as thromboxane A_2, exposure of submucosal cholinergic receptors, and release of neuropeptides, which promote bronchospasm.

Airway injury usually precedes damage to the alveolar capillary membrane. Increased alveolar microvascular permeability usually does not occur during the first 24 hours after smoke inhalation except in cases of massive smoke exposure. Subsequent damage to the alveolar capillary membrane can lead to interstitial pulmonary edema and alveolar flooding. Interstitial and alveolar edema reduce static compliance, increase the work of breathing, and impair gas exchange. Altered surfactant activity adds to alveolar instability and leads to atelectasis and hypoxemia.

EVALUATION OF THE PATIENT WITH SMOKE INHALATION INJURY

The diagnosis of smoke inhalation must be established on clinical grounds. No single diagnostic feature or laboratory test exists that can predict its presence or severity. Certain presenting features, however, suggest the possibility of smoke inhalation injury. These features include a history of a

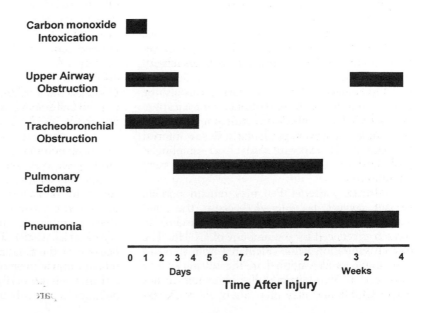

Figure 25–3
Time course of respiratory abnormalities occurring after smoke inhalation injury. (Modified from Haponik E: Clinical smoke inhalation injury: Pulmonary effects. Occup Med 8:431–468, 1993. With permission.)

closed-space exposure to smoke and the presence of a facial burn with a concomitant large body surface burn (Shirani et al, 1986). Other clinical signs such as dyspnea, cough, hoarseness, chest pain, bronchorrhea, and wheezing usually have a delayed onset, although they are eventually observed in up to 75% of victims. When these respiratory signs and symptoms are evident on presentation they strongly suggest smoke inhalation injury. Expectoration of carbonaceous sputum is seen in only 10 to 20% of patients, perhaps because of rapid clearance of secretions or variation in the extent or type of smoke exposure. Accordingly, the presence of carbonaceous sputum is not correlated with the presence or severity of inhalation injury and does not predict prognosis. Hoarseness or change in the quality of the voice or painful swallowing may be clues to severe upper airway injury and impending obstruction. Stridor from pharyngeal edema is a respiratory emergency that may not be apparent during quiet breathing and may be evident only during hyperventilation. Facial burns, especially those involving the nose, lips, and circumoral region as well as the upper cervical areas, are considered high-risk burns because they may be associated with upper airway injury. Associated large cutaneous burns imply an inability to escape from a fire with resultant prolonged thermal and smoke exposure. The presence of large cutaneous burns is also correlated with acute upper airway edema and delayed-onset pulmonary edema or pneumonia.

The possibility of systemic injury from asphyxiants with tissue hypoxia must always be considered in the evaluation of the patient with suspected inhalation injury. Because of the association of smoke inhalation and COHb intoxication, determination of the COHb level is necessary during the initial evaluation of smoke inhalation victims. Testing entails analysis of venous or arterial blood for COHb by differential spectrophotometry or co-oximetry. Measurement of end-expiratory CO concentration can also be utilized to evaluate the extent of CO intoxication. Normal COHb levels do not rule out an inhalation injury, however, particularly if the interval between smoke exposure and blood sampling is prolonged or if supplemental oxygen has been administered.

Although arterial PO_2 may remain normal, oxygen *content* is reduced because the total amount of hemoglobin available for binding to oxygen is reduced by the amount of COHb. The oxygen saturation value calculated from standard nomograms is also normal in the setting of CO intoxication. In addition, pulse oximeters do not detect COHb and may give falsely elevated oxygen saturation readings. Therapy for CO intoxication entails administration of a high inspired oxygen concentration, which increases the clearance rate of CO from hemoglobin. Hyperbaric oxygen therapy further increases the rate of clearance of CO but is difficult to administer and impedes provision of medical care owing to isolation of the patient in a hyperbaric chamber. Hyperbaric therapy is most beneficial in the setting of altered consciousness or COHb levels in excess of 25 to 40% (Jain, 1990).

Elevated COHb levels also suggest an increased likelihood of coexistent toxicity with CN. Unfortunately, the lack of a rapid screening laboratory test hinders detection of this agent. Because CN inhibits cytochrome function and interferes with aerobic glycolysis, however, a persistent metabolic acidosis in the setting of smoke exposure suggests CN toxicity. CN intoxication is usually treated with agents that increase methemoglobin (MetHb), which then binds CN. This treatment poses a theoretical risk in smoke inhalation victims, however, because concomitant CO intoxication with increased COHb levels is likely. Increasing MetHb formation in this setting may further detract from the oxygen-carrying capacity of blood and may exacerbate tissue hypoxia. Because of this concern, specific therapy for CN intoxication with MetHb-forming agents is usually avoided in smoke inhalation victims. If such therapy is necessary, sodium thiosulfate, which binds CN-forming thiocyanate, should be used initially, and sodium nitrite, which induces a state of methemoglobinemia, should be withheld until hyperbaric oxygen can be provided (Hall et al, 1989).

Smoke inhalation may cause a widened alveolar-arterial gradient with reduced arterial PO_2 and oxygen saturation as a result of atelectasis and ventilation-perfusion mismatching. Because of the delayed onset of alveolar capillary leak and pulmonary edema, early measurements of oxygenation may be normal. Thus, the initial arterial blood gas value is an insensitive predictor of subsequent pulmonary dysfunction from smoke inhalation.

The chest radiograph is also insensitive in detecting pulmonary injury in the early post-inhalation period. A study of chest radiographs taken on the day of injury demonstrated false-negative results in 92% of 106 patients who subsequently developed clinical evidence of pulmonary parenchymal injury secondary to smoke inhalation (Clark et al, 1989). This result most likely occurs because of the time course of the pattern of pulmonary injury in smoke inhalation, in which initial injury is primarily to the airways, not to the pulmonary parenchyma. Radiographic changes of atelectasis, pulmonary edema, and focal infiltrates usually do not become apparent until after the initial 24- to 48-hour post-injury period. Thus, serial chest radiographic evaluations are necessary to assess for the possible development of pulmonary parenchymal injury.

Radionuclide scanning, which is generally performed with radiolabeled xenon, has also been used in the evaluation of patients with smoke inhalation injury. Inhomogeneous lung uptake of radionuclide or delayed clearance (>90 sec) of the radiolabeled gas from the lung fields is characteristic of distal airway obstruction from tracheobronchial injury. False-positive scans can occur, however, in patients with pre-existing cardiopulmonary disorders.

Early airway injury in smoke inhalation may be detected by pulmonary function testing, which may demonstrate obstructive airways dysfunction manifested by reduction in expiratory flow rates and FEV_1/FVC ratio. Parenchymal lung injury including pulmonary edema, atelectasis, and pneumonia may produce a restrictive ventilatory defect. In fact, development of a restrictive pattern on pulmonary function testing usually precedes radiographic or gas exchange abnormalities and therefore may be a useful early marker for the development of pulmonary parenchymal injury. Serial pulmonary function measurement may also be a helpful tool to assess physiologic improvement. Abnormal flow-volume curve patterns may also be helpful because they can detect the presence of extrathoracic, intrathoracic, or fixed upper airway obstruction. Limitation of inspiratory flow suggests upper airway obstruction due to pharyngeal edema and may indicate the need for endotracheal intubation or tracheostomy (Haponik et al, 1984).

Serial measures of inspiratory flow rates have been demonstrated to parallel the development of upper airway injury and edema as visualized by nasopharyngoscopy. A "saw-tooth" pattern of the inspiratory limb of the flow-volume curve may also reflect upper airway edema and instability. The high negative predictive value of a normal pulmonary function study early in the course of smoke inhalation also adds to its clinical usefulness. In a study performed at the Baltimore Regional Burn Center, only 1 of 60 smoke inhalation and burn victims with normal pulmonary function studies required endotracheal intubation during the initial management phase (Haponik, 1993). Pulmonary function testing also has a role in detecting late sequelae of smoke inhalation. Delayed-onset subglottic stenosis may be detected. The presence of residual obstructive or restrictive ventilatory defects or increased bronchial hyper-

responsiveness from irritant-induced asthma may also be detected with serial pulmonary function measurement.

Bronchoscopic examination of the airways has been employed to detect impending airway obstruction and to assess the extent of respiratory system injury resulting from smoke inhalation. Most studies have found that supraglottic airway injury is more severe than infraglottic damage because of the protective effects of upper airway structures. Bronchoscopic demonstration of airway edema, hyperemia, and viscid secretions in the upper or lower airways provides confirmation of airway injury from smoke inhalation. Although normal endoscopic findings in the upper airway suggest that major lower airway injury is absent, such findings do not preclude the possibility of injury. Additionally, particulate matter in smoke with a diameter of less than 0.5 μm may bypass upper airway protective mechanisms and deposit in terminal bronchioles and alveoli, where adherent oxidants and other toxic substances may cause pulmonary parenchymal injury. Bronchoscopy may fail to detect such inhalational injury. Xenon ventilation scanning may be a good adjunct to bronchoscopy to detect this form of lung injury.

The necessity for bronchoscopic examination of the airways in all suspected smoke inhalation victims is controversial. Less invasive tests may provide sufficient evidence in many cases to establish a diagnosis. Furthermore, abnormal findings on the initial bronchoscopic evaluation do not predict the degree of airway injury and subsequent gas exchange impairment, need for mechanical ventilation, or ultimate prognosis (Bingham et al, 1987). Bronchoscopy does play an important role in defining chronic airway complications such as tracheal or bronchial stenosis and can demonstrate development of airway polyps, which can be treated with bronchoscopic laser ablation therapy, if necessary.

MANAGEMENT OF SMOKE INHALATION INJURY

Because of difficulties in predicting deterioration of respiratory status after smoke inhalation, a low threshold for hospitalization and close monitoring in an intensive care unit are indicated. Patients with a history of entrapment in a closed space, early neurologic dysfunction, high levels of asphyxiants (CO and CN), underlying cardiopulmonary disorders, advanced age, or young age are at greatest risk for deterioration. Patients who present with objective signs of injury, abnormal gas exchange, abnormal pulmonary function tests, cutaneous burns, or concomitant systemic abnormalities are also at high risk and should be observed closely in an intensive care unit. Healthier patients and those with low-risk exposures who do not demonstrate objective signs of injury, physiologic dysfunction, or significant surface burns can be followed on an outpatient basis.

The most urgent and treatable problem in the initial management of smoke inhalation injury is the potential for development of acute upper airway obstruction. Patients whose condition initially appears stable may rapidly develop pharyngeal edema during fluid resuscitation, which can lead to total airway occlusion. Edema not only compromises the airway lumen but can also limit the ability to extend the neck, open the mouth, and handle secretions without aspiration.

About 50% of patients with a smoke inhalation injury require intubation (Clark et al, 1989). Forty percent of these intubations are necessary because of compromise of the upper airway. Bronchoscopy may be necessary to guide placement of the endotracheal tube in patients unable to extend the neck owing to edema or cervical burns. The largest possible size of endotracheal tube should be used to facilitate adequate pulmonary toilet and diagnostic or therapeutic bronchoscopy. Subsequent development of facial or circumoral edema should be considered before trimming the length of the endotracheal tube. Endotracheal tube cuff pressures should be kept at minimal levels to prevent further damage to smoke injured tracheal mucosa. If endotracheal intubation is not possible, a cricothyroidotomy is the procedure of choice to secure the airway because emergency tracheotomy is potentially hazardous in burn victims. In patients who are intubated solely for upper airway obstruction, extubation can usually be performed after 72 hours because pharyngeal edema usually improves by that time. Concomitant tracheobronchial or pulmonary parenchymal damage prolongs the need for mechanical ventilation.

Progressive development of gas exchange abnormalities early in the course of smoke inhalation injury usually is due to occlusion of small airways, alveolar collapse and atelectasis resulting from airway edema, desquamation of mucosal cells, and accumulation of secretions and debris in the airway lumen. Because of the need to maintain pulmonary toilet and prevent atelectasis and alveolar collapse, early elective intubation with mechanical ventilation has been shown to decrease the incidence of respiratory failure in smoke inhalation victims with evolving gas exchange abnormalities (Venus et al, 1981). Humidification of inspired gases and frequent endotra-

cheal suctioning and position changes are important in the ventilatory management of these patients. Fiberoptic bronchoscopy may be necessary to clear the airway of accumulated casts, mucous plugs, and debris. Therapeutic bronchoscopy may also be helpful in the setting of extensive surface burns, which prevent adequate chest percussion and postural drainage.

Many theoretical reasons exist to support positive end-expiratory pressure (PEEP) in smoke inhalation injury victims requiring mechanical ventilation. PEEP may decrease the need for high inspired oxygen concentrations, which may limit lung injury because oxygen-derived free radicals play an important role in the pathogenesis of smoke inhalation injury. PEEP may also prevent alveolar collapse by increasing functional residual capacity and end-expiratory airway diameter. Increased airway diameter may decrease the propensity of intraluminal debris to form obstructing endobronchial casts (Cox et al, 1992). Additionally, PEEP has been demonstrated to decrease bronchial blood flow with consequent reduction in bronchial hyperemia and edema in an ovine model of smoke inhalation injury (Venus et al, 1981). Despite these theoretical advantages, no prospective controlled study exists to support prophylactic PEEP in clinical settings. Although some have advocated prophylactic administration of PEEP, most use PEEP only in established hypoxemic respiratory failure.

New modes of mechanical ventilation, in particular high-frequency ventilation, have been advocated in this setting (Nieman et al, 1994). No prospective controlled trials currently exist, however, to evaluate outcome with high-frequency ventilation. One study suggested that high-frequency percussive ventilation decreased the incidence of pneumonia and enhanced survival in smoke inhalation injury, but comparison was only with historic controls (Cioffi et al, 1991). Another study showed that although high-frequency ventilation decreased airway pressure excursions compared with conventional mechanical ventilation, it did not decrease development of pulmonary edema or improve other measures of pulmonary function (Nieman et al, 1994). Thus, routine high-frequency ventilation cannot be advocated at this time. Chapter 18 provides a thorough review of these modes of ventilation in the setting of acute lung injury.

The optimal approach to fluid management in smoke inhalation injury remains controversial. In animal models, after the initial 24 hours post-injury, smoke inhalation has been shown to increase permeability of the pulmonary microvasculature. In this setting, overhydration can theoretically lead to increased lung water with alveolar flooding and further impairment of gas exchange. Clinically, however, the effects of fluid resuscitation are variable. One study demonstrated no increase in extravascular lung water with fluid resuscitation after smoke inhalation injury in patients without concomitant sepsis or pneumonia (Tranbaugh et al, 1983). In the absence of cutaneous burns, a reasonable approach may be to provide only the minimal amounts of fluid necessary to maintain end-organ perfusion. Hemodynamic measurements obtained from right heart catheterization may provide needed information to achieve this goal. No improvement in outcome has been demonstrated in smoke inhalation patients with pulmonary parenchymal injury using this strategy, however.

When concomitant cutaneous burns are present, other factors must be considered in the approach to fluid resuscitation. The combination of smoke inhalation injuries and cutaneous burns has been demonstrated in an ovine model to triple the fluid requirement needed to maintain cardiac output and blood pressure during the first 6 hours of resuscitation compared with that needed in burn injury alone (Lalonde et al, 1995). This increase in fluid requirement is not the result of lung water accumulation but may be related to the increase in burn and nonburn tissue interstitial edema formation. Decreased vasomotor tone and increased venous capacitance may contribute to this phenomenon. Interestingly, the initial increase in fluid requirements and oxygen consumption has been demonstrated to reflect the degree of airway injury evident at 24 hours post-inhalation in this model. Thus, the extent of injury and resultant inflammatory response may be reflected in early increases in oxygen consumption and fluid requirements.

Burn patients with inhalation injury typically require about 30% more intravenous fluid during the resuscitative phase than patients without cutaneous burn injury (Navar et al, 1985). Formulas for fluid resuscitation in burn patients are therefore based on the percentage of body surface area burned, body weight, and urine output. Limiting fluid administration in this setting in an effort to minimize alveolar flooding has been shown to compromise tissue oxygen delivery and increase mortality (Dries and Waxman, 1991).

Tracheobronchitis with necrosis and sloughing of mucosa may worsen by 3 to 4 days after injury, which may contribute to an increased risk of pneumonia. Impairment of host defenses due to altered immune function and abnormal local pulmonary defenses may also contribute to development of nosocomial pneumonia, which may

occur in as many as 50% of cases (Shirani et al, 1986). Although pneumonia and sepsis may complicate the later stages of recovery from smoke inhalation injury, prophylactic antibiotic therapy has not been demonstrated to improve outcome and may increase the prevalence of resistant organisms.

Prophylactic use of aerosolized antibiotics in an attempt to decrease the incidence of pneumonia has received considerable attention. A study of aerosolized gentamicin prophylaxis in smoke inhalation injury, however, demonstrated no improvement in the incidence of pneumonia or sepsis, need for mechanical ventilation, or mortality (Levine et al, 1978). Thus, antibiotic therapy should be given only in the setting of established pulmonary or systemic infections

Bronchospasm may occur in the setting of smoke inhalation injury. Bronchospasm generally is best treated by administration of an aerosolized β-agonist such as albuterol or systemic administration of aminophylline (Pruitt et al, 1990). Treatment with steroids should be reserved for severe or intractable bronchospasm, because steroids have the potential to increase the incidence of infectious complications and mortality in smoke inhalation (Levine et al, 1978). Steroids may be helpful in the management of upper airway edema, particularly after failed attempts at extubation.

Because lipid peroxidation is an important part of the pathophysiology of smoke-induced injury to the airways and pulmonary parenchyma, antioxidants may be useful. Animal models of smoke inhalation have demonstrated protective effects of superoxide dismutase, catalase, glutathione reductase, allopurinol, ibuprofen, deferoxamine, and vitamin E, as well as other antioxidants (Haponik, 1993). These therapies have not yet been proven beneficial in the clinical setting.

LATE SEQUELAE OF SMOKE INHALATION INJURY

Even severe smoke-induced injury to the upper airway, tracheobronchial tree, and alveolar capillary membrane generally heals completely with few residual effects (Haponik, 1993). In one study of 28 smoke inhalation victims, no impairment of resting arterial blood gases or FEV_1 was noted 8 years after injury (Nylen et al, 1995). Few long-term studies exist regarding late sequelae of smoke inhalation injury, however. Most of the available information comes from pulmonary function measurements in firefighters. Mild nonspecific and self-limited symptoms such as productive cough, nasopharyngitis, and sinusitis often persist for some time after smoke inhalation. Reactive airways dysfunction syndrome or irritant-induced asthma, as well as subclinical bronchial hyperresponsiveness, may occur after smoke inhalation.

In a study of 13 patients with smoke inhalation, increased airway hyperreactivity was demonstrated within 3 days of injury (Kinsella et al, 1991), and reductions of FEV_1 and airway conductance persisted for several months. The degree of obstructive airways dysfunction observed was correlated with initial blood COHb concentration, which presumably reflects the degree of smoke exposure. Other studies have demonstrated development of severe and irreversible airflow obstruction in the post-inhalation period (Cooke et al, 1982; Moisan, 1991).

Additional late-appearing sequelae of smoke inhalation injury are less common. These include development of tracheobronchial polyps and stenosis, bronchiectasis, pulmonary fibrosis, and bronchiolitis obliterans (Wright, 1993; Tasaka et al, 1995). Steroids are usually effective in the treatment of bronchiolitis obliterans. Pulmonary arterial hypertension and cor pulmonale have also been demonstrated in association with chronic domestic wood smoke inhalation (Sandoval et al, 1993). Clinical experience has shown that patients who sustain more severe acute inhalation injuries and therefore require more prolonged mechanical ventilatory support have more frequent and severe residual pulmonary dysfunction.

REFERENCES

Abdi S, Herndon D, Maguire J, et al: Time course of alterations in lung lymph and bronchial blood flows after inhalation injury. J Burn Care Rehabil 11:510–515, 1990.

Abdi S, Herndon D, Traber L, et al: Lung edema formation following inhalation injury: Role of the bronchial blood flow. J Appl Physiol 71:727–734, 1991.

Anderson RA, Watson AA, and Harland WA: Fire deaths in the Glasgow area: II. The role of carbon monoxide. Med Sci Law 21:288–294, 1981.

Ashley K, Stothert D, Traber L, et al: Airway blood flow following light and heavy smoke inhalation injury. Surg Forum 41:293–295, 1990.

Aub JC, Pittman H, and Brues AM: Symposium on management of Cocoanut Grove burns at Massachusetts General Hospital: the pulmonary complications: a clinical description. Ann Surg 117:834–841, 1943.

Balis JU, Paterson JF, Haller EM, et al: Ozone-induced lamellar body responses in a rat model for alveolar injury and repair. Am J Pathol 132:330–344, 1988.

Bingham H, Gallagher TJ, and Powel MD: Early bronchoscopy as a predictor of ventilatory support for burned patients. J Trauma 27:1286–1288, 1987.

Birky M, Malek D, and Pazbo M: Study of biological samples obtained from victims of MGM Grand Hotel fire. J Anal Toxicol 7:265–271, 1983.

Cahalane M, and Demling R: Early respiratory abnormalities from smoke inhalation. JAMA 251:771–773, 1984.

Cioffi WG, Rue LW, Graves TA, et al: Prophylactic use of high frequency percussive ventilation in patients with inhalation injury. Ann Surg 213:575–582, 1991.

Clark WR: Smoke inhalation: Diagnosis and treatment. World J Surg 16:24–29, 1992.

Clark WR, Bonaventura M, and Myers W: Smoke inhalation and airway management at a regional burn unit: 1974–1983 I. Diagnosis and consequences of smoke inhalation. J Burn Care Rehabil 10:52–62, 1989.

Colatta F, Fabio R, Polentarutti N, et al: Modulation of granulocyte survival and programmed cell death by cytokines and bacterial products. Blood 80:2012–2020, 1992.

Cooke N, Cobley A, and Armstrong R: Airflow obstruction after smoke inhalation. Anaesthesia 37:830–833, 1982.

Cosgrove J, Barish E, Church D, and Pryor W: The metal-mediated formation of hydroxyl radical by aqueous extracts of cigarette tar. Biochem Res Commun 132:390–396, 1985.

Cox CS Jr, Zwischenberger JB, Traber DL, et al: Immediate positive pressure ventilation with positive end expiratory pressure (PEEP) improves survival in ovine smoke inhalation injury. J Trauma 33:821–827, 1992.

Crapo JB, Barry BE, Chang LY, and Mercer RR: Alterations in lung structure caused by inhalation of oxidants. J Toxicol Environ Health 13:301–321, 1984.

Demling R, and Lalonde C: Early post burn lipid peroxidation: Effect of ibuprofen and allopurinol. Surgery 107:85–90, 1990.

Demling R, Lalonde C, and Heron P: Initial effect of smoke inhalation injury on oxygen consumption (response to positive pressure ventilation). Surgery 115:563–569, 1994.

Demling R, Picard L, Campbell C, and Lalonde C: Relationship of burn-induced lung lipid peroxidation on the degree of injury after smoke inhalation and a body burn. Crit Care Med 21:1935–1943, 1993.

Dethloff L, Gilmore L, and Hook G: The relationship between intra- and extra-cellular surfactant phospholipids in the lungs of rabbits and the effects of silica-induced lung injury. Biochem J 239:59–67, 1986.

Dressler DP: Laboratory background on smoke inhalation. J Trauma 19:913–915, 1979.

Dries DJ, and Waxman K: Adequate resuscitation of burn patients may not be measured by urine output and vital signs. Crit Care Med 19:327–329, 1991.

Eskelson C, Chvapil M, and Strom K: Pulmonary phospholiposis in rats respiring air containing diesel particulates. Environ Res 44:260–271, 1987.

Ghio A, Kennedy T, Hatch G, and Tepper J: Reduction of neutrophil influx diminishes lung injury and mortality following phosgene inhalation. J Appl Physiol 71:657–665, 1991.

Gross N, and Narine R: Surfactant subtypes of mice: Metabolic relationships and conversion in vitro. J Appl Physiol 67:414–421, 1989.

Hales C, Musto S, Janssens W, et al: Smoke aldehyde component influences pulmonary edema. J Appl Physiol 72:555–561, 1992.

Hall AH, Kulig KW, and Rumack BH: Suspected cyanide poisoning in smoke inhalation: Complications of sodium nitrite therapy. J Toxicol Clin Exp 9:3–9, 1989.

Haponik E: Clinical smoke inhalation injury: Pulmonary effects. Occup Med 8:431–468, 1993.

Haponik EF, Munster AM, Wise RA, et al: Upper airway function in burn patients: Correlation of flow-volume curves and nasopharyngoscopy. Am Rev Respir Dis 129:251–257, 1984.

Herlihy J, Vermeulen P, Joseph P, and Hales C: Impaired alveolar macrophage function in smoke inhalation injury. J Cell Physiol 163:1–8, 1995.

Herndon D, Barrow R, Traber D, et al: Extravascular lung water changes following smoke inhalation and massive burn injury. Surgery 102:341–348, 1987.

Ikeuchi H, Sakano T, Sanchez J, et al: The effects of platelet activating factor (PAF) and a PAF antagonist (CV-3988) on smoke inhalation injury in an ovine model. J Trauma 32:344–349, 1992.

Isago T, Noshima S, Traber L, et al: Analysis of pulmonary microvascular permeability after smoke inhalation. J Appl Physiol 71:1403–1408, 1991.

Jain KK: Carbon Monoxide Poisoning. St. Louis, Warren H. Green, 1990.

Kinsella J, Carter R, Reid WH, et al: Increased airways reactivity after smoke inhalation. Lancet 337:595–597, 1991.

Kjellstrom B, and Risberg B: High dose corticosteroids and cell-cell interactions. Acta Chir Scand 526[Suppl]:37, 1985.

Kono Y, and Fridovich I: Superoxide radical inhibits catalase. J Biol Chem 257:5751–5754, 1982.

Kramer G, Herndon H, Linares A, et al: Effects of inhalation injury on airway blood flow and edema formation. J Burn Care Rehabil 10:45–51, 1989.

Kulle PJ, Sauder LR, Hebel JR, et al: Pulmonary effects of sulfur dioxide and respirable carbon aerosol. Environ Res 41:239–250, 1986.

Lachocki TM, Church DF, and Pryor WA: Persistent free radicals in wood smoke: An ESR spin trapping study. Free Radic Biol Med 7:17–21, 1989.

Lachocki TM, Church DF, and Pryor WA: Persistent free radicals in the smoke of common household

materials: Biological and clinical implications. Environ Res 45:127–139, 1988.

Lalonde C, Demling R, Brian J, and Blanchard H: Smoke inhalation injury in sheep is caused by the particle phase, not the gas phase. J Appl Physiol 77:15–22, 1994a.

Lalonde C, Ikegami K, and Demling R: Aerosolized deferoxamine prevents lung and systemic injury caused by smoke inhalation. J Appl Physiol 77:2057–2064, 1994b.

Lalonde C, Picard L, Campbell C, and Demling R: Lung and systemic oxidant and antioxidant activity after graded smoke exposure in the rat. Circ Shock 42:7–13, 1994c.

Lalonde C, Picard L, Youn Y, and Demling R: Increased early postburn fluid requirements and oxygen demands are predictive of the degree of airways injury by smoke inhalation. J Trauma 38:175–184, 1995.

Lansing MW, Mansour E, Ahmed A, et al: Lipid mediators contribute to oxygen-radical-induced airways response in sheep. Am Rev Respir Dis 144:1291–1296, 1991.

Levine BA, Petroff PA, Slade CL, et al: Prospective trials of dexamethasone and aerosolized gentamicin in the treatment of inhalation injury in the burned patient. J Trauma 18:188–193, 1978.

Lykens MG, Haponik EF, Meredith JW, and Bass DA: Bronchial epithelial cell damage after inhalation injury: Assessment by bronchoalveolar lavage. Chest 100:12S, 1991.

Marchal W, and Dimick A: The natural history of major burns with multiple subsystem failure. J Trauma 23:102–105, 1983.

Moisan T: Prolonged asthma after smoke inhalation: A report of three cases and a review of previous reports. J Occup Med 33:458–461, 1991.

Moritz AR, Henriques FC, and MacLean R: The effects of inhaled heat on the air passages and lungs, an experimental investigation. Am J Pathol 21:311–331, 1945.

Navar PD, Affle JR, and Warden GD: Effect of inhalation injury on fluid resuscitation requirements after thermal injury. Am J Surg 150:716–720, 1985.

Nieman G, Clark W, Paskanik A, et al: Segmental pulmonary vascular resistance following wood smoke inhalation. Crit Care Med 23:1264–1271, 1995a.

Nieman G, Paskanik A, and Fluck R: Comparison of exogenous surfactants in the treatment of wood smoke inhalation. Am J Respir Crit Care Med 152:597–602, 1995b.

Nieman GF, Cigada M, Paskanik AM, et al: Comparison of high frequency jet to conventional mechanical ventilation in the treatment of severe smoke inhalation injury. Burns 20:157–162, 1994.

Nylen E, Jeng J, Jordan M, et al: Late pulmonary sequelae following burns: Persistence of hyperprocalcitonemia using a 1–57 amino acid

N-terminal flanking peptide assay. Respir Med 89:41–46, 1995.

Ogura H, Cioffi W, and Jordan B: The effect of inhaled nitric oxide on smoke inhalation injury in an ovine model. J Trauma 37:294–301, 1994.

Oulton M, Janigan D, Josee M, et al: Effects of smoke inhalation on alveolar surfactant subtypes in mice. Am J Pathol 145:941–950, 1994.

Oulton M, Moorkes HK, Scott J, et al: Effects of smoke inhalation on surfactant phospholipids and phospholipase A2 activity in mouse lung. Am J Pathol 138:195–202, 1991.

Pruitt BA, Flemma RJ, DiVincent FC, et al: Pulmonary complications in burn patients. J Thorac Cardiovasc Surg 59:7, 1970.

Pruitt BA Jr, Cioffi WG, Shimazu T, et al: Evaluation and management of patients with inhalation injury, advances in understanding trauma and burn injury. J Trauma 30:S63–S69, 1990.

Quin D, DeHoyos A, and Hales C: Role of sulfidopeptide leukotrienes in synthetic smoke inhalation in sheep. J Appl Physiol 68:1962–1969, 1990.

Sandoval J, Salas J, Martinez-Guerra ML, et al: Pulmonary arterial hypertension and cor pulmonale associated with chronic domestic wood smoke inhalation. Chest 103:12–20, 1993.

Scharf SM, Thames M, and Sargeant K: Transmural myocardial infarction after exposure to carbon monoxide in coronary artery disease. N Engl J Med 291:85–86, 1974.

Shirani K, Pruitt B, and Mason A: The influence of inhalation injury and pneumonia on burn mortality. Ann Surg 205:82–86, 1986.

Tasaka S, Kanazawa M, Mori M, et al: Long term course of bronchiectasis and bronchiolitis obliterans as late complication of smoke inhalation. Respiration 62:40–42, 1995.

Thom S, Mendiguren I, van Winkle T, et al: Smoke inhalation with a concurrent systemic stress results in lung alveolar injury. Am J Respir Crit Care Med 149:220–226, 1994.

Traber L, Herndon J, Turner G, et al: Peptide mediation of the bronchial blood flow elevation following inhalation injury. Circ Shock 31:13, 1990.

Tranbaugh RF, Elings VB, Christensen JM, and Lewis FR: Effect of inhalation injury on lung water accumulation. J Trauma 23:597–604, 1983.

Venus B, Matsuda T, Copiozo JB, et al: Prophylactic intubation and continuous positive airway pressure in the management of inhalation injury in burn victims. Crit Care Med 9:519–523, 1981.

Watanabe K, and Makino K: The role of carbon monoxide poisoning in the production of inhalation burns. Ann Plast Surg 14:284–294, 1985.

Wetherell HR: The occurrence of cyanide in the blood of fire victims. J Forensic Sci 11:167–173, 1966.

Whyte M, Meagher L, MacDermot J, and Haslett C: Impairment of function in aging neutrophils is associated with apoptosis. J Immunol 150:5124–5134, 1993.

Wright JL: Inhalational lung injury causing bronchiolitis. Clin Chest Med 14:635–644, 1993.

Zikria BA, Weston GC, Chodoff M, and Ferrer JM: Smoke and carbon monoxide poisoning in fire victims. J Trauma 12:641–645, 1972.

C H A P T E R

Hyperbaric Medicine

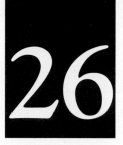

Irving Jacoby, M.D.

Stephen R. Hayden, M.D.

The first reported therapeutic use of oxygen under pressure was in 1935 when Behnke employed hyperbaric oxygen (HBO_2) for decompression sickness; significantly improved results were demonstrated compared with increased ambient air pressure alone (Behnke, 1935). The role of HBO_2 continues to evolve through the last decade of the 20th century, with the delineation of the numerous physiologic processes that are amplified, modified, and otherwise affected by such treatments. In all instances, hyperbaric oxygen therapy as discussed here refers only to systemic delivery of 100% oxygen to a patient totally enclosed in a hyperbaric chamber. Topical oxygen is useless and should never be considered an option as a therapeutic intervention.

At this writing, there are more than a dozen indications approved for clinical usage by the Hyperbaric Therapy Committee of the Undersea and Hyperbaric Medical Society, based on the 1996 report (Hyperbaric Oxygen Therapy, 1996). These are listed in Table 26–1. HBO_2 in these clinical settings is well described. A number of newer uses of HBO_2 are being investigated, however, and research continues into basic mechanisms of action of HBO_2.

In this chapter we review the kinds of hyperbaric chambers in use today, and the basic physiology leading to and caused by hyperbaric hyperoxia. We also examine the current state of knowledge regarding HBO_2 and the mechanisms relevant to cardiopulmonary critical care. We make particular reference to HBO_2 and its effects on reperfusion injury; myocardial infarction; neurotoxicity of carbon monoxide poisoning; and cerebral edema reduction in the head-injured patient.

The physiologic mechanisms by which HBO_2 leads to improvement in each clinical situation may vary markedly. The number of demonstrated physiologic effects of HBO_2 continues to increase. In decompression sickness, nitrogen gas is redissolved back into tissue from the bubble phase by the increased pressure during recompression. Then, during slow decompression, nitrogen is allowed to exit (offgas) from all tissue compartments in a controlled manner, avoiding the generation of further bubbles. Arterial gas embolism

Table 26–1
Currently Accepted Medical Indications for Hyperbaric Therapy

Diving-related
  Decompression sickness
  Arterial gas embolism secondary to pulmonary
    overinflation syndrome
Nondiving-related
  Iatrogenic or traumatic venous or arterial gas
    embolism
  Infectious diseases
    Clostridial myositis and myonecrosis (gas
      gangrene)
    Mixed aerobic/anaerobic necrotizing cellulitis
    Fournier's gangrene and necrotizing fasciitis
    Chronic refractory osteomyelitis
    Selected brain abscesses
  Carbon monoxide poisoning
  Cyanide poisoning
  Selected chronic problem nonhealing hypoxic soft
    tissue wounds, such as
    Nonhealing wounds in patients with diabetes
      mellitus, peripheral vascular disease, sickle cell
      disease, or vasculitis
  Radiation tissue damage
    Prophylaxis for and treatment of
      osteoradionecrosis
    Treatment of soft tissue radionecrosis, including
      radiation cystitis and enteritis
  Crush injury, compartment syndrome, and other
    acute traumatic ischemias
  Exceptional blood loss anemia
  Compromised skin grafts and flaps
  Thermal burns

Modified from Hyperbaric Oxygen Therapy: A Committee Report. Kensington, MD, Undersea and Hyperbaric Medical Society, 1996.

may result from pulmonary overinflation in scuba divers making a rapid ascent without exhaling, in patients with penetrating chest trauma, or in patients affected by iatrogenic causes, such as an air leak during insertion of a central line. In these cases the function of hyperbaric recompression is to reduce air bubbles to smaller sizes so that they may be resorbed more readily.

In clostridial myositis and myonecrosis, several effects of HBO_2 come into play, including the ability of HBO_2 at 3.0 atm absolute (abs), but not at 2.4 atm abs, to shut off the production of alpha toxin by clostridial species (Van Unnik 1965). This cut off production combined with clearance of extant toxin by the kidneys leads to detoxification of the patient, even in the presence of live organisms and oxygenation of tissue in the advancing border of necrosis, thereby decreasing the state of tissue reduction that allows proliferation

of anaerobes. This mechanism preserves viable tissue and helps demarcate necrotic tissue borders, thus reducing the amount of tissue requiring débridement. HBO_2 also enhances phagocytosis by supplementing oxygen substrate and increasing production of free radicals, which are the final mediators of bacterial killing by white blood cells.

In most clinical situations studied, HBO_2 treatment leads to constriction of blood vessels, with reduction of blood flow by 20 to 30%. In clinical situations associated with localized edema, such as in compartment syndrome, or in increased intracranial pressure with autoregulation intact, the reduced blood flow induced by HBO_2 often leads to reduced edema.

KINDS OF HYPERBARIC CHAMBERS

Two kinds of hyperbaric oxygen chambers are currently in use: the monoplace and the multiplace chambers. The monoplace chamber, which has a place for a single patient, is normally pressurized with 100% oxygen. The attendant controlling the chamber is on the outside. Because of the 100% oxygen environment, there is an increased risk of fire or explosion. The standard multiplace chamber is pressurized with air, and the oxygen is delivered to the patient either via a plastic hood over the patient's head and shoulders or via a tight-fitting aviation-type mask over the patient's nose and mouth, which is connected to the pure oxygen source. The multiplace chamber has room for multiple patients and a tender. Tenders are usually hyperbaric technicians or nurses. They assist patients with their air breaks (which are given to decrease the risk of oxygen toxicity), monitor for premonitory signs of oxygen toxicity, and assist in any other way necessary. When treating a critically ill patient, the tender should be a nurse with critical care training and skills. A respiratory therapist often accompanies such a patient to manage the ventilator. Almost all modalities that can be utilized to support a patient in an ICU setting can be utilized in a multiplace chamber setting.

Examples of the kinds of patients who would normally require such intensive care in the chamber setting are (1) those with sepsis with anaerobic necrotizing soft tissue infection, perhaps coming from the operating room and going to the chamber for an immediate treatment; (2) those with severe carbon monoxide poisoning, perhaps with myocardial depression, shock, and acidosis; (3) those with neurologic compromise, perhaps requiring ventilatory support to protect the airway, following a large air embolism from a surgical procedure, such as a transthoracic percutaneous needle biopsy of the lung. Although a few hyperbaric chambers are located at outpatient facilities, away from inpatient centers, most are located in hospitals, sometimes even within critical care areas, such as burn units and neurologic ICUs. Because multiplace chambers are mostly located outside the ICU setting, careful and competent patient transport is necessary to manage transfer from the ICU to hyperbaric chamber and back.

OXYGEN TRANSPORT UNDER HYPERBARIC HYPEROXIC CONDITIONS

Chapter 2 reviews the principles of gas transport in detail, and the reader is referred there. Briefly, oxygen is transported from the alveolus by two mechanisms: (1) chemical binding of four molecules of oxygen to each molecule of hemoglobin, at the alveolocapillary interface, and its subsequent circulation to cellular destinations with unloading of the oxygen; and (2) physical dissolution of oxygen in the plasma fraction of blood, independent of hemoglobin (Fife and Camporesi, 1991). Each gram of oxygen-saturated hemoglobin carries 1.34 ml of oxygen. Hence, 15 g of hemoglobin can transport approximately 20 ml of oxygen per 100 ml of blood. At the same time, the amount of oxygen dissolved in the plasma is physiologically negligible, amounting to only 0.0003 ml of oxygen per milliliter of blood, at a normal arterial oxygen partial pressure of 100 mm Hg. Once hemoglobin is fully saturated, further increases in the partial pressure of oxygen cannot cause any significant increase in the oxygen content of the blood unless the oxygen can be dissolved in the plasma fraction. The oxyhemoglobin dissociation curve modified to include hyperbaric conditions can be seen in Figure 26–1.

For each atmosphere increase in inspired oxygen pressure, arterial Po_2 rises approximately 700 mm Hg or approximately 2 vol%. At 3 atm abs, approximately 6 vol% of oxygen can be carried in plasma, which exceeds the normal tissue extraction of oxygen of 5 vol%. This increase in the oxygen-carrying capacity of blood has been used with success for transient treatment of severely anemic patients who cannot be immediately transfused (Hart et al, 1987).

EFFECT OF HYPERBARIC OXYGEN ON VENTILATION

Because the density of air increases as pressure increases, pulmonary work also increases during a hyperbaric treatment. Of the major flow regimens in the lung, turbulent and laminar, turbulent flow is the regimen in which resistance to airflow is dependent on gas density. Thus, work of breathing increases primarily because of elevated resistive work of breathing in large airways during HBO_2 treatment. This resistive work elevation is usually tolerated. There may be an occasional patient with chronic lung disease for whom the extra work of breathing may cause the sensation of breathlessness. In a situation in which the airway lumen in larger airways is narrowed, the increase in work of breathing is amplified, and respiratory distress may develop. This effect may occur with small-lumen endotracheal tubes or with increased respiratory rate.

There is also a net increase in resting ventilation during the hyperoxia experienced in the chamber, because the venous hemoglobin is fully saturated, displacing the fraction of CO_2 normally transported on deoxyhemoglobin as $HbCO_2$ (Gelfand et al 1987). Approximately 0.4 mmol of CO_2 is liberated, which causes an increased mixed venous Pco_2 of approximately 5 mm Hg, resulting in a slight acidosis (Lambertsen et al, 1953).

Because of the risk of fire in the hyperbaric oxygen environment, constraints exist on the type and design of mechanical ventilators that may be utilized in HBO_2 treatment facilities. The ability to scavenge excess oxygen and CO_2 buildup must be present. Moon and coworkers have provided guidelines for the Monaghan ventilator in HBO_2 treatment (Moon et al, 1986)

EFFECT OF HYPERBARIC OXYGEN ON THE POLYMORPHONUCLEAR LEUKOCYTE

Although there is still an incomplete understanding of all the physiologic effects of hyperoxia, one of the underlying mechanisms appears to involve the effect of HBO_2 on the polymorphonuclear leukocyte (PMN). Leukocytes depend on several mechanisms to kill bacteria. The first, and slower, nonoxidative mechanism involves phagocytosis of bacteria and degranulation of prepackaged enzymes within phagosomes to destroy microorganisms. The second mechanism, known as *oxidative killing*, is directly proportional to the available molecular oxygen, which is converted by leukocytes to oxygen radicals such as superoxide, hydroxyl, peroxide, and hypochlorite (Weiss, 1989). Badwey and Karnovsky also demonstrated this relationship between tissue oxygen tension and PMN oxidative burst after phagocytosis, and they determined that HBO_2 results in increased neutro-

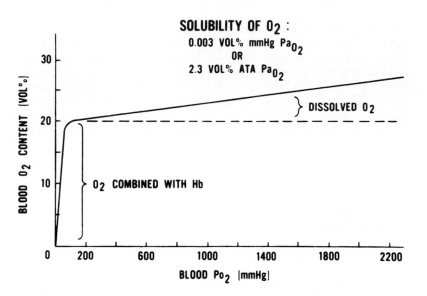

Figure 26–1
Extension of oxygen-hemoglobin dissociation curve. Blood oxygen content (vol%) available at high levels of blood oxygen pressure, assuming a normal hemoglobin level of 15 g/100 ml of blood. (From: Bassett BE, and Bennett PB: Introduction to the physical and physiological bases of hyperbaric therapy. In Davis JC, and Hunt TK (eds): Hyperbaric Oxygen Therapy. Bethesda, MD, Undersea Medical Society, 1977, p 20. Reprinted with permission of the Undersea and Hyperbaric Medical Society.)

phil microbial killing (Badwey and Karnovsky, 1980). Mader has demonstrated the synergistic effect of oxygen on the phagocytic killing of *Staphylococcus aureus* by neutrophils and opsonin (Mader et al, 1980).

ISCHEMIA-REPERFUSION INJURY

When tissue is subjected to a prolonged decrease in perfusion, a sequence of events is initiated that ultimately can result in dysfunction and even necrosis at the cellular level.

During this phase, the predominant injury is produced by hypoxia. Upon reperfusion of the tissue, secondary cellular injury can occur, which is thought to be mediated by cytotoxic oxidants. One of the pathways that produce oxygen radicals is that of xanthine oxidase (XO). Xanthine dehydrogenase (XD) is present in endothelial cells. During prolonged ischemia, XD is converted to XO, and upon reperfusion XO then converts hypoxanthine to xanthine and the toxic superoxide radical (Inauen et al, 1989). This process can be prevented by pretreatment with xanthine oxidase inhibitors such as allopurinol, as well as by treatment with free radical scavengers such as superoxide dismutase or deferoxamine mesylate (Thom, 1992). These XO-derived radicals can produce direct tissue damage but are very short-lived. More importantly, they may play a role in attracting neutrophils into post-ischemic tissue (Thom, 1992).

The PMN has been identified as a potential source of cytotoxic oxidants produced after reperfusion (Weiss, 1989). Neutrophils contain NADPH oxidase that reduces oxygen to the su-

peroxide anion. Leukocytes also produce hypochlorite via the myeloperoxidase pathway (Zamboni et al, 1993). This release of oxygen radicals occurs after the neutrophils adhere to the endothelium in post-ischemic tissue and become activated. Thom showed that this persistent leukocyte adherence is mediated by neutrophil cell surface proteins known as β_2-integrins (Thom, 1993). Once the PMN is firmly attached to the microvascular endothelium and begins to release oxygen free radicals as well as other vasoactive substances, endothelial injury results and allows extravasation of toxic metabolites into surrounding tissue. This extravasation produces the patchy necrosis characteristic of secondary reperfusion injury (Zamboni et al, 1993). Release of these same mediators by the leukocyte seems to cause further conversion of XD to XO, and a vicious cycle of free radical production may ensue. Beta$_2$-integrin–mediated neutrophil adherence can be blocked with hyperbaric oxygen.

THE OXYGEN PARADOX

It was initially thought that hyperoxia fueled the fire of reperfusion injury and resulted in an increased production of oxygen radicals. HBO$_2$, however, seems to have a net opposite effect. HBO$_2$ increases activity of superoxide dismutase, which is a potent free radical scavenger (Kaelin et al, 1990). Furthermore, HBO$_2$ seems to stimulate "quenching radicals" that neutralize oxygen free radicals and reduce lipid peroxidation and subsequent cellular injury (Thom and Elbuken, 1991). This observation is correlated with numerous experimental studies that demonstrate improved outcome of flaps and extremities exposed to ischemia-reperfusion injuries after treatment with HBO_2.

THE ROLE OF HYPERBARIC OXYGEN IN REPERFUSION INJURY

Although many studies have shown a benefit from HBO_2 in tissues in which the final common pathway is reperfusion injury, it has been only since 1993 that the mechanism became apparent. Using electron microscopy in an *in vivo* skeletal muscle preparation, Zamboni and coworkers (1993) demonstrated that leukocyte adherence to microvascular endothelium was significantly reduced by HBO_2 treatment performed for up to 1 hour after reperfusion. Additionally, progressive arteriolar vasoconstriction and patchy necrosis were also prevented. The decreased neutrophil adherence with HBO_2 results from selective inhibition of β_2-integrin function, which prevents persistent PMN adherence to the endothelium (Thom, 1993). It appears that other PMN functions are preserved and possibly enhanced so that the host does not become functionally neutropenic. Preventing persistent leukocyte adherence interrupts the production of free radicals at an early stage and can thus lead to significantly reduced tissue injury from reperfusion following ischemia. The decreased endothelial adherence of neutrophils seen with HBO_2 therapy has potential application in situations where ischemia-reperfusion plays a role in tissue injury. Thomas and Brown, for example, showed that the combination of recombinant tissue plasminogen activator (rTPA) and HBO_2 restored 97% oxidative enzyme activity in ischemic myocardial tissue—an effect that was significantly greater than that of rTPA or HBO_2 alone (Thomas et al, 1990).

CLINICAL THERAPEUTICS USING HYPERBARIC OXYGEN

The amount of material published in the area of hyperbaric oxygen therapy is overwhelming, with large numbers of papers, workshops, and peer-reviewed journals all within the fields of diving and hyperbaric medicine. Numerous texts have appeared over the years that accurately review the literature, clinical syndromes, and physiologic mechanisms related to hyperbaric medicine, with Kindwall's textbook being quite reliable (Kindwall, 1994). In the following section, those aspects of hyperbaric medicine that are of practical interest to the practicing cardiopulmonary critical care specialist are surveyed.

ARTERIAL AND VENOUS GAS EMBOLISM

Pulmonary overinflation syndrome (POS) is a result of ascent during scuba diving with breath-holding against a closed glottis resulting in a tear to the lung. Because air is delivered from the scuba regulator at ambient pressure underwater, as ambient pressure is reduced (the diver ascends), according to Boyle's law, intrapulmonary air expands if divers hold their breath. This can lead to air dissecting into one or more of three anatomic spaces: the pleural space, causing pneumothorax; the mediastinum, causing pneumomediastinum; or the alveolar circulation, causing arterial gas emboli. POS can result from any rapid ascent that causes a gradient of greater than 60 to 80 mm Hg across an alveolar wall. Such pressures can occur on ascent from as little as 6 or 7 feet of sea water (FSW.) In the scuba diver with pulmonary overinflation syndrome resulting in an arterial gas embolism, the clinical presentation usually includes loss of consciousness upon reaching the surface or within just a few minutes. In extreme cases the diver may sustain cardiac arrest.

POS often occurs in the situation of a panic ascent, such as when a diver loses a regulator, runs out of air, or lacks experience. Less extreme but nevertheless severe symptoms can include an acute confusional state, or any set of central neurologic deficits including dizziness, paralysis, muscle weakness, vision blurriness, or seizures. Other pulmonary syndromes associated with POS may also be present and should be sought. Pulmonary hemorrhage, which at times can be massive, may occur. A study reports the frequent finding of elevated creatine phosphokinase (CPK) enzyme levels in patients with arterial gas embolism, suggesting that gas emboli caused by a diving accident are distributed widely through the systemic vascular bed, inducing injury to skeletal muscle and possibly to the coronary circulation. In this study of 22 divers with arterial gas embolism, all had elevated serum CPK levels, often to very high levels, whereas the MB isoenzyme was greater than 4% of total activity in only 6 of the 20 patients in whom isoenzymes were measured (Smith and Neuman, 1994). The MM fraction predominated in the others. This test may be helpful in the differentiation of arterial gas embolism from decompression sickness in unusual cases. Furthermore, the degree of elevation of the CPK was correlated with the extent of the neurologic deficit. Radiologic manifestations of arterial gas embolism in the sport scuba diver have been reported (Harker et al, 1993) and may include pneumomediastinum, subcutaneous emphysema, pneumocardium without pneumopericardium, pneumoperitoneum, pneumothorax, and pulmonary hemorrhage with infiltrates. In over-whelming cases, air can be seen within the great vessels and major vessels beneath the diaphragm (Neuman et al, 1994).

In critical care situations, air embolism can occur following central line placement, and the condition can be fatal (Flanagan et al, 1969). It should also be suspected in the patient who "doesn't wake up" from general anesthesia after a surgical procedure. We have seen a case following transthoracic needle biopsy of the lung. The pa-tient presented with acute onset of confusion, slurred speech, and hemiparesis. The immediate treatment before entry into a hyperbaric chamber consists of high-flow oxygen, as close to 100% as possible. The increased oxygen tension in tissues is likely to hasten inert gas elimination and bub-ble resolution, even before recompression. Addi-tionally, in divers there may be other mechanisms present that exacerbate hypoxia, such as emesis or sea water aspiration, or the "chokes" (see later), each of which may also lead to hypoxia.

Placing the patient in a head-down position has been advocated in the past but is no longer recommended. Although anecdotal reports sug-gest that symptoms of arterial gas embolism some-times improve when the patient is placed in steep Trendelenburg position or with the head down on the left side to prevent ongoing embolization from trapped bubbles in the pulmonary circulation or the heart, there is currently more concern about exacerbating cerebral edema, particularly if the head-down position is maintained for more than 30 minutes (Van Meter, 1990). Nothing should delay the transfer of a patient to a chamber for definitive therapy.

Once a patient arrives at a hyperbaric facility, transfer into the chamber is appropriate if the patient is still alive and has cardiac rhythm. The treatment of choice is on the US Navy Table 6A, which is essentially a compression to 165 FSW, or 6 atm abs, in an attempt to "crush bubbles" to the smallest size. This pressure is maintained for 20 minutes, usually on a 50-to-50 oxygen-to-nitrogen mix to avoid oxygen toxicity. The pa-tient is then decompressed to 60 FSW (2.8 atm abs), and the rest of the treatment is carried out as in US Navy Table 6, which is a series of 3 to 6 breathing periods of 20 minutes each on 100% oxygen, with air breaks between each oxygen treatment period to reduce the risk of oxygen toxicity. This table allows the hyperbaricist to follow the progress of the response of the patient's symptoms and to extend the table further for symptoms that are slow to respond. The duration of treatment ranges from approximately 5 to 12 hours. Treatment on a standard Table 6 without the initial compression to 6.0 atm abs is also acceptable. Details of this and other tables are available in the standard reference (US Navy Diving Manual, 1993).

DECOMPRESSION SICKNESS

Decompression sickness (DCS) results from the emergence from solution of nitrogen bubbles in the circulation or within the tissues of the body in a quantity, and large enough size, to cause clinical symptoms. During scuba diving, as ambi-ent pressure increases at depth, the partial pres-sure of the inspired nitrogen also increases. This effect results in the accumulation of excess nitro-gen in peripheral tissues. When the diver ascends, the diver needs adequate time to "offload" the accumulated nitrogen. Sport divers generally dive within depth-time limits that allow for residual nitrogen to be offloaded without the necessity for undergoing decompression stops during ascent. DCS may occur in scuba divers who remain at depth too long, however, and either exceed their no-decompression limit without adequate decom-pression at shallower depths, or those who have dived close to the no-decompression limit without exceeding it, but have some other predisposition to DCS, such as being in cold water or being dehydrated.

Diving at higher altitudes is also a greater risk for DCS, as is flying after diving or traveling to a higher altitude within 12 hours of a dive. DCS also may occur at high altitude in pilots and astronauts.

It is known from Doppler studies that bubble formation is not uncommon in asymptomatic scuba divers. The majority of cases of silent bub-bles are filtered by the pulmonary capillaries and are not associated with symptoms. It is only when the number and size of the bubbles reach a certain level that symptoms of DCS appear more fre-quently. The exact pathologic steps are still to be completely defined. Despite numerous observa-tions of various phenomena associated with bub-ble formation in humans, including hemoconcen-tration, changes in blood viscosity, platelet aggregation and clumping, complement activa-tion, changes in protein structure, and changes in pulmonary hemodynamics, their roles in DCS are not yet well understood.

In a study by Moon and coworkers (1989), 30 divers with DCS were studied by echocardiog-raphy, and in the 18 divers with serious DCS, 61% had evidence of shunting through a patent foramen ovale (PFO) during the Valsalva maneu-ver. The incidence rate of PFO was in excess of that expected in a normal population and suggested the possibility of asymptomatic bubbles entering the arterial circulation by right-to-left shunting. Other intracardiac right-to-left shunts would be expected to have the same effect, resulting in symptomatic bubbles even when low levels of bubbles are present on the venous side, resulting in DCS from a non-decompression profile. Normally such affected candidates are disqualified from diving.

Symptoms of DCS range from minor joint pains, skin rash, and fatigue to neurologic decompression sickness, with weakness and paresthesias. The latter may progress rather suddenly to paralysis and bowel and bladder dysfunction. The neurologic manifestations of neurologic DCS do not fit the usual neurotomal patterns of deficit seen in trauma, because the pathophysiology is unique to this syndrome. Venous bubbles form in the low-pressure venous plexus draining the spinal cord, causing venous back pressure, edema, and infarction of the spinal cord. The deficits are usually patchy and are not necessarily symmetric. This pattern has been demonstrated in an animal model of DCS (Hallenbeck et al, 1975).

Pulmonary manifestations of DCS include the "chokes," which is a severe form of DCS thought to be due to gas emboli within the pulmonary capillaries, with release of vasoactive mediators in the pulmonary circulation. It is often associated with pleuritic chest pain. Nonproductive cough and shallow respirations may occur. Prehospital treatment consists of airway management and administration of oxygen and intravenous fluids. The definitive treatment remains recompression, on US Navy Table 6. Repetitive treatments are also sometimes used. The reader is referred elsewhere for further discussion on this topic.

CARBON MONOXIDE POISONING

Carbon monoxide (CO) is an odorless, colorless, noncaustic gas produced by incomplete combustion, as well as by methylene chloride metabolism. CO poisoning is responsible for many deaths per year in the United States and is seen commonly in cold weather areas with the use of defective heating systems and charcoal indoors, particularly by indigent populations, and with the use of hydrocarbon-burning machinery indoors. Patients may be asymptomatic, even with significant levels of carboxyhemoglobin (COHb), or they may have severe headaches, nausea and vomiting, confusion, ataxia, syncopal episodes, or loss of consciousness. Chest pain may be present, along with increased frequency, severity, or duration of angina or myocardial infarction. Other symptoms that may appear later, from 2 to 3 days to 2 or 3 weeks, are characterized by personality changes; return of prior symptoms; and other neuropsychiatric symptoms, including memory problems, inability to concentrate, and loss of interest in usual activities. These symptoms occurring together are often called *the delayed neurologic sequelae syndrome*.

Carboxyhemoglobin levels are used only as a marker for exposure, inasmuch as the level of COHb does not correlate well with symptoms. Development of neurologic and cardiac symptoms appears to be related to duration of exposure as well as the dose of CO. The neurotoxicity may be related to the β_2-integrin–mediated white blood cell clumping in the vasculature caused by CO, rather than the decrease in oxygen content of blood caused by the displacement of oxygen by CO in the hemoglobin. The additional effects of CO on the cytochrome system, including cytochrome P450, and on other enzyme systems are still not well understood.

Current literature appears to support the notion that HBO_2 in the acute poisoning period decreases the incidence of the delayed neurologic sequelae syndrome; however, this position is not without controversy. Differences in study design, patient selection, timing of hyperbaric treatments, and dosing pressure of HBO_2 all lead to different conclusions. There appears to be a trend toward reduced incidence of the delayed neurologic sequelae if patients are treated within 6 hours of exposure (Thom et al, 1995). A current ongoing double-blind multicenter study may answer many questions in the near future regarding correct dose and timing for successful treatment.

HBO_2 is currently recommended within 6 hours for any patient who has sustained loss of consciousness; has documented neurologic findings, including abnormalities on psychometric testing; has an absolute level of COHb greater than 25 to 30% (even if asymptomatic); or, in a pregnant patient, a level greater than 15%. Patients with cardiac symptoms of chest pain, hypotension, congestive heart failure, or electrocardiographic changes should also be treated. Treatment is in the range of 2.4 to 3.0 atm abs. The half life of COHb is markedly reduced with HBO_2, from approximately 4.5 hours breathing air and approximately 90 minutes breathing 100% oxygen at 1 atm, to approximately 20 minutes at 2.8 to 3.0 atm abs.

WOUND HEALING

Any wound requires a PO_2 level higher than 30 to 40 mm Hg for fibroblasts to undergo mitosis and for collagen deposition and capillary ingrowth into the wound site. In the presence of thickened basement membranes, as in diabetes or old age, or inflamed vasculature, as in vasculitis or radiation injury, if the depth of a wound is hypoxic, there is a high risk of nonhealing. Such conditions also occur in the presence of peripheral vascular disease and are often seen in nonhealing wounds where there is venous insufficiency, such as following saphenous vein graft donation, in the extremities. Extensive and complete discussions of the mechanisms involved in wound healing are found in Davis and Hunt (1988).

In treating such problem wounds, HBO$_2$ is an adjunct to standard therapy and does not substitute for standard wound care practices, such as the drainage of abscesses, débridement of necrotic tissue, appropriate antibiotic coverage for treatment of intercurrent infection, evaluation of extremities for fixed bypassable arterial lesions, correction of hypovolemia, maintenance of good nutrition, control of hyperglycemia and acidosis, and removal of sequestra of dead bone when chronic osteomyelitis is present. A typical treatment course consists of a 2.4-atm abs treatment pressure, with 90 minutes of 100% oxygen per 2-hour treatment. Treatment course duration is variable, depending on the size of the wound and individual wound healing factors. A typical foot ulcer may take 20 to 30 treatments, given on a once- or twice-daily protocol, whereas more extensive open wounds can require up to 60 or more treatments for resolution. Generation of a granulation bed covering a wound is the usual goal, so that grafting or flaps creation will be successful.

The role of HBO$_2$ in limb salvage for diabetics has been demonstrated in several studies (Baroni et al, 1987; Oriani et al, 1990), and its cost-effectiveness has been documented (Cianci et al, 1988).

HYPERBARIC OXYGEN AND MYOCARDIAL ISCHEMIA

Currently the use of HBO$_2$ for myocardial ischemia remains at a research level only. Animal model studies have shown that HBO$_2$ treatment leads to reduced mortality from ventricular fibrillation (Smith and Lawson, 1962); infarct size is reduced (Trapp and Creighton, 1964; Sterling et al, 1993); and myocardial injury is reduced in a reversible occlusion model (Kawamura et al, 1976). The Thomas and Brown study showing the synergistic protective effect of HBO$_2$ when combined with TPA was discussed earlier.

Despite these and other animal studies, data from human studies are less impressive and not as plentiful. The first successful use of HBO$_2$ in a human patient with myocardial ischemia was over 30 years ago (Moon et al, 1964), whereas a large controlled human study found little benefit from HBO$_2$ (Thurston et al, 1973). The interest in HBO$_2$ therapy in the 60s and 70s was attenuated by the rapid progress in anatomic reperfusion procedures, both surgical and biochemical. Once the roles of coronary artery bypass grafting, angioplasty, and thrombolysis began to be sorted out, however, the possibility of utilizing HBO$_2$ as an adjunct to the other methods was entertained. Interim data have been presented from a multicenter study comparing tPA with tPA plus HBO$_2$, which has been called the "hot MI" study (Ellestad and Hart, 1994). Patients in the HBO$_2$-treated group had a lower peak CPK, faster resolution of chest pain and ST segment elevation compared with the tPA-alone group. Survival and left ventricular ejection fraction were not statistically significantly improved. Further studies appear warranted.

Another area in which HBO$_2$ may have a role is as a component of assessment of reversibility of myocardial dysfunction. Swift and others (1992) reported on their evaluation of the potential for HBO$_2$ to produce transient improvement in function of areas of hibernating myocardium, defined as ischemic viable muscle with the potential to resume contraction if reperfused. Twenty-four patients were studied within 1 week of acute myocardial infarction, with transesophageal echocardiography (TEE), transthoracic echocardiography (TTE), and submaximal exercise thallium scintigraphy following an HBO$_2$ treatment of only 30 minutes. They were compared with 10 patients who received hyperbaric air alone. Segments of resting wall motion abnormalities were identified with TEE pre-HBO$_2$ and were reassessed following HBO$_2$ treatment. Perfusion-contraction matching with concordance for myocardial viability was present in 77% of segments. In 10 control patients, 25 abnormally contracting segments were identified, and none improved with hyperbaric air. Improvement was noted in 20 of 62 segments identified in 12 of the 24 study patients who received hyperbaric oxygen (p<.0005). These researchers advised that the technique of HBO$_2$ treatment and echocardiography may identify hibernating myocardium and may have the potential to predict improvement in left ventricular function with early intervention post-infarction. Further validation studies are required to correlate the findings with early interventions of bypass grafting or angioplasty.

INCREASED INTRACRANIAL PRESSURE AND SEVERE HEAD INJURY

A number of studies examine the effects of HBO_2 on severe head injury and increased intracranial pressure and its clinical correlates. Despite the outcome of the studies, the use of HBO_2 has not been approved for such an indication by the Undersea and Hyperbaric Medical Society, because its specific role and indications have not yet become clear. In certain critical clinical scenarios, however, it may be helpful to consider such treatment at times and report the results.

Pathophysiologically, inadequate oxygen supply to traumatized brain results in conversion of aerobic glucose metabolism to anaerobic metabolism and resultant acidosis. This process in turn leads to loss of ability to maintain normal electrolyte concentrations intracellularly, and as a result calcium levels increase. This effect, together with acidosis, may lead to a cascade of proteolytic enzymes, which further damages cells. HBO_2 treatment may improve oxygen delivery to brain cells sufficiently to enhance aerobic metabolism and stave off the anaerobic cascade. The benefit of HBO_2 is a reduction in cerebral blood flow, by 20 to 30%, which is due to cerebral vasoconstriction dependent on the persistence of autoregulation (Jacobson et al, 1963), as well as hyperoxygenation of hypoxic areas. A result of the decrease in cerebral blood flow is a decrease in intracranial pressure.

The most comprehensive study is by Rockswold (1994) at Hennepin County Medical Center, Minneapolis, MN. Between 1983 and 1989, this investigator randomized groups among 168 patients with closed-head injury for a prospective trial to evaluate the effect of HBO_2 in the treatment of brain injury. For admission to the study, Glasgow Coma Score (GCS) had to be 9 or less for at least 6 hours. Randomization was done, and stratification was made by GCS and age into treatment groups and control groups. HBO_2 was delivered at 1.5 atm abs for 1 hour every 8 hours, and continued for 2 weeks or until the patient was awake or brain-dead. The Glasgow Outcome Scale (GOS) was employed to assess recovery. Average number of treatments was 21. Only two patients were lost to follow-up by 12 months.

Mortality for the 84 HBO_2-treated patients was 17% versus 32% for the control group. Among the 80 patients with Glasgow scores of 4, 5, or 6, there was a 17% mortality rate for the HBO_2-treated group versus 42% for controls. These differences were statistically significant. For patients with peak intracranial pressures greater than 20 mm Hg, mortality rates were 21% in the HBO_2-treated group versus 48% in the controls. The difference in mortality between HBO_2-treated and control-group patients with surgical mass lesions was not statistically significant by two-tailed Chi-square analysis, but it was significant when probability of survival was compared using the log rank (Mantel-Haenszel) test. The functional recovery of the salvaged patients was not satisfactory, however, despite the increased survival rate, in any of the groups examined (GCS 4–6; GCS 7–9; presence of mass lesion, contusion or fixed pupils; and intracranial pressure level). The poor functional recovery rate may be a result of the severity of the brain injury, leaving the brain incapable of further recovery.

In addition, although this lengthy controlled study was a remarkable achievement, the HBO_2 treatment table was at 1.5 atm abs, and the outcomes may be different at different treatment pressures. The pressure level, and probably the frequency, duration, and timing of HBO_2 treatments, are likely to be important factors in determining clinical response to HBO_2. Further studies will likely study combining HBO_2 with antioxidants or other adjunctive therapies, in the hope of improving the outcome of the increased numbers of survivors.

CONTRAINDICATIONS TO USE OF HYPERBARIC OXYGEN

The only absolute contraindication to placing a patient in a hyperbaric chamber is the presence of an untreated pneumothorax. With an increase in the ambient pressure during HBO_2 treatment, the volume of the lung that was collapsed may increase back to normal as the pneumothorax, a closed air-containing compartment, decreases in size. This outcome occurs both because of the effects of Boyle's law and because nitrogen present in the pneumothorax is eliminated during 100% oxygen breathing at depth. On ascent, however, the pneumothorax may expand and may even lead to tension with cardiopulmonary decompensation. Accordingly, most patients undergoing elective care are cleared for treatment with a recent chest radiograph, as are patients with pulmonary overinflation syndrome. A chest tube should always be placed for control of the pleural space in the patient with pneumothorax before HBO_2 therapy. A chest film should always be obtained before a treatment if a recent central line insertion or an attempt at one has been made. Theoretically, patients with bullous lesions of the lung that have poor or slow rates of emptying during ventilation are also at risk for the development of a pneumothorax during hyperbaric treatments, although this occurrence has not been observed to be a problem and "rate of ascent" from treatment pressure can be controlled.

A number of unusual situations appear to make hyperbaric treatments relatively contraindicated. Examples of such situations include the patient who has problems with chronic CO_2 retention, who breathes owing to only hypoxic drive, and who may lose the drive to breathe during the condition of marked hyperoxia during an HBO_2 treatment. In such a situation, it is important to decide how critical the hyperbaric treatment is, and whether it is reasonable to intubate and ventilate the patient to attain the hyperbaric treatments.

The cardiac toxicity of doxorubicin (Adriamycin) chemotherapy appears to be enhanced with HBO_2 therapy in an animal model, and thus some hyperbaricists recommend waiting a week after a prior dose of doxorubicin before using HBO_2.

THE FUTURE OF HYPERBARIC MEDICINE

The field of hyperbaric medicine is a burgeoning one, with the elucidation of new mechanisms of action of HBO_2 appearing frequently. Hyperbaric oxygen therapy has often been criticized, however, because of the lack of controlled, double-blind studies. The number of controlled studies is higher than many estimate and the attempts of the Undersea and Hyperbaric Medical Society to scrutinize each new indication and ensure a sound scientific basis before approving a proposed new indication serve as a check and balance for those who wish to use HBO_2 treatment in every setting. HBO_2 should be thought of as a treatment modality whenever hypoxia or necrosis is implicated as a cause or component of pathology, and hyperbaric consultation should be sought. Entry of patients into ongoing studies and preparation of new protocols in conjunction with the hyperbaric community are essential parts of the evolution of the field of hyperbaric medicine and medicine in general. It is incumbent upon the practitioners of cardiopulmonary critical care to be familiar with the indications for and uses of HBO_2 therapy, as it becomes a greater part of mainstream medicine.

REFERENCES

Badwey JA and Karnovsky ML: Active oxygen species and the functions of phagocytic leukocytes. Annu Rev Biochem 49:695–726, 1980.

Baroni G, Porro T, Faglia E, et al: Hyperbaric oxygen in diabetic gangrene treatment. Diabetes Care 10:81–86, 1987.

Bassett BE and Bennett PB: Introduction to the physical and physiological bases of hyperbaric therapy. In Davis JC, and Hunt TK (eds): Hyperbaric Oxygen Therapy. Bethesda, MD, Undersea Medical Society, Inc., 1977, p 920.

Behnke AR: Decompression sickness. Am J Physiol 110:565–572, 1935.

Cianci P, Petrone G, Drager S, et al: Salvage of the problem wound and potential amputation with wound care and adjunctive hyperbaric oxygen therapy: An economic analysis. J Hyperbaric Med 3:127–141, 1988.

Davis JC and Hunt TK: Problem Wounds: The Role of Oxygen. New York, Elsevier Science Publishing, 1988.

Ellestad MH and Hart GB: The use of hyperbaric oxygen in the treatment of acute myocardial infarction in animals and man. In Kindwall EP (ed): Hyperbaric Medicine Practice. Flagstaff, AZ, Best Publishing, 1994, pp 657–659.

Fife CE and Camporesi EM: Physiologic effects of hyperbaric hyperoxia. In Moon RE and Camporesi EM (eds): Problems in Respiratory Care: Clinical Applications of Hyperbaric Oxygen 4:(2):142–149, 1991.

Flanagan JP, Gradisar IA, Gross RJ, and Kelly TR: Air embolus—a lethal complication of subclavian venipuncture. N Engl J Med 281:488–489, 1969.

Gelfand R, Clark JM, Lambertsen CJ, et al: Effects on respiratory homeostasis of prolonged, continuous hyperoxia at 1.5 to 1.0 ATA in predictive studies V. In Bove AA, Bachrach AJ, Greenbaum LJ Jr (eds): Underwater and Hyperbaric Physiology IX: Proceedings of the 9th International Symposium on Underwater and Hyperbaric Physiology. Bethesda, MD, Undersea and Hyperbaric Medical Society Inc., 1987, pp 751–761.

Hallenbeck JM, Bove AA, and Elliott DH. Mechanisms underlying spinal cord damage in decompression sickness. Neurology 25:308–316, 1975.

Harker CP, Neuman TS, Olson LK, et al: The roentgenographic findings associated with air embolism in sport scuba divers. J Emerg Med 11(4):443–449, 1993.

Hart GB, Lennon PA, and Strauss MD: Hyperbaric oxygen in exceptional acute blood loss anemia. J Hyperbaric Med 2:205–210, 1987.

Hyperbaric Oxygen Therapy: A Committee Report. Kensington, MD, Undersea and Hyperbaric Medical Society, 1996.

Inauen W, Suzuki M, and Granger DN: Mechanisms of cellular injury: Potential sources of oxygen free radicals in ischemia/reperfusion. Microcirc Endothelium Lymphatics 5:143–155, 1989.

Jacobson K, Harper AM, and McDowall DG: The effects of oxygen under pressure on cerebral blood-flow and cerebral venous oxygen tension. Lancet 2:549, 1963.

Kaelin CM, Im MJ, Myers RA, et al: The effects of

hyperbaric oxygen on free flaps in rats. Arch Surg 125(5):607–609, 1990.

Kawamura M, Sakakibara K, Sakakibara B, et al: Protective effect of hyperbaric oxygen for the temporary ischemic myocardium: Macroscopic and histologic data. Cardiovasc Res 10:599–604, 1976.

Kindwall EP (ed): Hyperbaric Medicine Practice. Flagstaff, AZ, Best Publishing, 1994.

Lambertsen CJ, Kough RH, Cooper DY, et al: Oxygen toxicity. Effects in man of oxygen inhalation at 1 and 3.5 atmospheres upon blood gas transport, cerebral circulation, and cerebral metabolism. J Appl Physiol 5(9):471–486, 1953.

Mader JT, Brown GL, Guckian JC, et al: A mechanism for the amelioration by hyperbaric oxygen of experimental staphylococcal osteomyelitis in rabbits. J Infect Dis 142(6):915–922, 1980.

Moon AJ, Williams KG, and Hopkinson WI: A patient with coronary thrombosis treated with hyperbaric oxygen. Lancet 1:18, 1964.

Moon RE, Bergquist LV, Conklin B, et al. Monaghan 225 ventilator use under hyperbaric conditions. Chest 89:846–851, 1986.

Moon RE, Camporesi EM, and Kisslo JA: Patent foramen ovale and decompression sickness in divers. Lancet 1:513–514, 1989.

Neuman TS, Jacoby I, and Olson L: Fatal diving related arterial gas embolism associated with complete filling of the central vascular bed. Undersea and Hyperbaric Medicine 21[Suppl]:101, 1994.

Oriani G, Meazza D, Favales F, et al: Hyperbaric oxygen therapy in diabetic gangrene treatment. J Hyperbaric Med 5(3):171–175, 1990.

Rockswold GL: The treatment of severe head injury with hyperbaric oxygen. In Kindwall EP (ed): Hyperbaric Medicine Practice. Flagstaff, AZ, Best Publishing, 1994, pp 641–648.

Smith G and Lawson DD: The protective effect of inhalation of oxygen at two atmospheres absolute pressure in acute coronary arterial occlusion. Surg Gynecol Obstet 114:320, 1962.

Smith RM and Neuman TS: Elevation of serum creatinine in divers with arterial gas embolization. N Engl J Med 330(1):19–24, 1994.

Sterling DL, Thornton JD, Swafford A, et al: Hyperbaric oxygen limits infarct size in ischemic rabbit myocardium in vivo, part 1. Circulation 88:1931–1936, 1993.

Swift PC, Turner JH, Oxer HF, et al: Myocardial hibernation identified by hyperbaric oxygen treatment and echocardiography in postinfarction patients: Comparison with exercise thallium scintigraphy. Am Heart J 124:1151–1158, 1992.

Thom SR: Dehydrogenase conversion to oxidase and lipid peroxidation in brain after carbon monoxide poisoning. J Appl Physiol 73(4):1584–1589, 1992.

Thom SR: Functional inhibition of leukocyte beta$_2$-integrins by hyperbaric oxygen in carbon monoxide mediated brain injury in rats. Toxicol Appl Pharmacol 123:248–256, 1993.

Thom SR and Elbuken ME: Oxygen-dependent antagonism of lipid peroxidation. Free Radic Biol Med 10(6):413–426, 1991.

Thom SR, Taber RL, Mendiguren II, et al: Delayed neuropsychologic sequelae after treatment with carbon monoxide poisoning: Prevention by treatment with hyperbaric oxygen. Ann Emerg Med 25(4):474–480, 1995.

Thomas MP, Brown LA, Sponseller DR, et al: Myocardial infarct size reduction by the synergistic effect of hyperbaric oxygen and recombinant tissue plasminogen activator. Am Heart J 120:791–800, 1990.

Thurston JGB, Greenwood TW, Berding MR, et al: A controlled investigation into the effects of hyperbaric oxygen on mortality following acute myocardial infarction. Q J Med 42(168):751–770, 1973.

Trapp WG and Creighton R: Experimental studies of increased atmospheric pressure on myocardial ischemia after coronary ligation. J Thorac Cardiovasc Surg 47:687, 1964.

U.S. Navy Diving Manual. Document 0994-LP-001-9010, revision 3. U.S. Naval Sea Systems Command, 15 February 1993.

Van Meter K: Diving accident management—first aid and medical evaluation. In Bennett PB, and Moon RE (eds): Diving Accident Management: 41st Undersea and Hyperbaric Medical Society Workshop. Bethesda, MD, Undersea and Hyperbaric Medical Society, 1990, pp 162–193.

Van Unnik AJM: Inhibition of toxin production in Clostridium perfringens in vitro by hyperbaric oxygen. Antonie van Leeuwenhoek J 31:181–186, 1965.

Weiss SJ: Tissue destruction by neutrophils. N Engl J Med 320(6):365–375, 1989.

Zamboni WA, Roth AC, Russell RC, et al: Morphologic analysis of the microcirculation during reperfusion of ischemic skeletal muscle and the effect of hyperbaric oxygen. Plast Reconstr Surg 91(6):1110–1123, 1993.

C H A P T E R

Pulmonary Failure Caused by High Altitude

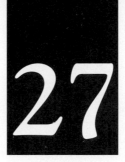

Robert B. Schoene, M.D.

Hypoxemic respiratory failure results from many etiologies, but in the context of normal alveolar ventilation, it results from impaired gas exchange with areas of low ventilation and perfusion matching and/or shunt. Atelectasis, airway narrowing from a number of causes, and alveolar edema are pathologic entities with physiologic consequences of hypoxemia. The problem worsens with a lower inspired partial pressure of oxygen, such as that at high altitude. No worse scenario exists than that of a patient with pulmonary edema at high altitude. The clinical entity of high altitude pulmonary edema (HAPE), which occurs in a previously healthy person, is a potentially fatal disease. To take care of the patient requires proper recognition and all the skill of an astute clinician with an understanding of physiology.

HAPE must be distinguished from acute mountain sickness (AMS), a milder form of altitude illness that develops at lower altitudes within the first 12 to 48 hours of ascent. AMS usually resolves with rest at the same altitude. It is marked by headache, malaise, anorexia, insomnia, periodic breathing, and nausea and vomiting in severe cases (Singh et al, 1969).

The purpose of this chapter is to review the historical, clinical, and physiologic aspects of HAPE to gain perspective of this disease as one that fulfills all the criteria for respiratory failure. Additionally, treatment modalities and directions for research to unravel the mechanism of fluid from the intravascular to extravascular space in the lung are discussed.

HISTORY

The history of all high-altitude maladies provides a rich saga that parallels that of modern medicine. Travelers over the last 2000 years traversed high mountain passes. Descriptions of illnesses that explorers and traders attributed to noxious gases and other demons appear in remote literature. These illnesses were in many cases either acute mountain sickness (AMS) or high-altitude pulmonary or cerebral edema. In 1891, high above the Chamonix Valley in the French Alps, Dr. Henri Jacottet climbed Mont Blanc to make scientific observations. He became ill but remained on the mountain to document his own acclimatization, which resulted in his death. Pathologic examination revealed gross pulmonary edema (Mosso, 1898.)

A few years later a young Italian soldier ascended to the newly built Campana Regina Margherita hut on the summit of Monte Rosa in the Italian Alps (4559 meters). He developed respiratory distress and became critically ill but recovered in a few days. His case appears in *Life of Man in the High Alps*, written by the eminent physiologist, Angelo Mosso (1898).

Europeans flocked to the Andes Mountains of South America for mining, and in 1913 an English physician, Dr. Thomas Ravenhill, clearly described several cases of high-altitude illness and HAPE (1913). But for many years clinicians attributed most of the cases of HAPE to pneumonia or congestive heart failure. Further cases from South America (Hurtado, 1937; Lizaraga, 1955), which in hindsight must have been HAPE, appeared in the literature. It was not until the 1960s that Hultgren and Houston (1961) in separate reports described cases of respiratory failure at high altitude, which they recognized as being noncardiogenic and noninfectious in origin. More detailed reports followed (Hultgren et al, 1961; Marticorena, 1979; Maldonado, 1978), and clinical investigations began.

CLINICAL PRESENTATION

A number of excellent reviews of HAPE are available (Hultgren, 1978; Schoene, 1985; Hackett and Roach, 1990), and from these one can gain a sense of the clinical and physiologic correlation. HAPE occurs in the context of rapid ascent to high altitude before normal acclimatization takes place. It can occur at a point as low as 2500 meters, as in recreational mountain areas in the United States, as well as in higher mountain areas of the world, and is more common above 3000 meters. HAPE occurs more frequently during rapid ascent, during higher levels of physical activity, more in men than women, and in individuals who are "susceptible." HAPE usually follows acute mountain sickness (AMS), which is a milder form of altitude illness. The symptoms progress to dyspnea at rest, marked limitation to exercise, and a dry cough. If not recognized and treated, severe dyspnea; a cough productive of pink, frothy sputum; obtundations; and death may ensue. Neurologic signs, particularly in more severe cases, such as ataxia and confusion, may accompany HAPE, suggesting the concom-

itant existence of high-altitude cerebral edema (HACE).

On physical examination, patients have crackles, usually beginning in the right middle lobe area and spreading diffusely; tachycardia; tachypnea; and cyanosis. Many have low-grade fevers. There are a few findings of cardiac dysfunction (i.e., no S_3 gallop, although an accentuated pulmonic component of S_2 is often present).

The laboratory examination reveals a mild leukocytosis and a wide range of arterial oxygen saturations (SaO_2), which depend on the severity of the disease and the altitude. For instance, on Mt. McKinley (Denali) in Alaska at 4300 meters, climbers with HAPE are more severely ill and SaO_2 values average slightly above 50% (Schoene et al, 1986; 1988); whereas in Keystone, Colorado, at a ski resort at 2928 meters, patients reporting to the local clinic had average SaO_2 values of 74%, but here too there was a wide range (38–93%), depending on the severity of the disease (Hultgren et al, 1996). Corresponding blood gas results showed a widened A-a O_2 gradient and respiratory alkalosis.

Radiographic examinations (Fig. 27–1) demonstrate a wide variety of presentations (Hultgren et al, 1962; Menon, 1965; Singh et al, 1965; Maldonado, 1978; Kobayashi et al, 1987; Vock et

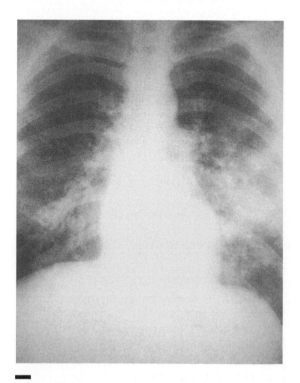

Figure 27–1
The radiograph in HAPE shows a normal cardiac silhouette with diffuse patchy infiltrates.

al, 1989, 1991; Koizumi et al, 1994). The cardiac silhouette is normal, except that there may be a prominent right ventricular shadow. Many times the infiltrates begin in the right middle lobe, progressing to patchy infiltrates that are predominantly in the mid-lung fields, but can be anywhere. They do not present in a bat wing–like pattern as in congestive heart failure. The pulmonary arteries may be enlarged. The infiltrates resolve within 48 to 72 hours when the patient recovers.

The electrocardiogram (ECG) shows sinus tachycardia, and some patients have signs of right heart strain and hypertrophy with right axis deviation, right bundle branch block, and peaked P waves in the anterior precordium (Hultgren et al, 1961; Hultgren et al, 1962; Menon, 1965; Singh et al, 1965; Marticorena et al, 1979). With recovery, the ECG returns to normal, but some of the signs of right heart strain may persist if patients stay at altitude. This observation has also been noted in normal individuals at high altitude, which is presumably a reflection of pulmonary hypertension that is a normal response to high altitude exposure and not of HAPE *per se.*

PATHOLOGIC FINDINGS

Autopsy data are scant. Several reports (Arias-Stella and Kruger, 1963; Heath et al, 1973; Marticorena et al, 1979; Kobayashi et al, 1987) give consistent findings of severe pulmonary edema with hemorrhagic, frothy, proteinaceous fluid in the airspace with right atrial and ventricular distention but no left ventricular pathology. The pulmonary microvasculature is congested, and thrombi have been reported in the arterioles. Hyaline membranes are present in some of the cases, and some patients have patchy bronchopneumonia (Arias-Stella and Kruger, 1963; Martocorena et al, 1979).

Because these are postmortem findings of the most severe cases, it is difficult to attribute all of them to the underlying mechanism of HAPE. For instance, are the thrombi and the assumed coagulation abnormalities pathogenic or merely postmortem effects? Are all cases of HAPE associated with underlying pneumonias or were the pneumonias present in the most severely ill? Most experts believe that these autopsy data are a reflection of the condition of the most ill individuals and are not common denominators in all those with HAPE.

PATHOPHYSIOLOGY

Most of the understanding of HAPE necessarily comes from human clinical investigations and observations. From these studies three areas emerge that are important in helping to determine the underlying mechanism of fluid into the alveolar space: the control of ventilation, the hemodynamic response, and the cellular and biochemical nature of alveolar fluid in HAPE.

The *hypoxic ventilatory response* (HVR) is the primary physiologic response that defends alveolar and subsequently arterial oxygen level upon ascent to high altitude (Weil, 1971; 1986). The HVR occurs immediately upon ascent and continues to increase during a stay at any given altitude for approximately two weeks, during which time the arterial oxygen saturation (SaO_2) continues to climb. This process is called *ventilatory acclimatization* and is essential to survival at high altitude. There is a wide range of responses with a normal bell-shaped distribution (Weil et al, 1971).

Of interest is the association of altitude illnesses with individuals who have blunted ventilatory responses upon ascent to high altitude (Hu et al, 1982; Masuda et al, 1992). These individuals have lower SaO_2 values and relatively higher $PaCO_2$ values. Researchers on Mt. McKinley (Denali) studied a group of climbers during and after HAPE as well as a group of controls (Hackett et al, 1988). The HAPE patients have substantially lower HVR values both during and after HAPE (Fig. 27–2), suggesting that they are not able to defend and maintain normal levels of oxygenation compared with control subjects. Other studies support this contention (Matsuzawa et al, 1989; Selland et al, 1993). A blunted HVR is, therefore, thought to be a permissive physiologic characteristic.

Over the last three decades, investigators have focused on the effect of the *hemodynamic* response on the pulmonary vasculature (see Chapter 3 for detailed discussion of the pulmonary vasculature). In the 1960s and 1970s, pioneering work was done to describe the pulmonary vascular and cardiac response in patients with HAPE. The first hemodynamic data in a patient with HAPE were reported in 1962 (Fred et al, 1962). Using a cardiac catheter, the researchers found pulmonary artery pressures of 68/39, which decreased with 100% oxygen breathing, whereas left atrial and pulmonary venous pressure levels were normal. This was the first paper to establish that left ventricular function was normal. Hultgren and coworkers (1964a,b) and Roy and coworkers (1969) studied the larger groups of patients, confirmed the earlier findings, and reported normal pulmonary wedge pressures, which substantiated that cardiac function was normal and that global pulmonary venoconstriction was not an etiologic factor in HAPE. As HAPE and gas exchange

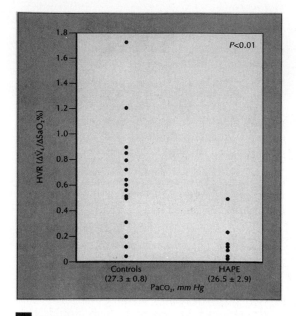

Figure 27–2
The hypoxic ventilatory response (HVR) (V̇E/SaO₂) is lower in subjects with HAPE than in control subjects when measured at 4300 meters, which suggests that a blunted HVR upon ascent to high altitude results in more profound hypoxemia. (From Hackett PH, Roach RC, Schoene RB, et al: Abnormal control of ventilation in high-altitude pulmonary edema. J Appl Physiol 64(3):1268–1272, 1988. With permission.)

improve, pulmonary hypertension decreases (Kobayashi et al, 1987).

Investigators have used cardiac echocardiography to assess the pulmonary vasculature in HAPE (Kawashima et al, 1989; Oelz et al, 1989; Hackett et al, 1992; Vachiery et al, 1995). The HAPE-susceptible subjects provide a fertile population for study. All of these studies have shown that pulmonary artery pressures are very elevated in most patients with HAPE, and these data lend further credence to the hypothesis that stress on the pulmonary microvasculature plays a role in the development of HAPE.

In an elegant field study, Bartsch and coworkers (1991) tested the hypothesis that accentuated pulmonary vascular responses to altitude played a role in the development of HAPE in HAPE-susceptible subjects. They used nifedipine, a pulmonary vasodilator, as a prophylactic measure in these subjects upon ascent to the Monte Rosa research station in the Italian Alps (4559 meters) and used Doppler measurements of pulmonary vasoreactivity, chest radiographs, and clinical evaluations. Nifedipine essentially prevented HAPE in these susceptible subjects, giving more evidence that pulmonary hypertension plays a role in ini-

tiating the permeability leak into the lung. At the same site, these same investigators gave nitric oxide (NO) in a similar group of subjects and found that NO improved gas exchange and increased perfusion to the nonedematous areas of the lung (Scherrer et al, 1996). Their observation suggests that pulmonary vasoconstriction may be patchy rather than homogeneous.

The question of patchy versus homogeneous hypoxic pulmonary vasoconstriction is a critical one that begs for an answer. Much of the theory at this time is based on circumstantial evidence and speculation. From a radiographic standpoint, HAPE is patchy (Hultgren et al, 1961; Menon, 1965; Singh et al, 1965; Maldanado, 1978; Kobayashi et al, 1987; Vock et al, 1989; Vock et al, 1991; Koizumi et al, 1994). Perfusion scans suggest that HAPE-susceptible subjects when exposed to hypoxia have patchy distribution of perfusion compared with controls (Viswnathan et al, 1979). Several patterns of leak can, therefore, be hypothesized (Fig. 27–3).

If alveolar hypoxia results in homogeneous pulmonary vasoconstriction, intravascular pressures are increased in the precapillary arterioles, resulting in stress on the endothelial layer. This observation suggests that the entire vascular bed is the site of the leak of fluid into the interstitium and eventually into the alveoli. In contrast, if it is patchy, vasoconstriction protects some alveoli while other alveoli undergo increased flow and stress. Conceivably, stress on two vascular beds, the precapillary arterioles and the overperfused pulmonary capillaries *per se*, can result in two sites of leak.

The concept of overperfusion gains some support from observations reported by Hackett and coworkers (1980). They described four cases of patients with congenital absence of a pulmonary artery who developed HAPE at modest altitudes, which suggests that overperfusion of a compromised pulmonary capillary bed can lead to leak into the alveoli. Hultgren (1978) reported an experiment in a dog model in which he sequentially ligated all but one of the lobar pulmonary arteries, thus placing all of the cardiac output into an isolated pulmonary vascular bed, which resulted in an edematous lobe.

West (1991, 1992, 1993) has explored the concept that the pulmonary capillaries can withstand only so much mechanical stress. In a rabbit model, he and colleagues elevated the pulmonary capillary pressure acutely and demonstrated on electron microscopy fractures in the endothelial barrier with leak of proteinaceous fluid and some erythrocytes. The researchers contend that this

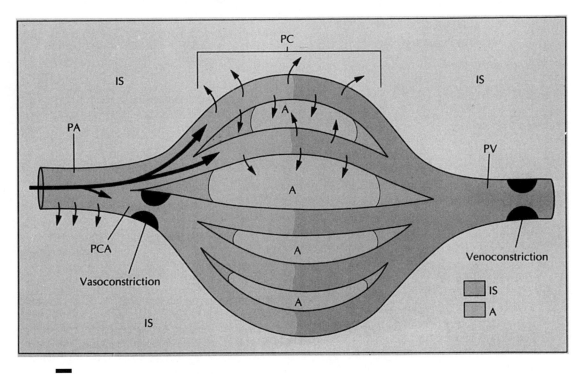

Figure 27–3
Sites of possible hypoxic pulmonary vasoconstriction at which high intravascular pressure may lead to extravascular leak. (Schoene RB: In Braunwald E (ed): Atlas of Heart Disease, Vol III, Cardiopulmonary Diseases and Tumors. Saint Louis, Mosby-Year Book, 1995 © Current Medicine.)

model has similarities to HAPE and may explain a vulnerability of this thin membrane to leak.

Another scenario emanates from the possibility of hypoxic pulmonary venoconstriction, which results in increased pulmonary capillary pressures, and these result in fluid leak directly into the alveolar space.

Mechanical stresses are not the only forces that lead to leak of fluid from the intra- to extravascular space. The classic definition of a "permeability" leak involves *inflammation*, which leads to increased permeability of the endothelial barrier to proteins (Fig. 27–4). Although it is clear that high intravascular pressures play a role in HAPE, investigators have found markers of inflammation in blood, urine, and alveolar fluid (Fig. 27–5). Utilizing bronchoalveolar lavage in climbers with HAPE at 4300 meters on Mt. Mc-Kinley, Schoene and coworkers (1986; 1988) found high concentrations of proteins, including high molecular weight protein, as well as chemotactic (leukotriene B_4, C_3) and vasoactive mediators (thromboxane B_2) compared with controls. High levels of cells, primarily alveolar macrophages (although higher levels than normal of neutrophils), were present. These results were compared with those in patients with adult respiratory distress syndrome (ARDS) whose protein levels were elevated but not as high as in patients with HAPE. In addition, the cells were predominately neutrophils. These results give some insight into the clinical picture of the two syndromes, in that HAPE usually resolves quickly without clinical or functional sequelae, whereas ARDS may last for weeks with an intense inflammatory response. This presumably results from the neutrophilic content of the alveolar and interstitial space, which may leave the lung impaired with scarring.

Richalet and coworkers (1991) also found evidence of inflammatory mediators (leukotrienes B_4 and C_4, and prostaglandin E_2) in blood of subjects with AMS, the levels of which paralleled the course of the disease. In 38 patients with HAPE at a moderate altitude, Kaminsky and coworkers (in press) found elevated levels of urinary leukotriene E_4, the stable metabolite of the inflammatory arachidonic acid cascade. This substance was not found in control subjects at the same altitude. Additionally, a majority of the patients had a prior or concomitant viral illness, mostly upper respiratory, which suggests that inflammation preceding the altitude exposure may prime the endothelium, making it more vulnerable to the stress of higher pressures.

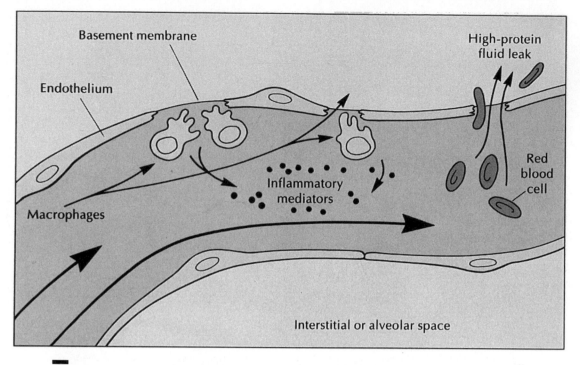

Figure 27–4

The potential relationship between inflammation and the pulmonary vascular endothelium. Hypoxia *per se* and/or stress on the endothelium may incite a chemotactic response for both polymorphonuclear leukocytes and macrophages. (Schoene RB: In Braunwald E (ed): Atlas of Heart Disease, Vol III, Cardiopulmonary Diseases and Tumors. Saint Louis, Mosby-Year Book, 1995 © Current Medicine.)

E-selectin and P-selectin are adhesion molecules that have been found in the blood of patients with various inflammatory processes (see Chapter 1). If present, they indicate that chemotaxis, followed by adhesion and activation of neutrophils, has taken place. E-selectin is elevated in subjects going to high altitude (Eldridge et al, 1994), some of whom develop AMS and HAPE. These findings suggest that hypoxia *per se* may set off a cascade of events in some susceptible individuals that instigates inflammation and affects the permeability of the endothelium.

From the evidence mentioned, the relative contribution of inflammation versus mechanical stresses on the pulmonary vascular beds is not clear (Fig. 27–6). Questions for future investigation remain unanswered. Do the forces of high pressures lead to stretching of the endothelium, an early leak of proteins, and a subsequent inflammatory response that accentuates and perpetuates the leak until the stress has been relieved? Or is inflammation necessary at the onset to permit the high pressures to violate the endothelium? The sequence of these events is not known and is difficult to ascertain in the clinical setting. Future research in an animal model may afford a

better understanding of the biochemical and cellular events so that therapy can be tailored precisely to prevent or treat HAPE.

PREVENTION AND TREATMENT

HAPE should be treated as acute respiratory failure that is encountered in a unique and challenging environment, often without medical personnel present. Knowledge of adaptation to high altitude and recognition of symptoms of maladaptation (i.e., altitude illnesses) are essential to both medical and nonmedical personnel going to high altitude for recreation or work. Unless severe accompanying orthopedic injuries or impenetrable weather conditions are present, either or both preventing evacuation, no one should die of HAPE.

Starting with that premise, early signs of HAPE must be recognized before patients become too ill to help themselves, at which point they become a danger to others, and the difficulty of descent is compounded. If medical help is available, such as in a recreational ski area, and if patients can be observed by family or friends (and

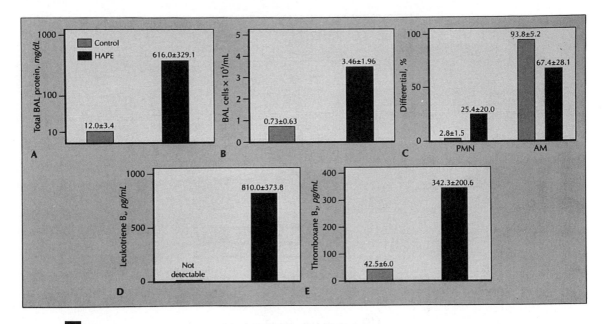

Figure 27–5
The results of bronchoalveolar lavage fluid in patients with HAPE compared with fluid in healthy controls at 4300 meters show (A) high protein concentrations; (B) a high cell count consisting primarily of alveolar macrophages but also (C) a higher overall count of both neutrophils and macrophages; (D) a high concentration of the chemotactic mediator leukotriene B_4; and (E) vasoactive mediator thromboxane B_2. These results suggest the presence of a larger permeability leak, an inflammatory and vasoactive response, but they do not tell when in the evolution of the syndrome each of these plays a role.

maintained with an arterial oxygen saturation of more than 90% on low-flow oxygen), and if judged clinically stable, patients can be sent back to their accommodations and seen on a daily basis until well (Zafren et al, 1996). This approach reduces logistic and financial difficulties and leads to a minimal disruption of work or vacation. Of course, if the patient's condition is unstable and if the patient cannot be oxygenated adequately, evacuation and hospitalization are essential. The patient may need intensive care observation.

If a patient is in a remote setting, the party must be prepared to take care of the patient primarily by descent of 500 to 1000 meters or more. Recovery usually follows. Other modalities, if available, should be considered.

Nonpharmacologic interventions are quite helpful and have ranged from bed rest alone (Singh et al, 1965; Marticorena and Hultgren, 1979), to the use of supplemental oxygen, which is quite effective even in some of the most sick individuals. In remote settings, oxygen is usually not available and, if so, the supply cannot be renewed when depleted. A lightweight continuous positive airway pressure (CPAP) mask can be applied in the end-positive airway pressure

(EPAP) mode as a temporizing measure, which is effective in improving gas exchange (Schoene et al, 1985). Portable hyperbaric chambers are now available and have been employed on treks and expeditions (Tabor, 1990; King and Greenlee, 1990). They work well, as a temporizing measure, allowing the victim to descend to lower altitude until improved. None of these measures should delay or supersede descent, if possible.

Because of the low incidence and unpredictability of HAPE, pharmacologic therapy for the most part has been inadequately studied (Hackett and Roach, 1987). If HAPE is a continuum of less severe altitude illness, drugs such as acetazolamide (Forwand et al, 1968; Larson et al, 1982) and dexamethasone (Johnson et al, 1984; Rock et al, 1989; Ellsworth et al, 1991), which are effective by different mechanisms in preventing and treating AMS, may be effective in the same manner for HAPE. But neither has been studied, and, except in desperate situations, each has little place in treatment. Acetazolamide is a carbonic anhydrase inhibitor that acts in a number of ways to facilitate the normal acclimatization process to minimize the chances of AMS. The drug acts to stimulate ventilation (Cain and Dunn, 1965),

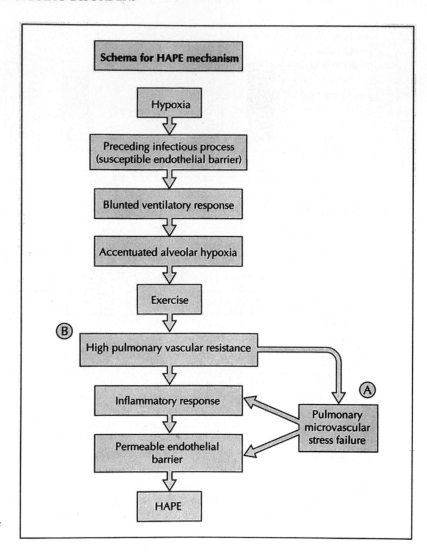

Figure 27–6
A hypothetical schema for the
pathogenesis of HAPE.

eradicate periodic breathing during sleep (Sutton et al, 1979), and promote renal excretion of bicarbonate in compensation for the respiratory alkalosis of high altitude (Swenson et al, 1991). All of these are probably effective in preventing or treating altitude maladaptation. Dexamethasone, in contrast, may promote the integrity of the microvascular endothelium and thus may minimize leak of fluid into the extravascular space. Many other drugs, such as diuretics, morphine, digitalis, and antibiotics, have been tried but with little rationale; their use is not without risk.

A pulmonary vasodilator, nifedipine, was tested for efficacy in preventing HAPE and found to be effective and safe in HAPE-susceptible individuals (Bartsch et al, 1991). Two other studies (Oelz et al, 1989; Hackett et al, 1990) showed that giving sublingual nifedipine resulted in improved gas exchange in most but not all of the

patients with HAPE who were at high altitude. The present recommendation for nifedipine is as follows. For individuals who have had a history of documented HAPE who are returning to high altitude, it is reasonable for them to start taking a long-acting (20–30 mg qd or bid) preparation at the beginning of their ascent and continue the dose until returning to low altitude. Side effects are rare, but patients should be knowledgeable about the drug and the symptoms of HAPE. Nifedipine as adjunctive therapy to oxygen and rest to treat HAPE may be helpful but is usually not necessary.

CONCLUSIONS

HAPE is a noncardiogenic form of pulmonary edema and acute hypoxic respiratory failure that can be fatal. It is associated with rapid ascent from high altitude before normal acclimatization is possible. Accentuated pulmonary vascular pressures are common and along with an inflammatory response may play a critical role in the pathogenesis of the disease. Future research is aimed at ascertaining the mechanism of the permeability leak into the lung. Prevention is allowing enough time for normal acclimatization. Treatment is aimed at providing adequate oxygen to the patient either by descent or supplemental oxygen and other measures, such as pulmonary vasodilators, which help to decrease the severe pulmonary hypertension.

REFERENCES

Arias-Stella J and Kruger H: Pathology of high altitude pulmonary edema. Arch Pathol 76:147–157, 1963.

Bartsch P, Maggiorini M, Ritter M, et al: Prevention of high altitude pulmonary edema by nifedipine. N Engl J Med 325:1284–1289, 1991.

Cain SM and Dunn JE: Increase of arterial oxygen tension at altitude by carbonic anhydrase inhibition. J Appl Physiol 20:882–884, 1965.

Eldridge MW, Johnson DH, Podolsky A, et al: Evidence of immunological mediator activation with exposure to high altitude (abstract). Am J Respir Crit Care Med 149(4):A 298, 1994.

Ellsworth AJ, Meyer EF, and Larson EB: Acetazolamide or dexamethasone use versus placebo to prevent acute mountain sickness on Mount Rainier. West J Med 154:289–293, 1991.

Forwand SA, Landoune M, Follansbee JN, and Hansen JE: Effect of acetazolamide on acute mountain sickness. N Engl J Med 279:839–845, 1968.

Fred H, Schmidt A, Bates T, and Hecht H: Acute pulmonary edema of altitude: Clinical and physiologic observations. Circulation 25:929–937, 1962.

Hackett P, Creagh C, Grover R, et al: High-altitude pulmonary edema in persons without the right pulmonary artery. N Engl J Med 302:1070–1073, 1980.

Hackett P, Greene E, Roach P, et al: Nifedipine and hydralazine for treatment of high altitude pulmonary edema (abstract). In Sutton J, Coates G, and Remmers J (eds): Hypoxia: The Adaptations. Toronto, B.C. Decker, 1990; pp. 219.

Hackett PH and Roach RC: Medical therapy of altitude illness. Ann Emerg Med 16:980–986, 1987.

Hackett PH and Roach RC: High altitude pulmonary edema. J Wilderness Med 1:3–26, 1990.

Hackett PH, Roach RC, Hartig GS, et al: The effect of vasodilators on pulmonary hemodynamics in high altitude pulmonary edema: A comparison. Int J Sports Med 13[Suppl 1]:S68–S71, 1992.

Hackett PH, Roach RC, Schoene RB, et al: Abnormal control of ventilation in high-altitude pulmonary edema. J Appl Physiol 64(3):1268–1272, 1988.

Heath D, Moosavi H, and Smith P: Ultra structure of high altitude pulmonary edema. Thorax 28:694–700, 1973.

Houston C: Acute pulmonary edema of high altitude. N Engl J Med 253:478–480, 1960.

Hu ST, Huang WY, Chu SC, and Pa CF: Chemoreflexive ventilatory response at sea level in subjects with past history of good acclimatization and severe acute mountain sickness. In Brendel W, and Zink RA (eds): High Altitude Physiology and Medicine. New York, Springer-Verlag, 1982, pp 28–32.

Hultgren H: High altitude pulmonary edema. In Staub N (ed): Water and Solute Exchange. New York Marcel Dekker, 1978, pp 437–464.

Hultgren HN, Grover RF, and Hartley LH: Abnormal circulatory responses to high altitude in subjects with a previous history of high-altitude pulmonary edema. Circulation 44:759–770, 1964a.

Hultgren HN, Honigman B, Theis K, and Nicholas R: High altitude pulmonary edema at a ski resort. West J Med 164:222–227, 1996.

Hultgren H, Lopez C, Lundberg E, and Miller H: Physiologic studies of pulmonary edema at high altitude. Circulation 29:393–408, 1964b.

Hultgren H and Marticorena E: High altitude pulmonary edema: Epidemiologic observations in Peru. Chest 74:372, 1978.

Hultgren H, Spickard W, Hellriegel K, and Houston C. High altitude pulmonary edema. Medicine 40:289–313, 1961.

Hultgren H, Spickard W, and Lopez D: Further studies of high altitude pulmonary edema. Br Heart J 24:95–102, 1962.

Hurtado A: Aspectos Fisicos y Patologicos de la Vida en Las Alturas. Lima, Imprenta Rimac, 1937.

Johnson TS, Rock PB, Fulco CS, et al: Prevention of acute mountain sickness by dexamethasone. N Engl J Med 310:683–686, 1984.

Kaminsky DA, Schoene RB, and Voelkel NF: Urinary leukotriene E4 levels in high altitude pulmonary edema: A possible role for inflammation. Chest (in press).

Kawashima A, Kubo K, Kobayashi T, and Sekiguchi M. Hemodynamic responses to acute hypoxia, hyperbaria, and exercise in subjects susceptible to high-altitude pulmonary edema. J Appl Physiol 67(5):1982–1989, 1989.

King SI and Greenlee RR: Successful use of the Gamow Hyperbaric Bag in the treatment of altitude illness at Mount Everest. J Wilderness Med 1:193–202, 1990.

Kobayashi T, Koyama S, Lubo K, et al: Clinical features of patients with high-altitude pulmonary edema in Japan. Chest 92:814–821, 1987.

Koizumi T, Kawashima A, Kubo K, et al: Radiographic

and hemodynamic changes during recovery from high-altitude pulmonary edema. Intern Med 33:525–528, 1994.

Larson EB, Roach RC, Schoene RB, and Hornbein TF: Acute mountain sickness and acetazolamide: Clinical efficacy and effect on ventilation. JAMA 248:328–332, 1982.

Lizarraga L: Soroche Agudo: Edema agudo del pulmon. An Fac Med (Lima) 38:244, 1955.

Maldonado D: High altitude pulmonary edema. Radiol Clin North Am 16:537–549, 1978.

Marticorena E and Hultgren HN: Evaluation of therapeutic methods in high altitude pulmonary edema. Am J Cardiol 43:307–312, 1979.

Masuda A, Kobayashi T, Honda Y, et al: Effect of high altitude on respiration chemosensitivity. Jpn J Mtn-Med 12:177–181, 1992.

Matsuzawa Y, Fujimoto K, Kobayashki T, et al: Blunted hypoxic ventilatory drive in subjects susceptible to high-altitude pulmonary edema. J Appl Physiol 66:1152–1157, 1989.

Menon N: High altitude pulmonary edema. A clinical study. N Engl J Med 273:66–73, 1965.

Mosso A: Life of Man in the High Alps. London, T. Fisher Unwin, 1898.

Oelz O, Maggiorini M, Ritter M, et al: Nifedipine for high altitude pulmonary edema. Lancet 2:1241–1244, 1989.

Ravenhill TH: Some experience of mountain sickness in the Andes. J Trop Med Hyg 20:313–320, 1913.

Richalet JP, Hornych A, Rathat C, et al: Plasma prostaglandin, leukotrienes and thromboxane in acute high altitude hypoxia. Respir Physiol 85:205–215, 1991.

Rock PB, Johnson TS, Larsen RF, et al: Dexamethasone prophylaxis for acute mountain sickness. Chest 95:568–573, 1989.

Roy SB, Guleria JS, Khanna PK, et al: Hemodynamic studies in high altitude pulmonary oedema. Br Heart J 31:52–58, 1969.

Scherrer U, Vollenweider L, Delabays A, et al: Inhaled nitric oxide for high altitude pulmonary edema. N Engl J Med 334:624–629, 1996.

Schoene RB: In Braunwald E (ed): Atlas of Heart Disease, Vol III, Cardiopulmonary Diseases and Tumors. St. Louis, Mosby-YearBook, 1995, pp 512–516.

Schoene RB: Pulmonary edema at high altitude: Review, pathophysiology, and update. Clin Chest Med 6(3):491–507, 1985.

Schoene RB: High altitude pulmonary edema: Pathophysiology and clinical review. Ann Emerg Med 16:987–992, 1987.

Schoene RB, Hackett PH, Henderson WR, et al: High-altitude pulmonary edema: Characteristics of lung lavage fluid. JAMA 256:63–69, 1986.

Schoene R, Roach R, Hackett P, et al: High altitude pulmonary edema and exercise at 4,400 meters on Mount McKinley: Effect of expiratory positive airway pressure. Chest 87:330–333, 1985.

Schoene RB, Swenson ER, Pizza CJ, et al: The lung at high altitude: Bronchoalveolar lavage in acute mountain sickness and pulmonary edema. J Appl Physiol 64(6):2605–2613, 1988.

Selland MA, Stelzner TJ, Stevens T, et al: Pulmonary function and hypoxic ventilatory response in subjects susceptible to high-altitude pulmonary edema. Chest 103:111–116, 1993.

Singh I, Kapila C, Khanna P, et al: High altitude pulmonary edema. Lancet 1:229–234, 1965.

Singh I, Khanna P, Srivastava M, et al: Acute mountain sickness. N Engl J Med 280:175–184, 1969.

Sutton JR, Houston CS, Mansell AL, et al: Effect of acetazolamide on hypoxemia during sleep at high altitude. N Engl J Med 301(24):1329–1331, 1979.

Swenson ER, Leatham RL, Roach RC, et al: Renal carbonic anhydrase inhibition reduces high altitude sleep periodic breathing. Respir Physiol 86:333–343, 1991.

Tabor R: Protocols for the use of a portable hyperbaric chamber for the treatment of high altitude disorders. J Wilderness Med 1:181–192, 1990.

Vachiery JL, McDonagh T, Moraine JJ, et al: Doppler assessment of hypoxic pulmonary vasoconstriction and susceptibility to high altitude pulmonary oedema. Thorax 50:22–27, 1995.

Viswanathan R, Subramanian S, and Radha T: Effect of hypoxia on regional lung perfusion by scanning. Respiration 37:142–144, 1979.

Vock P, Brutsche MH, Nanzer A, and Bartsch P: Variable radiomorphologic data of high altitude pulmonary edema. Features from 60 patients. Chest 100:1306–1311, 1991.

Vock P, Fretz C, Franciolli M, et al: High altitude pulmonary edema: Findings at high-altitude chest radiography and physical examination. Radiology 170:661–666, 1989.

Weil JV: Ventilatory control at high altitude. Handbook of Physiology: The Respiratory System II. Bethesda, MD, American Physiologic Society, 1986.

Weil JV, Bryne-Quinn E, Sodal IE, et al: Acquired attenuation of chemoreceptor function in chronically hypoxic man at high altitude. J Clin Invest 50:186–195, 1971.

West JB and Mathieu-Costello O: High altitude pulmonary edema is caused by stress failure of pulmonary capillaries. Int J Sports Med 13[Suppl 1]:S54–S58, 1992.

West JB and Mathieu-Costello O: Pulmonary blood-gas barrier: A physiological dilemma. News Physiol Sci 8:249–253, 1993.

West J, Tsukimoto K, Mathieu-Costello O, and Prediletto R: Stress failure in pulmonary capillaries. J Appl Physiol 70:1731–1742, 1991.

Zafren K, Reeves JT and Schoene RB: Treatment of high altitude pulmonary edema by bed rest and supplemental oxygen. J Wilderness Environ Med 7:127–132, 1996.

Index

Note: Page numbers in *italics* refer to illustrations; page numbers followed by t refer to tables.